# Pathology of the Breast

Fattaneh A. Tavassoli, MD

Assistant Chairman
Department of Gynecologic and Breast Pathology
Armed Forces Institute of Pathology
Washington DC

Adjunct Professor of Pathology
Uniformed Services University of Health Sciences
Bethesda, Maryland

Consultant in Pathology
National Cancer Institute
Bethesda, Maryland

**Chapter 3 Specimen Processing**

Contributed by

Stuart J. Schnitt, MD
Associate Director of Surgical Pathology
Beth Israel Hospital
Assistant Professor of Pathology
Harvard Medical School
Boston, Massachusetts

APPLETON & LANGE
Norwalk, Connecticut

93 94 95 96 97 / 10 9 8 7 6 5 4 3 2 1

Prentice Hall International (UK) Limited, *London*
Prentice Hall of Australia Pty. Limited, *Sydney*
Prentice Hall Canada, Inc., *Toronto*
Prentice Hall Hispanoamericana, S.A., *Mexico*
Prentice Hall of India Private Limited, *New Delhi*
Prentice Hall of Japan, Inc., *Tokyo*
Simon & Schuster Asia Pte. Ltd., *Singapore*
Editora Prentice Hall do Brasil Ltda., *Rio de Janeiro*
Prentice Hall, *Englewood Cliffs, New Jersey*

ISBN 0-8385-7702-4

90000

9 780838 577028

Library of Congress Catalog Card Number: 93-070153

PRINTED IN THE UNITED STATES OF AMERICA

*To my family—Bahman, Shahab, and Homa*

# Preface

The widespread use of screening mammography has led to the detection of an increasing number of early malignant and proliferative lesions. These include small invasive carcinomas, in situ cancers, and an overwhelming number of proliferative lesions which are believed to be associated with an increased risk for the subsequent development of carcinoma. Coupled with the trend toward more conservative surgical treatment of breast carcinoma, these developments have dramatically altered the type of information a pathologist has to include in the pathology report. Today pathologists not only have to determine the status of the axillary nodes, but are also required to provide information regarding the size, grade, and extent of the carcinoma, proportion of the in situ component associated with an invasive carcinoma, and assess the tumor margins for adequacy of excision.

Currently, the optimal management of patients with breast disease requires close cooperation of a team of radiologist, surgeon, pathologist, and oncologist. This approach is not limited to the area of breast cancer, but also involves the management of patients at increased risk for the development of breast carcinoma. The major responsibility for providing the precise diagnosis which serves as the basis of all treatment rests with the pathologist.

With due consideration to the expanding role of the pathologist and the increasing demand for a variety of information regarding the lesion, this book focuses on the morphologic features (criteria), discussion of differential diagnosis, and illustration of the wide variety of breast lesions. The immunohistochemical and ultrastructural characteristics of some lesions are included and their role in the diagnostic process discussed when indicated. Whenever appropriate, the historic background regarding the initial description of the lesion is presented, followed by the clinical signs and symptoms of the disease, pathologic features, prognostic factors, and finally the treatment. The discussion of therapeutic options is more limited in its scope compared to books that focus mainly on the treatment of breast disease; but nonetheless, some of the traditional views are addressed, as well as the more recent consensus regarding the treatment of early stage breast carcinoma and a wide range of other lesions.

A comprehensive reference list has been provided at the end of every chapter. Reports of historic interest, the best discussions of the subject, and those which are themselves a useful source of references have been highlighted with an asterisk. While I have freely drawn upon the superb work of many authors, the contents of the chapters reflect primarily my personal viewpoints based on the 4,000 to 5,000 breast lesions reviewed annually in the Department of Gynecologic and Breast Pathology at the Armed Forces Institute of Pathology over the past 15 years. The incredible variety and quality of this large number of breast lesions are unique assets of the Armed Forces Institute of Pathology, and I am grateful for the access to this national treasure.

It is a pleasure to acknowledge the advice, comments, and encouragements of Drs. Lauren V. Ackerman and Robert E. Fechner throughout the preparation of this book. I am also grateful to Dr. Franz Enzinger for his review and comments on selected chapters. My indebtedness and gratitude extend to the many contributing pathologists who referred their challenging cases to the Armed Forces Institute of Pathology; without them, this work would not have been possible.

I have been fortunate to have assistance from Robin-Anne V. Ferris, MFS, and Luther Duckett in photography; Steven A. Kruger, B.J. Jones, and F.R. Hincherick in the printing of the illustrations; and the Armed Forces Institute of Pathology's Medical Illustration Department. I also wish to thank my publisher, Elsevier, for their cooperation during the production of this book.

More important, I wish to thank my family, Bahman, Shahab, and Homa, for their understanding and patience.

*Fattaneh A. Tavassoli, MD*

# Contents

# 1

# Normal Development and Anomalies



## NORMAL BREAST

Mammary glands are modified sweat glands with the specialized function of providing nutrients for the newborn infant. Located in the anterior chest wall, they serve as target organs for a variety of hormones (20). These hormones either have an active or a passive role in the physiology of mammary glands. Hormones that actively influence breast physiology are prolactin (PRL), estrogen and progesterone. Estrogen promotes the growth and development of the duct system and progesterone stimulates lobular development. For estrogen and progesterone to exert their effect, the presence of PRL is necessary (25). Estrogen initiates mammary epithelial stem cell division, but PRL, insulin and growth hormone are necessary for the process to continue (31). A variety of other hormones including human placental lactogen and thyroxine influence DNA synthesis in the ductal epithelial cells (20).

The various hormones act in concert to promote morphologic and functional development of the breast through the establishment of the duct system and production of milk. These dynamic processes of mammogenesis and galactopoeisis commence during fetal life, continue throughout puberty and the reproductive years, and end following menopause. The ultimate function of the breast is realized during lactation in a normal pregnancy. Following lactation, the altered functional units (lobules) revert to the resting state. The end stage results in involutional and regressive changes in the duct system after menopause. Salazar et al (27) have provided an excellent account of the morphologic and ultrastructural changes of the human breast during development, gestation and postgestational involution.

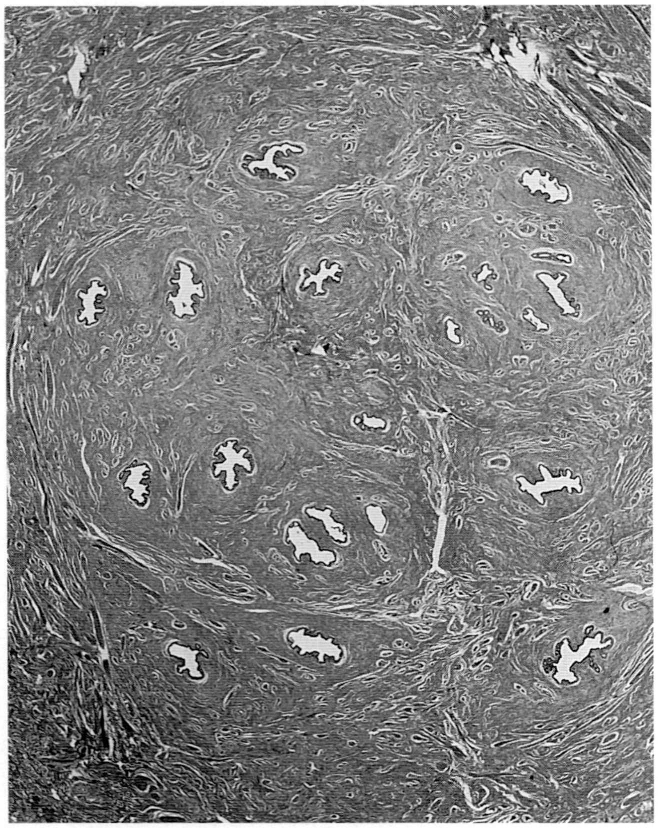

**Figure 1.1(a)** Cross-section of the nipple. Approximately 20 collecting ducts are apparent in the densely muscular nipple stroma. (H&E, X15)

## Fetal Mammary Development

The primitive milk streak (milk line) appears in the human embryo during the fifth week of gestation (11,13). The pair of milk lines extend from the axilla to the groin. Shortly after its formation, most of the band regresses except for a small segment which remains in the thoracic region where it forms the mammary ridge. By the seventh to eighth week of gestation the mammary anlagen has been established as a thickening of the milk line. This is followed by the development of the nipple. The smooth muscle of the nipple and areola form through differentiation of the mesenchymal cells in the chest wall between 12th and 16th week. Subsequently, epithelial buds appear and form 15 to 20 epithelial strips about the 16th week of gestation. It is believed that this initial stage of mammary development is independent of hormones. Sex differences become apparent towards the end of the first trimester under the influence of estrogen and testosterone. Any antiandrogenic interference at this stage or absence of testosterone receptors (ie, testicular feminization syndrome) can result in the female pattern of mammary growth.

During the third trimester, placental hormones initiate canalization of the epithelial strips; this process continues from the 20th to the 32nd week of gestation. The development of the mammary lobules between the 32nd to 40th week results in a multifold increase in the mammary tissue. Meanwhile, the pigmented nipple-areolar complex develops.

## Postnatal Stage

### *Childhood to Puberty*

A transient mammary hyperplasia is observed in some newborn infants as a result of transplacental transfer of the maternal hormones. A colostrum-like fluid may appear in the nipples of newborn males or females up to a week postpartum. The hyperplastic breast tissue involutes by the third to fourth postpartum week.

During childhood, some branching of the pri-

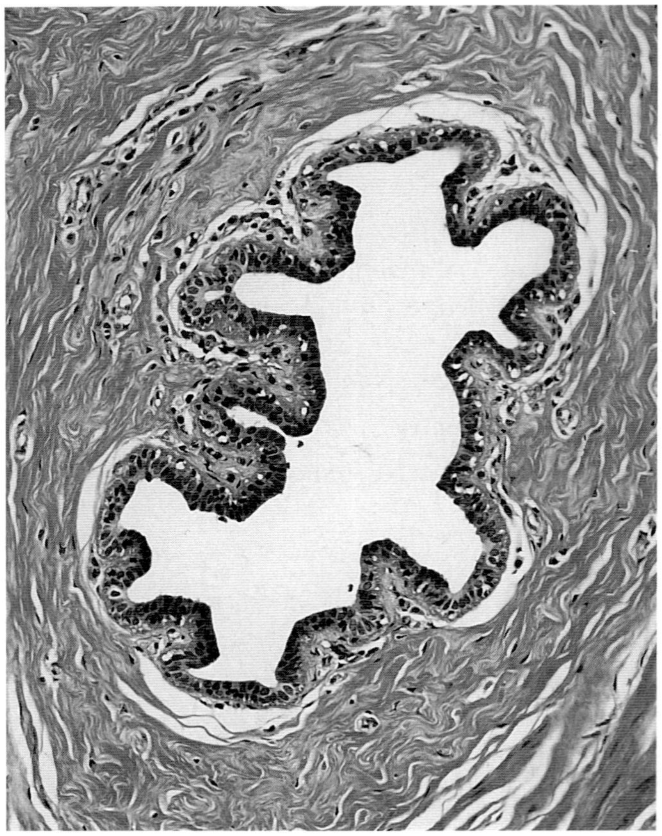

**Figure 1.1(b)** Cross-section of a collecting duct. Note the typical undulating outline. Epithelial and myoepithelial (note vacuoles) cells line the duct. (H&E, X200)

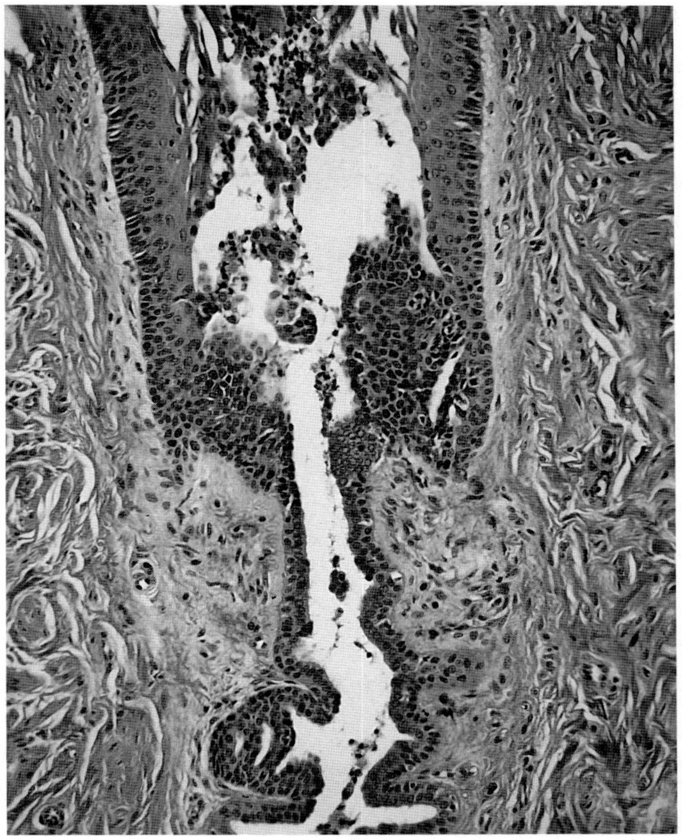

**Figure 1.1(c)** Nipple-collecting duct close to the orifice displaying transition from two cell layers to squamous epithelium. (H&E, X160)

mary duct system occurs but significant changes do not become apparent until puberty.

The changes taking place during puberty and adolescence result from a surge of hormonal activity by the pituitary gland and the ovaries. The ovarian follicles secrete estrogenic hormones which stimulate further growth and branching of the duct system simultaneously with proliferation of the periductal stroma. Along with progesterone, the estrogen secretion results in development of the lobular units.

The adult breast assumes its final protuberant appearance with pigmented nipple and areola about three to four years following the initial surge of the hormonal activity. The average adult breast is 10 to 12 cm in diameter and about 5 to 7 cm thick. The vertical axis of the adult breast extends from the second to the sixth rib; its horizontal axis lies between the midaxillary line and the sternal edge. A small portion of the breast extends into the axilla and is known as the "axillary tail" of the breast.

## *Nipple-Areolar Complex*

The nipple, rich in sensory nerve endings, is located in the center of the complex surrounded by the areola and elevated above it over the fourth intercostal space. The initial development of the primitive nipples which appears as a narrow crest of ectodermal cells precedes that of the mammary gland (14). The nipple nodule is composed of bundles of smooth muscle and elastic tissue traversed by lactiferous ducts which have their orifice at the tip of the nipple (Figs. 1.1a, b, c). Lobules have been identified in about 17% of nipples routinely examined from mastectomies performed for breast carcinoma (26). The

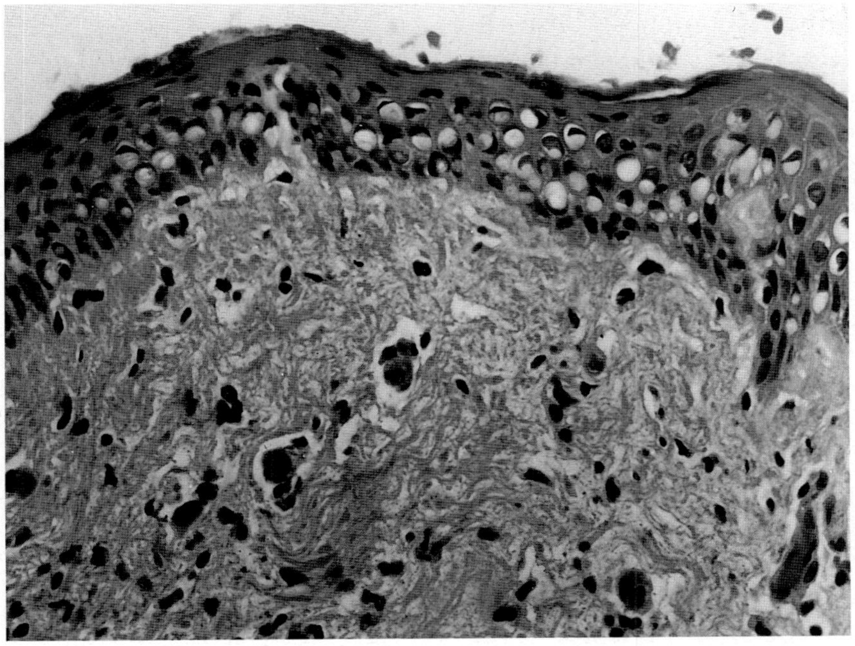

**Figure 1.2** Nipple-surface epithelium. Clear cells were particularly abundant in this case and they closely simulate signet ring cells. (H&E, X400)

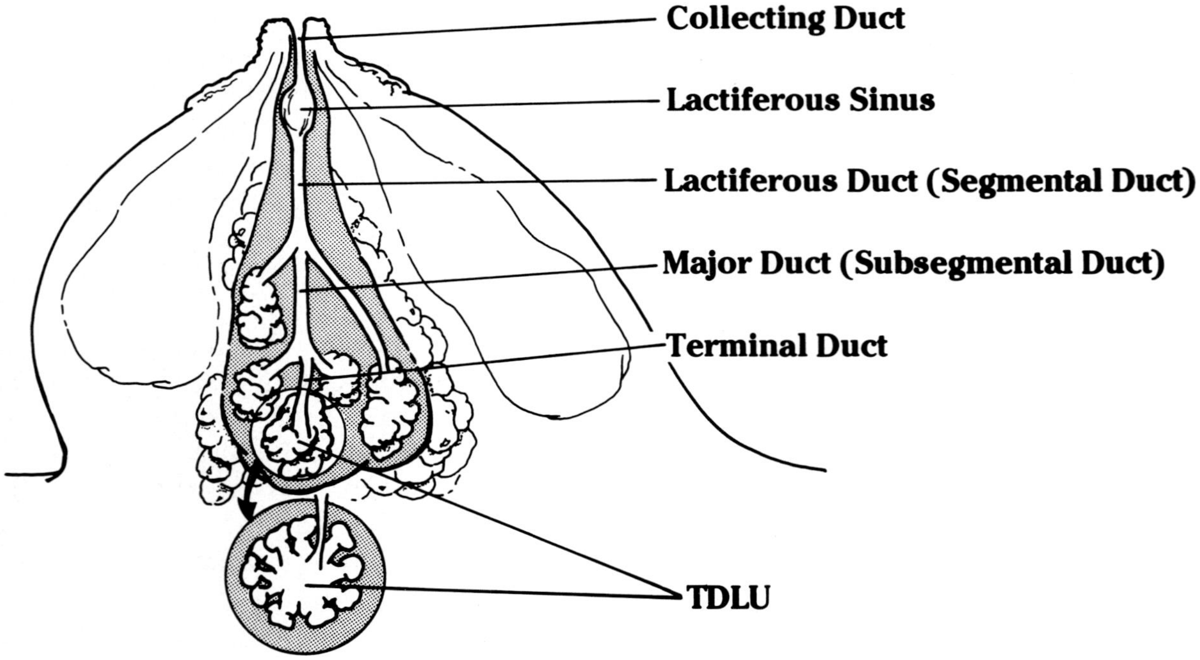


**Figure 1.3** A diagrammatic presentation of the duct system with the different parts specified. TDLU = Terminal duct-lobular unit.

surrounding circular areola varies from 2 to 6 cm in diameter. Stratified squamous epithelium covers the nipple and areola. Clear cells may be present in the surface epithelium (Fig. 1.2). These cells lack intracytoplasmic mucin, have normal nuclei, fail to react with carcinoembryonic antigen (CEA) and should not be mistaken for Paget's cells. Sebaceous and apocrine glands are present in the nipple and areola, but hair follicles are found only in the periphery of the areola. The areolar surface is punctated by rounded elevations known as tubercles of Montgomery—these reflect the openings of the ducts of large sebaceous glands known as glands of Montgomery. The areola enlarges and becomes more pigmented during pregnancy; these changes are permanent.

## Structure of the Adult Duct System

The breast consists of 15 to 20 segments or lobes. Each lobe is drained by a collecting duct, but the lobes are ill-defined and not appreciated on gross inspection. The collecting ducts converge on the nipple with the majority opening at the nipple. The different parts of the duct system are assigned specific designations to help communicate the site of a lesion (Fig. 1.3). Also referred to as the terminal duct-lobular unit

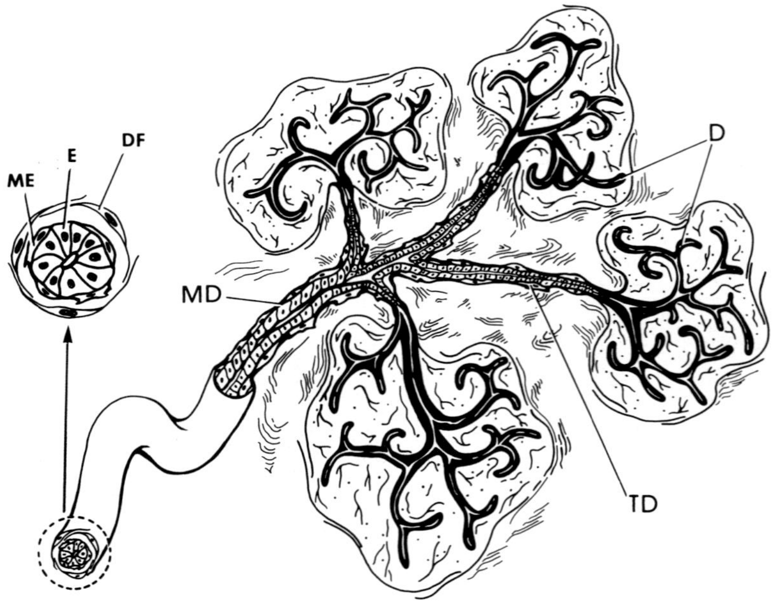


**Figure 1.4(a)** A schematic diagram of a major duct (MD) leading to terminal ducts (TD) and ending in ductules (D), which are also referred to as acini. Because of the small caliber of the ductules (acini), the two cell layers are not illustrated. The terminal duct-lobular unit (TDLU) consists of a small segment of terminal duct and the cluster of ductules. On the left side, cross section of the major duct displays the unit structure of the breast with a continuous layer of luminal epithelial cells (E), surrounded by an interrupted layer of spindled, myoepithelial cells (ME). These two cell layers are in turn invested by basal lamina and surrounded by delimiting fibroblasts (DF). These layers and relationships persist through the entire duct system including the ductules within the lobule.

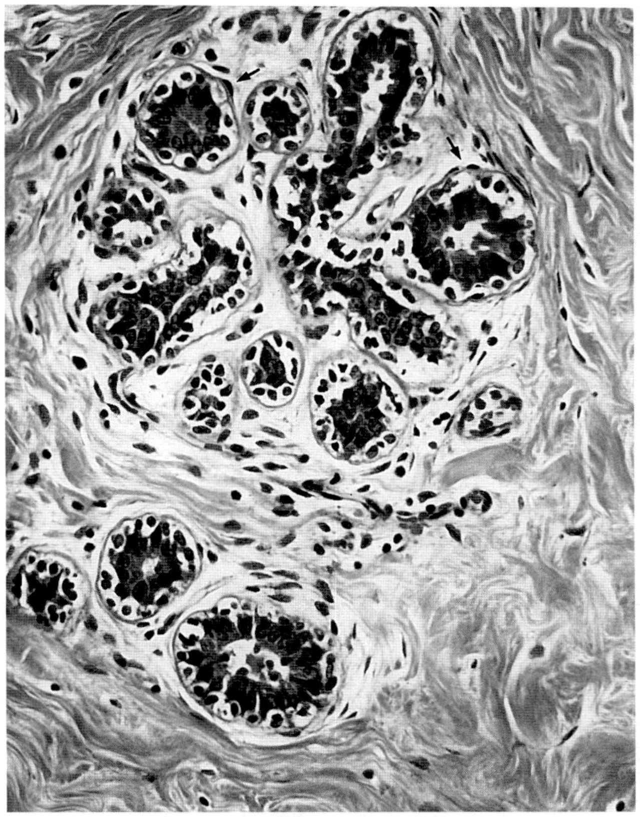

**Figure 1.4(b)** A lobule composed of multiple ductules, each perfectly displaying the unit structure components. The luminal epithelial cells surrounded by the ME cells with clear cytoplasm, and the basal lamina are quite conspicuous in all ductules. Even the nucleus of a delimiting fibroblast is readily evident peripheral to the basal lamina around some of the ductules (arrows). (H&E, X250)

(TDLU), a small portion of the terminal duct together with the acini constitutes the lobule (37).

## *Microscopic Anatomy*

The duct system constitutes the functional component of the breast. The fibroadipose tissue surrounding the duct system accounts for the major bulk of the breast, however.

Except for a small segment of the collecting ducts at the nipple orifice where squamous epithelium lines the duct, the entire duct system is lined by two cell layers, the inner epithelial cell layer along the luminal side surrounded by an interrupted layer of myoepithelial (ME) cells (Figs. 1.4a, b). The long axis of the epithelial cell is perpendicular to that of the myoepithelial cell. The two cell layers are surrounded by a layer of basal lamina. This entire structure is enveloped by one or more "delimiting fibroblast" depending on the caliber of the duct; this constitutes the unit structure of the breast. Any alteration in the number of these cell layers constitutes a pathologic change.

The existence of an intermediate (basal, clear) cell type has been suggested (30) in some studies. Considering the various appearances that either the epithelial or the myoepithelial may assume, it is doubtful that a third cell population exists in the adult female breast. The cell illustrated by Smith et al (30) appears similar to the cells described in clear cell change (Fig. 1.5) in the breast (1,34) and is probably a reflection of a metaplastic alteration which occurs mainly in the epithelial cells but can also involve the myoepithelial cells to a lesser degree. Lobules adjacent to those showing diffuse clear cell metaplasia often show isolated cells with similar features; these cells are identical to the so-called "intermediate" cell.

The intralobular stroma is loose and more cellular than the interlobular stroma. A thin rim of similarly loose stroma surrounds the entire duct system but it is most conspicuous in the lobule where a cluster of ductules is present (Figs. 1.6a, b, c). This stroma is believed to be the specialized, hormone sensitive component of the mammary stroma.

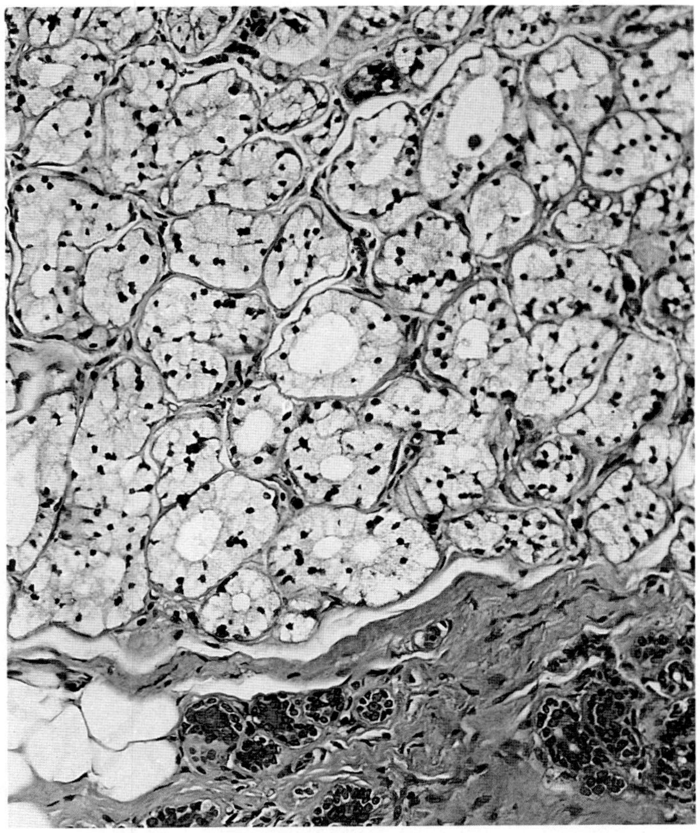

**Figure 1.5** The cells with clear cytoplasm reflect a metaplastic change (H&E, X160). Note the enlargement of the metaplastic cells compared to the cells in the adjacent normal lobules below.

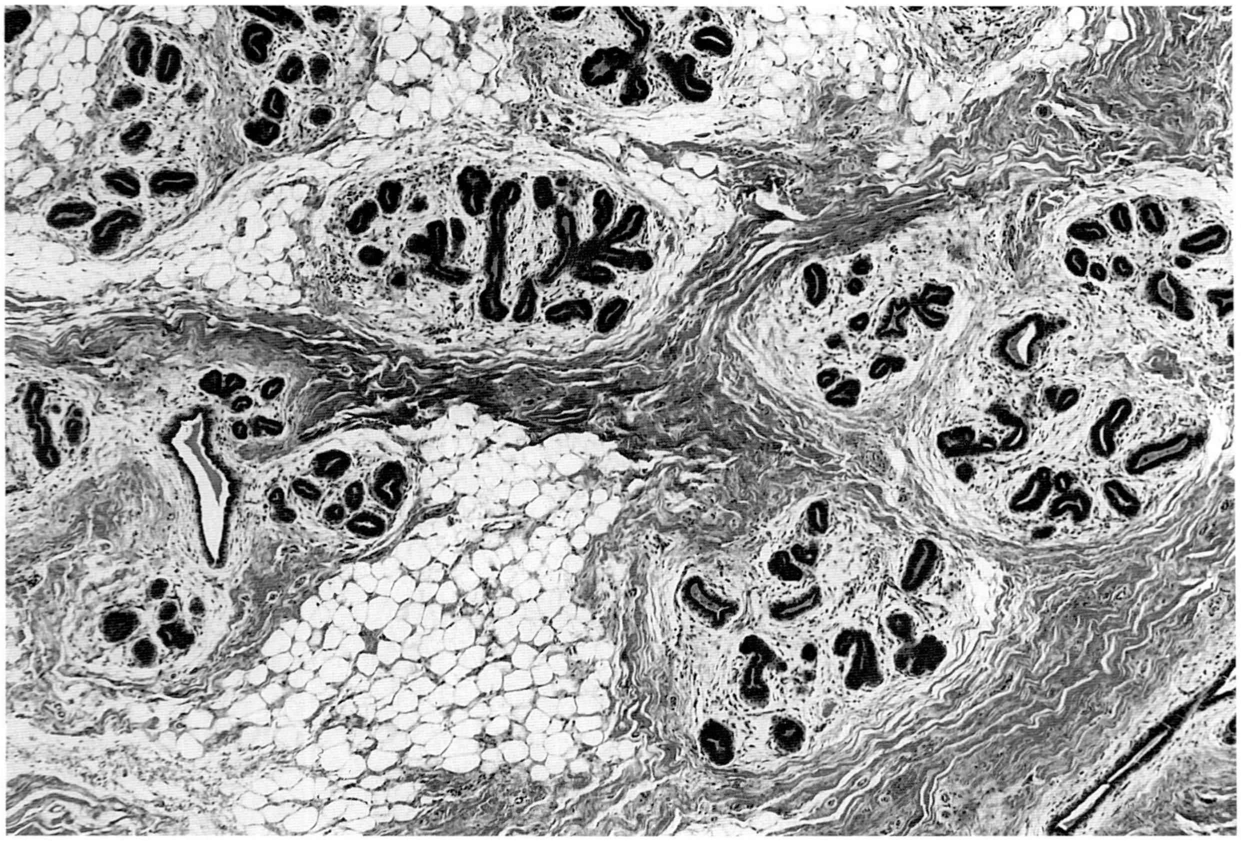

**Figure 1.6(a)** A number of lobules from a mature resting breast (38-year-old). Note the loose intralobular stroma in contrast to the dense, collagenous interlobular stroma. (H&E, X40)

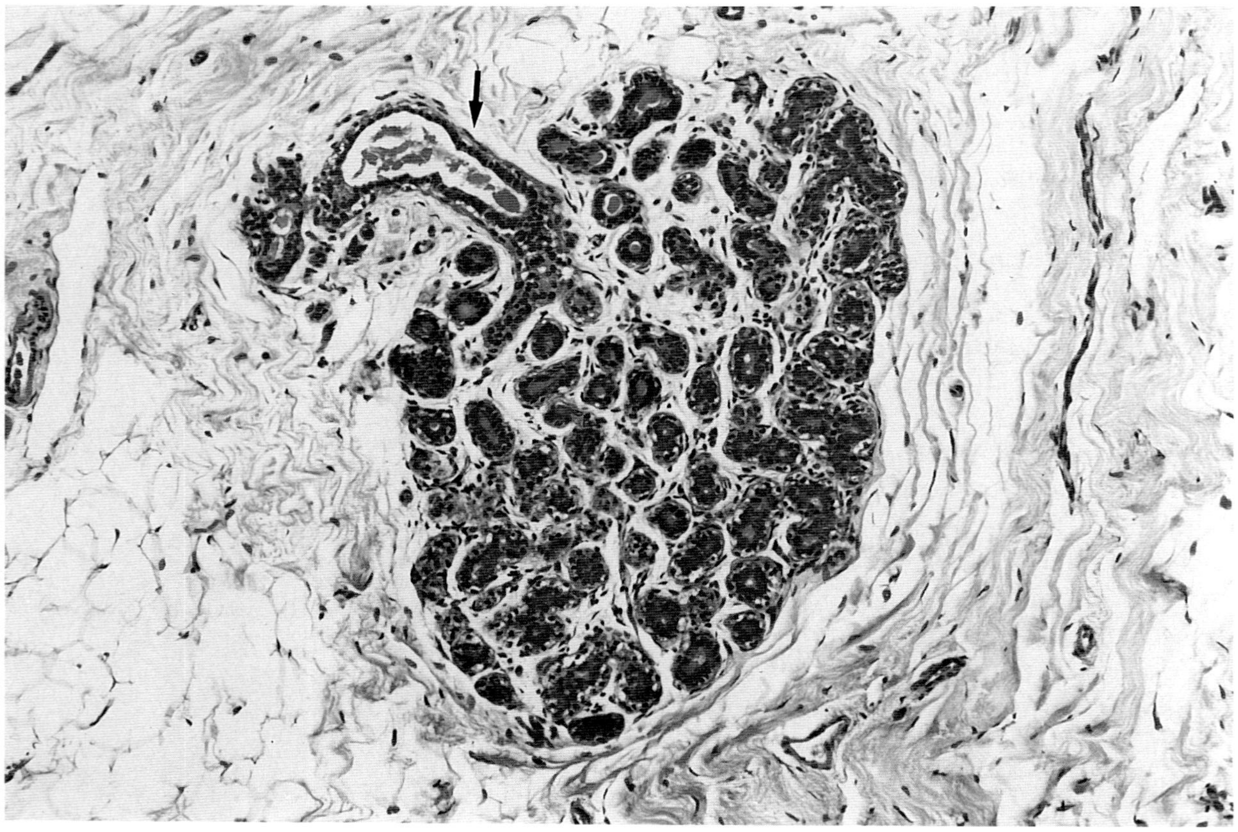

**Figure 1.6(b)** A lobule from a 26-year-old woman showing a terminal duct (arrow) leading to the lobule; the lobular stroma is not as distinctive in some lobules. (H&E, X100).

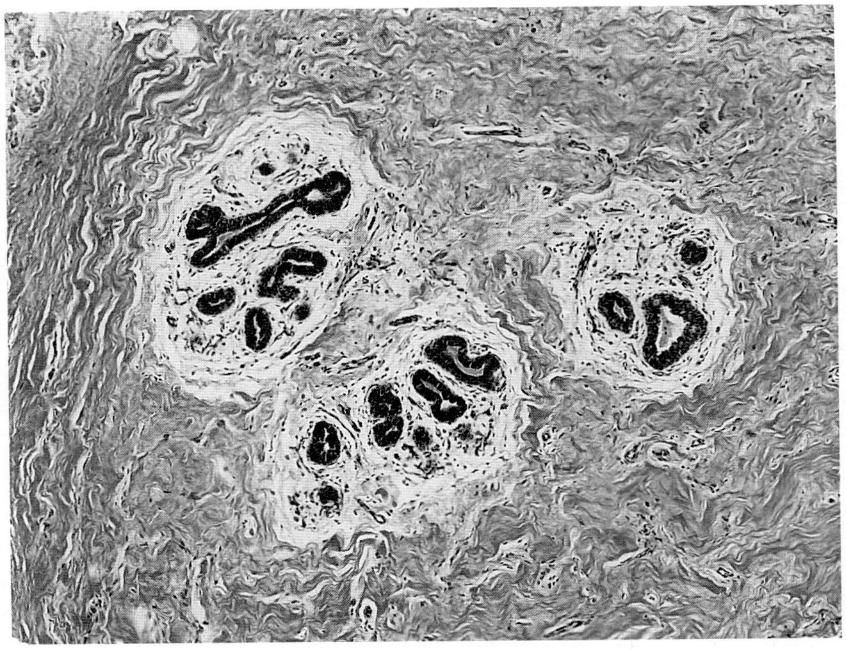

**Figure 1.6(c)** For comparison, note the loose lobular stroma in this underdeveloped lobule from a 13-year-old girl (H&E, X40).

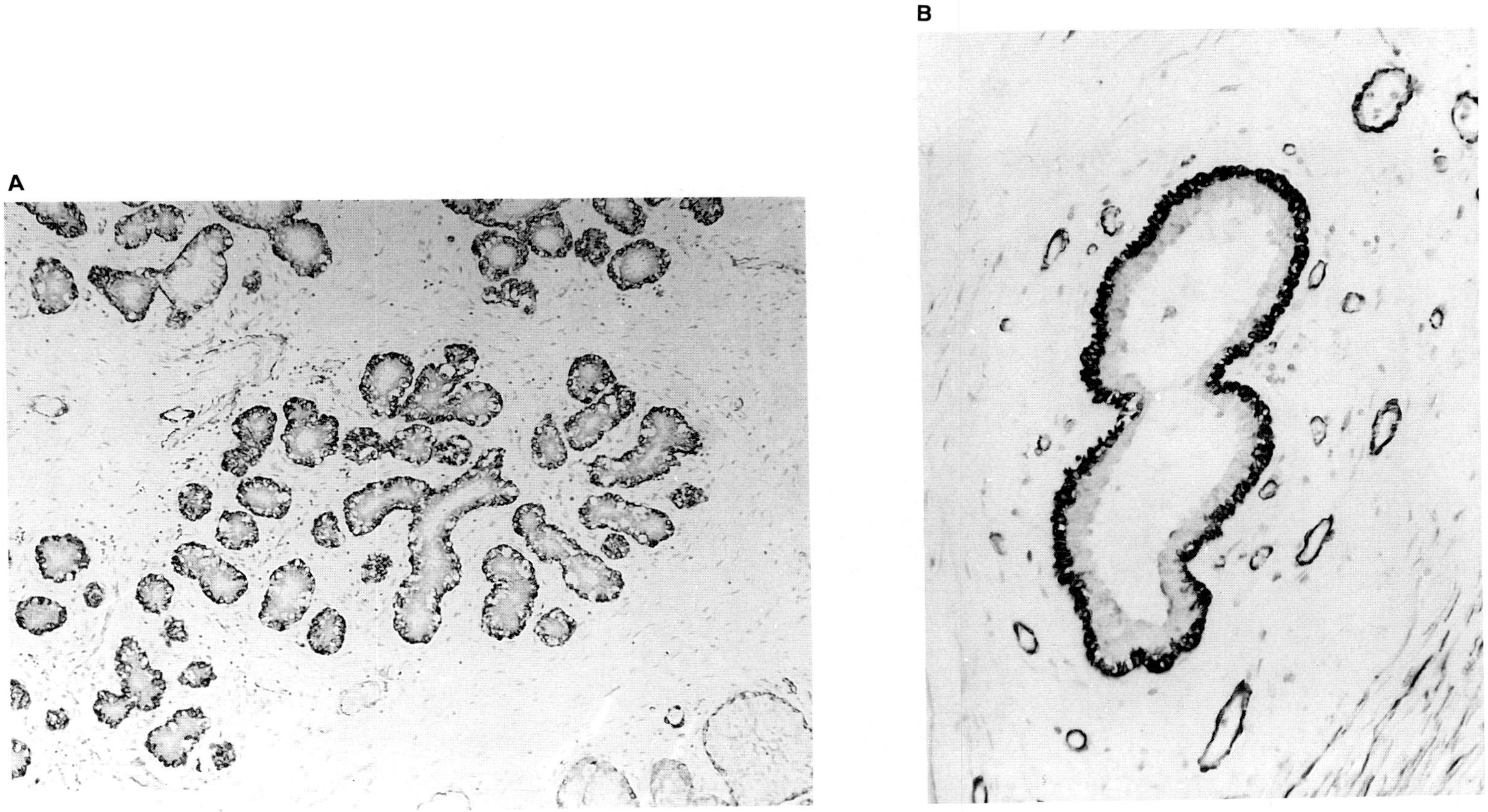


**Figure 1.7** (a) Lobule; (b) Normal duct. The myoepithelial cells in both regions of the duct system display a strongly positive reaction for actin, while the epithelial cells fail to react. (Immunoreaction for actin, (a) X100; (b) X160)

### *Immunohistochemical Features of the Unit Structure Components*

The epithelial and myoepithelial cells have distinctive immunohistochemical and ultrastructural characteristics. The epithelial cells display a strongly positive reaction for various cytokeratins. Positivity for alpha-lactalbumin is evident in the epithelial cells during secretory activity; the positivity is not as strong and uniform in the resting epithelial cells. The myoepithelial cells show a strongly positive reaction for actin and a more variable degree of positivity for S-100 protein and cytokeratins. These two cell types can be easily distinguished based on their immunoreactivity for actin (Figs. 1.7a, b). A positive reaction for actin indicates a myoepithelial cell type in the mammary duct system. Since epithelial cells also display a sporadic positivity for S-100 protein, this antibody is not as useful as actin in discriminating the two cell types.

The basal lamina shows positive reaction for laminin and type IV collagen (6).

### *Ultrastructural Features*

As mentioned before, the epithelial cells form a continuous, luminal cell layer and are surrounded by an interrupted layer of myoepithelial cells. The epithelial cells which are for the most part separated from the basal lamina by the ME cells come in direct contact with the basal lamina wherever there is a gap between the ME cells (Fig. 1.8).

Both the epithelial and myoepithelial cells show a tremendous range of appearances. The myoepithelial cell generally has a more elongated to spindled configuration and the cytoplasm appears more electron dense. The myoepithelial cells contain intracytoplasmic myofibrils with dense bodies and pinocytotic vesicles; a few bundles of tonofilaments are seen in some ME cells. Both cell types adhere to adjacent cells by desmosomes or well formed tight junctions. The myoepithelial cells display basal laminar investiture when directly apposing stroma. Secretory and lactational changes take place primarily in the epithelial cells but the myoepithelial cells also show a few

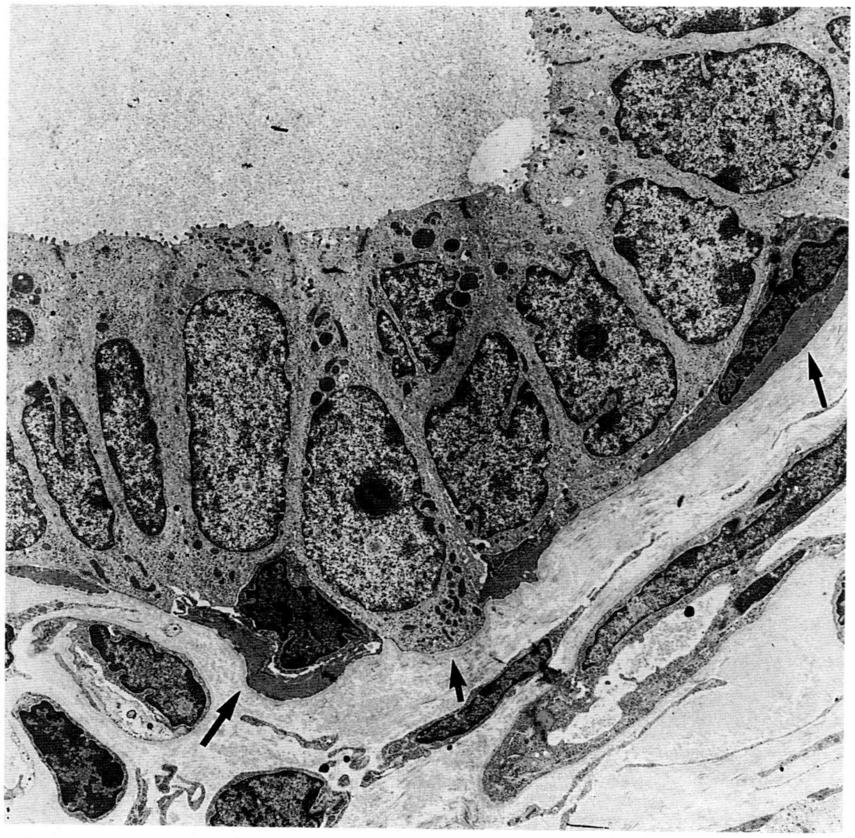

**Figure 1.8** Portion of a terminal duct showing the epithelial cells with their long axis perpendicular to that of the ME cells (long arrows). Note the gaps between the ME cells where the epithelial cells lie directly on the basal lamina (short arrow). A delimiting fibroblast with its elongated cytoplasmic processes extending around the duct is evident at the base of the short arrow. Endothelial lined vascular spaces are located outside the delimiting fibroblastic layer. (Uranyl acetate-lead citrate, X3,450)

A

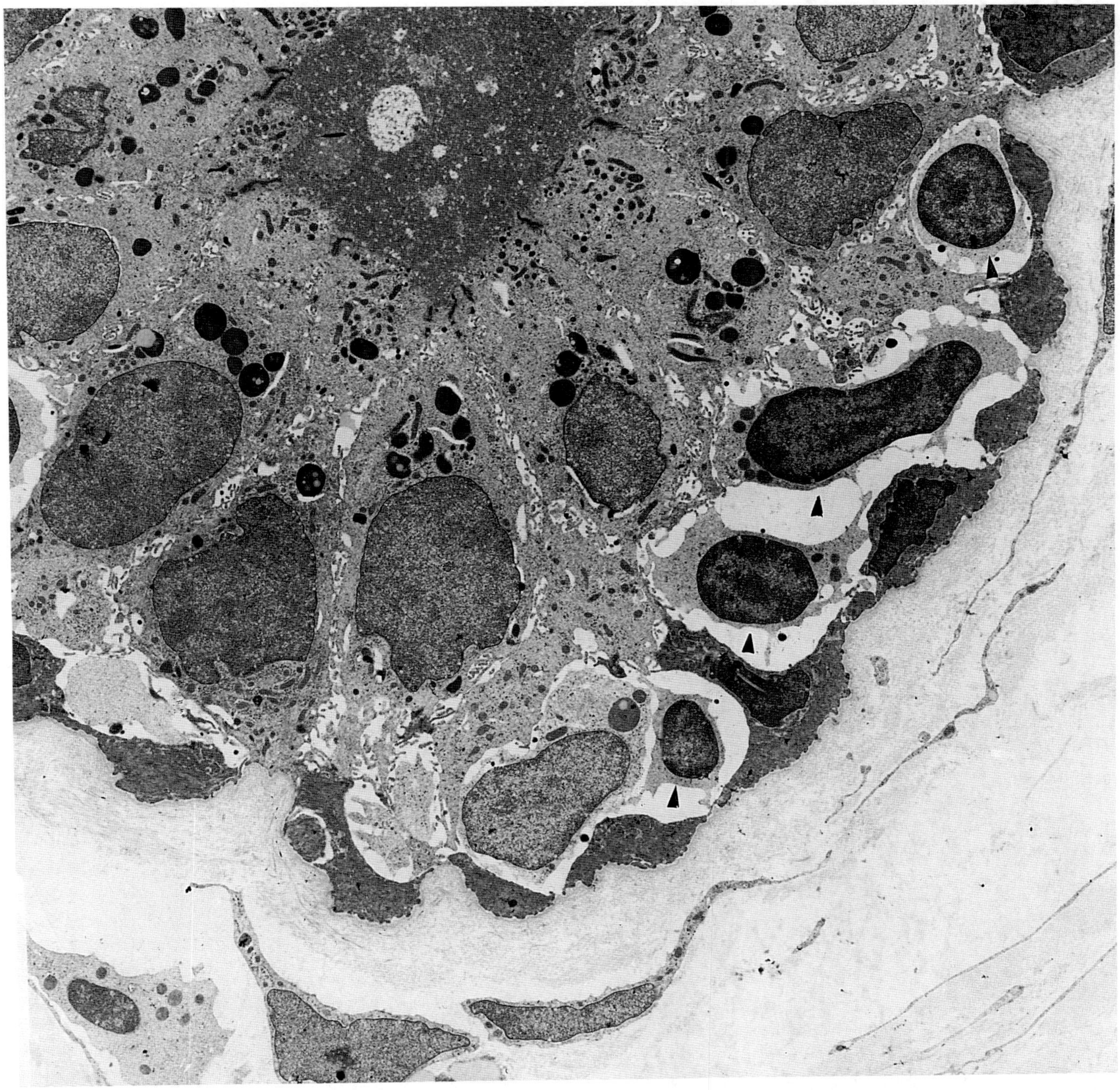

**Figure 1.9(a)** Portion of a ductule (acinus). Multiple migrating lymphocytes are present (arrows) between the epithelial and ME cells. (Uranyl acetate-lead citrate, X3,300)

B

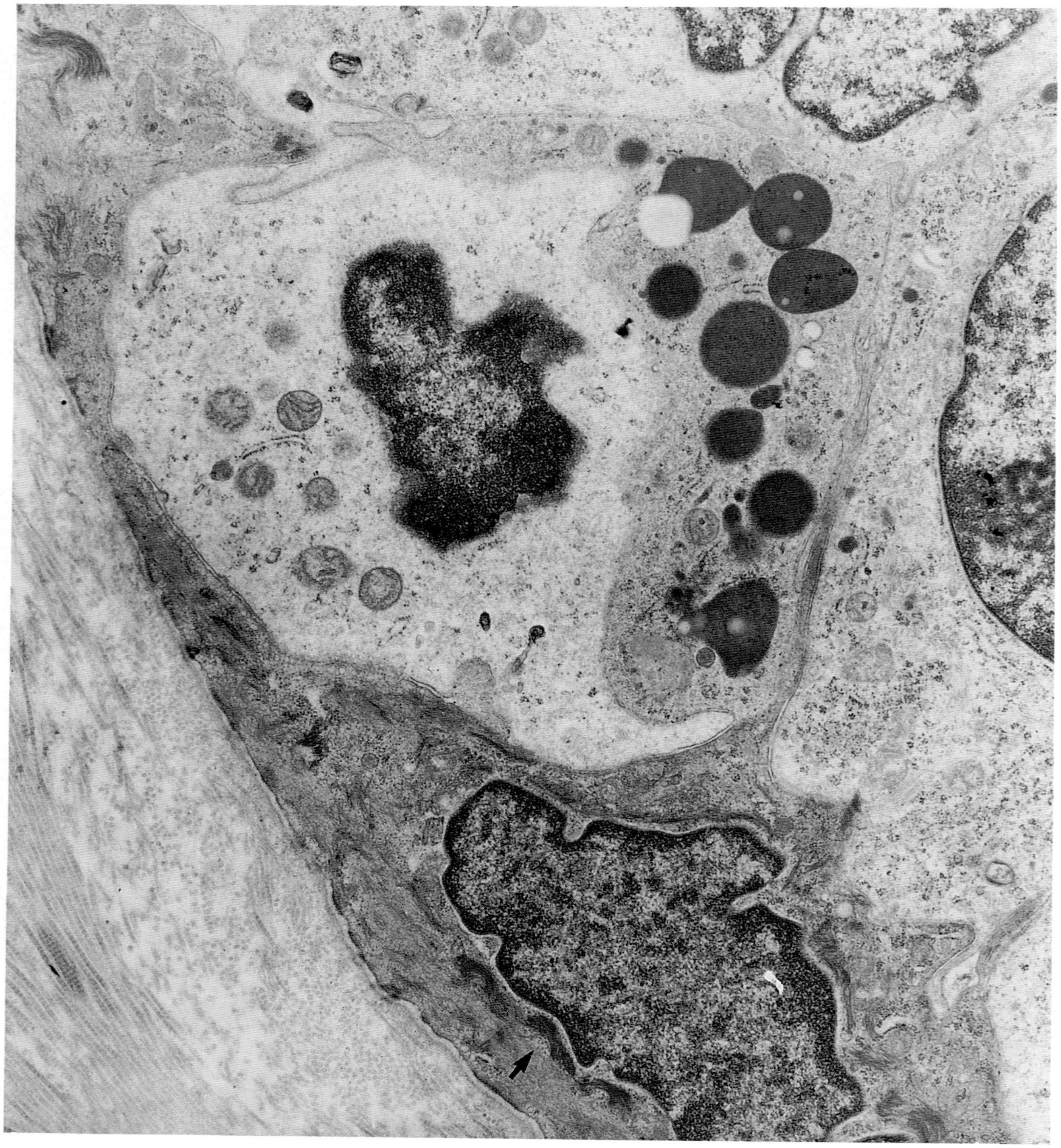

**Figure 1.9(b)** Portion of a ductule (acinus). A myoepithelial cell shows myofibrils with dense bodies peripherally and bundles of tonofilaments in the perinuclear position (arrow); pinocytotic vesicles are not readily apparent. The ME cell is attached to the basal lamina by hemidesmosomes and surrounded by basal lamina. (Uranyl acetate-lead citrate, X4,990)

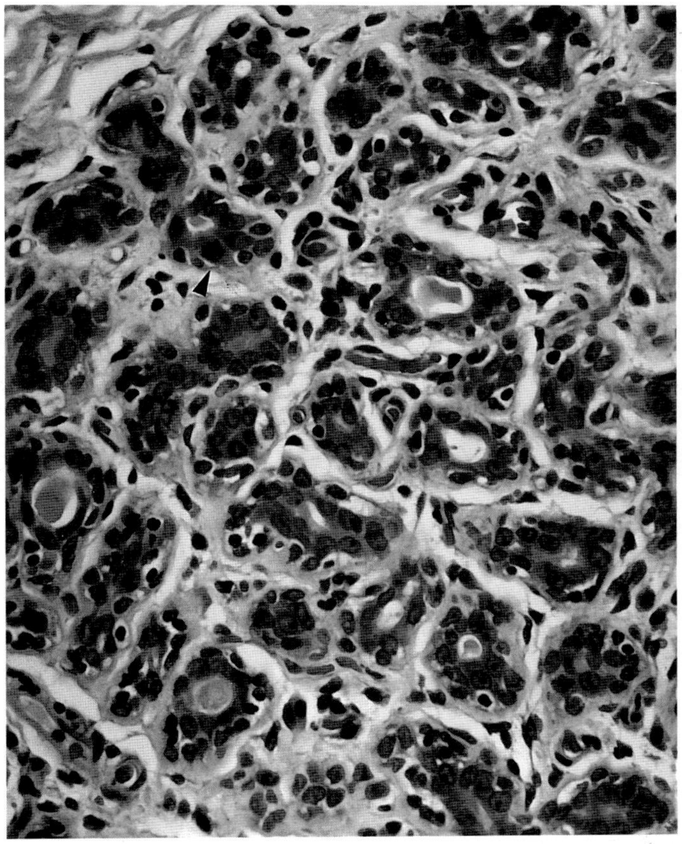

**Figure 1.10** Ductular (acinar) appearance during the proliferative phase. Note admixture of closed lumens with some that are open and contain secretory material. The luminal margin of the epithelial cells is truncated. A mitotic figure is apparent (arrow). Myoepithelial cells show minimal, if any, vacuolization. (H&E, X250)

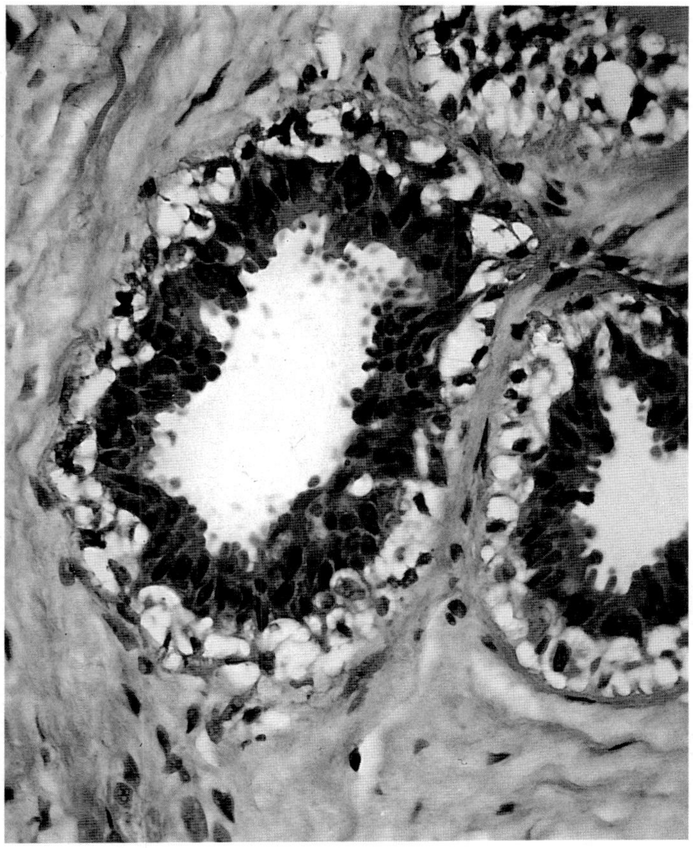

**Figure 1.11** Secretory phase: The epithelial and myoepithelial cells are quite distinctive. Note the open lumen of the ductules and the apical snout (cytoplasmic projections) along the luminal margin of the epithelial cells. The epithelial cells have a densely staining cytoplasm. The myoepithelial cells, in contrast, appear as naked nuclei surrounded by clear, or vacuolated cytoplasm. (H&E, X400)

secretory droplets during secretory and gestational alterations. Not infrequently, migrating lymphocytes and macrophages are present within the epithelial cell layer (9,32). These cells are most frequently seen adjacent to myoepithelial cells or between epithelial and myoepithelial cells and should not be mistaken for a third cell population native to the duct system (Fig. 1.9).

## Reproductive Years

### *Cyclic Morphologic Changes*

While exogenous sex steroids have been shown to profoundly influence the mammary gland morphology in experimental animals (2), the influence of cyclic hormonal changes on the morphology of the so-called "resting" breast is not well recognized.

The resting breast undergoes cyclic changes reflecting the hormonal alterations of the menstrual cycle (19,36). The changes are not as uniform and distinct as the changes observed in the endometrium, however. Based on the appearance of the intralobular stroma, luminal content, orientation, mitotic and secretory activity of the epithelial cells and the appearance of the myoepithelial cells, Vogel et al (36) divided these morphologic alterations into five phases to correspond to the five stages of the menstrual cycle. They designated these phases of mammary cyclic change as proliferative (days 3–7), follicular (days 8–14), luteal (days 15–20), secretory (days 21–27), and menstrual (days 28–2).

The most obvious differences between the pre- and postovulatory phases are the presence of a densely cellular stroma, closed lumens, epithelial mitotic activity and nonvacuolated myoepithelial cells during the proliferative phase (Fig. 1.10) in contrast to a loose, edematous stroma, open lumens with varying amounts of secretory material, absence of

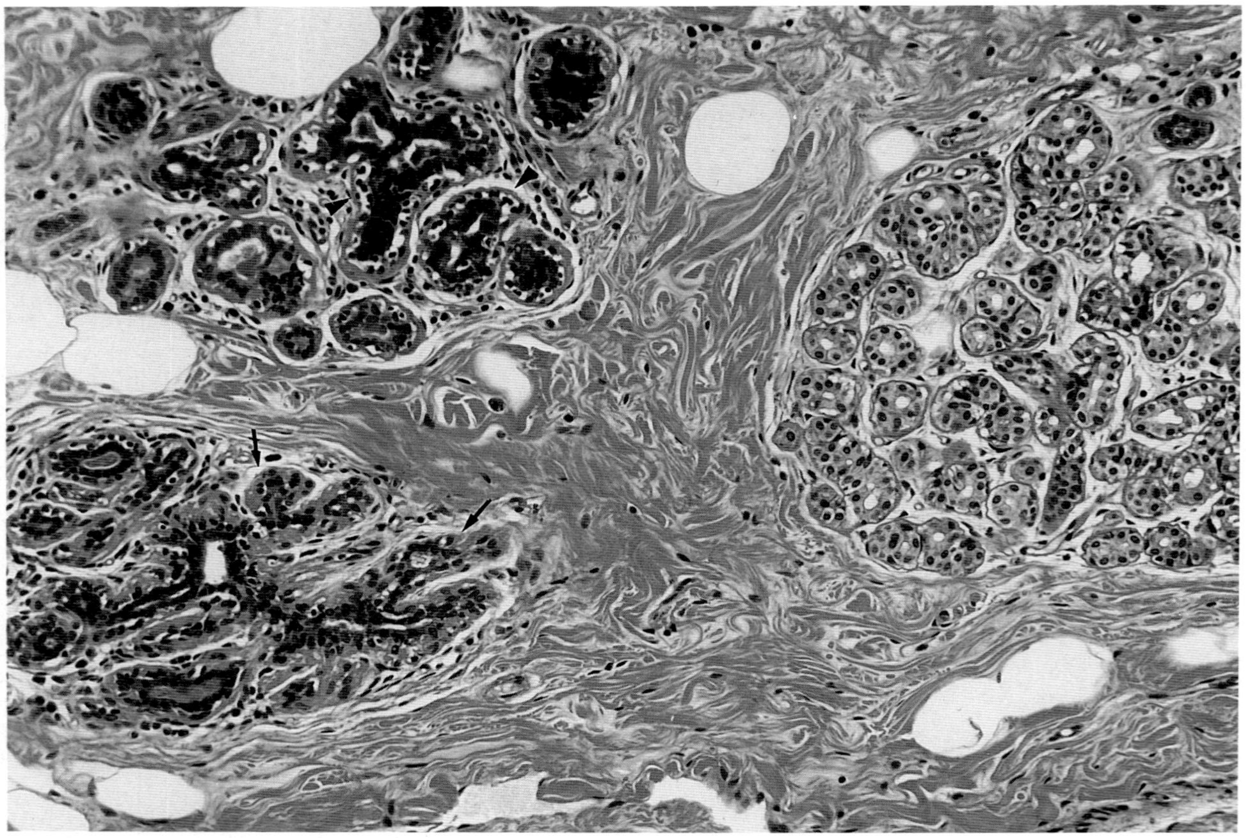

**Figure 1.12** Three adjacent lobules displaying ME cells with totally different appearances. One lobule shows clear ME cells (short arrows), the other displays an eosinophilic, myoid appearance (long arrows), and the ME cells are inconspicuous in the remaining lobule on the right. (H&E, X120)

epithelial mitotic activity and vacuolated myoepithelial cells in the secretory (postovulatory) phase (Fig. 1.11). Initially, the luminal appearance and content along with the appearance of the myoepithelial cells are the most helpful features. With practice and complete clinical information, Vogel et al's criteria can easily separate the preovulatory from the postovulatory phase of the cycle. It should be emphasized that the appearance of both the epithelial and ME cells is highly variable even in adjacent lobules within a single sample (Fig. 1.12). In general, however, one cell variant dominates throughout a sample. Furthermore, a mild secretory activity is present even in the resting breast as evident from the presence of secretory material within ductular lumens even during the proliferative phase. This mild secretory activity is generally balanced by the continuous process of resorption which prevents accumulation.

At the ultrastructural level, the epithelial cells of the proliferative phase lack microvillous prominence and organelles necessary for production of secretory material while those of the secretory phase show prominent luminal microvilli as well as glycogen, marked increase in rough endoplasmic reticulum and secretory vacuoles indicative of protein synthesis (8).

## *Cyclic Changes in Sex Steroid Receptor Level*

Epithelial enriched "normal" breast tissues of premenopausal women demonstrate menstrual cycle dependent variations in cytosol levels of estrogen (ER) and progesterone receptors (PR) (28). The mean ER level (7.5 + 2.9 fmole/mg protein) and the number of samples with ER > 3 fmole/mg protein (57%) are highest during the proliferative phase (using the five phases described by Vogel et al (36); the highest mean level of PR (36 + 27.8 fmole/mg protein) and the largest number of samples with PR > 3 fmole/mg protein (33%) have been noted during the follicular phase (28).

## *Pregnancy*

During gestation, significant hormonal alterations take place. The corpus luteum and the placenta produce large amounts of estrogen and progesterone

A

B

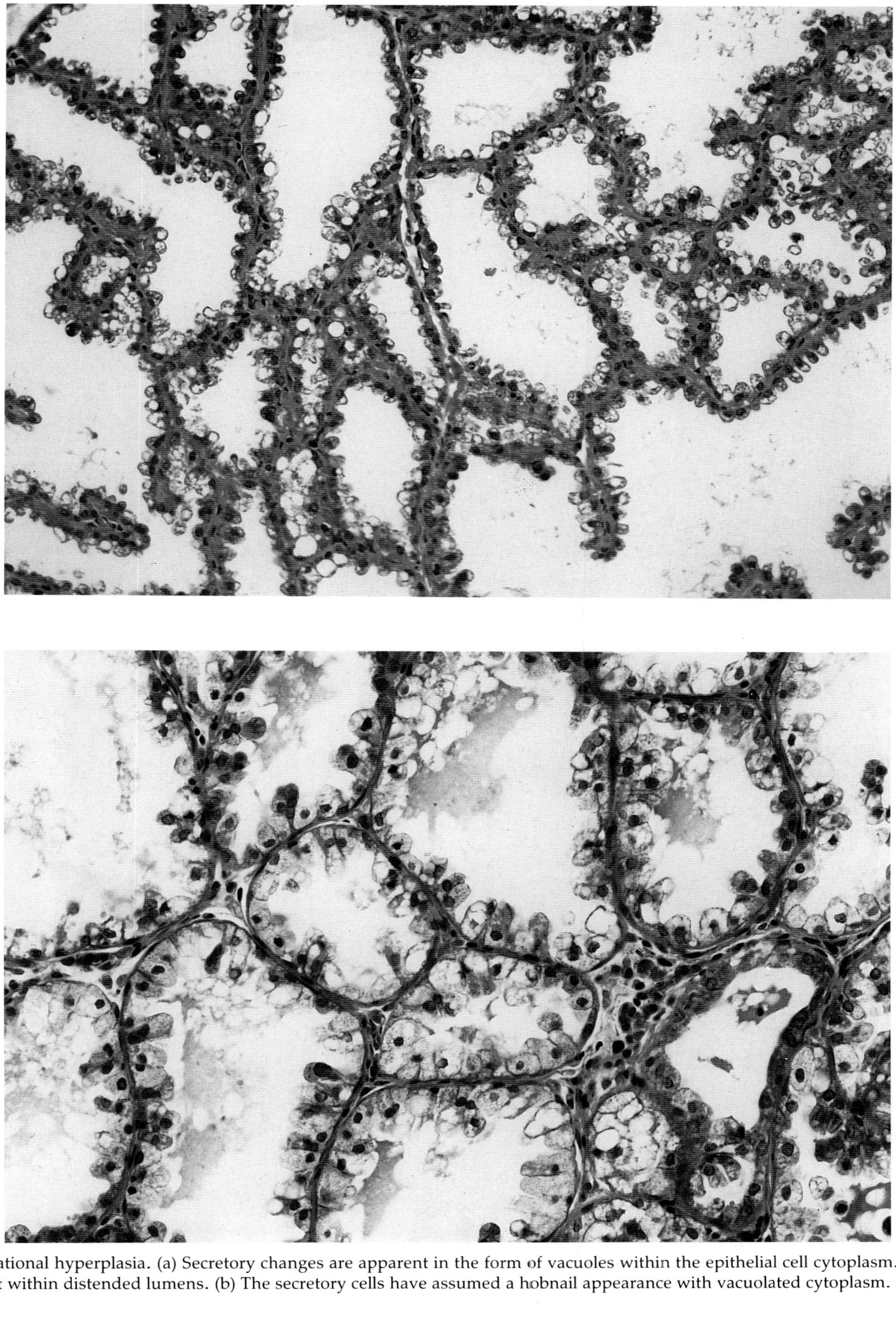

**Figure 1.13** Lactational hyperplasia. (a) Secretory changes are apparent in the form of vacuoles within the epithelial cell cytoplasm. Some secretory material is present within distended lumens. (b) The secretory cells have assumed a hobnail appearance with vacuolated cytoplasm. (H&E, (a), X160; (b), X200)

A

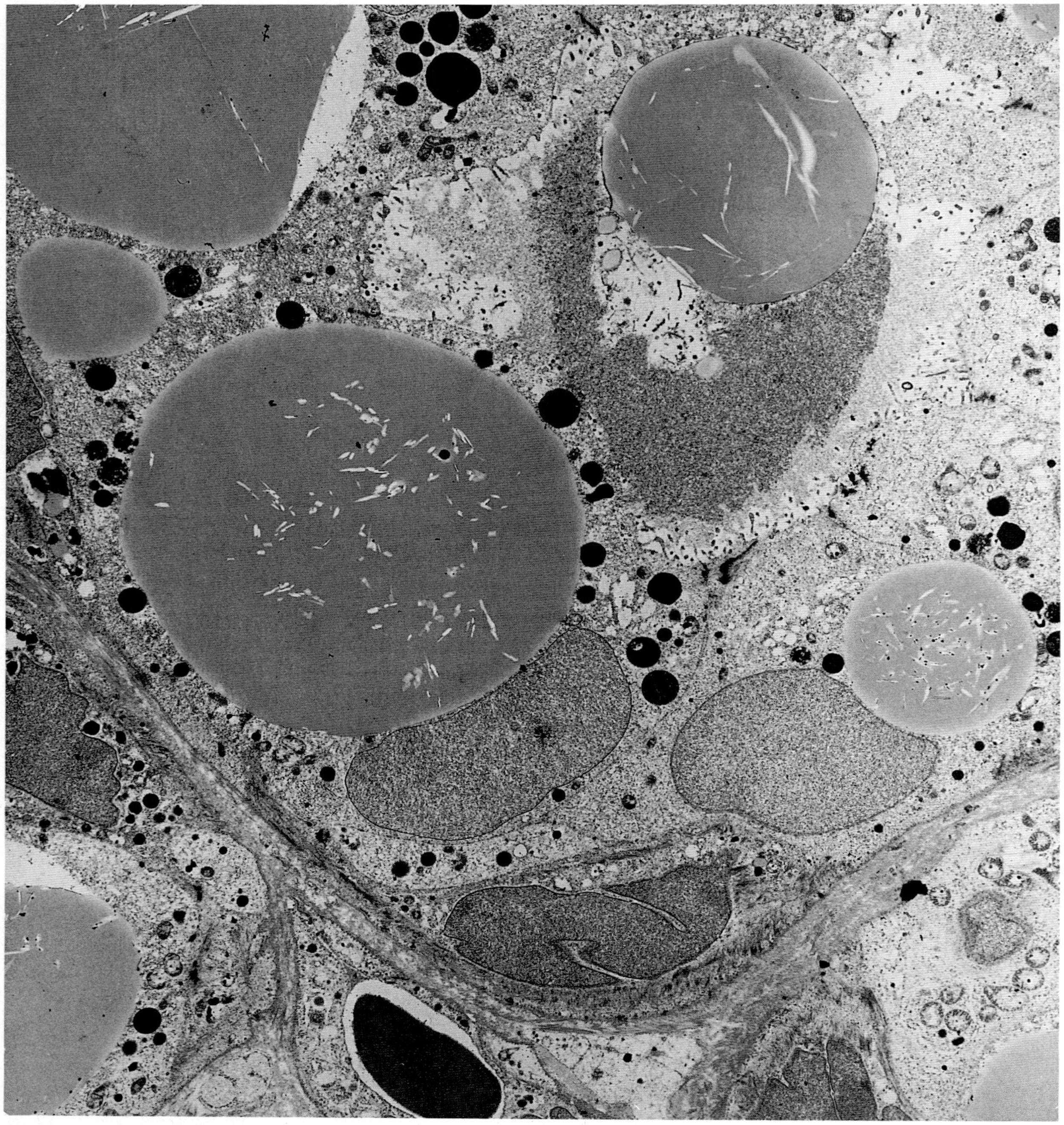

**Figure 1.14(a)** Lactational change. Ultrastructurally, abundant secretory material is apparent within the ductular (acinar) epithelial cytoplasm and the lumen; the acinar cells contain both lipid and electron dense secretory granules. (Uranyl acetate-lead citrate, X1,930)

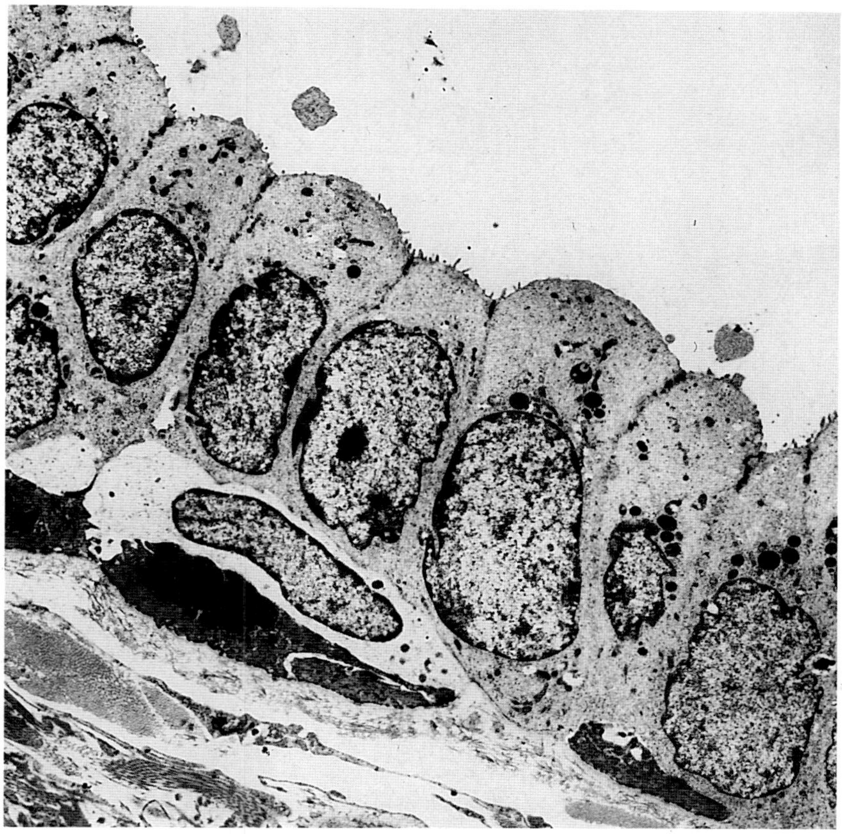

**Figure 1.14(b)** Lactational change. At the same time, a terminal duct shows only a few electron dense secretory granules and no evidence of lipid droplets. (Uranyl acetate-lead citrate, X2,700)

**Figure 1.15** Post-lactational involution (a–e). Various lobules from the same breast.

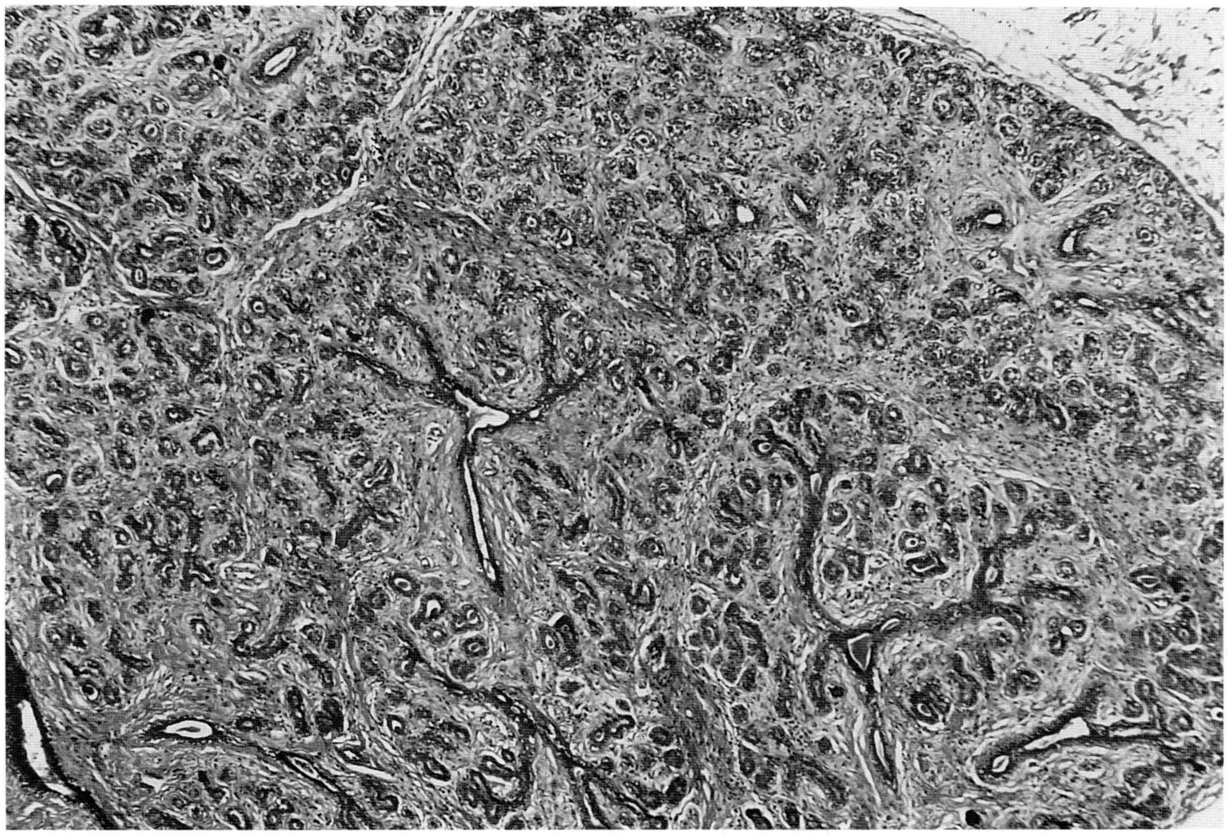

**Figure 1.15(a)** There is still evidence of gestational hyperplasia with massively enlarged lobules due to increased number of ductules. (H&E, X25)

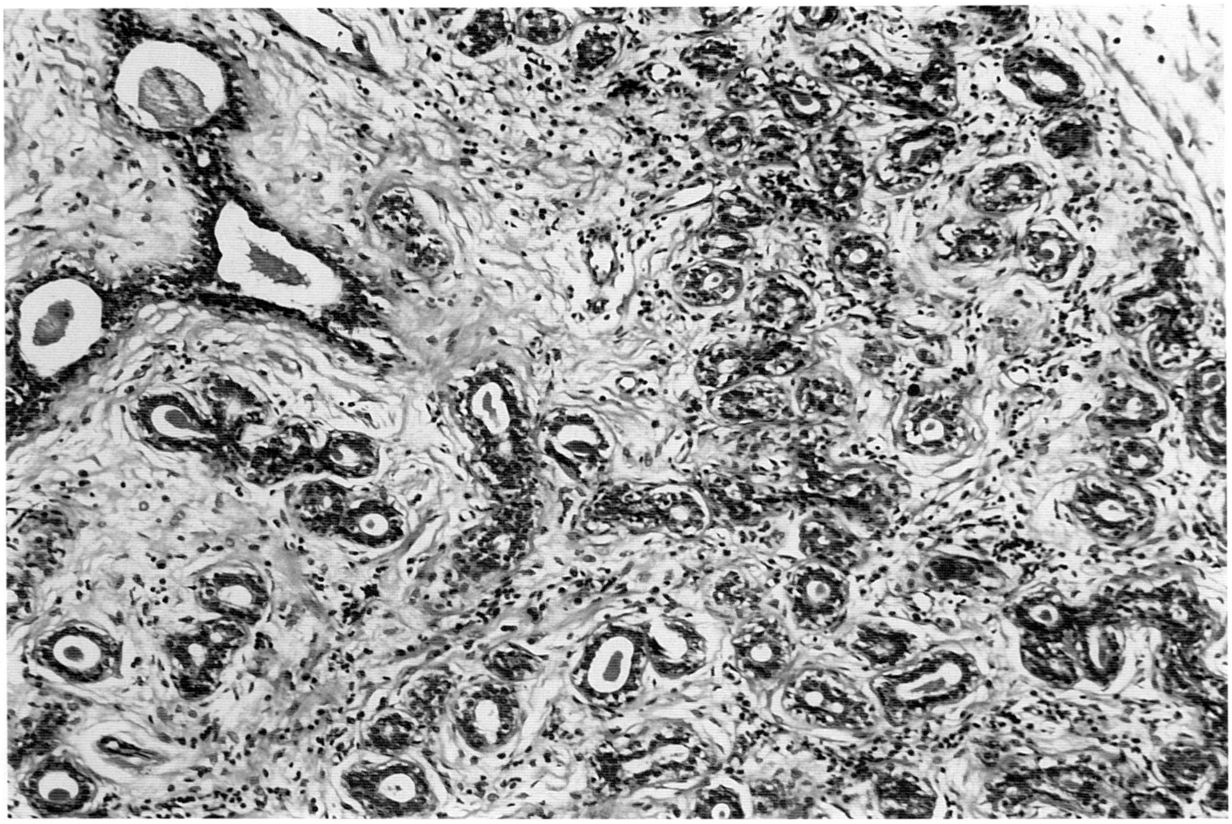

**Figure 1.15(b)** The intralobular stroma is infiltrated by lymphocytes, rare plasma cells, and macrophages. (H&E, X100)

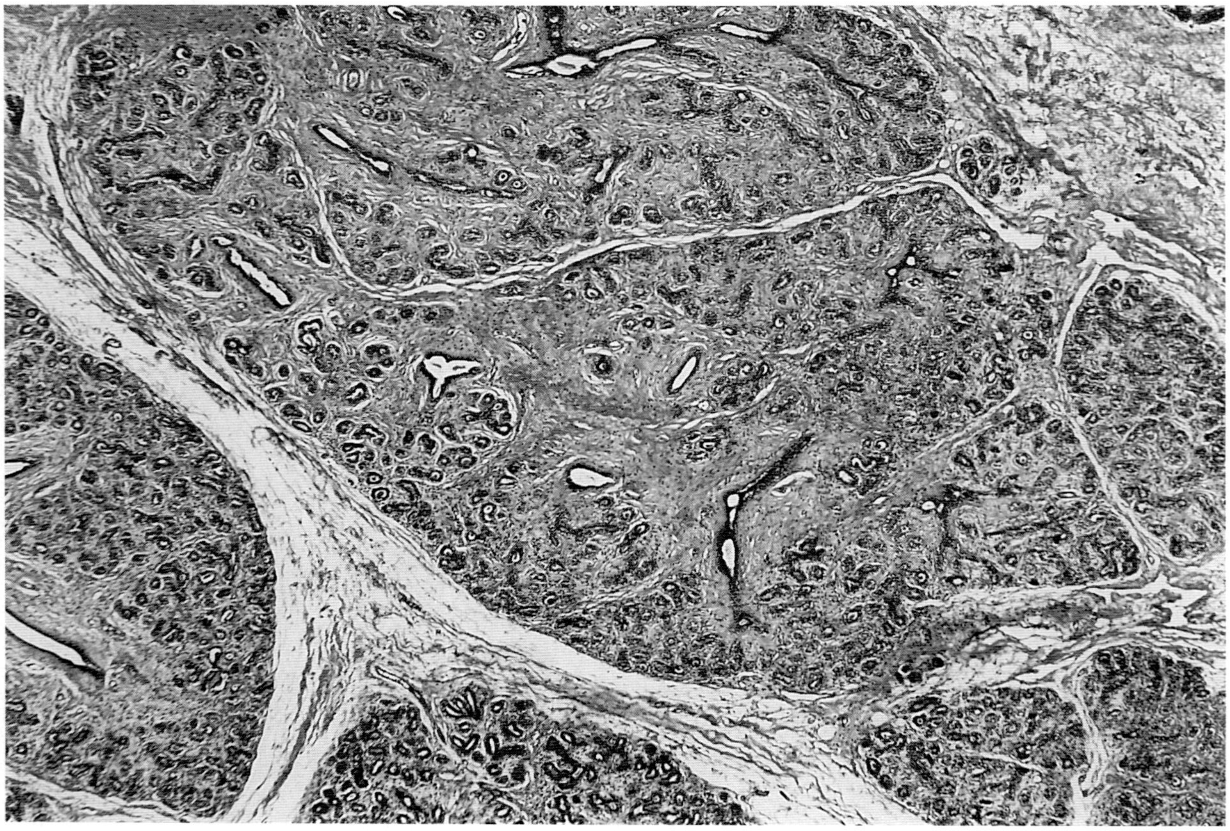

**Figure 1.15(c)** Early fibrosis and involution is evident around some of the ductules. (H&E, X40)

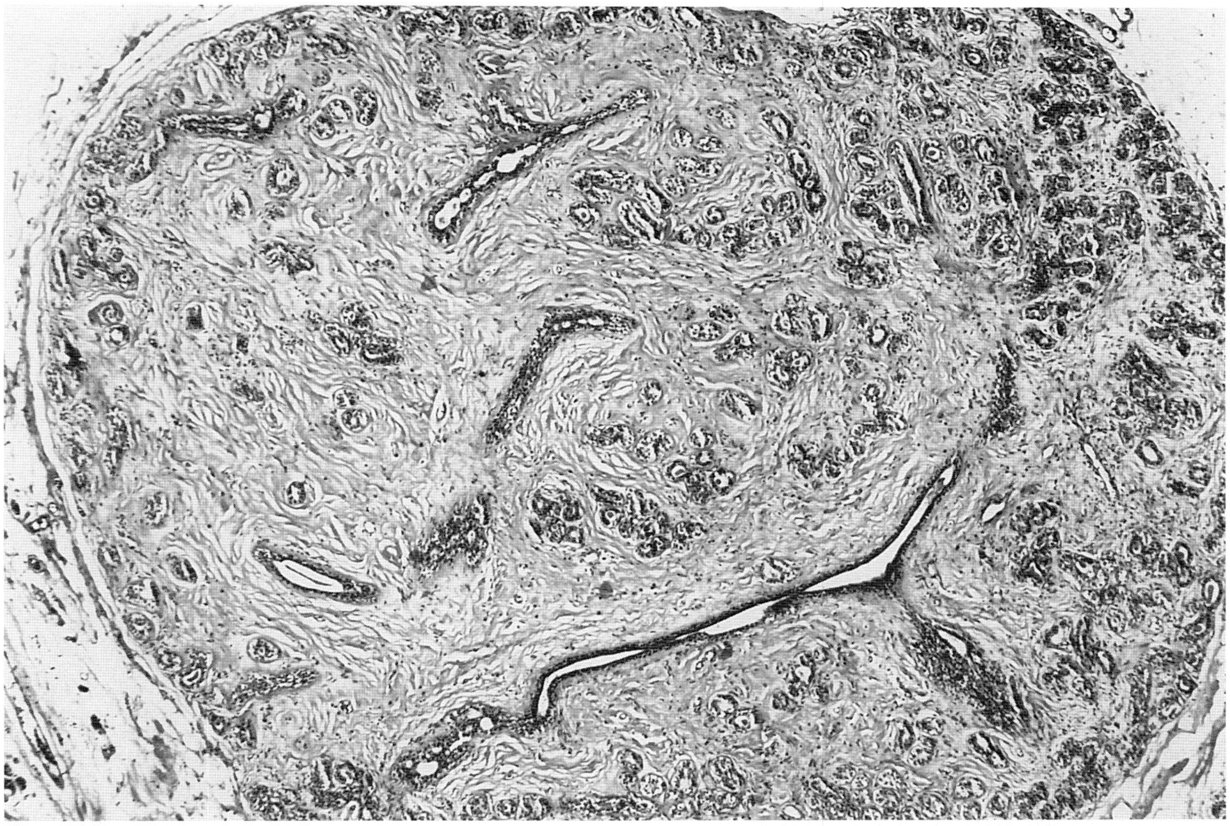

**Figure 1.15(d)** A more advanced stage of involution is displayed here with irregular distribution of the ductules (acini) and increasing lobular fibrosis; this should not be mistaken for a fibroadenoma. (H&E, X60)

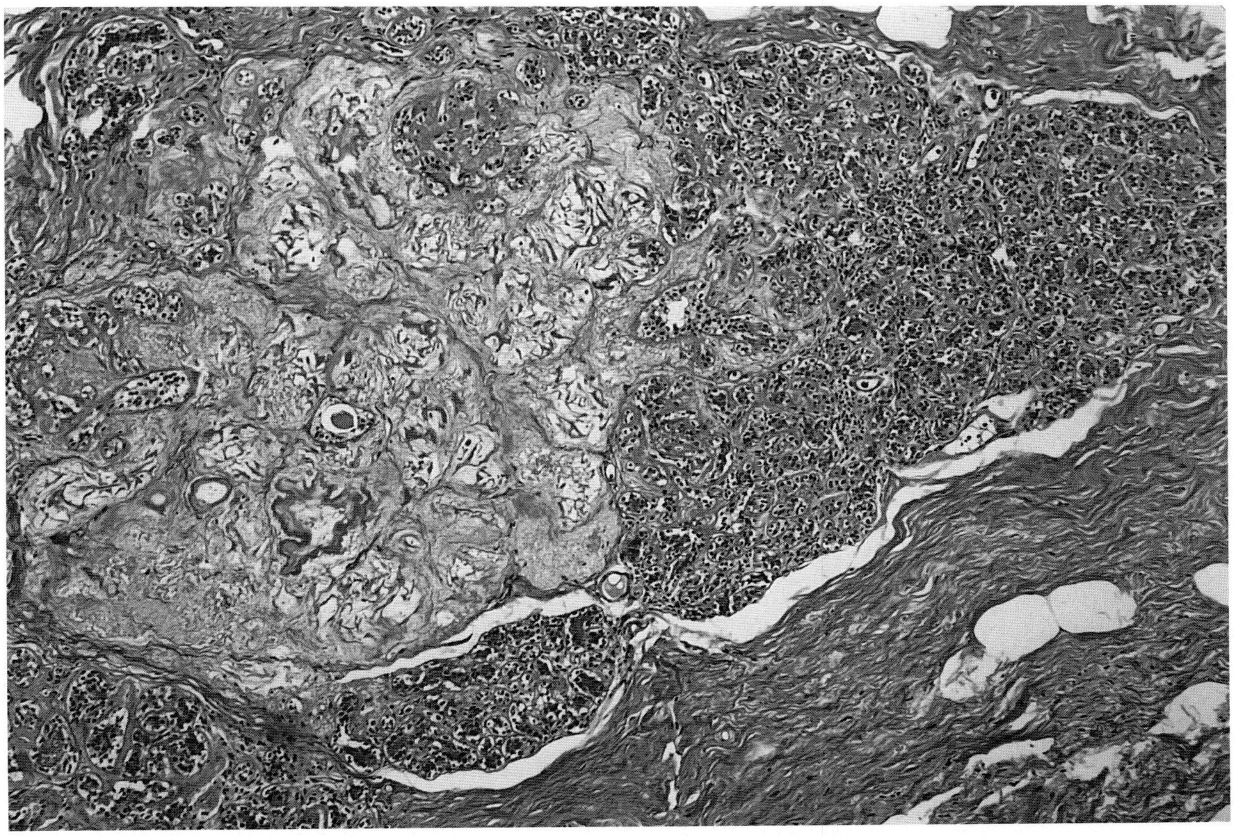

**Figure 1.15(e)** Almost half of the ductules in this lobule have been replaced by a fibroelastotic, degenerative change—a less frequent method of involution. (H&E, X60)

A

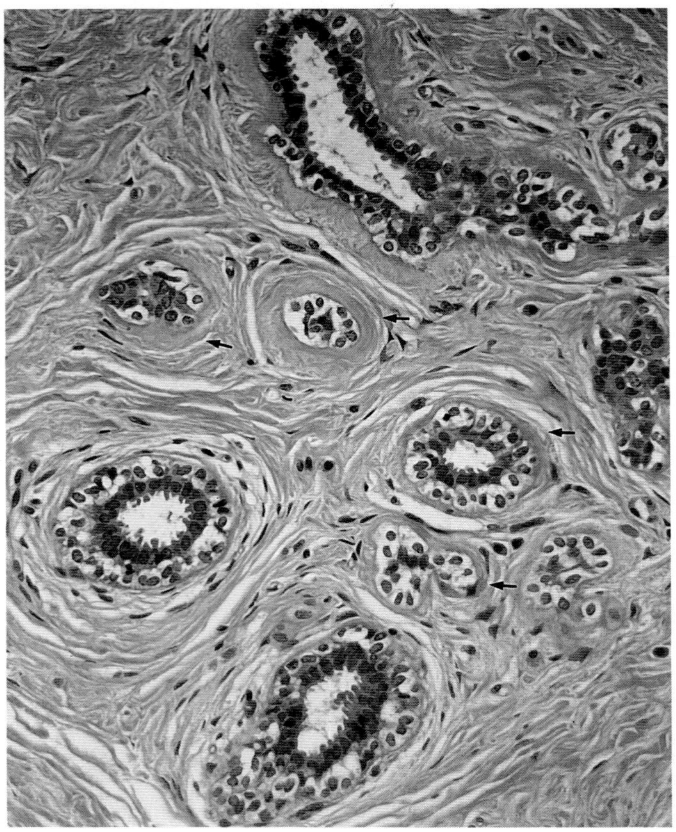

B

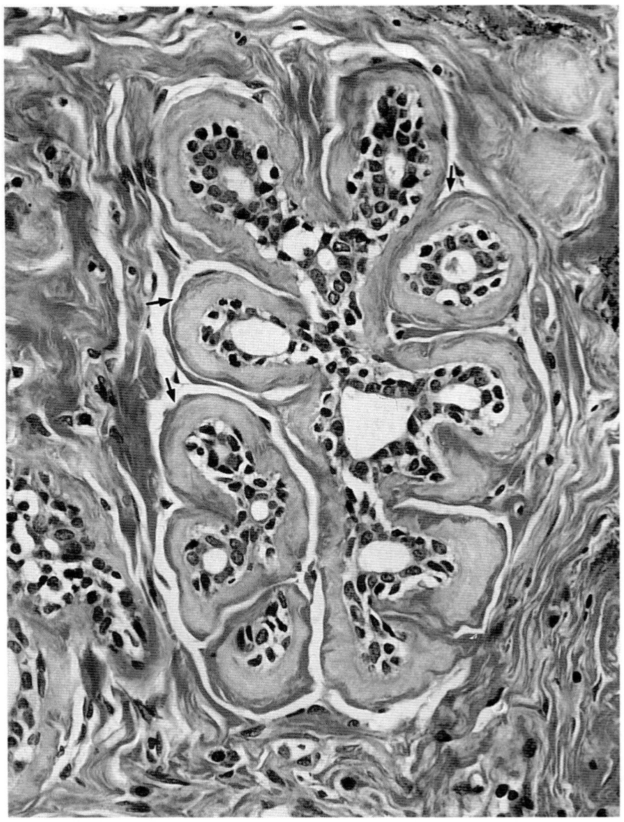

Figure 1.16(b)

**Figure 1.16** Post-menopausal involution-atrophy. (a, b) This process begins with a thickening of the basal lamina (arrows) around the ductules and gradual diminution of the ductular lumens in the lobules. (c) The acini within this lobule show various stages of involution from a basal laminar thickening (arrows) to complete fibrosis or hyalinization of the acini. (d–f) There is progressive decrease in the number of acini within lobules and hyalinization of the ductules. (g) The ghost of the lobule (arrows) blends with the surrounding hyalinized stroma. (H&E, (a, b) X250; (c) X160; (d–f) X100; (g) X75)

C

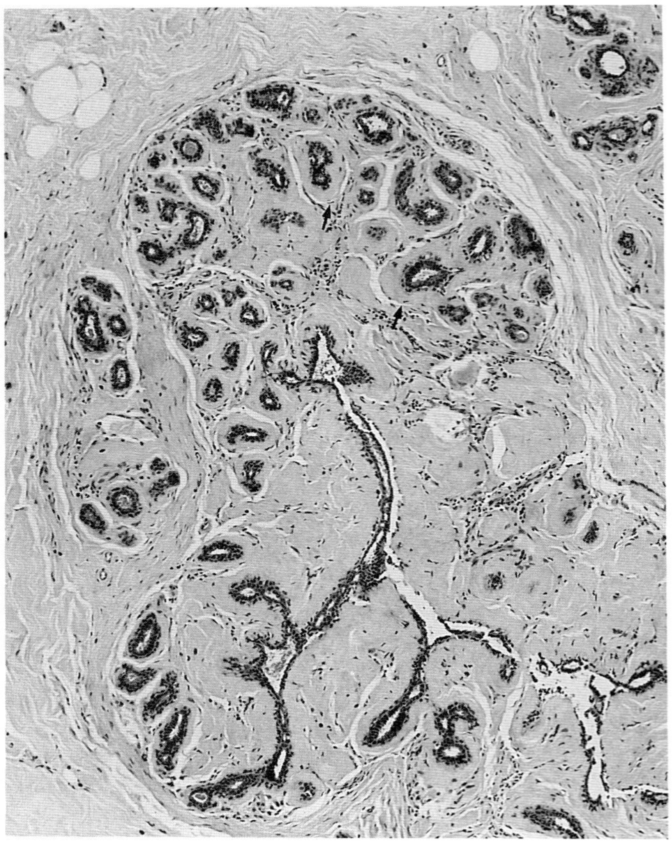

Figure 1.16(c)

resulting in a progressive rise of prolactin levels throughout gestation (25). The secretion of human placental lactogen and human chorionic somatomammotropin (HCS) by the placenta (intermediate trophoblasts) associated with the large amounts of estrogen and progesterone cause a remarkable growth and induction of secretory activity in the breast. The most significant morphologic effect of gestation is observed in the lobules. The number of acini per lobule increases tremendously and as pregnancy progresses, there is progressive accumulation of secretory material in the lobular epithelial cells generally beginning during the second trimester. The myoepithelial cells become attenuated. The proliferative activity is at its highest during the first 20 weeks of gestation reflected by the presence of numerous mitotic figures and an elevated Thymidine labelling index; during the second half of gestation, prolifera-

D

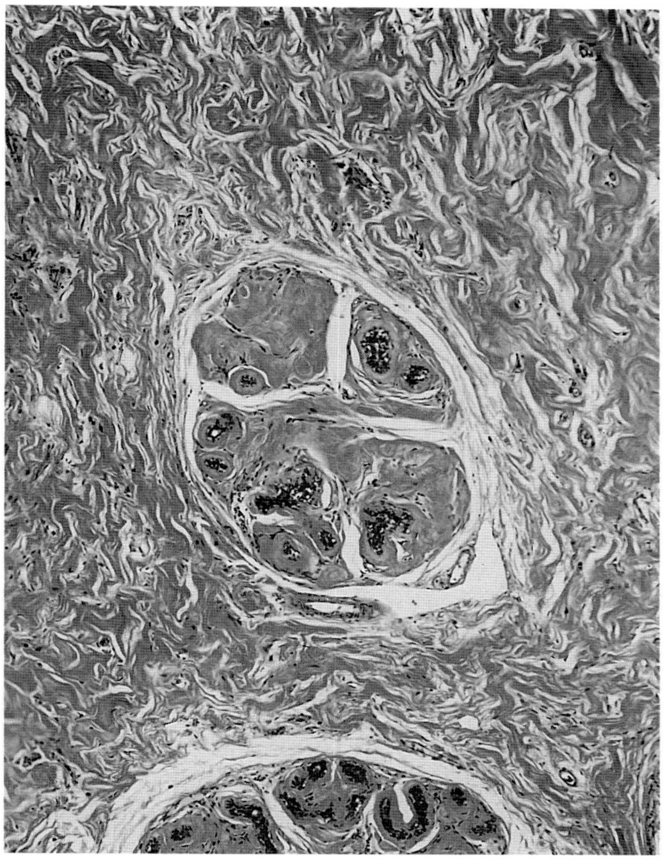

Figure 1.16(d)

E

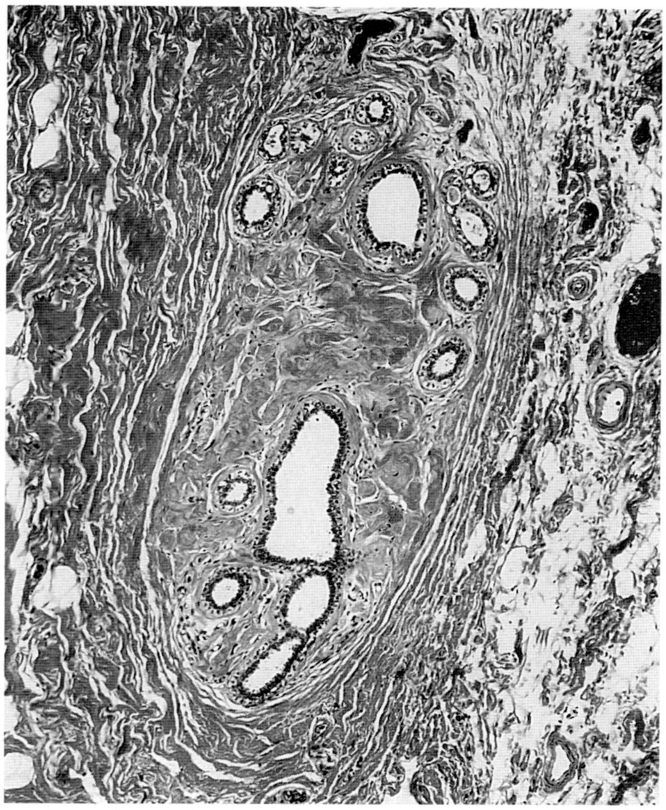

Figure 1.16(e)

F

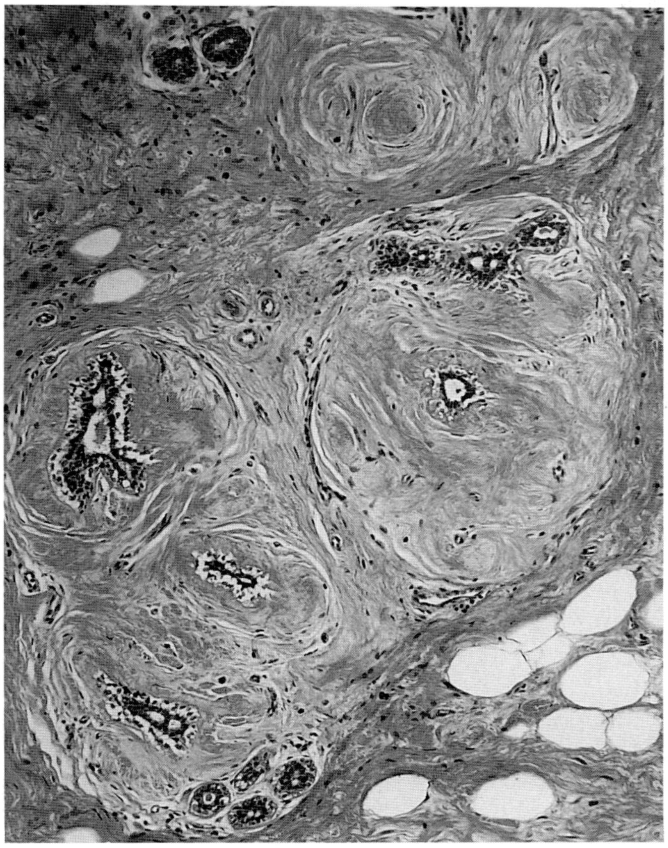

Figure 1.16(f)

G

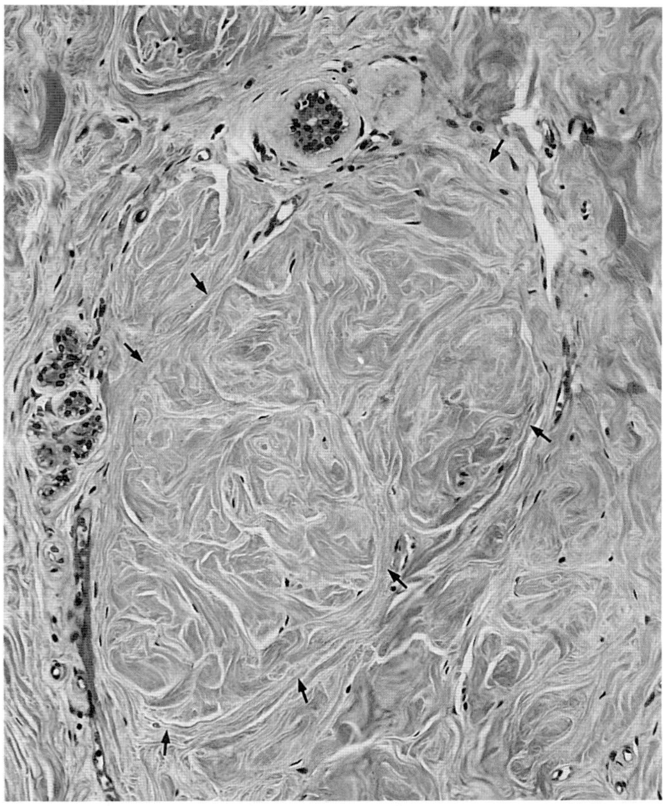

Figure 1.16(g)

Legends on opposite page.

tive activity diminishes while secretory and lactational changes increase (4). The interlobular stroma becomes inconspicuous as the lobules expand. While there is no morphologic difference between the epithelial cells lining the ductules (acini) and those lining the ducts during the resting (non-gestational) state, significant differences develop during gestation with accumulation of secretory material mainly in the ductular (acinar) epithelial cells of the lobule.

Galactopoeisis takes place after parturition and removal of the inhibitory effects of estrogen and protesterone on prolactin; it is well established between the second and fifth day after delivery. The lactating breast shows distension of acini with abundant secretory material in the lumen as well as the epithelial cytoplasm (Figs. 1.13, 1.14a, b). Myoepithelial cells are particularly inconspicuous at this time. The lactation process ceases within seven to ten days when nipple stimulation (suckling) is discontinued.

On the average, it takes three to four months for the breast to return to the resting state after lactation, but the rate is highly variable and the process is not uniform (Figs. 1.15a, b, c, d, e). During the early stages of lobular regression or involution, the lobules display an irregular, tapered shape, with disordered distribution of angulated ductules and ductular remnants (3). The epithelium appears flattened or angular and the basement membrane becomes crenulated, while the intralobular stroma is infiltrated by lymphocytes and rare plasma cells (3). In my opinion, the latter feature is the most notable in helping to distinguish lobules in a postpartum breast from those of a resting breast. Postgestational involution eventually results in an increase in the amount of fat and fibrous tissue. Lobules undergo fibrous replacement and hyalinization. The process of involution is a gradual one and most probably accomplished by phagocytic activity leading to the reduction and reformation of the lobules (18). A reduction in prolactin levels is believed to play a major role in this transformation, but the extent of contribution of cellular (phagocytic), hormonal or vascular factors to postgestational involution following lactation is not known.

## Postmenopausal Involution (Atrophy)

Following menopause, the breast undergoes involution characterized by diminution and eventual atrophy of the parenchymal elements (16,22). Within lobules, the ductular epithelial and ME cell layers become attentuated, while the lumens become practically obliterated and the basal lamina thicken significantly. Simultaneously, the surrounding specialized lobular stroma is transformed into a dense hyaline tissue which blends with the thickened basal lamina. As involution progresses, the epithelial component completely atrophies and the lobule becomes entirely hyalinized forming a hyaline nodule (Figs. 1.16a, b, c, d, e, f, g). Eventually, the hyaline nodule looses its circumscription and fades into the background stroma. The number of ductules (acini) in persisting lobules decreases to about one third of the number present during the reproductive years (12), with only three to four acini per lobule persisting in some elderly women. Mild to moderate dilatation of the ductules known as cystic atrophy occurs in some atrophic breasts (Fig. 1.17). In many aging breasts, the myoepithelial cells become more conspicuous and actually become hypertrophic or hyperplastic (Figs. 1.18a, b). This change has been referred to as myoepithelial atrophy (10), a term which is inappropriate considering the prominence of the ME cells in this alteration.

The breast stroma also undergoes involutional change. Alterations occur in the elastic and collagen fibers resulting in loss of supporting connective tissue. The adipose tissue, on the other hand, increases.

Involution does not take place as a uniform process throughout the breast. Therefore, a sample of postmenopausal breast tissue will display lobules and stroma at different stages of involution. As a result, variations are often noted in the consistency and firmness of the breast on palpation.

## Anatomic Relations, Blood Supply, and Lymphatic Drainage

### *Anatomic Relations*

The breast is surrounded by fascial tissues. The superficial pectoral fascia envelops the breast. The undersurface of breast lies over the deep pectoral fascia which covers the pectoralis major. Fibrous bands (Cooper's accessory ligament) connect the fascial layers representing the natural means of support for the breast.

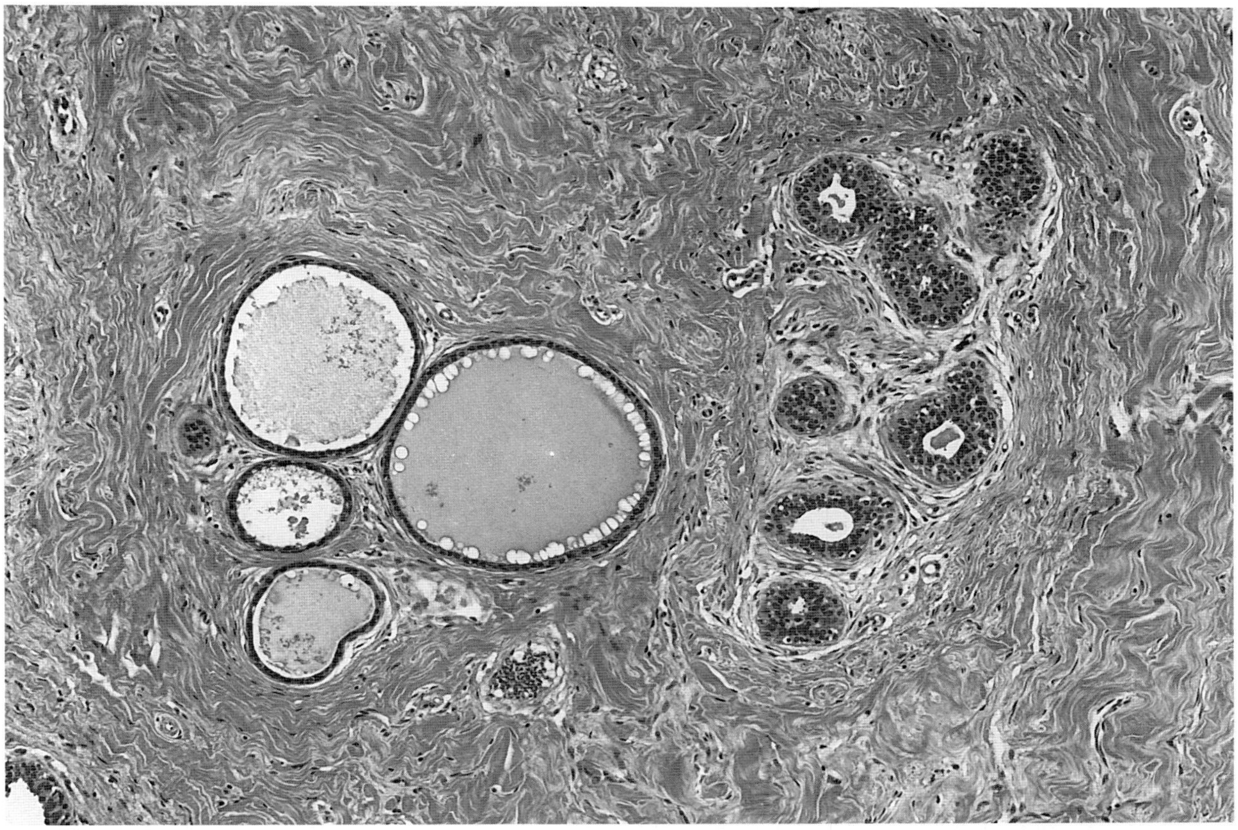

**Figure 1.17** Postmenopausal involution. The lobular stroma is dense in the lobule on the right, and there is cystic atrophy of the ductules in the lobule on the left. (H&E, X30)

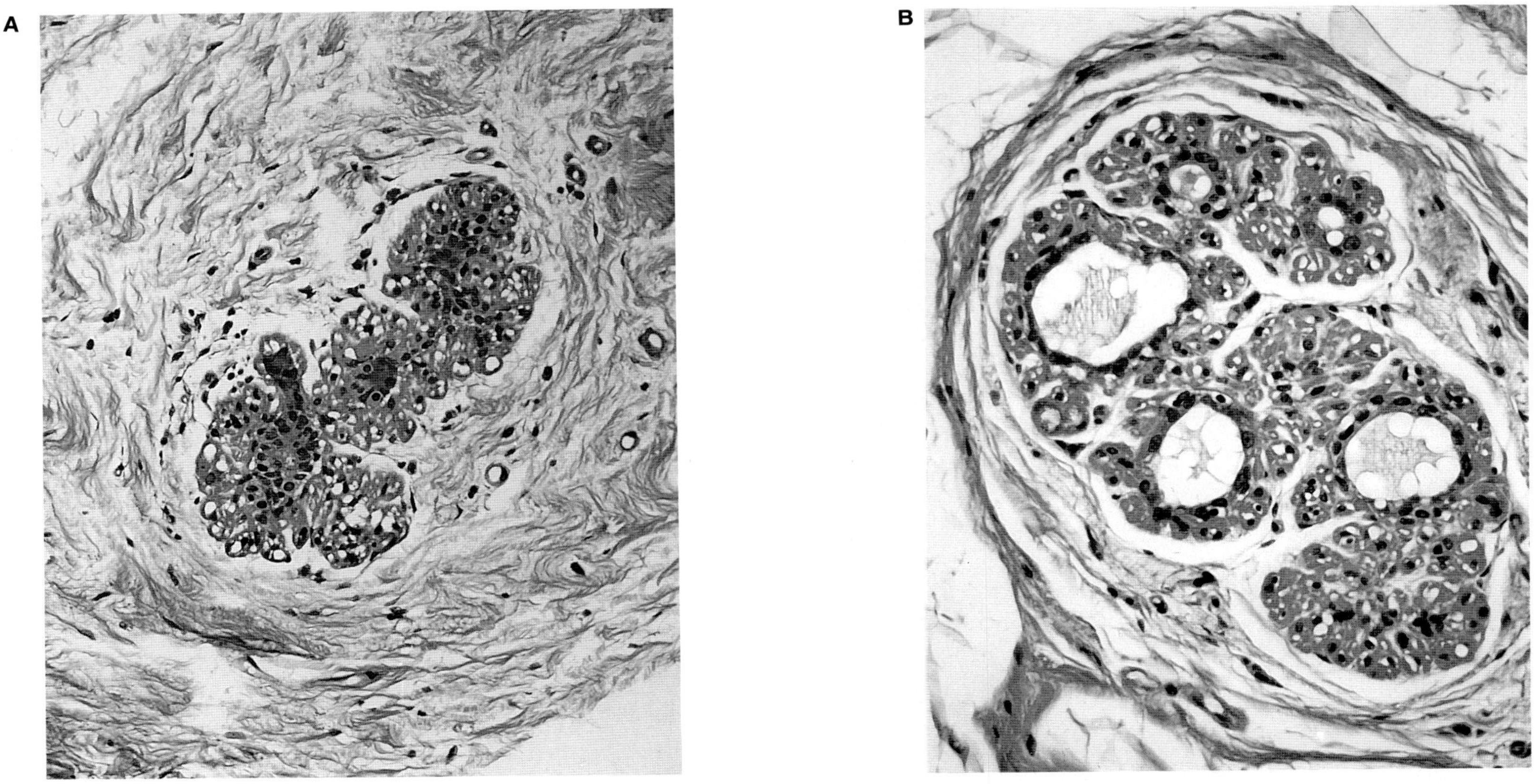


**Figure 1.18** Myoepithelial hyperplasia in a postmenopausal woman (a&b) The lobule shows significant prominence and hyperplasia of the myoepithelial cells. (H&E, (a) X200; (b) X250)

### *Blood Supply*

The internal mammary and lateral thoracic arteries provide the major blood supply to the breast. The anterior perforating branches of internal mammary artery feed 60% of the breast—the medial and central parts—, while the upper outer quadrant is supplied by the lateral thoracic artery.

### *Lymphatic Drainage*

About 97% of lymph from the breast flows to the axillary nodes while about three percent goes to the internal mammary chain (15).

## Axillary and Other Nodes

The axillary nodes serve as the major pathway for the spread of mammary carcinoma (21).

Axillary nodes are subdivided into apical or subclavicular nodes which lie medial to the pectoralis muscle, those along the axillary vein lateral to the lateral border of pectoralis minor, and finally the central group lying below the pectoralis minor muscle. There is also the interpectoral Rotter's node lying between pectoralis major and minor.

For determining metastatic progression, the axillary nodes are divided into levels corresponding to their location along the theoretic path of axillary lymphatic drainage from the breast (5). The level 1 lymph nodes lie lateral to the lateral border of the

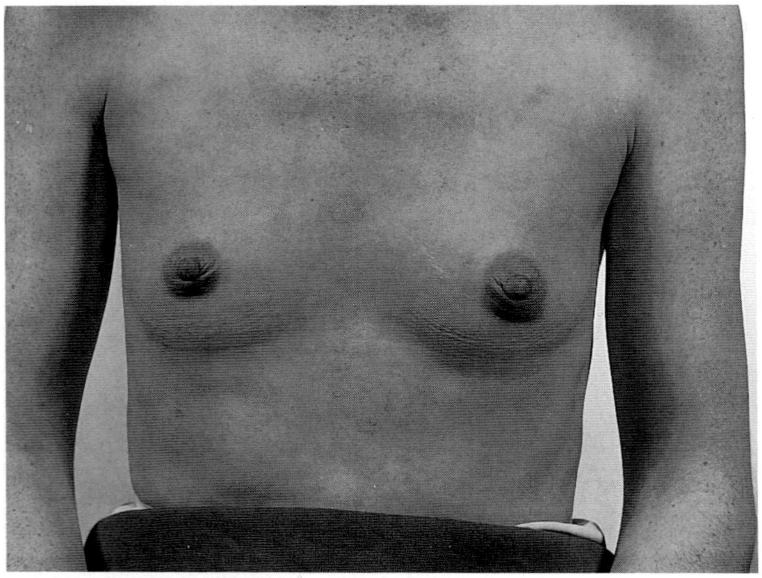

**Figure 1.19** Bilateral Hypoplasia. Both breasts are underdeveloped.

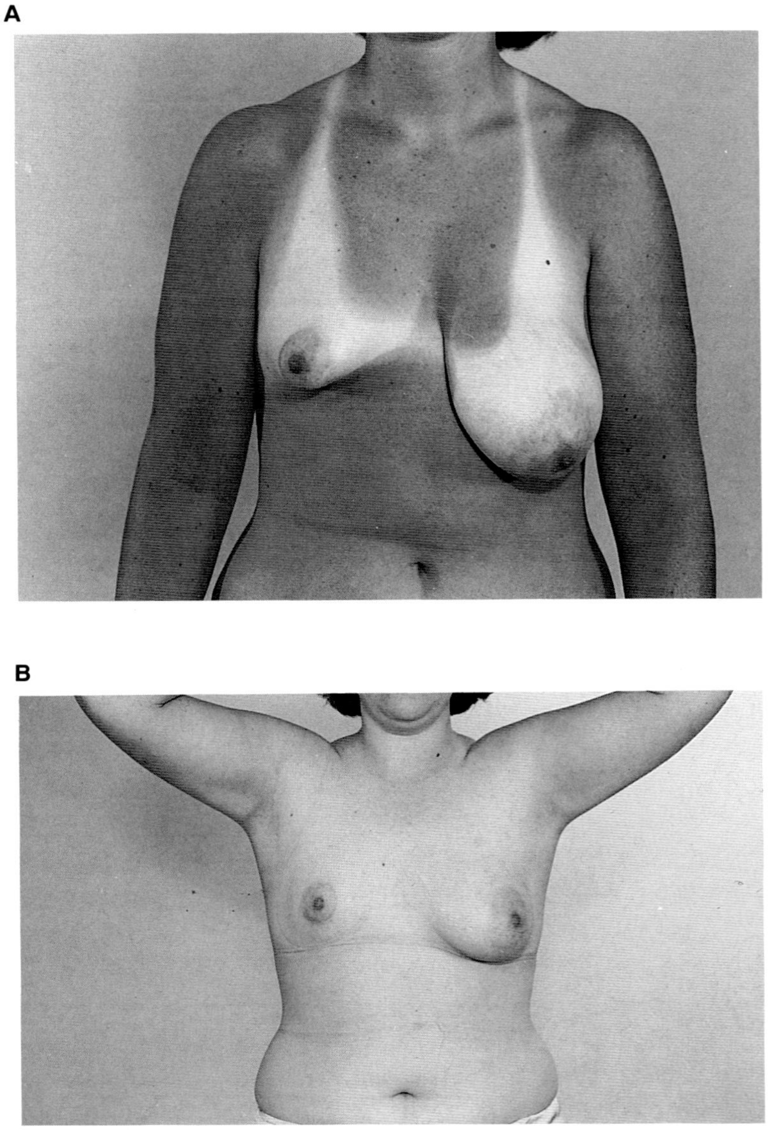

**Figure 1.20** Unilateral hypoplasia (a&b). Two examples of unilateral hypoplasia or asymmetry. In both cases, it is the right breast that is hypoplastic.

pectoralis minor, the level II lymph nodes lie behind the pectoralis minor, and level III nodes are located medial to the medial border and superior to the pectoralis minor muscle.

The internal mammary nodes lie in the intercostal spaces in the parasternal region—medial to the internal mammary vessels.

## CONGENITAL ANOMALIES

Deaver and McFarland (7) noted that complete or partial suppression of the breast anlagen in the em-

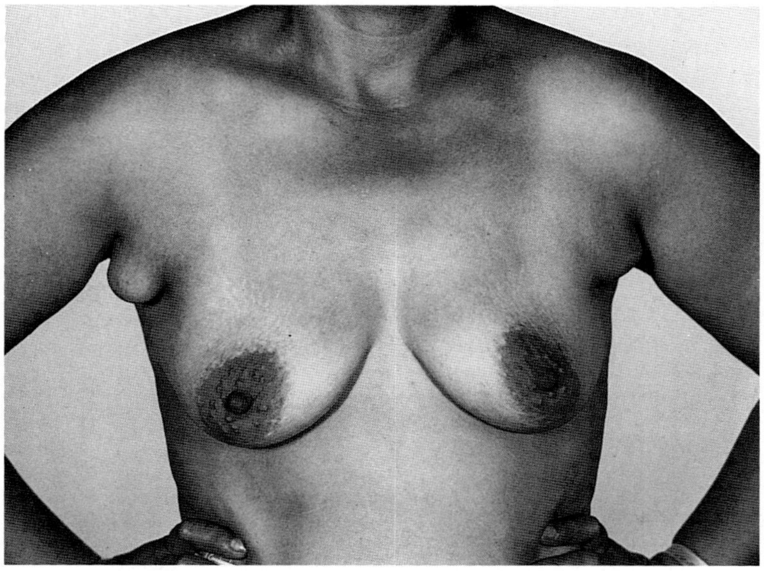

**Figure 1.21** Polymastia. Accessory breast tissue is most often found in the axillary region.

bryo would result in incomplete development or absence of breasts. Underdevelopment of the breast (hypoplasia) when marked is associated with hypoplasia of pectoral muscles in 90% of cases (35). Hypoplasia may be unilateral or bilateral (Fig. 1.19). Minor variation in size of the two breasts (asymmetry) is relatively common. While believed to be uncommon, the incidence of more severe asymmetry (Fig. 1.20a, b) is unknown. It is probably much higher than commonly believed, however, since a significant number of patients do not seek corrective treatment (29). Congenital absence of the breast, also designated as amastia, is quite rare (24).

Incomplete regression and persistence of portions of the milk line results in accessory mammary tissue in 2% to 3% of adult women. Accessory mammary glands (polymastia) are most often located in the axilla (Fig. 1.21). In Haagensen's experience (12), accessory breast tissue was found most frequently just below the normal breast. Radner et al (23) have thoroughly reviewed previously reported cases of polymastia and added a most interesting case of dorsal interscapular supernumerary mammary gland complete with nipple. Accessory mammary tissue sometimes becomes apparent for the first time during pregnancy when gestational hyperplasia causes enlargement of the mammary tissue. Accessory mammary tissue and polymastia are observed more frequently in Orientals, having been noted in 5.19% of Japanese females and 1.68% of Japanese males (17). It is also seen in 3.6% of Chinese males (33).

Accessory nipple is the most commonly observed abnormality in both sexes. Accessory nipples occur anywhere along the milk line (Fig. 1.22). Because of its pigmentation, the accessory nipple may be mistaken for a nevus. Absence of the nipple, on the other hand, is the rarest of all anomalies.

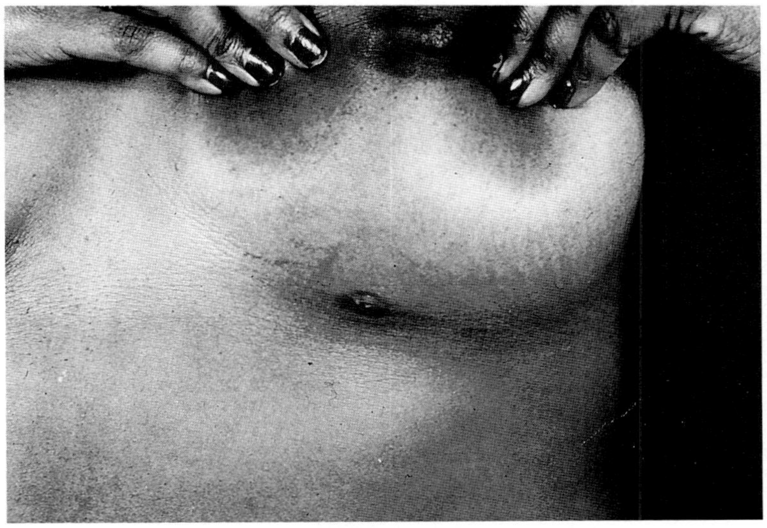

**Figure 1.22** Supernumerary nipple in the mammary fold.

## ACQUIRED MAMMARY HYPOPLASIA OR APLASIA

The mammary bud can be damaged by unnecessary biopsies of precociously developing breast, trauma from severe cutaneous burns and radiation to the thoracic wall.

### REFERENCES


* 1. Barwick K, Kashgarian M, Rosen PP: "Clear cell" change within duct and lobular epithelium of the human breast. *Path Annual* 1982;17(Pt 2):319–328.

* 2. Bassler R: The morphology of hormone-induced structural changes in the female breast. *Curr Top Pathol* 1970;53:1–89.

* 3. Battersby S, Anderson TJ: Histologic changes in breast tissue that characterize recent pregnancy. Histopathology 1989;15:415–433.

4. Battersby S, Anderson TJ: Proliferative and secretory activity in the pregnant and lactating human breast. *Virchows Archiv A (Pathol Anat)* 1988;413:189–196.

5. Berg JW: The significance of axillary node levels in the study of breast carcinoma. *Cancer* 1955;8:776–778.

6. Charpin C, Lissitzky JC, Jacquemier J, et al: Immunohistochemical detection of Laminin in 98 human breast carcinomas: a light and electron microscopic study. *Hum Pathol* 1986;17:355–365.
7. Deaver JB, McFarland J: *The Breast*. Philadelphia, P. Blakiston's Son & Co., 1917.
* 8. Fanager H, Ree HJ: Cyclic changes of human mammary gland epithelium in relation to the menstrual cycle—an ultrastructural study. *Cancer* 1974;34:574–585.
* 9. Ferguson DJP: Intraepithelial lymphocytes and macrophages in the breast. *Virchows Archiv A (Pathol Anat)* 1985; 407:369–378.
* 10. Foote FW, Stewart FW: Comparative studies of cancerous vs noncancerous breasts. *Ann Surg* 1945;121:6–53.
* 11. Geschickter CF: *Diseases of the Breast. Diagnosis. Pathology. Treatment*, ed 2. Philadelphia, JB Lippincott Company, 1945.
* 12. Haagensen CD: *Diseases of the Breast*, ed 3. Philadelphia. W.B. Saunders, 1986. p 50.
* 13. Hamilton NJ, Boyd JD, Mossman HW: *Human Embryology*. Cambridge, Mass, Heffer, 1968, p 428.
* 14. Hughes ESR: The development of the mammary gland. *Ann R Col Surg Engl* 1950;6:99–119.
15. Hultborn KA, Larsson LG, Ragnhult I: The lymph drainage from the breast to the axillary and parasternal lymph nodes: studied with the aid of colloid Au 198. *Act Radiol* 1955;43: 52–64.
* 16. Hutson SW, Cowen PN, Bird CC: Morphologic studies of age related changes in normal human breasts and their significance in the evolution of mammary cancer. *J Clin Pathol* 1985;38:281–287.
17. Iwai T: A statistical study on the polymastia of the Japanese. *Lancet* 1907;2:753–759.
18. Lascelles AK, Lee CS: Involution of the mammary glands. In: Larson BL (ed). *Lactation. A Comprehensive Treatise*. New York, Academic Press. 1978.
* 19. Longacre TA, Bartow SA: A correlative morphologic study of human breast and endometrium in the menstrual cycle. *Am J Surg Pathol* 1986;10:382–393.
20. McManus MJ, Welsch CW: The effect of estrogen, progesterone, thyroxine and human placental lactogen on DNA synthesis of human breast ductal epithelium maintained in athymic nude mice. *Cancer* 1984;54:1920–1927.
21. Pickren JW: Lymph node metastases in carcinoma of the female mammary gland. *Bull Roswell Park Meml Inst* 1956;1: 79–90.
22. Prechtel K: Mastopathic und Altersabhangige Brustdrusen Verandernagen. *Fortschr Med* 1971;89:1312–1315.
23. Radner H, Berger A, Schmid KO: Mamma supernumeraria dorsalis interscapularis (paravertebralis). *Pathologe* 1987;8: 310–315.
24. Rees TD: Mammary asymmetry. *Clin Plast Surg* 1975;2:371–374.
25. Reyniak JV: Endocrine physiology of the breast. *J Reprod Med* 1979;22:303–309.
26. Rosen PP, Tench W: Lobules in the nipple. Frequency and significance for breast cancer treatment. *Path Annual* 1985; 20(Pt 2):317–322.
* 27. Salazar H, Tobon H, Josimovich JB: Developmental, gestational and postgestational modifications of the human breast. *Clin Obstet & Gynecol* 1975;18:113–137.
* 28. Silva JS, Georgiade GS, Dilley WG, McCarty KS Sr, Wells SA, McCarty KS Jr: Menstrual cycle-dependent variations of breast cyst fluid protein and sex steroid receptors in the normal human breast. *Cancer* 1983;51:1297–1302.
29. Simon BE, Hoffman S, Kahn S: Treatment of asymmetry of the breasts. *Clin Plast Surg* 1975;2:375–390.
30. Smith CA, Monaghan P, Munro Nurelle A: Basal clear cells of the normal human breast. *Virchows Archiv A (Pathol Anat)* 1984;402:319–329.
31. Speroff L, Glass RH, Kase NG: *Clinical Gynecologic Endocrinology and Infertility*. Baltimore, Williams & Wilkins Co., 1973.
32. Stirling JW, Chandler JA: The fine structure of the normal, resting terminal ductal-lobular unit of the female breast. *Virch Arch* (A) 1976;372:205–226.
33. Takeya S: Ueber die uberzahligen Brustwarzen bei Chinesen. *J Orient Med* 1934;20:32.
* 34. Tavassoli FA, Yeh IT: Lactational and clear cell changes of the breast in nonlactating, nonpregnant women. *Am J Clin Pathol* 1987;87:23–79.
* 35. Trier WC: Complete breast absence. Case report and review of literature. *Plastic Reconstr Surg* 1965;36:430–439.
* 36. Vogel PM, Georgiade NG, Fetter BF, et al: The correlation of histologic changes in the human breast with the menstrual cycle. *Am J Pathol* 1981;104:23–34.
* 37. Wellings SR, Jensen HM, Marcum RG: An atlas of subgross pathology of the human breast with special reference to possible precancerous lesions. *J Natl Cancer Inst* 1975;55:231–273.

# 2

# General Considerations



This chapter will briefly cover some issues that are important as background information in our understanding of current discussions related to the diseases of the breast. In addition to the presentation of a variety of factors known to influence the manifestation of breast cancer, some of the features that are thought to influence the behavior and management of mammary carcinoma will be discussed.

## EPIDEMIOLOGY

Breast cancer has been the subject of extensive epidemiologic studies. These studies have provided insight to the magnitude of this problem and identified factors that place a woman at increased risk for the development of carcinoma. Despite the volume of accumulated information, it remains impossible to predict with accuracy which women in a given population will develop breast cancer. This is undoubtedly due in part to the multifactorial nature of the disease. If there is a single factor, the presence of which will invariably and consistently lead to manifestation of breast carcinoma, we have not yet been able to identify it.

Breast cancer is the most common malignancy in women in the United States, estimated to account for close to 32% of all cancers that will develop in women in the United States in 1992 (10). It is second only to lung cancer in the 1992 estimated cancer deaths, being responsible for 18.8% of deaths from cancer in women. In 1992, it has been estimated that 181,000 new cases of invasive breast cancer will develop in women in the United States and an additional 1,000 cases will develop in men. Furthermore, of women with breast carcinoma, an estimated 46,000 will die of their disease in 1992, compared to 300 of the men (10).

Based on the 1986–1988 data for cancer around

the world, the age-adjusted death rate for breast carcinoma is 22.4 per 100,000 population (10) in the United States.

While the worldwide number of new cases of in situ carcinoma (CIS) has not been documented as precisely as that of invasive tumors, it has been estimated that there are about 20,000 new cases of CIS annually in the United States (10). Some information is available regarding the frequency of in situ carcinoma from autopsy and reduction mammoplasty specimen in other countries. The breasts in 110 consecutive autopsies of Danish women 20 to 54 years of age were studied by an extensive histopathologic method and correlated with specimen mammography (138). Noninvasive carcinoma was identified in 18% of the women—14% intraductal carcinoma, 3% lobular carcinoma in situ, and 1% both intraductal and lobular carcinoma in situ (138). In another series, 5.9% of breasts examined in toto from random autopsies had intraductal carcinoma, but no lobular in situ carcinomas were identified (86). In a thorough evaluation of specimen from 200 consecutive cases of bilateral breast reduction mammoplasties, none of the patients younger than 30 years of age (85 women) were found to have significant abnormalities. In the older group, of those over 40 years of age (70 patients), 8% had lobular carcinoma in situ (94). In a study of 83 consecutive unselected autopsies, two of six women who were known to have had previous breast carcinoma were found to have contralateral breast carcinoma (137). Of the 77 remaining women who had no history of previous breast carcinoma, one was found to have infiltrating carcinoma, and 14 had carcinoma in situ. Based on these findings, Nielsen et al concluded that about one third of in situ carcinomas progress to infiltrating cancers (137).

The demographic features of black and caucasian women with breast carcinoma has been compared in several studies (28,43,51,65). The incidence of breast cancer has been somewhat lower in black women compared to caucasian women. The age-adjusted incidence rate was 71.9 per 100,000 for black women, compared to 85.6 per 100,000 for caucasian women for the years 1978 to 1981 (52). This gap appears to be closing, however. Spratt et al (57) speculated that the reduction in the gap that previously existed may reflect environmental influences or increasing affluence of the black population in the United States. Comparative studies have shown that the risk factor profile for breast cancer in black women is similar to that observed in caucasians (21,28,52).

### Geographic Influence

The death rate for breast carcinoma varies in different countries (10). For the period of 1986–1988, the highest death rate from breast carcinoma was found in England and Wales (29.3/100,000), followed by Denmark (28.3/100,000) and Scotland (27.5/100,000). The United States is 16th with a rate of 22.4/100,000. The countries at the bottom of the list of 50 nations for which this information is available are Thailand, ranking 50th (1.0/100,000), Korean Republic (6.0/100,000; data for 1986–1987 only), and China with 4.7 deaths per 100,000 population.

Interestingly, Japanese who have emigrated to the continental United States have a higher mortality rate than those living in Japan and the rates are higher for Japanese born in the United States (Nisei) than for immigrants who were born in Japan (Issei), (53). Second generation immigrants to the United States have rates closely approaching those observed in the native white population (16).

While the mortality rate has remained constant over the past 40 years, the incidence of breast carcinoma increased by 50% between 1965 and 1975 (20) and it is expected to increase at a rate of 2%–3% annually (39). Only 40% of the women with a diagnosis of breast carcinoma between 1965–1975 had a fatal disease, however; the remaining 60% had morphologically malignant lesions that behaved less aggressively within the follow-up period (20).

## RISK FACTORS

Berg (6) defined risk factor as the characteristic of individual patients that increased their chances of developing breast cancer above the level of risk in the general population. He classified risk factors as genetic (family history), hormonal, nutritional, morphologic, and radiation related. More importantly, he noted that even in women who lack these risk factors, there is a substantial risk for developing breast cancer.

It is important to keep in mind that the absence of known risk factors does not preclude the development of cancer. Seidman and associates (54) calculated that the available information on risk factors accounts for 20% of the risk in younger women and less than 30% in older women in the United States. In 1984, the overall probability of an American woman developing breast carcinoma by age 75 years was about 1 in 12, while a woman with no known risk factors had a 1 in 17 chance of developing the disease (6). Apparently, the absence of recognized risk factors does not eradicate the chances of developing breast carcinoma. It would be interesting to study women who do not develop breast carcinoma despite having a majority of the risk factors.

Based on the U.S. incidence and mortality data for 1973–1977 (67), white women had the highest probability (8.2% or 1 in 12) of developing breast carcinoma by age 75 years among various ethnic and racial groups in the United States. In comparison, the probability for black women was 7% (1 in 14), Chinese-Americans, 6.1% (1 in 16), Japanese-Americans, 5.4% (1 in 19), New-Mexican Hispanics, 4.8% (1 in 21), and New-Mexican American Indians, 2.5% (1 in 40). For a woman in the United States, the overall probability of developing breast carcinoma at some point in her life has increased to 1 in 9 in 1991.

## Genetic Factor (Family History)

The trend for breast carcinoma to develop in some families has been identified for many years. It is now recognized that a positive family history of breast carcinoma constitutes a major risk factor. The risk is significant mainly when the diagnosis of breast cancer is in a first degree relative (mother, daughter, sister), however. This increase, which is about two- to threefold for women with a single postmenopausal first degree relative with breast cancer, increases to ninefold if the first-degree relative is premenopausal, with bilateral breast cancer. The lifetime risk for a woman with a first-degree relative with premenopausal onset of bilateral carcinoma is 50% (1,3,4). It is noteworthy that only about 15% of women have a positive family history of breast carcinoma, while 85% of all breast cancers develop in women without known family history of breast cancer (31).

Patients from families prone to breast cancer tend to be younger and have a higher frequency of bilaterality (2,24). The risk of breast cancer in relatives of patients with bilateral disease is three to four times higher than that in relatives of patients with unilateral disease (2).

### *Li-Fraumeni Syndrome*

There is a higher frequency of breast carcinoma in patients with this autosomal dominant syndrome characterized by a defect in the tumor suppressor gene p53. Multiple cancers (breast, brain, sarcomas, and adrenal cortical tumors) are observed in the kindred (8,30,34).

## Hormonal Influence

Risk factors that implicate reproductive steroid hormones in the development of mammary carcinoma include the female sex, menstrual and reproductive history. The influence of these hormones is thought to be exerted on the first stage in the two-stage model for human carcinogenesis proposed by Moolgavkar and Knudson (40). In this model, it is postulated that human carcinomas arise from epithelial stem cells following a series of two or more errors in normal cell division. The errors probably result from damage to the deoxyribonucleic acid (DNA) caused by initiators such as ionizing radiation, chemicals or viruses. Initiating factors are more likely to cause carcinoma if there is proliferation or an increase in the number of the susceptible undifferentiated stem cells, and less likely to do so if the stem cells are either killed or encouraged to differentiate. Ionizing radiation is thought to initiate the development of cancer by damaging the DNA in the stem cells (61). Reproductive steroid hormones, on the other hand, are most likely to exert an influence on carcinogenesis by altering the kinetics of proliferation, differentiation or atrophy of the stem cell resulting in an increase in the number of susceptible cells (60).

Estrogens and progestins are the most likely hormones involved in the pathologic cellular changes, but prolactin and androgens may also play a role (60). Estrogens promote growth and proliferative activity of the duct system, and would be expected to increase the risk of breast cancer by stimulating proliferation of the undifferentiated cells. Progestins cause growth and differentiation of the cells; the latter has a protective influence. Androgens depress mammary epithelial proliferation and would have a protective effect. Prolactin stimulates and maintains lactation of the estrogen-primed cell and is associated with the function of a differentiated cell. Therefore, it is not expected to increase the risk of cancer (60).

Thomas hypothesized that prolonged exposure to normal levels of cyclic estrogen and progestins act at an early stage in the development of breast cancer by stimulating epithelial proliferative activity (60,61). Excess endogenous estrogens resulting from early menarche, late menopause, and nulliparity are thought to stimulate proliferation of cells that have undergone "malignant transformation" and result in some increased risk of breast cancer (60).

### *Menstrual and Reproductive History*

The age at menarche is inversely related to the risk for development of breast carcinoma. Women who begin menstruating before age 13 years have a twofold increase in relative risk compared to those who start menses at age 13 years or older (50).

Age at menopause bears a direct relationship to the risk. Women whose natural menopause occurs after age 55 have twice the risk for breast cancer, as compared to those whose menopause occurs before age 45.

Parity is another important factor. Nulliparous women have a relative risk of 1 compared to 0.5 for women who have their first child before age 20, and 1.4 for women who give birth to their first child after age 37 (33). A full term pregnancy causes an initial proliferation followed by a specialized secretory differentiation of the epithelial stem cells. While the initial proliferative activity increases the number of susceptible cells, the subsequent differentiation removes them from the pool of susceptible cells (55).

Oophorectomy provides a protection inversely related to age at oophorectomy.

### *Exogenous Reproductive Steroid Hormones*

Numerous studies have provided divergent viewpoints regarding the relation between oral contraceptive steroid use and the risk of breast carcinoma. Earlier studies had refuted any association between the two, but subsequent reports suggest an increased risk for breast carcinoma in long-term users of oral contraceptives, as well as in women on estrogen-progestogen replacement therapy (7,37,39,50). Confirmation of these findings is needed.

Interestingly, other studies have reported a reduced risk of benign breast disease among women using oral contraceptive hormones (24,44,66). The reduction in risk for fibrocystic changes has been related to the progestin content of the pill (11).

It is possible that high doses of exogenous estrogens increase the risk of breast carcinoma, but smaller amounts do not (60). Dupont et al (18) reported that exogenous estrogens actually lowered the observed breast cancer risk in women with atypical hyperplasia, proliferative disease without atypia, and in women without proliferative disease. They concluded that exogenous estrogens are not associated with increased breast cancer risk in women with benign breast disease, and noted that a previous history of benign breast disease does not contraindicate replacement estrogen therapy.

The length of exposure to estrogenic stimulation may also be a factor is assessing the influence of these hormones as a risk factor. The relative risk estimate of developing breast cancer before age 45 for women with less than ten years of exogenous steroid use approximates 2.0; for women with ten or more years of use, it is 4.1 (39). Miller et al's (39) findings suggest that those with very long-term use of oral contraceptive steroids may be at increased risk for development of breast cancer.

Several studies have also reported relative risks of 1.5 to 2.0 in association with long-term use of estrogens or estrogen/progestogen regimens as replacement therapy (7,12,25,29).

Support relating high doses of estrogens to the development of breast cancer comes from a report of breast carcinoma developing in two transsexual men who were treated with massive doses of estrogen for the induction of breast development (58).

In rhesus monkeys, long-term use of a variety of synthetic oral contraceptive steroids causes proliferative epithelial changes identical to atypical hyperplasia, intraductal carcinoma, and invasive carcinoma of the human breast (59). In an evaluation of 213 rhesus monkeys, 12 of which served as controls, 45% of the animals treated with long-term synthetic oral contraceptive steroids developed proliferative atypia (atypical intraductal hyperplasia, intraductal carcinoma, and invasive carcinoma), compared to 12% of the control animals (59). The atypia in the control animals was focal and mild compared to the more extensive and severe atypia of treated animals. Contrary to expectations, the most severe atypias, the intraductal carcinomas and the invasive carcinomas, developed in animals receiving high doses of progestins alone or in combination with mestranol. These animals also displayed secretory changes, sometimes of a pronounced lactational type, in the same terminal duct-lobular units (TDLU) where the atypias and carcinomas were present simultaneously. Nonetheless, the atypical and carcinoma cells developing amongst the secretory cells of the TDLU, failed to show similar secretory activity. Carcinogenesis in these cells either occurred prior to the development of functional, secretory activity, or it arrested functional differentiation of the altered cell population. Pure mestranol induced a maximum of moderate atypia. These findings support a role for steroid hormones in either initiation or promotion of breast carcinoma.

## Diet—Nutritional Influences

There is an increasing interest regarding the role of nutrition as a risk factor for breast carcinoma as more information is collected at a variety of settings in different countries around the world (69,73–76,78,79,81,83–85). This interest is valid since certain risk factors such as obesity (80) and age at menarche (82) are nutritionally mediated. In postmenopausal women, obesity—body weight of greater than 70 kg—approximately doubles a woman's risk, compared to those weighing less than 60 kg (77). Furthermore, a number of population studies have correlated the incidence and mortality of breast carcinoma with total dietary fat (72); serum cholesterol levels have also been linked to breast cancer (25). Attention has been focused on specific components of diet such as fat and animal proteins (81), as well as meat and coffee (83). In 1982, a panel convened by the National Research Council (United States) recommended reduction in fat intake when comparisons on an international scale suggested a strong correlation between dietary fat intake and breast cancer (70). It is important to emphasize that subsequent comparisons even within a relatively homogenous population at three levels of risk (low for Japanese in Japan, intermediate for Japanese in Hawaii, and high for whites in Hawaii) have not supported the dietary fat hypothesis (74,75). Others have suggested no dietary fat influence for women in the premenopausal age group, but a modest effect for women older than 50 years (81). Another case control study in several countries also failed to confirm a real association between increased fat intake and breast cancer risk (69); interestingly, the investigator found the emergence of a new hypothesis that related alcohol intake to breast cancer risk.

Changes in dietary habits may also be partly responsible for the changes observed in the incidence and mortality of breast carcinoma in migrant populations (68,71). This is an area that requires in-depth study. Considering the inconsistency of human diet in general, and the fact that isolated populations with strict dietary habits may experience other genetic or environmental influences (socioeconomic and ethnic influences), the best that can be expected from a retrospective study of dietary habits is identification of trends. It would be of interest to know if the type of diet prior to menarche, during reproductive years and following menopause exerts a different influence on the magnitude of any risk associated with dietary habits. The influence of additives and preservatives in canned and packaged goods, as well as the use of steroids in raising cattle destined for general consumption may be worth further evaluation as this is another general aspect of a food consumption pattern that is more typical of Western affluent countries.

## Morphologic Factors<br>An Explanation of Relative Risk

The significance of a variety of morphologic changes as risk factors for development of breast carcinoma has been established relatively recently (13,17,27,45–48). Lesions that constitute a risk factor for the subsequent development of invasive breast carcinoma include intraductal hyperplasia (IDH), atypical intraductal hyperplasia (AIDH) and atypical lobular hyperplasia or lobular neoplasia and, to a lesser degree, sclerosing adenosis. Fibrocystic changes without proliferative activity do not constitute a significant risk factor; because of their prevalence in the general population, these changes are no longer considered a disease (129). Prior to the extensive use of mammography, about 25% of women who had breast biopsies were found to have IDH (47); this finding increased their relative risk for subsequent development of invasive carcinoma to 1.5 to 2.0 times that of general population during the 10 to 15 years following their initial diagnosis. During the same period about 3% to 5% of the women had AIDH in their biopsies. Atypical intraductal hyperplasia is associated with a moderately increased (4.6) relative risk for the subsequent development of carcinoma (48). The presence of a family history of breast carci-

**Table 2.1** Relative Risk for Invasive Breast Carcinoma Associated with Various Lesions

| Risk, if any, Not Established | Slight Risk | Moderate Risk | High Risk |
|---|---|---|---|
| Mild/minimal Hyperplasia | Regular IDH (1.5–2X) | IDH + Pos FH (4.3X) | IDCA (8–10X) |
| | SA & FA (≈1.7X) | AIDH (4.6X) | AIDH + Pos FH (9X) |
| | Gross CD | ALH* (4–5X) | LCIS* (8–10X) |

Abbreviations: IDH = intraductal hyperplasia; Pos FH = positive family history breast carcinoma; IDCA = intraductal carcinoma; SA = sclerosing adenosis; FA = fibroadenoma; AIDH = atypical intraductal hyperplasia; CD = cystic disease; ALH = atypical lobular hyperplasia; LCIS = lobular carcinoma in situ; * = as defined by Page et al (142).

noma in a sister, mother, or daughter of a patient with either IDH or AIDH doubles the relative risk in either group (48). In effect, a woman with AIDH and a family history of breast carcinoma has the same relative risk as one with intraductal carcinoma.

Sclerosing adenosis is thought to be associated with a slightly increased risk for subsequent development of breast carcinoma (27,35,46,59). Gross cystic disease has also been reported to be associated with a slight increase in the relative risk of breast carcinoma (13). The relative risk associated with a variety of morphologic changes in the breast is listed in Table 2.1.

The relative risk as determined in these reports indicates the number of cancers observed in the study group compared to the number expected in the general population of comparable age within a given time interval (generally a follow-up period of 10 to 20 years) after the diagnosis (19). The absolute risk reflects the probability of developing breast carcinoma over a specified time interval after the diagnosis and is related to the patient's age, relative risk, and the age specific incidence of breast carcinoma and death from other causes in the general population. The relative risk of 4.5 for a 40-year-old woman with AIDH translates to an absolute risk of about 8% to 10% of such a woman developing invasive breast carcinoma over a period of 10 to 20 years following the diagnostic procedure; for a 60-year-old woman with AIDH, the absolute risk over a 20-year period is about 25% (19). Considering that the age-specific incidence of invasive breast carcinoma for a 30-year-old American woman is 27.5/100,000 women/year, a relative risk of 10 would increase her chances of developing invasive carcinoma to 275/100,000 women/year at age 30 years (19).

## Radiation Exposure

Radiation is thought to influence the early stages of carcinogenesis by causing damage to the DNA (15). Radiation-induced breast carcinomas are generally characterized by a latent period of about 10 to 15 years. Follow-up of the Japanese atomic bomb survivors, patients who received radiation therapy for postpartum mastitis, and those who had multiple fluoroscopy has shown an increased incidence of breast carcinoma following exposure to external radiation (62,63). Most of these findings have been restricted to women exposed to radiation during adolescence or adult life. Initial evaluation of atomic bomb survivors had suggested that radiation exposure prior to an age of ten years does not alter the risk for subsequent development of breast cancer (36,64). Later, however, it was suggested that the development of breast cancer may be a long-term consequence of prepubertal radiation exposure (26,63). Those first exposed to radiation prior to nine years of age display the strongest sensitivity to induction of breast carcinoma (26). The significance of radiation exposure during early life was evaluated by comparing the incidence of breast carcinoma in 1,201 women who had received radiation therapy for an enlarged thymus during infancy with that of their 2,469 nonirradiated sisters. Twenty breast cancers developed in the irradiated women and 12 among their nonirradiated sisters after an average of 36 years of follow-up (26). The estimated absorbed dose of radiation to the breast was 0.69 Gy, and the first breast cancer was diagnosed 28 years after irradiation. As a result of these findings, it was concluded that exposure of the breast to ionizing radiation during infancy increases the risk for subsequent development of breast cancer.

The carcinogenicity of ionizing radiation became a major concern in assessing the benefits versus the risks of mammography. When wide scale mammographic screening was initiated in the late 1960s and early 1970s, there was limited information available on the long-term effects of periodic exposure to small doses of ionizing radiation. Mackenzie (32) had observed an increased number of breast carcinomas in tuberculous women subjected to repeated fluoroscopic examinations. His observations were confirmed in several subsequent studies (14,22,41,42). Boice and Monson (9) noted the greatest absolute excess breast cancer risk among women who had their first therapy between the ages of 15 and 19 years. With an average follow-up of 31.5 years, the ratio of observed to expected carcinomas among 1,115 women treated with ionizing radiation for various non-neoplastic conditions of the breast at Radiumhemmet was 4:1 in the irradiated breast; furthermore, patients irradiated at lower ages were at considerably higher risk of developing breast carcinoma (5).

An increased incidence of breast cancer has also been reported in women with a history of radiation therapy for acute mastitis (38). The incidence of mammary neoplasms in women treated with X rays for acute postpartum mastitis was compared to that of three control groups—nonirradiated sisters of these women, women with postpartum mastitis not treated with X rays, and their untreated sisters. With up to 34 years of follow-up, the overall risk of developing breast carcinoma was comparable to an increase of 0.5% per rad (55). Furthermore, the study results suggested radiation exposure up to age 45 years induces carcinoma, and that the fractionated doses are cumulative. There is, however, a long latency period between exposure and cancer development of up to two to three decades. Synergism between radiation and other risk factors has been studied (56), but needs further evaluation. Current practice suggests that the benefits of early detection of carcinoma by mammography in women over 45 and particularly those with other risk factors outweigh its risk.

## PROGNOSTIC INDICATORS

A variety of features have been evaluated as prognostic indicators for breast carcinoma and several reviews of this topic have appeared in the literature (93,97,98,102,125,126,135,141,152,156). Some of the more important prognostic factors and those that potentially could influence the management of breast carcinoma are presented here. These factors can be used to divide breast carcinomas into those with a good or a poor prognosis. (See Table 2.2).

**Table 2.2** The Influence of Various Prognostic Indicators on the Prognosis of Breast Carcinoma

| | Good Prognosis | Poor Prognosis |
|---|---|---|
| Size | <1 cm | >5 cm |
| Local Extension | Absent | Present |
| Grade | Low | High |
| Receptor status | ER+, PR+ | ER−, PR− |
| Axillary nodes | Tumor − | Tumor + |

## Staging

Staging of breast cancer is essential in the evaluation of the tumor and determination of the type of treatment. Breast carcinoma is classified on the basis of the anatomic extent of the lesion into four stages; each stage identifies a group of tumors that have approximately similar prognoses.

The stage of the carcinoma alone or incorporated into a prognostic index is an important predictor of survival (105,118,123,147), and its assessment is crucial in the management of the patient (107,108). Staging may be purely clinical and based on a combination of physical examination, mammograms, and scans (90,105). The physical examination should include evaluation of the size, mobility, and associated skin changes of the primary tumor, assessment of the size and mobility of regional lymph nodes, and any evidence of distant metastases.

A pathologic stage, in contrast, requires actual examination of tissue specimen from the primary tumor, axillary nodes, and other distinct sites (when warranted) to confirm the presence of a tumor and size of the lesion (105).

The clinical and pathologic stages do not always correlate. For example, inflammatory changes in the skin of the breast do not necessarily reflect dermal lymphatic invasion (inflammatory carcinoma), and clinical estimation of the presence or absence of nodal involvement is incorrect in about one third of the cases (115). The Yorkshire Breast Cancer Group (166) found that pathologists and surgeons agree on tumor size in 54% of cases, while surgeons and radiologists agreed in 59% of cases. Nonetheless, since clinical evaluation takes place prior to any therapeutic intervention, it can be more helpful in the initial management of the patient. The advantage of pathologic staging is in the certainty it provides regarding the true extent of the lesion in the sampled areas.

A system of staging of breast cancer based on a meticulous evaluation of the primary tumor (T), the regional lymph nodes (N), and distant metastases (M) was first proposed in 1954 (107) by the International Union Against Cancer (UICC). Metastases to nodes other than axillary, transpectoral, or internal mammary lymph nodes are considered distant metastases for staging purposes. Involvement of the supraclavicular, cervical, or contralateral internal mammary lymph nodes qualifies as distant metastases, while involvement of intramammary nodes is considered axillary involvement for purposes of staging. Various combinations of the subcategories of T, N, and M define four stages that are designated as I, II, III, and IV in ascending order of gravity, and the system is currently referred to as the TNM system of staging. The American Joint Committee for Cancer Staging and End Results Reporting (AJC) adopted a modified version of the TNM concept shortly after its introduction. The TNM classification has undergone several revisions and the 1989 version is presented in Table 2.3 (89,122,157).

Other systems of classification (Manchester and Columbia Clinical Classification) are also used in different institutions (121,165), but will not be discussed in this chapter.

## Stromal Invasion

Among morphologic parameters, the presence of stromal invasion is the most significant prognostic indicator since the in situ or noninvasive carcinomas are almost invariably cured by mastectomy. Actually, breast cancer statistics and epidemiologic studies report only on the invasive carcinomas (10). Furthermore, when intraductal proliferative lesions have been studied for determination of the associated relative risk for subsequent development of carcinoma, only the development of subsequent invasive carcinoma has been recorded and utilized for analytic purposes in some studies (48).

Although identification of invasion is of utmost importance, determination of the extent of in situ disease within and beyond the invasive component is quite useful when breast conservation is contemplated (154,155).

## Nodal Metastases

### *Axillary Lymph Node Metastases*

The number of positive axillary nodes is of paramount importance as a prognostic factor in cases of invasive carcinoma treated by mastectomy. Survival, recurrence, speed of recurrence, and treatment failure all correlate with the number of positive axillary nodes (164). The number of nodes obtained per axillary dissection varies. The larger the number of nodes identified, the greater is the number of positive nodes (112). When there is no evidence of axillary node metastases, the ten year surgical failure is 24%; the presence of any positive nodes increases the failure rate to 75%; 64.5% of those with one to three positive nodes and 86.5% of those with four or more positive nodes manifest treatment failure (113).

The presence of gross rather than microscopic tumor in the axillary nodes adversely affects the prognosis (88). Opinions vary regarding the significance of micro (occult and clandestine, or small in size) metastases which are identified either routinely or by gross or microscopic serial sections in 9% to 33% of cases in different series (87,91,95,111,114,117,136, 145,149,153,158,159,162,163). Some studies (mainly those from the United States) have suggested that patients with axillary node metastases smaller than 0.2 cm have survival rates comparable to women with no evidence of nodal metastases (111,124,163). Finally, patients with fixed axillary nodes have a worse prognosis compared to those with non-palpable or mobile axillary nodes (104).

European studies attach great prognostic significance to the presence of axillary micro (occult) metastases. Friedman et al (117) found that the presence of tumor emboli in the subcapsular marginal sinuses of one axillary node ("clandestine" metastasis) discovered by serial sectioning is associated with a relative risk of distant metastases of 1.7 compared to patients without axillary node metastases. They con-

**Table 2.3** 1989 TNM Classification

**Measuring the Size of the Primary Cancer**

The tumor size is a measure of the invasive component. If there is a large in situ component (eg, 4.0 cm) and a small invasive component (eg, 0.5 cm), the tumor is coded $T_{1a}$.

**Multiple, Simultaneous Cancers**

The following guidelines should be used when staging multiple, simultaneous primary (grossly measurable, infiltrating) cancers within the same breast. These criteria do not apply to multiple microscopic lesions (since they may represent intramammary spread).

Use the largest primary cancer to stage the case.

Enter on the record that the case is one of the simultaneous, multiple primary cancers in one breast. These cases should be analyzed separately; the tumor with the highest T category should be used for classification.

Include in breast checklist (pathology) simultaneous, multiple, primary infiltrating cancers.

Simultaneous bilateral breast cancers: Each should be staged independently.

**Inflammatory Carcinoma**

Inflammatory carcinoma of the breast is characterized by diffuse, brawny induration of the skin, with an erysipeloid edge, usually with no underlying palpable mass. This clinical presentation is due to tumor embolization of dermal lymphatics. The tumor of inflammatory carcinoma is coded $T_{4d}$.

**Primary Tumor (T)**

The size of the intact tumor should be measured before any tissue is removed for special studies, such as estrogen-binding studies.

$T_X$ The primary tumor cannot be assessed.

$T_0$ No evidence of primary tumor.

$T_{IS}$ Carcinoma in situ: intraductal carcinoma, lobular carcinoma in situ, or Paget's disease of the nipple with no tumor. Paget's disease associated with a tumor is classified according to the size of the tumor.

$T_1$ Tumor is 2.0 cm or smaller in greatest dimension.
- $T_{1a}$ 0.5 cm or smaller
- $T_{1b}$ Larger than 0.5 cm but not larger than 1.0 cm
- $T_{1c}$ Larger than 1.0 cm but not larger than 2.0 cm

$T_2$ Tumor is larger than 2.0 cm but not larger than 5.0 cm in greatest dimension.

$T_3$ Tumor is larger than 5.0 cm in greatest dimension.

$T_4$ Tumor of any size with direct extension to chest wall or skin. (Chest wall includes ribs, intercostal muscles, and serratus anterior muscle, but not pectoral muscle).

$T_{4a}$ Extension to chest wall.

$T_{4b}$ Edema (including peau d'orange), ulceration of the skin of the breast, or satellite skin nodules confined to the same breast.

$T_{4c}$ Both a and b above.

$T_{4d}$* Inflammatory carcinoma (as defined in introductory comments).

*Note:* Dimpling of the skin, nipple retraction, or other changes, except those in $T_4$, may occur in $T_1$, $T_2$, and $T_3$ without affecting the classification.

**Regional Lymph Nodes (N)**

*Axillary (ipsilateral) and interpectoral (Rotter's nodes):* lymph nodes along the axillary vein and its tributaries, which may be divided into the following levels:

Level I (low axilla): lymph nodes located lateral to the lateral border of the pectoralis major muscle.

Level II (mid axilla): lymph nodes located between the medial and lateral borders of the pectoralis minor muscle and the interpectoral (Rotter's) lymph nodes.

Level III (apical axilla): lymph nodes medial to the medial margin of the pectoralis minor, including those designated as the subclavicular, or apical lymph nodes.

*Intramammary* lymph nodes are coded as axillary lymph nodes.

*Internal mammary* (ipsilateral): lymph nodes located in the intercostal spaces along the edge of the sternum in the endothoracic fascia. All other lymph node metastases are coded as distinct metastases ($M_1$), including supraclavicular, cervical, or contralateral internal mammary lymph nodes.

*(continued)*

**Table 2.3** 1989 TNM Classification *continued*

**Regional Lymph Nodes, Clinical Classification (N)**

| | |
|---|---|
| $N_X$ | Regional lymph nodes cannot be assessed (eg, previously removed) |
| $N_0$ | No regional lymph node metastasis |
| $N_1$ | Metastasis to movable ipsilateral axillary lymph node(s) |
| $N_2$ | Metastasis to ipsilateral axillary lymph nodes(s) fixed to one another or to other structures |
| $N_3$ | Metastasis to ipsilateral internal mammary lymph node(s) |

**Regional Lymph Nodes, Pathologic Classification (pN)**

| | |
|---|---|
| $pN_X$ | The regional lymph nodes cannot be assessed (eg, previously removed, or not removed for pathologic study). |
| $pN_0$ | No regional lymph node metastases. |
| $pN_1$ | Metastasis to moveable ipsilateral axillary lymph node(s). |
| $N_{1a}$ | Only micrometastases (none larger than 0.2 cm) |
| $N_{1b}$ | Metastases lymph node(s), any one larger than 0.2 cm. |
| $pN_{1bi}$ | Metastasis in 1 to 3 lymph nodes, any more than 0.2 cm and all less than 2 cm in greatest dimension |
| $pN_{1bii}$ | Metastasis to 4 or more lymph nodes, any more than 0.2 cm and all less than 2 cm in greatest dimension. |
| $pN_{1biii}$ | Extension of tumor of tumor beyond the capsule of a lymph node metastasis less than 2 cm in greatest dimension. |
| $pN_{1biv}$ | Metastasis to a lymph node 2 cm or more in greatest dimension. |
| $pN_2$ | Metastases to ipsilateral axillary lymph nodes that are fixed to one another or to other structures. |
| $pN_3$ | Metastasis in any ipsilateral internal mammary lymph node(s). |

**Distant Metastasis (M)**

| | |
|---|---|
| $M_x$ | Distant metastasis cannot be assessed. |
| $M_0$ | No distant metastasis. |
| $M_1$ | Distant metastasis (includes metastasis to ipsilateral supraclavicular lymph node(s). |

**Clinical Staging**

Clinical staging includes the following: physical examination, including careful inspection and palpation of the skin, the mammary glands, and the lymph nodes (axillary, supraclavicular, and cervical). Pathologic examination of the breast or other tissues to establish the diagnosis of breast cancer. The extent of tissue examined pathologically for clinical staging is less than that required for pathologic staging (see Pathologic Staging below). Appropriate operative findings are elements of clinical staging, including size and chest wall invasion of the primary cancer and the presence or absence of regional or distant metastasis.

**Pathologic Staging**

Pathologic staging includes the following:

All data used for clinical staging.

Surgical resection and pathologic examination of the primary cancer, including not less than excision of the primary carcinoma with no tumor in any margin of resection by *gross* pathologic examination. A case can be included in the pathologic stage if there is only microscopic, but not gross, involvement in a margin. If there is tumor in the margin of resection by gross examination, it is coded $T_x$. Resection of least the low axillary lymph nodes (Level I), that is, those lymph nodes located lateral to the lateral border of the pectoralis minor muscle should be carried out. Such a resection ordinarily includes 6 or more lymph nodes.

**R Classification**

The absence or presence of residual tumor after treatment may be described by the symbol R:

| | |
|---|---|
| $R_X$ | Presence of residual tumor cannot be assessed |
| $R_0$ | No residual tumor |
| $R_1$ | Microscopic residual tumor |
| $R_2$ | Macroscopic residual tumor |

**Table 2.3** (continued)

**Stage Groupings**

| | | | |
|---|---|---|---|
| Stage O | $T_{IS}$ | $N_0$ | $M_0$ |
| Stage I | $T_1$ | $N_0$ | $M_0$ |
| Stage II | | | |
| IIa | $T_0$ | $N_1$ | $M_0$ |
| | $T_1$ | $N_1$** | $M_0$ |
| | $T_2$ | $N_0$ | $M_0$ |
| IIb | $T_2$ | $N_1$ | $M_0$ |
| | $T_3$ | $N_0$ | $M_0$ |
| Stage III | | | |
| IIIa | $T_3$ | $N_1$ | $M_0$ |
| | $T_1,T_2,T_3,$ | $N_2$ | $M_0$ |
| IIIb | $T_4$ | Any N | $M_0$ |
| | Any T | $N_3$ | $M_0$ |
| Stage IV | Any T | Any N | $M_1$ |

* If the skin biopsy is negative and there is no localized, measurable primary cancer, the T category is $pT_x$ when pathologically staging a clinical inflammatory carcinoma, $cT_{4d}$.

** The prognosis of patients with $pN_{1a}$ is similar to that of patients with $pN_0$.

From Beahrs et al (89), Hermanek and Sobin (122), and Spiessl et al (157).

cluded that the presence of occult or micrometastases does influence the likelihood of distant metastases and should be taken into account in the management of the patient and consideration of adjuvant chemotherapy. In a prospective study by the International (Ludwig) Breast Cancer Study Group, evaluation of the lymph nodes by serial sections in 921 breast cancer patients initially thought to be node-negative identified micrometastases in 9% of the axillary nodes (92,136). Patients with micrometastases had a poorer disease-free and overall survival after five and six years of follow-up compared to women in whom no axillary micrometastases were found after serial sectioning (136). The presence of micrometastases correlated with the presence of peritumoral vascular invasion and tumor size; tumors with vascular invasion and those larger than 2 cm were more likely to have micrometastases. The disease-free survival for those who converted to node-positive was 58%, compared to 74% for those who remained node-negative; the overall five-year survival was 79% and 88% for the two groups respectively (92). At six years of follow-up, the disease-free survival was 53% for those who converted to node-positive after serial sections, compared to 71% for those who remained node-negative; the overall survival was 70% and 86% for the two groups respectively (136). Immunostains have been helpful in detecting nodal metastases overlooked by the routine single slice technique (158). Studies by immunohistochemical methods for the detection of occult metastases have also reported higher recurrence and poorer survival rates for those women with infiltrating duct carcinoma who converted to node-positive as a result of the special studies (158), but not for women with infiltrating lobular carcinoma (158).

Some of our European colleagues have concluded that the pathologic examination of a single H&E stained section is probably no longer tenable clinically. While the optimum approach to the evaluation of the lymph node is under study, it has been proposed that division of the axillary node into 2 mm slices, as proposed by Wilkinson et al (163), and staining of the sections by immunohistochemical methods (95,162), along with evaluation of the bone marrow aspirates by immunohistochemical markers for epithelial cells (101,132), and measurement of tumor markers (ploidy, growth rate, oncogenes, etc) may help identify the poor risk patients in the "presumed node-negative" group.

### *Involvement of the Rotter's, Supraclavicular, and Internal Mammary Nodes*

The involvement of Rotter's node by metastatic carcinoma does not influence the prognosis independent of the axillary node status (127). The Rotter's node is involved in 0.5% of cases with negative axillary nodes and 8.2% of axillary node positive patients (100). The presence of metastatic tumor in the internal mammary nodes, particularly when untreated, is associated with a poor ten-year survival (108,121). The outlook is particularly ominous for patients who have metastases in both axillary and internal mammary nodes. The five-year survival of patients with either axillary or internal mammary node metastases alone is 56% and 52% respectively, but it drops to 24% when both nodal regions are involved (96). In another study, when axillary nodes were negative, and the internal mammary nodes were positive, the ten-year survival was 62.4%; when axillary nodes were positive, and the internal mammary nodes were negative, the ten-year survival was 59.6%. With nodes from both groups positive, the ten-year survival dropped to 37.3% (160).

The involvement of the supraclavicular nodes portends a particularly ominous outlook because these nodes are generally reached after invasion of axillary or internal mammary nodes (109,144,160). Other features associated with unfavorable prognosis include spilling of the tumor to the extranodal tissue in patients with three or fewer involved nodes (130), and involvement of the apical lymph nodes (107, 121).

## Tumor Size

In repeated studies from different centers, the gross size (maximum diameter) of the invasive primary neoplasms has emerged as one of the most important prognostic factors (97,141), and together with nodal involvement constitutes two of the three features used for staging. There is actually a direct relationship between increasing tumor size and the probability of axillary node metastases (121); axillary node metastases is present in 26% of tumors 1 cm or less in diameter, compared to 78% of those over 10 cm in diameter. Patients whose tumors are 2 cm or smaller in maximum diameter have a significantly better prognosis and survival compared to those with larger tumors (143). Among women with $T_1$ tumors, those with tumors 1 cm or smaller had a 20-year recurrence-free survival of 86%; the survival dropped to 69% for those with tumors over 1 to 2 cm in size (148). Provision of the tumor size should be considered mandatory in surgical pathology reports.

## Tumor Type

Breast carcinomas have been divided into prognostically favorable and unfavorable types (13). Tumor type, though important, does not influence the stage of the tumor. Certain types of breast carcinoma—medullary, tubular, mucinous (colloid), and adenoid cystic carcinoma—are low grade cancers and associated with a low frequency or absence of axillary node metastases and a relatively good prognosis. Poorly-differentiated, signet-ring, and inflammatory carcinoma, as well as carcinosarcomas are generally considered aggressive neoplasms. One of the most aggressive breast carcinomas is inflammatory carcinoma with a five-year survival of only 11%. With the use of chemotherapy, survival rates of patients with inflammatory carcinoma may improve. As a rule, low grade carcinomas have a better prognosis than high grade carcinomas. In a review of 950 women diagnosed as axillary node negative (ANN), stage I invasive breast carcinoma with eight years of follow-up, mucinous (colloid), tubular, and papillary carcinomas were associated with the most favorable prognosis (108). Contrary to expectation, the prognosis of medullary carcinomas was similar to that of infiltrating carcinomas, not otherwise specified (NOS), and lobular invasive types in a 1990 study by Fisher et al (116). In another study of 767 $T_1N_0M_0$ and $T_2N_0M_0$ breast carcinomas, recurrences were significantly less frequent among patients with tubular, medullary, invasive papillary, and colloid carcinoma (147).

## Tumor Grade

Tumor grade is another important prognostic indicator though it is not used as a parameter in staging the tumor. Grading systems that use tubule formation as a parameter are best suited for grading infiltrating duct carcinomas (see also infiltrating duct carcinoma, Chapter 9). Though some special types of breast carcinoma also lend themselves to such grading systems with good survival correlation, others—particularly medullary carcinomas—do not.

Even as early as the 1920s (183,190) and 1930s (184), a clear association between tumor grade and survival was demonstrated. Nonetheless, grading invasive breast carcinomas did not gain much popularity, probably due to the rather complex system initially recommended by Greenhough (183) which was based on the evaluation of eight histologic features. The histologic grade correlated with the five year "cure." Of patients with a grade I carcinoma, 68% were cured at five years, compared to 33% of patients with grade II carcinoma, and 0% of women with grade III neoplasms.

Haagensen (184) evaluated 164 mastectomy specimen to determine the prognostic significance of various histologic parameters. The 15 features evaluated were categorized under the growth pattern, cell morphology, and the reaction of the surrounding stroma. He found six of the 15 features to correlate with survival, and subdivided the tumors into three grades. The five-year survival for grade I tumors was 80%, compared to 38% for grade II, and 13% for grade III carcinomas.

In 1950, Bloom (170,171) reviewed the literature, examined the various grading systems used, and proposed a method that emphasized three factors: 1) the degree of tubule formation, 2) regularity in the size, shape and staining character of the nuclei, and 3) nuclear hyperchromasia and mitotic activity. Based on a subjective evaluation of these features, the tumors were graded as a low, moderate, or high grade malignancy. Applying this grading system in the evaluation of 470 tumors, he found that the five-year survival was 79% for grade I tumors compared to 25% for grade III tumors. At ten years, the survival dropped to 45% for the grade I, and 13% for grade III tumors.

Several years later, Bloom and Richardson (172) provided a modified version of the grading method which utilized a scoring system to facilitate the grading effort. Each of the three features were examined and given a score of 1 to 3, corresponding to their presence in slight, moderate or marked degree. A total score of 3 to 9 would be attainable by a given tumor. A score of 3 to 5 qualified the carcinoma as a grade I tumor, 6 or 7, as grade II, and 8 or 9, as grade III. Subsequent modification of this scoring has been introduced based on multivariate analysis of 1,262 invasive ductal carcinomas (189).

Black et al (103,167–169) evaluated the prognostic significance of tubule formation and the nuclear features separately, and concluded that only nuclear morphology is a significant prognostic factor. They proposed a nuclear grading system with five grades. Contrary to common practice, grades 0 and I were used to designate the most poorly-differentiated or anaplastic neoplasms, while grade IV reflected the well-differentiated tumors. This reversal of the numerical order remained a disturbing aspect of this nuclear grading system, and contributed to a lack of wide support for its application.

Hartveit (185) introduced a grading system based on an assessment of cytologic factors including nuclear crowding, nuclear diameter, nuclear lobulation, and cell border definition. Grade I tumors had clearly defined borders, minimal nuclear crowding and lobulation, along with a nuclear/cytoplasmic ratio less than one half. Grade III tumors displayed cells with undefined cell margins, marked nuclear crowding and lobulation, along with a nuclear/cytoplasmic ratio more than one half.

Fisher et al (182) devised a grading method combining features of Bloom and Richardson (172), and Black and Speer's (169) approaches. But first, they modified Black and Speer's nuclear grading system by reducing it from five to three grades after combining grades 0 and I into one group, and grades III and IV into another. Furthermore, they reversed the numerical order so that grade I corresponded to the well-differentiated carcinomas and grade III reflected the most poorly-differentiated tumors. After assigning a nuclear grade to a tumor, they checked for the presence of tubular or adenocystic arrangement by the tumor cells. The histologic grade of a tumor was determined by combining the nuclear grade with presence or absence of tubular or adenocystic features. Fisher et al found that 2.3% of 1,000 breast carcinomas in one of the National Surgical Adjuvant Breast Projects qualified as grade I, compared to 28.1% as grade II, and 69.6% as grade III. They also found consistent correlation between the histologic grade and various pathological and clinical features.

In an attempt to improve the objective aspect of the grading system, Elston (178–181) has proposed a modified version of the Bloom and Richardson's method (179, 181). He emphasized the importance of tissue preparation, proper fixation, and sections of appropriate thickness ranging from 4 to 6 microns. Furthermore, he pointed out that grading is carried out for invasive duct carcinomas and that special types of invasive breast carcinoma (ie, colloid carcinoma, medullary carcinoma, etc) are not generally graded. The most significant change introduced by Elston is in the evaluation of the features grouped as "nuclear hyperchromasia and mitotic activity." Because of the difficulties in recognition of true hyperchromasia and its distinction from pyknotic nuclei, Elston deleted this feature. He also refined the method of counting the mitotic figures.

In Elston's method, *tubule formation* is given a score of one, when an overall evaluation of the tumor shows formation of tubules with visible lumens in a majority (>75%) of the lesion. When solid areas of tumor growth are admixed with a moderate degree of the tubular arrangements (10% to 75%), the tumor is given a score of two. When the tumor shows minimal or no tubule formation (<10%), it gets three points.

In the assessment of *nuclear pleomorphism*, variation in the size and shape of the tumor nuclei is evaluated. A score of one is given to tumors with uniform or regular, small nuclei and those exhibiting minimal variation. Tumors with a moderate degree of variation in nuclear size and shape and occasional nucleoli are given two points. Those with marked variation and containing bizzare nuclei, often with one or more prominent nucleoli, are given three points.

In the determination of *mitotic rate*, at least ten fields in the periphery of the most mitotically active part of the tumor are evaluated. The tumor is scored 1 to 3 depending on the number of mitotic figures per 10 high power fields (HPF). The number of mitotic figures required for each point varies with the size of the high power field for a given microscope. In the original study (180), using a microscopic field with a diameter of 0.59 mm and an area of 0.274 $mm^2$ (Leitz Ortholux microscope with wide angle eyepieces and X25 objective), tumors with a count of 0 to 9 mitotic figures per 10 HPF, were given one point, with 10 to 19 mitotic figures per 10 HPF score two, and those with 20 or more mitotic figures per 10 HPF got three points. Using a Nikon Labophot microscope with a X40 objective and a field diameter of 0.44 mm, the field area would be 0.152 $mm^2$; therefore, the point scoring system would be modified to one point for 0 to 5 mitotic figures per 10 HPF, two points for 6 to 10 mitotic figures per 10 HPF, and three points for 11 or more mitotic figures per 10 HPF (180). For a Leitz Diaplan microscope with a X40 objective and a field diameter of 0.63 mm, the field area would be 0.312; therefore, the number of mitotic figures required per 10 HPF would be 0 to 11 for one point, 12 to 22 for two points, and 23 or more for three points (180).

In an excellent study of 1,010 patients with solitary, unilateral, nonmetastatic carcinomas treated at the Institut Gustave-Roussy (173), the histologic grade (using a modification of Scarff and Handley/ Bloom and Richardson system) was found to be an important and independent prognostic factor. The number of histologically positive nodes and the histologic grade were found to be the most valuable predictors for 612 patients with operable disease. In their modification of the grading system, Contesso et al (173) have also abandoned evaluation of nuclear hyperchromatism and rather assess the variation in nuclear size (anisonucleosis). Code 1 is given to tumors with nuclei that are uniform in size and shape. Tumors with highly variable, giant, and bizarre nuclei get a code of 3, while those with moderately unequal nuclei get a code of 2. In evaluating the architecture of the lesion, tumors with tubular or papillary arrangements throughout, are given one point, those with occasional tubules or papillae, get two points, and those without any such arrangements get three points. Contesso et al (173) quantify the mitotic activity by expressing the maximum number of mitotic figures in a single field at 400X magnification (a field of 0.159 $mm^2$), after examining 20 successive fields for the highest value, rather than taking an average of mitotic figures per 10 HPF. Tumors with a maximum of one mitotic figure in any given field are given one point, those with a maximum of two mitotic figures in any of the 20 successive fields are given two points, and those with three or more in any one of the fields get three points.

Comparing Contesso et al's modification to that of Elston, both have abandoned evaluation of nuclear hyperchromatism. The evaluation of nuclear features (anisonucleosis) in Contesso et al's approach is similar to Elston's, except that the latter also incorporates the nucleolar appearance. In the evaluation of the architectural arrangement of the tumor, Contesso et al evaluated formation of tubular or papillary arrangements throughout the lesion, while Elston assessed tubular arrangement only. Assessment of the mitotic count also differs in the two modifications. Contesso et al use a 400X magnification (a field of 0.159 $mm^2$), while Elston uses a 300X magnification (a field of 0.274 $mm^2$). Contesso et al, use the highest number in any given field among 20 successive ones, while Elston uses the number of mitotic figures in ten high power fields mainly in the periphery of the tumor, or the most mitotically active areas of the carcinoma. Contesso et al found that 21% of 612 carcinomas qualified as grade I, 50% as grade II, and 29% as grade III. In Elston's system, 17% of carcinomas were designated as grade I, 37% as grade II, and 46% as grade III; the ten-year survival of patients with grade I tumor was 85% compared to 43% for those with grade III carcinomas in a study of 2,000 women with primary operable cancer (179).

Regardless of which modification is used (Contesso et al's or Elston's), the grade of the tumor would depend on the total score from the three features evaluated.

**A**

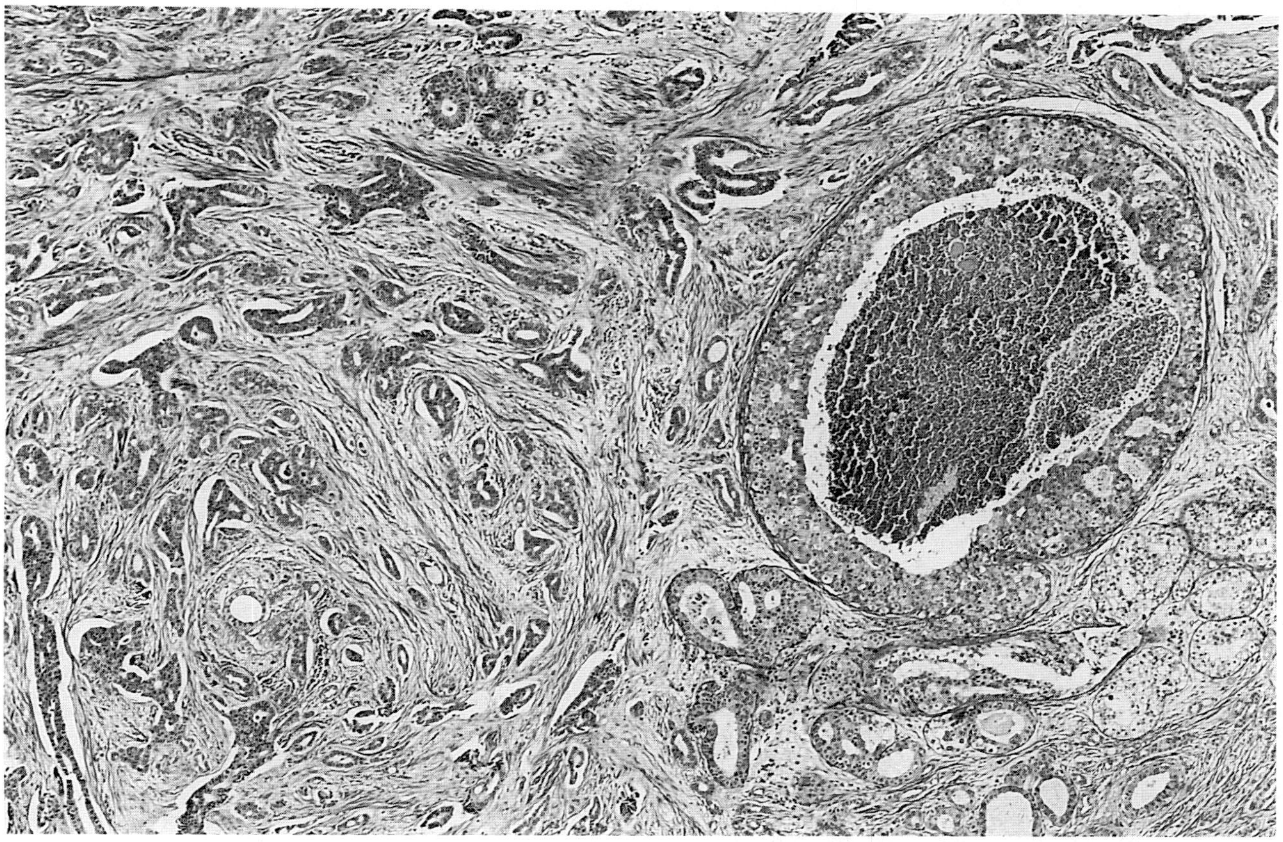

**B**

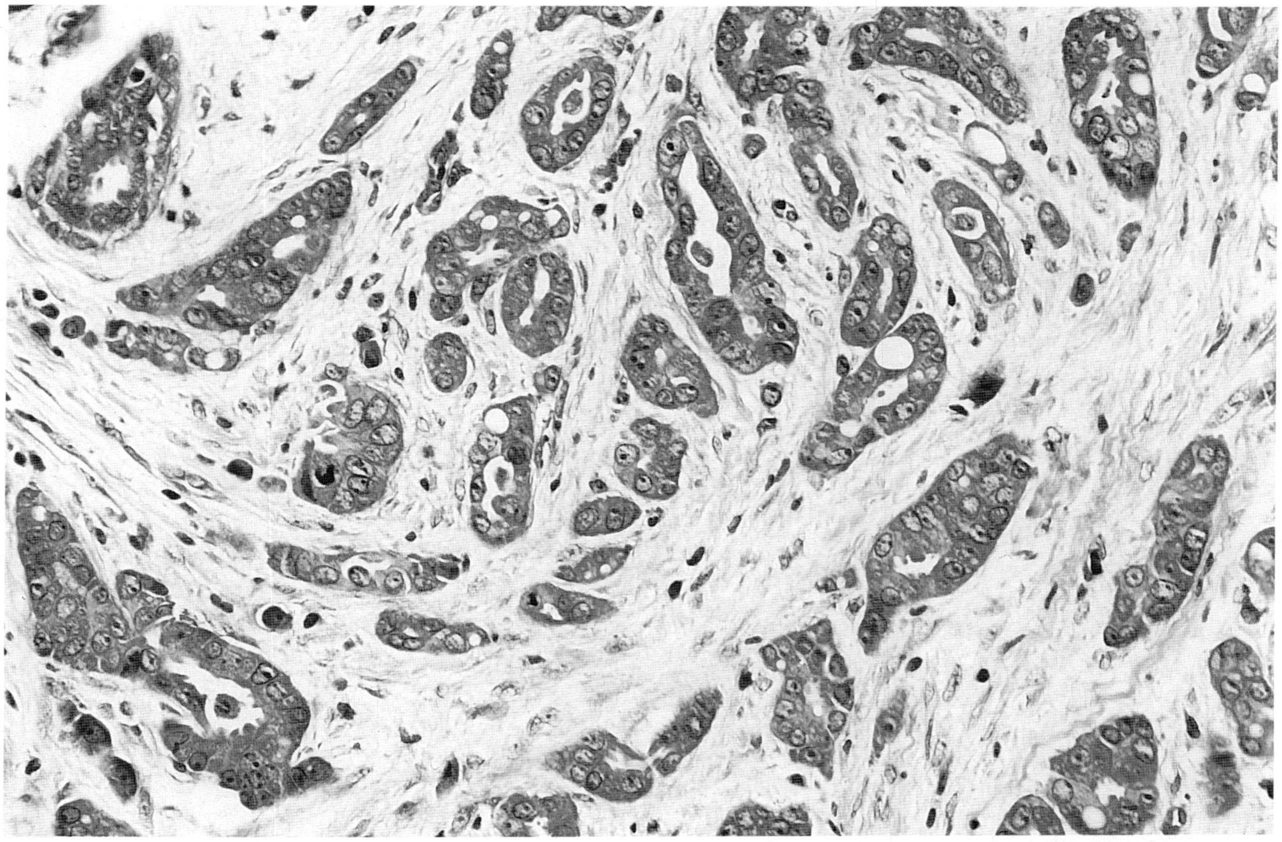

**Figure 2.1** Well differentiated carcinoma. (a&b) There is prominent tubule formation, moderate cytologic atypia, and rare mitotic figures. Tubule formation = 1, atypia = 2, mitotic figures = 1; total score = 4. (H&E, (a) X300; (b) X400)

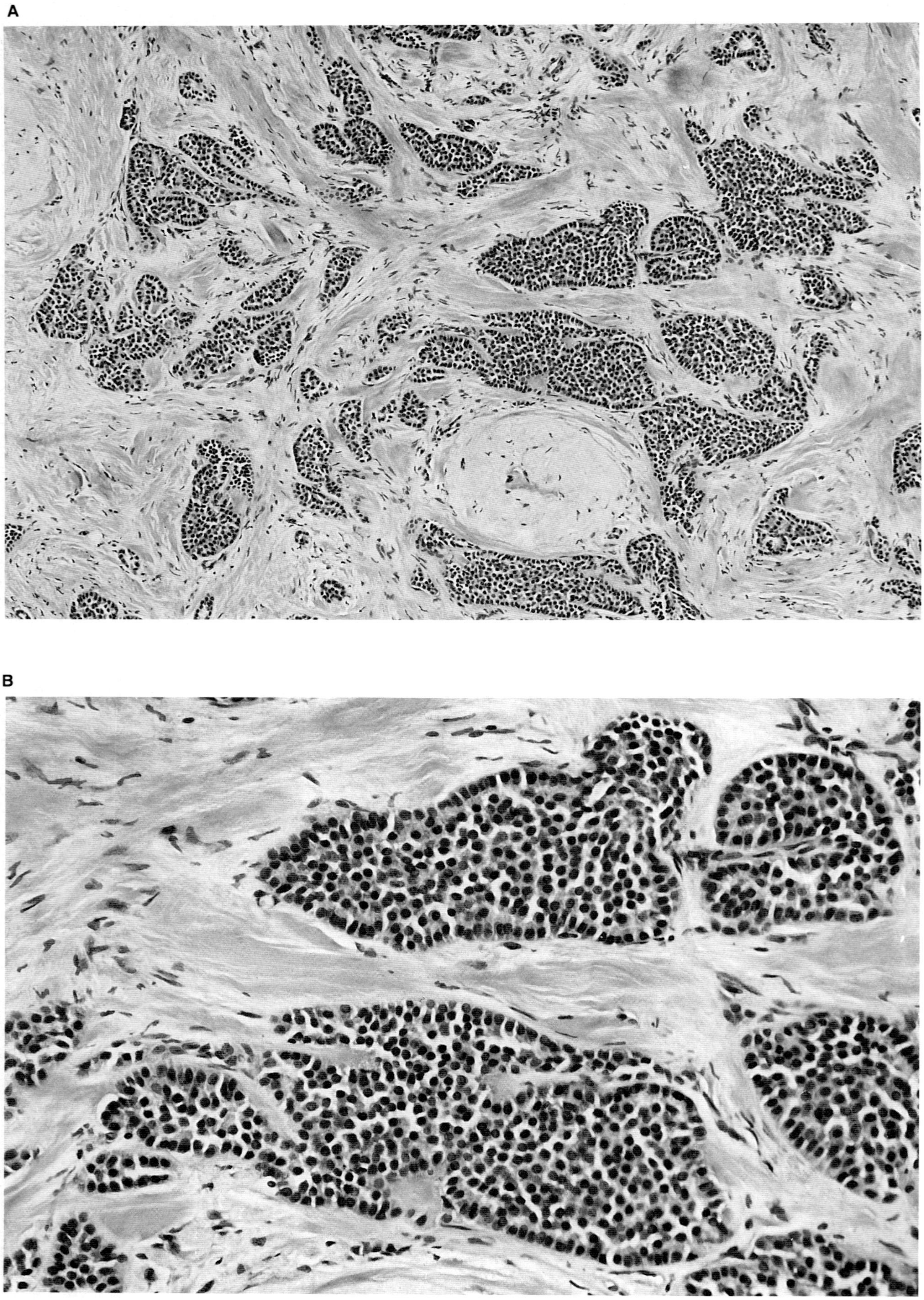


**Figure 2.2** Well differentiated carcinoma. Tubule formation = 3, atypia = 1, mitotic figures = 1; total score = 5. (H&E, (a) X60; (b) X300)

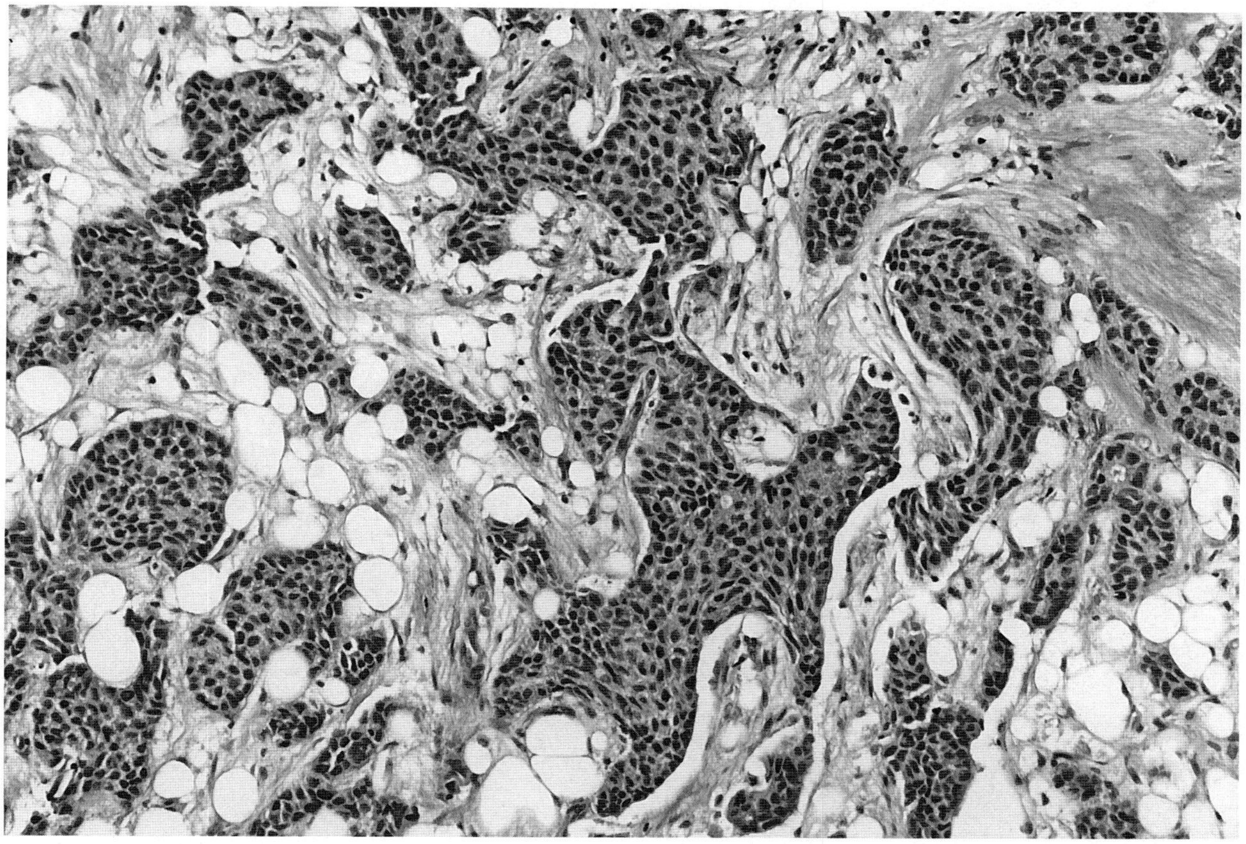

**Figure 2.3** Moderately differentiated carcinoma. The tumor is basically composed of solid cell clusters with few lumens forming within the clusters. The cells lack significant pleomorphism or atypia, and mitotic figures are not conspicuous. Tubule formation = 3, atypia = 2, mitotic figures = 1; total score = 6. (H&E, X240)

Grade I: 3–5 points, well differentiated (Figs. 2.1, 2.2).

Grade II: 6–7 points, moderately differentiated (Figs. 2.3, 2.4).

Grade III: 8–9 points, poorly differentiated (Fig. 2.5).

Finally, Helpap (186) has proposed a modification of Bloom & Richardson's grading method to include nucleolar features such as its frequency, size, number, and localization.

Obviously, the grading system is still undergoing evolution and the ultimate system has not yet been devised. Though not identical, both the histologic method of Bloom and Richardson (172) and the nuclear grading system of Black et al (168,169) have been found to be useful in predicting prognosis (176). The absence of tubule formation in one study (49), and a high mitotic count in another (99) have been shown to be the most significant predictors of survival in women with node-negative infiltrating duct carcinoma; using a combination of features is more appealing to me, however. It may be beneficial to incorporate the presence of necrosis, a feature common in some high grade invasive carcinomas, into the grading system.

In order to further simplify the grading system, we have witnessed not only a reduction in the number of features evaluated, but also a reversal of Black et al's original numerical order for nuclear grades by many who rely on nuclear grading. A reversal of Black's original numerical order has been necessary to prevent confusion and facilitate communication. Furthermore, there is also a trend toward reducing the number of grades from three to two in the evaluation or grouping of patients for determining survival rates. Utilizing two nuclear grades, Fisher et al (116) found that stage I, node negative tumors with good nuclear grade have an 86% survival at eight years compared to a 64% survival for those with a poor nuclear grade. Questions have been raised, however, regarding the two grades that have been combined by Fisher et al. Obviously, some favor combining grades 1 and 2, while others prefer combining grades 2 and 3. If a two-grade system is used,

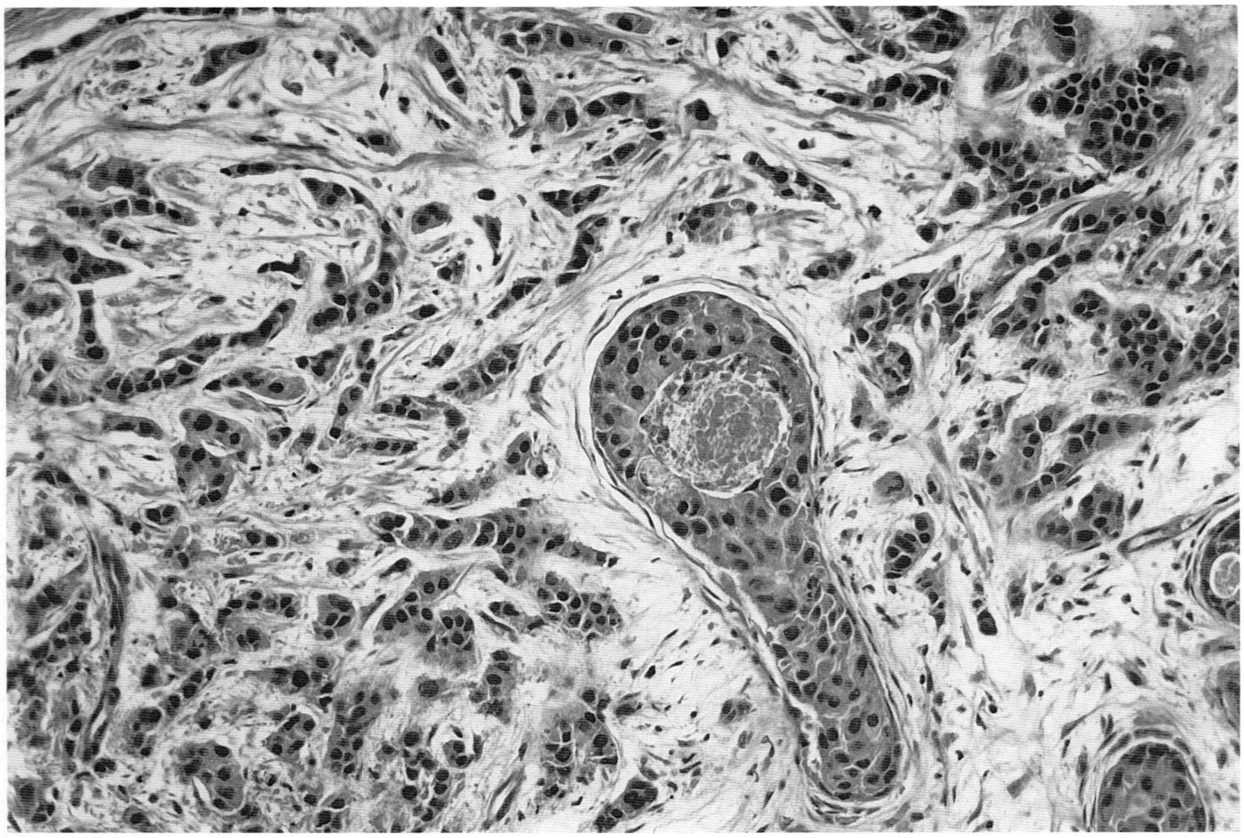

**Figure 2.4** Moderately differentiated carcinoma. Tubule formation = 3, atypia = 2, mitotic figures = 2; total score = 7. (H&E, X300)

I propose that consideration be given to inclusion of tumor necrosis in the invasive areas as one of the features to be evaluated; a simple two-grade system could be designed to include the variety of features of known prognostic significance and necrosis (Table 2.4). This approach needs to be tested.

All pathologists should learn and make an effort to grade tumors preferably using a uniform approach. My personal preference and approach to grading has been quite similar to Elston's. Although I also assess the number of mitotic figures per 10 HPF and have adhered to the same numbers for scoring as recommended by Elston, I feel that the maximum number of mitotic figures allowed for giving the tumor one point (up to 9 per 10 HPF), or two points (10 to 19 per 10 HPF) is too high. Most tumors that have ten or more mitotic figures per 10 HPF have been rather high-grade carcinomas in my experience, making the utility of a group with 20 or more mitotic figures per 10 HPF in this system somewhat questionable. Contesso et al's system appears simple to apply, but the methodology for obtaining the mitotic count is different from that used for most tumors. Furthermore, the inclusion of a papillary pattern, in addition to the formation of tubular structures in the assessment of the tumor architecture, is a rather novel approach, the reason for which is not explained. Most papillary carcinomas do not have a classic invasive component, and they can get very large but remain confined to a duct. Also, invasive carcinomas that retain complete or partial papillary arrangement are quite rare in the United States. Therefore, it is difficult to explain why this feature has been included in the assessment of the tumor architecture unless the tumors observed in France differ significantly in their morphology from those occurring in the United States.

### *Reproducibility of the Grading Systems*

One of the major problems with grading breast carcinomas is in its reproducibility. A 70% intraobserver agreement between two independent readings by the same experienced observer has been reported (174). Fisher et al (182) have reported a 94% intraobserver and 90% interobserver consistency. Theissig et al (194) found a satisfactory correlation of histopathologic grades assessed by three pathologists in 72.3%

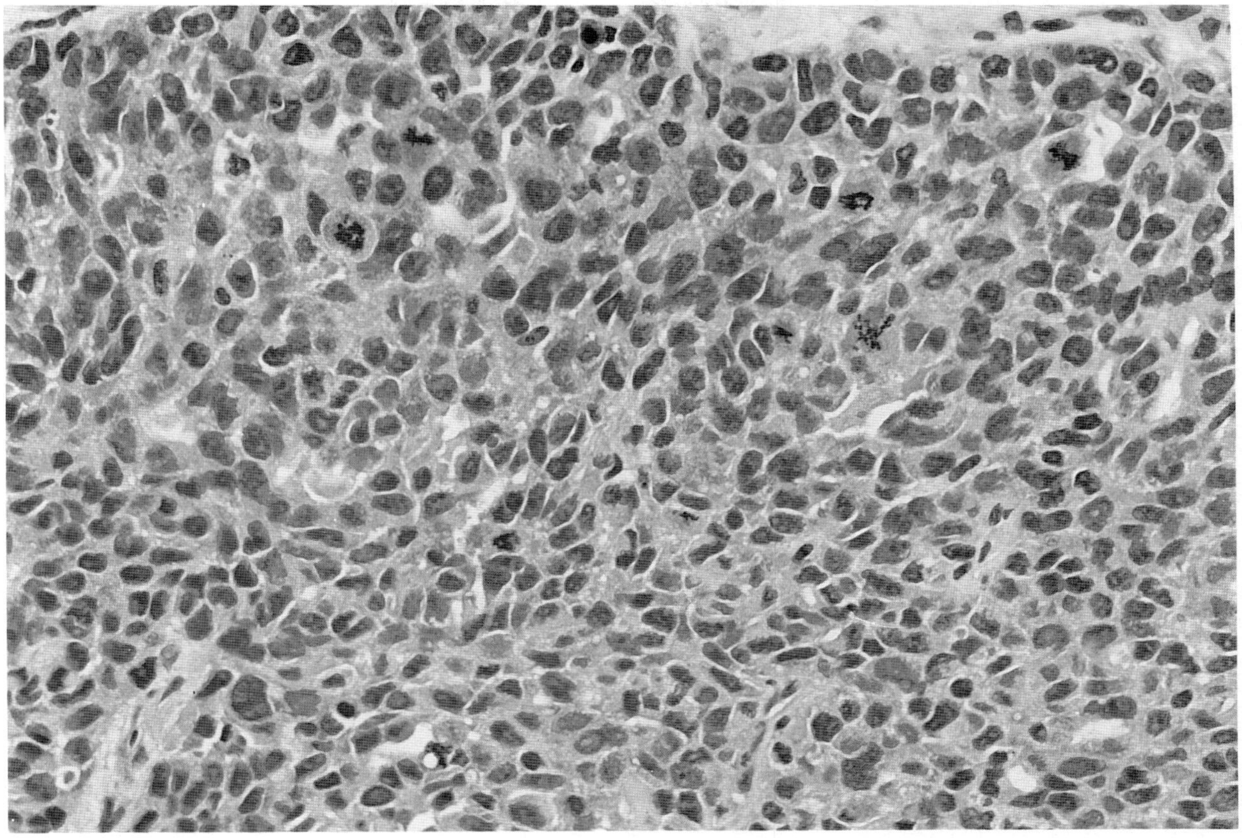

**Figure 2.5** Poorly differentiated carcinoma. There is no evidence of tubule or lumen formation within this solid cluster of cells; significant pleomorphism and atypia are evident along with numerous mitotic figures. Tubule formation = 3, atypia = 2, mitotic figures = 3; total score = 8. (H&E, X400)

of cases using Bloom and Richardson's system. Obviously, none of the systems proposed to date is perfect; all rely, at least in part, on a subjective estimation of cytologic and/or histologic features under study. This subjective aspect is a major reason for problems in reproducibility of any of the grading systems. Therefore, interobserver variation (175,192) and reproducibility will continue to remain problems. As Henson has pointed out, however, grading provides an estimation of prognosis which is very useful information despite the variations inherent in its subjective nature (187,188). With increased experience and training, it is hoped that there will be an improvement in the reproducibility of grading.

**Table 2.4** Two Grade System of Classification of Breast Carcinoma

| Low Grade | High Grade |
|---|---|
| Tubules or secondary lumen formation (75% or more) | Tubules or secondary lumen formation (25% or less) |
| Nuclear uniformity ± minimal variation | Nuclear pleomorphism |
| Nucleoli inconspicuous | May have prominent and/or multiple nucleoli |
| <5 MF/10 HPF* | 5 or more MF/ 10 HPF |
| No Necrosis | ±Necrosis |

* = Based on high power field on an American Optical Microstar, X40 objective, 0.66 mm field diameter.

## The Nottingham Prognostic Index

Based on the finding that size, lymph node status, and histologic grade are the most important prognostic features of a tumor, a relatively simple index has been derived by the Nottingham group (177) and designated and the Nottingham Prognostic Index (NPI). The formula for obtaining this index is as follows:

$$\text{NPI} = 0.2\text{X tumor size (cm)} + \text{lymph node stage (1,2,3)} + \text{tumor grade (1,2,3)}.$$

The lower the NPI value, the better the prognosis. This index has been used to correctly assign 86%

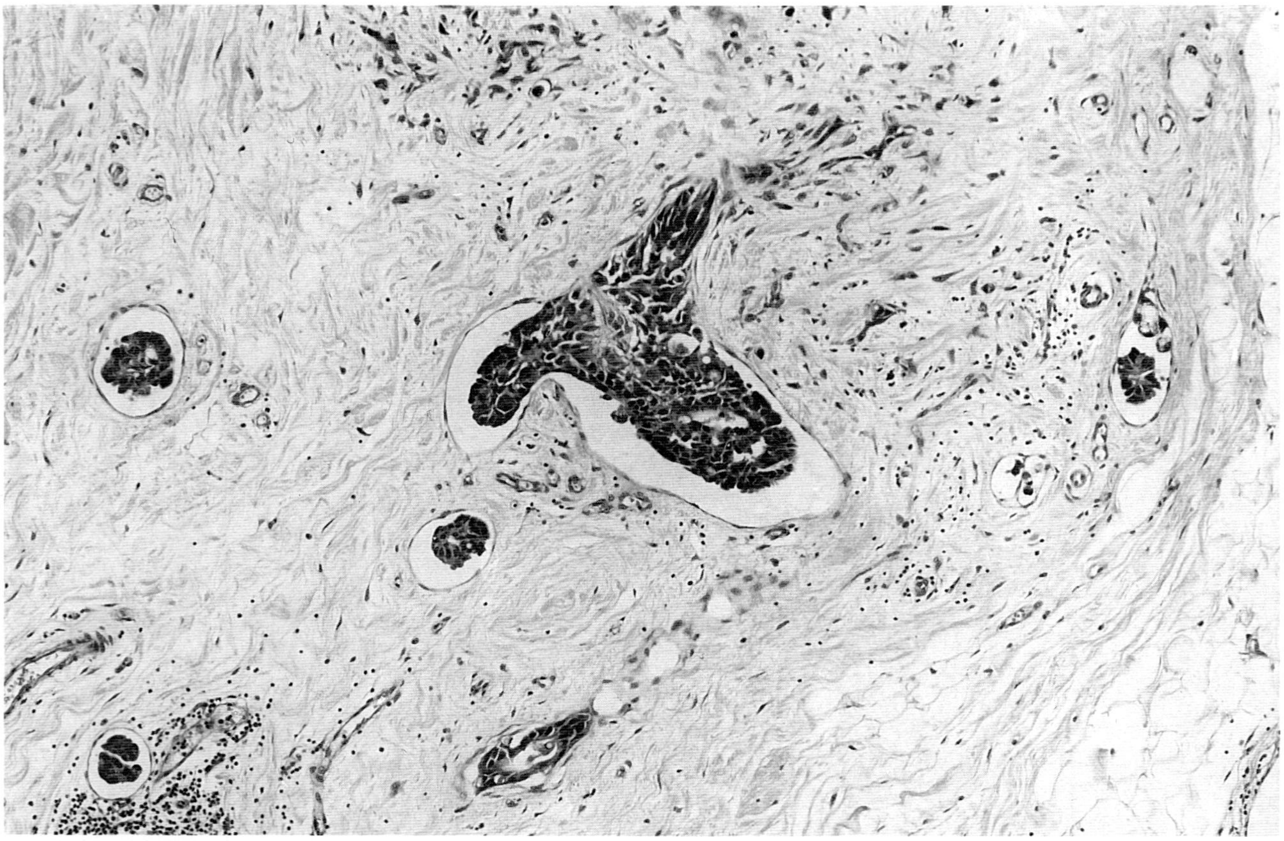

**Figure 2.6** Intravascular carcinoma is present in several vascular spaces of various sizes. (H&E, X240)

of women into either an exceedingly poor prognosis group, or one with a very good prognosis (123). Over 15 years of follow-up, the patients in the good prognosis group have a survival rate of 81%, compared to a 16% survival rate for those in the poor prognosis group.

## Vascular Invasion

Blood vessel and lymphatic spaces both within and around the invasive carcinoma may be invaded by tumor cells (Fig. 2.6). The location of tumor emboli relative to the invasive tumor was thought to be of little significance (140). The specific type of vascular space involved is not always readily recognizable. The identification of vascular invasion around the invasive carcinoma is important, however, as it is a significant predictor of early local recurrence and distant metastases (91,106,139,146,150,151). Of 33 patients with axillary node metastases, 69% had vascular invasion, compared to 26% of 30 women who had no evidence of axillary node involvement (131). The presence of vascular invasion also indicates a greater likelihood of treatment failure (106,149). In Davis et al's study (106), 27% of tumors with vascular invasion developed distant recurrences, compared to 18% of those without vascular invasion; in another study recurrences developed in 32% of patients with lymphatic invasion, compared to 10.3% of those without lymphatic invasion (151). Following a review of 95 breast carcinomas, 23 of which had lymphatic vessel invasion, Orbo et al (140) concluded that lymphatic vessel involvement is a more powerful predictor of lymph node status than tumor size, tumor contour, histologic grade, and type.

Because of interobserver variation in identification of vascular or lymphatic invasion by tumor cells on H&E stained sections (120), immunostains for Factor VIII-related antigen or Ulex Europeus can be used to confirm this finding (91,128,131).

## Cell Kinetics

As a prognostic parameter, cell kinetics analysis of breast carcinomas has the advantage of being quantifiable, objective, independent of axillary node status, and applicable to node-negative patients (197, 201). This feature can be evaluated by either thymidine labeling or DNA analysis by flow cytometry. The former relies on uptake of tritiated thymidine, a specific DNA precursor, by cells in the process of replicating their chromosomes in preparation for division. The incorporated tritiated thymidine is detectable in tissue sections by autoradiographic methods. In effect, the labelled cells reflect cells that are in the S-phase (DNA synthesis).

### *Thymidine Labelling Index (TLI)*

The thymidine labelling index (TLI) indicates the proportion (percent) of cells within the tumor that are in the S-phase. The median TLI for breast carcinomas is approximately 5%. In general, low-grade carcinomas such as mucinous and adenoid cystic carcinoma, have low TLI. Medullary and atypical medullary carcinoma, however, have above median TLIs. Carcinomas with high TLIs have the potential to grow rapidly and recur early. TLI correlates weakly with the clinical stage of the tumor, it correlates inversely with ER content (202,203), and it is directly related to the histologic grade (204). It may be helpful to select patients at risk of early relapse for adjuvant chemotherapy. The heterogeneity of the patients, tumors evaluated within and in between various studies, along with differences in methodology, analytical approach, small number of patients, short follow-up, and different therapeutic approaches have resulted in highly diverse findings (196).

### *Flow Cytometry*

The cells in S-phase can be identified by the intensity of their fluorescent pulses after having been stained with a DNA-specific dye using flow cytometry (194). The fluorescence of cells in the S-phase is more than the fluorescence of cells in the G1 phase and less than those in the G2 phase. The S-phase fraction (SPF) determined by flow cytometry is generally considered equivalent to the TLI, but a consistent excess of SPF values over the TLI was noted in early studies; the mean SPFs of breast carcinoma ranged from 9% to 13%, compared to 5% to 7% for TLIs (200). Subsequent studies have reported a mean SPF value of 8%, and a mean TLI of 7.5, showing a decrease in the gap between the two values (133).

In addition to providing SPF values, flow cytometry can provide a DNA index, comparing tumor cell DNA content to that of a benign cell. A DNA index of 1.0 indicates that the DNA content of the tumor cells and that of the benign cell are similar. A DNA index of 2.0 indicates a hyperdiploid tumor cell population.

It has been suggested that abnormal ploidy or elevated SPF identifies patients with shorter survival, and worsened disease-free survival, as well as being associated with poor outcome in locoregional control of the disease (199). Clark et al (195) measured ploidy and SPF on 345 tumors from node negative breast cancer patients. Of these, 32% were diploid, and the remaining 68% were aneuploid. The probability of disease-free survival at five years was 88% for patients with diploid tumor and 74% for those with aneuploid lesions. The probability of disease-free survival at five years for patients with diploid tumors and low S-phase was 90% compared to 70% for those with diploid tumors and high S-phase. With improved techniques, S-phase may also be able to discriminate between aneuploid tumors with high or low probability of relapse.

Flow cytometry can be applied successfully to paraffin-embedded tumor specimen permitting retrospective evaluation of archival material. Merkel and McGuire (199) have listed some of the complications associated with the use of paraffin-embedded material which should be kept in mind during analysis of generated data. Due to fixation-induced changes in fluorochrome binding, external diploid standards often cannot be used to determine which G0–1 peak in a mixed histogram reflects the diploid cell population. Despite this problem, since a majority of tumor specimen also contain some nonmalignant tissue, aneuploidy can be reliably identified, except for hypodiploid tumors.

Another problem associated with the use of paraffin-embedded material is superimposition of variable amounts of debris on the DNA histogram which results from the enzymatic digestion required to obtain a nuclear suspension. If this debris is not taken into account and mathematically subtracted from the histogram before cell cycle analysis, it can result in an overestimation of the S-phase fraction. Correction for this source of error would bring the SPF values into closer agreement with TLI.

Finally, the resolution of G0–1 peaks obtained from paraffin-embedded specimen is usually inferior to that obtained from fresh tissue. This could result in misclassification of aneuploid tumors with a near-diploid DNA content.

In comparison with TLI, flow cytometry provides an automated and more speedy analysis of cell kinetics, while it can also determine the ploidy of the tumor.

While tumor ploidy and SPF may eventually prove to be important prognostic indicators that may assist in selecting patients who may benefit from systemic treatment, the disease-free survival and overall survival of women has not differed significantly on the basis of tumor ploidy (196,198,205). Furthermore, ploidy and SPF by flow cytometry appear to be of borderline clinical significance in node-positive women (198).

## Steroid Receptors

Determination of estrogen receptors (ER) and progestin receptors (PR) on biopsies of invasive carcinomas prior to therapeutic manipulations has become standard practice in the management of patients with breast carcinoma. The clinical utility of these steroid receptors was suspected around 15 to 20 years ago (229,256); their correlation with the degree of tumor differentiation was confirmed subsequently (231).

Identification of women who are likely to respond to hormonal manipulations was a serious problem for the clinician treating patients with breast carcinomas until recently when hormone receptor analysis became part of the routine evaluation of breast carcinomas. Approximately 55% to 65% of primary breast carcinomas and 45% to 55% of the metastases from breast carcinomas have been found to be ER positive (ER+) and contain more than 10 femtomoles/mg cytosol protein of ER. Studies have shown that 55% to 60% of women with ER+ tumors respond to additive or ablative hormone therapy compared to about 8% of women with ER negative (ER−) tumors. Furthermore, ER− tumors show a better response to cytotoxic chemotherapy. Tumors that are better differentiated are more likely to be ER+, and ER+ carcinomas have a relatively better prognosis (230).

Approximately 45% to 60% of primary and metastatic breast cancers contain PR. The presence of both ER and PR in the tumor increases the likelihood of response to endocrine manipulations from the 55% observed in patients with ER+ tumors to 75% to 80% (247,256). Progesterone receptors are at least as valuable in predicting the behavior of breast carcinomas as estrogen receptors, and the loss of PR by tumor cells is associated with a worse prognosis (232).

The correlation of ER with prognosis and survival in patients with breast carcinoma is controversial. Some studies suggest that ER positive tumors have better prognosis (206,210,216,223,224,238,240), while others fail to show this relationship (221,244, 245). It is noteworthy that a strong correlation between the histologic grade and hormone receptors has been observed (211,213). At present, the determination of ER and PR is considered one of the most important features of the tumor to be assessed; the results are used in making therapeutic decisions and regarded as an independent prognostic indicator (225) following different procedures (222).

### *Immunocytochemical Determination of ER and PR*

Several reports have confirmed an acceptable to excellent correlation of immunocytochemically determined ER with ER values determined by dextran-coated charcoal assay (242,253), with an average concordance of 84% and a range of 66% to 98%. O'Keane et al (236) have shown that when nuclear staining alone is considered as the parameter of a positive immunoreaction, the immunocytochemical assay of ER with anti–17 beta-estradiol antibody in routinely processed, formalin fixed, archival material is an accurate and specific method for the determination of the ER status of breast carcinoma. They found that greater than 30% nuclear positivity as a cut-off point yielded a sensitivity of 76% and a specificity of 82%. Pertschuk et al (242) concluded that immunocytochemically assessed ER does correlate with survival and disease-free survival in patients with stage I or II breast carcinoma, but PR is a better predictor of survival. They also found excellent correlation of the immunocytochemical results and biochemically determined values. More important, they concluded that immunocytochemically determined ER and PR are more predictive of prognosis than biochemically assessed ER and PR assays.

While evaluation of ER assays in fresh tissue should be given first priority, if there is no fresh tissue or the tissue is small, immunocytochemical assessment of ER in paraffin-embedded tissue offers a reasonably good alternative both as a prognostic factor and as a predictor of response to endocrine manipulations (207). While this procedure needs to be more standardized, it would be most valuable when the diagnosis of carcinoma comes as a surprise during microscopic review.

### *Steroid Receptors in Male Breast Carcinoma*

Everson et al (214) found ER positivity in 90% of male breast carcinomas. A negative correlation was observed between patient's age and ER concentration. Progesterone receptor positivity was identified in 9 of 14 breast carcinomas from the patients in the same group. In contrast few examples of gynecomastia are ER+ and these are usually of the 4S species as detected by sucrose gradient centrifugation (256).

## Ancillary Prognosticators

Currently, the treatment of patients with breast carcinoma is based mainly on the stage of the tumor at diagnosis, number of axillary nodes with metastases, tumor size, and the status of estrogen and progesterone receptors. Tumor grade, obtained on the basis of a uniform approach is another invaluable prognostic indicator that has been used successfully as an accurate predictor of prognosis in many European medical centers (118,123,173,177), but it has never been widely accepted or utilized in the United States. Also considered significant in the therapeutic decision-making process are the ploidy and S-phase fraction of the tumor. Nonetheless, it is practically impossible to determine the course of disease even for patients who have no evidence of axillary node metastases. The tumor will relapse in approximately 30% of node-negative women, and some have proposed that all patients, including those who are node-negative, receive systemic adjuvant therapy (226). However, since adjuvant therapy is not without harm (233), the identification of biomarkers that would separate patients with a good prognosis who will need no additional therapy from those who are more likely to develop recurrences and metastases and who are more likely to benefit from adjuvant therapy has become a major goal of breast cancer research.

At this time there is no biomarker—material elaborated exclusively or in abnormal amounts by cancer cells—that is unique to breast carcinoma. A number of markers that have shown promise as prognosticators will be presented. The application of a variety of monoclonal antibodies along with more established parameters as an aid in the diagnosis, prognostication, and therapeutic management of breast carcinoma has been discussed in several review articles (125,212,234).

### *c-erbB-2 (HER-2/neu or HER-2) Oncogene*

Initially considered to be genetic material from a retrovirus resulting in malignant transformation when incorporated into normal cells, the majority of HER-2 oncogenes are now thought to be activated homologues of protooncogenes which have persisted in the normal cell (215). HER-2/neu, also known as c-erbB-2, is a member of the erbB oncogene family, and is related to, but distinct from, epidermal growth factors. It is found to be amplified (two or more folds) in about 30% of human breast carcinomas; this amplification was found to be an independent predictor of overall survival and time to relapse in patients with lymph node-positive breast cancer (246). The expression of this protein has been associated with poor histologic grade (208), spread to axillary nodes, and number of nodes involved (246); a negative association between c-erbB-2 expression and ER and PR has been noted (257). No significant association has been found between c-erbB-2 expression and ploidy (250). In axillary node-positive patients, there is a significant correlation between amplification of HER-2 protein and shorter disease-free and overall survival (248). HER-2 oncogene amplification correlates with absence of estrogen and progesterone receptors. In node-negative patients, Paik et al (239) found an association between HER-2 overexpression with decreased survival only among women with tumors that displayed a good nuclear grade; HER-2 overexpression in these women was associated with an almost five-fold increase in mortality rates. In 1991, four papers that appeared simultaneously along with an editorial on c-erbB-2 oncogene have provided excellent discussions and additional support for the significance of expression of this oncogene in tumors of advanced stage and those that are more poorly differentiated (208,220,228,237,241).

Thus far, the published studies, have all been retrospective in nature. Prospective studies with a large number of patients are necessary to properly determine the prognostic significance of this biologic variable. It is possible that HER-2 overexpression may identify the few women with small (<2 cm), ER+, and low grade tumors in the node-negative group of patients who are likely to develop early recurrence. Amplification of c-erbB-2 strongly correlates with each element (architectural pattern, nuclear atypia, and number of mitotic figures) of the histologic grade (251). Even if a primary tumor does not express c-erbB-2 protein, subsequent metastases may express the protein; in contrast, if a primary tumor expresses c-erbB-2 protein, this capacity is retained in all tumor metastases (235).

### *Cathepsin D*

The acidic lysosomal protease, cathepsin D is produced and secreted by breast cancer cells. It is one of the latest markers being currently evaluated as a prognostic indicator. In normal cells, cathepsin D is secreted as a 52-Kd precursor and has a growth-promoting and extracellular proteolytic activity; these activities may have prognostic significance in breast cancer (243). Overexpression of this enzyme (>70 pmole/mg protein of tumor cytosol) appears to be associated with aggressive tumor behavior and shortened relapse-free survival. The actuarial five-year recurrence rate of axillary node-negative, aneuploid tumors with overexpression of cathepsin D is 60% (249).

The relationship of cathepsin D with HER-2 (c-erbB-2) and c-myc oncogene amplification was studied by Brouillet et al (209). They concluded that cathepsin D does not correlate with HER-2 oncogene expression, but it does correlate with c-myc amplification. Expression of c-myc is generally related to cell proliferation, and patients whose tumor DNA shows amplified c-myc gene have a decreased short-term survival (219,252).

Since lysosomal proteases are also present in phagocytic cells, the presence of a large number of such cells in the tumor tissue may influence the cytosol levels of cathepsin D.

### *Ki67*

In Germany, Gerdes et al (217,218) developed a monoclonal antibody Ki67 that reacts with an undefined nuclear antigen present in all non-G0 cells of the cell cycle. Therefore, Ki67 identifies the proliferating cells within a tumor. Since cells from any phase of the cycle can enter the G0 phase regardless of their DNA content, determination of the Ki67 fraction could reflect more significant information regarding the proliferating cell component of a tumor compared to the DNA content (227).

Using immunocytochemistry, the Ki67 "growth fraction" reflects the percent of positively stained cells in a tumor. The higher the Ki67 growth fraction, the more aggressive the tumor. Positive Ki67 correlates with the tumor's degree of differentiation, vascular invasion, lymph node metastases, and it relates inversely to the presence of steroid hormone receptors. Node-negative breast carcinomas have an average Ki67 growth fraction of 13%, while node-positive tumors with less than four involved nodes have an average Ki67 growth fraction of 20%.

Regardless of the current enthusiasm concerning the variety of monoclonal antibodies, it is important to maintain a healthy skepticism. Only a few, if any, of these antibodies may pass the test of time and find their way from the shelves of research laboratories to that of the diagnostic laboratories. Eventually, a battery of antibodies, rather than a single antibody, may provide the best prognostic information. Standardization of methods and quality control is required prior to widespread use. At present, an accurate diagnosis, typing and grading of the carcinoma on H&E stained sections, remains the most valuable source of information on which therapeutic decisions are based.

### *Prognosis of Pregnancy-Associated Breast Cancer*

Pregnancy-associated (PA) breast carcinoma is defined clinically as a carcinoma diagnosed simultaneously or within one year after pregnancy. It appears that these carcinomas grow despite, rather than because of, the pregnancy (264). Only 9% of women develop a carcinoma during their first pregnancy (264). The carcinomas present with equal frequency within the three trimesters of pregnancy (264). Traditionally, it has been thought that, stage for stage, PA breast carcinomas have either an equivalent or worse prognosis compared to non-pregnancy associated cancers (259,265,271,272). Petrek et al (272), however, found no significant difference in the survival of the two groups when they reviewed 56 PA breast carcinomas and compared their survival with that of nonpregnant women with breast carcinoma.

A high proportion of these patients have axillary node metastases at the time of presentation. The incidence of axillary node metastases ranges from 53% to 81% (258–263,266–269,273). Delay in diagnosis and treatment may be responsible for the higher

**Table 2.5** Results of Various Studies on Breast Cancer Multicentricity According to Different Evaluation Techniques

| Reference | No. of Cases Studied | Method | Multicentricity (%) |
|---|---|---|---|
| 290 | 157 | Large tissue paraffin sections | 54 |
| 297 | 64 | 2–5 histologic sections/quadrant | 26 |
| 295 | 508 | Routine laboratory | 59 |
| 278 | 904 | 1 random section per quadrant | 13.4 |
| 287 | 500 | 2 random sections per quadrant and any suspicious areas | 42 |
| 291 | 203 | 2–3 sections per quadrant | 65 |
| 281 | 85 | Correlated serial subgross, radiographic, & histologic | 21 |
| 289 | 156 | Screening of asymptomatic women | Not specified |
| 294 | 53 | Histologic sections from each quadrant | 39.6 |
| 282 | 211 | Serial subgross and correlated radiographic | 56 |
| 293 | 43 | 4 histologic sections from each quadrant | 44 |
| 298 | 173 | Suspicious and random sections per quadrant | 30 |
| 284 | 53 | Serial subgross and correlated radiographic | 32 |
| 277 | 118 | Serial subgross and correlated radiographic | 60 |
| 285 | 880 | 2 histologic sections per quadrant | 30 |
| 292 | 100 | Submacroscopic selection from 5 slices/quadrant | 36 |

Modified with permission from Sarnelli and Squartini, (292).

stages of PA breast carcinomas at presentation. About 70% of the carcinomas are ER− (264) providing further evidence that PA breast carcinomas tend to be more aggressive.

The treatment of PA breast carcinoma depends on the stage of the pregnancy and the patient's concern regarding breast conservation (252). Fentiman (264) has suggested a treatment plan for operable breast carcinomas after limited staging. In his plan, women in the first or second trimester of pregnancy are offered mastectomy. If they accept and the nodes are negative, no further treatment is necessary and the pregnancy is allowed to progress. If the nodes are positive, pregnancy is terminated and adjuvant chemotherapy initiated. If the woman refuses to have a mastectomy, the pregnancy is either terminated or early delivery is undertaken. The patient will undergo breast conservation and radiotherapy with adjuvant chemotherapy if the nodes are positive.

For third trimester pregnancy, either early delivery or modified radical mastectomy is the first step. Early delivery precedes breast conservation and radiotherapy since radiotherapy is contraindicated during pregnancy. If there are positive nodes, adjuvant chemotherapy is administered; if not, the patient is observed for completion of gestation. For women who choose mastectomy and have positive nodes, early delivery is necessary prior to administration of chemotherapy. The pregnancy is not interfered with if the nodes are negative.

## MULTICENTRICITY

While the terms multicentric and multifocal are used synonymously by some pathologists, I believe a distinction should be made between these two terms. I use the term multifocal to refer to the presence of more than a single focus of either intraductal carcinoma, lobular neoplasia, or invasive carcinoma within a slide or a biopsy not larger than 5 cm in its maximum dimension. For example, multiple lobules within a 1 cm tissue section may show lobular neoplasia; therefore, the lesion would be multifocal. To qualify as multicentric, a lesion (lobular neoplasia, in situ or invasive carcinoma) should be separated from a similar (lobular neoplasia, in situ or invasive carcinoma) focus elsewhere in the biopsy or the breast by a distance of 5 cm from the border or periphery of the reference lesions. In most cases, this implies presence of lesions in different quadrants or in the subareolar-central region.

The frequency of multicentricity in the literature ranges from 9% to 75% (278,279). This considerable variation is observed because of 1) lack of a uniform definition, 2) variation in the tissue evaluation techniques, and 3) differences in the amount or extent of tissue sampling. The results of numerous studies, their method of evaluation, and their findings are listed in Table 2.5. Reviewing the data available on this topic, McDivitt (286) concluded that the overall rate of multicentricity is in the range of 25% to 50%;

the incidence of multicentric invasive carcinoma is 5% to 10%.

Defining multicentricity as the presence of two separate and independent foci of carcinoma at 5 cm or more distant from each other, Lagios et al (284) studied 286 total mastectomies and found multicentric lesions in 28% of the cases. The second site may be invasive also, noninvasive or reflect Paget's disease. Using a similar definition, Lagios et al evaluated the presence of multicentricity in 41 intraductal carcinomas. When the extent of intraductal carcinoma was less than 2.5 cm, multicentricity was found in 17% of the cases. Intraductal carcinomas that extended beyond 2.5 cm, displayed multicentricity in 47% of the cases. Interestingly, occult invasive carcinoma was absent in all intraductal carcinomas less than 2.5 cm in extent, but it was present in 47% of those larger than 2.5 cm. Holland et al (280) found no difference in the occurrence of multicentric carcinoma whether the reference carcinoma was less than 2 cm or from 2 to 4 cm in size.

The concept of multicentricity is of particular importance in the conservative management of patients with breast carcinoma. While currently, multicentricity does not appear to be a deterrent to conservative surgery in some centers, this concept was and remains a significant rational for preference of mastectomy in the treatment of breast carcinoma by many surgeons. Crile et al (276) found that 12% of women with breast cancer 2 cm or smaller develop local recurrence following partial mastectomy and an additional 3% develop cancer elsewhere in the breast during a follow-up period of at least five years; these tumors were not detectable at the time the reference carcinoma was detected and could be multicentric lesions not detected simultaneously. Since ten-year follow-up results of lumpectomy with radiation as the primary treatment of women with intraductal carcinoma has proven quite promising, conservative treatment seems justified with proper patient selection (296). About 16% to 20% of women with various types of intraductal carcinoma treated conservatively—lumpectomy with or without radiation—develop recurrent disease (275,296). The type of intraductal carcinoma appears to be a predictor of the likelihood for the development of recurrent disease. When the patients for conservative treatment were carefully selected based on the presence of clinically occult, mammographically-detected lesions which did not extend beyond 2.5 cm, and stratified according to the type of intraductal carcinoma, none of the women with the micropapillary variant of intraductal carcinoma developed recurrences, whereas 19% of those with comedocarcinoma and 10% of those with atypical cribriform carcinoma recurred (332). It appears paradoxical that there is general acceptance of conservative surgery in the treatment of early invasive carcinoma (288), while there remains a great diversity of opinions regarding conservative surgery in the management of women with intraductal carcinoma. In effect, a woman with intraductal carcinoma is more likely to lose her breast, compared to a woman with early invasive carcinoma. It is not clear whether the subsequent carcinoma in these conservatively treated women reflects residual foci of in situ carcinoma that progressed, or de novo lesions developing in the remaining normal duct system.

## BILATERALITY

Women with breast carcinoma are at an increased risk of developing carcinoma in the contralateral breast (308,316,322). The risk for the development of a metachronous contralateral breast carcinoma is approximately 1% per year after mastectomy (309,315, 322), while the risk of synchronous bilateral breast carcinoma ranges from 0.2% to 2% (311,328). Expressed in comparison to the general population, the relative risk of developing an invasive carcinoma in the contralateral breast is four to seven times the incidence of a first primary invasive breast carcinoma in the general population (307,322).

The frequency of contralateral carcinoma reported from various centers differs because of differences in study design, patient selection, and sampling technique. Studies relying upon clinically diagnosed lesions yield the lower frequencies, whereas those based upon random or mirror image biopsy with or without mammography, and prophylactic mastectomy provide the higher frequencies (310,321,327,328). Chaudary et al (307) found simultaneous breast carcinoma in 3% of women in their study; the use of mammography enhanced the detection of synchronous bilateral breast carcinomas by five-fold. Identification of in situ carcinomas and occult invasive carcinomas histopathologically contribute to the higher frequencies obtained in some studies (319,321). In autopsy studies, the contralateral breast has been found to harbor an invasive carcinoma in 12% (314) to 21% (303) of women with invasive breast carcinoma.

In order to provide a reliable estimate of the lifelong risk for the development of contralateral breast carcinoma, and assess its impact on survival, Nielsen et al (318) used a thorough histopathologic approach to evaluate 86 consecutive autopsies of Danish women with a clinical diagnosis of invasive breast carcinoma. Thirty-three percent of these women were found to have a second invasive carcinoma in the contralateral breast, while 35% had an in situ carcinoma in the contralateral breast. Only in eight patients was the presence of the contralateral carcinoma either diagnosed or suspected clinically. Of those women with an invasive contralateral carcinoma, 71% had axillary node metastases. A higher proportion of women with contralateral invasive carcinoma died from disseminated disease, but the mean survival time was similar for women with or without contralateral breast carcinoma. In comparison, in a previous autopsy study of 77 unselected Danish women without any clinical evidence of invasive breast carcinoma and with an age distribution similar to the patients in Nielsen et al's 1986 study, Nielsen and colleagues found 14 examples of in situ and one invasive breast carcinoma. Considering the similarity of histopathologic methods in the two studies, women with an invasive breast carcinoma appear to have a significantly greater risk of a second in situ or invasive primary lesion.

Features of the first primary carcinoma that may be associated with increasing the risk for a contralateral breast carcinoma include tumor size, degree of anaplasia, location and clinical stage (308,309,315,322, 324). A family history of breast carcinoma may be associated with a greater frequency of bilateral carcinoma (300,301,312), though some studies do not support this viewpoint (299,302). Multicentricity of the first carcinoma is another parameter implicated in increasing the likelihood of a subsequent contralateral carcinoma (315,317,322); Wanebo et al (328) consider bilateral breast carcinoma as a special reflection of multicentricity. Finally, the tubular and lobular variants of breast carcinoma are more commonly bilateral (303,313,316,329). Several studies have reported a greater incidence of bilaterality in premenopausal women (315,316,322,324). Bilateral breast carcinoma has also been reported in patients with Peutz-Jeghers syndrome (304,320,325).

While some studies have reported a decreased survival rate for women with bilateral carcinoma compared to those with unilateral cancer (322,328), others have shown no significant difference (306), specifically in the 10-year (309,311) or the 20-year (323) survival of these two groups.

## CLASSIFICATION OF BREAST TUMORS

The histologic classification of breast tumors is a descriptive one, and probably the most widely used classification is the one proposed by the World Health Organization (WHO) (330). The most recent revision of the classification took place in 1982, and is presented in Table 2.6. While this classification is the basis for the presentations in this book, modifications were necessary in practically all areas, most significantly in the areas of metaplastic carcinoma, myoepithelial tumors, and mammary dysplasia and fibrocystic changes.

For those interested in examining other classifications, Bassler's handbook (331) provides details of his classification, while the approach proposed by Linell and Rank (333) is discussed in a monograph on breast cancer. A major criticism that I have of the latter classification is that they have lumped together all types of intraductal carcinoma (solid, cribriform, papillary, bridging, mural, or clinging) into one: comedo carcinoma in situ. Classically, the term intraductal comedo carcinoma has been used for those lesions that display not only central necrosis, but also significant cytologic atypia and pleomorphism. Furthermore, it has been shown that this subtype of intraductal carcinoma is associated with a greater frequency of local recurrence following tylectomy (332). Therefore, it seems inappropriate to designate all intraductal carcinomas as comedo type when there are distinctive morphologic and clinical differences among them. The WHO designation of intraductal carcinoma without further qualification is more logical since it would allow for further subdivision according to the subtype.

### Ductal vs Lobular Carcinoma

In most systems of classification, ductal carcinomas are separated from lobular carcinomas at both the in situ and invasive levels. The designation of ductal vs

**Table 2.6** WHO Histologic Classification of Breast Tumors

I. Epithelial Tumors

A. Benign
- 1. Intraductal papilloma
- 2. Adenoma of the nipple
- 3. Adenoma
  - a. Tubular
  - b. Lactating

B. Malignant
- 1. Noninvasive
  - a. Intraductal carcinoma
  - b. Lobular carcinoma in situ
- 2. Invasive
  - a. Invasive ductal carcinoma
  - b. Invasive ductal carcinoma with a predominant intraductal component
  - c. Invasive lobular carcinoma
  - d. Mucinous carcinoma
  - e. Medullary carcinoma
  - f. Papillary carcinoma
  - g. Tubular carcinoma
  - h. Adenoid cystic carcinoma
  - i. Secretory (juvenile) carcinoma
  - j. Apocrine carcinoma
  - k. Carcinoma with metaplasia
    - i. Squamous type
    - ii. Spindle cell type
    - iii. Cartilaginous and osseous type
    - iv. Mixed type
  - l. Others
- 3. Paget's disease of the nipple

II. Mixed Connective Tissue And Epithelial Tumors

A. Fibroadenoma
B. Phyllodes Tumor (cystosarcoma phyllodes)
C. Carcinosarcoma

III. Miscellaneous Tumors

A. Soft Tissue Tumors
B. Skin Tumors
C. Tumors of Hematopoeitic and Lymphoid Tissues

IV. Unclassified Tumors

V. Mammary Dysplasia/Fibrocystic Disease

VI. Tumor-like Lesions

A. Duct Ectasia
B. Inflammatory Pseudotumors
C. Hamartoma
D. Gynecomastia
E. Others

From Azzopardi et al (330).

lobular carcinoma may give the erroneous impression that one group originates in the ducts, while the other has its origin in the lobules. It is important to emphasize that these terms do not necessarily imply the site of origin since the studies of Wellings et al (334) have shown that a majority of breast carcinomas of both ductal and lobular type originate in the terminal duct-lobular unit (TDLU). It is the growth pattern that generally determines whether a lesion is classified as ductal or lobular. What we designate as lobular neoplasia or lobular carcinoma in situ is a lesion that originates in the TDLU and is characterized by a solid, occlusive proliferation of a relatively uniform cell population. What is designated as intraductal carcinoma also originates in the TDLU, but the proliferating cells form non-occlusive layers, or epithelial bridges and secondary lumens. As this proliferation progresses within the acini, it causes an unfolding of the lobules and their transformation into duct-like structures. The proliferating cells of intraductal carcinoma may be highly pleomorphic or quite uniform and even small, similar to those of classic lobular neoplasia. Likewise, small and large cell variants of lobular neoplasia (ALH, LCIS) have been described. Finally, even intracytoplasmic lumens (ICL) which occur most frequently in lobular disease, are not exclusive to this group of lesions and have also been reported in ductal proliferations as well as a variety of adenocarcinomas in other organs. It is, therefore, predominantly the growth pattern that distinguishes what is designated as ductal from a lobular lesion and not the site of origin. There are carcinomas and other proliferative lesions that originate in the major and lactiferous ducts, but a large majority of proliferative lesions in the breast begin in the TDLU.

The concentration of proliferative activity in the TDLU is understandable considering the normal physiologic changes in the mammary gland. Much of the potential for both proliferation and functional activity appears to reside in the TDLU segment of the duct system judging from the development of physiological and gestational hyperplasia as well as lactational and secretory activity in this region. As mentioned in Chapter 1 on the normal breast, during gestation and lactation there is an increase in the number of acini per lobule, and the cells in the acini within the TDLU show a large amount of intracytoplasmic secretory droplets reflecting both proliferative and functional capacity by these cells. The cells lining the portion of the duct system away from the TDLU, however, display minimal if any secretory droplets within their cytoplasm, and there is no readily apparent evidence of significant expansion of this portion of the duct system during gestation and lactation. Since the cells in the TDLU are the ones that more frequently divide, multiply, and differentiate to meet the physiologic requirements of the mammary gland, they are more prone to errors that may occur during any of these stages leading to abnormal proliferative activity and neoplasia compared to the relatively less active cells elsewhere in the duct system.

The invasive carcinomas are also classified predominantly according to the growth patterns that they assume. The major subdivision is into ductal and lobular carcinomas, with the former accounting for 75% of the infiltrating carcinomas diagnosed in the United States after all special types are set aside. There are many variants of ductal carcinoma, some of which are considered among the special types, but variants of infiltrating lobular carcinoma are also recognized. When the differential has been narrowed down to a lobular versus ductal type of invasive carcinoma, my preference is to designate a lesion as ductal if it forms any tubules or secondary lumens within a cluster of tumor cells even if the cells are small and uniform with some cord-like arrangements and regardless of the cell type and nature of any associated in situ component, which should be recorded separately.

## REFERENCES

### Epidemiology and Risk Factors


* 1. Anderson DE: Breast cancer in families. *Cancer* 1977;40: 1855–1860.

2. Anderson DE: Some characteristics of familial breast cancer. *Cancer* 1971;28:1500–1504.

3. Anderson DE, Badzioch MD: Survival in familial breast cancer patients. *Cancer* 1986;58:360–365.

4. Anderson DE, Williams WR: Implications of family history of breast or colon cancer, in Chaganti RSK, German JL (eds): *Genetics in Clinical Oncology*. Oxford University Press, 1985, pp 241–256.

* 5. Baral E, Larsson L, Mattson B: Breast cancer following irradiation of the breast. *Cancer* 1977;40:2905–2910.

* 6. Berg JW: Clinical implications of risk factors for breast cancer. *Cancer* 1984;53:589–591.

* 7. Bergkvist L, Adami HO, Persson I, et al: The risk of breast cancer after estrogen and estrogen-progestin replacement. *N Eng J Med* 1989;321:293–297.

8. Birch JM: The Li-Fraumeni cancer family syndrome. *J Pathol* 1990;161:1–2.

* 9. Boice JD, Monson RR: Breast cancer in women after repeated fluoroscopic examinations of the chest. *J Natl Cancer Inst* 1977;59:823–832.

* 10. Boring CC, Squires TS, Tong T: Cancer statistics, 1992. *CA* 1992;42:19–38.

11. Brinton LA, Hoover RN, Szklo M, et al: Menopausal estrogen and risk of breast cancer. *Cancer* 1981;47:2517–2522.

* 12. Brinton LA, Hoover R, Fraumeni JF Jr: Menopausal estrogens and breast cancer risk: an expanded case control study. *Br J Cancer* 1986;54:825–832.

13. Ciatto S, Biggeri A, Del Turco MR, et al: Risk of breast cancer subsequent to proven gross cystic disease. *Eur J Cancer* 1990;26:555–557.

14. Cook DC, Dent O, Hewitt D: Breast cancer following multiple chest fluoroscopy: the Ontario experience. *Can Med Assoc J* 1974;111:406–409,412.

15. Day NE, Brown C: Multistage models and primary prevention of cancer. *J Natl Cancer Inst* 1980;64:977–989.

16. Dunn JE: Breast cancer among American Japanese in the San Francisco Bay area. *Natl Cancer Inst Monogr* 1977;47: 157–166.

17. Dupont WD, Page DL: Risk factors for breast cancer in women with proliferative breast disease. *N Engl J Med* 1985;312:146–151.

* 18. Dupont WD, Page DL, Rogers LW, et al: Influence of exogenous estrogens, proliferative breast disease, and other variables on breast cancer risk. *Cancer* 1989;63:948–957.

19. Dupont WD, Page DL: Relative risk of breast cancer varies with time since diagnosis of atypical hyperplasia. *Hum Pathol* 1989;20:723–725.

20. Fox MS: The diagnosis and treatment of breast cancer. *JAMA* 1979;241:489–494.

21. Funderburk WW, Rosero E, Leffal LD: Breast lesions in blacks. *Surg Gynecol Obstet* 1972;135:58–60.

22. Grundy GW, Uzman BG: Breast cancer associated with repeated fluoroscopy. *J Natl Cancer Inst* 1973;51:1339–1340.

23. Harris JR, Hellman S, Kinne DW: Limited surgery and radiotherapy for early breast cancer. *J Clin Oncol* 1985;313: 1365–1368.

24. Harris RE, Lynch HT, Giurgis HA: Familial breast cancer: risk to the contralateral breast. *J Natl Cancer Inst* 1978;60: 955–960.

25. Hiatt RA, Friedman GD, Bawol RD, et al: Breast cancer and serum cholesterol. *J Natl Cancer Inst* 1982;68:885–889.

* 26. Hildreth NC, Shore RE, Dvoretsky PM: The risk of breast cancer after irradiation of the thymus in infancy. *N Engl J Med* 1989;321:1281–1284.

* 27. Jensen RA, Page DL, Dupont WD, et al: Invasive breast cancer (IBC) risk in women with sclerosing adenosis (SA). *Cancer* 1989;64:1977–1983.

28. Kovi J, Mohla S, Norris HJ, et al: Breast lesions in black women. *Pathol Annu* 1989;24 (pt 1):199–218.

* 29. La Vecchia C, Decarli A, Parazzini F, et al: Noncontraceptive oestrogens and the risk of breast cancer in women. *Int J Cancer* 1986;38:853–858.

* 30. Li FP, Fraumeni JF Jr, Mulvihill JJ, et al: A cancer family syndrome in twenty-four kindred. *Cancer Res* 1988;48: 5358–5362.

31. Lippmann ME: Epidemiology of breast cancer, in Danforth D, Lichter AS, Lippmann ME (eds): *Diagnosis and Management of Breast Cancer*. Philadelphia, WB Saunders, 1988, pp 1–9.

32. MacKenzie I: Breast cancer following multiple fluoroscopies. *Br J Cancer*. 1965;19:1–8.

33. MacMahon B, Cole P, Lin TM, et al: Age at first birth and cancer of the breast. A summary of an international study. *Bull WHO* 1970;43:209–217.

34. Malkin D, Li FP, Strong LC, et al: Germ line p53 mutations in a familial syndrome of breast cancer, sarcomas, and other neoplasms. *Science* 1990;250:1233–1238.

35. McDivitt RW, Stevens JA, Lee NC, et al: Benign breast disease histology and the risk for breast cancer. *Cancer* 1992;69:1408–1414.

36. McGregor H, Land CE, Choi K, et al: Breast cancer incidence among atomic bomb survivors, Hiroshima and Nagasaki, 1950–69. *J Natl Cancer Inst* 1977;59:799–811.

37. McPherson K, Neil A, Vessey MP, et al: Oral contraceptives and breast cancer. *Lancet* 1983;17:1414–1415.

38. Mettler FA Jr, Hemplemann LH, Dutton M, et al: Breast neoplasms in women treated with X-rays for acute postpartum mastitis. A pilot study. *J Natl Cancer Inst* 1969;43: 803–811.

39. Miller AB, How GR, Sherman GJ, et al: Mortality from breast cancer after irradiation during fluoroscopic examinations in patients being treated for tuberculosis. *N Engl J Med* 1989;321:1285–1289.

* 40. Moolgavkar SH, Knudson AG Jr: Mutation and cancer: a model for human carcinogenesis. *J Natl Cancer Inst* 1981;66: 1037–1052.

* 41. Myrden JA, Hiltz JE: Breast cancer following multiple fluoroscopies during artificial pneumothorax treatment of pulmonary tuberculosis. *Can Med Assoc J* 1969;100:1032–1034.

* 42. Myrden JA, Quinlan JJ: Breast carcinoma following multiple fluoroscopies with pneumothorax treatment of pulmonary tuberculosis. *Ann R Coll Physicians Surg Can* 1974; 7:45–48.

* 43. Natarajan N, Nemoto T, Metllin C, et al: Race-related differences in breast cancer patients. Results of the 1982 national survey of breast cancer by the American College of Surgeons. *Cancer* 1985;56:1704–1709.

44. Ory H, Cole P, MacMahon B, et al: Oral contraceptives and reduced risk of benign breast diseases. *N Engl J Med* 1976;294:419–422.

* 45. Page DL: Cancer risk assessment in benign breast biopsies. *Human Pathol* 1986;17:871–873.

* 46. Page DL, Dupont WD: Anatomic markers of human premalignancy and risk of breast cancer. *Cancer* 1990;66:1326–1335.

47. Page DL, Dupont WD: Histopathologic risk factors for breast cancer in women with benign breast disease. *Sem Surg Pathol* 1988;4:213–217.

* 48. Page DL, Dupont WD, Rogers LW, et al: Atypical hyperplastic lesions of the female breast. *Cancer* 1985;55:2698–2708.

49. Parl FF, Dupont WD: A retrospective cohort of histologic risk factors in breast cancer patients. *Cancer* 1982;50:2410–2416.

* 50. Pike MC, Henderson BE, Casagrande JT, et al: Oral contraceptive use and early abortion risk as factors for breast cancer in young women. *Br J Cancer* 1981;43:72–76.

51. Polednak AP: Breast cancer in black and white women in New York state. Case distribution and incidence rates by clinical stage at diagnosis. *Cancer* 1986;57:807–815.

* 52. Schatzkin A, Jones Y, Hoover R, et al: Alcohol consumption and breast cancer in the epidemiologic followup study of the First National Health and Nutrition Examination Survey. *N Engl J Med* 1987;316:1169–1173.

* 53. Seidman H: *Cancer of the Breast*. Statistical and epidemiological data. New York, American Cancer Society, 1972.

* 54. Seidman H, Stellman SD, Mushinski MH: A different perspective on breast cancer risk factors. Some implications of the nonattributable risk. *CA* 1982;32:301–313.

* 55. Shore RE, Hempelmann LH, Kowaluk E, et al: Breast neoplasms in women treated with Xrays for acute postpartum mastitis. *J Natl Cancer Inst* 1977;59:813–822.

56. Shore RE, Woodard ED, Hemplemann LH, et al: Synergism between radiation and other risk factors for breast cancer. *Prev Med* 1980;9:815–822.

* 57. Spratt JS, Donegan WL, Greenberg RA: Epidemiology and Etiology, in Donegan WL & Spratt JS (eds): *Cancer of the Breast*. Philadelphia, WB Saunders, 1988, pp 46–73.

58. Symmers WS: Carcinoma of the breast in transsexual individuals after surgical and hormonal interference with the primary and secondary sex characteristics. *Br Med J* 1968;2:82.

* 59. Tavassoli FA, Casey HW, Norris HJ: The morphologic effects of synthetic reproductive steroids on the mammary gland of rhesus monkeys. Mestranol, ethynerone, mestranol-ethynerone, chlorethynyl Norgestrel-mestranol, and anagestone acetate-mestranol combinations. *Am J Pathol* 1988;131:213–234.

* 60. Thomas DB: Do hormones cause breast cancer? *Cancer* 1984;53:595–604.

61. Thomas DB: Factors that promote the development of human breast cancer. *Environ Health Perspect* 1983;50:209–218.

* 62. Tokunaga M, Land CE, Yamamoto T, et al: Breast cancer among atomic bomb survivors, in Boice JDjr, Fraumeni JFjr (eds): *Radiation Carcinogenesis Epidemiology and Biologic Significance*. New York, Raven Press, 1984, pp 45–46.

* 63. Tokunaga M, Land CE, Yamamoto T, et al: Incidence of female breast cancer among atomic bomb survivors, Hiroshima and Nagasaki. *Radiat Res* 1987;112:243–272.

64. Tokunaga M, Norman JE Jr, Asano M, et al: Malignant breast tumors among atomic bomb survivors, Hiroshima and Nagasaki. *J Natl Cancer Inst* 1979;62:1347–1359.

* 65. Vernon SW, Tilley BC, Neale V, et al: Ethnicity, survival,

and delay in seeking treatment for symptoms of breast cancer. *Cancer* 1985;55:1563–1571.

66. Vessey MP, Doll R, Peto R, et al: A long-term follow-up study of women using different methods of contraception. An interim report. *J Biosoc Sci* 1976;8:373–427.

67. Young JL Jr, Percy CL, Asire AJ (eds): *Surveillance, Epidemiology, and End Results: Incidence and Mortality Data, 1973–1977*. NCI monograph 57. Bethesda, US Department of Health and Human Services, 1981.

### Diet

* 68. Buell P: Changing incidence of breast cancer in Japanese-American women. *J Natl Cancer Inst* 1973;51:1479–1483.

69. Byers T: Diet and cancer: any progress in the "interim?" *Cancer* 1988;62:1713–1724.

70. Committee on Diet, Nutrition and Cancer, Assembly of Life Sciences, National Research Council: *Diet, Nutrition and Cancer*. Washington DC, National Academy Press, 1982, pp 1–16.

* 71. Dunn JE: Breast cancer among American Japanese in the San Francisco Bay area. *Natl Cancer Inst Monogr* 1977;47: 157–160.

72. Enig MG, Munn RJ, Keeney M: Dietary fats and cancer trends—a critique. *Fed Proc* 1978;37:2215–2220.

73. Graham S, Marshall J, Mettlin C, et al: Diet in the epidemiology of breast cancer. *Am J Epidemiol* 1982;116:68–75.

* 74. Hirohata T, Nomura AMY, Hankin JH, et al: An epidemiologic study on the association between diet and breast cancer. *J Natl Cancer Inst* 1987;78:595–600.

75. Hirohata T, Shigematsu T, Nomura AMY, et al: The occurrence of breast cancer in relation to diet and reproductive history: A case-control study in Fukuoka, Japan. *NCI Monog* 1985;69:187–190.

* 76. Katsouyanni K, Boyle P, Trichopoulou A, et al: Diet and breast cancer: A case-control study in Greece. *Int J Cancer* 1986;38:815–820.

77. Kelsey JL: A review of the epidemiology of human breast cancer. *Epidemiol Rev* 1979;1:74–109.

78. La Vecchia C, Decarli A, Franceschi S, et al: Dietary factors and the risk of breast cancer. *Nutri Cancer* 1987;10:205–214.

* 79. La Vecchia C, Decarli A, Negri E, et al: Epidemiological aspects of diet and cancer: A summary review of case-control studies from northern Italy. *Oncology* 1988;45:364–370.

80. Lubin F, Ruder AM, Wax Y, et al: Overweight and changes in weight throughout adult life in breast cancer etiology. *Am J Epidemiol* 1985;122:579–588.

* 81. Lubin F, Wax Y, Modan B: Role of fat, animal protein, and dietary fiber in breast cancer etiology: A case-control study. *J Natl Cancer Inst* 1986;77:605–612.

* 82. Miller AB, Bulbrock RD: Special report: The epidemiology and etiology of breast cancer. *N Engl J Med* 1980;303:1246–1248.

83. Phillips RL, Snowdon DA: Association of meat and coffee use with cancers of the large bowel, breast, and prostate among Seventh Day Adventists. Preliminary results. *Cancer Res* 1983;43(Suppl):2403–2408.

84. Talamini R, LaVecchia C, Becarli A, et al: Social factors, diet and breast cancer in a northern Italian population. *Br J Cancer* 1984;49:723–729.

* 85. Willet WC, McMahon B: Diet and cancer—an overview. (second of two parts). *N Engl J Med* 1984;310:697–703.

### Staging and Prognostic Factors

86. Alpers CE, Wellings SR: The prevalence of carcinoma in situ in normal and cancer-associated breasts. *Hum Pathol* 1985;16:796–807.

87. Apostolikas N, Petraki C, Agnantis NJ: The reliability of histologically negative axillary lymph nodes in breast cancer. *Path Res Pract* 1989;184:35–38.

88. Attiyeh FF, Jensen M, Huvos AG, et al: Axillary micrometastases and macrometastases in carcinoma of the breast. *Surg Gynecol Obstet* 1977;144:839–842.

* 89. Beahrs OH, Henson DE, Hutter RVP, Myers MH (eds): *Manual for Staging of Cancer: American Joint Committee on Cancer*, ed 3. Philadelphia, J. B. Lippincott, 1988, pp 145–148.

90. Berndt H, Titze U: TNM clinical stage classification of breast cancer. *Int J Cancer* 1969;4:837–844.

91. Bettelheim R, Penman HG, Thorton-Jones H, et al: Prognostic significance of peritumoral vascular invasion in breast cancer. *Br J Cancer* 1984;50:771–777.

* 92. Bettelheim R, Price KN, Gelber RD, et al: International (Ludwig) Breast Cancer Study Group. Prognostic importance of occult axillary lymph node micrometastases from breast cancers. *Lancet* 1990;335:1565–1568.

* 93. Bonadonna G: Conceptual and practical advances in the management of breast cancer. *J Clin Oncol* 1989;7:1380–1397.

94. Bondeson L, Linell F, Ringberg A: Breast reductions: what to do with all the tissue specimens. *Histopathology* 1985;9: 281–285.

95. Bussolati G, Gugliotta P, Morra I, et al: The immunohistochemical detection of lymph node metastases in breast cancer. *Br J Cancer* 1986;54:631–636.

96. Caceras E. An evaluation of radical mastectomy and extended radical mastectomy for cancer of the breast. *Surg Gynecol Obstet* 1967;125:337–341.

* 97. Carter CL, Allen C, Henson DE: Relation of tumor size, lymph node status, and survival in 24,740 breast cancer cases. *Cancer* 1989;63:181–187.

98. Clark GM, McGuire WL: New biologic prognostic factors in breast cancer. *Oncology* 1989;3:49–54.

99. Clayton F: Pathologic correlates of survival in 378 lymph node-negative infiltrating ductal breast carcinomas. Mitotic count is single predictor. *Cancer* 1991;68:1309–1317.

* 100. Cody HS III, Egeli RA, Urban JA: Rotter's node metastases. Therapeutic and prognostic considerations in early breast carcinoma. *Ann Surg* 1984;199:266–270.

101. Cote RJ, Rosen PP, Hakes TB, et al: Monoclonal antibodies detect occult breast carcinoma metastases in the bone marrow of patients with early stage disease. *Am J Surg Pathol* 1988;12:333–340.

* 102. Contesso G, Mouriesse H: Facteurs anatomo-patho-

logiques du prognostic des cancers du sein. *Path Biol* 1990;38:834–835.

103. Cutler SJ, Black MM, Mork T, et al: Further observations on prognostic factors in cancer of the female breast. *Cancer* 1969;24:653–667.
104. Cutler SJ, Zipin C, Asire AJ: The prognostic significance of palpable lymph nodes in cancer of the breast. *Cancer* 1969;23:243–250.
105. Danforth D, Lichter AS, Lippmann ME: The diagnosis of breast cancer, in Lippmann ME, Lichter AS, Danforth D (eds): *Diagnosis and Management of Breast Cancer*. Philadelphia, WB Saunders, 1988, pp 50–94.
106. Davis BW, Gelber R, Goldhirsh A, et al: Prognostic significance of peritumoral vessel invasion in clinical trials of adjuvant therapy for breast cancer with axillary lymph node metastasis. *Hum Pathol* 1985;16:1212–1218.
107. Donegan WL: Staging and primary treatment, in Donegan WL, Spratt JS (eds): *Cancer of the Breast*. Philadelphia, WB Saunders, 1988, chap 12, pp 336–402.
108. Donegan WL: The influence of untreated internal mammary metastases upon the course of mammary cancer. *Cancer* 1977;39:533–538.
*109. Fentiman IS, Lavelle MA, Caplan D, et al: The significance of supraclavicular fossa node recurrence after radical mastectomy. *Cancer* 1986;57:908–910.
110. Ferguson DJ, Meier P, Karrison T, et al: Staging of breast cancer and survival rates. Node assessment based on 50 years of experience with radical mastectomy. *JAMA* 1982; 248:1337–1341.
*111. Fisher ER, Palekar A, Rockette H, et al. Pathologic findings from the National Surgical Adjuvant Breast Project (Protocol No. 4). V. Significance of axillary nodal micro- and macrometastases. *Cancer* 1978;42:2032–2038.
112. Fisher B, Slack NH: Number of lymph nodes examined and the prognosis of breast carcinoma. *Surg Gynecol Obstet* 1970;131:79–88.
113. Fisher B, Slack N, Katrych D, et al: Ten year follow-up results of patients with carcinoma of the breast in a cooperative clinical trial evaluating surgical adjuvant chemotherapy. *Surg Gynecol Obstet* 1975;140:528–534.
114. Fisher ER, Swamidoss S, Lee CH, et al: Detection and significance of occult axillary node metastases in patients with invasive breast cancer. *Cancer* 1978;42:2025–2031.
*115. Fisher B, Wolmark N, Bauer M, et al: The accuracy of clinical nodal staging and of limited axillary dissection as a determinant of histologic nodal status in carcinoma of the breast. *Surg Gynecol Obstet* 1981;152:765–772.
*116. Fisher ER, Redmond C, Fisher B, et al: Pathologic findings from the National Surgical Adjuvant Breast and Bowel Projects. Prognostic discriminants for 8-year survival for node-negative invasive breast cancer patients. *Cancer* 1990; 65:2121–2128.
*117. Friedman S, Bertin F, Mouriesse H, et al: Importance of tumor cells in axillary node sinus margins (clandestine metastases) discovered by serial sectioning in operable breast carcinoma. *Acta Oncologica* 1988;27:483–487.
*118. Fuster E, Garcia-Vilanova A, Narbona B, et al: A statistical approach to an individualized index (IPI) for breast cancer survivability. *Cancer* 1983;52:728–736.
*119. Gallager HS: Pathologic types of breast cancer: Their prognoses. *Cancer* 1984;53:623–629.
120. Gilchrist KW, Gould VE, Hirschl S, et al: Interobserver variation in the identification of breast carcinoma in intramammary lymphatics. *Hum Pathol* 1982;13:170–172.
121. Haagensen CD: *Diseases of the Breast*, ed 3, Philadelphia, WB Saunders, 1986, p 656.
*122. Hermanek P, LH Sobin (eds): *TNM Classification of Malignant Tumours. UICC International Union Against Cancer*. New York, Springer-Verlag, 1987, pp 93–99.
*123. Haybittle JL, Blamey RW, Elston CW, et al: A prognostic index in primary breast cancer. *Br J Cancer* 1982;45:361–366.
*124. Huvos AG, Hutter RV, Berg JW: Significance of axillary macrometastases and micrometastases in mammary cancer. *Ann Surg* 1971;173:44–46.
125. Ingle JN: Assessing the risk of recurrence in breast cancer. *N Engl J Med* 1990;322:329–331.
126. Jotti GS: New prognostic indicators in resectable breast cancer. *Anticancer Res* 1989;9:1227–1232.
*127. Kay S: Evaluation of Rotter's lymph nodes in radical mastectomy specimens as a guide to prognosis. *Cancer* 1965;18:1441–1444.
128. Lee AKC, DeLellis RA, Silverman ML, et al: Lymphatic and blood vessel invasion in breast carcinoma: A useful prognostic indicator? *Hum Pathol* 1986;17:984–987.
129. Love SM, Gelman RS, Silen W: Fibrocystic "disease" of the breast—a nondisease. *N Engl J Med* 1982;307:1010–1014.
*130. Mambo NC, Gallager HS: Carcinoma of the breast. The prognostic significance of axillary disease. *Cancer* 1977;39: 2280–2285.
131. McGuire WL: Prognostic factors in primary breast cancer. *Cancer Surv* 1986;5:527–536.
*132. Martin SA, Perez-Reyes M, Mendelsohn G: Angioinvasion in breast carcinoma. An immunohistochemical study of Factor VIII-related antigen. *Cancer* 1987;59:1918–1922.
133. Mathiew M-C, Friedman S, Bosq J, et al: Immunohistochemical staining of bone marrow biopsies for detection of occult metastasis in breast cancer. *Br Ca Res Treat* 1990;15: 21–26.
134. McDivitt RW, Stone KR, Craig RB, et al: A proposed classification of breast based on kinetic information: derived from a comparison of risk factors in 168 primary operable breast cancers. *Cancer* 1986;57:269–276.
135. Merkel DE, Osborne CK: Prognostic factors in breast cancer. *Hematol Oncol Clin North Am* 1989;3:641–652.
136. Neville AM, Price KN, Gleber RD, et al: Axillary node micrometastases and breast cancer. *Lancet* 1991;337:1110.
137. Nielsen M, Jensen J, Andersen J: Precancerous and cancerous breast lesions during lifetime and at autopsy. A study of 83 women. *Cancer* 1984;54:612–615.

138. Nielsen M, Thomsen JL, Primdahl S, et al: Breast cancer and atypia among young women and middle-aged women: A study of 110 medicolegal autopsies. *Br J Cancer* 1987;56:814–819.

* 139. Nime F, Rosen PP, Thaler H, et al: Prognostic significance of tumor emboli in intramammary lymphatics in patients with mammary carcinoma. *Am J Surg Pathol* 1977;1:25–30.

* 140. Orbo A, Stalsberg H, Kunde D: Topographic criteria in the diagnosis of tumor emboli in intramammary lymphatics. *Cancer* 1990;66:972–977.

* 141. Page DL: Prognosis and breast cancer. Recognition of lethal and favorable prognostic types. *Am J Surg Pathol* 1991;15:334–349.

142. Page DL, Kidd TE, Dupont WD, et al: Lobular neoplasia of the breast: Higher risk for subsequent invasive cancer predicted by more extensive disease. *Hum Pathol* 1991;22: 1232–1239.

143. Palmer MK, Lythgoe JP, Smith A: Prognostic factors in breast cancer. *Br J Surg* 1982;69:697–698.

144. Papaioannou A, Urban JA: Scalene node biopsy in locally advanced primary breast cancer of questionable operability. *Cancer* 1964;17:1006–1011.

145. Pickren JW: Significance of occult metastases. A study of breast cancer. *Cancer* 1961;14:1266–1271.

* 146. Rosen PP: Tumor emboli in intramammary lymphatics in breast carcinoma: pathologic criteria for diagnosis and clinical significance, in Sommers S, Rosen PP (eds): *Pathology Annual*. Norwalk, Connecticut, Appleton-Century-Crofts, 1983, pt 2, pp 215–232.

147. Rosen PP, Goshen S, Saigo PE, et al: A long-term follow-up of survival in Stage I (T1N0M0) and Stage II (T1N1M0) breast carcinoma. *J Clin Oncol* 1989;7:355–366.

* 148. Rosen PP, Goshen S, Saigo PE, et al: Pathologic prognostic factors in stage I (T1N0M0) and stage II (T1N1M0) breast carcinoma: a study of 655 patients with median follow-up of 18 years. *J Clin Oncol* 1989;7:1239–1251.

* 149. Rosen PP, Saigo PE, Braun DW Jr, et al: Occult axillary lymph node metastases from breast cancers with intramammary lymphatic tumor emboli. *Am J Surg Pathol* 1982; 6:639–641.

150. Rosen PP, Saigo PE, Braun DW, et al: Predictors of recurrence in stage I (T1N0M0) breast carcinoma. *Ann Surg* 1981;193:15–25.

151. Roses DF, Bell DA, Flotte TJ, et al: Pathologic predictors of recurrence in stage I (T1N0M0) breast cancer. *Am J Clin Pathol* 1982;78:817–820.

152. Saccanijotti G, Bonadonna G: The pathologist and the clinical oncologist: a new effective partnership in assessing tumor prognosis. *Eur J Cancer Clin Oncol* 1989;25:585–598.

153. Saphir O, Amromin GD: Obscure axillary lymph-node metastasis in carcinoma of the breast. *Cancer* 1948;1:238–241.

* 154. Schnitt SJ, Connoly JL, Harris JR, et al: Pathologic predictors of early local recurrence in stage I and II breast cancer treated by primary radiation therapy. *Cancer* 1984;53:1049–1057.

* 155. Schnitt SJ, Connolly JL, Khettry U: Pathologic findings on re-excision of the primary site in breast cancer patients considered for treatment by primary radiation therapy. *Cancer* 1987;59:675–681.

156. Sigurdsson H, Baldetorp B, Borg A, et al: Indicators of prognosis in node-negative breast cancer. *N Engl J Med* 1990;322:1045–1053.

* 157. Spiessl B, Beahrs OH, Hermanek P, et al: *TNM Atlas. Illustrated Guide to the TNP/pTNM-Classification of Malignant Tumours. UICC International Union Against Cancer*, 3 ed., New York, Springer-Verlag, 1989, pp 173–183.

158. Trojani M, de Mascarel I, Bonichon F, et al: Micrometastases to axillary lymph nodes from carcinoma of breast. Detection by immunohistochemistry and prognostic significance. *Br J Cancer* 1987;55:303–306.

159. Trojani M, de Mascarel I, Coindre JM, et al: Micrometastases to axillary lymph nodes from invasive lobular carcinoma of breast: Detection by immunohistochemistry and prognostic significance. *Cancer* 1987;56:838–839.

* 160. Urban JA, Marjani MA: Significance of internal mammary lymph node metastases in breast cancer. *AJR* 1971;111:130–136.

* 161. Veronesi U, Cascinelli N, Bufalino R, et al: Risk of internal mammary lymph node metastases and its relevance on prognosis of breast cancer patients. *Ann Surg* 1983;198:681–684.

162. Wells CA, Heryet A, Brochier J, et al: The immunocytochemical detection of axillary micrometastases in breast cancer. *Br J Cancer* 1984;50:193–197.

* 163. Wilkinson EJ, Hause LL, Hoffman RG, et al: Occult axillary lymph node metastases in invasive breast carcinoma: characteristics of the primary tumor and significance of the metastases. *Pathol Annu* 1982;17:670–691.

164. Wilson RE, Donegan WL, Mettlin C, et al: The 1982 national survey of carcinoma of the breast in the United States by the American College of Surgeons. *Surg Gynecol Obstet* 1984;159:309–318.

165. Windeyer BW: Cancer of the breast. *Am J Roentgenol Radium Ther Nucl Med* 1949;62:345–354.

166. Yorkshire Breast Cancer Group: Critical assessment of the clinical TNM system in breast cancer. *Br Med J* 1980;281: 134–136.


## Grading


* 167. Black MM, Barclay THC, Hankey BF: Prognosis in breast cancer utilizing histologic characteristics of the primary tumor. *Cancer* 1975;36:2048–2055.

* 168. Black MM, Opler SR, Speer FD: Survival in breast cancer cases in relation to structure of the primary tumor and regional lymph nodes. *Surg Gynecol Obstet* 1955;100:543–551.

* 169. Black MM, Speer FD: Nuclear structure in cancer tissues. *Surg Gynecol Obstet* 1957;105:97–102.

* 170. Bloom HJG: Prognosis in carcinoma of the breast. *Br J Cancer* 1950;4:259–288.

* 171. Bloom HJG: Further studies on prognosis of breast carcinoma. *Br J Cancer* 1950;4:347–367.

* 172. Bloom HJG, Richardson WW: Histologic grading and prognosis in breast cancer: A study of 1,709 cases of which 359 have been followed for 15 years. *Br J Cancer* 1957;2:353–377.

* 173. Contesso G, Mouriesse H, Friedman S, et al: The importance of histologic grade in long-term prognosis of breast cancer. A study of 1,010 patients, uniformly treated at the Institut Gustave-Roussy. *J Clin Oncol* 1987;5:1378–1386.

174. Cutler SJ, Black MM, Friedell GH, et al: Prognostic factors in cancer of the female breast. II. Reproducibility of histopathologic classification. *Cancer* 1966;19:75–82.

175. Delides GS, Garas G, Georgouli G, et al: Intralaboratory variations in the grading of breast carcinoma. *Arch Pathol Lab Med* 1982;106:126–128.

176. Eichner WJ, Lemon HM, Friedell GH: Tumor grade in the prognosis of breast cancer. *Nebr Med J* 1970;55:405–409.

* 177. Ellis IO, Elston CW, Blamey RW: The Nottingham prognostic index (NPI) a combination of multiple prognostic factors derived from the Nottingham Tenovus primary cancer study. *Mod Pathol* 1991;4:11A.

* 178. Elston CW. Grading of invasive carcinoma of the breast, in Page DL, Anderson TJ (eds): *Diagnostic Histopathology of the Breast*. New York, Churchill Livingstone, 1987. pp 300–311.

* 179. Elston CW. The assessment of histological grade in breast cancer. *Aust N Z J Surg* 1984;54:11–15.

* 180. Elston CW, Ellis IO: Pathological prognostic factors in breast cancer. I. The value of histological grade in breast cancer: experience from a large study with long-term follow-up. *Histopathology* 1991;19:403–410.

181. Elston CW, Gresham GA, Rao GS, et al: The cancer research campaign (Kings/Cambridge) trial for early breast cancer—pathological aspects. *Br J Cancer* 1982;45:655–669.

* 182. Fisher ER, Redmond C, Fisher B: Histologic grading of breast cancer. *Pathol Annu* 1980;15:239–251.

* 183. Greenhough RB: Varying degrees of malignancy in cancer of the breast. *Cancer Res* 1925;9:452–463.

* 184. Haagensen CD: The basis for histologic grading of carcinoma of the breast. *Am J Cancer* 1933;1:285–327.

185. Hartveit F: Prognostic typing in breast cancer. *Br Med J* 1971;4:253–257.

186. Helpap B: Nucleolar grading of breast cancer. *Virchows Archiv A Pathol Anat* 1989;415:501–508.

187. Henson DE: The histological grading of neoplasms. *Archiv Pathol Lab Med* 1988;112:1091–1096.

188. Henson DE: Endpoints and significance of reproducibility in pathology. *Arch Pathol Lab Med* 1989;113:830–831.

189. Le Doussal V, Tubiana-Hulin M, Friedman S, et al: Prognostic value of histologic grade nuclear components of Scarff-Bloom-Richardson (SBR): An improved score modification based on a multivariate analysis of 1262 invasive ductal breast carcinomas. *Cancer* 1989;64:1914–1921.

190. Patey DH, Scarff RW: The position of histology in the prognosis of carcinoma of the breast. *Lancet* 1928;1:801–804.

191. Rosen PP: The pathological classification of human mammary carcinoma: Past, present and future. *Ann Clin Lab Sci* 1979;9:144–156.

192. Stenkvist B, Westman-Naeser S, Vegelius J, et al: Analysis of reproducibility of subjective grading systems for breast carcinoma. *J Clin Pathol* 1979;32:979–985.

193. Theissig F, Kunze KD, Haroske G, et al: Histological grading of breast cancer. Interobserver, reproducibility and prognostic significance. *Path Res Pract* 1990;186:732–736.


## Tumor Cell Kinetics


194. Braylan RC: Flow cytometry. *Arch Pathol Lab Med* 1983;107:1–6.

195. Clark GM, Dressler LG, Owens MA, et al: Prediction of relapse or survival in patients with node-negative breast cancer by flow cytometry. *N Engl J Med* 1989;320:627–633.

196. Fisher B, Gunduz N, Costantino J, et al: DNA flow cytometric analysis of primary operable breast cancer. *Cancer* 1991;68:1465–1475.

* 197. Gentili C, Sanfilippo O, Silvestrini R: Cell proliferation and its relationship to clinical features and relapse in breast cancers. *Cancer* 1981;48:974–979.

198. Kute TE, Muss HB, Anderson D, et al: Relationship of steroid receptor, cell kinetics and clinical status in patients with breast cancer. *Cancer Res* 1981;41:3524–3529.

* 199. Merkel E, McGuire WL: Ploidy, proliferative activity and prognosis. DNA flow cytometry of solid tumors. *Cancer* 1990;65:1194–1205.

* 200. Meyer JS: Cell kinetics analysis of human breast carcinomas, Chapter 3. in McDivitt RW, Oberman HA, Ozzello L, et al (eds): *The Breast*. Baltimore, Williams & Wilkins, 1984.

201. Meyer JS: Cytokinetic analysis of breast carcinoma. Implications for adjuvant cytotoxic therapy of node-negative patients, in Blumenschein, GR (ed): *Current Controversies in Breast Cancer*. 26th Annual Clinical Conference, the University of Texas, MD Anderson Hospital and Tumor Institute, 1983.

* 202. Meyer JS, Bauer WC, Rao BR: Subpopulations of breast carcinoma defined by S-phase fraction, morphology, and estrogen receptor content. *Lab Invest* 1978;39:225–235.

203. Silvestrini R, Sanfilippor O, Tedesco G: Kinetics of human mammary carcinomas and their correlation with the cancer and the host characteristics. *Cancer* 1974;34:1252–1258.

204. Tubiana M, Pejovic MH, Renaud A, et al: Kinetic parameters and the course of the disease in breast cancer. *Cancer* 1981;47:937–943.

205. Witzig TE, Gonchoroff NJ, Therneau T, et al: DNA content flow cytometry as a prognostic factor for node-positive breast cancer. *Cancer* 1991;68:1781–1788.


## Estrogen and Progesterone Receptors and Other Markers


206. Allegra JC, Lippman ME, Simon R, et al: Association between steroid hormone receptor status and disease-free interval in breast cancer. *Cancer Treat Rep* 1979;63:1271–1277.

207. Andersen J, Thorpe SM, King WJ, et al: The prognostic value of immunohistochemical estrogen receptor analysis in paraffin-embedded and frozen sections versus that of steroid-binding assays. *Eur J Cancer* 1990;26:442–449.

208. Berger MS, Locher GW, Saurer S, et al: Correlation of c-erb-B-2 gene amplification and protein expression in human breast carcinoma with nodal status and nuclear grading. *Cancer Res* 1988;48:1238–1243.

* 209. Brouillet J-P, Theillet C, Maudelonde T, et al: Cathepsin D assay in primary breast cancer and lymph nodes: Relationship with c-myc, c-erb-B-2 and int-2 oncogene amplification and node invasiveness. *Eur J Cancer* 1990;26:437–441.

* 210. Chevallier B, Heintzmann F, Mosseri V, et al: Prognostic value of estrogen and progesterone receptors in operable breast cancer: Results of a univariate and multivariate analysis. *Cancer* 1988;62:2517–2524.

* 211. Contesso G, Delarue JC, Mouriesse H, et al: Anatomopathologie du cancer du sein et recepteurs hormonaux. *Pathol Biol* 1983;31:747–754.

212. Ellis GK, Gown AM: New applications of monoclonal antibodies to the diagnosis and prognosis of breast cancer, in Rosen PP, Fechner, RE (eds): *Pathology Annual*. Norwalk, Connecticut, Appleton & Lange, vol 25, pt 2, pp 193–235.

213. Elton CW, Blamey RW, Johnson J, et al: The relationship of oestradiol receptors (ER) and histological tumor differentiation with prognosis in human primary breast carcinoma, in Mouridsen, Palshof, (eds): *Breast Cancer: Experimental and Clinical Aspects*. Oxford, Pergamon, 1980, pp 59–62.

* 214. Everson RB, Lippmann ME, Thompson EB, et al: The relationship between estrogen receptors and response to cytotoxic chemotherapy in metastatic breast cancer. *N Engl J Med* 1978;298:1223–1228.

* 215. Friend SH, Dryja TP, Weinberg RA: Oncogenes and tumor suppressing genes. *N Engl J Med* 1988;308:618–622.

216. Furmanski P, Saunder E, Brooks SR, et al: The prognostic value of estrogen receptor determinations in patients with primary breast cancer. *Cancer* 1980;46:2794–2796.

* 217. Gerdes J, Lemke H, Baisch H, et al: Cell cycle analysis of a cell proliferation-associated human nuclear antigen defined by the monoclonal antibody Ki67. *Immunol* 1984;133: 1710–1715.

* 218. Gerdes J, Schwab U, Lemke H, et al: Production of a mouse monoclonal antibody reactive with a human nuclear antigen associated with cell proliferation. *Int J Cancer* 1983;31: 13–20.

219. Guerin M, Barrois M, Terrier MJ, et al: Overexpression of either c-myc or c-erb-B-2/neu protooncogenes in human breast carcinomas: correlation with poor prognosis. *Oncogene Res* 1988;3:21–31.

* 220. Gullick WJ, Love SB, Wright C, et al: C-erb-B-2 protein overexpression in breast cancer is a risk factor in patients with involved and uninvolved lymph nodes. *Br J Cancer* 1991;63:434–438.

221. Hilf R, Feldstein ML, Savlov ED, et al: The lack of relationship between estrogen receptor status and response to chemotherapy. *Cancer* 1980;46:2797–2800.

222. Jensen EV, Block GE, Smith S, et al: Estrogen receptors and breast cancer response to adrenalectomy. *Natl Cancer Inst Monogr* 1971;34:55–79.

223. Kinne DW, Ashikari R, Butler A, et al: Estrogen receptor protein in breast cancer as a predictor of recurrence. *Cancer* 1981;47:2364–2367.

* 224. Kinne DW, Butler JA, Kimmel M, et al: Estrogen receptor protein of breast cancer in patients with positive nodes: High recurrence rates in the postmenopausal estrogen receptor-negative group. *Arch Surg* 1987;122:1303–1306.

* 225. Knight WA, Livingston RB, Gregory BH, et al: Estrogen receptor as an independent prognostic factor for early recurrence in breast cancer. *Cancer Res* 1977;37:4669–4771.

226. Lee KC, DeVita V: The "clinical alert" from the National Cancer Institute. *N Engl J Med* 1988;319:948–949.

* 227. Lelle RJ, Heidenreich W, Stauch G, et al: Determination of growth fraction in benign breast diseases (BBD) with monoclonal antibody Ki67. *J Cancer Res Clin Oncol* 1987;113: 73–77.

* 228. Lovekin C, Ellis IO, Locker A, et al: C-erbB-2 oncoprotein expression in primary and advanced breast cancer. *Br J Cancer* 1991;63:439–443.

229. Maas H, Engle B, Trams G: Steroid hormone receptors in human breast cancer and the clinical significance. *J Steroid Biochem* 1975;6:743–749.

230. Maynard PV, Davis CJ, Blamey RW, et al: Relationship between estrogen-receptor content and histological grade in human primary breast tumors. *Br J Cancer* 1978;38:745–748.

231. McCarty KS Jr, McCarty KS Sr: Steroid hormone receptors in the regulation of differentiation. *Am J Pathol* 1977;86:705–744.

232. McGuire WL, Clark GM: The role of progesterone receptors in breast cancer. *Semin Oncol* 1985;12(Suppl):12–16.

233. McGuire WL, Clark GM, Fisher ER, et al: Predicting recurrence and survival in breast cancer: a panel discussion. *Breast Cancer Res Treat* 1987;9:27–38.

234. McGuire WL, Tandon AK, Allred DC, et al: How to use prognostic factors in axillary node-negative breast cancer patients. *J Natl Cancer Inst* 1990;82:1006–1015.

235. Nesland JM, Ottestad L, Borresen A-L, et al: The c-erbB-2 protein in primary and metastatic breast carcinomas. *Ultrastruct Pathol* 1991;15:281–289.

236. O'Keane JC, Okon E, Moroz K, et al: Anti-estradiol immunoperoxidase labeling of nuclei, not cytoplasm in paraffin sections, determines estrogen receptor status of breast cancer. *Am J Surg Pathol* 1990;14:121–127.

* 237. O'Reilly SM, Barnes DM, Camplejohn RS, et al: The relationship between c-erbB-2 expression, S-phase fraction and prognosis in breast cancer. *Br J Cancer* 1991;63:444–446.

* 238. Osborne CK, Yochomowitz MG, Knight WA, et al: The value of estrogen and progesterone receptors in the treatment of breast cancer. *Cancer* 1980;46:2884–2888.

* 239. Paik S, Hagan R, Fisher ER, et al. Pathologic findings of the

National Surgical Adjuvant Breast and Bowel Project: Prognostic significance of erb B-2 protein overexpression in primary breast cancer. *J Clin Oncol* 1990;18:103–112.

*240. Parl FP, Schmidt BP, DuPont WD, et al: Prognostic significance of estrogen receptor status in breast cancer in relation to tumor stage, axillary node metastasis and histopathologic grading. *Cancer* 1984;54:2237–2242.

*241. Perren TJ: C-erbB-2 oncogene as a prognostic marker in breast cancer. *Br J Cancer* 1991;63:328–332.

242. Pertshuck LP, Kim DS, Nayer K, et al: Immunocytochemical estrogen and progestin receptor assays in breast cancer with monoclonal antibodies. *Cancer* 1990;66:1663–1670.

*243. Rochefort H, Capony E, Augereau P, et al: The estrogen-regulated 52-K-cathepsin-D in breast cancer: From biology to clinical application. *Int J Rad Appl Instrum* 1987;14(B):377–384.

244. Sears HF, Janus C, Levy W, et al: Breast cancer without axillary metastases: Are there high risk biologic subpopulations? *Cancer* 1982;1820–1827.

245. Shapiro CM, Schiffeling D, Bitran JD, et al: Prognostic value of the estrogen receptor value in pathologic stage I and II adenocarcinoma of the breast. *J Surg Oncol* 1982;19: 119–121.

*246. Slamon DJ, Clark GM, Wong SG, et al: Human breast cancer—correlation of relapse and survival with amplification of the HER-2/neu oncogene. *Science* 1987;235:177–182.

247. Stanford JL, Szklo M, Brinton LA: Estrogen receptor and breast cancer. *Epidemiol Rev* 1986;8:42–56.

*248. Tandon AK, Clark GM, Chamness GC, et al: HER-2/neu oncogene protein and prognosis in breast cancer. *J Clin Oncol* 1989;7:1120–1128.

*249. Tandon AK, Clark GM, Chamness GC, et al: Cathepsin D and prognosis in breast cancer. *N Engl J Med* 1990;322:297–302.

250. Tavassoli M, Quirke P, Farzaneh F, et al: C-erbB-2/c-erbBA co-amplification indicative of lymph node metastasis, and c-myc amplification of high tumour grade, in human breast carcinoma. *Br J Cancer* 1989;60:505–510.

251. Tsuda H, Hirohashi S, Shimosato Y, et al: Correlation between histologic grade of malignancy and copy number of c-erbB-2 gene in breast carcinoma: A retrospective analysis of 176 cases. *Cancer* 1990;65:1794–1800.

252. Varley JM, Swallow J, Brammer WJ, et al: Alterations to either c-erb B-2 or c-myc protooncogenes in breast carcinomas correlate with poor short term prognosis. *Oncogene* 1987;1:423–440.

253. Wilbur DC, Willis J, Mooney RA, et al: Estrogen and progesterone receptor detection in archival formalin-fixed, paraffin-embedded tissue from breast carcinoma: A comparison of immunohistochemistry with the Dextran-coated charcoal assay. *Mod Pathol* 1992;5:79–84.

*254. Winstanley J, Cooke T, Murray GD, et al: The long-term prognostic significance of c-erbB-2 in primary breast cancer. *Br J Cancer* 1991;63:447–450.

255. Wittliff JL: Specific receptors of the steroid hormones in breast cancer. *Semin Oncol* 1974;1:109–118.

256. Wittliff JL: Steroid hormone receptors in breast cancer. *Cancer* 1984;53:630–643.

*257. Zeillinger R, Kury F, Czerwenska K, et al: HER-2 amplification, steroid receptors and epidermal growth factor receptor in primary breast cancer. *Oncogene* 1989;4:109–114.

### Pregnancy-Associated Breast Cancer

258. Applewhite RR, Smith LR, DiVincenti F: Carcinoma of the breast associated with pregnancy and lactation. *Am Surg* 1973;39:101–104.

259. Bunker ML, Peters MV: Breast cancer associated with pregnancy or lactation. *Am J Obstet Gynecol* 1963;85:312–321.

260. Byrd BE, Bayer DS, Robertson JC, et al: Treatment of breast tumors associated with pregnancy and lactation. *Ann Surg* 1962;155:940–947.

261. Clark RM, Reid J: Carcinoma of the breast in pregnancy and lactation. *Int J Radiat Oncol Biol Phys* 1978;4:693–698.

262. Crosby CH, Barclay THC. Carcinoma of the breast: Surgical management of patients with special conditions. *Cancer* 1971;28:1628–1636.

263. DeVitt JE, Beattie WG, Stoddart TG: Carcinoma of the breast and pregnancy. *Can J Surg* 1964;7:124–128.

264. Fentiman IS: *Detection and Treatment of Early Breast Cancer*. Philadelphia, JB Lippincott, 1990, pp 154–173.

*265. Haagensen CD: The treatment of breast carcinoma occurring during pregnancy or lactation, in Haagensen CD: *Diseases of the Breast*, ed 3. Philadelphia, WB Saunders, 1986, pp 927–928.

*266. Holleb AI, Farrow JH: The relation of carcinoma of the breast and pregnancy in 283 patients. *Surg Gynecol Obstet* 1962;115:65–71.

267. Mickal A, Torres JE, Mule JG: Carcinoma of the breast in pregnancy and lactation. *Am Surg* 1963;29:509–514.

268. Miller HK: Cancer of the breast during pregnancy and lactation. *Am J Obstet Gynecol* 1962;83:607–611.

269. Montgomery TL: Detection and disposal of breast cancer in pregnancy. *Am J Obstet Gynecol* 1961;81:926–933.

270. Peete CH, Honeycutt HC, Cherny WB: Cancer of the breast in pregnancy. *NC Med* 1966;27:514–520.

271. Peters MV: The effect of pregnancy in breast cancer, in Forrest APM, Kunkler PB, (eds): *Prognostic Factors in Breast Cancer*. Baltimore, William & Wilkins, 1968, pp 65–80.

*272. Petrek JA, Dukoff R, Rogatko A: Prognosis of pregnancy-associated breast cancer. *Cancer* 1991;67:869–872.

273. Ribeiro G, Jones DA, Jones M: Carcinoma of the breast associated with pregnancy. *Br J Surg* 1986;73:607–609.

274. Rosemond GP: Carcinoma of the breast during pregnancy. *Clin Obstet Gynecol* 1963;6:994–1001.

### Multicentricity

*275. Bornstein BA, Recht A, Connoly JL, et al: Results of

treating ductal carcinoma in situ of the breast with conservative surgery and radiation therapy. *Cancer* 1991;67:7–13.

276. Crile G Jr, Cooperman A, Esselstyn CB Jr, et al: Results of partial mastectomy in 1,973 patients followed for from five to ten years. *Surg Gynecol Obstet* 1980;150:563–566.

*277. Egan RL: Multicentric breast carcinomas: Clinical-radiographic-pathologic whole organ studies and 10-year survival. *Cancer* 1982;49:1123–1130.

*278. Fisher ER, Gregorio R, Redmond C, et al: Pathologic findings from the national surgical adjuvant breast project (Protocol No. 4). I. Observations concerning the multicentricity of mammary cancer. *Cancer* 1975;35:247–254.

279. Gallager HS, Martin JE: Early phases in the development of breast cancer. *Cancer* 1969;24:1170–1178.

280. Holland R, Velig Solke HJ, Mravunac M, et al: Histologic multifocality of T1s, T1-2 breast carcinomas. Implications for clinical trials of breast conserving surgery. *Cancer* 1985; 56:979–990.

*281. Lagios MD: Multicentricity of breast carcinoma demonstrated by routine correlated serial subgross and radiographic examination. *Cancer* 1977;40:1726–1734.

282. Lagios MD, Rose MR, Margolin FR: Tubular carcinoma of the breast. Association with multicentricity, bilaterality, and family history of mammary carcinoma. *Am J Clin Pathol* 1980;73:25–30.

283. Lagios MS, Westdahl PR, Rose MR: The concept and implications of multicentricity in breast carcinoma. *Pathol Annu* 1981;16(2):83–102.

*284. Lagios MD, Westdahl PR, Margolin FR, et al: Duct carcinoma in situ. Relationship of extent of non-invasive disease to the frequency of occult invasion, multicentricity, lymph node metastases, and short-term failures. *Cancer* 1982;50:1309–1314.

*285. Lesser ML, Rosen PP, Kinne DW: Multicentricity and bilaterality in invasive breast carcinoma. *Surgery* 1982;91: 234–240.

286. McDivitt RW: Breast cancer multicentricity, in McDivitt RW, Oberman HA, Ozzello L, et al (eds): *The Breast*. Baltimore, Williams & Wilkins, pp 139–148.

287. Morgenstern L, Kaufman PA, Friedman NB: The cases against tylectomy for carcinoma of the breast. The factor of multicentricity. *Am J Surg* 1975;130:251–258.

*288. NIH Consensus Conference. Treatment of early-stage breast cancer. *JAMA* 1991;265(3):391–395.

289. Patchefsky AS, Shaber GS, Schwartz GF, et al: The pathology of breast cancer detected by mass population screening. *Cancer* 1977;40:1659–1670.

290. Qualheim RE, Gall EA: Breast carcinoma with multiple sites of origin. *Cancer* 1957;10:460–468.

*291. Rosen PP, Fracchia AA, Urban JA, et al: "Residual" mammary carcinoma following simulated partial mastectomy. *Cancer* 1975;35:739–747.

*292. Sarnelli R, Squartini F: Multicentricity in breast cancer: A submicroscopic study, in Sommers SC, Rosen PP, Fechner RE (eds): *Pathology Annual*, Norwalk, Connecticut, Appleton-Century-Crofts, 1986, 21(pt 1) pp 143–158.

293. Schwartz GF, Patchefsky AS, Feig SA, et al: Clinically occult breast cancer. Multicentricity and implications for treatment. *Ann Surg* 1980;191:8–12.

*294. Schwartz GF, Patchefsky AS, Feig SA, et al: Multicentricity of non-palpable breast cancer. *Cancer* 1980;45:2913–2916.

295. Shah JP, Rosen PP, Robins GF: Pitfalls of local excision in the treatment of carcinoma of the breast. *Surg Gynecol Obstet* 1973;136:721–725.

296. Solin LJ, Recht A, Fourquet A, et al: Ten-year results of breast-conserving surgery and irradiation for intraductal carcinoma (ductal carcinoma in situ) of the breast. *Cancer* 1991;68:2337–2344.

297. Tellem M, Prive L, Meranze DR: Four-quadrant study of breasts removed for carcinoma. *Cancer* 1962;15:10–17.

298. Westman-Naeser S, Bengtsson E, Eriksson O, et al: Multifocal breast carcinoma. *Am J Surg* 1981;142:255–257.

**Bilaterality**

*299. Adami H, Bergstrom R, Hansen J: Age at first primary as a determinant of incidence of bilateral breast cancer. Cumulative and relative risks in a population-based case-control study. *Cancer* 1985;55:643–647.

300. Anderson DE: Some characteristics of familial breast cancer. *Cancer* 1971;28:1500–1504.

*301. Anderson DE, Bazdiock MD: Bilaterality in familial breast cancer patients. *Cancer* 1985;56:2090–2098.

302. Bailey MJ, Royce C, Sloana JP, et al: Bilateral carcinoma of the breast. *Br J Surg* 1980;67:514–516.

303. Berge T, Ostberg G: Bilateral carcinoma of the female breast. *Acta Chir Scand* 1974;140:27–32.

304. Besson A, Delacretaz F, Pescia S, et al: Peutz-Jeghers syndrome, intessusception and associated malignancies. *Chirurgie* 1978;104:117–130.

*305. Bodian C, Haagensen CD: Bilateral carcinoma of the breast, in Haagensen CD: *Diseases of the Breast*. ed 3. Philadelphia, WB Saunders, 1986, chap 31, pp 440–461.

*306. Burns PE, Dabbs K, May C, et al: Bilateral breast cancer in northern Alberta: risk factors and survival patterns. *Can Med Assoc J* 1984;130:881–886.

*307. Chaudary MA, Millis RR, Hoskins EOL, et al: Bilateral primary breast cancer: a prospective study of disease incidence. *Br J Surg* 1984;71:711–714.

308. Farrow JH: Bilateral mammary cancer. *Cancer* 1956;9:1182–1188.

309. Fisher ER, Fisher B, Sass R, et al: Pathologic findings from the national surgical adjuvant breast project (Protocol No. 4). XI. Bilateral breast cancer. *Cancer* 1984;54:3002–3011.

310. Guiss LW: The problem of bilateral independent mammary carcinoma. *Am J Surg* 1954;88:171–177.

311. Haagensen CD: *Diseases of the Breast*, ed 3. Philadelphia, WB Saunders, 1986, p 450.

312. Harris RE, Lynch HT, Guirgis HA: Familial breast cancer: Risk to the contralateral breast. *J Natl Cancer Inst* 1978;60: 955–960.

313. Lagios MD, Rose MR, Margolin FR: Tubular carcinoma of the breast: Association with multicentricity, bilaterality,

and family history of mammary carcinoma. *Am J Clin Pathol* 1980;73:25–30.

314. Lawson R: Mammary cancer: The other breast. *Can Med Assoc J.* 1955;73:676–677.

315. Leis HP: Managing the remaining breast. *Cancer* 1980;46: 1026–1030.

316. Lewison EF, Neto AS: Bilateral breast cancer at the Johns Hopkins Hospital. *Cancer* 1971;28:1297–1301.

317. Martin JK, van Heerden JA, Gaffey TA: Synchronous and metachronous carcinoma of the breast. *Surgery* 1982;91:12–16.

*318. Nielsen M, Christensen L, Andersen J: Contralateral cancerous breast lesions in women with clinical invasive breast carcinoma. *Cancer* 1986;57:897–903.

*319. Nielsen M, Jensen J, Andersen J: Precancerous and cancerous breast lesions during lifetime and at autopsy. *Cancer* 1984;54:612–615.

320. Riley E, Swift M: A family with Peutz-Jeghers syndrome and bilateral breast cancer. *Cancer* 1980;46:815–817.

321. Ringberg A, Palmer B, Linnel F: The contralateral breast at reconstructive surgery after breast cancer operation: A histopathological study. *Breast Cancer Res Treat* 1982;2:151–161.

322. Robbins GF, Berg JW: Bilateral primary breast cancers. *Cancer* 1964;17:1501–1527.

*323. Schell SR, Montague ED, Spanos WJ, et al: Bilateral breast cancer in patients with initial stage I and II disease. *Cancer* 1982;50:1191–1194.

*324. Slack NH, Bross IDJ, Nemoto T, et al: Experiences with bilateral primary carcinoma of the breast. *Surg Gynecol Obstet* 1973;136:433–440.

325. Trau H, Schewach-Millet M, Fisher BK, et al: Peutz-Jeghers syndrome and bilateral breast carcinoma. *Cancer* 1982;50: 788–792.

326. Urban JA: Bilateral breast cancer. *Cancer* 1969;24:1310–1313.

*327. Urban JA, Papachristou D, Taylor J: Bilateral breast cancer. *Cancer* 1977;40:1968–1973.

*328. Wanebo HJ, Senofsky GM, Fechner RE, et al: Bilateral breast cancer. *Ann Surg* 1985;201:667–677.

329. Webber BL, Heise H, Neifeld JP, et al: Risk of subsequent contralateral breast carcinoma in a population of patients with in situ breast carcinoma. *Cancer* 1981;47:2928–2932.

## Classification

*330. Azzopardi JG, Chepick OF, Hartmann WH, et al: The World Health Organization histological typing of breast tumors—second edition. *Am J Clin Pathol* 1982;78:806–816.

331. Bassler R: *Pathologie der Brustdruse*. Berlin, Springer, 1978.

332. Lagios MD, Margolin FR, Westdahl PR, et al: Mammographically detected duct carcinoma in situ: Frequency of local recurrence following tylectomy and prognostic effect of nuclear grade on local recurrence. *Cancer* 1989;63:618–624.

333. Linell F, Rank F: *Breast Cancer*. Comments on histologic classifications with reference to histogenesis and prognosis. *Dialogos*, Lund, 1989, chapt 2, pp 12–14.

*334. Welling SR, Jensen HM, Marcum RG. Atlas of subgross pathology of the human breast with special reference to possible precancerous lesions. *J Natl Cancer Inst* 1975;55: 231–273.

# 3

# Specimen Processing

Stuart J. Schnitt, MD



## INTRODUCTION

Breast specimens are among the most commonly encountered specimens in the clinical practice of pathology. As a result, most pathologists consider such specimens to be "routine" and are confident in their ability to evaluate them. However, several recent developments have created the need for pathologists to reevaluate critically the manner in which breast specimens are processed and examined. These developments include:

1. ***Changes in the therapeutic approach for patients with breast cancer:*** With the increasing use of conservative surgery (CS) and radiation therapy (RT) for the treatment of many breast cancer patients, it is no longer sufficient for a pathologist to merely determine whether a breast mass is or is not carcinoma. Successful implementation of CS and RT requires careful pathologic evaluation to determine the adequacy of excision and histologic features of potential prognostic significance (9). In addition, the use of preoperative radiation therapy, chemotherapy, or both (including so-called neoadjuvant chemotherapy) for some patients with locally advanced breast cancer requires that the pathologist evaluate such specimens to determine the therapeutic response.
2. ***The increasing use of mammographic screening:*** An increasing number of breast biopsies are performed because of a mammographic abnormality in the absence of a palpable mass. Such specimens require careful mammographic-pathologic correlation for accurate evaluation.
3. ***The increasing requirement for cost-containment:*** With the increasing pressure to reduce the cost of medical care, pathologists must develop cost-effective methods for examining breast biopsies, many of which are large specimens consisting of fibrofatty tissue without grossly evident abnormalities.
4. ***New techniques for the analysis of breast tumors:*** In addition to routine histologic examination and determination of estrogen and progesterone receptor status, flow cytometric, immunohistochemical, morphometric, and molecular biologic studies are considered by many to be useful for the characterization of breast tumors.

In this chapter, methods for the processing and evaluation of breast specimens will be described.

Particular emphasis will be placed upon the processing of breast excision specimens and upon clinically relevant and cost-effective methods of specimen handling. In addition, methods for the examination of axillary lymph nodes will be considered.

## TYPES OF SPECIMENS

A variety of types of breast specimens are encountered by the pathologist on a daily basis. These include needle biopsies, incisional biopsies, excision specimens, re-excision specimens, mastectomies, and mammary reductions. In addition, patients with operable breast cancer usually have some type of surgical procedure to procure axillary lymph nodes for pathologic evaluation.

### Needle Biopsies

#### *Fine Needle Aspiration (FNA) Biopsies*

A detailed discussion of breast FNA is beyond the scope of this chapter and the interested reader is referred to two recent monographs on this subject (19,24). However, a few brief comments regarding FNA of the breast are in order.

At many institutions, FNA constitutes the initial diagnostic procedure for palpable breast masses. More recently, this technique has also been used to evaluate non-palpable, mammographically-detected lesions. FNA can both permit the distinction between a cyst and a solid tumor and produce material for cytologic evaluation. In addition, specimens obtained by FNA may be suitable for immunohistochemical determination of estrogen and progesterone receptor analysis, flow cytometric studies, and morphometric analysis. The accuracy of breast FNA depends upon the skill and experience of the personnel who perform the aspiration, prepare the slides, and interpret the results. However, most studies indicate that with experience, the frequency of false-negative and false-positive results can be minimized.

It is essential that the pathologist who interprets a breast FNA obtain all relevant clinical information. A number of benign lesions such as fibroadenomas, lactational change, fat necrosis, and radiation effects are well-known causes for false-positive interpretations of breast FNA; the risk of erroneously categorizing such lesions can be minimized if adequate clinical information is provided. One major limitation of FNA is the inability to permit a reliable distinction between in situ and invasive ductal carcinomas (43,47). Since the therapeutic approach to these two types of lesions may differ at some institutions, awareness of this limitation is important for both the pathologist and the clinician.

#### *Core Needle Biopsies*

In contrast to FNA which provides material for cytologic evaluation, core needle biopsies yield tissue fragments suitable for histologic examination. The amount of tissue obtained is usually insufficient for routine biochemical analysis for estrogen and progesterone receptors but may be suitable for immunohistochemical evaluation of these hormone receptors, either on frozen sections or paraffin sections. Core needle biopsy specimens should be submitted for microscopic evaluation in their entirety, and drying and distortion of the specimens should be avoided. In some cases, multiple levels of the paraffin blocks will be necessary to obtain sections which contain the diagnostic lesion.

### Incisional Biopsies

The manner in which an incisional biopsy is processed depends upon the reason for which the procedure was performed. Incisional biopsies may be performed to obtain tissue for diagnosis, for steroid hormone receptor assays or for both. Consultation with the surgeon prior to specimen processing is imperative so that the maximum amount of clinically useful information is obtained from the specimen.

### Excision Specimens

#### *General Considerations*

Breast excisions are most commonly performed because of the presence of a palpable mass, an abnormality detected by mammography or both. Occasionally, breast tissue is excised because of the presence

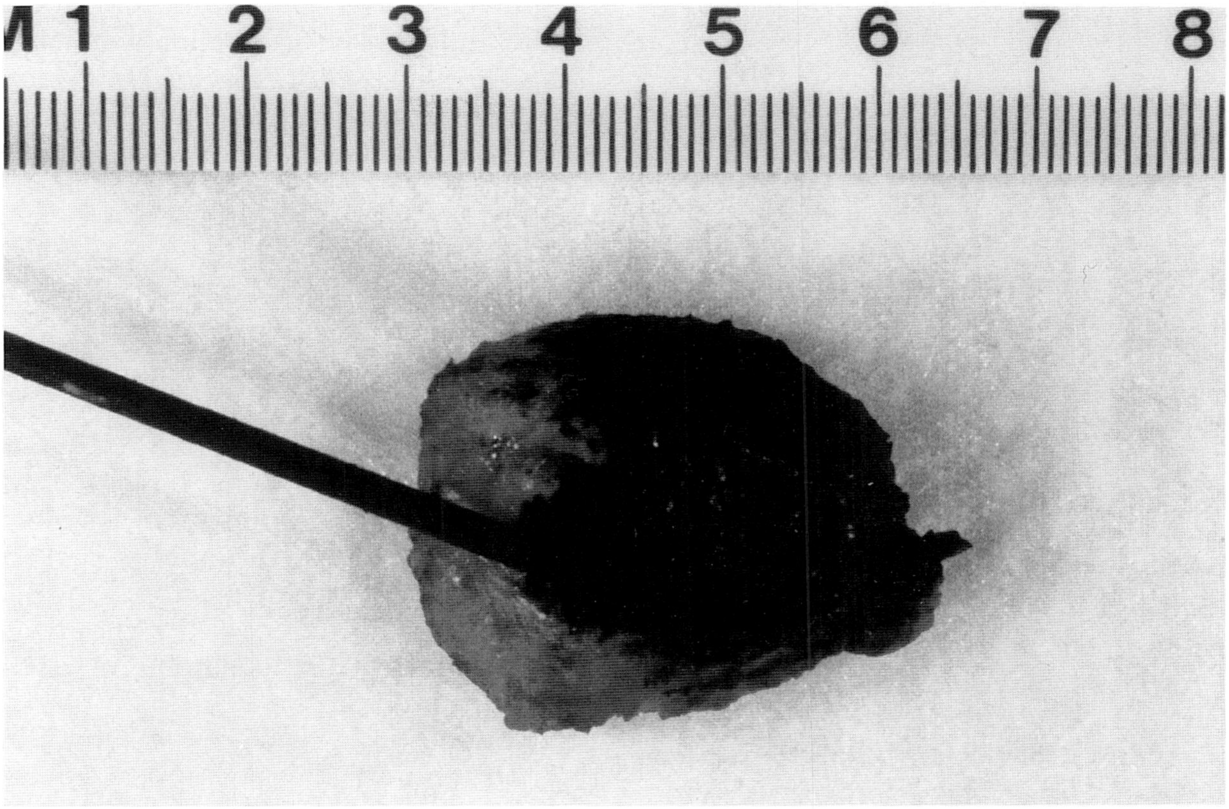


**Figure 3.1** Breast excision specimen partially painted with India ink which is used to permit identification of the margins of excision.

of nipple discharge. While the processing of these three types of specimens differs in some respects, it is worthwhile to briefly discuss the examination of breast excision specimens in general.

As noted earlier, the combination of conservative surgery and radiation therapy is becoming increasingly common for the treatment of patients with stage I and II breast cancer. It has become clear that pathologic evaluation of the breast excision specimen is an important component in the selection and implementation of this form of therapy (9). Since the ultimate method of treatment of a patient with breast cancer may be determined on the basis of the pathologic findings in the excision specimen, the pathologist should approach every breast excision with the view that if the specimen reveals carcinoma, the patient may desire breast-conserving therapy. To this end, a careful macroscopic examination of the excised tissue is essential. The specimen should be presented to the pathologist intact and should then be inspected, palpated, and measured in three dimensions. The presence of skin, fascia and/or skeletal muscle should be noted. If a palpable tumor is present, it should be measured in three dimensions and its relationship to overlying skin and underlying fascia or muscle, if present, should be recorded. If the specimen contains a grossly suspicious lesion which extends to the surface of the specimen, the surgeon, if still operating, should be informed immediately so that additional tissue may be obtained from the involved area.

Prior to incising any breast excision specimen, the surface should be blotted dry and then painted with a marker which will be visible on the permanent sections. This will facilitate the microscopic evaluation of the resection margins should the specimen contain carcinoma. A number of substances are available in a variety of colors but a very satisfactory one is India ink (Fig. 3.1). After applying the ink, the surface should again be blotted dry. An alternative method is to apply the ink to the specimen's surface and immediately immerse the inked specimen into Bouin's solution for a brief period of time (e.g., 30 seconds). This serves to fix the ink to the specimen's surface. The specimen should then be briefly rinsed in cold water and blotted dry. The subsequent steps in processing will depend upon the nature of the specimen, i.e., whether it is obtained because of the presence of a palpable mass, a mammographic abnormality or nipple discharge.

## *Specimens Excised Because of the Presence of a Palpable Mass*

Following gross inspection of the intact specimen, palpation, measurement of the specimen, and inking of margins as described above, the specimen should be incised. However, the subsequent method used for incising the specimen should depend upon the information already obtained from the clinical impression and examination of the intact specimen.

**Fibroadenoma suspected.** If the lesion present is likely to be a fibroadenoma, the specimen may be bisected or sectioned at 3 to 5 mm intervals in order to examine the cut surface. If the impression of fibroadenoma is confirmed and the lesion has been enucleated, one or two blocks should be submitted for permanent sections. If there is breast tissue surrounding the lesion, it is reasonable to submit a block of this tissue for histologic examination as well.

**Grossly benign fibrofatty tissue.** Many breast excision specimens lack a discrete lesion on palpation. Such specimens should be sectioned ("breadloafed") at 3 to 5 mm intervals. If gross examination of the cut specimen fails to reveal a discrete lesion and consists exclusively of unremarkable fibrofatty tissue (with or without small cysts), the pathologist must decide how thoroughly the specimen should be sampled for microscopic examination. At some institutions, only a few "representative" areas are selected for histologic evaluation, whereas at others, such specimens are submitted for microscopic examination in their entirety, regardless of specimen size. Examining such specimens in their entirety provides the highest level of detection of clinically significant lesions (26). However, such exhaustive microscopic examination of these often large specimens is not feasible at many institutions. Although the extent to which grossly unremarkable fibrofatty breast specimens should be sampled for histologic examination ultimately depends upon the judgment of the individual pathologist, a possible cost-effective method for sampling such specimens has recently been suggested (39). Schnitt and Wang studied 384 breast biopsies performed because of a palpable mass in which gross examination revealed only benign fibrofatty tissue, and in which all tissue was submitted for histologic examination. Carcinoma or atypical hyperplasia was identified in 26 of these cases (6.7%). The most common type of carcinoma was lobular carcinoma in situ (12 cases), but examples of ductal carcinoma in situ and invasive carcinoma were also detected (four and three cases, respectively). Among the atypical hyperplasias, four were lobular and three were ductal in type. The salient findings of this study were as follows:

1. In 25 of the 26 cases of carcinoma and atypical hyperplasia, at least a portion of the lesion was identified in the fibrous parenchymal component of the specimen. In only one case of atypical lobular hyperplasia was the lesion present exclusively in grossly fatty tissue. Therefore, submitting the grossly fatty component of such specimens appears to be unnecessary. Restricting histologic examination to the fibrous parenchymal component is a useful means for reducing the number of tissue blocks processed without significantly compromising the likelihood of detecting clinically significant lesions.
2. Submitting every grossly benign breast biopsy in its entirety did not appear to be cost-effective. However, it was also shown that submitting only a predetermined small number of blocks (such as two or five) regardless of specimen size can result in the failure to detect clinically significant lesions. For example, if as a maximum, five tissue blocks had been submitted for each case, 41% fewer blocks would have been processed, but six (23%) of the carcinomas or atypical hyperplasias would have gone undetected. In contrast, submitting a maximum of ten blocks for each case would have resulted in 18% fewer blocks submitted and in the detection of all cases of carcinoma and atypical hyperplasia except for a single focus of lobular carcinoma in situ in one case. Thus, if a breast specimen, after careful macroscopic examination, reveals only grossly benign fibrofatty tissue, it is reasonable to submit a *maximum* of ten blocks of fibrous parenchyma as a screening step regardless of the size of the specimen. If no carcinoma or atypical hyperplasia is identified among these blocks, the likelihood of finding such lesions in additional blocks is extremely low. In contrast, if carcinoma or atypical hyperplasia is detected among these first ten blocks, the remainder of the specimen should be examined microscopically to determine the extent of the lesion, to identify other associated lesions, and to evaluate margins of excision in cases in which carcinoma is present.

**Carcinoma suspected.** If carcinoma is suspected clinically and/or on gross examination of the intact specimen, the specimen should be cut in such a way as to permit examination of the resection margins on histologic sections, since many clinicians use this information in the selection of breast cancer patients for breast-conserving therapy. At some institutions, it is considered desirable to have the final pathologic report reflect the relationship of the tumor to particular margins of resection, and sutures or other suitable markers are used by the surgeon to orient the specimen for the pathologist. Specimen orientation may be of particular value in directing further surgery. For example, if the superficial margin of excision is involved by tumor, re-excision which includes a segment of skin overlying the tumor site may be desirable. In contrast, for a tumor deep within the breast abutting the pectoral fascia, if the deep margin of excision is involved, removal of additional breast tissue will not improve the margin of concern. It should be noted that if the tumor has been grossly excised, the importance of obtaining microscopically "negative" margins of excision is an unresolved issue at this time. At many institutions, clinicians insist on microscopically negative margins prior to radiation therapy whereas at others, tumor-free microscopic margins are not considered mandatory in all cases. Given the uncertainly regarding the need for microscopically tumor-free margins, it seems prudent for the pathologist to attempt a careful evaluation of margins until additional data on this subject becomes available.

As noted by Carter (6), the margins of breast excision specimens containing carcinomas are technically among the most difficult type of margins to evaluate. This is in large part related to the fact that the tumor is commonly associated with subclinical carcinoma extending imperceptibly into the surrounding soft tissue in three dimensions. This situation is complicated by the fact that this extension away from the tumor is not uniform but more root-like in its character. Certain types of breast carcinomas, e.g., medullary, mucinous, and some infiltrating ductal carcinomas, are relatively well-circumscribed and usually not associated with much in situ carcinoma, rendering evaluation of margins relatively easy. In contrast, most infiltrating ductal carcinomas have irregular borders and are associated with variable amounts of ductal carcinoma in situ in the adjacent tissue. The ease with which the margins of these types of specimens can be evaluated varies greatly, depending primarily upon how close the infiltrating lesion is to the margin and the extent of associated ductal carcinoma in situ.

An optimal method to section the specimen to permit evaluation of the margins has not been established. There are several options for the examination of margins and, to some degree, the approach depends upon the size of the excised tissue. It should be noted, however, that in all methods, there is an element of sampling error. For example, Carter notes that a complete evaluation of the margins of 2 cm carcinoma cut through the equatorial plane would require more than 3,000 sections; this clearly is not feasible (6). One approach to margin evaluation proposed by Fisher et al (13), involves orientation of the specimen and sectioning it in different planes to obtain a representative sampling of the tumor and the various margins of resection (Fig. 3.2). Another method, proposed by Carter (6), involves inking the surface of the specimen, peeling off the margins in their entirety and embedding the inked surface for sectioning (Fig. 3.3). However, given the highly irregular surface of most specimens, this too has its inherent difficulties.

At our institution (Beth Israel Hospital, Boston), the method of sectioning varies, depending upon the size of the excised specimen. For small excisions (i.e., 3 cm or less in greatest diameter), after inking the specimen, it is palpated to determine the closest margin and cut at 3 to 5 mm intervals, perpendicular to the closest margin (Fig. 3.4). The size and appearance of the gross tumor mass, the location of the mass within the excision specimen, the distance to the nearest gross margin, and the location of that margin (if the specimen has been previously oriented) are described. The remaining tissue is then macroscopically examined for additional tumor nodules, areas suspicious for in situ carcinoma, or other abnormalities. In general, unless the surgeon or the patient are extremely anxious to obtain an immediate diagnosis, frozen sections are not performed on the tumor to confirm the diagnosis of malignancy if gross examination suggests that the lesion is likely to be carcinoma. After obtaining an aliquot of tumor for hormone receptor studies and DNA analysis, the entire specimen is submitted for permanent sections. There is little role for frozen section evaluation of resection margins which are grossly free of tumor. Because of the inherent sampling error, the fatty nature of the margins, and the number of sections necessary for a thorough study, this evaluation is best performed on

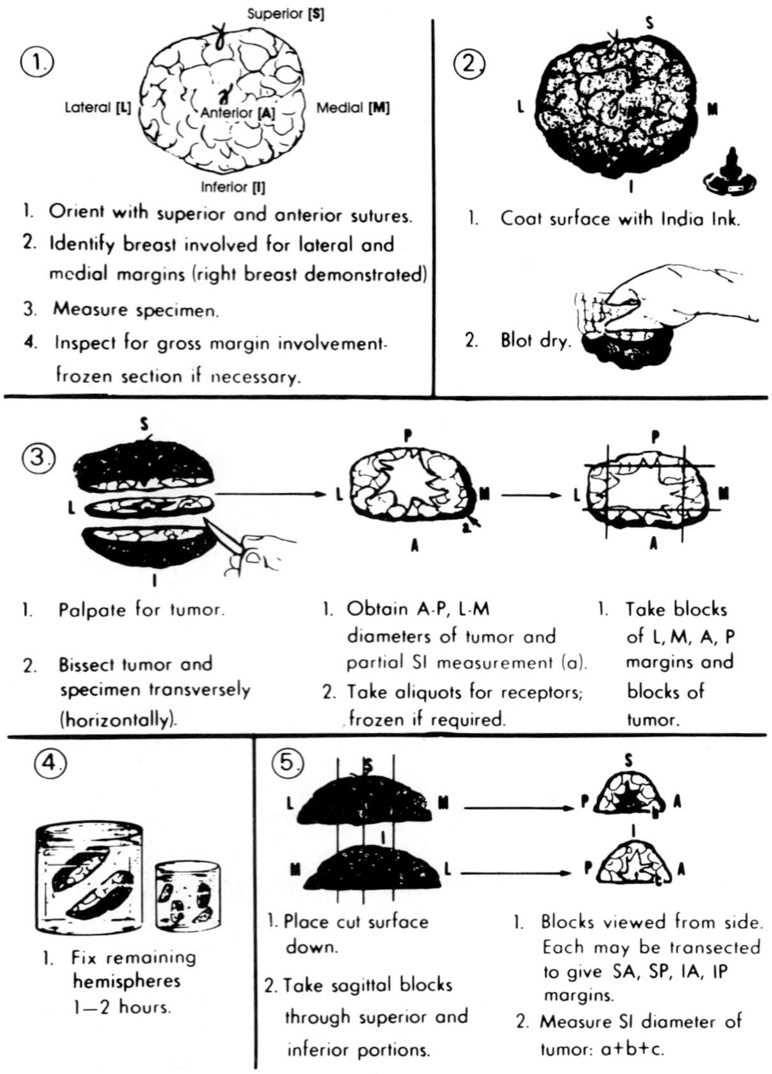


**Figure 3.2** In this method of evaluating the margins of a breast excision specimen, the specimen is oriented, the margins are painted with India ink, and the specimen is sectioned in various planes. (Reprinted from Fisher ER, Sass R, Fisher B, et al: *Cancer* 1986;57:1717–1724, with permission.)

the permanent sections. If there is a specific area of concern to the surgeon or if on gross sectioning, the tumor appears to approach a margin, a frozen section of that particular area may be indicated.

For larger specimens (i.e., larger than 3 cm in greatest dimension), this procedure is modified. After inking the specimen, a single incision is made through the center of the palpable mass where it most closely approaches the margin. In this way, the size of the tumor and the relationship to the nearest margin can be quickly determined, and an aliquot can be obtained for hormone receptor assays and DNA analysis. As indicated above, at our institution frozen sections on the margins of excision are usually not performed, but sections to demonstrate the relationship of the tumor to the closest margin of excision should be submitted for paraffin-embedding. The remaining margins can then be entirely removed from the specimen and submitted for permanent sections as described by Carter (6), or may be sampled by shaving off representative sections from each of the six surfaces of the specimen (i.e., medial, lateral, anterior, posterior, superior, and inferior) as illustrated in Figure 3.5. Multiple sections can then be made through the remainder of the specimen at 3 to 5 mm intervals and several sections of the tumor and the adjacent parenchyma or fat should be submitted for microscopic evaluation.

If a segment of skin is included with the specimen, a section should be taken to demonstrate the relationship of the tumor to the skin. If this cannot be accomplished because the tumor is at a considerable distance from the skin, a random section of the skin should be obtained. Similarly, if a portion of muscle is present at the deep aspect of the specimen, this too should be sampled.

## *Specimens Excised Because of the Presence of Mammographic Abnormality*

With the increasing use of mammographic screening, a growing number of breast excisions are performed because of an abnormality detected by mammography in the absence of a palpable mass (3,4,8–10, 12,16,21,23,28–30,32–35,41,42). The most frequent mammographic abnormalities prompting biopsy are microcalcifications, a soft tissue density, or a soft tissue density with associated microcalcifications. These specimens are usually excised using the hookwire or needle localization technique. Specimen radiography is a crucial component in the evaluation of these specimens in order to both document the presence of the lesion detected by mammography and localize the suspicious area for histologic examination. Therefore, close cooperation among the surgeon, radiologist, and pathologist is essential.

At some institutions, the specimen is transported from the operating room to the radiology department where a radiograph of the intact specimen is obtained. The specimen and radiograph are then submitted together to the pathologist for examination. At other institutions, the intact specimen is submitted to the pathologist who performs specimen radiography using a self-contained, portable x-ray unit. Regardless of where it is performed, several aspects of specimen radiography merit comment. First, the

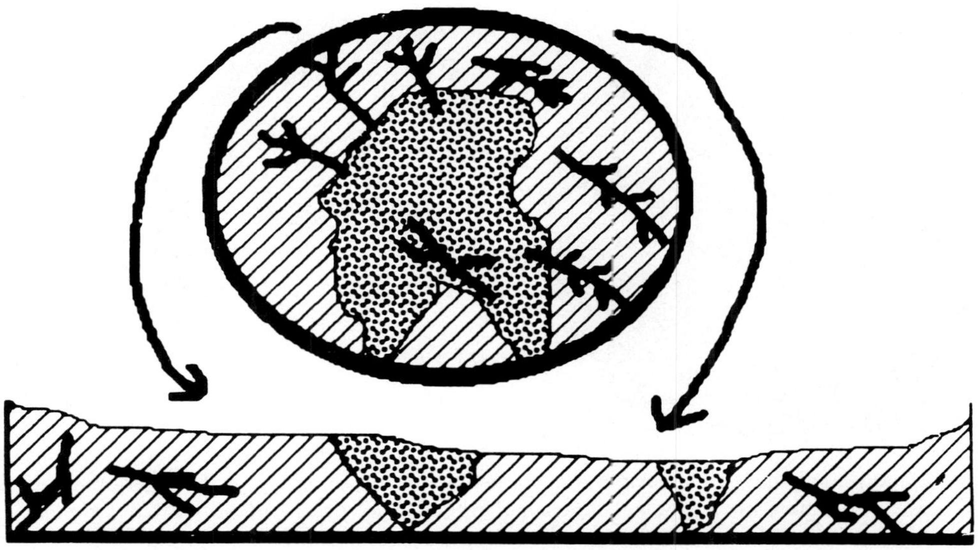

**Figure 3.3** This diagram illustrates a breast excision specimen containing an infiltrating ductal carcinoma (stippled area) with associated intraductal carcinoma (branched structures). The black area at the periphery represents the inked margin of excision. In this method of examining the margins, the margin of the specimen is peeled off and submitted for sectioning with the inked surface down; the histologic sections are then cut parallel to this surface. When examined in this manner, the margin is considered involved if tumor is present anywhere on the sections, even though it may not be at an inked surface, since the sections have been cut parallel to the inked margin. (Reprinted from Carter D: *Hum Pathol* 1986;17:330–332, with permission.)

value of magnification views cannot be over-emphasized. This frequently permits the identification of mammographic abnormalities (particularly microcalcifications) that are not well-demonstrated using standard non-magnified radiographs. Second, many radiologists consider specimen compression an essential component of specimen radiography, especially for cases in which the mammographic abnormality is a soft tissue density without microcalcifications. Finally, specimen radiographs should always be compared with the preoperative mammograms to be certain that the lesion of concern has been excised.

After radiography of the intact specimen has been performed, the surgeon should be notified as to whether or not the suspicious area has been removed. If the lesion is contained within the specimen, the area in question must then be identified by the pathologist. Some specimens excised because of a mammographic abnormality will, on initial macroscopic examination, contain a grossly evident tumor; such specimens should be processed as if they were palpable masses, as described above. If, however, no lesion is apparent on initial gross examination, a number of methods can be used to identify the lesion within the specimen. One simple method consists of comparing the gross specimen with the specimen radiograph and placing a safety pin or needle into the specimen at the site of the mammographic lesion to permit the identification of its location by the prosector. Another involves slicing the specimen at 3 to 5 mm intervals and obtaining a radiograph of the sliced specimen. The slices on the radiograph can then be

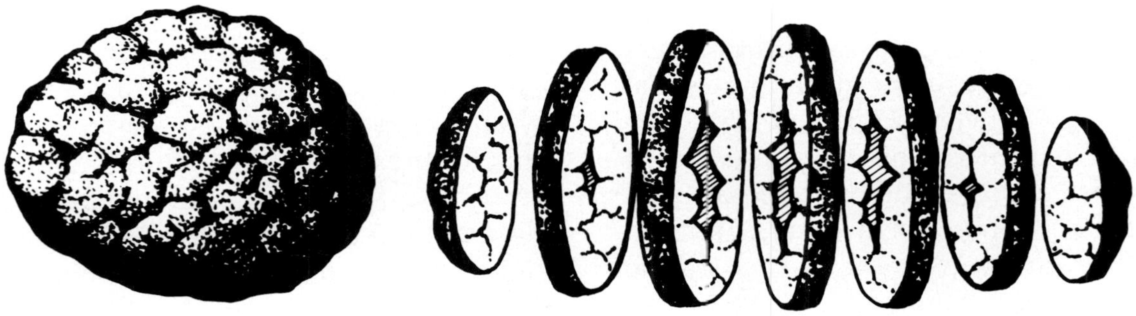

**Figure 3.4** This method of sectioning a breast excision specimen is suitable for smaller specimens (generally 3 cm or less). The margin of excision is inked and the specimen is sectioned using parallel cuts 3 to 5 mm apart. (Reprinted from Connolly JL, Schnitt SJ: *Pathol Annu* 1988;(pt 1):1–23, with permission.)

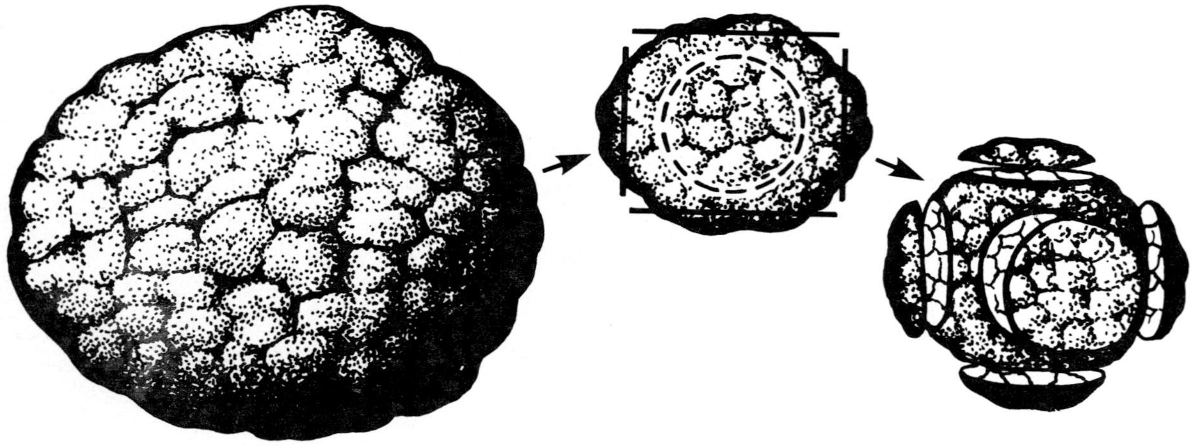

**Figure 3.5** In this method of evaluating the margins of larger specimens, representative areas of the margins from the inferior, superior, anterior, posterior, medial, and lateral surfaces are shaved from the specimen and embedded with the inked surface down as in the method illustrated in Fig. 3.3. (Reprinted from Connolly JL, Schnitt SJ: *Pathol Annu* 1988;(pt 1):1–23, with permission.)

labeled and the tissue slices placed in correspondingly labelled tissue cassettes to permit correlation between the histologic sections and the radiograph of the sliced specimen (25). A third method consists of performing the initial specimen radiograph after placing the tissue in a specimen holder which incorporates a grid which is visible on the radiograph. The holder containing the specimen and the specimen radiograph are then compared to precisely locate the target lesion using the X and Y coordinates of the grid (1). In any case, as for palpable masses, the specimen *should not* be incised before the surface is painted with ink.

Beyond submitting the breast tissue containing the mammographically detected lesion, the extent to which the remaining breast tissue is sampled for microscopic evaluation varies. At some centers, only the areas of the specimen containing the mammographic lesion are submitted, whereas at other institutions a variable amount of the remaining breast tissue is also examined microscopically. A number of studies have indicated that in some breast biopsies performed for the presence of microcalcifications and in which carcinoma is identified, the calcifications are identified histologically exclusively in benign breast tissue adjacent to the cancer (8,23,29,30,35). The implication of this is that microscopic examination of such specimens must include not only the area of mammographic calcifications, but also an unknown quantity of the surrounding breast tissue. While submitting such specimens for histologic evaluation in their entirety would permit the highest level of detection of clinically significant lesions, such exhaustive examination is not feasible at many institutions. A recent prospective mammographic-pathologic correlative study of breast biopsies performed because of mammographic microcalcifications sought to address this issue (25). In this study, 157 consecutive breast biopsies performed because of the mammographic finding of microcalcifications without a soft tissue density were examined in their entirety using a technique in which the radiographic findings in sectioned specimens were correlated with the histologic findings. Microscopic examination revealed carcinoma in 32%, atypical hyperplasia in 12%, and benign breast tissue without atypia in 56% of the cases. It is noteworthy that, 49 of the 50 cancers (98%) and 14 of the 19 atypical hyperplasias (74%) were associated with the radiographic calcifications. If histologic examination had been restricted to the areas of the specimen containing the radiographic microcalcifications, 38% fewer tissue blocks would have been processed, but one case of noncomedo ductal carcinoma in situ and five cases of atypical hyperplasia would have gone undetected. If microscopic evaluation had also included all additional tissue consisting of fibrous parenchyma, all 50 carcinomas and 17 of the 19 atypical hyperplasias would have been detected, and 20% fewer tissue blocks would have been processed. These findings indicate that for breast biopsies containing microcalcifications, restricting histologic examination to the areas of radiographic calcifications results in a high level of detection of clinically significant lesions and a considerable reduction in the amount of tissue processed. Additionally, submitting the fibrous parenchymal tissue component of the specimen further improves the likelihood of detecting such lesions. In the event

A

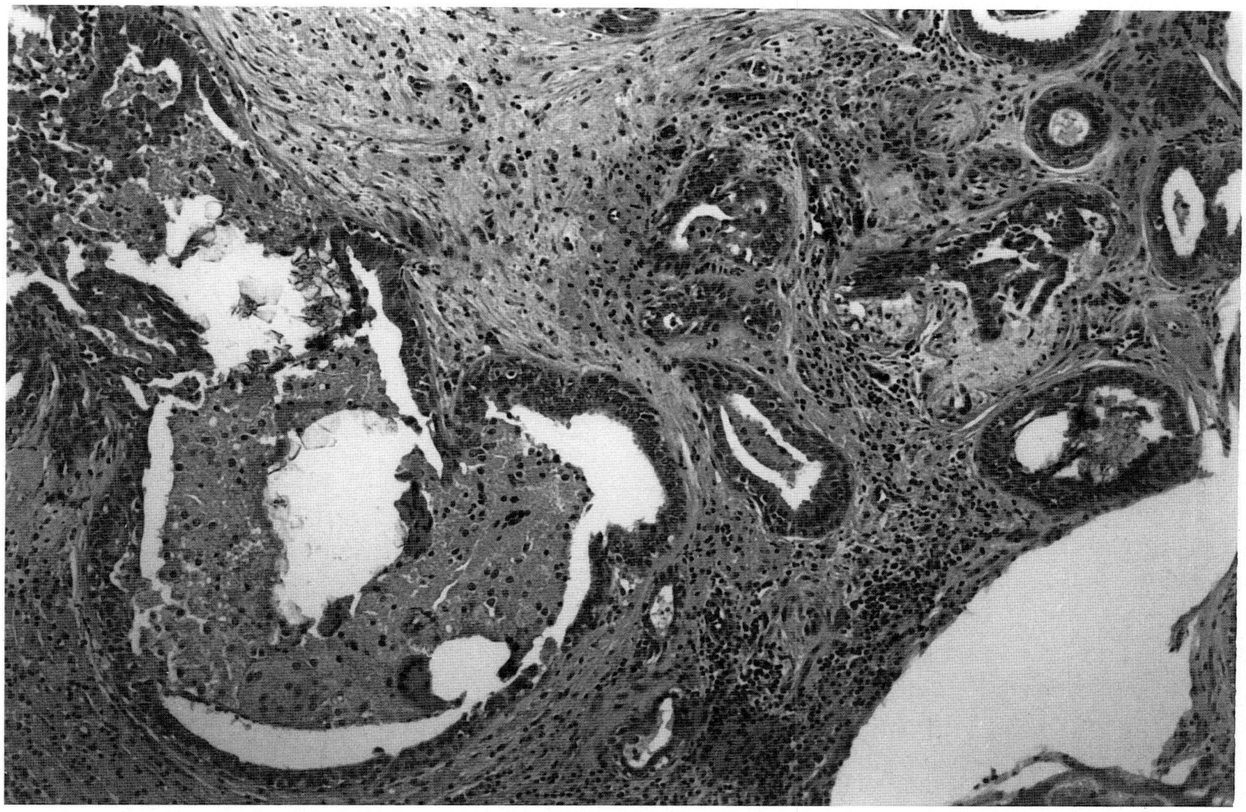

B

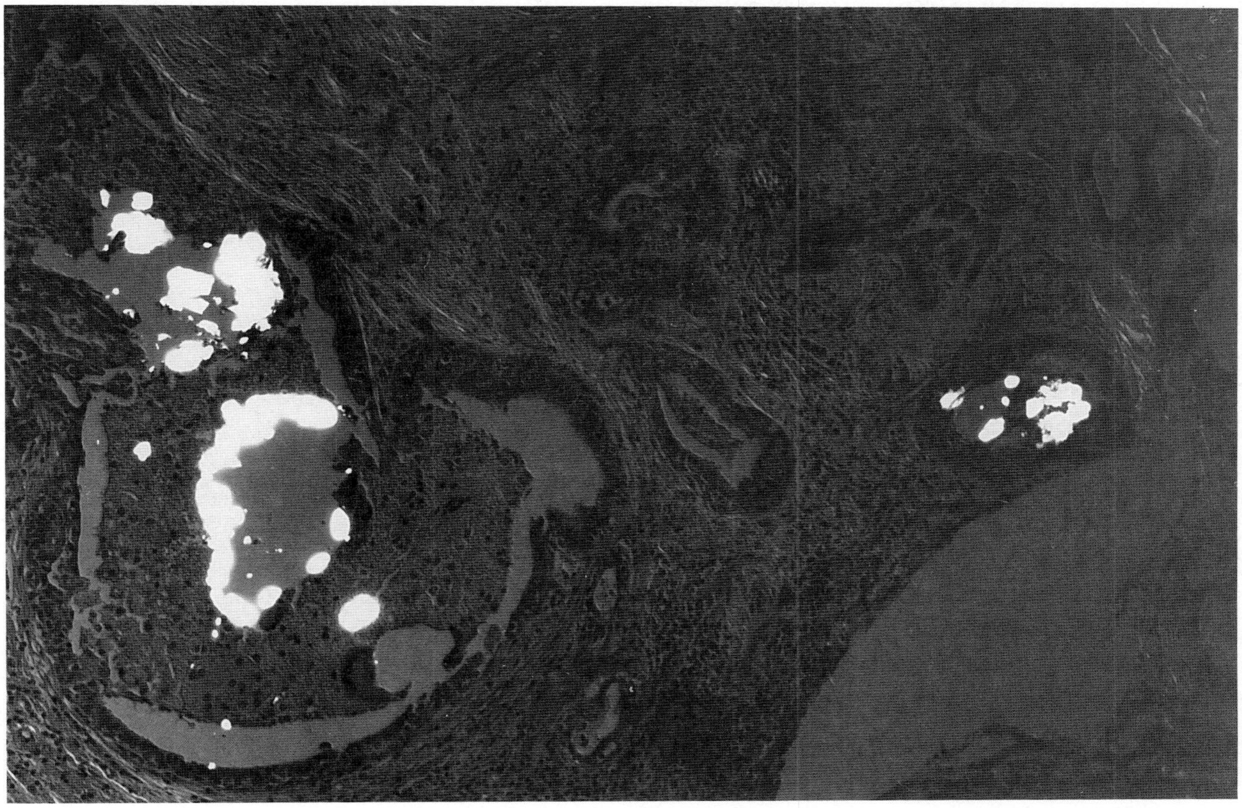

**Figure 3.6** (a) Hematoxylin and eosin stained section of a breast excision specimen removed because of mammographic microcalcifications. Although the microcalcifications were clearly present on the specimen radiograph, no calcifications were evident on routine examination of the histologic sections which revealed duct stasis and mild stromal inflammation. (b) Examination of the same section under polarized light revealed numerous polarizable crystals consistent with calcium oxalate.

that carcinoma is detected in the specimen, the margins will be evaluable on microscopic examination since the outer surface of the specimen will have been inked prior to sectioning.

In some cases, the initial histologic sections of breast specimens containing radiographic calcifications fail to reveal microscopic calcifications, even when the specimen radiograph clearly indicated that the calcifications are contained within the specimen. There are several possible explanations for this. First, the calcifications may be composed of calcium oxalate rather than the usual calcium phosphate (31,46). Both types of calcium deposits produce the mammographic appearance of microcalcifications but appear different histologically. The basophilic nature of calcium phosphate deposits is well-known and easily recognized by pathologists. In contrast, calcium oxalate deposits, on hematoxylin-eosin sections, are pale and refractile and may be difficult to identify using routine microscopy. Examination of such specimens under polarized light, however, readily demonstrates this type of calcification (Fig. 3.6). If, after examination under polarized light, there is still no microscopic evidence of calcifications, other possibilities must be considered. For example, the paraffin blocks may not have been cut deeply enough to provide histologic sections which demonstrate the calcifications. To investigate this possibility, the blocks may themselves be radiographed (48); any blocks containing radiographic calcifications should be cut more deeply until the calcifications are microscopically identified. Finally, in some cases, larger calcifications may shatter out of the block during sectioning and will, therefore, not be demonstrable on histologic sections. It should be emphasized that it is incumbent upon the pathologist to make every effort to identify histologically the lesion for which the surgical excision was performed.

The use of frozen sections to examine breast excision specimens removed because of mammographic calcifications should be discouraged. Many of these lesions are small and it may not be possible to both perform a frozen section and retain a sufficient amount of lesional tissue for permanent sections. Moreover, artifacts resulting from freezing the specimen may make it extremely difficult or impossible to accurately evaluate the permanent sections. Frozen sections may be indicated in specimens excised because of a mammographic soft tissue density which on gross examination is suspicious for carcinoma. However, since many of these lesions are also quite small, it may be more prudent to obtain an aliquot of the tumor for hormone receptor studies and DNA analysis, if feasible. The remainder of the lesion is then submitted for permanent sections.

### *Specimens Excised Because of the Presence of Nipple Discharge*

Some breast excision specimens from women with unilateral nipple discharge are submitted to the pathologist with a presumptive diagnosis of "intraductal papilloma." The best approach to this type of specimen is to attempt to open the involved duct using a fine pair of scissors until the lesion is exposed. Identification of the lesion may be facilitated by the surgeon placing a suture at the end of the involved duct nearest the nipple. Serially sectioning ("breadloafing") the excised tissue is not recommended as the initial approach since a small intraductal lesion may be overlooked or destroyed. However, if no lesion is identified after carefully dissecting the duct in question, it may be necessary to breadloaf the specimen in an attempt to identify any abnormality. If a grossly evident papillary lesion is present, it should be submitted for permanent sections. Frozen sections of grossly papillary breast lesions are not recommended since the frozen sections may be difficult to interpret and freezing of the specimen may render accurate interpretation of the subsequent permanent sections difficult if not impossible.

## Re-Excision Specimens

Some patients with breast cancer who are considered candidates for conservative surgery and radiotherapy undergo a re-excision of the tumor site for one or more of the following reasons: 1) an initial biopsy which did not remove the tumor grossly, 2) the presence of microcalcifications in the vicinity of the tumor site on post-biopsy mammograms, 3) tumor involvement of margins of the initial excision, 4) unknown or unassessable margins of the initial excision, and 5) the presence of certain histologic features of the primary tumor associated with an increased risk of local recurrence after conservative surgery and radiotherapy (e.g., an extensive intraductal component) (9).

The sizes of the re-excision specimens are quite

variable. At our institution they have ranged from 2 cm to over 20 cm in greatest dimension, averaging approximately 6 cm. This variation depends upon the location of the primary site (it is difficult to obtain a wide margin around a very superficial or a very deep tumor), the ease with which the surgeon can identify the tumor site, and the size of the breast. As is the case for primary excision specimens, the surgeon should present the re-excision specimen to the pathologist intact, and sutures may be used by the surgeon to orient the specimen. The surface of the specimen should be examined for defects which might suggest that the previous biopsy site has been cut across, and therefore, has not been entirely removed. Before incising the specimen, the outer surface of the re-excision should be inked as it is for primary excisions. Subsequent processing is similar to that described for primary excisions and depends upon the size of the specimen. In most cases, hemorrhage, fat necrosis, and fibrosis in the vicinity of the tumor site render accurate gross evaluation for the presence or absence of residual neoplasm extremely difficult if not impossible. This judgment is best deferred to the permanent sections. Frozen sections on re-excision specimens are usually not necessary and should be performed only on the rare occasion when a margin of excision is grossly suspicious for involvement by malignancy. If the re-excision is performed because the initial biopsy was incisional and gross residual tumor is evident in the re-excision specimen, an aliquot of tumor should be obtained for estrogen and progesterone receptor assays and DNA analysis if this had not been done at the time of the initial biopsy.

The extent of sampling of re-excision specimens for permanent sections depends upon the size of the tissue excised. Smaller specimens (i.e., less than 3 cm in greatest dimension) should be breadloafed and submitted in their entirety. With larger specimens, the margins of excision should be removed as demonstrated for primary excisions in Figures 3.3 or 3.5, and the biopsy site should be extensively sampled. Patients in whom the re-excision specimen shows little or no residual tumor are considered to be good candidates for subsequent radiotherapy. In contrast, if there is a prominent component of residual carcinoma (particularly extensive residual intraductal carcinoma) or involvement of the new margins of excision or both, a mastectomy may be more prudent (9).

## Microscopic Evaluation of Margins in Excision and Re-Excision Specimens of Patients with Breast Cancer

Microscopic sections demonstrating the margins of excision and re-excision specimens should be evaluated for the presence of both invasive and in situ carcinoma. Unfortunately, there is no generally accepted definition as to how close the tumor must be to an inked surface to render the margin "positive." For example, Fisher et al (13) reported that the referring pathologists considered margins of excision specimens to be involved by tumor in 52 patients in National Surgical Adjuvant Breast Project (NSABP) Protocol 6. However, review of these cases by the NSABP headquarters pathologists revealed disagreement with the initial evaluation of the margins in 69% of the cases. This discrepancy was related to the fact that the NSABP headquarters pathologists required the presence of invasive or in situ tumor directly at an inked surface to consider the margin involved. A few adipocytes or a few strands of collagen between the edge of the tumor and the margin of excision was sufficient for those investigators to regard a margin as negative, whereas many of the referring pathologists considered such a margin to be involved. At this time there are no definitive data to indicate what constitutes an involved margin or "how close is too close." In our experience (9) and as noted by Fisher et al (13), microscopic involvement of resection margins is subject to considerable sampling error. Furthermore, "involved" microscopic margins do not guarantee the presence of residual carcinoma and "uninvolved" margins do not preclude its presence. In several recent studies, positive microscopic margins were associated with residual carcinoma in only 51% to 69% of cases whereas residual carcinoma was seen in 26% to 33% of cases with negative microscopic margins (14,20,37,38,44). In the absence of objective definitions, we believe it reasonable to report a margin as involved if tumor is present at an inked surface (Fig. 3.7), and to specify the extent of that involvement (i.e., focal or extensive). If the tumor cells are not present at an inked surface, we indicate the distance from the edge of the tumor to the inked margin as measured with an ocular micrometer or, for larger distances, a ruler. The biologic and prognostic significance of tumor at or close to the margins remains to be determined.

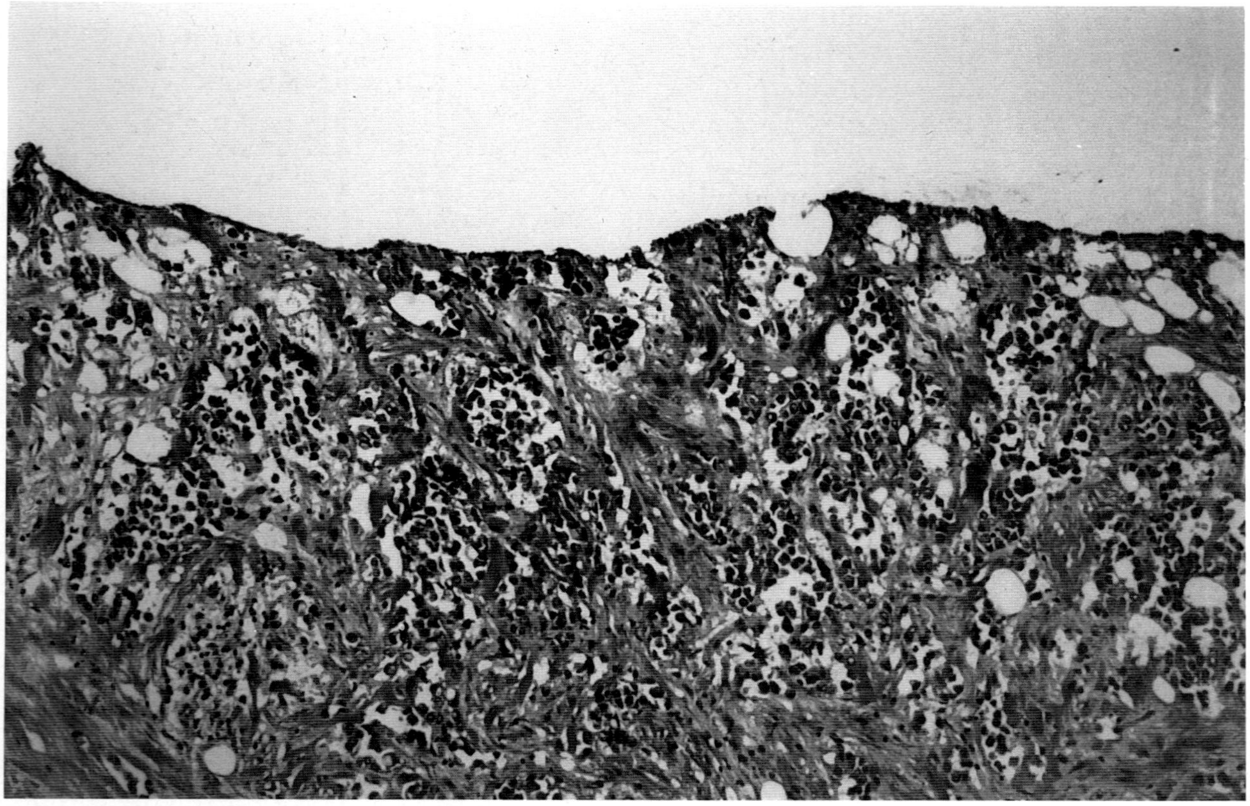

**Figure 3.7** Histologic section demonstrating an infiltrating carcinoma extending to the inked margin of excision.

A major pitfall in the microscopic evaluation of margins is the tendency of ink to flow into defects in the surface of the specimen. These defects vary from nicks made by the surgeon or pathologist to open cysts and dilated ducts. Commonly, the adipose tissue around the tumor is inadvertently torn as the specimen is removed from the patient, providing another route for ink to run into the specimen. Microscopic sections of such areas may demonstrate tumor close to ink, but this may not represent a true margin of excision. Therefore, careful evaluation of the location of the inked surface on low power microscopic examination should be undertaken.

## Mastectomy Specimens

The methods used for examination of a mastectomy specimen as well as the extent of sampling depend, in part, upon the type of surgical procedure and the reasons for which the procedure was performed. Nonetheless, several aspects of the examination apply to all mastectomy specimens. Ideally, the specimen should be oriented for the pathologist by the surgeon, particularly for mastectomy specimens which do not have a contiguous axillary tail. The following features should be recorded before any mastectomy specimen is incised: the overall dimensions; descriptions and measurements of the skin, areola, nipple, and any incisions or scars; composition of the deep margin, (i.e., presence of fascia or muscle); description of the axillary tail (if present); and the location and size of any palpable tumor, with careful attention paid to its relationship to the overlying skin and deep margin.

Prior to incising the specimen, the deep margin should be painted with ink to facilitate its identification on histologic sections. Further examination of the specimen is best performed by placing the specimen skin side down and making multiple parallel incisions through the deep aspect 1 to 2 cm apart leaving the skin intact. The cut surfaces of each slice should be examined carefully for the presence of grossly evident tumor, biopsy site, or both. If a tumor is identified and tissue has not been previously obtained for hormone receptor and DNA analysis, an aliquot should be sequestered for these studies at this time. The nature of the remaining breast tissue should also be described.

Sampling for histologic examination should include sections of any grossly apparent tumor and/or biopsy site, the deep margin, the overlying skin (including scars), the nipple, and random sections of the grossly unremarkable quadrants of breast tissue. If the specimen is a radical mastectomy (which is uncommon in current practice), the interpectoral fascia should be examined for the presence of Rotter's node.

In a number of situations, more extensive examination of a mastectomy specimen may be required. In patients with ductal carcinoma in situ, particularly those with larger lesions, many sections may be required to determine the presence of stromal invasion, a finding which has major clinical importance. Similarly, extensive sampling may be required to identify a carcinoma in the breast in patients with Paget's disease of the nipple and in patients who present with metastatic carcinoma in an axillary lymph node and an "occult" primary tumor. In these situations, radiography of the mastectomy specimen (either intact or after it has been sectioned) may be of value in directing histologic sampling. Finally, some patients with locally advanced breast cancer undergo chemotherapy and/or radiation therapy prior to mastectomy. It is important for the pathologist to carefully examine the mastectomy specimen to assess the therapeutic response and to document the morphologic effects of treatment on the tumor and on the non-tumorous breast tissue (17).

The interested reader should consult references 36 and 45 for a more detailed account of processing mastectomy specimens.

## Axillary Lymph Nodes

Pathologic evaluation of axillary lymph nodes in patients with breast cancer serves two purposes: to assess prognosis and to determine the need for adjuvant systemic therapy.

A number of different types of axillary lymph node specimens may be encountered by the pathologist. Radical mastectomy and modified radical mastectomy specimens consist of the breast and contiguous axillary tail. Some specimens designated "simple" or "total" mastectomies may also include lower axillary tissue. In most patients treated with breast-conserving therapy, an axillary dissection usually comprises a specimen which is separate from the breast excision specimen. Unless the specimen is a classical radical mastectomy, it is not possible for the pathologist to identify the anatomic location (level) of the lymph nodes received. If it is considered desirable that the final pathology report include this information, the location of the lymph nodes must be designated by the surgeon or lymph nodes from different groups must be submitted as separate specimens.

Any axillary dissection specimen should initially be inspected and palpated. Lymph nodes which are grossly suspicious for metastatic carcinoma should be bisected and a portion obtained for hormone receptor and DNA analysis. A variety of methods are available for further examination of the axillary specimen. The most simple method consists of carefully dissecting the axillary adipose tissue in the fresh state. The number and size range of apparent lymph nodes should be recorded. An alternative method consists of immersing the axillary adipose tissue in Bouin's solution for several hours before attempting to locate the lymph nodes. Using this method, the lymph nodes appear white, in contrast to the adipose tissue which stains yellow. Some investigators have advocated radiographic imaging of the axillary dissection specimen (2,15) or clearing of the axillary adipose tissue with substances such as methyl salicylate to assist in the identification of axillary lymph nodes (11). Although these methods do increase the number of lymph nodes identified, the additional information obtained is of questionable clinical significance. For example, Morrow et al (22) found that by clearing the fat in 42 axillary dissections, there was a 30% increase in the number of lymph nodes identified. However, among 31 patients considered to be node-negative after routine manual nodal dissection, none of the additional lymph nodes identified by clearing the specimen contained metastases. The only patients in whom clearing the axillary fat yielded lymph nodes containing metastases were those already categorized as node-positive by routine nodal dissection. Thus, in this study, clearing the axillary fat added no additional prognostic information. Similar results have been reported by others (18). It can, therefore, be concluded that it is difficult to justify the time and expense required to clear the axillary adipose tissue.

Once lymph nodes have been grossly identified, the pathologist must decide to what extent they should be sampled for microscopic evaluation. In general, small nodes may be bisected and submitted in their entirety. For larger lymph nodes, one representative section per lymph node is the standard of practice at most institutions (36). The clinical value of more extensive microscopic examination of lymph nodes (such as by serial sectioning or by immunohistochemical staining using epithelial cell markers) is an unresolved issue at the present time.

## Mammary Reduction Specimens

Mammary reduction procedures commonly result in hundreds of grams of tissue submitted to the pathologist. The extent to which such specimens should be evaluated microscopically is, in part, a philosophical decision. It could be argued that since the procedure is performed solely for cosmetic reasons, it is unnecessary to submit tissue for microscopic examination. On the other hand, many pathologists consider it prudent to submit some tissue for histologic evaluation. However, the extent to which such specimens should be sampled is unknown since there are few available data on this subject. In one study of 400 mammary reduction specimens from 200 patients, no pathologic abnormalities were found among the specimens from 85 patients less than 30 years of age. In contrast, lobular carcinoma in situ was seen in 8% of the 70 patients over 40 years of age (5). These findings suggest that the extent to which breast reduction specimens should be examined microscopically should, at least in part, be influenced by the patient's age.

## SPECIAL STUDIES

In addition to histologic examination, a number of special studies can be used to evaluate breast tumors. These include estrogen and progesterone receptor analysis, electron microscopy, flow cytometry and other methods to assess DNA content and proliferative rate, immunohistochemical studies for the identification of a broad range of antigens, studies of oncogenes and their products, and morphometric analysis. Nonetheless, careful histologic evaluation remains the cornerstone of diagnosis, and the first priority in processing a breast tumor is to be certain that there is adequate tissue submitted for histologic assessment. In recent years, this has become a considerable practical problem since at many institutions the size of the average breast carcinoma is decreasing at a time when the number of available methods to evaluate these tumors is increasing.

A discussion of each of these special methods and their clinical value is beyond the scope of this chapter, but a few comments regarding estrogen and progesterone receptor analysis are in order since this is currently the most widely applied of these special studies. At this time, the biochemical method for determination of estrogen and progesterone receptor content remains the gold standard. Therefore, if a breast cancer is of sufficient size, an aliquot of tissue should be obtained for this type of analysis. This usually requires 300 to 350 mg of tumor. If the tumor is too small to provide adequate tissue for the biochemical assay, a small portion should be frozen for immunohistochemical evaluation for the presence of these receptors. An alternative method to freezing a portion of the specimen is to obtain a fine needle aspirate or imprint (touch preparation) of the tumor and perform the immunohistochemical receptor assays on these specimens. Although immunohistochemical analysis for estrogen and progesterone receptors can be performed on routinely fixed paraffin sections, the risk of a false negative result is greater than when this procedure is performed on frozen sections or cytologic preparations (7,27,40). Therefore, paraffin sections should be used for estrogen and progesterone receptor analysis only in situations in which there is insufficient tissue for biochemical evaluation and frozen tissue or cytologic preparations are not available.

## REFERENCES

1. Alberhasky MT: Mammographic and gross pathologic analysis of breast needle localization specimens. Use of a tissue analysis device. *Am J Clin Pathol* 1989;92:452–457.
2. Andersen J, Jensen J: Lymph node identification. Specimen radiography of tissue predominated by fat. *Am J Clin Pathol* 1977;68:511–512.
3. Bauermeister DE, McClure HH: Specimen radiography—a mandatory adjunct to mammography. *Am J Clin Pathol* 1973;59:782–789.
4. Bigelow R, Smith R, Goodman PA, et al: Needle localization of nonpalpable breast masses. *Arch Surg* 1985;120:565–569.
5. Bondeson L, Linell F, Ringberg A: Breast reductions: What to do with all the tissue specimens? *Histopathology* 1985;9: 281–285.

6. Carter D: Margins of "lumpectomy" for breast cancer. *Hum Pathol* 1986;17:330–332.
7. Cheng L, Binder SW, Fu YS, Lewin KJ: Demonstration of estrogen receptors by monoclonal antibody in formalin-fixed breast tumors. *Lab Invest* 1988;58:346–353.
8. Colbassani HJ, Feller WF, Cigtay OS, et al: Mammographic and pathologic correlation of microcalcification in disease of the breast. *Surg Gynecol Obstet* 1982;155:689–696.
9. Connolly JL, Schnitt SJ: Evaluation of breast biopsy specimens in patients considered for treatment by conservative surgery and radiation therapy for early breast cancer. *Pathol Annu* 1988;(pt I):1–23.
10. Dershaw DD: Nonpalpable, needle-localized mammographic abnormalities: Pathologic correlation in 219 patients. *Cancer Invest* 1986;4:1–4.
11. Durkin K, Haagensen CD: An improved technique for the study of lymph nodes in surgical specimens. *Ann Surg* 1980;191:419–429.
12. Egan RL, McSweeney MB, Sewell CW: Intramammary calcifications without an associated mass in benign and malignant diseases. *Radiology* 1980;137:1–7.
13. Fisher ER, Sass R, Fisher B, et al: Pathologic findings from the National Surgical Adjuvant Breast Project (Protocol 6). II. Relation of local breast recurrence to multicentricity. *Cancer* 1986;57:1717–1724.
14. Frazier TE, Wong R, Rose D: Implications of accurate pathologic margins in the treatment of primary breast cancer. *Arch Surg* 1989;124:37–38.
15. Groofe AD, Oosterhuis JW, Molenaar WM, et al: Radiographic imaging of lymph nodes in surgical specimens. *Lab Invest* 1985;52:326–329.
16. Hall FM, Storella JM, Silverstone DZ, et al: Nonpalpable breast lesions: recommendations for biopsy based on suspicion of carcinoma at mammography. *Radiology* 1988;167:353–358.
17. Kennedy S, Merino MJ, Swain SM, et al: The effects of hormonal and chemotherapy on tumoral and nonneoplastic breast tissue. *Hum Pathol* 1990;21:192–198.
18. Kingsley WB, Peters GN, Cheek JH: What constitutes adequate study of axillary lymph nodes in breast cancer? *Ann Surg* 1985;201:311–314.
19. Kline TS, Kline IK: *Guides to Clinical Aspiration Biopsy. Breast.* New York, Igaku-Shoin, 1989.
20. McCormick B, Kinne D, Petrek J, et al: Limited reaction for breast cancer: A study of inked specimen margins before radiotherapy. *Int J Radiat Oncol Biol Phys* 1987;13:1667–1671.
21. Meyer JE, Kopans DB, Stomper PC, et al: Occult breast abnormalities: percutaneous preoperative needle localization. *Radiology* 1984;150:335–337.
22. Morrow M, Evans J, Rosen PP, et al: Does clearing of axillary lymph nodes contribute to accurate staging of breast carcinoma? *Cancer* 1984;53:1329–1332.
23. Murphy WA, DeSchryver-Kecskemeti K: Isolated clustered microcalcifications in the breast: radiologic-pathologic correlation. *Radiology* 1978;127:335–341.
24. Oertel YC: *Fine Needle Aspiration of the Breast.* Boston, Butterworths, 1987.
25. Owings D, Hann L, Schnitt SJ: How thoroughly should needle localization breast biopsies be sampled for microscopic examination? A prospective mammographic-pathologic correlative study. *Am J Surg Pathol* 1990;14:578–583.
26. Pathchefsky AS, Potok J, Hoch WS, et al: Increased detection of occult breast carcinoma after more thorough histologic examination of breast biopsies. *Am J Clin Pathol* 1973;60:799–804.
27. Perrot-Applanat M, Groyer-Picard M-T, Hai M, et al: Immunocytochemical staining of progesterone receptor in paraffin sections of human breast cancers. *Am J Pathol* 1989;135:457–468.
28. Powell LW, McSweeney MB, Wilson CE: X-ray calcifications as the only basis for breast biopsy. *Ann Surg* 1983;197:555–559.
29. Price JL, Gibbs NM: The relationship between microcalcification and in situ carcinoma of the breast. *Clin Radiol* 1978;29:447–452.
30. Prorok JJ, Trostle DR, Scarlato M, et al: Excisional breast biopsy and roentgenographic examination for mammographically detected microcalcification. *Am J Surg* 1983;145:684–686.
31. Radi MJ: Calcium oxalate crystals in breast biopsies. An overlooked form of microcalcification associated with benign breast disease. *Arch Pathol Lab Med* 1989;113:1367–1369.
32. Rogers JV, Powell RW: Mammographic indications for biopsy of clinically normal breasts: Correlation with pathologic findings in 72 cases. *AJR* 1972;115:794–800.
33. Rosen PP, Snyder RE: Nonpalpable breast lesions detected by mammography and confirmed by specimen radiography—recent experience. *Breast* 1977;3:13–16.
34. Rosen PP, Snyder RE, Robbins G: Specimen radiography for nonpalpable breast lesions found by mammography: Procedures and results. *Cancer* 1974;34:2028–2033.
35. Roses DF, Harris MN, Gorstein F, et al: Biopsy for microcalcification detected by mammography. *Surgery* 1980;87:248–252.
36. Schmidt WA: *Principles and Techniques of Surgical Pathology.* Menlo Park, Addison-Wesley, 1983, p 362–388.
37. Schmidt-Ullrich R, Wazer DE, Tercilla O, et al: Tumor margin assessment as a guide to optimal conservation surgery and irradiation in early stage breast carcinoma. *Int J Radiat Oncol Biol Phys* 1989;17:733–738.
38. Schnitt SJ, Connolly JL, Khettry U, et al: Pathologic findings on re-excision of the primary site in breast cancer patients considered for treatment by primary radiation therapy. *Cancer* 1987;59:675–681.
39. Schnitt SJ, Wang HH: Histologic sampling of grossly benign breast biopsies. How much is enough? *Am J Surg Pathol* 1989;13:505–512.
40. Shintaku IP, Said JW: Detection of estrogen receptors with monoclonal antibodies in routinely processed formalin-fixed paraffin sections of breast carcinoma. Use of DNase pre-

treatment to enhance sensitivity of the reaction. *Am J Clin Pathol* 1987;87:161–167.

41. Sickles EA: Mammographic features of 300 consecutive nonpalpable breast cancers. *AJR* 1986;146:661–663.
42. Silverstein MJ, Gamagami P, Rosser RJ, et al: Hooked-wire-directed breast biopsy and overpenetrated mammography. *Cancer* 1987;59:715–722.
43. Sneige N, White VA, Katz RL, et al: Ductal carcinoma in situ of the breast: Fine-needle aspiration cytology of 12 cases. *Diag Cytopathol* 1989;5:371–377.
44. Solin LJ, Fowble B, Marz K, et al: Results of re-excisional biopsy of the primary tumor in preparation for definitive irradiation of patients with early stage breast cancer. *Int J Radiat Oncol Biol Phys* 1986;12:721–725.
45. Standardized management of breast specimens. Recommended by pathology working group, breast cancer task force. *Am J Clin Pathol* 1973;60:789–798.
46. Tornos C, Silva EG, El-Naggar A, et al: Calcium oxalate crystals in breast biopsies: The missing microcalcifications. *Am J Surg Pathol* 1990;14:961–968.
47. Wang HH, Ducatman BS, Eick D: Comparative features of ductal carcinoma in situ and infiltrating ductal carcinoma of the breast on fine-needle aspiration biopsy. *Am J Clin Pathol* 1989;92:736–740.
48. Wilkinson EJ, Gnadt JT, Milbrath J, et al: Breast biopsy evaluation by paraffin-block radiography. *Arch Pathol Lab Med* 1978;102:470–473.

# 4

# Benign Lesions



## FIBROCYSTIC CHANGES

### Definition

The term fibrocystic changes (FCC) as used currently refers to a variety of benign mammary alterations which are considered exaggerated physiological phenomena rather than diseases (63). These alterations include gross and microscopic cysts, apocrine metaplasia and hyperplasia, stromal alterations, mild epithelial hyperplasia, and mild degrees of adenosis.

### Historical Perspective

Close to 40 different designations have been used to describe this complex of benign alterations which constitute the most common changes in the female breast. Included in the long list of terms are chronic cystic mastitis, fibrous mastopathy (89), fibroadenosis cystica (107), Schimmelbusch's disease (107), cystiphorous hyperplasia, fibrocystic disease, and mammary displasia, none of which is particularly appropriate. The designation used most commonly in the United States until recently has been "fibrocystic disease;" this term referred not only to the variety of changes listed above in the definition of FCC, but also included proliferative lesions such as sclerosing adenosis, intraductal hyperplasia (ordinary and atypical), and papillomatosis. Unfortunately, this practice implies that all these various alterations develop through the same pathophysiologic process (79). For many years, these proliferative changes have been listed separately in the diagnosis at the Armed Forces Institute of Pathology (AFIP).

It is believed that Sir Benjamin Brodie (22) provided the first detailed clinical and gross pathologic description of FCC in 1846, using the term "benign cystic disease." He gave credit to Sir Astley Cooper for having previously described the same changes. Subsequently, several reports elaborated on these alterations and separated gross cystic changes from nodular adenosis, as well as the clinical pain syndrome (14,23,120). Reclus (102) designated the changes as "Maladie kystique des mammelles" and pointed out the multiplicity and generalized distribution of the cysts, along with either simultaneous or consecutive bilateral involvement of the breasts. Schimmelbusch (107) and Reclus (102) emphasized the histopathologic features of the "disease," and included epithelial hyperplasia as a component of FCC. In the 1920s, because of concern that the epithelial hyperplasia may be a precursor of carcinoma, and possibly due to misinterpretation of some of these proliferative changes as carcinoma, it was not uncommon to perform mastectomy when epithelial proliferation was found in cystic disease. Bloodgood, having reviewed his experience with 1,200 cases of carcinoma and 900 benign breast lesions, concluded that chronic cystic changes are not invariably linked with proliferative changes, and that only infrequently is "chronic cystic mastitis" in any of its forms (purely cystic, proliferative, or mixed patterns) followed by carcinoma (17). Though some of Bloodgood's observations have been questioned (46), he deserves special credit for averting surgeons from performing unnecessary mastectomies, and prompting not only a more conservative approach to the treatment of fibrocystic changes, but also more in depth studies of fibrocystic changes and their components. Almost a decade later, Cheatle and Cutler (25) also pointed out that nodularity in the breast of women with FCC is not necessarily pathologic, but a reflection of cyclic physiologic changes. Separation of the clinical and various pathologic forms of FCC was suggested by various investigators (3,48,98).

Several decades later, Haagensen maintained that microcysts, apocrine metaplasia, and blunt duct adenosis are variations in changes that are normally seen in the breasts of women, while many continued to regard these changes as components of fibrocystic "disease." After many years of debate over the significance of these changes by both pathologists and surgeons (29,32) all over the world, the Cancer Committee of the College of American Pathologists finally proposed in 1986, that "the fibrocystic process in the breast is not a disease, but rather an exaggerated physiologic phenomenon" because of its frequent occurrence in a high proportion of both surgical and autopsy breast specimen (65). Furthermore, the committee suggested separation of these changes from proliferative lesions that are associated with an increased risk for subsequent development of carcinoma (65).

## Incidence

While it is impossible to give a precise incidence of FCC, it has been estimated that over one third of women between 20 to 45 years of age have some clinical evidence of FCC on routine physical examination (73,74,75). Histologic evidence of FCC has been identified in 54% of autopsies of clinically normal breasts (47), 34% of breast biopsies (76), and 40% of all cancer-bearing breasts (110). Interestingly, histologic evidence of cystic changes has been identified in not only 61% of autopsy specimen with grossly evident FCC, but also in 58% of breasts with a grossly normal appearance (11).

## Clinical Features

Fibrocystic changes or cystic disease of the breast generally affects premenopausal women, between 20 and 50 years of age. About 70% to 75% of the women are in their mid-30s to 40s (124). There is cessation of FCC symptomatology about one to two years after menopause unless estrogen replacement therapy is initiated. Fibrocystic changes may involve one breast partially or diffusely. More frequently, it is a multifocal, bilateral disease. Mammographically, the breasts may show a diffuse density secondary to extensive connective tissue proliferation. Many women with FCC have menstrual abnormalities, are nulliparous, give a history of spontaneous abortions, or take no oral contraceptive hormones. Women who have ever taken oral contraceptive hormones have been reported to be at reduced risk for, and less likely to develop, FCC (97). HLA typing of women with FCC has shown a decrease in the frequency of BW 35 antigen among these women (103).

Clinically, three stages or varieties of presentation have been observed, though frequently there is an overlap of the symptoms. In the first stage, referred to clinically as "mazoplasia," women in their mid to late 20s begin to complain of premenstrual breast swelling and/or tenderness of one week's duration (76,124). At this time, the breast tissue may be tender with increased density. During the second stage, clinically referred to as "the stage of adenosis," "the multinodular breast" or "Schimmelbusch's disease," there is gradual development of multiple hard, tender nodules, plaques, and 2 to 3 cm lumps as the patient enters her 30s; at the same time, the duration of the premenstrual pain and tenderness increases to two weeks or more. Finally, in the third stage and as the patient enters her 40s, the breast pain and tenderness becomes a permanent and debilitating problem. Single or multiple large cysts and lumps are easily palpated.

Approximately, 20% of women complain of axillary tenderness, and enlarged nodes are identifiable on palpation. This is thought to be a reaction to the inflammatory infiltrate around the ruptured cysts and their irritative content.

After menopause, the levels of ovarian estrogen secretion become negligible and fibrocystic changes involute, gradually being replaced with adipose and connective tissue. According to Bassler (13), approximately 25% of postmenopausal women between 60 and 80 years of age have FCC at autopsy, but only 10% are symptomatic. The postmenopausal FCC is generally due to the use of estrogen replacement therapy (118). In obese women, however, peripheral conversion of androstenedione to estrone in adipose tissue is an important source of estrogens that may sustain fibrocystic changes.

## Etiology, Pathophysiology, and Risk Factors

It appears that the hormonal milieu in which the breasts exist contributes significantly to the development of FCC (50). The risk of developing FCC appears to be increased in women with ovarian dysfunctions that result in a predominance or relative excess of estrogenic hormones. In 1941, Geschikter (48) postulated hyperestrogenism as the factor responsible for the development of breast nodularity. Based on animal studies, he subsequently suggested that hormonal imbalances causing a relative hyperestrogenism during the luteal phase is the crucial factor; he was able to induce adenosis in rats by giving them large doses of estrone. The role of hormonal alterations in the induction of FCC has been supported by subsequent investigators (69). Comparison of plasma estradiol (E2), progesterone (P), and prolactin levels of women with fibrocystic changes and women with normal ovulatory cycles, has shown elevated or normal E2, lowered P, and similar prolactin levels, suggesting that an imbalance of E2 and P levels may play a role in the induction of fibrocystic changes (111).

Estrogens induce proliferation of connective tissue and development of ductal epithelial cells, while progesterone brings about the development of normal lobular-ductal-alveolar structures. Ordinarily, the estrogenic influences over the connective tissues precede and predominate over the epithelial changes (124). Hyperestrogenism has also been implicated in the induction of extensive stromal fibrosis (119). The stromal fibrosis causes obstruction of ductules, and persistence of cyclic epithelial secretion results in gradual dilatation of the obstructed ductules and cyst formation. The cysts are most frequently microscopic, but gross cysts are observed in 20% to 40% of patients with fibrocystic changes (124). The cyst fluid contains proteins, a variety of steroid and polypeptide hormones, glucose, cholesterol, and minerals. The cyst fluid may be resorbed by phagocytic histiocytes; calcification of the contents occurs in 25% of cases (124).

Methylxanthines (coffee, tea, cola drinks, and chocolate) intake has also been implicated as playing a role in the development of fibrocystic changes by some (91), but avoidance of these substances appeared to have no influence on the development and course of fibrocystic changes in other studies (124).

## Macroscopic Features

The specimen generally shows several blue-domed or clear cysts, a majority of which do not exceed 1 to 2 mm in size. The cysts are randomly distributed in a fibrofatty tissue. Larger cysts about 1 to 2 cm in diameter are seen less frequently.

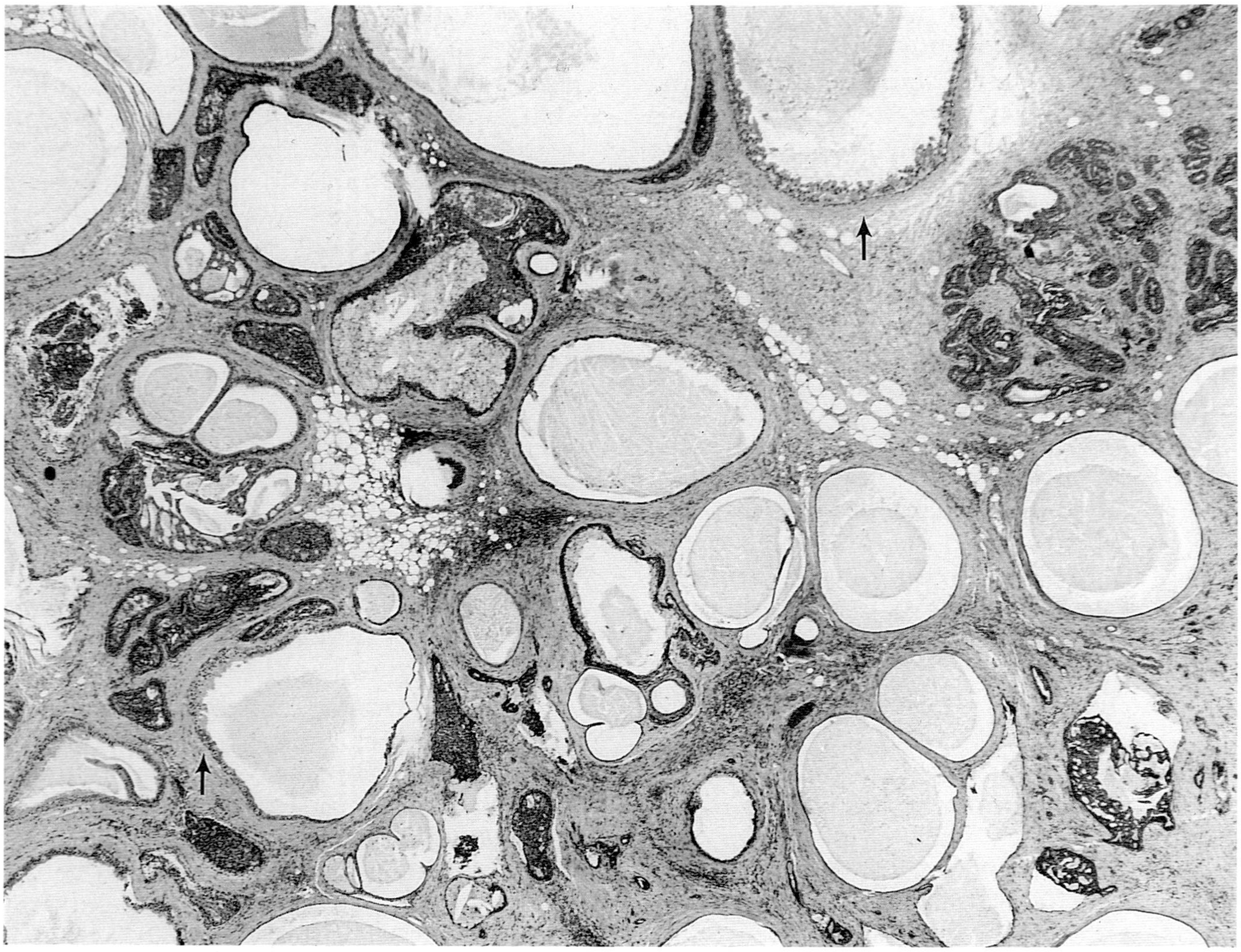

**Figure 4.1** Fibrocystic changes with intraductal hyperplasia (IDH). The presence of numerous dilated cysts is characteristic. Some of the cysts are lined by an attenuated epithelium, while others have a metaplastic apocrine (arrow) cell lining. There is also intraductal hyperplasia present in several ducts. (H&E, X20)

## Microscopic Features

Fibrocystic changes consist of a group of cystically dilated round to ovoid spaces lined by slightly attenuated epithelial and myoepithelial cell layers. The intralobular stroma is often sclerotic and indistinguishable from the surrounding interlobular stroma. The mild cystic changes in the TDLU are the equivalent of cystic lobular involution (9,60). As these cystic changes progress, there is gradual coalescence of the smaller cysts or actually unfolding of the lobule resulting in the formation of a larger cyst. These cysts are either lined by the native epithelial/myoepithelial lining, albeit in a more attenuated form, or they are lined by metaplastic apocrine cells (Fig. 4.1) which may simply replace the single epithelial cell layer or form epithelial tufts and papillae. The rupture of these cysts incites an inflammatory infiltrate and eventually the reparative changes cause fibrosis in the region. Adenosis, a microscopic expansion of the lobules by an increase in the number of ductules or acini per lobule, is also seen as part of the spectrum of changes in FCC. Adenosis often maintains a lobular outline, but sometimes it displays an irregular outline.

These cystic changes should be distinguished from cystic lobular involution and duct ectasia which also cause cystic structures in the breast. Both cystic lobular involution and cystic changes take place in the lobules, while duct ectasia is a disease of the extralobular ducts. The persistence of recognizable lobular stroma associated with cystic involution distinguishes involutional changes from early stages of cystic change, but this distinction is not always clearcut and may no longer be relevant since fibrocystic changes are now considered an exaggeration of physiologic changes anyway.

## Composition of Cyst Fluid

A variety of electrolytes, hormones, and proteins have been identified in the cyst fluid. The electrolyte concentration greatly exceeds that in plasma (19). The type of cyst lining correlates with the electrolyte composition of cyst fluid (36). Apocrine cysts have high potassium and low sodium concentrations, while cysts lined by attenuated cells contain a high concentration of sodium and low levels of potassium. The former contain IgA predominantly in the 11S form, while the latter contain IgA in the 7S form. IgG is also present in higher concentrations in the cysts lined by attenuated epithelium. Calcitonin, prolactin, human chorionic gonadotropin, androsterone, epiandrosterone, dehydroepiandrosterone, and its conjugates are all present in cyst fluid in higher levels compared to those in plasma (20). Carcinoembryonic antigen, progesterone binding protein, and a series of glycoproteins are also present in the cyst fluid in concentrations exceeding those in the plasma (34). A variety of proteins designated as gross cystic disease fluid protein (GCDFP) have also been isolated from these cysts; these will be discussed in more detail in the section on apocrine metaplasia.

## Relationship of Fibrocystic Changes to Breast Carcinoma

Many investigators in the past have looked at the relationship of cystic disease to cancer (39,53,59,64, 67,70,105,121). With few exceptions, much of the older published data regarding the relationship of fibrocystic changes to breast carcinoma is conflicting and confusing. One reason for the conflicting viewpoints is that, until recently, all degrees of intraductal epithelial hyperplasia were included in the spectrum of FCC. Therefore, depending on the proportion of cases with epithelial hyperplasia and their type (ordinary vs atypical), investigators arrived at different conclusions regarding the clinical significance of FCC as a cancer risk factor. According to a variety of reports, the risk for developing breast carcinoma in women with FCC is around 1.7 to 4.5 times that of the general population; and in many of these reports, the increasing incidence has been related to the presence of epithelial hyperplasia (29,54,59,64,67,76,96,105, 125). More recent studies (96,115) have confirmed that it is not necessarily the presence of cystic changes, but rather the presence of moderate to severe epithelial (non-apocrine) hyperplasia, with or without atypia, within the ducts and lobules that is associated with an increased risk for subsequent development of carcinoma. Mild degrees of hyperplasia (when the epithelial proliferation is more than two, but not more than four cells deep) are extremely common in the breast and do not constitute a risk factor (95).

The risk for subsequent development of breast carcinoma is very low for FCC with only mild or no epithelial hyperplasia, compared with the risk of women from Atlanta (Third National Cancer Survey). In Dupont & Page's study (39), women with nonproliferative changes had a relative risk of 0.89 overall. Those with nonproliferative changes and no family history of breast carcinoma in a first-degree relative (mother, sister, daughter) had a risk of 0.86; the risk increased to 1.2 with a positive family history. When gross cysts were present in patients with nonproliferative lesions, the relative risk was 1.5, but it increased to 3.0 in patients who had gross cysts and a positive family history of breast carcinoma. Ciatto et al (26) also noted that the presence of gross cysts is associated with an increased risk for subsequent development of carcinoma; the observed to expected subsequent carcinoma ratio was 1.77.

In response to the accumulated data regarding the risk associated with proliferative changes, the Cancer Committee of the College of American Pathologists (65) subdivided patients with benign breast diseases into three major risk categories compared with women having no biopsies: I. no increased risk; II. slightly increased risk (1.5 to 2.0×); III. moderately increased risk (4 to 5×). Fibrocystic changes with apocrine cysts and mild epithelial hyperplasia (as previously described) fall into category I. The presence of intraductal hyperplasia without atypia in the biopsy designates the patient in category II with a slightly increased risk for subsequent development of carcinoma; sclerosing adenosis is also associated with a slightly increased risk (142) and has been added to this category subsequent to the publication of the consensus report. Finally, the presence of atypical intraductal hyperplasia designates the patient at moderately increased risk and in category III.

Using these risk categories, Mongeau et al (91) found subsequent carcinoma in only 5% of category I lesions. The risk for subsequent development of carcinoma in women with FCC is considered to be similar to that of the general population; therefore, no special follow-up of these women is required.

## Explanation of Relative Risk

*(See Also Chapter 2)*

A woman's relative risk reflects the risk of developing invasive carcinoma in a given time interval compared to women of the same age in the general population; it does not represent the lifetime risk (40). The statistics indicating that one in nine women (11%) will develop breast carcinoma reflect a lifetime incidence. When a pathology report states that the presence of intraductal hyperplasia in a 30-year-old woman is associated with a relative risk of two times that of general population, it does not imply that the patient's absolute risk is $2 \times 1/9 = 22\%$. For women 30 or 60 years of age in the United States, the age-specific incidence of breast carcinoma is 27.5 and 292 cases per year, per 100,000 women, respectively. The relative risk for a 30-year-old woman with intraductal carcinoma to develop invasive carcinoma is ten times the general population. Therefore, the chance for developing invasive carcinoma is obtained by multiplying $10 \times 27.5 = 275$/year/100,000 women (40).

## Treatment of Fibrocystic Changes

Nonsurgical treatment of FCC is directed at providing symptomatic relief, and preventing progression of the disease, with eventual softening of the breast tissue. Since patients on oral contraceptives and those with regular menses and ovulation are protected from developing FCC (21), oral contraceptives have been used for treatment of FCC with success rates of up to 70% to 90% (7,21,43). Use of oral or percutaneous progesterone during the luteal phase of the cycle has also resulted in improvement of FCC in around 80% to 85% of the patients (71,79,85,124). Oral progesterone has been variably reported to be effective in management and relief of mastalgia (27,31), or worse than a placebo (101).

Other hormones have also been used with variable results in the treatment of FCC. Bromocriptine, a prolactin antagonist, has been used to restore the normal luteal phase and in the treatment of premenstrual syndrome with improvements in the breast symptoms (4,16,38,41,83,84,128). Unpleasant side effects including nausea and vomiting, dizziness, and headaches were observed in 30% of the patients in one report (40).

Danazol, a synthetic (2,3 isoxazol) derivative of 17-alpha-ethinyl-testosterone, has also been used for treatment of FCC (15,37,52,72,82,117). It directly affects the hypothalamic-pituitary function, several types of steroid receptors, and gonadal steroid production (10), but the precise mechanism by which it influences FCC is not clear. Side effects of danazol include menstrual irregularities, voice changes, increased facial hair, and weight gain.

Tamoxifen, known to compete for estrogen receptors in target tissue, has been used in treatment of patients with severe breast "dysplasia." A relatively high proportion of women treated with tamoxifen have experienced complete remission or showed improvements clinically (104,109).

Less commonly used hormones include thyroxine (45), human chorionic gonadotropin hormone (92), and androgens (8). In small studies, vitamin E was initially reported to reduce tenderness and cyst size and clinical improvement of symptoms (1,78,113), but subsequent randomized, double-blind, controlled studies failed to show any significant improvement with vitamin E therapy (44,80).

Total or subcutaneous mastectomy should rarely if ever be considered as a serious option in the management of patients with severe, nodular FCC. One of the reasons for considering prophylactic mastectomy has been that the density of the breast tissue along with the degree of nodularity preclude a reliable follow-up and assessment of the breasts for the development of subsequent carcinoma both clinically and mammographically. In this regard, it should be emphasized that menopause will cause mammary tissue changes that facilitate the follow-up process in patients with FCC unless the patients are put on estrogen replacement therapy. Furthermore, subcutaneous mastectomy does not remove all of the breast tissue; it has been estimated that 5% of the breast tissue remains after subcutaneous mastectomy (116).

Also, even the minimal amounts left behind following a careful subcutaneous mastectomy can give rise to carcinoma (42,49,51,62,99). This procedure might give the patient a false sense of security that may prevent her from paying careful attention to alterations in the residual breast tissue. A recent study has shown that even total mastectomy leaves behind breast tissue within the superficial pectoralis major muscle and the lower skin flap (116).

## METAPLASIAS
## APOCRINE METAPLASIA

Also referred to as pale cells (29), pink epithelium (77), and "pink cells" (18), apocrine cells reflect a metaplastic alteration of the native epithelial cells and are a component of fibrocystic changes. Metaplastic apocrine cells often display a columnar configuration with abundant granular, eosinophilic cytoplasm and luminal cytoplasmic projections or "apical snouts." Sometimes the cells contain crescents of coarse, PAS-positive, glycolipid granules slightly beneath the luminal margin of the cytoplasm (Fig. 4.2). Rarely, lipofucsin granules are found admixed with the glycolipid granules (9). More frequently a small vacuole occasionally containing a yellow-brown pigment is present in the supranuclear position; iron pigment has been identified in some of these vacuoles (18), or among the glycolipid granules (9). The nuclei are round, basally to centrally located, and often contain a prominent nucleolus.

Haagensen (53) actually believed that the apocrine breast epithelium is derived embryologically from the apocrine axillary sweat glands. It has now been established, however, that apocrine metaplasia has its origin in the terminal duct-lobular unit in most cases (9,122,127), and appears to be the progenitor of FCC (55). The presence of apocrine metaplasia in papillomas located within the lactiferous ducts, however, indicates that not all metaplastic apocrine cells are lobular in origin.

### Frequency of Apocrine Metaplasia

In histologic reviews of autopsy material from "normal" breasts, apocrine epithelium has been identified in 20% to 85% of women (28,47,94,112,126). The lowest figure of 20% was from an autopsy of 100 women aged 50 to 104 years; the highest figure of 85% is from an autopsy series of 88 women aged 20 to 54. Obviously apocrine metaplasia is far more common among the younger age group, but no apocrine change was found in women 13 to 19 years of age with clinically normal breasts in two separate autopsy studies (47,126).

### Apocrine Metaplasia and Hyperplasia as a Risk Factor

Wellings et al (126) studied apocrine metaplasia in 293 whole human breasts by a subgross sampling technique. They concluded that extensive apocrine metaplasia in papillary formations appears to be more common in breasts with cancer, and that it is a useful marker for tissue at a slightly increased risk for subsequent development of breast cancer, but metaplastic apocrine epithelium has little intrinsic malignant potential. Further assessment of the significance of apocrine metaplasia as a risk factor is needed to confirm Wellings et al's suggestions.

Cystic apocrine change has been noted more frequently (83%) in cancer-associated breasts, compared to 52% of normal breasts (126). Apocrine cysts are also more numerous in the cancer-associated breasts (126). Based on these findings, Wellings and Alpers concluded that metaplastic apocrine change reflects a significant epithelial unrest associated with carcinoma (126).

Apocrine metaplasia and grossly visible cysts are also present in a high proportion of biopsies with intraductal hyperplasia with or without atypia. Among 117 cases with ordinary intraductal hyperplasia, 87% had apocrine metaplasia, and 58% had grossly visible cysts; among 82 cases of atypical intraductal hyperplasia, 82% had apocrine metaplasia, and 56% had visible cysts (115). Because this study was designed to evaluate ordinary and atypical intraductal hyperplasias of the non-apocrine type, however, the apocrine changes were always found in association with other types of intraductal hyperplasia. Therefore, the risk of subsequent development of carcinoma related to apocrine metaplasia alone could not be assessed, although among 142 women with apocrine hyperplasia (which included women with

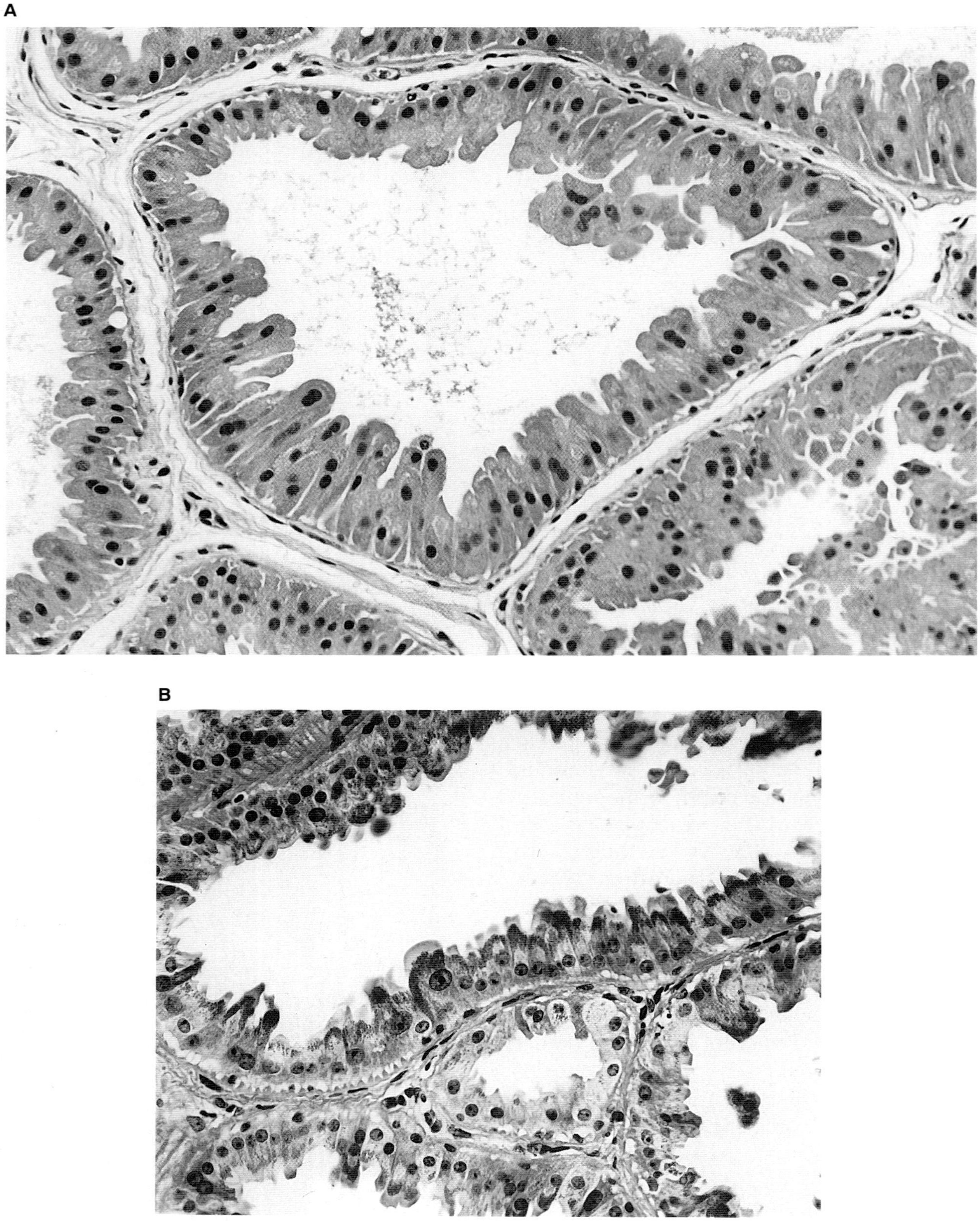


**Figure 4.2** Apocrine metaplasia. (a) The cells are columnar with abundant granular, pink cytoplasm and round, basally-located nuclei. Minimal tufting of the cells is evident. (b) The apocrine cells sometimes display a crescent of PAS-positive coarse granules close to the luminal margin. The nuclei show prominent nucleoli. (H&E, (a) X300; (b) PAS, X300)

c

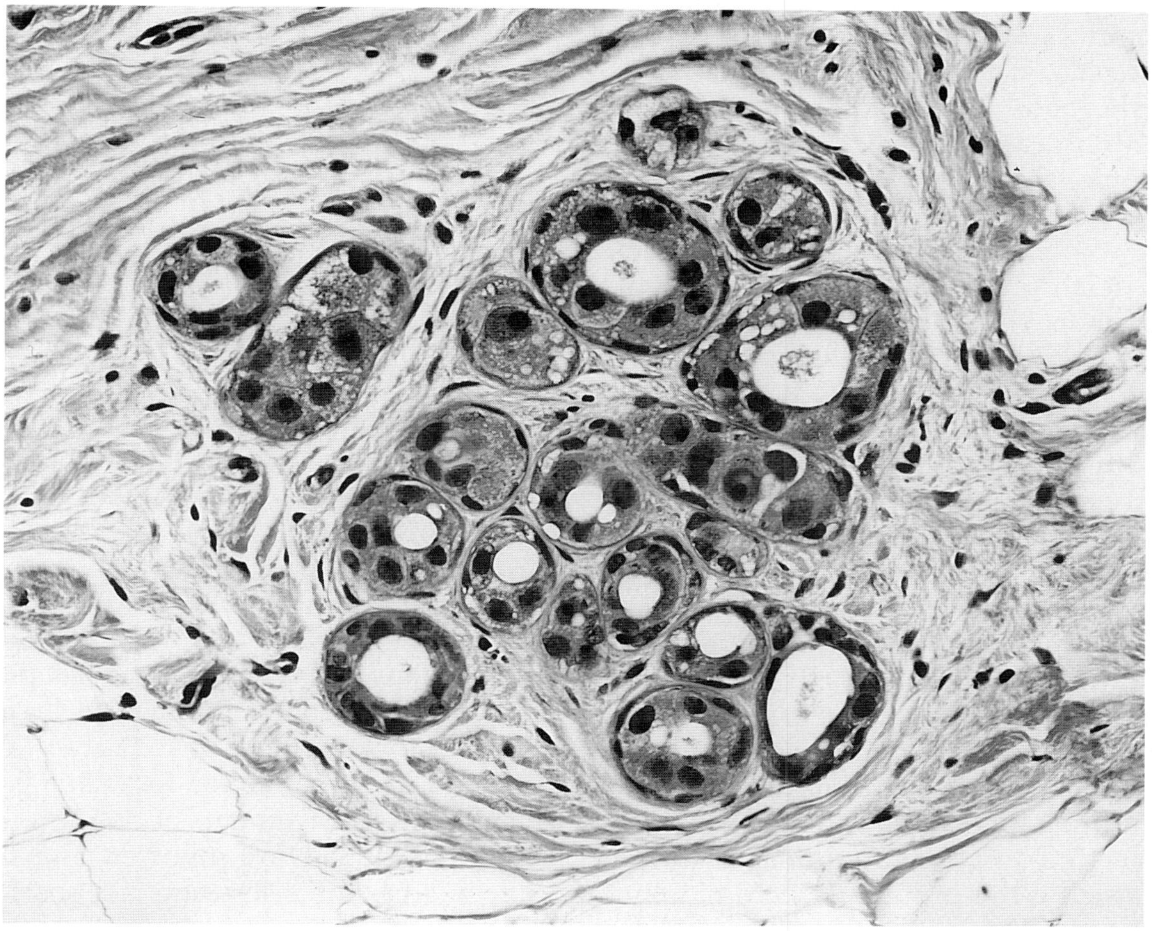

**Figure 4.2(c)** Apocrine metaplasia. Atypical apocrine metaplasia shows a three to fourfold variation in the size of the nuclei. (H&E, X480)

both ordinary and atypical non-apocrine hyperplasia), 4.1% subsequently developed carcinoma.

Haagensen (55) suggested three possible roles for apocrine metaplasia. First is that apocrine metaplasia may be a precursor to malignant transformation. The second possibility is that it reflects a response to the same stimulus that can also induce carcinoma. Finally, these changes may have a higher propensity for malignant changes.

## Atypical Apocrine Metaplasia

Either simple metaplastic or hyperplastic apocrine cells may display cytologic atypia. To qualify as atypical apocrine metaplasia or atypical apocrine hyperplasia, the nuclei should at least display a threefold variation in size (Fig. 4.2c). The presence of nucleolar prominence alone is not an indication of atypicality. Occasionally, mitotic figures are also present. Atypical apocrine metaplasia is most often encountered in the setting of a papilloma (frequently a sclerosing papilloma) and sclerosing adenosis (132).

Presence of papillary apocrine cell hyperplasia or tufting is not as worrisome as the finding of epithelial bridges formed by metaplastic apocrine cells. A cribriform arrangement by metaplastic apocrine cells is always worrisome and should be carefully assessed for the possibility of intraductal carcinoma; the cribriform pattern of intraductal apocrine carcinoma may not be associated with significant cytologic atypia. Follow-up of women with atypical metaplasia, as defined here, is advised.

## Gross Cystic Disease Fluid Protein (GCDFP)

A group of proteins between 15,000 to 44,000 kD in size and designated as gross cystic disease fluid protein (GCDFP) has been isolated from cyst fluid of the breast (56,57). Immunocytochemically, these proteins have been localized mainly in all normal apocrine glands in the body as well as in metaplastic apocrine cells of the breast (24,86,87). About 50% of mammary carcinomas also show a positive immunoreaction for GCDFP-15 (55). Since normal breast epithelium does not elaborate GCDFP-15, the hypothesis may be put forth that breast carcinomas that express this protein have either acquired apocrine-like functions or are derived from the metaplastic apocrine cells (55).

Normal apocrine glands in experimental animal are trophically stimulated by androgens and inhibited by estrogens. In cultures of breast cancer cells, estrogens decrease or inhibit the production of GCDFP-15, while they stimulate cell division, whereas, androgens inhibit cell division while stimulating the production of GCDFP-15. In clinical studies, Halostatin (androgen) most dramatically influences (increases) blood levels of GCDFP-15 in patients with metastatic breast carcinoma whose baseline levels of GCDFP-15 were abnormal from the start. This finding suggests that the androgenic stimulation is effective only for carcinomas that are capable of synthesizing the protein (33,58). Finally, it has been suggested that the selector gene controlling apocrine metaplasia may also coordinate cell kinetics and the response to specific hormones and growth factors (58). Therefore, one of the changes during the oncogenesis of breast carcinomas with apocrine features, probably involves activation of the selector gene for apocrine metaplasia (58). These findings are fascinating, and hopefully continued studies in this area will unravel some of the mysteries of carcinogenesis in the breast.

### Ultrastructural Features and Ploidy

At the ultrastructural level, apocrine cells have distinct cell margins with widely-spaced microvilli along the luminal margin. The mitochondria are of various sizes and shapes and are distributed throughout, dominating in the basal aspect of the cell; they display scant or incomplete cristae that do not extend into the central area (2,6,93,100).

The apocrine cells contain a tetraploid cell population; the proportion of the tetraploid cells increases with the degree of hyperplasia of the metaplastic cells (66).

## CLEAR CELL METAPLASIA

In 1980, attention was focused on the presence of clear cell change in mammary ducts and lobules by Barwick and Rosen (12). This change is characterized by extensive clearing of the epithelial cell cytoplasm, and its recognition is important to prevent its misinterpretation as clear cell carcinoma, primary or metastatic. Clear cell changes occur in about 1.6% of breast biopsies (123); patients range in age from 30 to 71 years with a median of 47 years.

### Pathologic Features

The lesions are generally microscopic in size and are therefore incidental findings in breast biopsies performed for other reasons. Microscopically, clear cell metaplasia presents as a focal change, with partial or complete involvement of lobules. In most cases, multiple lobules are involved and the changes also affect areas of sclerosing adenosis. The clear cell change does not alter the basic unit structure of the ductules within the acini. The lobules involved by clear cell metaplasia are often enlarged because these metaplastic cells are generally larger than the native epithelial cell population; clear cell metaplasia may also involve areas of sclerosing adenosis (Fig. 4.3). The cytoplasm of these cells is clear and abundant; rarely, it may appear foamy or vacuolated. A few PAS positive granules may be identified within the cytoplasm; these are partially removed by diastase predigestion. The cytoplasm is mucicarmine and alcian blue negative. The slightly eccentrically-located nuclei are small and round, without nucleolar prominence. The lumens of the ductules may be open or obliterated, but almost never distended. Sometimes these cells extend in a pagetoid fashion into adjacent ductules and in this setting can be easily confused with a myoepithelial cell layer; the cells fail to react with either actin or S-100 protein, however. The possibility that clear cell metaplasia reflects an eccrine type of differentiation has been suggested, but these clear cells look somewhat different from the eccrine clear cell population that is rarely seen in some breast adenomas.

At the ultrastructural level, multiple coalescing empty rounded spaces are present in the epithelial cells. The myoepithelial cell layer is retained and also shows similar empty spaces; the vacuoles are very small in number and size, however. The vacuoles sometimes indent the nucleus, but often simply push the nucleus aside. Glycogen granules are not identified in the vacuoles.

None of the patients with clear cell metaplasia is known to have had concurrent, or developed subsequent, clear cell carcinoma.

## LACTATIONAL METAPLASIA

### Lactational Changes in Nonlactating, Nonpregnant Women

Occasionally, lactational changes identical to those observed during pregnancy and lactation are seen in the breast of women who are neither pregnant nor lactating (88,114). Some of these patients have never been pregnant and may, in fact, be many years postmenopausal. Lactational metaplasia has been observed in both autopsy and surgical specimen in around 3% to 3.7% of cases (47,68,106). It occurs predominantly in women, but has also been reported in a 61-year-old man taking stilbestrol (114). The patients range in age from 21 to 87 years. The changes are generally incidental microscopic findings in biopsies performed for other lesions.

### Microscopic Features

Lactational metaplasia is a focal change that generally affects several lobules, and resembles the Arias-Stella (5) changes in the endometrium. It assumes two forms. In the first variety, there is abundant secretory material within the dilated acini which are lined by plump cells with notable cytoplasmic vacuolization and small rounded nuclei (Fig. 4.4). In the second (regressive) type, the cytoplasmic vacuolization is minimal, many cells show a hobnail appearance. The nuclei range from large and irregularly shaped to pyknotic and smudged in appearance. The acini are distended and contain detached cells and minimal amounts of secretory material (Fig. 4.5).

Both cell types are negative for mucicarmine and alcian blue except for the apical portions of the cells reflecting glycocalyceal staining. Both contain PAS positive granules before and after digestion with diastase. The intraluminal secretory material is mucin and PAS positive.

### Etiology

Three possible etiologies have been mentioned for lactational metaplasia: 1) persistent lactational changes from previous pregnancy; 2) exogenous hormonal induction; 3) "selective susceptibility" of mammary lobules (68). Though conceivable, it is unlikely that lactational changes would persist or only partially regress many years after a pregnancy in a dynamic tissue like breast that is subject to hormonal influences. Furthermore, the presence of lactational metaplasia in one male patient and a nulliparous woman indicates that at least some of the cases are definitely not residual lactational alterations from a previous pregnancy, and involve other mechanisms. It is quite likely, however, that breast lobules are selectively susceptible to developing sporadic lactational changes; some lobules may be more sensitive with a tendency to develop lactational changes even in response to the normal levels of nongravid endogenous hormones.

The potential of exogenous hormones to induce focal lactational changes is well known (63,100,127). Women receiving estrogens for advanced breast carcinoma develop lactational changes (63). The finding of lactational changes in a 61-year-old male on stilbestrol, supports the role of exogenous hormones in the induction of these changes in some patients (114). Furthermore, among patients showing lactational metaplasia, those who were taking premarin showed more diffuse changes (114).

Nonhormonal drugs have also been noted to cause lactational changes. Lactational changes have been observed more commonly in women taking digitalis, dilantin, and reserpine (127). Reserpine stimulates prolactin secretion, which influences the mammary morphology. Neuroleptic agents are also known for stimulating prolactin secretion (61), and inducing lactational changes in the rat mammary glands (100). Thioridazine has been reported to induce lactation in up to 26% of patients who take it (61).

A

B

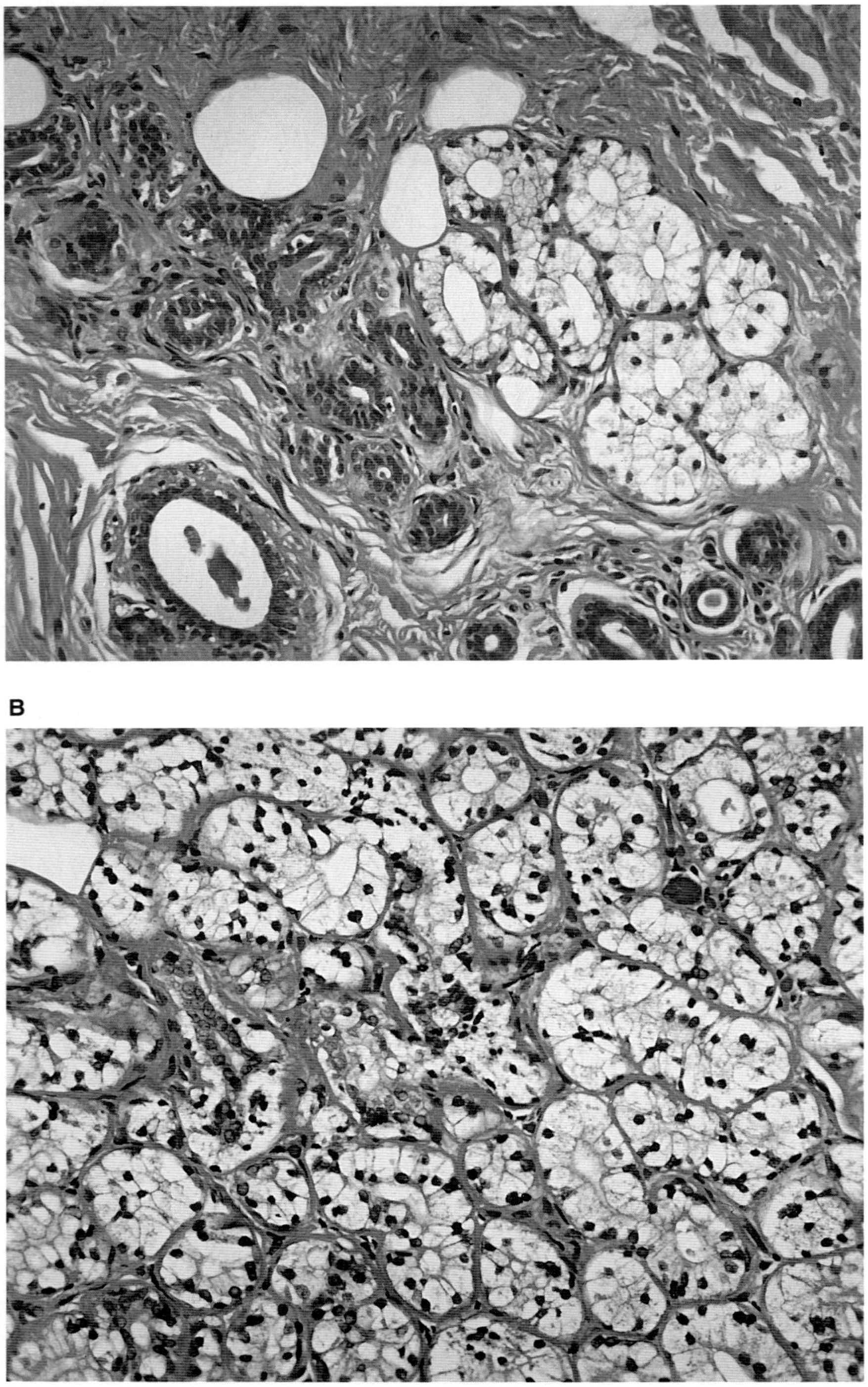

**Figure 4.3** Clear cell metaplasia. (a) The acinar epithelial cells are transformed to clear cells with abundant cytoplasm and small, rounded eccentrically or basally-located nuclei. (b) Clear cell metaplasia affecting an area of adenosis. (H&E, (a) X250; (b) X250) (Reproduced from Tavassoli FA, Yeh I: *Am J Clin Pathol* 1987;87:23–29, with permission.)

C

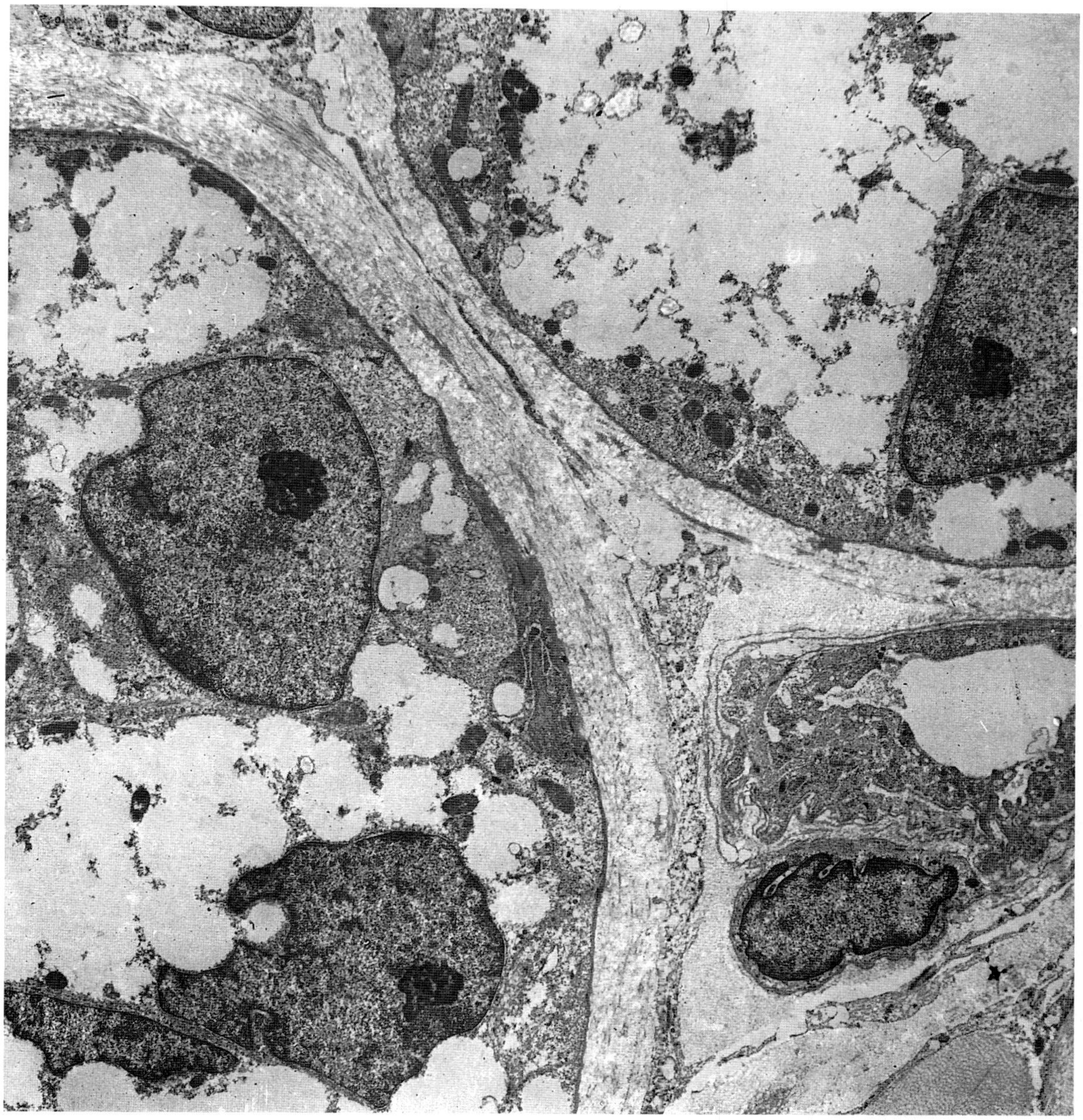

**Figure 4.3(c)** Clear cell metaplasia. At the ultrastructural level, there are numerous coalescing empty, rounded spaces in the epithelial cells; a small vacuole is present in a myoepithelial cell as well. (Uranyl acetate-lead citrate, X2,800)

## OTHER EPITHELIAL METAPLASIAS

Less commonly, the epithelial cells undergo squamous or mucinous metaplasia. The squamous metaplasia is often seen around areas of infarction in a papilloma, whereas mucinous metaplasia occurs most often within otherwise unaltered lobules.

## ADENOSIS

Adenosis in its most simple form reflects what appears as an expansion of the lobules with an increased number of ductules or acini within the lobule. Also referred to as blunt duct adenosis, this simple microscopic lesion is considered a component of

A

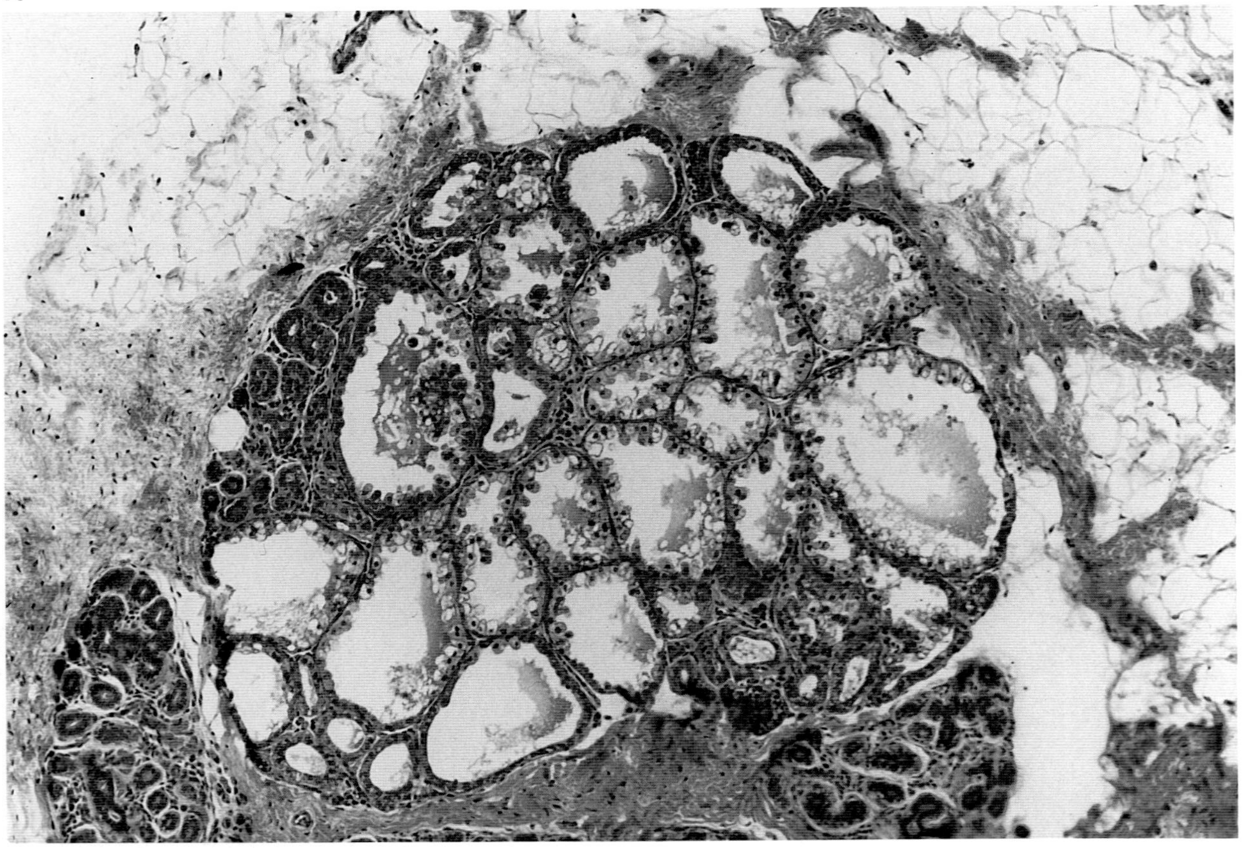

B

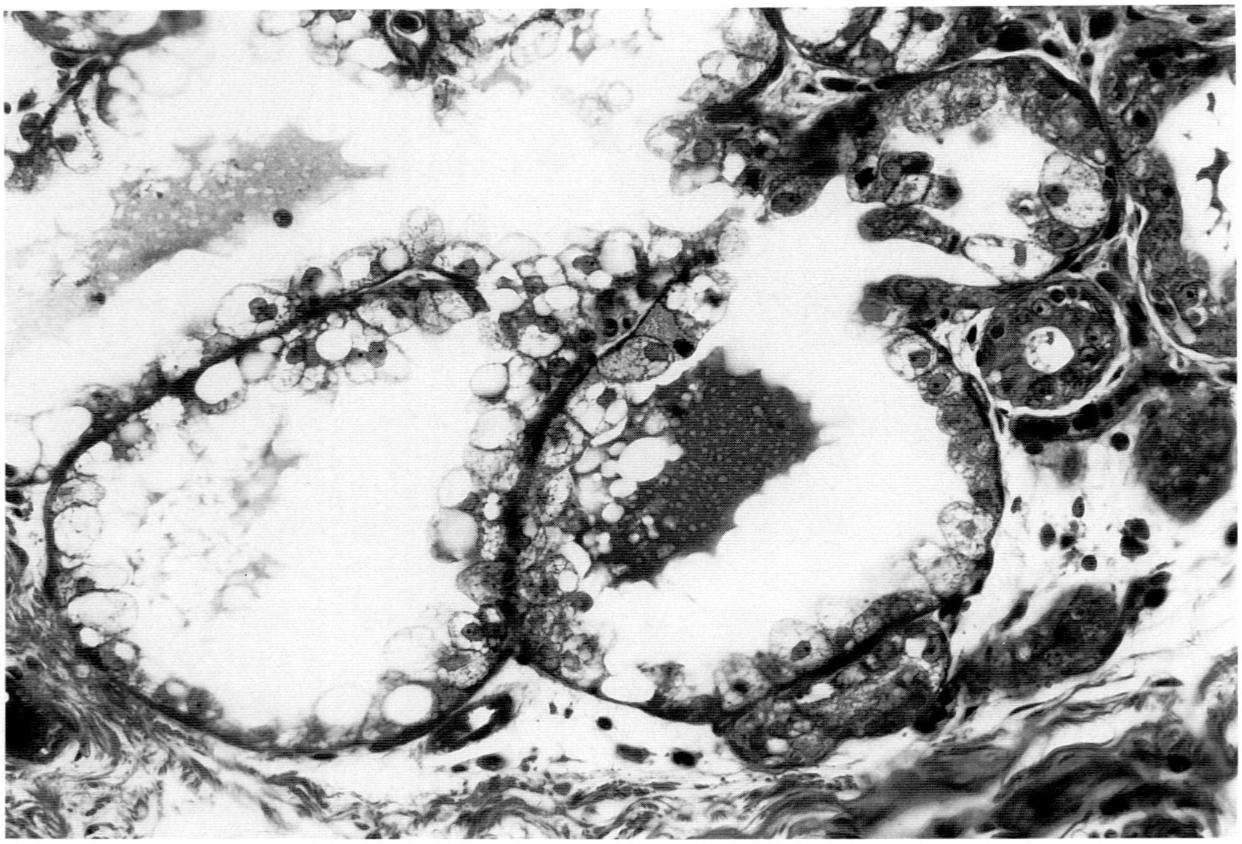

**Figure 4.4** (a) Lactational change partially involving a mammary lobule. (H&E, X150) (b) The distended acini contain secretory material and are lined by vacuolated secretory cells. (H&E, X600) (Figure (a) reproduced from Tavassoli FA, Yeh I: *Am J Clin Pathol* 1987;87:23–29, with permission.)

A

B

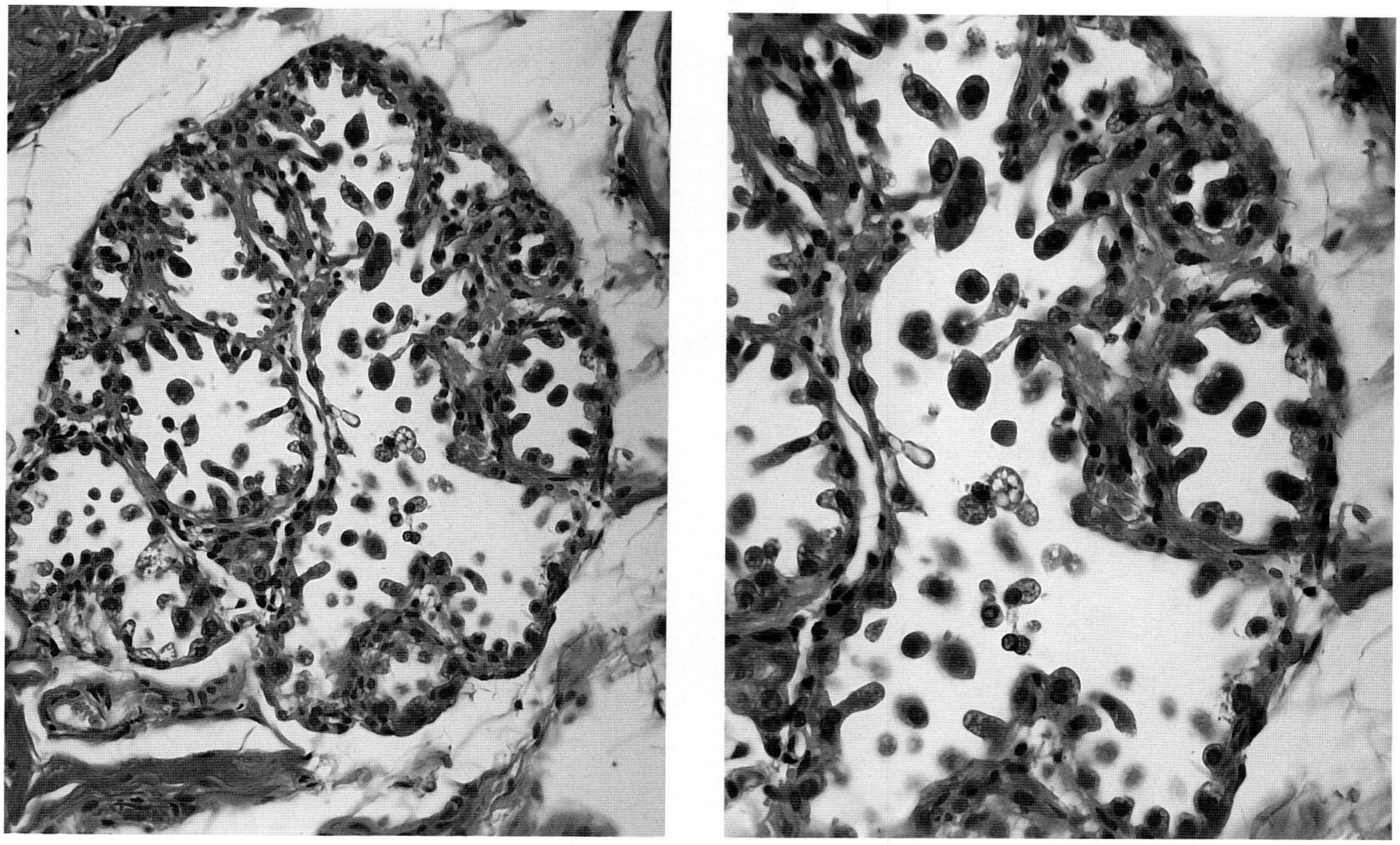

**Figure 4.5** Lactational change, regressive type. (a) The cells have a hobnail appearance. (H&E, X250) (b) The distended acini contain detached cells, some of which are multinucleated. (H&E, X400) (Figure (a) reproduced from Tavassoli FA, Yeh I: *Am J Clin Pathol* 1987;87:23–29, with permission.)

FCC. The reason for its inclusion in the complex of FCC is that it may reflect a failure of physiologic lobular hyperplasia of pregnancy to regress. It is found in 6.2% to 16.7% of female breasts in autopsy series (47,153). It may form conspicuous nodules for which the designation of nodular adenosis is appropriate (Fig. 4.6).

## SCLEROSING ADENOSIS

Recognized since the 1940s as a benign lobulocentric lesion (46,136,160), sclerosing adenosis is notable for its ability to mimic infiltrating carcinoma grossly and microscopically (140,160). Even its mammographic patterns of calcification may mimic that of carcinoma (145). Some have speculated that sclerosing adenosis (SA) reflects an abnormal pattern of age-related regression or an involutional process following lactation (131,156). Others consider SA to be a proliferative process (129,150,157). Using stereomicroscopic techniques with subsequent tissue correlation, Tanaka and Oota (157) suggested that SA consists of parallel arrays of ductules which sprout from a large duct and run parallel to the stem duct or curve around it, and end in bouquet-like structures simulating a lobule. These proliferating tubules often grow around the stem duct, may extend into the ducts, or may be distributed both around and in the ducts.

In its pure form, SA has been seen in 3.1% of female breasts at autopsy. Among surgical specimen, it has been observed in 12.2% to 12.5% of noncancerous, and 5.3% to 7% of cancerous breasts (46,154).

Occasionally, SA forms large nodules, around 2 to 2.5 cm in diameter that are either clinically palpable or grossly visible (141). At AFIP, we prefer to designate these lesions as nodular sclerosing adenosis. The term "adenosis tumor" (148) has also been used, among a variety of other designations, to refer to this type of lesion (130,140–142,149,154,156,160). Nodular sclerosing adenosis occurs in a wide age range, with a majority of the patients between 30 and 45 years of

A

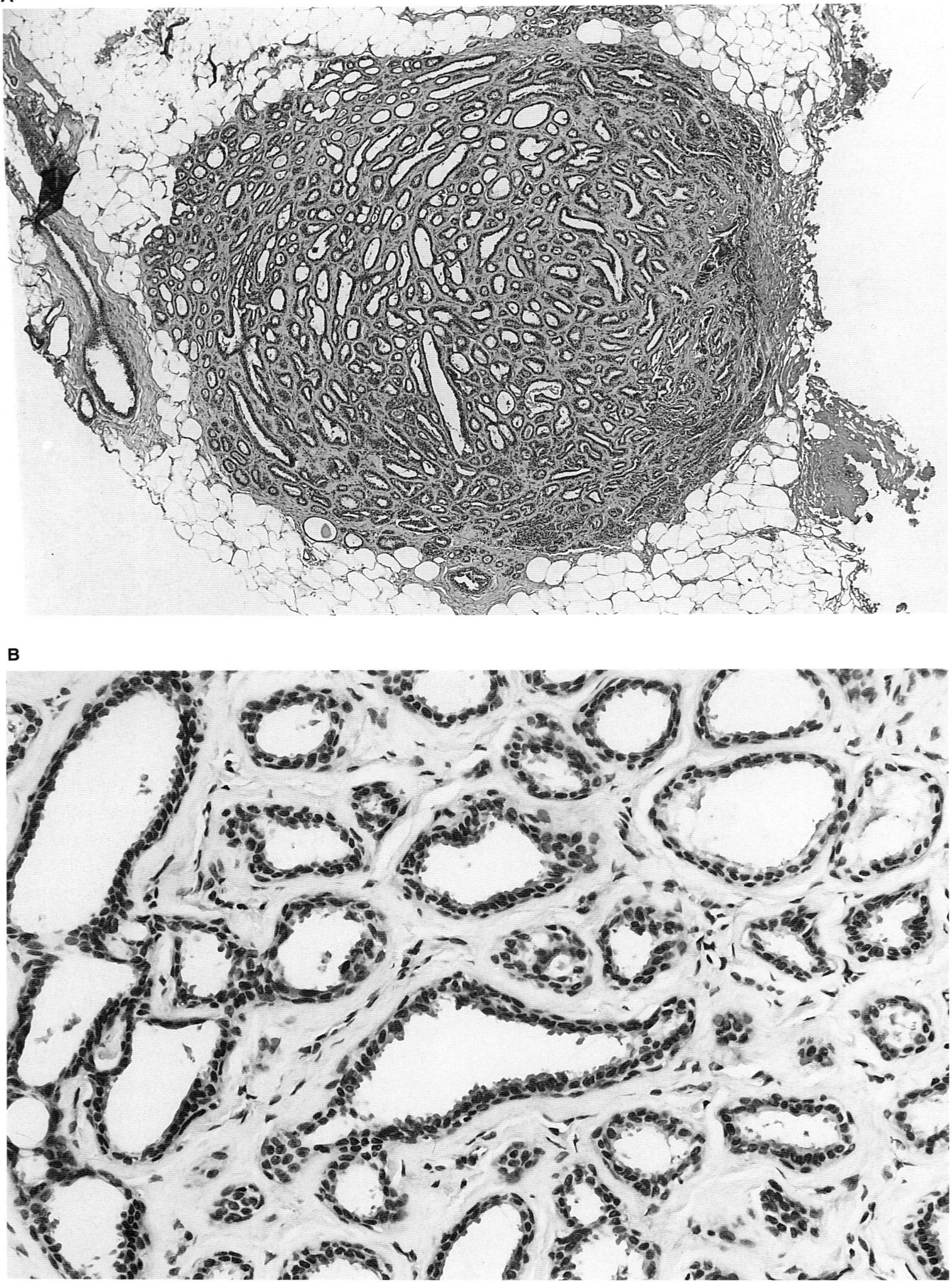

B

**Figure 4.6** Nodular adenosis. (a) A closely-packed aggregate of tubules many of which display open lumens. (b) The tubules are lined by epithelial and myoepithelial cell layers. (H&E, (a) X60; (b) X200)

A

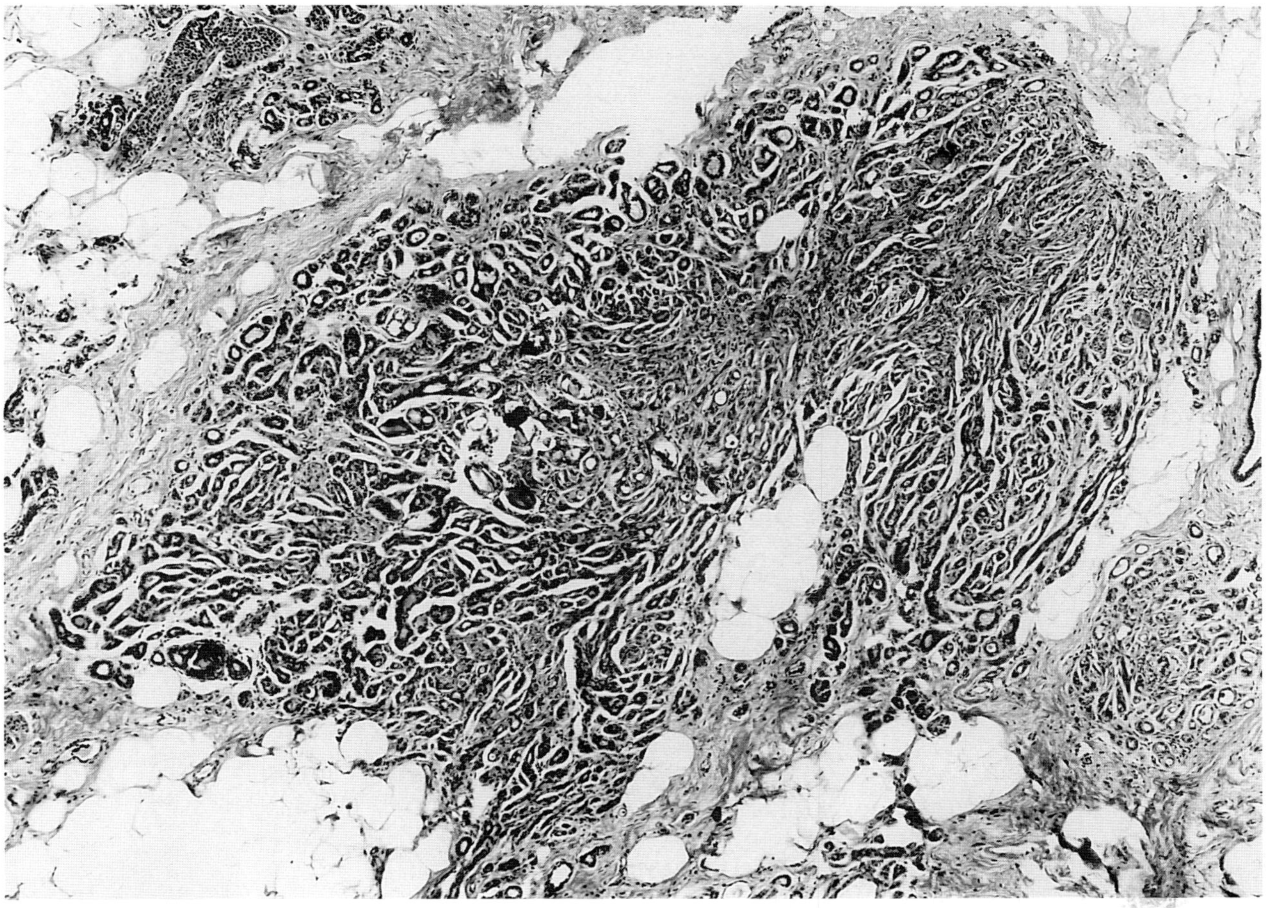

**Figure 4.7(a)** Sclerosing adenosis. An area of sclerosing adenosis characterized by a streaming tendency. (H&E, X80)

age. Regression of SA has been noted with menopause (140). Sandison (154) did not see SA in any of the 500 male breasts he examined and attributed this to the lobular origin of the lesion. These nodules may be very well delineated or ill defined on palpation. Sometimes they are associated with pain or tenderness.

## Microscopic Features

Sclerosing adenosis is classically characterized by an organoid, lobulated proliferation of closely-packed ductules that exhibit elongation and distortion due to compression by the collagen in the sparse background stroma (Fig. 4.7). The normal bicellular lining is retained in the ductules, but the myoepithelial cell layer is frequently prominent or hyperplastic. The central portion of the lesion generally reflects earlier stages, and is more cellular. In the periphery of the lesion, which reflects later stages, the cellularity is less, and the sclerosis dominates. When the myoepithelial cells dominate, which is rather common, the lesion assumes a variety of appearances ranging from an obviously myoid though tubular appearance to a solid, nodular and predominantly spindle cell proliferation (Fig. 4.8). More typical compressed or rounded ductules are often present in the periphery, even when the myoepithelial cells dominate, facilitating recognition of the lesion. Calcification is present in around 50% of the cases. Sclerosing adenosis may be focal, or rather diffuse and florid. Different stages of the lesion are generally evident in various foci within a biopsy. As noted by Tanaka and Oota (157), the tubules of SA proliferate parallel to the duct system, either around the duct of origin, extending into the duct lumen, or both (Fig. 4.9).

In some women, there is a massive proliferation of ductules in each focus of adenosis which may present as a distinctive, well delineated palpable nodule. Some of these massive nodules are formed

B

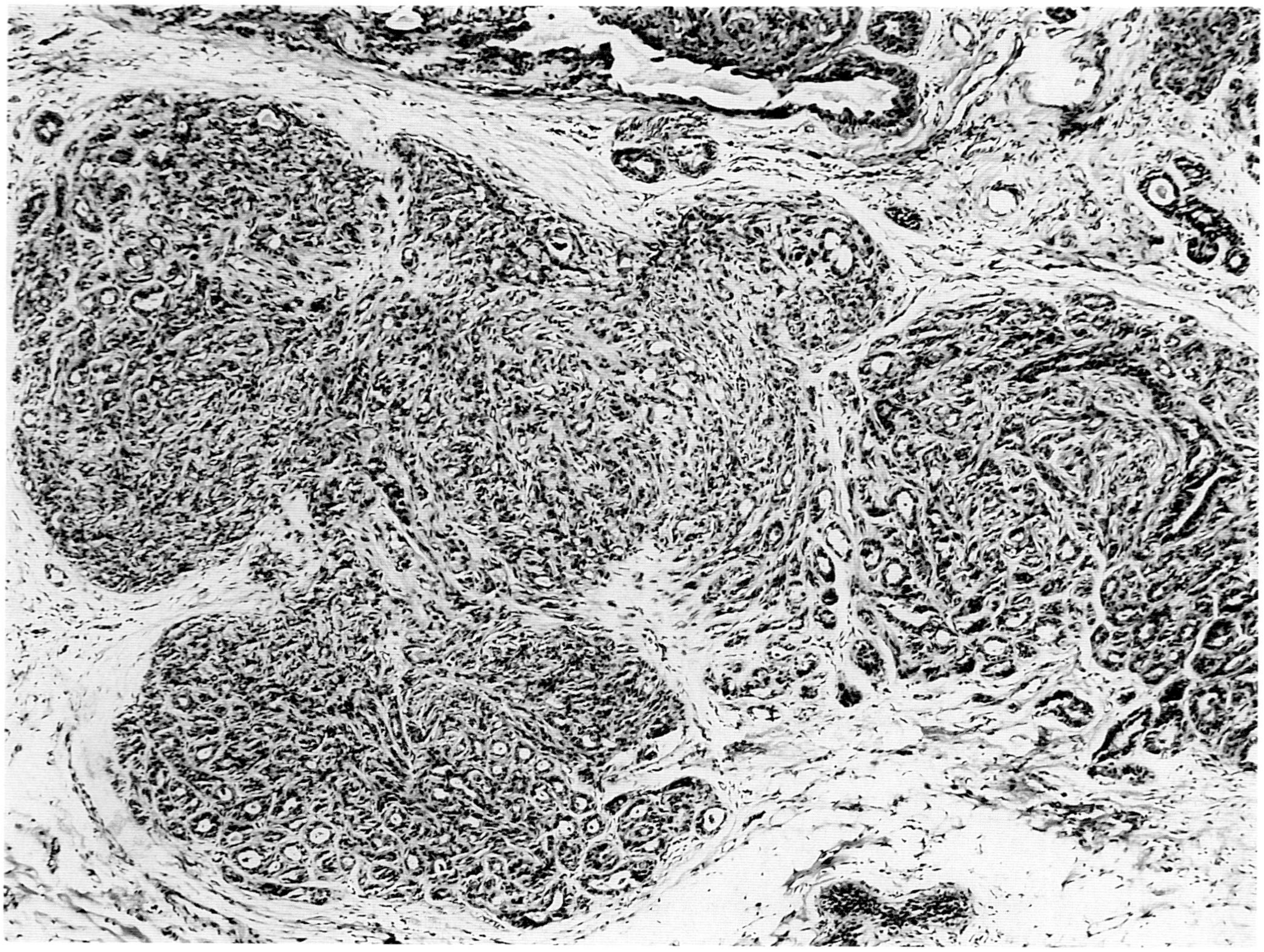

**Figure 4.7(b)** Sclerosing adenosis. Lobulated outline; myoepithelial predominance at the center. (H&E, X120)

by coalescence of adjacent foci of sclerosing adenosis. Anytime a distinct nodule forms, the term nodular sclerosing adenosis would be appropriate for the lesion.

In about 2% of cases, sclerosing adenosis extends into perineural spaces (135,139,159) (Fig. 4.9d).

The epithelial cells in sclerosing adenosis may show apocrine metaplasia; the metaplastic cells in this setting often show prominent nucleoli (132,155), which may be confused with a carcinoma. Apocrine adenosis is present in approximately 3% of benign breast biopsies (155). Atypicality may develop in either this metaplastic apocrine adenosis (Fig. 4.9e), or in areas of hyperplasia within the ductules. Lobular neoplasia (138) and intraductal carcinoma (133) may also develop in sclerosing adenosis and may be confined to SA when there is florid sclerosing adenosis in the biopsy.

When SA is florid, nodular, or displays atypia or involvement by lobular neoplasia or intraductal carcinoma, these findings should definitely be recorded in the diagnosis (see Chapter 7, Intraductal Carcinoma and Chapter 8, Lobular Neoplasia).

## Differential Diagnosis

The differential diagnosis of sclerosing adenosis includes tubular carcinoma, microglandular adenosis, and radial scar. At low magnification, the lobulated arrangement of the ductules is the most crucial feature that distinguishes SA from all other lesions. At higher magnification, the streaming effect and the obliteration of the lumens along with the presence of both epithelial and myoepithelial cell layers lining the ductules is in sharp contrast to the rounded or

C

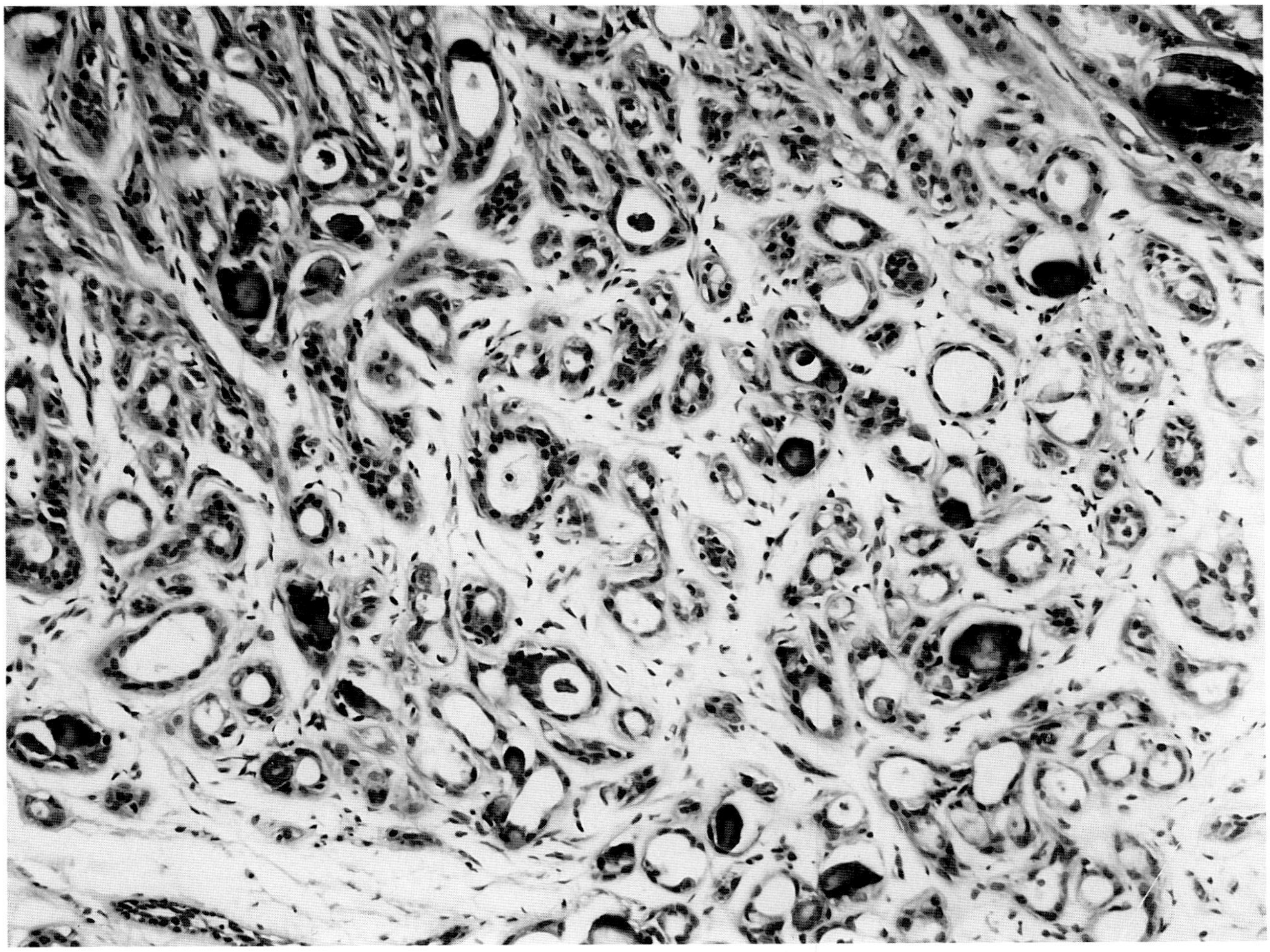

**Figure 4.7(c)** Sclerosing adenosis. Microcalcifications are evident in the tubules. (H&E, X240)

teardrop shape, open lumens, and the single layer of epithelial cells lining the tubules in both tubular carcinoma and microglandular adenosis. A PAS stain enhances the presence of basement membrane around the ductules which further distinguishes SA from tubular carcinoma. Features that are helpful in differentiating SA from tubular carcinoma and microglandular adenosis are listed in Table 4.1. Radial scars have a characteristic stellate appearance at low magnification and a central zone of fibrocollagenous scar tissue, in contrast to the lobulated pattern and absence of a central fibrocollagenous zone in SA.

## Prognostic Significance of Sclerosing Adenosis

While initial studies had suggested no increased or very minimal cancer risk associated with SA (39,96), several subsequent studies first suggested an increased risk when SA is present in association with intraductal hyperplasias (115,146). Finally, 349 women with SA were followed for an average of 17 years. The relative risk for infiltrating breast carcinoma was determined to be in the range of 1.7, independent of the presence of atypical intraductal hyperplasia and not influenced by the presence of a positive family history of breast carcinoma in a first-degree relative (143).

The clinical significance of atypical apocrine metaplasia in sclerosing adenosis has not been clearly established (132).

## MICROGLANDULAR ADENOSIS

Microglandular adenosis (MA) is an extremely rare variant of adenosis characterized by a proliferation of

A

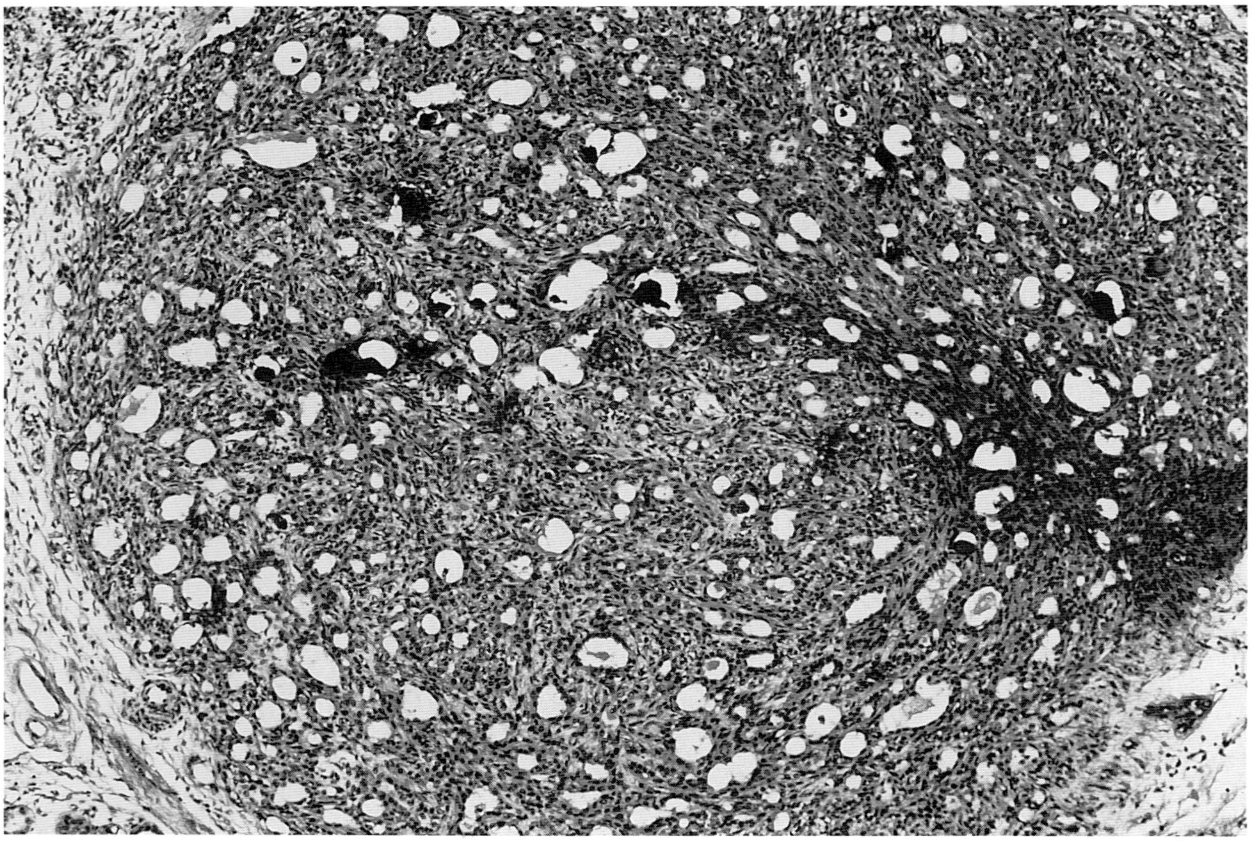

B

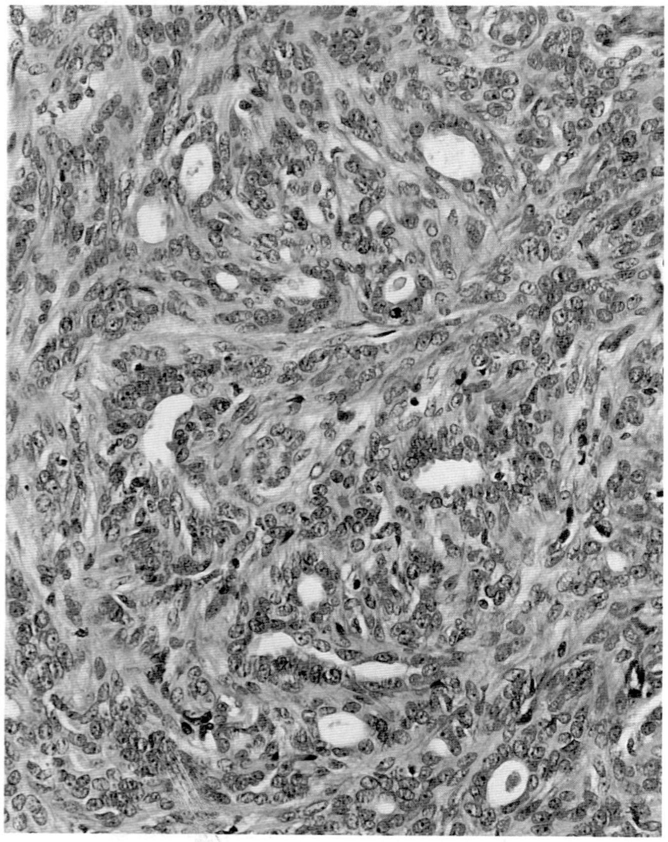

**Figure 4.8** Nodular sclerosing adenosis. (a) The nodule is rounded and there are microcalcifications. (b) The more solid areas reflect myoepithelial cell dominance and proliferation. (H&E, (a) X200; (b) X240)

A

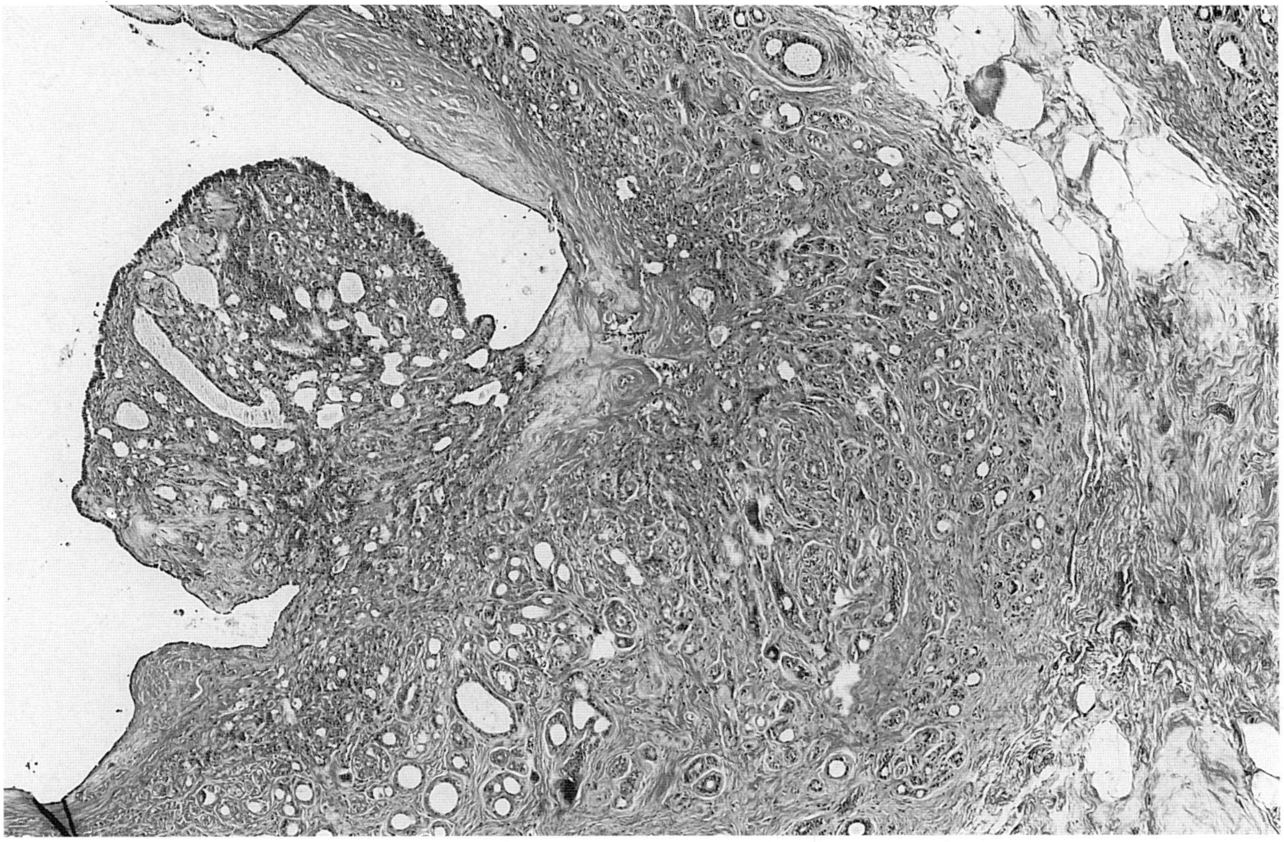

**Figure 4.9(a)** Sclerosing adenosis. Hundreds of small tubules are proliferating around and parallel to the distended duct, focally extending into the duct lumen. (H&E, X60)

small, round, duct-like structures in a generally collagenous background stroma (134,147,151,158). The patients, all women, range in age from 28 to 82 years, with a median of 51 years. While a majority of the patients present with a palpable mass, several reported cases have been incidental findings in biopsies performed for other lesions. There is no distinctive radiologic pattern of presentation for MA.

## Macroscopic Features

The appearance of microglandular hyperplasia varies from focal areas of irregular whitish-gray density to a vaguely circumscribed, firm and rubbery lesion. The size can only be approximated in most cases, and it ranges from 2 to 20 cm with a majority being around 3 to 4 cm.

## Microscopic Features

Classic microglandular hyperplasia is characterized by haphazardly distributed, round, gland-like structures accompanied by a distinctive fibrocollagenous stroma proliferating between the normal ducts and lobules and extending into adipose tissue (Fig. 4.10a). The glands are closely packed in some areas, and widely separated in other foci. They are rounded in configuration, with open lumens that contain a colloid-like secretory material at their center (Fig. 4.10b). The secretory material is strongly positive with periodic acid-Schiff (PAS) reaction and is not altered by diastase predigestion; it also stains with mucin and alcian blue, but the staining is not uniform with either one. Rarely, laminated calcospherules are present in the center of the secretory material. The glands are lined by a single layer of epithelial cells. These cells often appear cuboid with a truncated luminal margin lacking apical cytoplasmic projections. The nuclei are

B

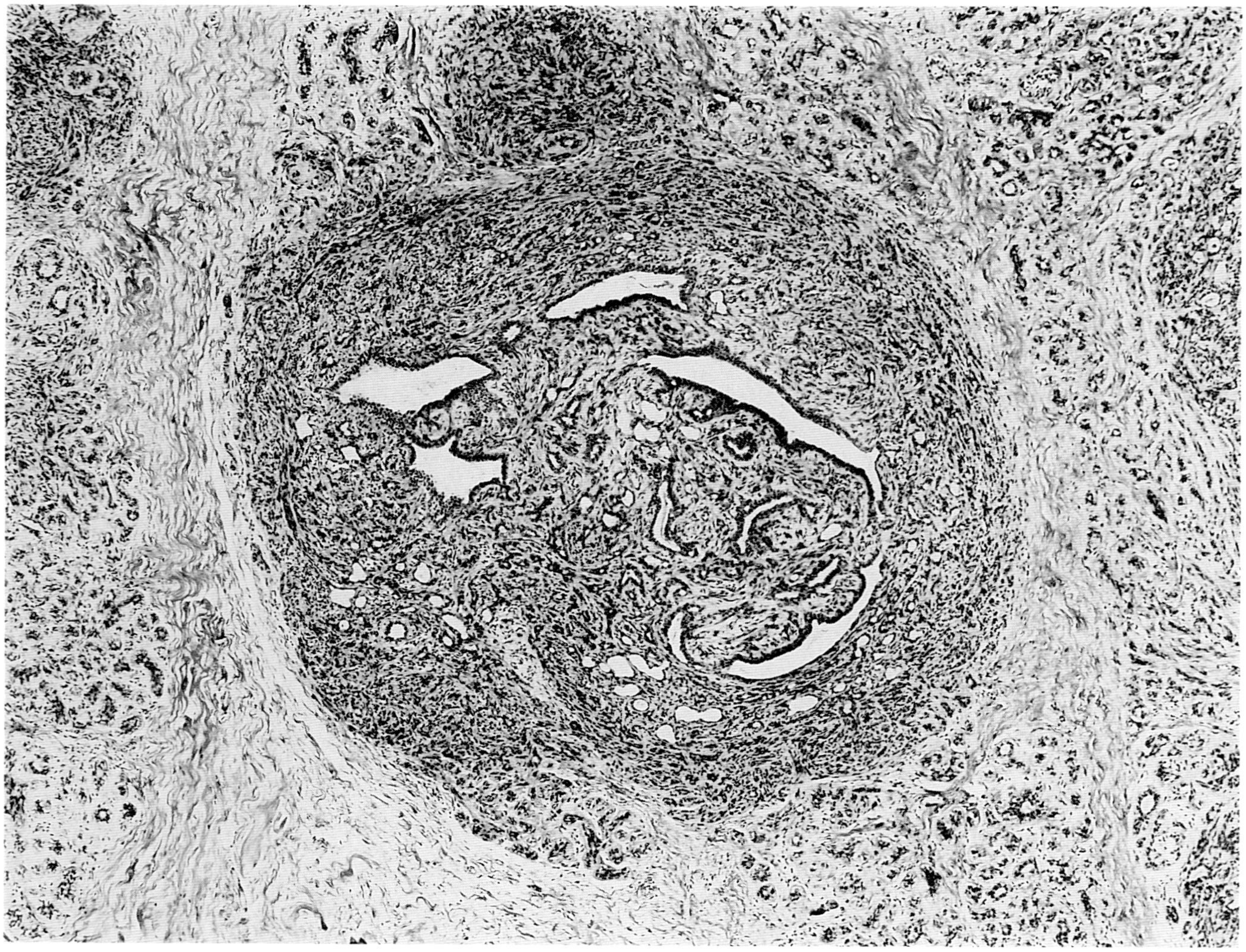

**Figure 4.9(b&c)** Sclerosing adenosis. A similar process has distorted the centrally located duct with numerous tubules growing around and into the duct lumen. (H&E, (b) X200; (c) X400)

round or ovoid, and quite bland in appearance. Nucleoli are generally small, but occasionally they do appear prominent. Mitotic figures are generally absent, and when observed do not exceed 4 to 5 per 10 high power fields. The lining cells have a clear or vacuolated cytoplasm, but may be finely granular and lightly eosinophilic. The clear cells are present in all cases, and in a majority of cases, they are the dominant cell population. Glycogen granules can be identified within the cytoplasm in most cases. While the glands frequently proliferate around normal or altered ducts and lobules, and often also extend into adipose tissue, perineural or intravascular extension has not been observed. The most important diagnostic feature of these glands is the absence of a myoepithelial cell layer.

The fibrocollagenous background stroma is distinctive and helps delineate the lesion from the adjacent uninvolved breast tissue. Its appearance varies from densely collagenous to loose and hypocellular.

## Immunohistochemical and Ultrastructural Features

Ten of the lesions evaluated at AFIP were stained with cytokeratin, S-100 protein, and actin; none of these cases showed any evidence of a myoepithelial cell layer.

At the ultrastructural level, the presence of a single layer of epithelial cells and the absence of a myoepithelial cell layer has been confirmed (158) (Fig.

c

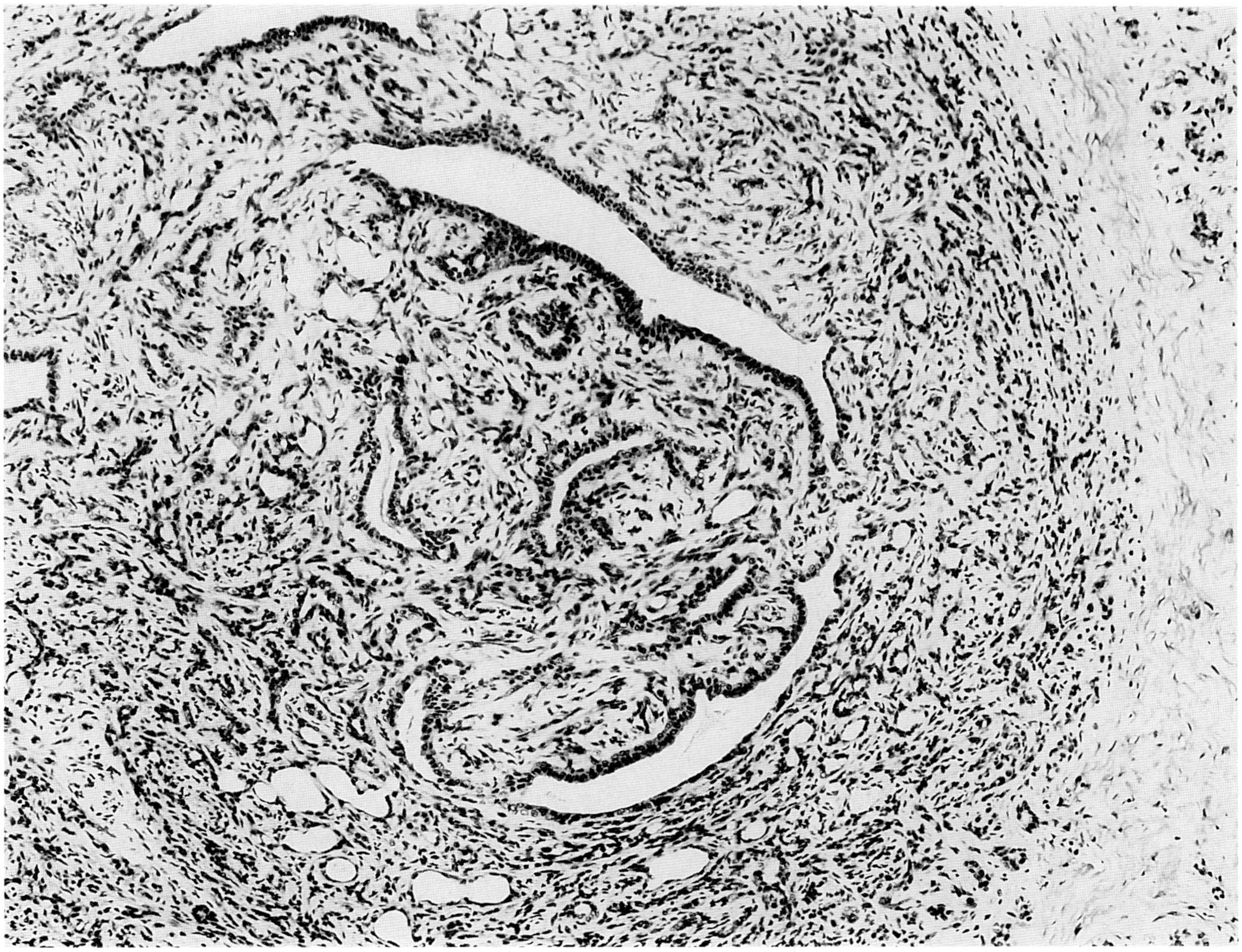

**Figure 4.9(c)** Legend on opposite page.

4.10c). A significant finding is the presence of a thick, multilayered basement membrane around the glandular structures and persistence of the delimiting fibroblastic cell layer. The epithelial cells display a truncated luminal margin which contains small secretory granules.

## Differential Diagnosis

Microglandular adenosis is most frequently confused with tubular carcinoma. The features distinguishing MA from tubular carcinoma are listed in Table 4.1. The major source of confusion is the presence of a single epithelial cell layer lining the glandular structures in both lesions; a myoepithelial cell layer is absent in both lesions. However, a comparison of the two demonstrates significant differences that can help distinguish these lesions. The tubules in tubular carcinoma are haphazardly distributed in a reactive appearing, moderately cellular, fibroblastic stroma, generally displacing normal or altered mammary ducts and lobules; a stellate overall appearance is common. The glands of MA are also haphazardly distributed but in a hypocellular, fibrocollagenous stroma, and almost invariably entrap normal or altered ducts and lobules within the lesion; the lesion lacks an overall stellate configuration. The tubules of tubular carcinoma have a tear-drop shape, lack intraluminal secretory material, and their lining cells may show apical snouts. The glands of MA are rounded, contain a colloid-like secretory material, and their lining cells have a truncated luminal margin. The epithelial cells in tubular carcinoma generally display an eosinophilic cytoplasm, in contrast to

D

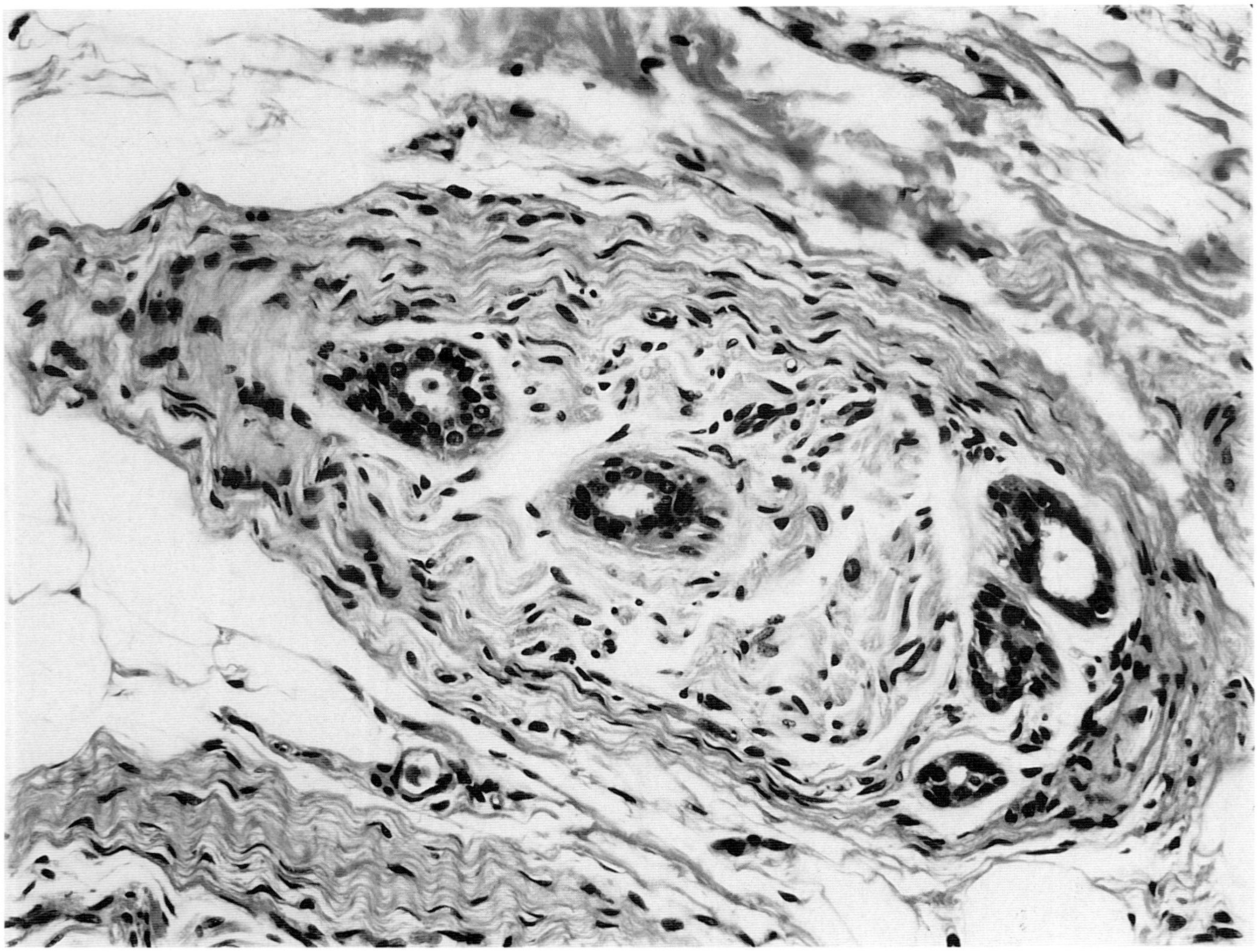

**Figure 4.9(d)** Sclerosing adenosis. The two cell layers characteristic of SA tubules persist even when they extend into the perineural space. (H&E, X160)

the clear or vacuolated cytoplasmic appearance of the cells in MA. The presence of basement membrane around the glands of MA, and its absence around the tubules of tubular carcinoma, cannot be readily assessed on H&E sections in all cases. Even the use of PAS stain to demonstrate the basement membrane is not very helpful. In MA the collagenous nature of the stroma, which is closely apposed to the glands, makes a delineation of the basement membrane from the surrounding stroma difficult. At the ultrastructural level, however, the multilayered basement membrane and well-retained delimiting fibroblastic cell layer characteristic of MA are clearly evident and in sharp contrast to the complete absence or patchy nature of the basement membrane and the disruption of the delimiting fibroblastic cell layer evident in tubular carcinoma.

Secretory adenosis is another lesion that has been confused with microglandular adenosis. On H&E stained section, secretory adenosis also shows rounded glands with secretory material within their lumens (Fig. 4.11a). The secretory material may very much resemble the colloid-like secretory material of MA (Fig. 4.11b), but may be more granular. The epithelial cells may also show cytoplasmic vacuolization in some cases. The crucial myoepithelial cell layer is often quite attenuated and may be missed by some pathologists on H&E stained slides, further contributing to the confusion with MA. An immunoreaction with actin or S-100 protein invariably demonstrates the myoepithelial cell layer which easily distinguishes secretory adenosis from MA (Fig. 4.11c). The lesions described by Diaz et al (137) and Kay (144), all of which had a ME cell layer, are undoubtedly examples of secretory adenosis.

E

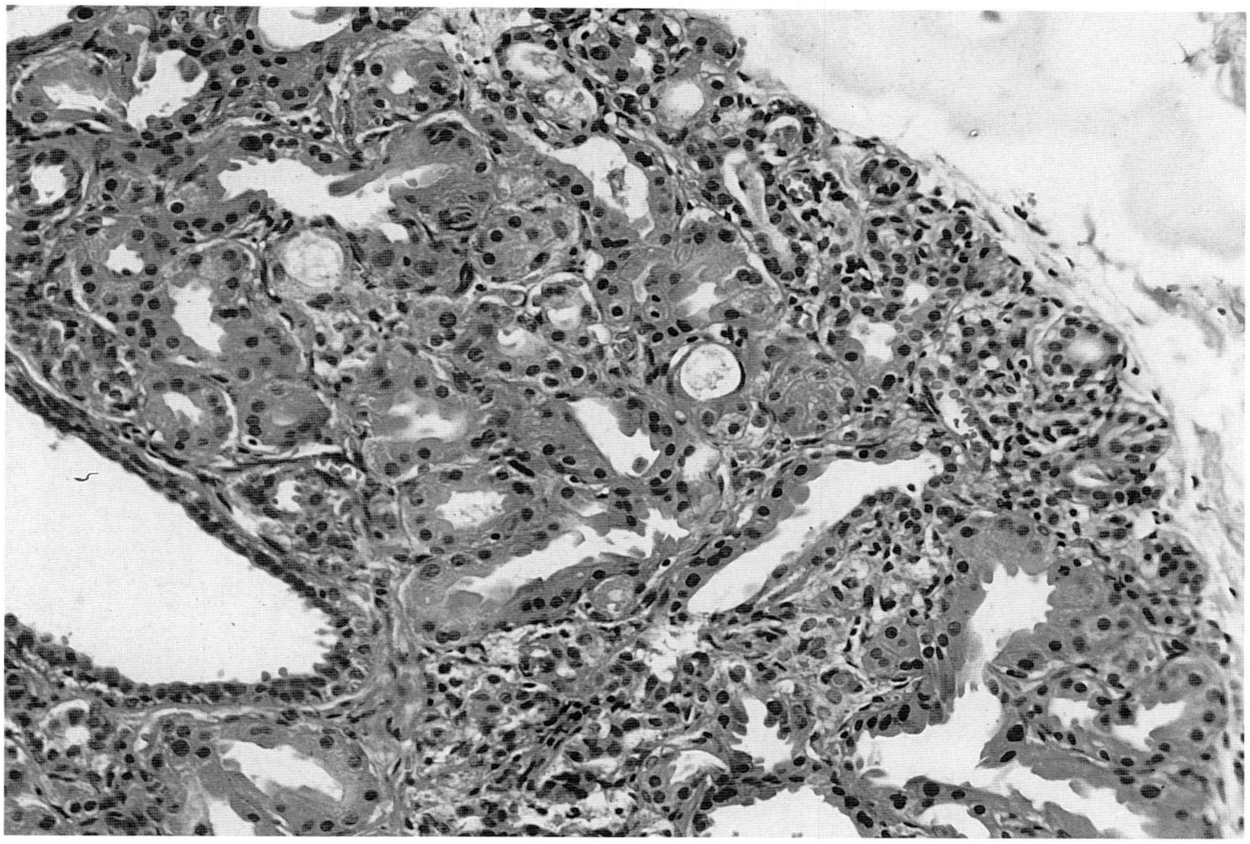

**Figure 4.9(e)** Sclerosing adenosis. Apocrine metaplasia may involve sclerosing adenosis. (H&E, X150)

## Behavior and Treatment

None of the 11 patients reported from AFIP had developed any recurrences at the time of the report (158). One patient who had presented with extensive MA involving a 12 cm biopsy developed two recurrences, 6 and 13 years after the initial diagnosis. Both recurrent lesions were extensive and involved up to 19 cm of biopsy tissue. The second recurrence

**Table 4.1** A Comparison of Morphologic Features of Microglandular Adenosis, Tubular Carcinoma, and Sclerosing Adenosis

| | **Microglandular Adenosis** | **Tubular Carcinoma** | **Sclerosing Adenosis*** |
|---|---|---|---|
| Glandular distribution | Haphazard | Haphazard, stellate | Lobular, rounded |
| Glandular shape | Round | Angulated | Round |
| Lumens | Open | Open | Small, compressed |
| Intraluminal secretion | +++(Colloid-like) | ± | ± |
| No. cell layers | Epithelial only, one layer | Epithelial only, one layer | Epithelial & myoepithelial, two layers |
| Cytoplasm | Vacuolated, clear, granular | Eosinophilic | Epithelial cell, granular<br>Myoepithelial cells, vacuolated |
| Cytoplasmic protrusions (apical snouts) | Absent | Present | ± |
| Basement membrane | +++(Multilayered) | ± | ++ |
| Stroma | Collagenous<br>Uniformly hypocellular<br>Distinctive, not zonal | Desmoplastic (reactive) and cellular | Zonal, sclerotic |

Note: ± generally absent; ++ = usually present; +++ = prominent.
*Based on direct observation and information gathered from various reports.
From Tavasolli and Norris (158), with permission.

A

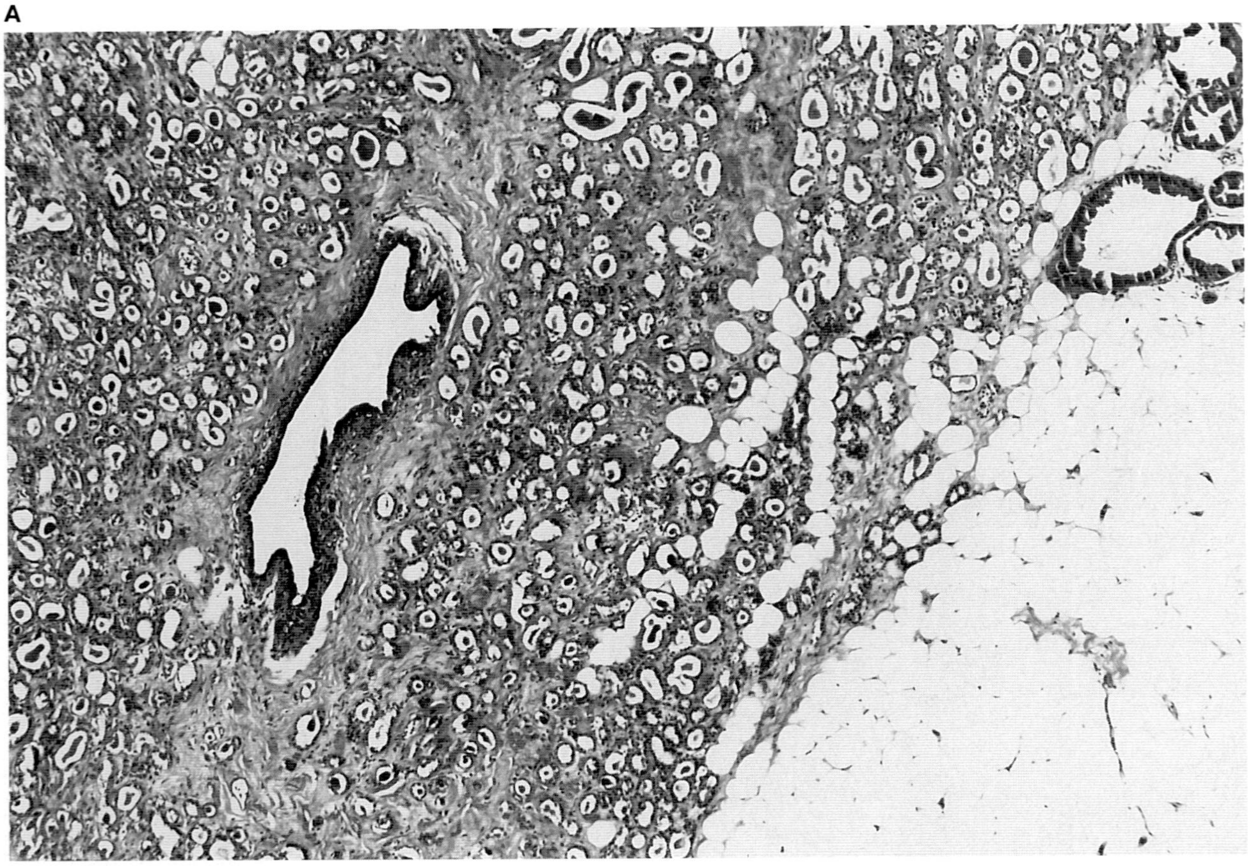

B

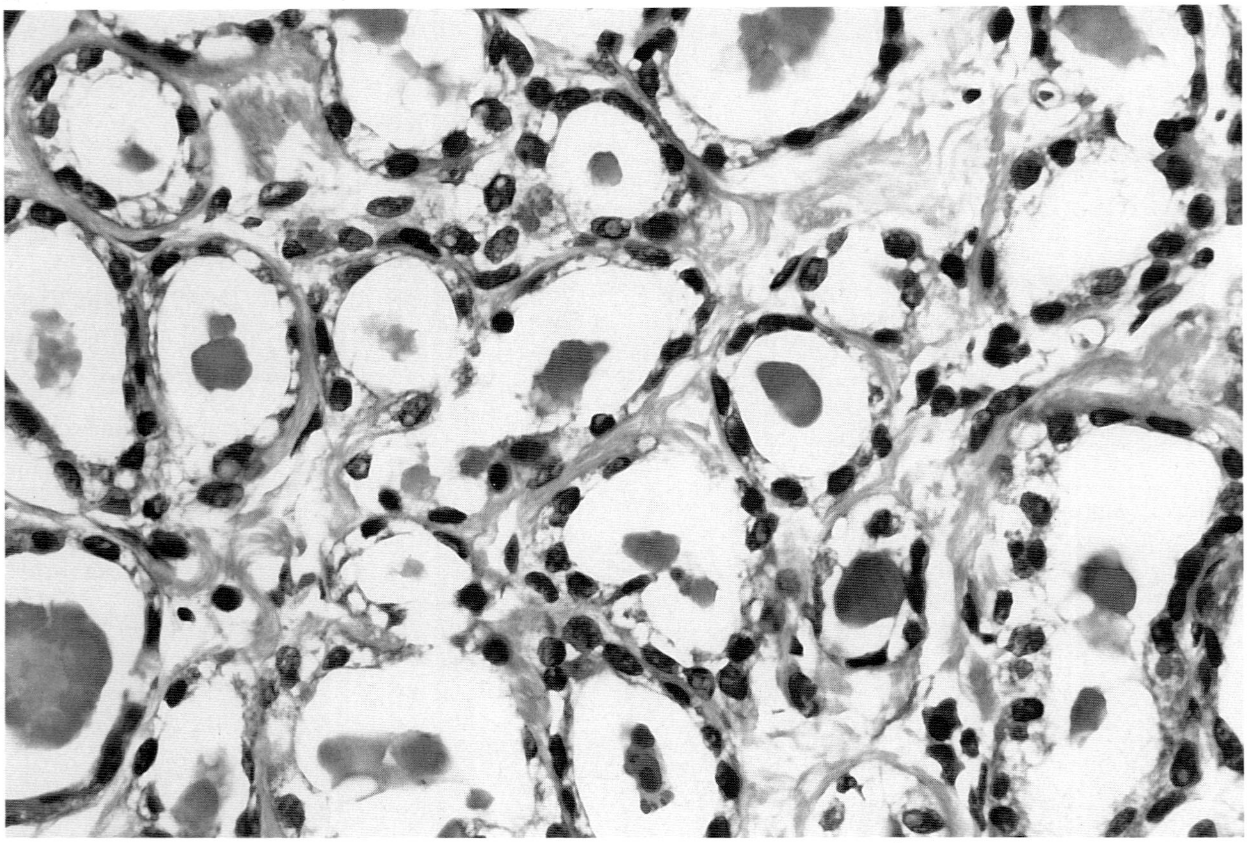

**Figure 4.10** Microglandular adenosis. (a) A dense background stroma defines the extent of this MA which is characterized by and irregular growth margin and proliferation around a duct. (H&E, X80) (b) A single layer of clear or vacuolated epithelial cells lines round tubules with open lumen filled with a colloid-like secretory material. (H&E, X200) (c) A thick basement membrane surrounds the tubules. (H&E, X480) (d) At the ultrastructural level, the myoepithelial cell layer is absent, but there is a thick multilayered basement membrane around the tubules. (Uranyl acetate-lead citrate, X2,300) (Figures (b&d) reproduced from Tavassoli FA, Norris HJ: *Am J Surg Pathol* 1983;7:731–737, with permission.)

C

D

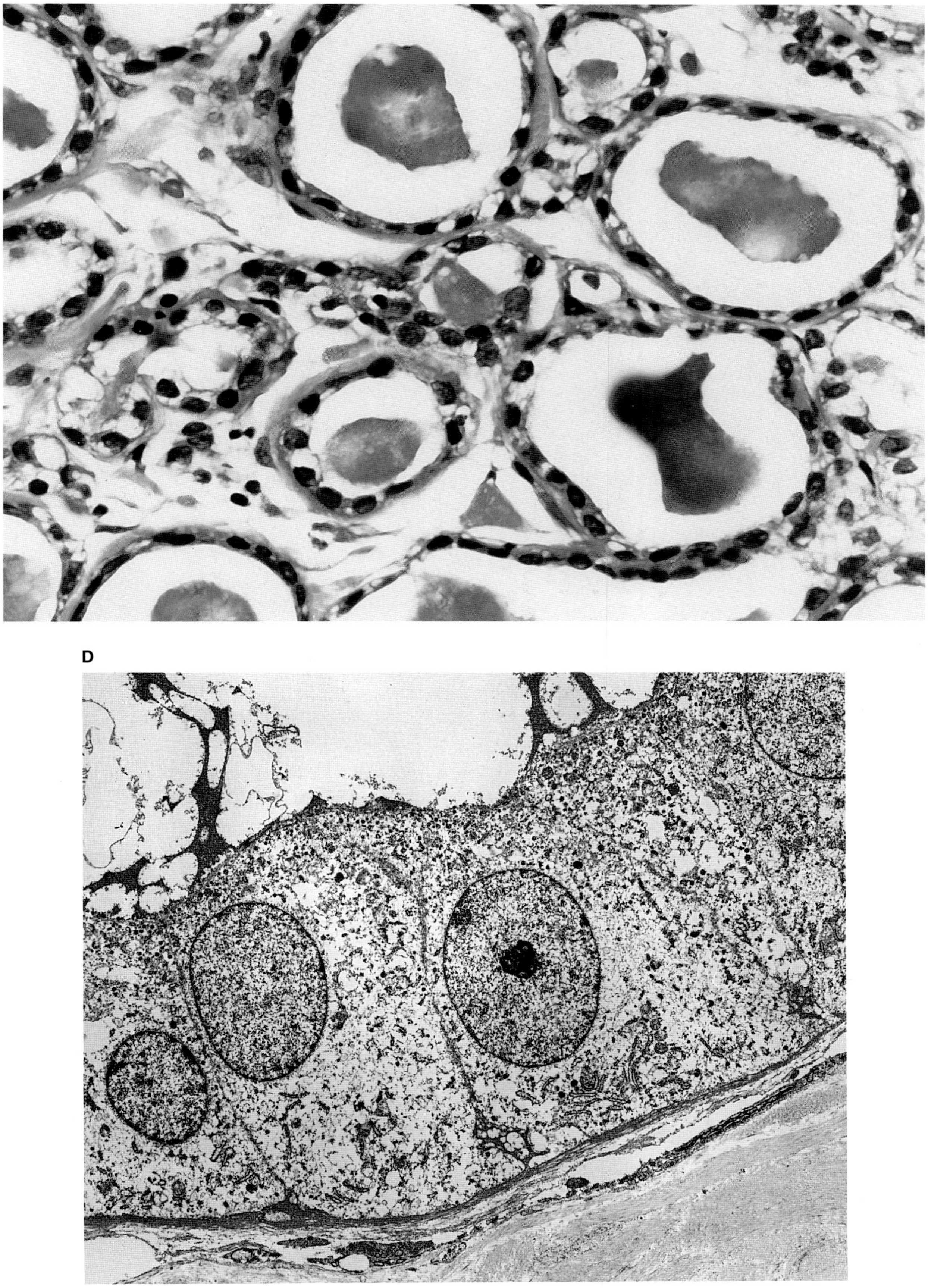

**Figure 4.10(c&d)** Legend on opposite page.

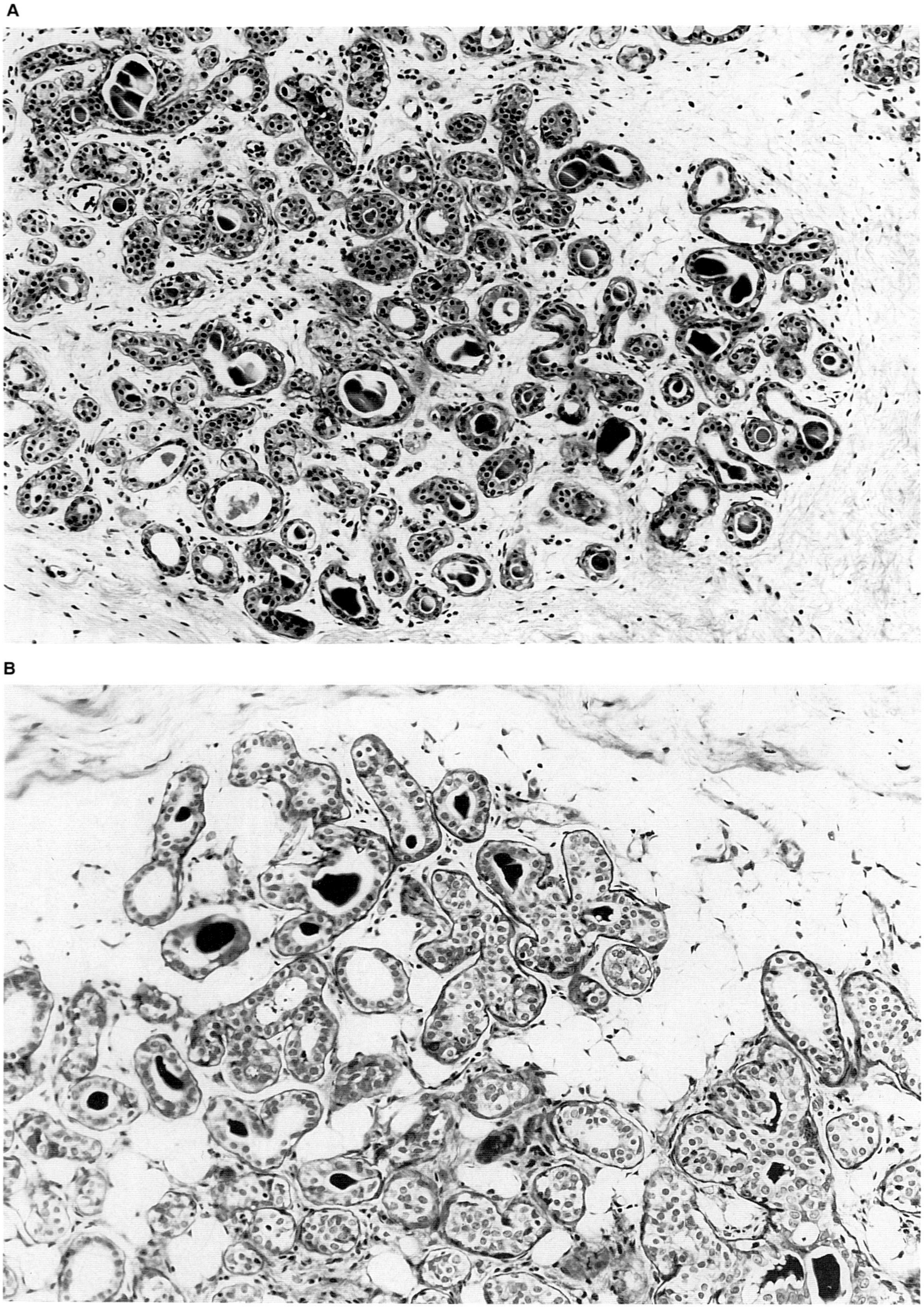


**Figure 4.11** Secretory adenosis. (a) The rounded tubules containing secretory material mimic microglandular adenosis, but the stroma is loose. (H&E, X160) (b) The secretory material is PAS positive, and a distinct basement membrane is evident on PAS stain. (X160)

C

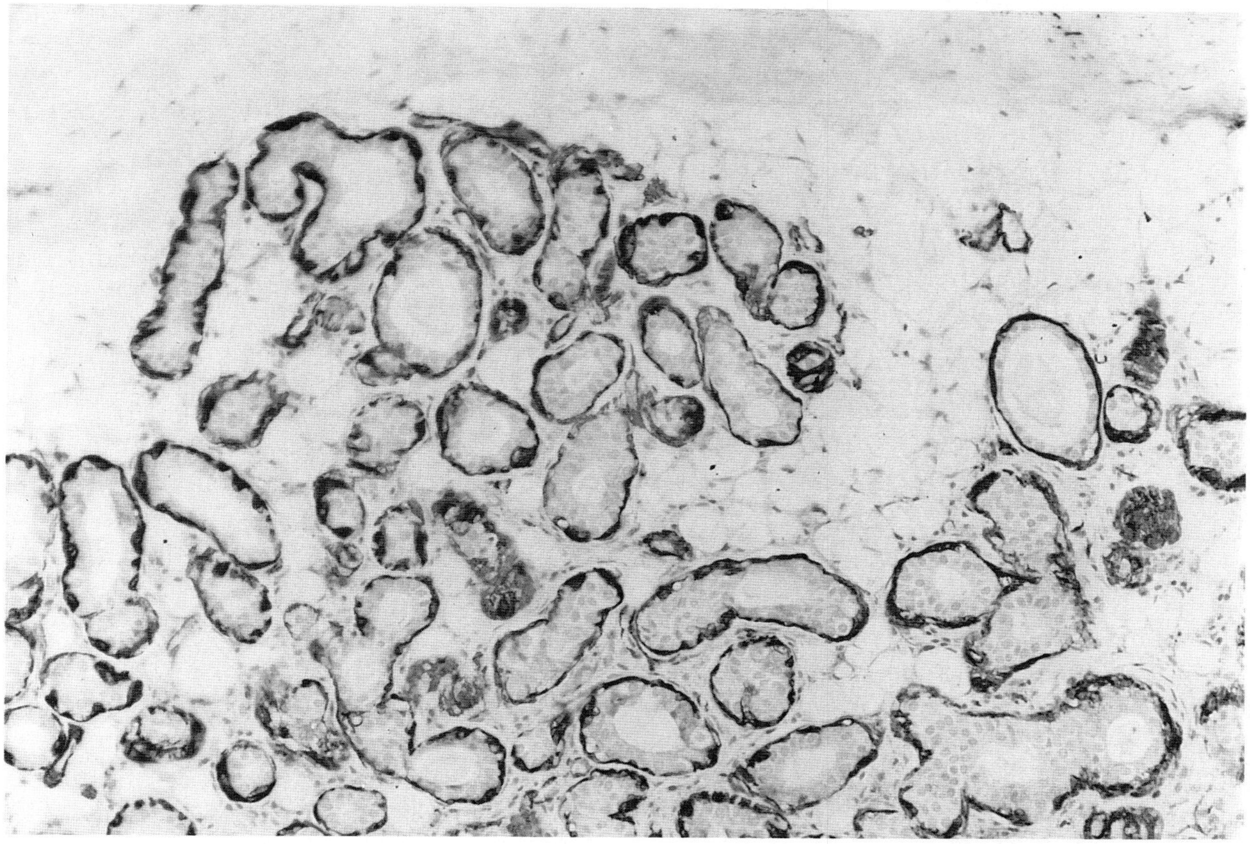

**Figure 4.11(c)** Secretory adenosis. An immunostain for actin demonstrates the presence of a myoepithelial cell layer excluding the possibility of MA. (X200)

showed transition from the typical bland cells lining the glands to a more atypical cell population in some parts of the lesion along with increased mitotic activity in these areas. Because of this change and the fact that the lesion had recurred twice, a mastectomy was performed. Abundant residual lesion was present in the mastectomy specimen, but there was no evidence of axillary node metastases in 19 nodes. The absence of any lymph node metastases despite the massive amounts of lesion and two recurrences over a 13-year period point to a benign lesion similar to sclerosing adenosis that also recurs and even develops atypia, but does not metastasize.

Complete excision of the lesion is adequate therapy. When the lesion is extensive and particularly if there is any evidence of atypia, the patient should be closely monitored with periodic follow-up.

## Relationship of MA to Carcinoma

Microglandular adenosis may coexist with infiltrating carcinoma in a biopsy, but in its usual form it is completely benign. As any other proliferative lesion, it may occasionally serve as the milieu for the development of subsequent carcinoma. The development of atypia in MA along with increased mitotic activity should be considered worrisome and deserving of periodic follow-up after complete excision of the mass. The lesion should not be designated as a carcinoma simply because of the presence of areas of cytologic atypia, however. If an unequivocal pattern of carcinoma is seen in continuity with, or transition from MA, there should be no hesitation in calling the lesion a carcinoma even if there are areas of benign MA around the carcinoma. Several patterns of carcinoma, including a clear cell carcinoma, have been reported as arising in MA (152).

## RADIAL SCAR

*Synonyms*: Rosette-like lesion (174), sclerosing ductal proliferation (177), non-encapsulated sclerosing lesion (168), le centre de proliferation d'Aschoff (165), and indurative mastopathy (173).

*Definition*: A radial scar consists of a fibroelastotic core surrounded by radiating ducts and lobules displaying various amounts and types of epithelial hyperplasia, adenosis or ectasia. The central core often shows entrapped tubular structures (161).

Though described more than 50 years ago (174) and referred to by a variety of designations in the past (164), radial scars (169–172) became the focus of renewed interest after a rather detailed report in English by Linell et al (170) suggested that it may have an association with tubular carcinoma, even though this possible association had been previously alluded to in the German and Italian literature (166,169). The term radial scar is a translation of "Strahlige Narben" which was first proposed by Hamperl (169). Clearly indicative of a benign process, this simple designation distinguishes radial scars from a variety of other sclerosing lesions that occur in the breast. I prefer the term "radial scar" regardless of the size and degree of complexity of the lesion.

Radial scar has been observed in women ranging in age from 47 to 72 with a mean of 55 years. It has been found in 28% of breasts from 83 consecutive, unselected autopsies (171). The lesion was multicentric in 67% and bilateral in 43% of cases. It was observed more frequently among women with fibrocystic changes (43%), compared to those women who had no evidence of these changes (17%). There was no evidence of difference in the frequency of radial scars in women with breast cancer and those with benign lesions or no pathology at all. Considering the relatively common occurrence of radial scars, it is not surprising that it has also been observed in breasts showing invasive carcinomas. Mammographically, radial scars appear as small speculated structures that mimic invasive carcinoma.

## Macroscopic Features

A majority of radial scars are not grossly visible. Those that are apparent to the naked eye often mimic a carcinoma because of the stellate or nodular appearance with central puckering, the firmness of the lesion, and the presence of creamy white streaks of elastica. Although the size often does not exceed a few millimeters, it is sometimes larger than 1 cm.

## Microscopic Features

The radial nature of the lesion is invariably evident, although the microscopic appearance varies depending on the degree of sclerosis, elastosis, amount of ductular entrapment in the central zone, and the presence and nature of proliferative changes in the surrounding ductules (Fig. 4.12). Characteristically, there is a stellate or radial arrangement of ductules around a central fibroelastotic or fibrocollagenous zone. The ductules surrounding the central scarred zone are either lined by both epithelial and myoepithelial cell layers, or exhibit intraluminal epithelial hyperplasia in a variety of patterns. The degree of radial arrangement and amount of elastosis in these lesions is highly variable. In some lesions, the central fibrocollagenous zone is rather small, while in others, almost the entire lesion may be sclerotic. The central zone may be surrounded by minimally altered clusters of ductules, or the surrounding region may display various patterns of adenosis, collagenous spherulosis, intraductal hyperplasia, atypical intraductal hyperplasia, intraductal carcinoma, or even lobular neoplasis. Rarely, an invasive carcinoma is present in and around the fibroelastotic core of a radial scar.

Radial scar occurs in association with both benign and malignant lesions (163). During the earlier stages of its formation, the central areas of the lesion contain a chronic inflammatory infiltrate and reactive appearing fibroblasts without significant distortion of the surrounding structures. During the later phases, the central portion is dominated by hyalinization and fibroelastosis, with considerable distortion. Entrapped ductules can be found during either stage and these have been a tremendous source of confusion with an invasive carcinoma. The surrounding ducts and ductules may display a variety of proliferative lesions including lobular neoplasia and intraductal carcinoma.

## Differential Diagnosis

The most important lesion from which a radial scar should be distinguished is a tubular carcinoma. The

A

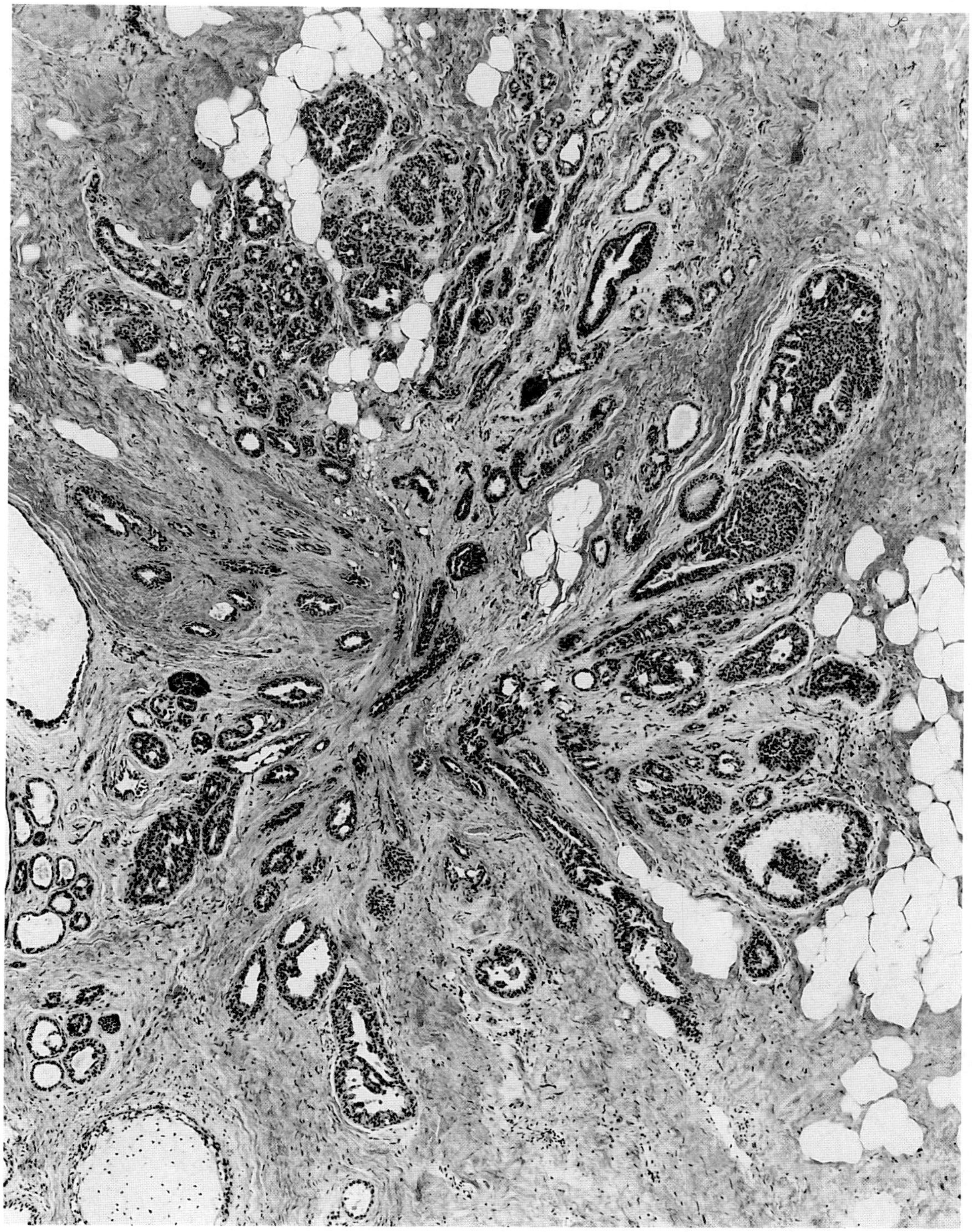

**Figure 4.12(a)** Radial scar. Early stage with a radial arrangement, but no significant scarring evident in this field; the surrounding ducts show IDH. (H&E, X120)

B

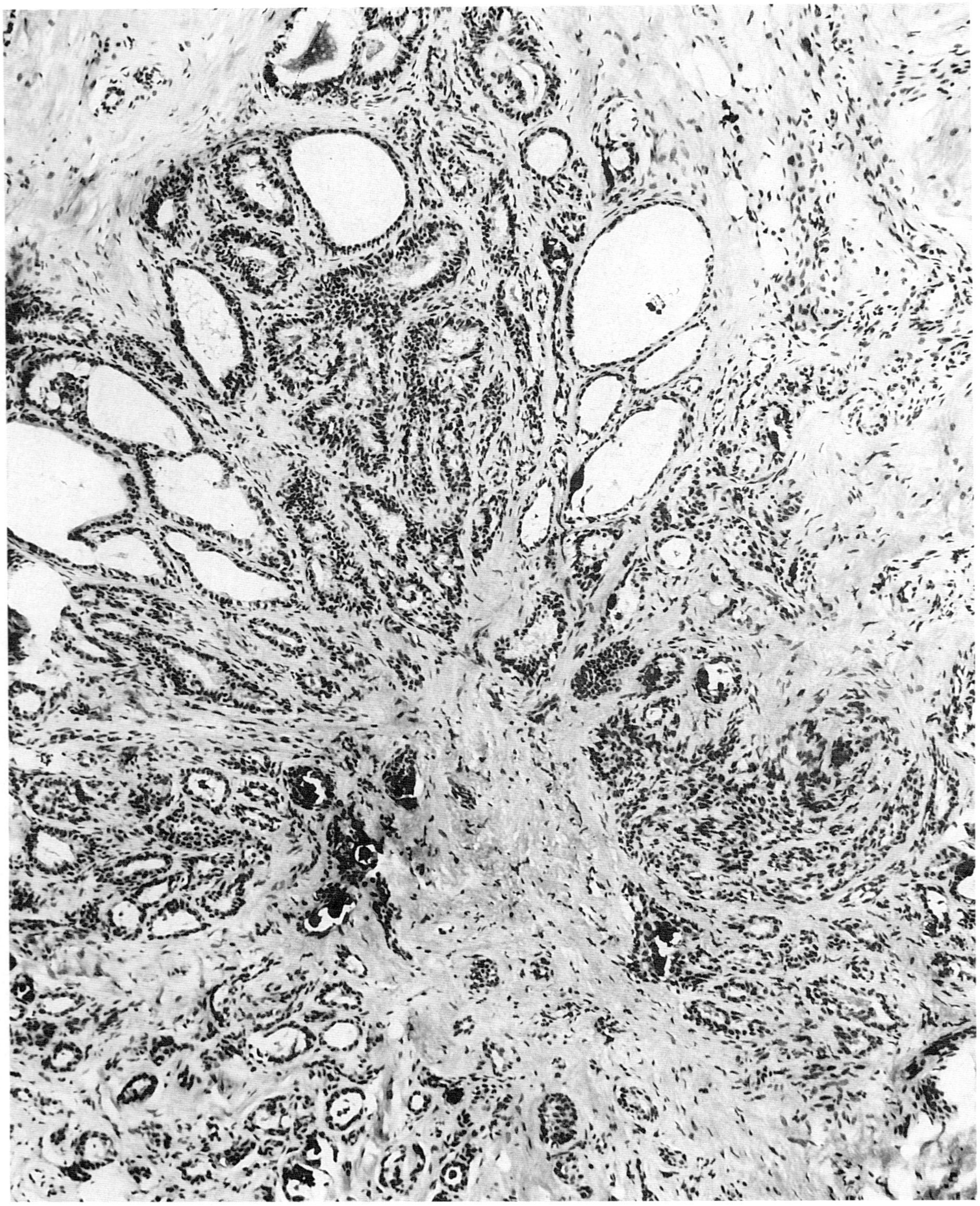

**Figure 4.12(b)** Radial scar. Minimal fibrosis and calcification are evident in the center. (H&E, X200)

c

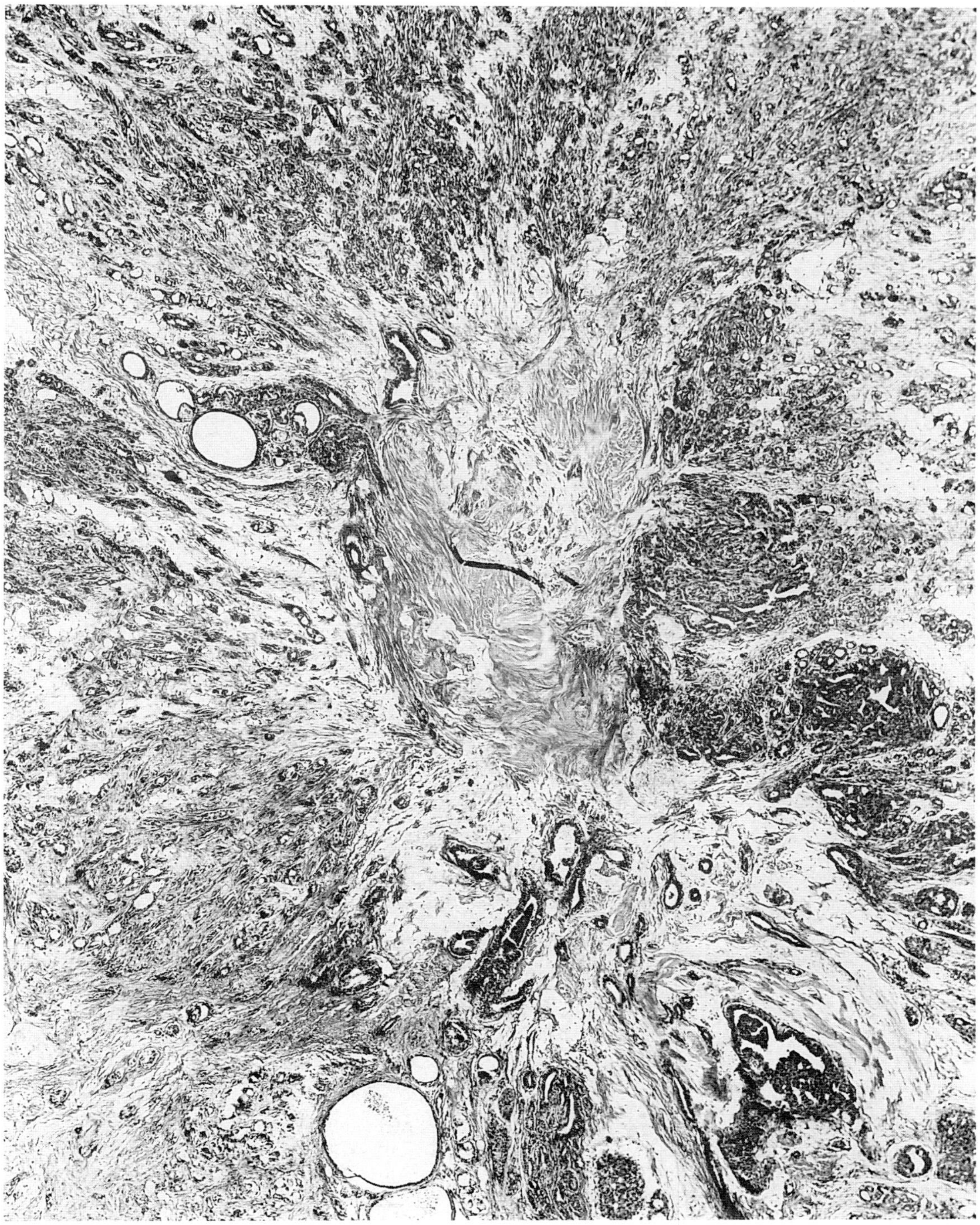

**Figure 4.12(c)** Radial scar. Central collagenous scar surrounded by radiating sclerosing adenosis. (H&E, X100)

D

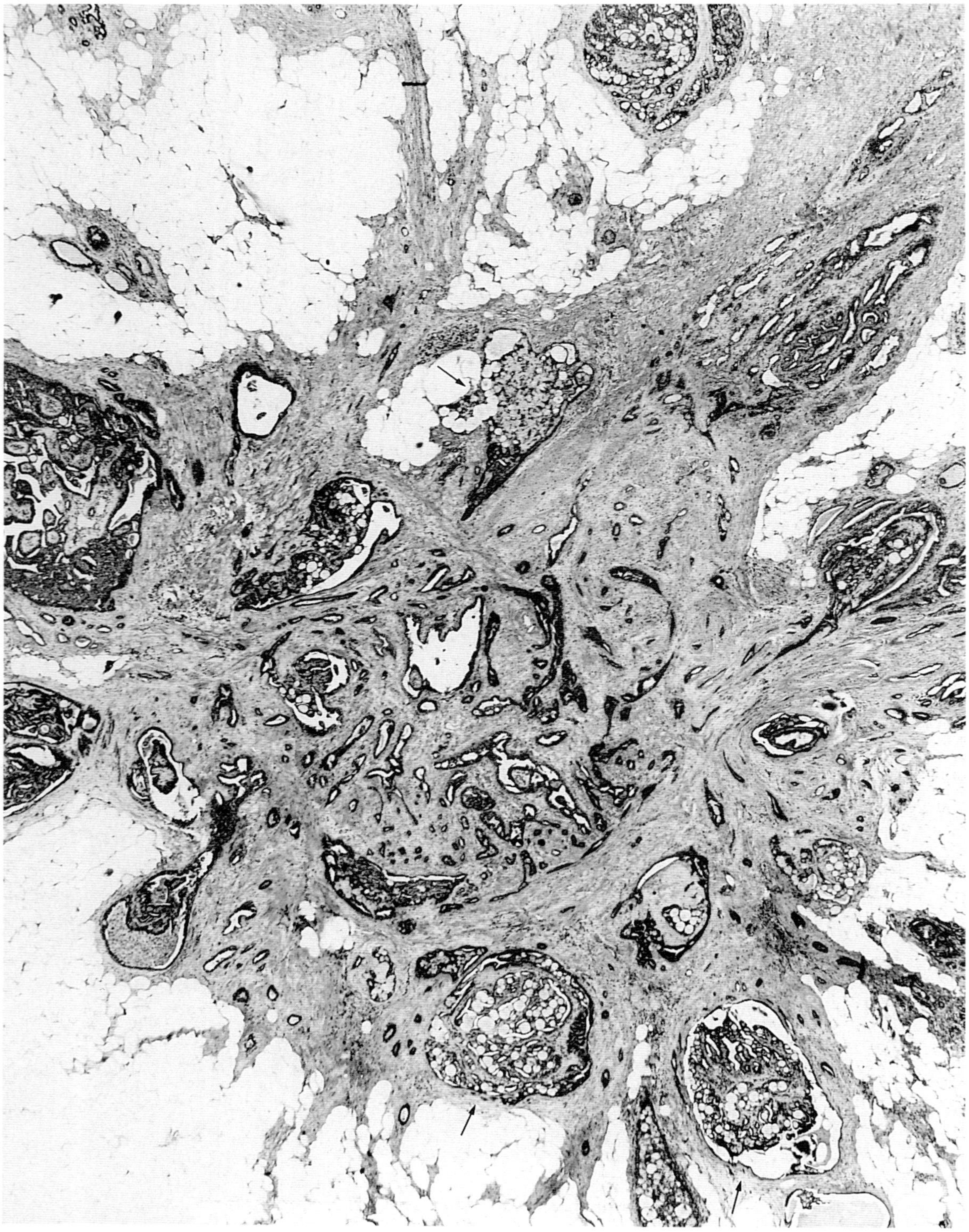

**Figure 4.12(d)** Radial scar. Entrapped hyperplastic ducts are evident in the center; collagenous spherulosis is present in several of the surrounding ducts (arrows). (H&E, X60)

E

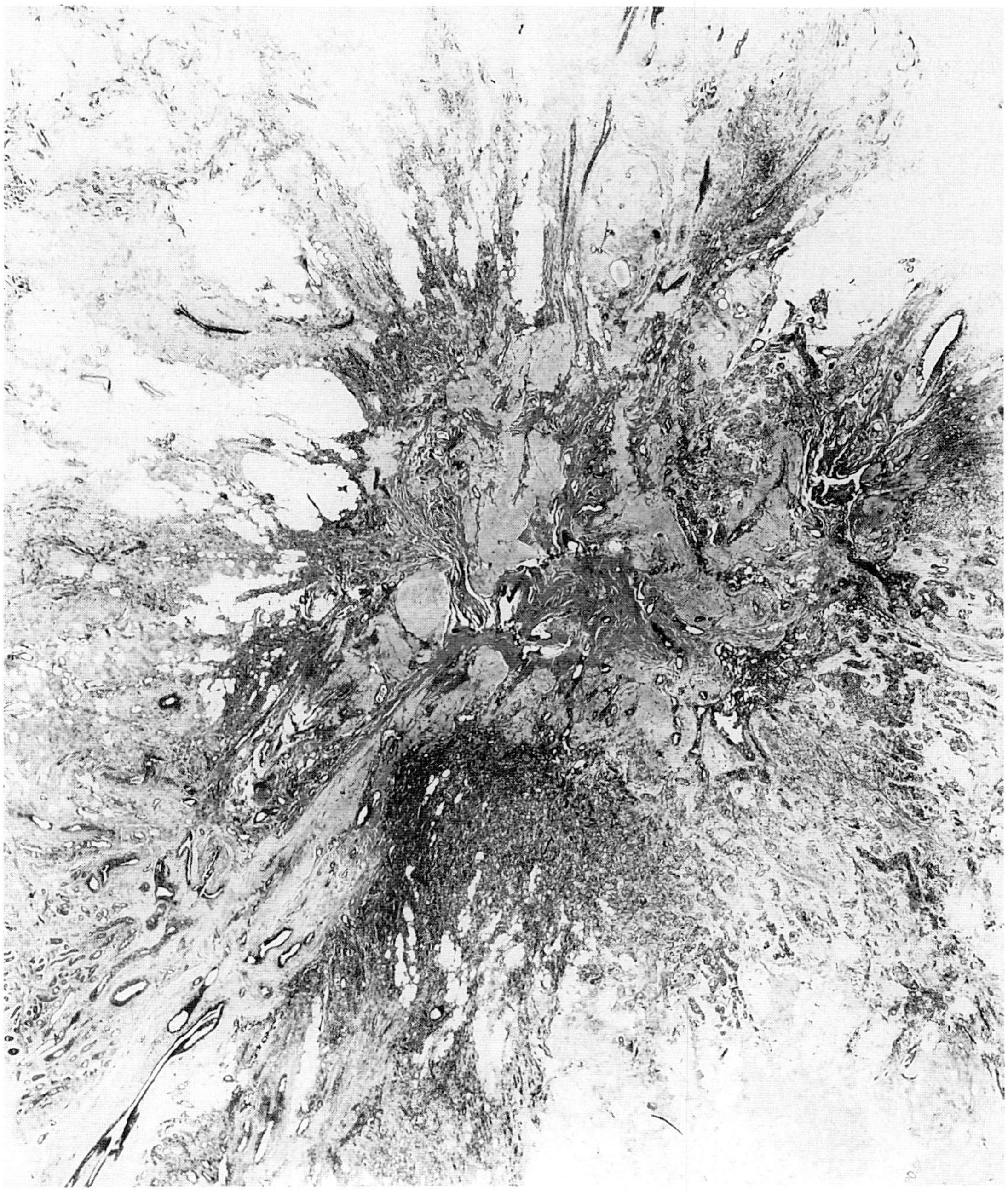

**Figure 4.12(e)** Radial scar. There is extensive fibroelastosis in this end-stage radial scar. (H&E, X60)

distinction is not terribly difficult, since the entrapped ductules that mimic a carcinoma at the center of radial scars are lined by both epithelial and myoepithelial cells which are often recognizable on H&E sections. When identification of the myoepithelial cells proves to be difficult on the H&E stained slide, immunostains for actin invariably resolve the problem. Furthermore, the entrapped benign ductules may display a circumferentially distributed basal lamina, a feature that is not observed in invasive carcinomas of any type.

### Relationship of Radial Scar to Carcinoma

Linell et al (170) had proposed that radial scars reflect stage 0 in the development of tubular carcinoma, but no additional support has been found for this concept that radial scars are premalignant. Two clinical follow-up studies have concluded that women with biopsy-treated radial scar are not at an increased risk for the subsequent development of invasive carcinoma (161,167). When there is either intraductal carcinoma or lobular neoplasia present in the surrounding ducts, the prognostic implications of the most aggressive lesion would prevail.

### Pathogenesis

The pathogenesis of radial scars remain speculative. Wellings and Alpers (176) hypothesized that radial scars start as a reaction to injury which heals and forms areas of fibrosis and elastosis. Theoretically, the increasing use of needle aspiration biopsy could result in formation of radial scars. The fibroelastotic core contracts, pulling the surrounding ducts and lobules into a radial arrangement. Proliferative changes may already be present in these surrounding structures or they may develop later.

Ductal obliteration has also been proposed as a factor in the histogenesis of radial scars (169). The sclerotic core seems to be derived from obliterating duct ectasia in some cases (161).

## DUCT ECTASIA (PERIDUCTAL MASTITIS)

Duct ectasia or periductal mastitis is a distinctive lesion characterized by dilatation of major ducts, generally in the subareolar region, associated with various degrees of inflammatory reaction around the duct and progressive fibrosis. Clinically, this lesion can mimic a carcinoma. Unfortunately, it has often been included histologically, as part of the spectrum of fibrocystic changes by many practicing pathologists. Despite many excellent descriptions of the lesion (177,178,180,183,186,189,190,193,196)—albeit under different designations in the older literature—many pathologists seem to have difficulty separating duct ectasia from cystic changes of lobular origin, though the clinical syndrome is very well recognized (195). The term duct ectasia was proposed by Haagensen (189) and remains the most widely used term for the lesion by those who do make a distinction between duct ectasia and cystic changes. Azzopardi (179), however, prefers the designation of "periductal mastitis" as more appropriate for the range of pathologic alterations observed in this lesion. The dilated ducts can be palpated as a worm-like mass beneath the areola, resulting in the designation of "varicocele tumor" (180). The abundant lymphoplasmacytic infiltrate around the duct along with reactive cells and changes within the duct have led to the erroneous interpretation of the lesion as plasma cell mastitis (178, 182), "comedomastitis" (196), and "mastitis obliterans" (191).

### Pathogenesis and Etiology

Neither the pathogenesis nor the etiology of duct ectasia has been established, and opinions vary regarding both. Some regard dilatation of the ducts and stasis of the contents as the initial phase of the disease, and the inflammatory changes as a consequence of leakage of the irritant duct content to the surrounding stroma (188,196). Others favor periductal inflammation as the initial stage of the disease, particularly since this manifestation predominates in the younger patients (181,184).

Pregnancy and lactation have been proposed as playing a role in the development of the disease possibly due to damage to the major ducts during suckling (181).

It is important to emphasize that duct ectasia is not a disease limited to parous women. It has been reported in virgins (193,197) as well as a male patient (194). Furthermore, not all cases of duct ectasia can be attributed to changes associated with aging and involution as suggested by Haagensen. Congenital inverted nipples (192) and ill-fitting garments have also been proposed as etiologic factors, but their role remains questionable and without confirmation.

## Clinical Features

The disease becomes clinically evident rather infrequently, but it has been identified in approximately 25% of supposedly normal female breasts at autopsy (187). Azzopardi noted that 30% to 40% of women over age 50 show evidence of duct ectasia. The clinically evident disease is seen mainly in the aging breast, around menopause or thereafter. The mean age of patients with duct ectasia in Haagensen's series was 54 years, with a range of 33 to 79 years. The patients may variably present with either nipple discharge, nipple retraction, pain and tenderness, abscess like features, or a tumor that may be mistaken for carcinoma. The nipple discharge is either serous, bloody, or pus-like; it may be of several years duration; and is not always associated with an underlying palpable mass. Exploration of the subareolar ducts is necessary in these patients and results in the identification of multiple dilated, ectatic ducts which appear as bluish cysts, 3 to 5 mm in size. The distended ducts are filled with secretory material which often escapes to the surrounding stroma and incites an inflammatory reaction. Acute pain and tenderness along with edema of the overlying skin and low grade fever heralds the recurrent, episodic acute inflammatory changes which clinically suggest an infection or abscess. These acute inflammatory episodes generally subside without intervention within a week to ten days. As the disease progresses, the inflammatory cells are replaced by fibrosis which thickens the duct wall and shortens the ducts at the same time. The contraction of fibrosed ducts lead to inversion, retraction, or tipping of the nipple (179,188,192). This nipple alteration is often mistaken for a manifestation of an underlying carcinoma, particularly when there is also axillary node enlargement due to reactive changes.

## Microscopic Features

In the early stages of the disease, the major or lactiferous ducts are dilated and surrounded by inflammatory cells (Fig. 4.13); they may be empty or filled with secretory material. As the lesion progresses, foamy histiocytes migrate into the duct lumen and replace all inflammatory cells (Fig. 4.14a). The basement membrane apparently develops widely open gaps, through which histiocytes easily migrate from the vascular channels surrounding the ducts into the duct lumen (Figs. 4.14b&c); the epithelium overlying these gaps folds over the adjacent intact epithelium giving the impression of hyperplasia. These epithelial folds may be lifted further, forming clumps and aggregates mimicking epithelial hyperplasia; there is no epithelial hyperplasia, however. In more advanced stages, the epithelial cell layer appears desquamated, flattened, or attenuated. The luminal content varies from simple granular secretory material sometimes with crystalline structures to a mass of histiocytes. The duct wall and the surrounding stroma display an intense inflammatory or histiocytic infiltrate. A granulomatous reaction with foreign body type giant cells may be present in the stroma surrounding the duct. Ochrocytes, which are histiocytes containing yellow to light brown ceroid pigment (185), are frequently present along with the usual histiocytes. The inflammatory infiltrate may almost completely disrupt the elastic layer around the involved duct, but often remnants of the elastica persist.

As the disease progresses, the type of the inflammatory infiltrate becomes more of the chronic lymphoplasmacytic type. Eventually, the inflammatory reaction is replaced by fibrosis and reparative changes. Once the periductal fibrosis becomes prominent, any remaining inflammatory infiltrate will be seen only beyond this fibrotic zone. Occasionally, lymphoid follicles with germinal centers encircle the fibrosed ectatic duct (Fig. 4.15). Azzopardi has also described the formation of fibrous "cushions" which present as eccentric fibrous plaques bulging into the duct lumen internal to the elastic coat. The extensive fibrosis can lead to complete obliteration and disap-

A

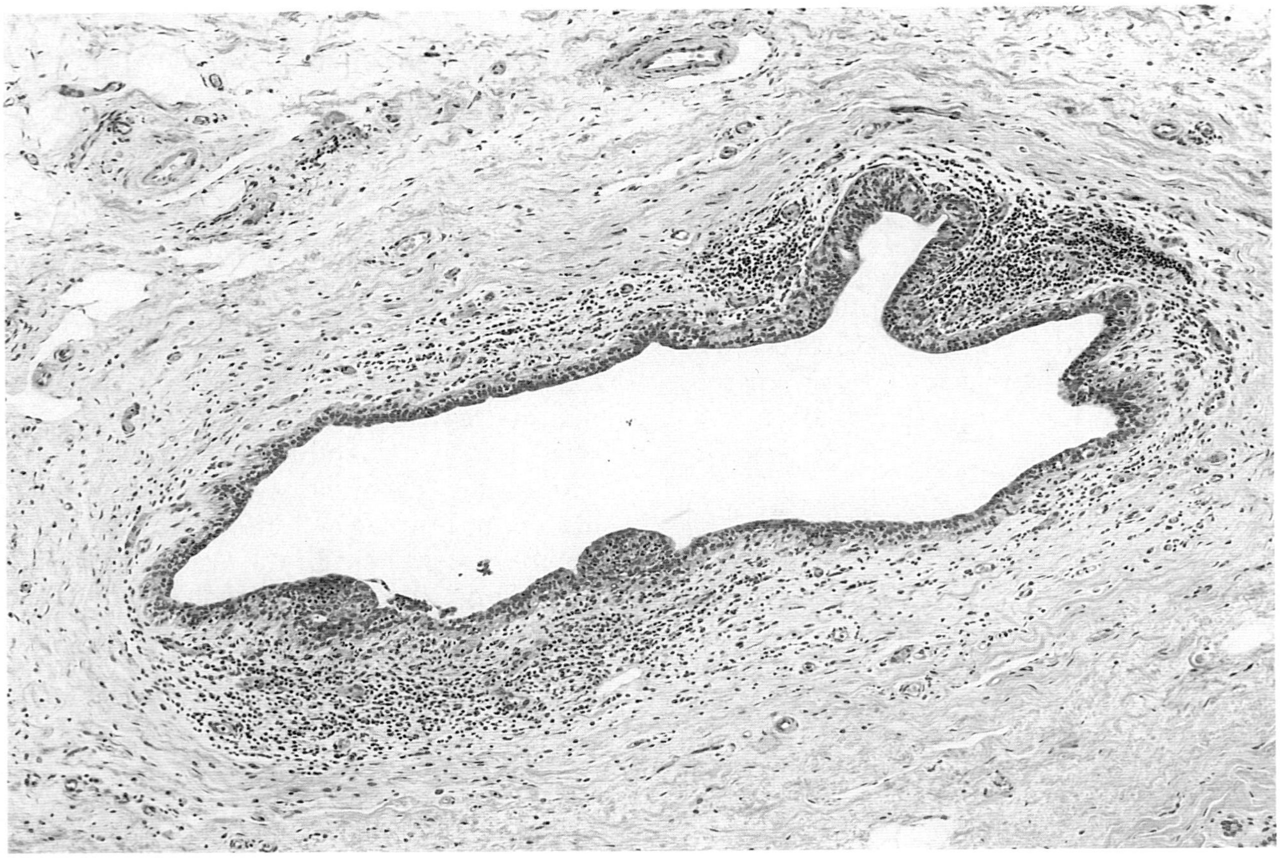

B

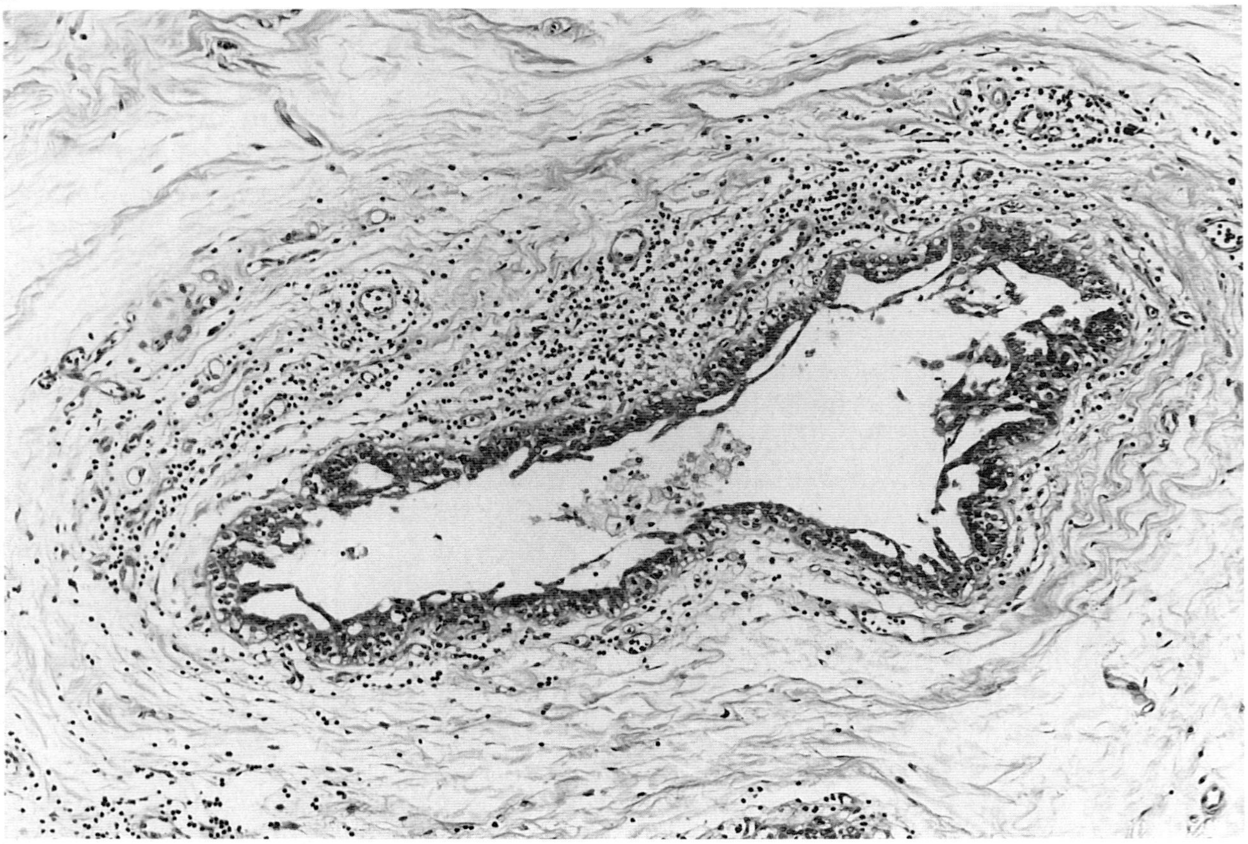

**Figure 4.13** Duct ectasia, early inflammatory phase. (a) A major duct is distended and surrounded by numerous inflammatory cells. (H&E, X40) (b) Lifting and folding over of the epithelial cell layer by the migrating histiocytes and inflammatory cells gives the false impression of epithelial hyperplasia (H&E, X80)

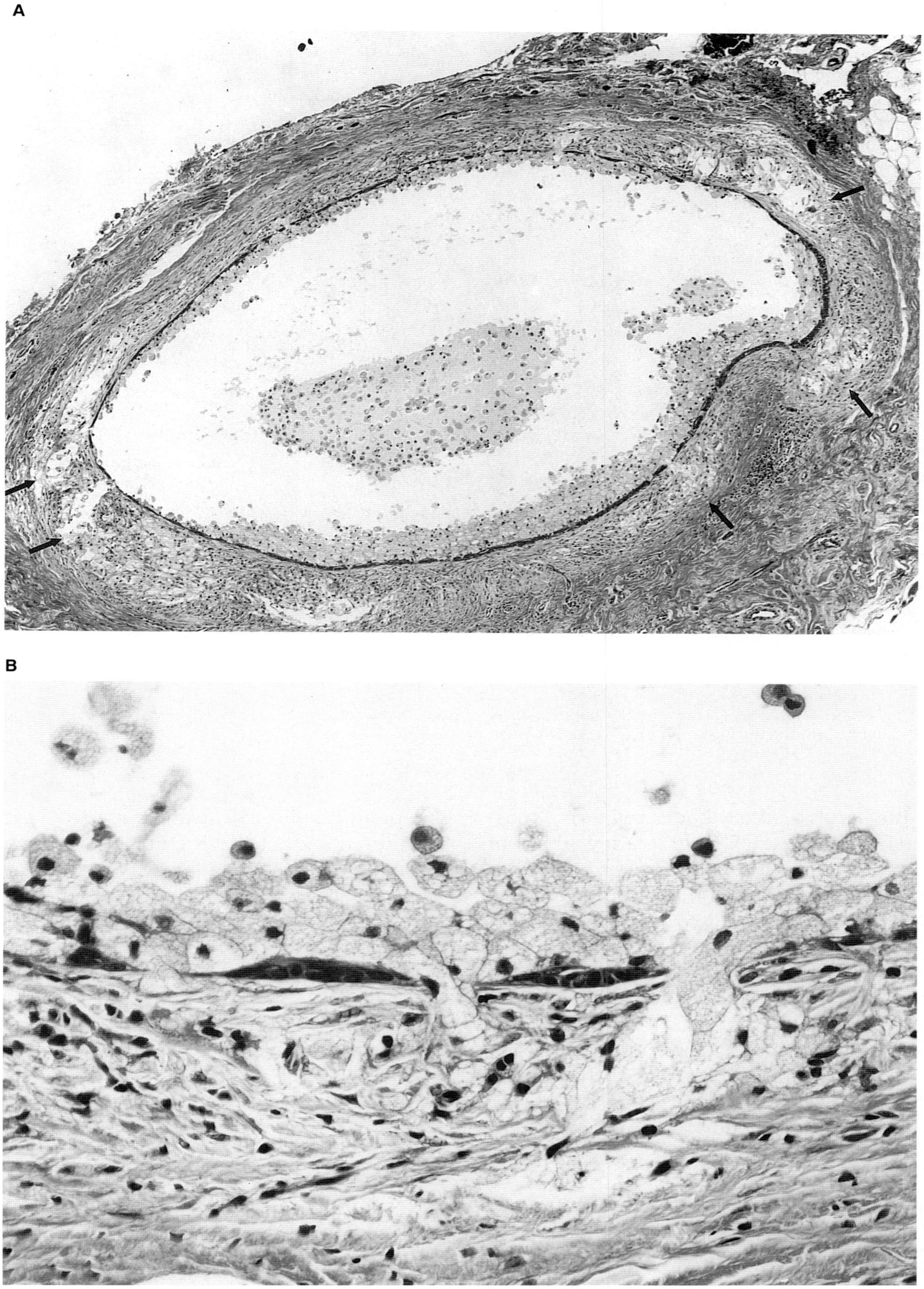

**Figure 4.14** Duct ectasia. (a) A distended ectatic duct lumen showing numerous foamy histiocytes overlying the epithelial lining and as a cluster in the center. The vascular network around the duct is also distended and filled with foamy histiocytes (arrows). (H&E, X40) (b) Areas of disruption in the duct wall show histiocytes migrating through these gaps into the duct lumen. (H&E, X400)

c

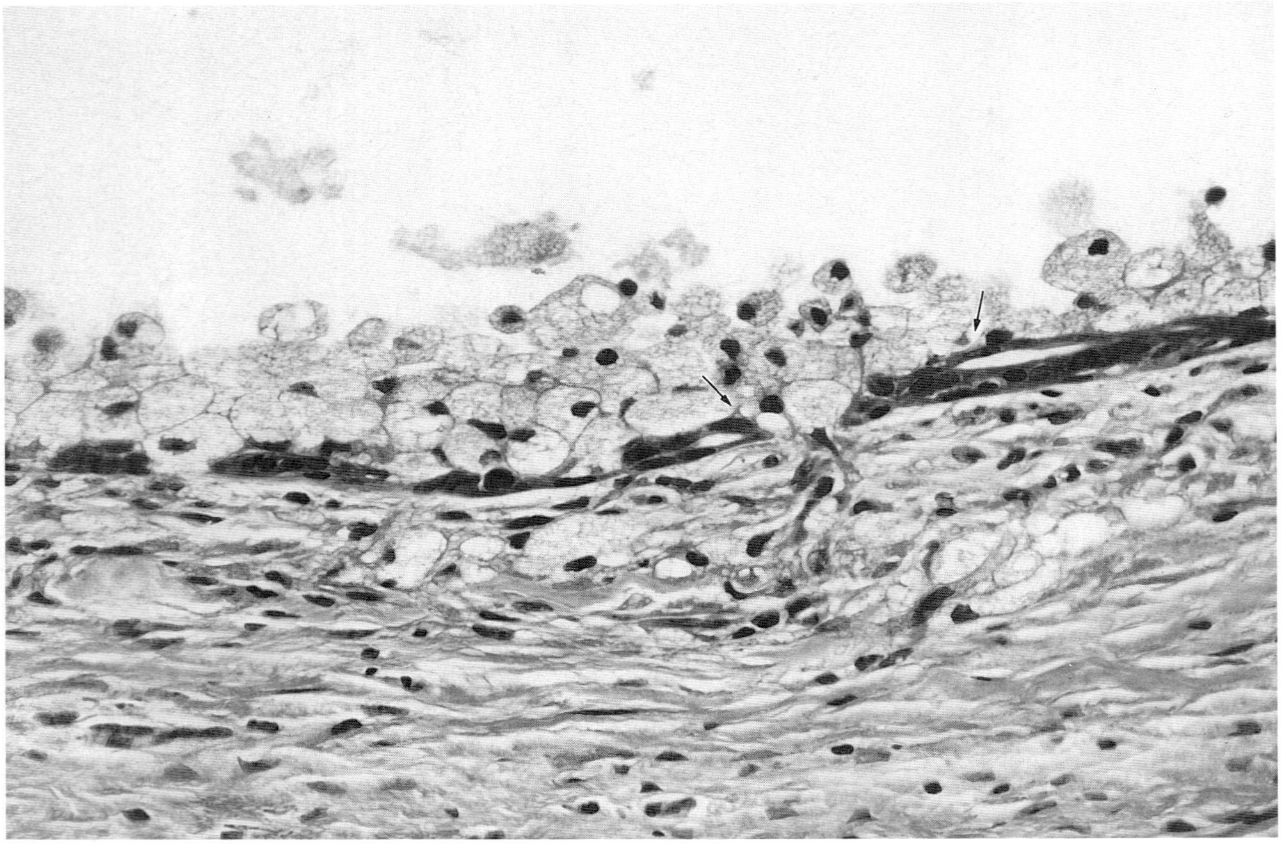

**Figure 4.14(c)** Duct ectasia. The epithelial lining of the gap region has folded over the adjacent epithelial cells covering the intact portions of the duct as the histiocytes migrate into the duct through gaps in the basement membrane. (H&E, X320)

pearance of the involved duct, hence the term "mastitis obliterans" (190–191). This obliterating phase of the lesion contradicts the term duct ectasia which has become the preferred designation for the entire spectrum of changes characterized by this process. Recanalization of the obliterated duct occurs rarely, producing a "garland" effect (180).

Duct ectasia can be distinguished from cysts of fibrocystic changes by its location within the subareolar region. When it extends deeper into the breast, the presence of elastica in the duct wall distinguishes ectatic ducts from cystically altered ductules within lobules which lack an elastic layer around them.

## Mammographic Features

Classically, duct ectasia shows a ring and tubular shadows on mammograms, due to the location of the calcification in the periductal fibrous tissue. Less frequently, the calcification may be present in the obliterating duct and the fibrous cushions. It appears that neoplasms are more easily detected in breasts previously affected by duct ectasia; this has led to a false impression of a relationship between duct ectasia and carcinoma (198).

## Treatment

For the early stages of the disease, Haagensen (188) suggested severence of all ducts at the base of the nipple and their excision along with a cone of surrounding breast tissue to include segments of ducts not involved by the disease process.

For advanced disease with fibrosis and tumor-like presentation of the affected ducts, Haagensen recommended local excision of the entire diseased area.

Since duct ectasia is generally a disease affecting

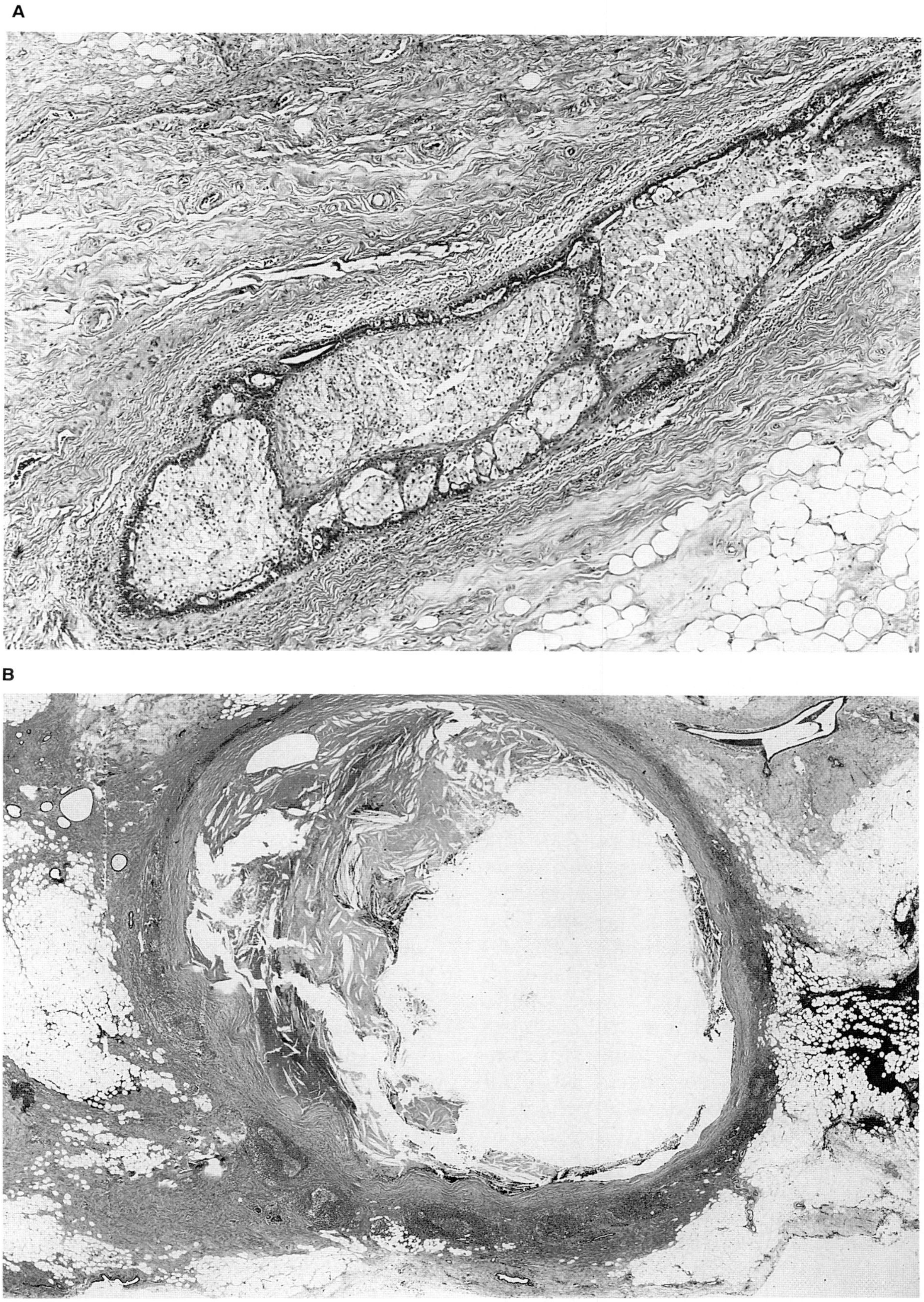


**Figure 4.15** Duct ectasia, late stages. (a) Obliterative variant—the lumen is obliterated by fibrocellular plug which may eventually hyalinize. (H&E, X200) (b) The duct wall is thickened by fibrosis; a band of lymphocytes focally forming germinal centers surrounds the fibrotic wall. (H&E, X30)

an elderly age group, preservation of a functioning duct system for breast feeding is not a consideration at the time of surgery.

## ADENOMAS

A variety of pure adenomas are observed in the breast (199,201,215,227,228,232). A pure adenoma is defined as a benign, well-delineated proliferation of epithelial/myoepithelial-lined tubular structures separated by sparse supportive stroma. The epithelial cell population may be identical to those of the resting breast, it may look similar to secretory and lactating cells, or it may display a variety of usual and unusual metaplastic changes (apocrine, clear cells, etc). The myoepithelial cell population may also display a variety of configurations and differentiations. Either cell type or its derivatives may show florid hyperplasia and areas of solid growth.

The most common adenomas are the lactating and tubular types, both of which occur during the reproductive years. The rare apocrine adenomas, pleomorphic adenomas, and those resembling skin adnexal tumors are also discussed in this chapter. Nipple duct and syringomatous adenomas are additional variants which are described in Chapter 14, Diseases of the Nipple, since they occur in the nipple. Adenomas in which the myoepithelial cells are the conspicuous or dominant proliferating cells while retaining their myoepithelial cell phenotype are discussed in Chapter 15, Miscellaneous Lesions. The lesion designated as ductal adenoma (200,203, 213,219) is discussed in Chapter 6, Papillary Lesions, because at the AFIP it is considered as one of the manifestations of sclerosing papilloma. Although the illustrations may be somewhat misleading, it is possible that some of the lesions designated as ductal adenomas (203) may reflect the tubular variant of adenomyoepithelioma (see Chapter 15, Miscellaneous Lesions). Fibroadenoma is excluded from this group because of its biphasic nature and since the dominant proliferation is by the stromal cells; fibroadenoma is discussed in Chapter 11, Biphasic Tumors.

Many of the cases recorded as breast "adenomas" in the older literature reflect fibroadenomas. Conversely, some tubular and lactating adenomas were reported as variants of fibradenoma (210). Only two of the previously reported cases in the older literature were accepted as true adenomas by Persaud et al (232), and they considered lactating adenoma as a fibroadenoma altered by the hormonal stimulation of pregnancy. In 1961, Le Gal (220) wrote an excellent review of mammary adenomas and described 21 pure adenomas which he subdivided into the tubular and the tubuloalvolar or lactating varieties, along with three examples of hidradenomas. The lactating adenomas occurred exclusively during pregnancy and lactation. The tubular adenomas also presented frequently during pregnancy, but also occurred in nonpregnant women including a 9-year-old girl and a 72-year-old woman. He concluded that both tubular and lactating adenomas may arise de novo or result from a glandular proliferation within a fibroadenoma. Hertel et al (214) considered these two adenomas as closely related and basically reflecting the same proliferative or neoplastic type of process, but presenting during different physiologic states.

## TUBULAR ADENOMA

Tubular adenomas are well-circumscribed aggregates of compact proliferating tubules lined by epithelial and myoepithelial cells with sparse intervening stroma. They may be poorly encapsulated or merely sharply demarcated. Patients with tubular adenoma are usually young and of the reproductive age, but they range in age from 9 to 76 years. Over a 15-year period from 1975 to the end of 1989, 142 cases of tubular adenoma were diagnosed at AFIP. Ninety percent of the patients were less than 40 years of age; the youngest was a 13-year-old girl and the oldest was a 76-year-old woman. One of the 142 patients was a 21-year-old black male.

Patients present with a well-defined, freely movable mass without skin or nipple alterations. About a quarter of the patients complain of tenderness to palpation. About 40% of the patients have noted the tumor initially during pregnancy. Multiple tubular adenomas have been reported occurring along with fibroadenomas in the contralateral breast in 16-year-old, black identical twins (220). Among the 142 previously noted cases reviewed at AFIP, five were bilateral, and two of these also presented as multiple lesions in one of the involved breasts. Clinically, the tubular adenoma most closely resembles a fibroadenoma.

A

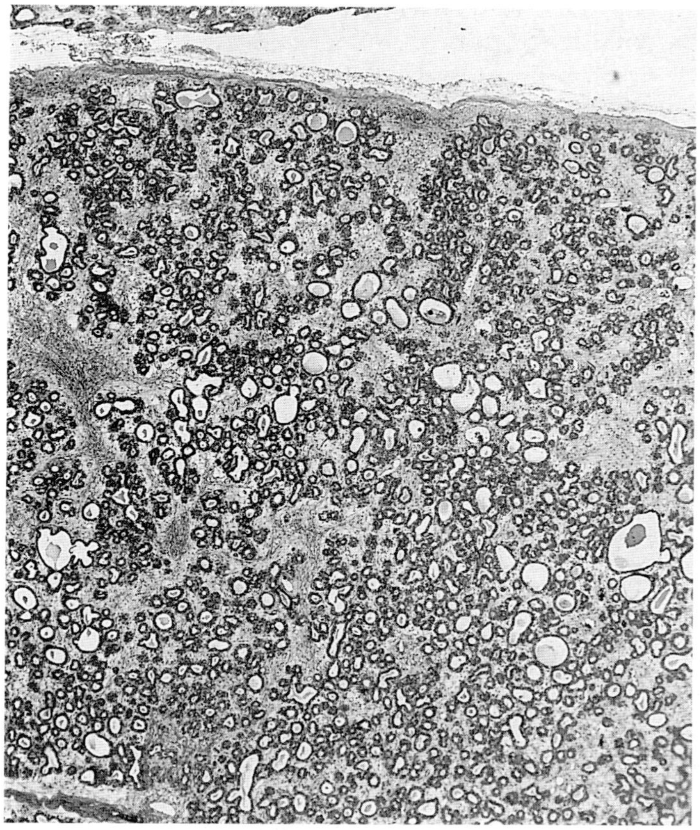

Figure 4.16 Tubular adenoma. (a) A delicate capsule surrounds this tubular adenoma from a 26-year-old woman, who was seven months postpartum. (H&E, X30) (b) Some tubules contain secretory material, but the epithelial cells are predominantly non-secretory with rare cells showing a few cytoplasmic vacuoles; the secretory changes probably reflect residue from the recent pregnancy. (H&E, X400)

B

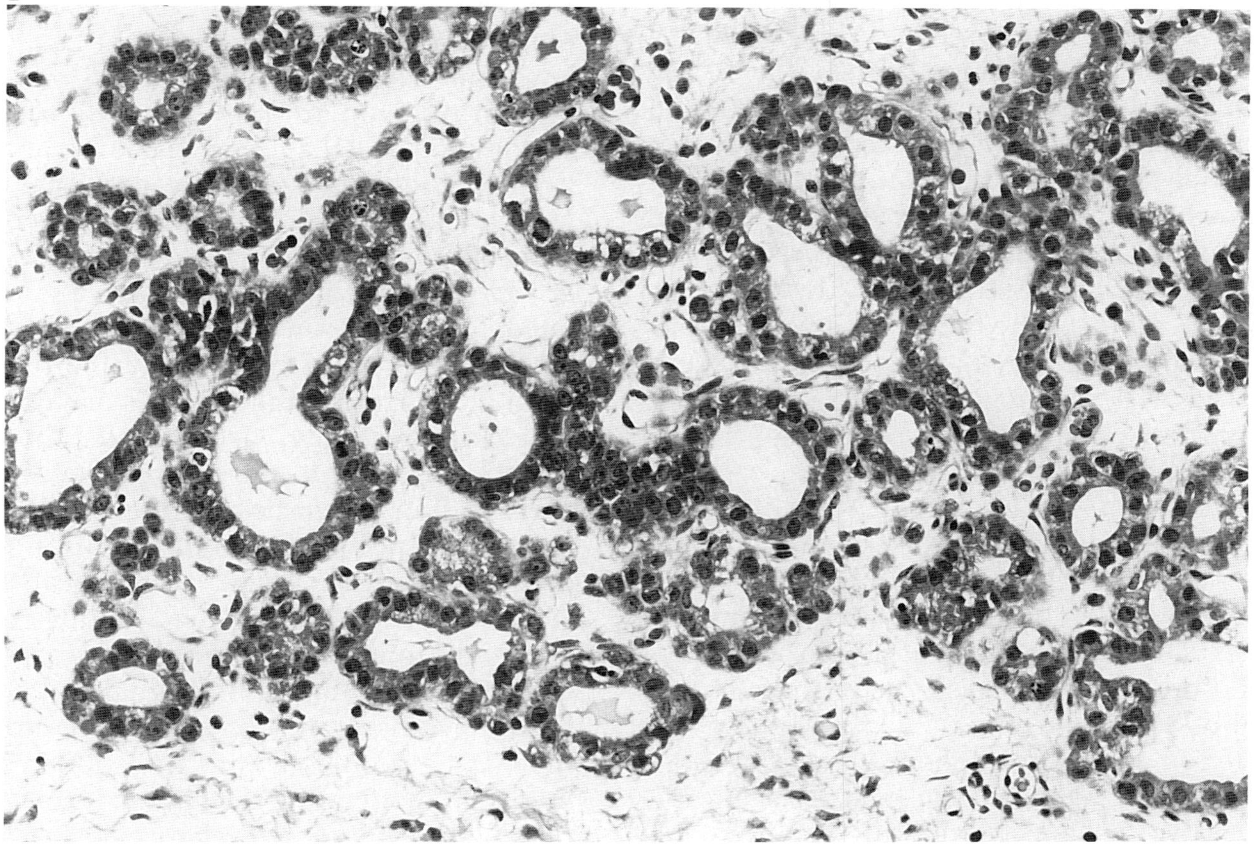

## Pathology

Grossly, the lesion is well circumscribed, with a solid, homogeneous to finely nodular, tan-yellow cut surface, and a firm consistency.

Microscopically, tubular adenomas are well circumscribed lesions, often displaying a delicate or poorly-formed capsule, and composed of a densely-packed cluster of small round tubules lined by epithelial and myopithelial cell layers (Fig. 4.16). The epithelial cells do not display atypia, but mitotic activity is observed and is occasionally abundant. The epithelial cells lack vacuolization and evidence of intracytoplasmic secretory material. The tubular lumens may contain an eosinophilic secretory material, but the lumens do not appear distended. Occasionally, the tubules manifest a tendency to form a lobulated arrangement; a larger duct is rarely observed in the lesion. The intervening stroma separating the tubules is sparse, and often infiltrated by lymphocytes. Rarely, the stroma may appear slightly more prominent, but it always appears as a supportive type of stroma in contrast to the actively proliferating, neoplastic stroma typical of fibroadenomas. Four of the 142 cases diagnosed at AFIP during a 15-year period showed focal to extensive areas of infarction. One of these adenomas had focal areas of apocrine metaplasia, two displayed focal intraductal hyperplasia, four showed atypical intraductal hyperplasia, and one had atypical lobular hyperplasia. Four of the five patients with atypical ductal or lobular hyperplasia were over 60 years of age; the fifth one was 35 years old. None of the five lesions with atypia were classic examples of tubular adenoma, however. Lactational and secretory changes were the most common alteration within tubular adenomas, being present in around 20% of the cases.

There are cases in which a combination of classic tubular and fibroadenoma patterns occur within a solitary mass; six of the 142 tubular adenomas diagnosed at AFIP had areas of fibroadenoma within the lesion. These should be designated as combined tubular and fibroadenomas (see also Chapter 11, Biphasic Tumors).

To qualify as a tubular adenoma, I require that the nodule should be at least 1 cm in size, or encapsulated if smaller in size. I find this requirement necessary because adenosis and nodular adenosis are commonly observed as a component of fibrocytic changes, and since gestational changes are associated with a tremendous increase in the number of acini per lobule as part of the physiologic hyperplasia.

## Clinical Behavior

Tubular adenomas are completely benign and are not known to be associated with any increased risk for subsequent development of breast carcinoma. Many of these tumors are found when the patients are too young for the cancer age group. Theoretically, however, it is not impossible to have a patient with tubular adenoma who also manifests simultaneous carcinoma. Total excision of the lesion is curative.

# LACTATING ADENOMA

Patients with lactating adenomas are also young and either pregnant or nursing (212,214,215). During a 15-year period between 1975 to the end of 1989, 68 lactating adenomas were diagnosed at AFIP. The oldest patient was 38 years of age. An unusual adenoma with lactational changes was also seen in a 53-year-old woman, however. The clinical presentation is similar to that of tubular adenomas, except that lactating adenomas may be multiple. Furthermore, lactating adenomas have also occurred in accessory breast tissue in the axilla and vulva (228). The tumors are grossly well-delineated, with a tan-yellow, lobulated appearance on cut surface (Fig. 4.17a). They are generally softer in consistency than tubular adenomas. Hemorrhage and necrosis are not observed.

Microscopically, lactating adenomas have a lobulated outline and are sharply delineated from the surrounding breast tissue, often without a true capsule (Fig. 4.17b). The lobulated arrangement is also evident within the lesion, with delicate fibrous bands separating the lobules. The amount of secretory activity within the lesion is highly variable and dependent on the duration of pregnancy and initiation of lactation. Therefore, during earlier months of pregnancy, the tubules within the adenoma may appear mildly to moderately distended with secretory material and the lining epithelial cells show simply small secretory intracytoplasmic vacuoles. On the other hand, tumors removed during breast feeding show

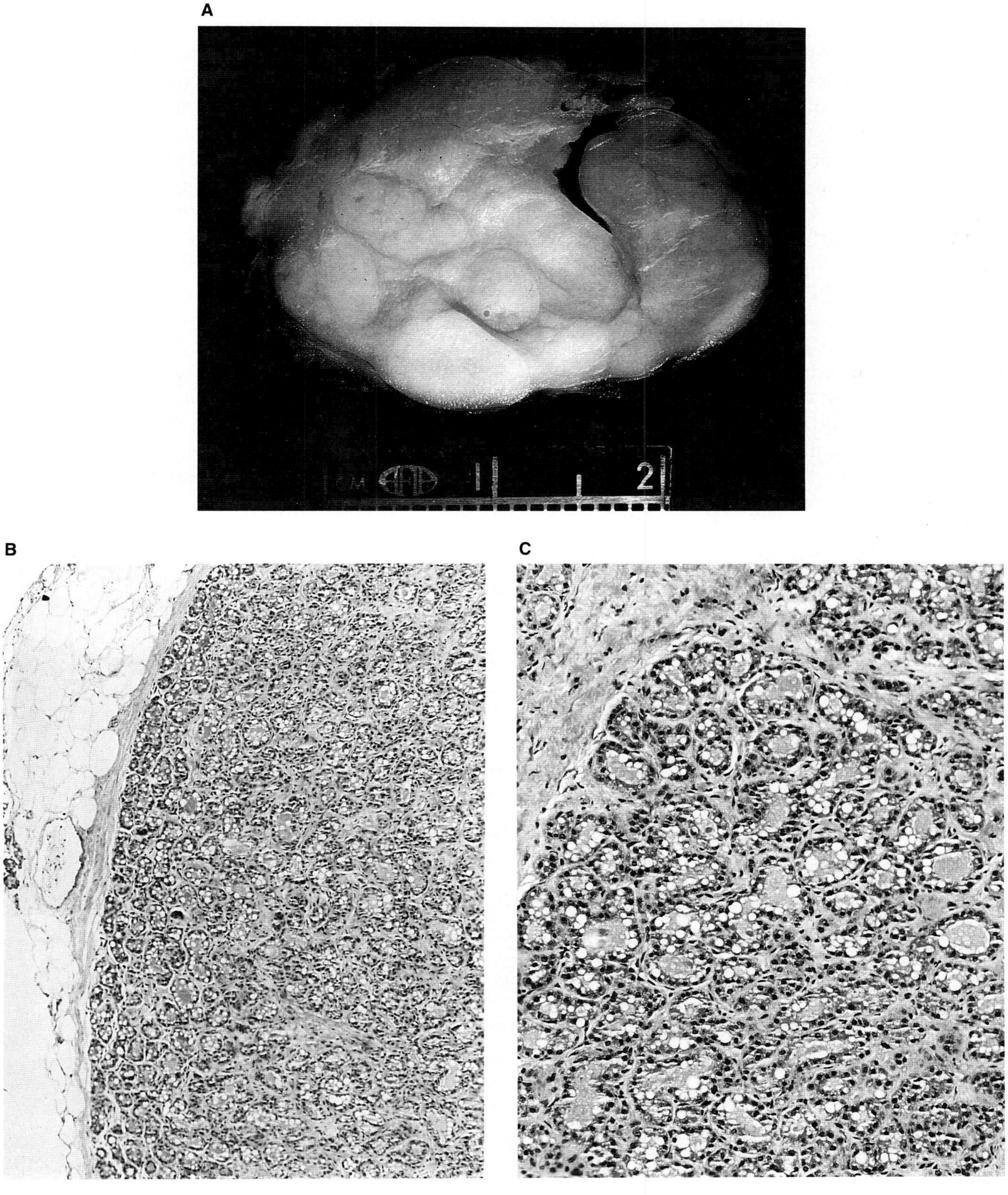


**Figure 4.17** Lactating adenoma. (a) The lobulated cut surface is typical. (b) The margin of the adenoma shows a delicate capsule. (H&E, X75) (c) The tubules are lined by vacuolated secretory cells and there is abundant secretory material in the lumens. (H&E, X150)

extensive distention of the tubules by secretory material. The epithelial lining cells show extensive vacuolization and show Arias-Stella-like features with a hobnail appearance as a reflection of the actively lactating cell population (Fig. 4.17c). The secretory material in lactating adenomas contains lipid. Mitotic activity is often abundant among the epithelial cells. Degenerating cells and cellular debris are readily found in the lumens during lactation. In contrast to the prominent secretory appearance of the epithelial cells, the myoepithelial cells become rather inconspicuous in lactating adenomas, but they continue to show a positive reaction for actin or S-100 protein. About 5% of lactating adenomas show evidence of infarction. The adjacent breast tissue also shows various degrees of gestational hyperplasia or lactational changes depending on the stage of the pregnancy.

Lactating adenomas are benign, but may occur simultaneously with a carcinoma (210,214) even though they are not considered a risk factor for the development of subsequent carcinoma.

### Ultrastructural Features

At the ultrastructural level, both tubular and lactating adenomas show retention of the epithelial and myoepithelial cell layers. The tubules are identical in their make-up to the unit structure of the normal duct system in the breast (see Chapter 1 for more detail). In my personal experience, it is impossible to distinguish the tubules of a tubular adenoma from those found in the lobules of a normal resting breast. The tubules of lactating adenoma are identical to the acini within the normal lactating breast. The epithelial stromal relationship is also similar to that of the normal breast.

## PLEOMORPHIC ADENOMA

Pleomorphic adenoma, also referred to as benign mixed tumor, is a rare and unusual breast adenoma with around 60 examples reported in the world literature (202,204,206,207,211,217,218,221–224,226, 229–231,233–235,237,238,240–242). Morphologically, it is identical to the pleomorphic adenomas that occur commonly in the salivary glands frequently with the presence of abundant osseous and particularly chondroid differentiation. Although bone and cartilage are occasionally noted in a variety of breast lesions including papillomas and sarcomas, as well as unusual metaplastic carcinomas (233,236), pleomorphic adenoma is often mistaken for metaplastic carcinoma because of the peculiar blending of the clearly epithelial elements with spindled myoepithelial cells, the chondromyxoid and osseous components in the lesion.

### Clinical Features

Patients with pleomorphic adenoma present with a palpable mass of several weeks to months duration. They range in age from 19 to 85 years with a median of 65 years. The lesion occurs predominantly in the female breast, but has also been reported in the male breast (211,221). About a third of the tumors are sub- or juxtaareolar in location. Nipple discharge has been observed only in three patients, however. The tumors are firm, nontender, and mobile in a majority of cases. Mammographically, calcifications are commonly present, and the tumors are interpreted as a benign lesion, fibroadenoma, or suspicious for malignancy (202,217,218,223,226,234,235,241). The presence of reactive axillary node enlargement at the time of presentation can increase the suspicion of a malignant process (240).

### Macroscopic Features

Pleomorphic adenomas are well circumscribed with a lobulated surface. The cut surface appears tan to gray-white, and varies depending on the amount of myxoid change, as well as the presence and quantity of osseous and chondroid differentiation. The tumors range in size from 7 mm to 17 cm, with a median of 2 cm. Occasionally, the tumor is multifocal (224).

### Microscopic Features

Histologically, pleomorphic adenomas are well circumscribed nodules with lobulations in some cases.

A

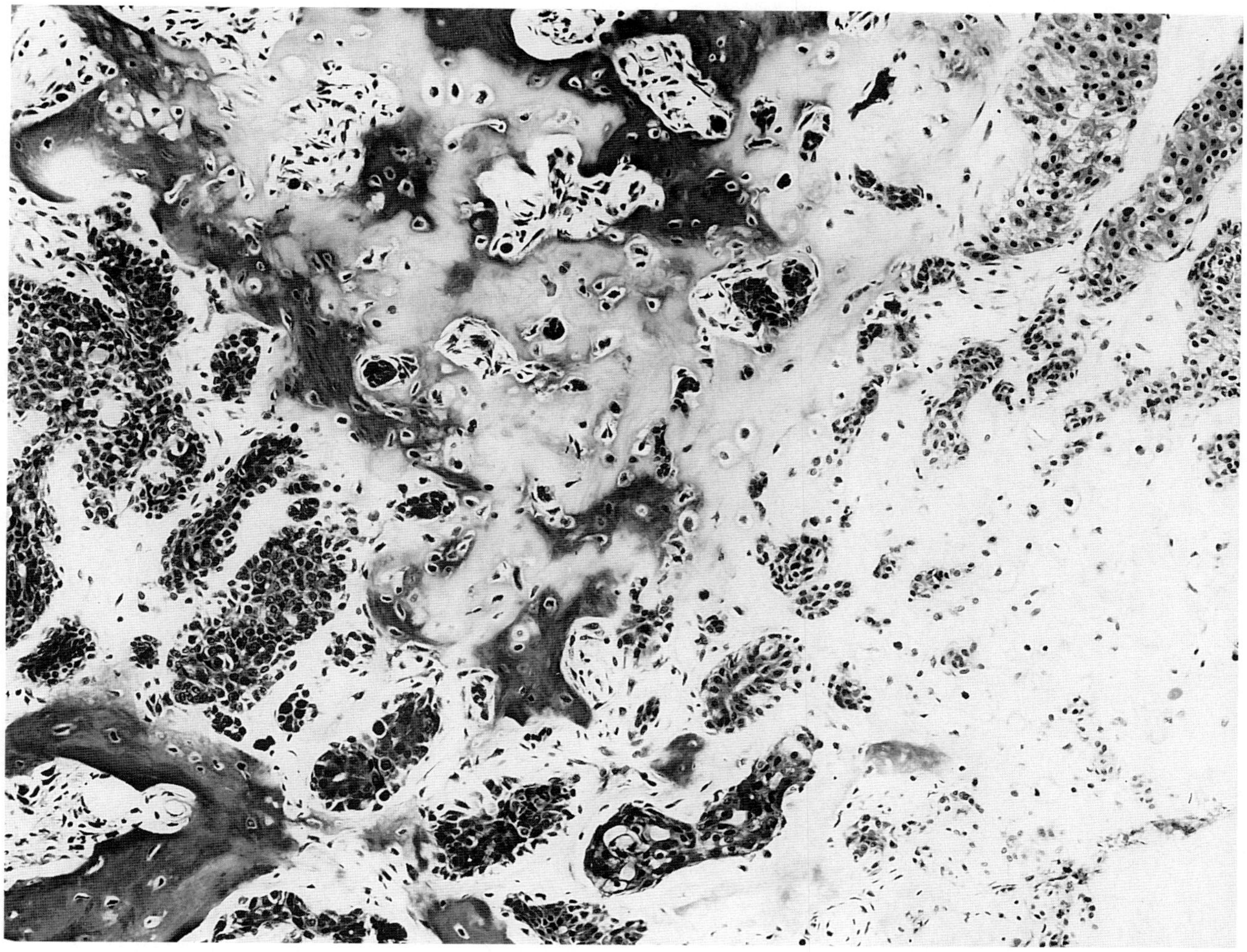

**Figure 4.18(a)** Pleomorphic adenoma. An intimate admixture of epithelial/myoepithelial islands surrounded by a chondro-osseous matrix is characteristic. (H&E, X100)

The tumor margins are generally pushing in nature. The adenoma consists of a variable admixture of epithelial/myoepithelial cell clusters in a chondromyxoid matrix, frequently admixed with areas of ossification (Fig. 4.18). Either the epithelial or the myoepithelial cells, or both, may appear hyperplastic in different cell clusters, but duct-like structures simply lined by epithelial and myoepithelial cell layers are also present. Large masses of spindled, myoid myoepithelial cells may be present adjacent to, and merging with the myxochondroid areas. Rarely, rosette-like radially-arranged crystals typical of tyrosine are found within the solid islands of myoepithelial cells. The epithelial cells are cytokeratin positive, while the myoepithelial cells and the chondrocytes show a positive reaction for S-100 protein. The myoepithelial cells also show a positive reaction for actin and at least focally for cytokeratin (224). The spindled myoepithelial cells and the myxochondroid elements have been reported to also show a positive reaction for glial fibrillary acidic protein (GFAP) (224); in our laboratories at AFIP, neither normal, nor neoplastic mammary myoepithelial cells have so far displayed a positive reaction for GFAP. Multifocal nodules are separated from each other by breast tissue containing other alterations such as intraductal hyperplasia or papillomatosis.

## Hormone Receptors and Ploidy

Estrogen and progesterone receptors have been evaluated in rare cases and have been reported to be

B

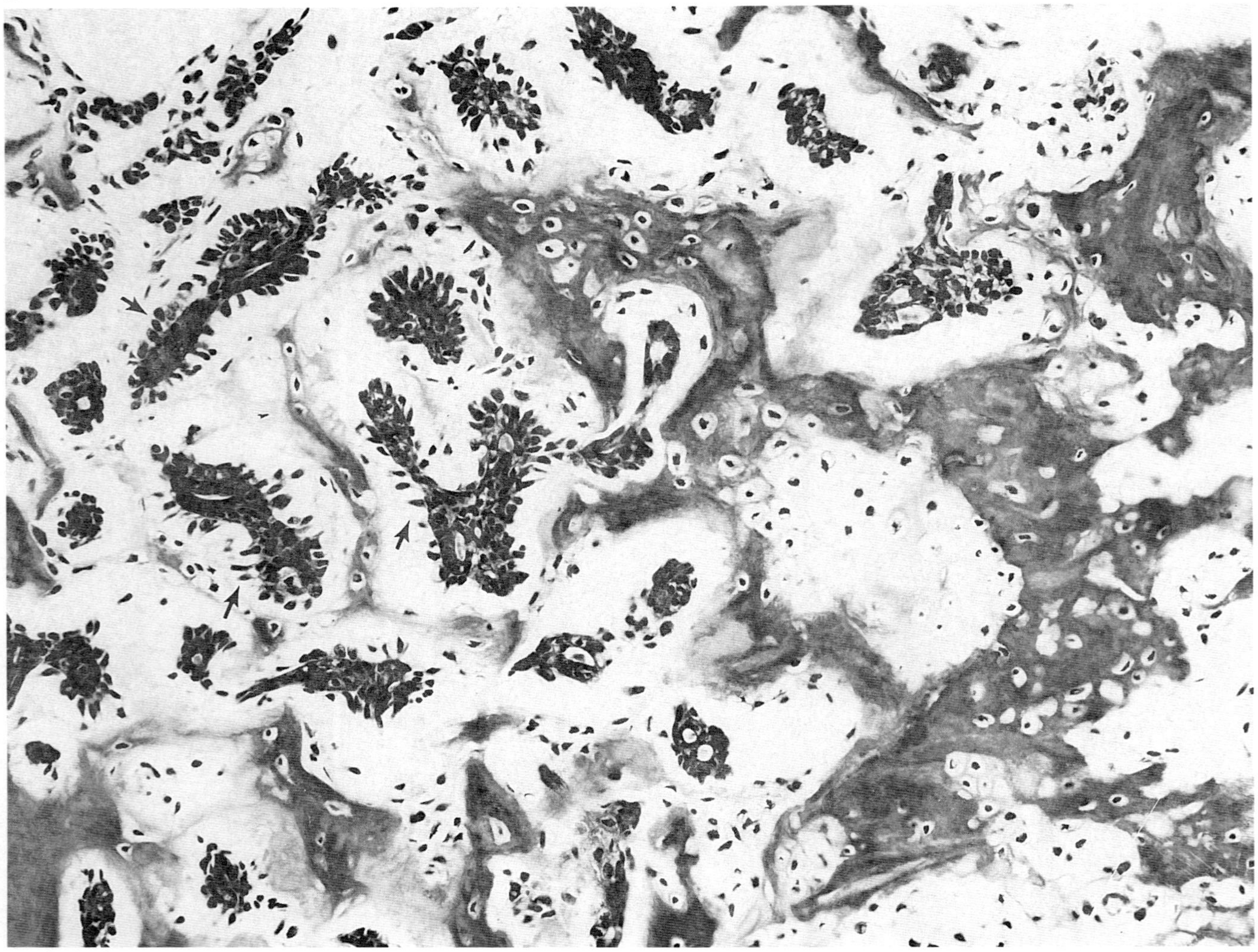

**Figure 4.18(b&c)** Pleomorphic adenoma. The presence of epithelial cells in the center and myoepithelial cells (arrows) in the periphery of the islands and tubules helps distinguish pleomorphic adenomas from a metaplastic carcinoma. (H&E, X150)

moderately positive at 46 and 33 fmol/mg protein, respectively, in one tumor (241); in another case, both assays were negative (204). Flow cytometric DNA analysis performed on one case showed a diploid pattern with low S-phase fraction (204).

## Ultrastructural Features

At the ultrastructural level, epithelial and myoepithelial cells, as well as chondrocytes along with areas of osseous differentiation, have been identified. The proliferating masses of spindle cells are myoepithelial in nature (202,206,222).

## Differential Diagnosis

Pleomorphic adenoma should be distinguished from metaplastic carcinomas with osseous and chondroid differentiation. The latter generally display unequivocal foci of an infiltrating carcinoma and lack the epithelial/myoepithelial islands so typical of mixed tumors. The abundant spindle cell myoepithelial cell proliferation present in most pleomorphic adenomas is another feature that helps distinguish the two. The bone and cartilage in pleomorphic adenoma are benign, whereas they may be malignant or atypical in appearance in metaplastic carcinomas.

Papillomas may also show areas of osseous or chondroid differentiation, but they lack the distinc-

c

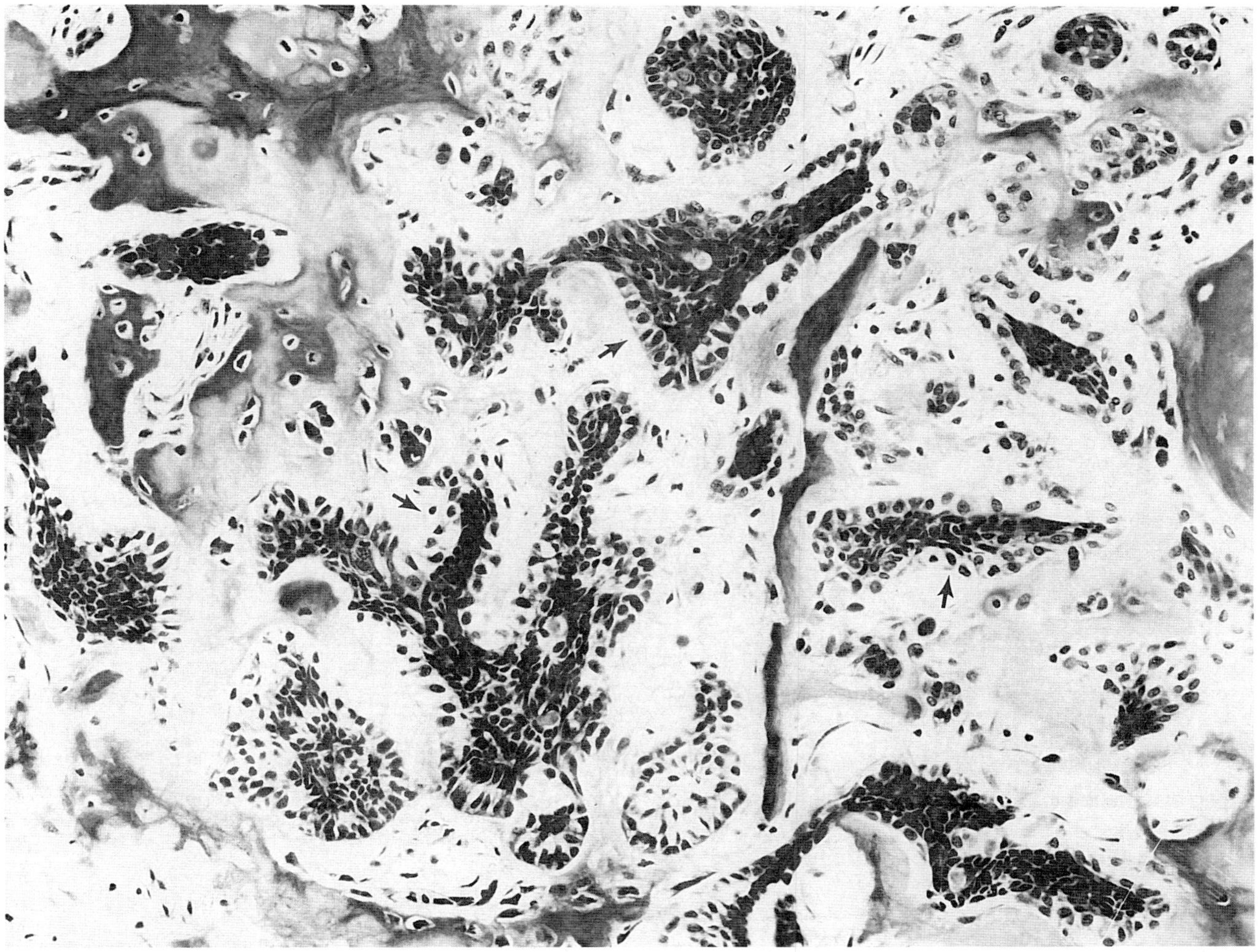

**Figure 4.18(c)** Legend on opposite page.

tive masses of spindled myoepithelial cells and the chondromyxoid martix typical of pleomorphic adenomas; seven of the nine cases reported by Smith and Taylor were simply papillomas with chondroid or osseous differentiation, rather than true pleomorphic adenomas (237).

## Behavior and Treatment

Pleomorphic adenomas are benign and are cured by simple excision. Care should be taken in excision of the multilobulated and multifocal lesions to prevent local recurrences. Although rare, recurrences have been reported in two cases and are probably due to incomplete excision of a multifocal lesion.

## Malignant Mixed Tumor

I have seen one case in which the epithelial and the chondroid elements of an otherwise typical pleomorphic adenoma showed obvious atypicality, mitotic activity, and invasive character. This lesion had been misinterpreted as a metaplastic carcinoma, but the presence of epithelial/myoepithelial cell clusters, tubules, and cords showing transition from benign to unequivocally malignant areas helped identify the

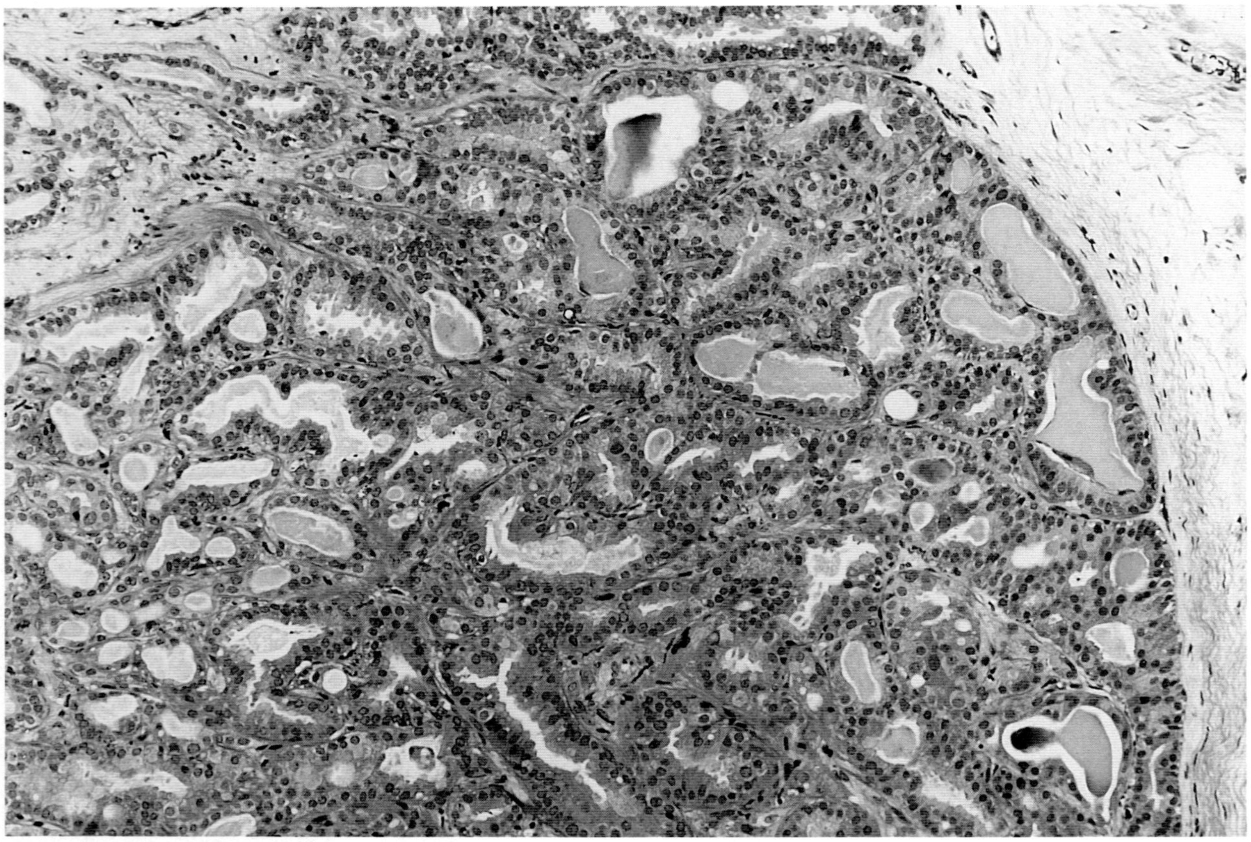

**Figure 4.19** Apocrine adenoma. A compact aggregate of tubules lined by apocrine cells without significant intervening stroma (H&E, X200)

lesion as a malignant counterpart of pleomorphic adenoma.

## APOCRINE ADENOMA

While apocrine metaplasia is one of the most common metaplastic changes in the breast, apocrine adenomas have rarely been described (205,239). Both reported cases have occurred in young women, one only 14 years of age (205), and the other 24 years of age (239). We have seen about ten examples of such adenomas at AFIP. Some are similar to tubular adenomas, but the epithelial cells are replaced by a single layer of metaplastic apocrine cells (Fig. 4.19); the nucleoli may appear unusually prominent in this group. Others show extensive tufting and papillary hyperplasia of the metaplastic apocrine cells distending the tubules.

## SWEAT GLAND TYPE ADENOMAS

Rare examples of mammary clear-cell hidradenoma, eccrine acrospiroma, and eccrine spiradenoma-like tumors, as well as combined eccrine and apocrine adenoma (243) have been either described or mentioned along with discussions of other types of adenoma (208,209,214,243). These are morphologically identical to their counterparts occurring in the skin. There are less than 25 such cases in AFIP files recorded as being primary in the breast proper, while many more occur related to the overlying skin of the breast.

## HAMARTOMA

The first description of hamartoma has been attributed to Hogeman and Ostberg (247) who, in 1968, described the lesion along with providing a clinical, radiologic and pathologic correlation. By definition, a hamartoma is a benign tumor-like nodule composed of an overgrowth of mature cells and tissue that normally occur in the affected part, but often with one element predominating. Hamartomas generally lack the structural organization of the tissue in which they proliferate. Furthermore, they lack the growth patterns attributed to any of the recognized entities arising in that tissue. Therefore, a fibroadenoma, or any other adenoma, and other distinct lesions such as juvenile hypertrophy, adenolipoma, myolipoma, myoma, and chondrolipoma do not qualify as a hamartoma. It is unfortunate and difficult to understand why some recent reviewers have included all these varieties of lesions under the category of hamartoma. Even more surprising is the inclusion of lesions containing cartilage, a tissue definitely heterologous to the breast, among hamartomas (248). Hamartomas present either as a palpable mass or as discrete lesions detected mammographically. With the increasing popularity of screening mammography over the past two decades, a number of reports of hamartomas have appeared in the radiologic literature. Radiographically, the lesion appears as a well-defined density, surrounded by a narrow zone of radiolucency and often gives the appearance of being encapsulated. Most tumors have a mottled appearance reflecting the admixture of fibroadipose tissue in the lesion.

## Clinical Features

Hamartomas are benign lesions that occur in patients ranging in age from 15 to 88 years with a mean age in the fourth or fifth decade of life (245,246,249,251,253). Generally, the patients present with a palpable mass identified during routine examination or detected by screening mammography. Occasionally, the mass is associated with tenderness; rarely, there is a history of nipple discharge. They are seldom multiple. All tumors have been unilateral. While initially it was thought that the development of hamartomas might be chronically related to pregnancy and lactation (247), this has not been substantiated in subsequent reports. Actually, it appears that the development of hamartomas is independent of the hormonal influences of pregnancy or lactation since they have been reported in women who have never been pregnant (244); pregnancy and lactation may increase the rate of growth, however.

## Macroscopic Features

The tumors are round, ovoid, or lense-shaped with the appearance of a fibroadenoma when intact. They vary greatly in size and weight, attaining a weight of 1,400 g in one case (249). They range in size from 1 to 13.5 cm, with a mean of about 3 cm. They are less firm than fibroadenomas, and may have a rubbery consistency. The cut surface ranges from gray-white to yellow-white depending on the amount of various components in the lesion; occasionally small cysts may be evident.

## Microscopic Features

Hamartomas are highly variable in appearance depending on the proportion of fibroadipose and glandular components within the lesion. Most frequently they consist of a completely or partially encapsulated nodule of sequestered normal or mildly altered breast tissue (Fig. 4.20), the alterations generally consist of fibrocystic changes and sclerosing adenosis.

## Behavior and Treatment

Hamartomas are benign lesions. Only one of the reported patients has developed recurrent tumors. She was 28 years of age at the time of her initial lesion which was enucleated. The recurrences developed 6 and 7.3 years following the initial diagnosis. All three tumors were well-circumscribed and morphologically similar; they were all enucleated without difficulty (249). It is possible that these lesions reflect multifocality rather than recurrences. Because they are encapsulated, they can be easily enucleated from the surrounding breast tissue. Goussot et al (245) do not consider surgical enucleation mandatory, unless the

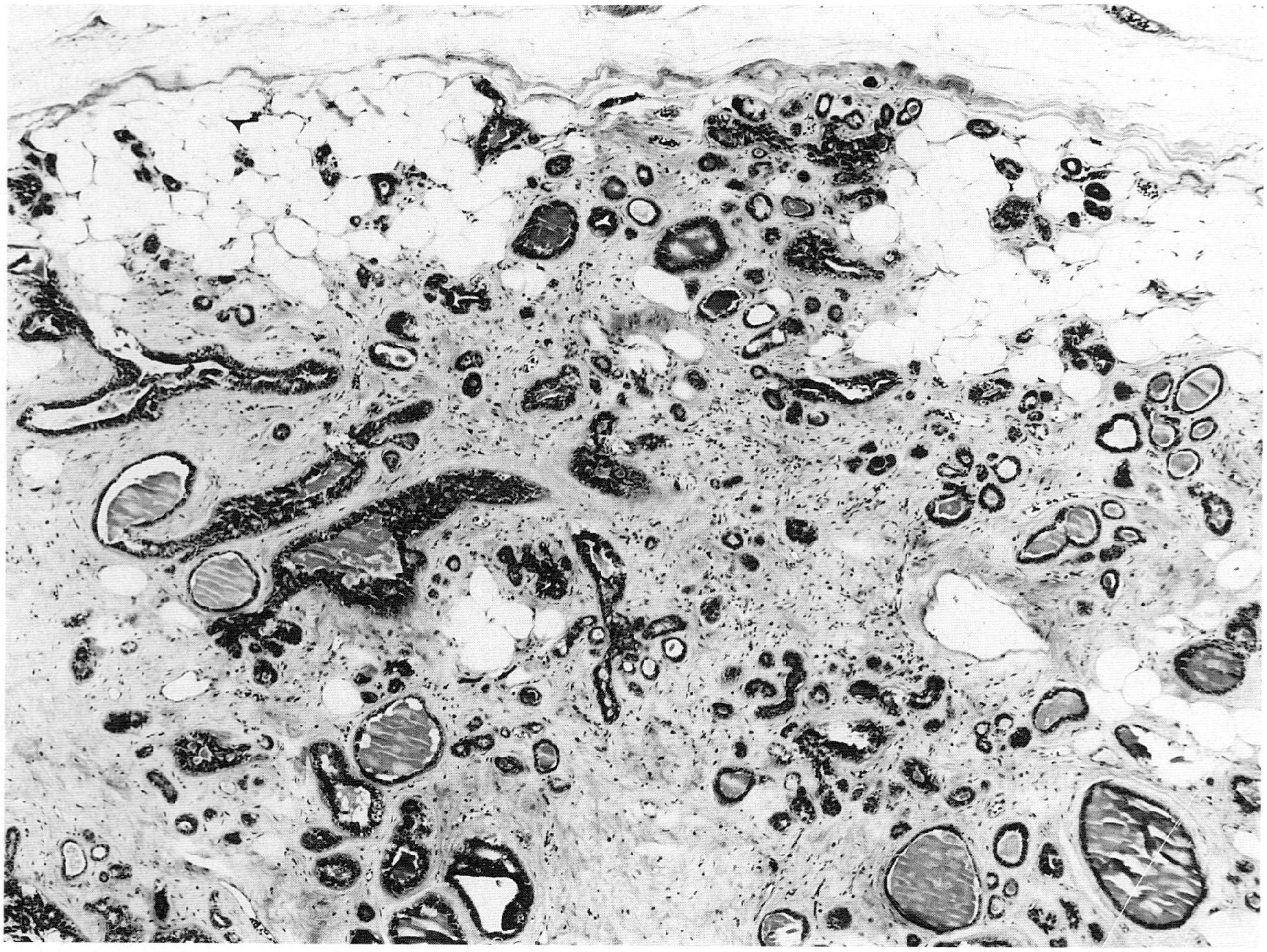

**Figure 4.20** Hamartoma. An admixture of fibroadipose tissue, irregularly distributed ducts and lobules are surrounded by a delicate capsule. (H&E, X40)

lesion is causing discomfort or appears unsightly. Since the clinical and radiologic findings are not specific or exclusive to hamartomas, however, it would be more prudent to excise any breast masses detected by palpation or mammography.

## CHORISTOMA

The term choristoma has been used to refer to a well-circumscribed mass of breast containing adipose tissue, ducts, smooth muscle, and cartilage (250). Since this mass contains normal breast parenchyma, it does not qualify as a true choristoma which should be composed of tissues normal for other organs but foreign to the site where it is found.

## JUVENILE HYPERTROPHY

Virginal or juvenile hypertrophy reflects the excessive and persistent enlargement of one or both breasts during adolescence which occurs predominantly in girls from 11 to 14 years of age (254,257,260–266). While in some young girls the onset of mammary enlargement precedes menarche by one to two years, it most often coincides with the first menstruation and continues for three to six months (260).

The breasts can become massive; Fisher reported a case in which each breast weighed 17.5 pounds (259). The enlargement causes severe back pain in some patients. Geschikter (260) noted unilateral and bilateral involvement of the breasts with equal frequency; Haagensen (262) also accepted unilateral

A

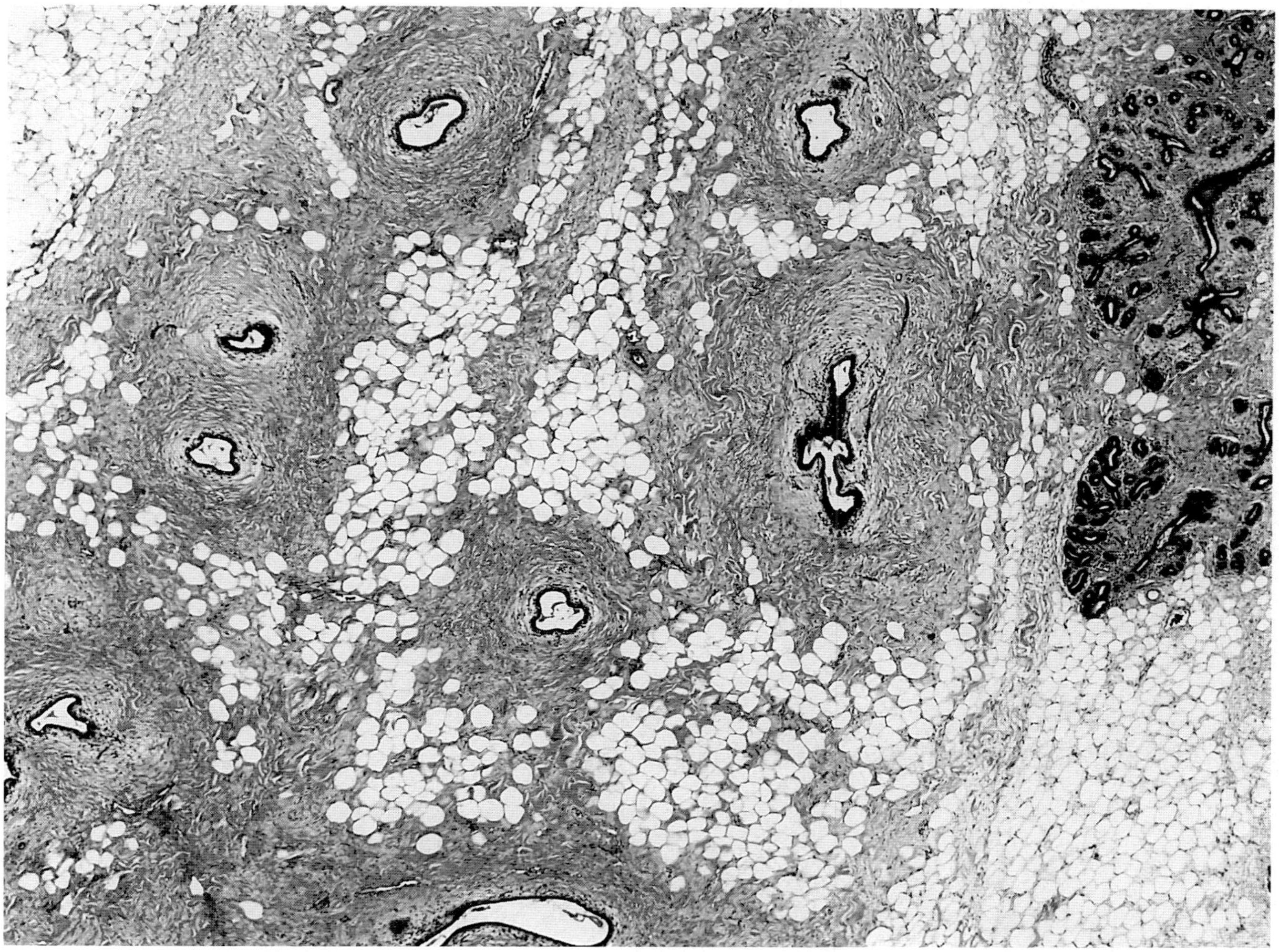

**Figure 4.21** Various patterns of juvenile hypertrophy. (a) A pattern similar to gynecomastia was present in a 14-year-old girl who presented with massive bilateral mammary enlargement 14 months after onset of menses. (H&E, X25)

development of juvenile hypertrophy and actually illustrated one in his textbook. Others regard juvenile hypertrophy as a bilateral process, and use this aspect to distinguish juvenile hypertrophy from juvenile fibroadenoma (258). I believe a distinction between juvenile fibroadenoma and juvenile hypertrophy is possible in most cases both clinically and on microscopic grounds. A majority of fibroadenomas are discrete nodules that easily shell out. They are more firm in consistency and look grossly different compared to the surrounding mammary tissue. Juvenile hypertrophy may look identical to the surrounding breast tissue and blends with it.

Microscopically, juvenile hypertrophy is characterized by proliferation of both connective tissue and tubular ductal structures. It lacks the organized stromal proliferation typical of juvenile fibroadenoma, but may manifest a variety of appearances (Fig. 4.21). Sometimes it is indistinguishable from the poorly-developed adjacent pubertal breast tissue. On other occasions, it forms a pattern identical to gynecomastia. Finally, it may display a proliferation of ductules in poorly-formed lobular arrangements and a densely collagenous stroma with diffuse pseudoangiomatous changes. While both lesions may be well delineated, fibroadenomas are more likely to form discrete nodules. On rare occasions I have seen bilateral hypertrophy in which the epithelial cells appear to be notably larger than those in the surrounding breast tissue (Fig. 4.21c); the myoepithelial cells were also particularly prominent. At the ultrastructural level, the myoepithelial cells were unusually plump, containing abundant myofibrils with dense bodies and numerous mitochondria (Fig. 4.21d).

B

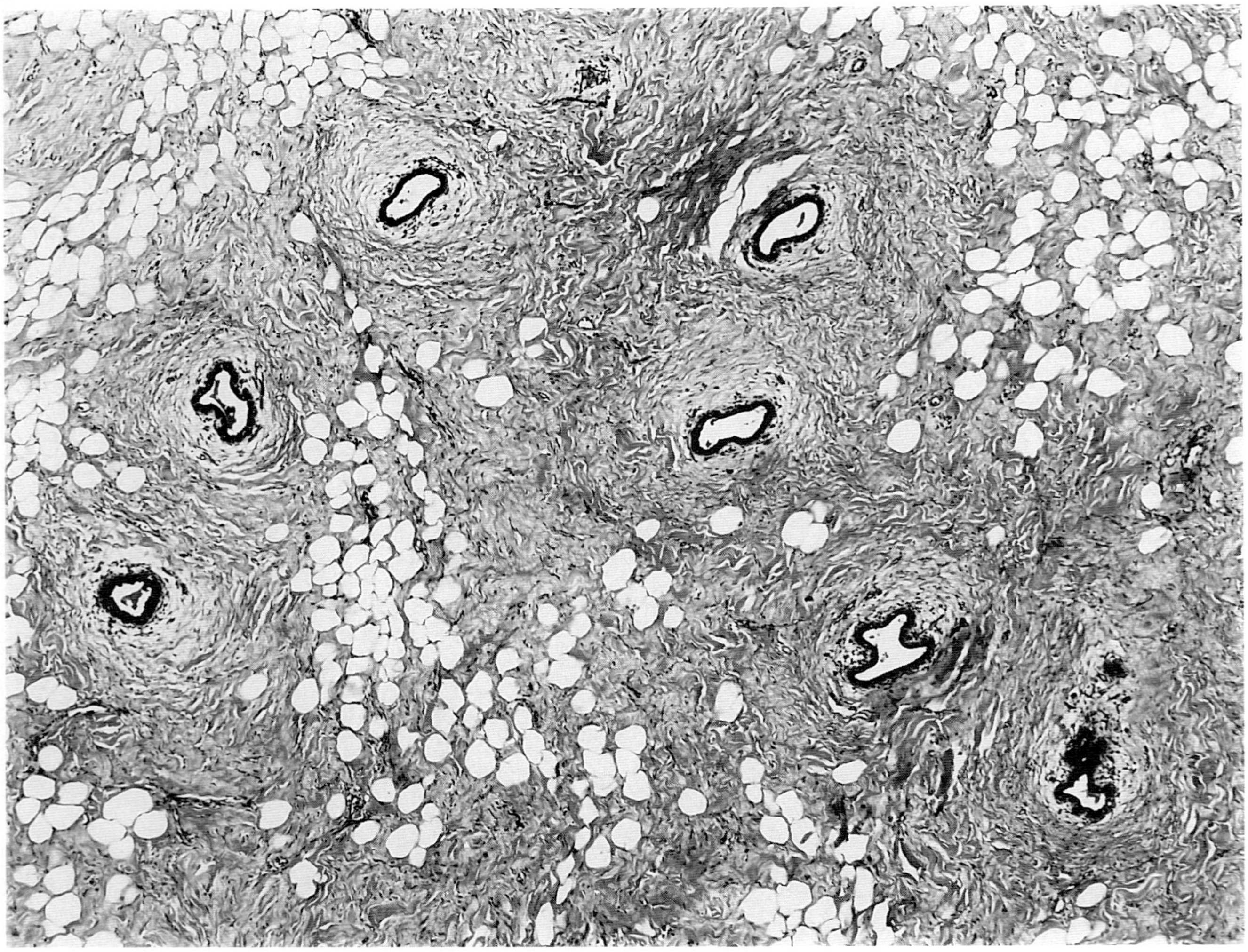

**Figure 4.21(b)** Juvenile hypertrophy. Gynecomastia-type pattern. (H&E, X60)

Barreto (255) reported an unusual presentation of juvenile hypertrophy. The patient, a 13-year-old Chilean girl, developed bilateral breast enlargement at age 13. At age 16 she had bilateral reduction mammoplasty. Six months later she became pregnant and developed massive mammary gestational enlargement involving both breasts as well as accessory mammary tissue in both axillae and beneath the mammary fold on one side. The mammary enlargement caused rupture of a superficial vein with sufficient blood loss to cause shock. The patient had repeat reduction mammoplasty and excision of the accessory breast tissues.

The hormone levels in these patients is often not abnormal (257,265). It has been proposed that the rapid enlargement is due to increased sensitivity of mammary tissue to hormonal alterations of puberty, mainly the estrogenic stimulation (260,265).

## MICROCALCIFICATION

Microcalcifications are an important feature of a variety of mammary lesions including carcinoma. Early in the twentieth century several authors noted microcalcifications in radiographs of the breast (302,314). Subsequently LeBorgne (294) observed that the presence of microcalcifications can be used for mammographic detection of breast carcinoma. In pathology specimen, however, Sandison noted laminated "calcospherites" in the breast of only four of 800 women evaluated at autopsy; these were either intraductal or intraacinar (303). Frantz et al (47) noted calcification in ten of their 225 autopsy cases. None of the calcifications in either study were observed in association with carcinomas. Depending on their appearance

C

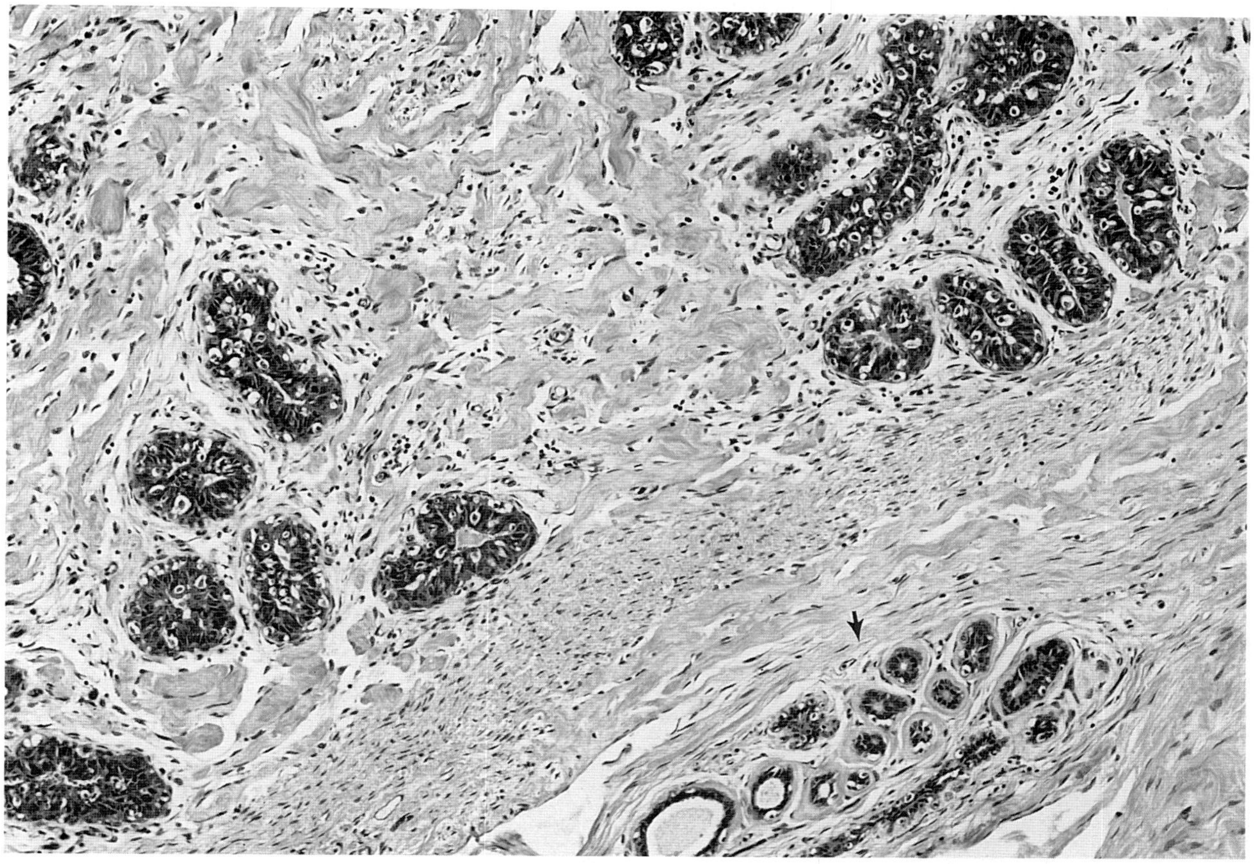

D

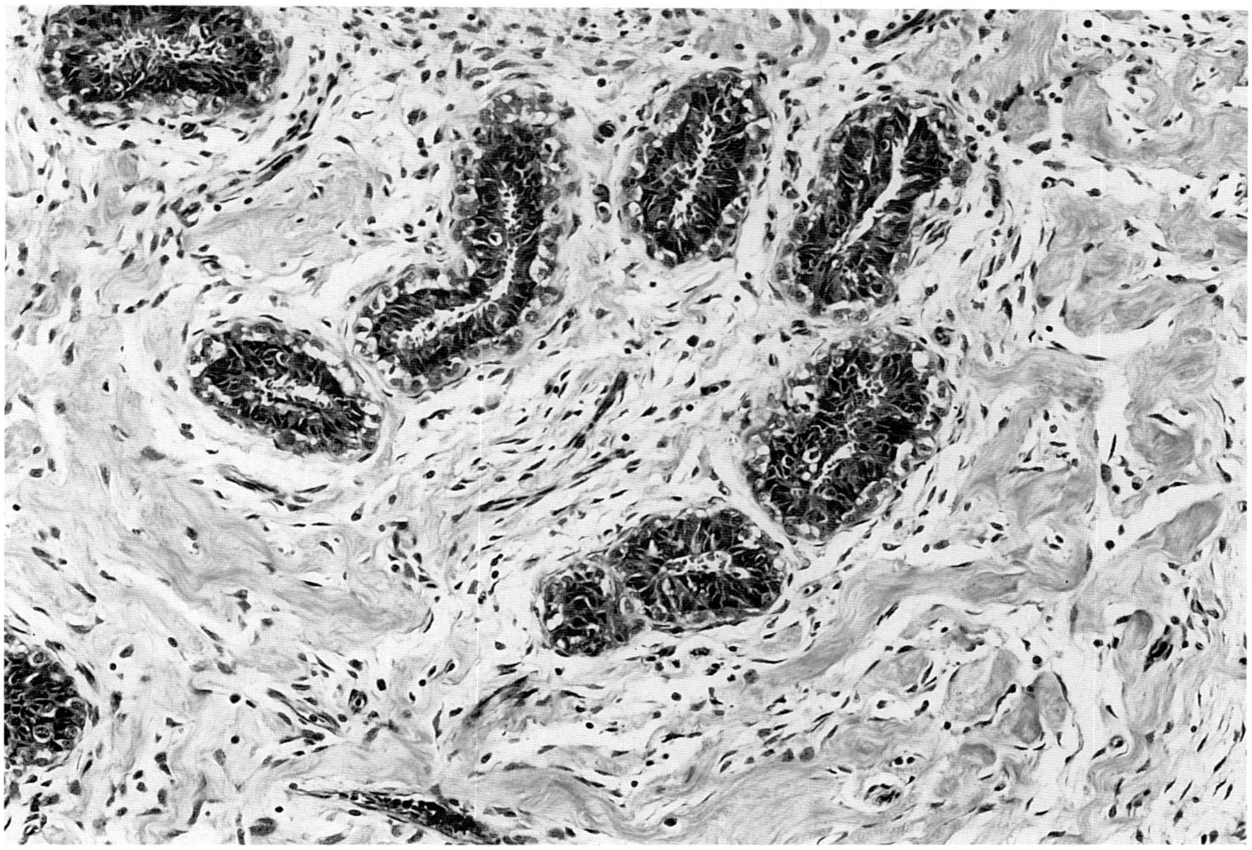

**Figure 4.21(c&d)** Juvenile hypertrophy in a 12-year-old girl. (c) The tubules and the epithelial cells in the areas of hypertrophy were quite large compared to the adjacent normal lobules. (H&E, X120) (d) The myoepithelial cells are very prominent. (H&E, X200)

E

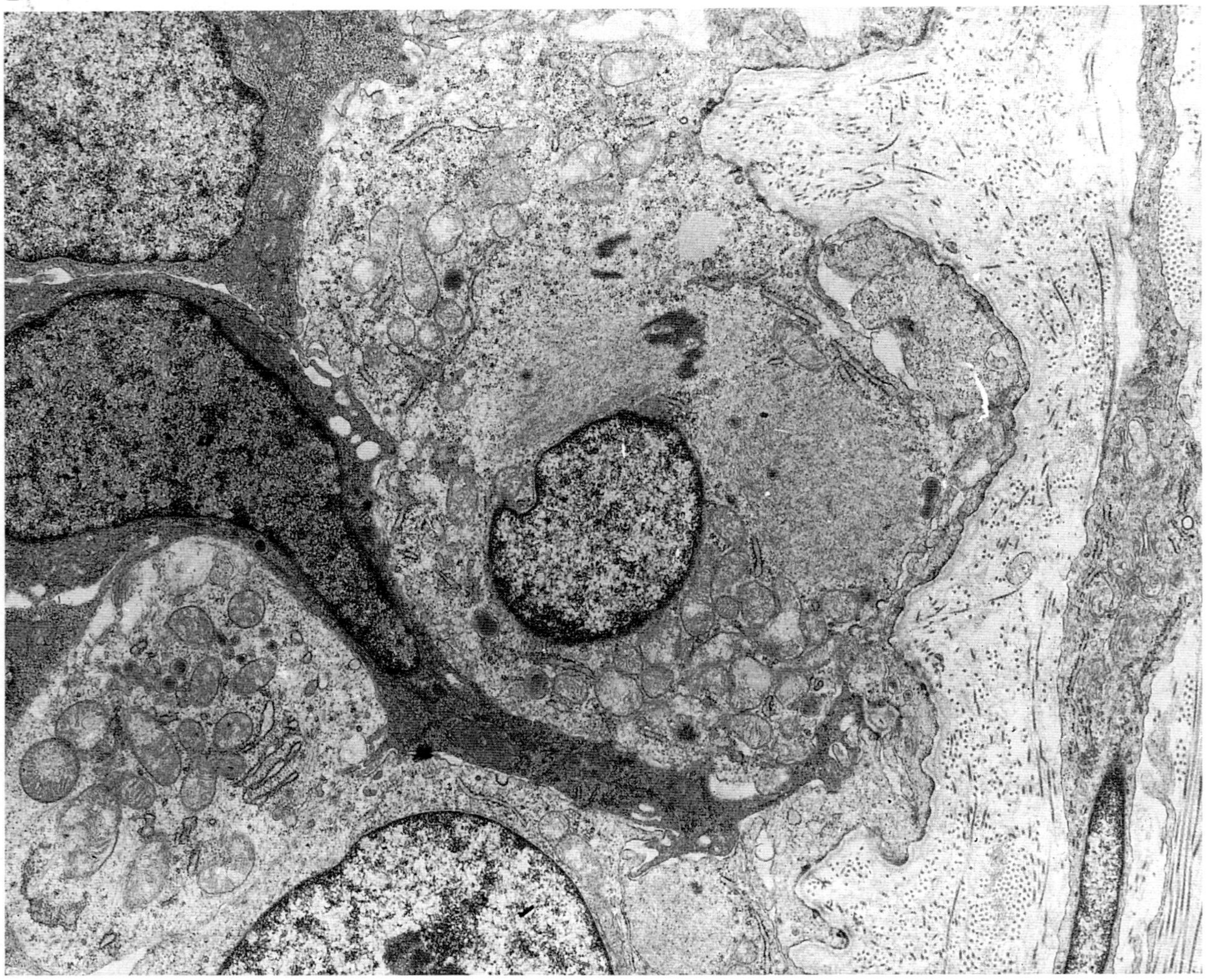

**Figure 4.21(e)** Juvenile hypertrophy in a 12-year-old girl. The prominent ME cells contained abundant mitochondria and microfilaments at the ultrastructural level. (Uranyl acetate-lead citrate, X3,200)

(size and shape), number, and pattern of distribution, microcalcifications have proved invaluable to radiologists in their efforts to determine the benign and malignant nature of a mammographically detected lesion.

Approximately 40% to 50% of mammary carcinomas have microcalcifications that are mammographically detectable (270,297,298). An increasing number of noncomedo intraductal carcinomas are also detected mammographically. The apparent mammographic distribution of microcalcification in these cases does not correlate well with the microscopic findings, however. Some studies have described an overestimation of the extent of the intraductal carcinoma (292) based on the mammographic distribution of microcalcifications. This error is due to the incorporation of microcalcification associated with surrounding benign lesions into the measurements (292). Other investigators have found that the intraductal carcinoma may actually extend beyond the mammographically defined area of involvement (288). These studies indicate that while current mammographic techniques can detect carcinomas, the extent of the malignancy cannot be assessed reliably. There are two major reasons for this problem. As mentioned earlier, microcalcification is not limited to areas of carcinoma and often involves benign areas around a malignant process as well. Furthermore, not all areas of carcinoma contain or are surrounded by microcalcification.

Among 213 asymptomatic women who had biopsies performed at Institut Gustave-Roussy because of mammographically detected microcalcifications, 65 women (31%) had carcinomas (275). Thirty-four of

F

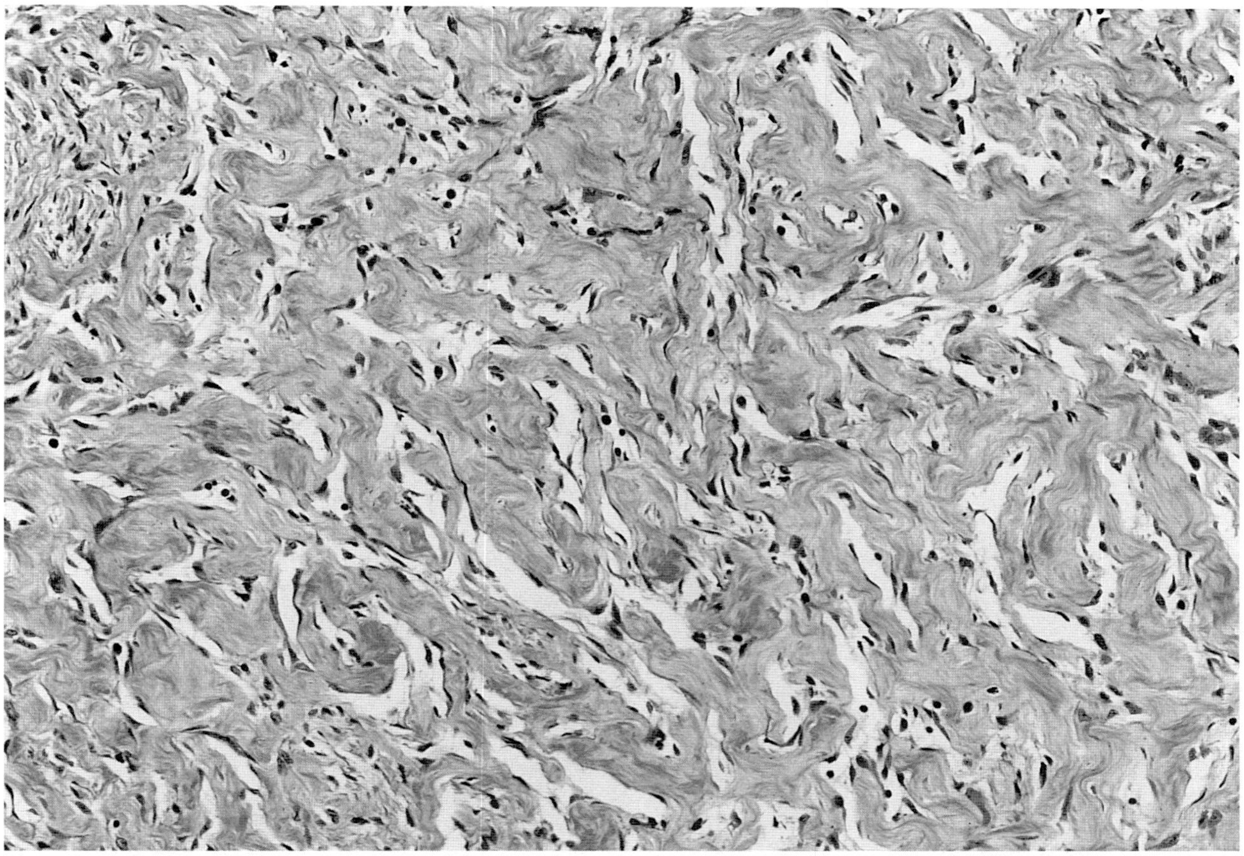

G

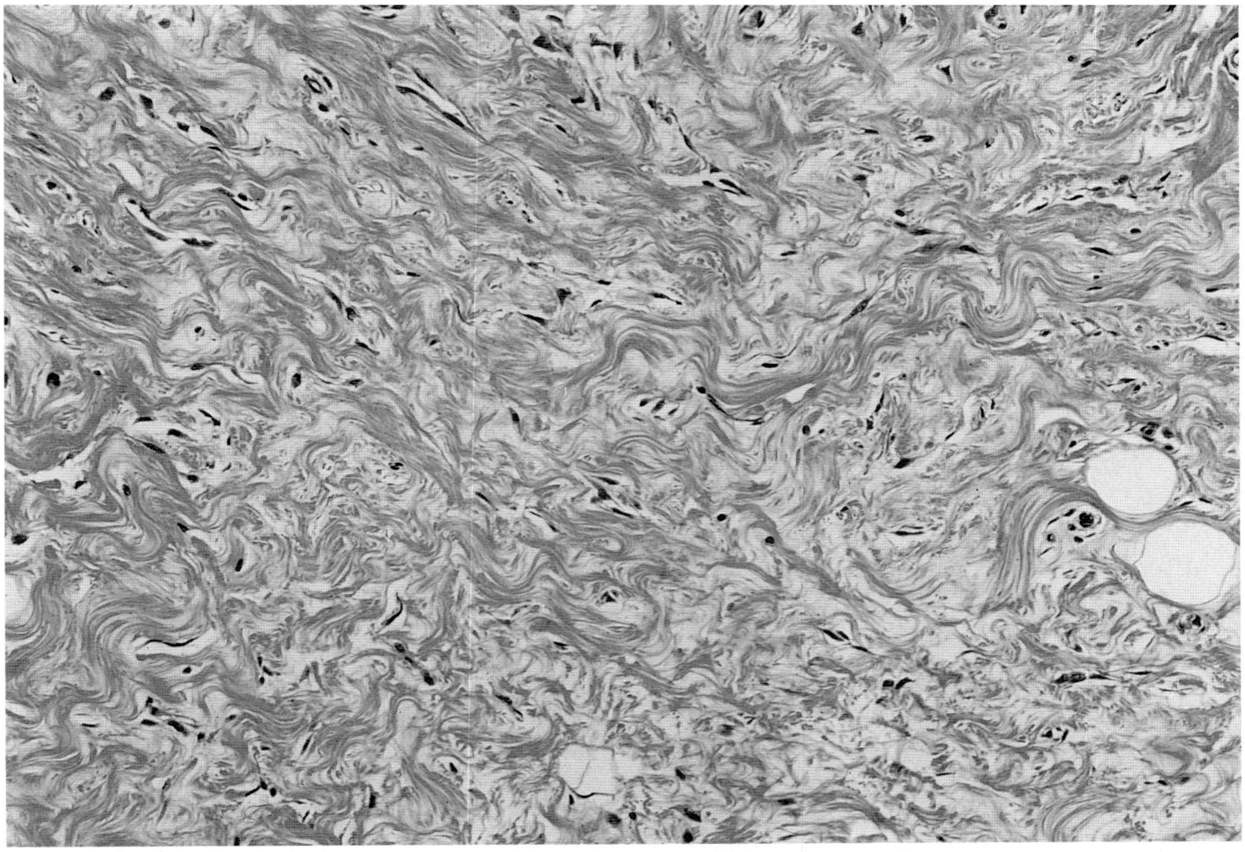

**Figure 4.21(f&g)** Juvenile hypertrophy in a 12-year-old girl. The stroma in the areas of hypertrophy had a pseudoangiomatous appearance compared to the (g) loose fibrocollagenous stroma of the surrounding breast tissue. (H&E, (f) X200; (g) X200)

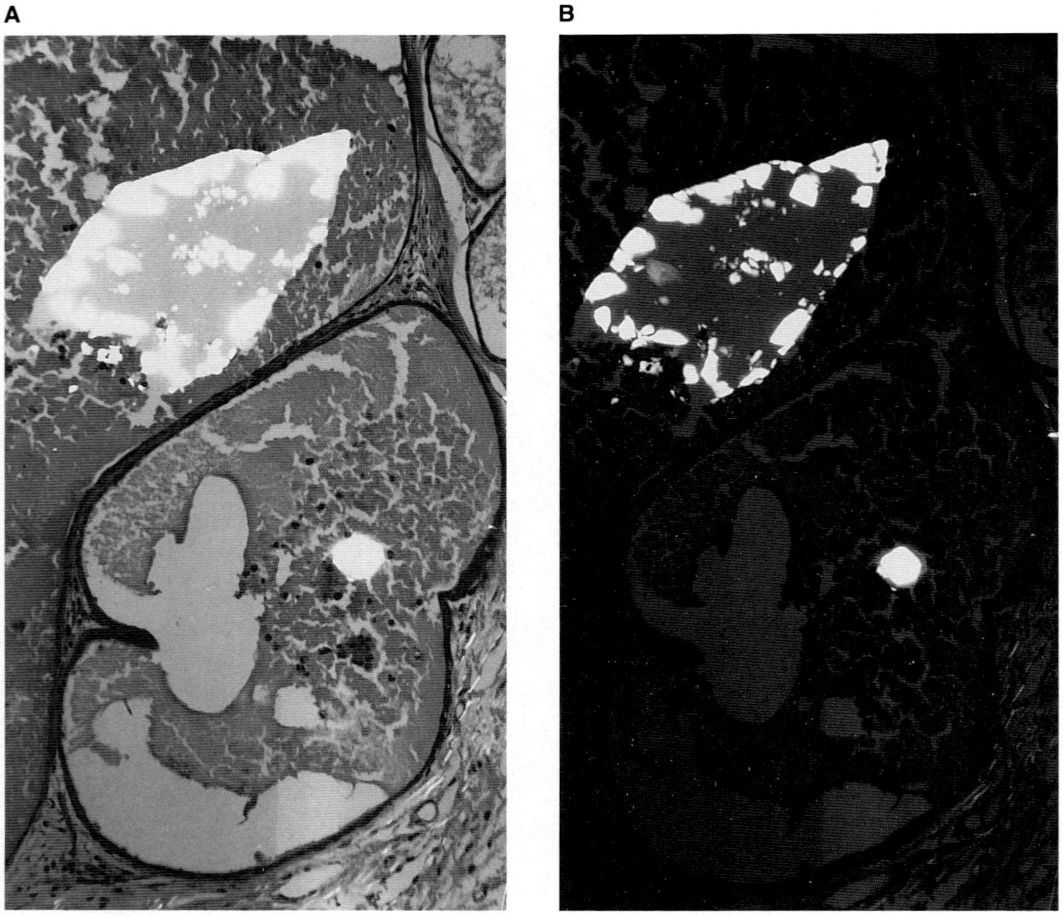


**Figure 4.22** Calcium oxalate crystals. (a) Two dilated ducts contain granular secretory material, degenerating cells and angulated structures. (b) Under polarized light, the latter show pronounced birefringence of crystals. (Courtesy of Dr. C. Tornos).

the carcinomas were in situ (27 ductal, 7 lobular), 16 were microinvasive, and 15 had infiltrating ductal carcinoma. The remaining 149 women had a variety of benign lesions. In this series, slightly less than one third of the mammographically detected microcalcifications in asymptomatic women from ages 26 to 76 years (median of 48.6 years) were due to carcinoma.

Microcalcifications in breast carcinomas have been described as being irregular and fine rather than coarse in appearance (281,295), while those in adenosis have been described as being smooth, minute, globular or spheroid-shaped (282). Calcifications in sclerosing adenosis are more often bilateral and widely scattered. Koehl et al (291) maintained that calcifications in fibrocystic changes and sclerosing adenosis are smaller, smoother and more uniform in size. Thin, curvilinear, or branching shapes of microcalcification in cluster form are often diagnostic of carcinoma (293), but many other patterns of microcalcification also occur in both benign and malignant processes. Identical patterns of microcalcification may be seen in benign and malignant lesions, and there is no particular pattern that is invariably pathognomonic of carcinoma or a benign lesion (314). A biopsy of the lesion is, therefore, necessary to establish the diagnosis with absolute certainty (304).

Many studies have tried to correlate the presence of mammographically-detected microcalcifications in the biopsy by specimen and paraffin block radiography or study of the histologic sections (270,273,277, 282,288,295,298,299,303). Pathologists are often responsible for identifying and correlating the presence of microcalcifications in the biopsy specimen to ascertain that the mammographically detected lesion has been excised. Despite exhaustive sampling and search, however, occasionally microcalcifications that were detected on mammograms and specimen radiographs or in paraffin blocks cannot be identified histologically.

It has become evident that several types of microcalcification occur in the breast, all of which are readily detected by mammographic techniques, but

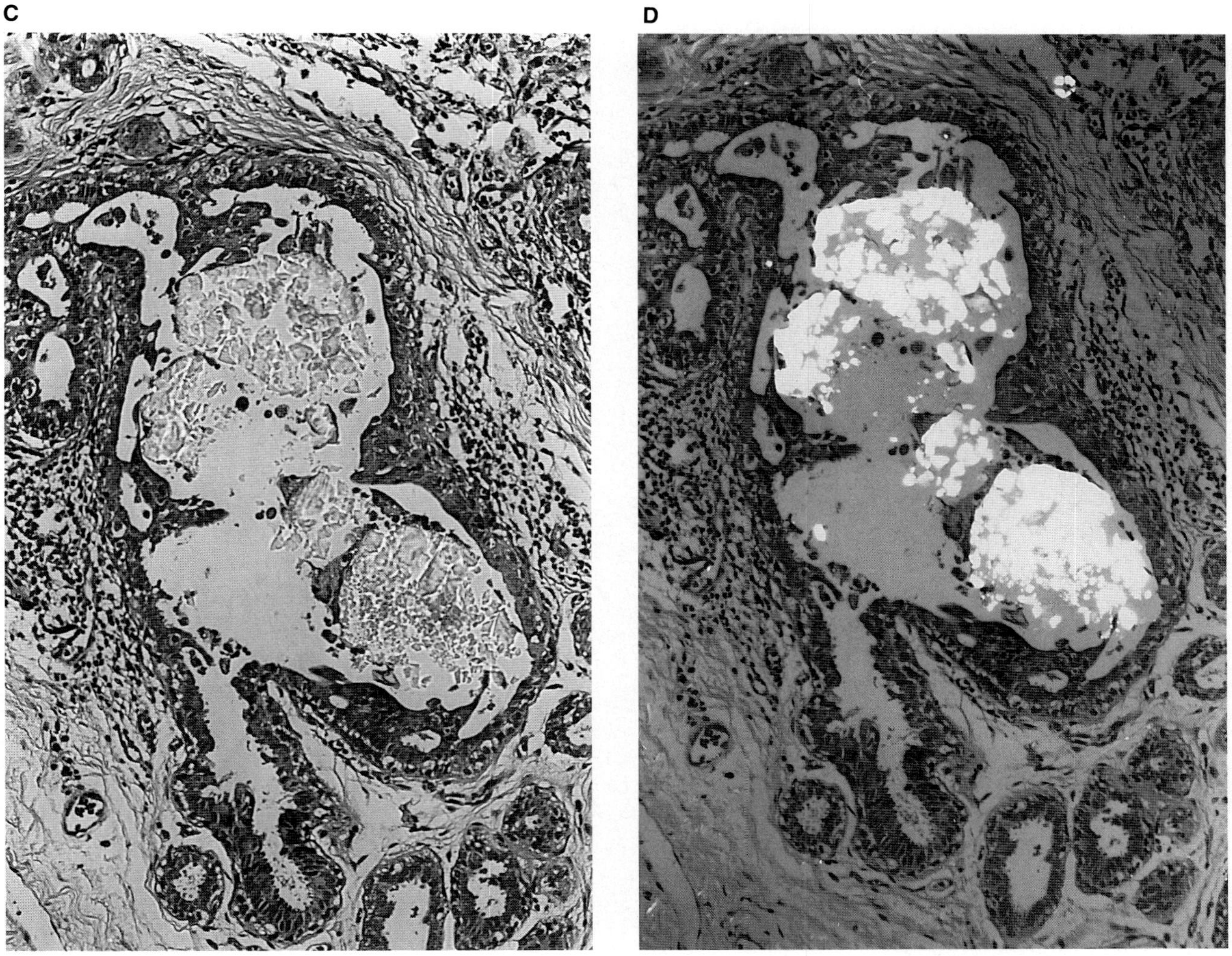

**Figure 4.22(c&d)** Calcium oxalate crystals. (c) Another duct showing irregularly-shaped crystalline material. (d) Same field under polarized light shows birefringence of the intraluminal calcium oxalate crystals. (Figs. 4.22(c,d) reprinted from Tornos C, et al: *Am J Surg Pathol* 1990;14:961–968, with permission.)

one of these (calcium oxalate or weddelite) is particularly difficult to detect on the routine hematoxylen and eosin (H&E) stained sections (286,300,312). In general, the various microcalcifications are deposited in areas where compound lipids are present (268,271), but differ in their chemical composition with some forming a crystal lattice (267,269,289,290). The laminated, psammoma body type of calcification generally reflects calcium phosphate in the form of hydroxyapatite. Sometimes the calcium deposits are within amorphous necrotic debris or a thick secretory material; this type of calcification often corresponds to calcium phosphate. Finally, there are amorphous, poorly stained, cloud-shaped intraluminal birefringent bodies which represent calcium oxalate (Fig. 4.22) mainly in the crystalline form of weddelite (286,300,301); these are easily missed on H&E stained sections and fail to react with von Kossa and alizarin red at pH 4.2, but do stain with silver nitrate/rubeanic acid with 5% acetic acid pretreatment (312). The acetic acid pretreatment dissolves both calcium phosphate and calcium carbonate, making the silver nitrate/rubeanic acid stain rather specific for calcium oxalate (315). The monohydrate calcium oxalate crystals are bipyramidal in shape though this appearance is generally not appreciated in tissue sections; these crystals are easily detected under polarized light. In guinea pigs, the intradermal injection of an aqueous suspension of the granular, dihydrate variant of calcium oxalate crystals has failed to incite a significant inflammatory reaction (301).

In addition to these more common calcium compositions, microcalcifications may be composed of calcium with very little phosporus, or admixed with

A

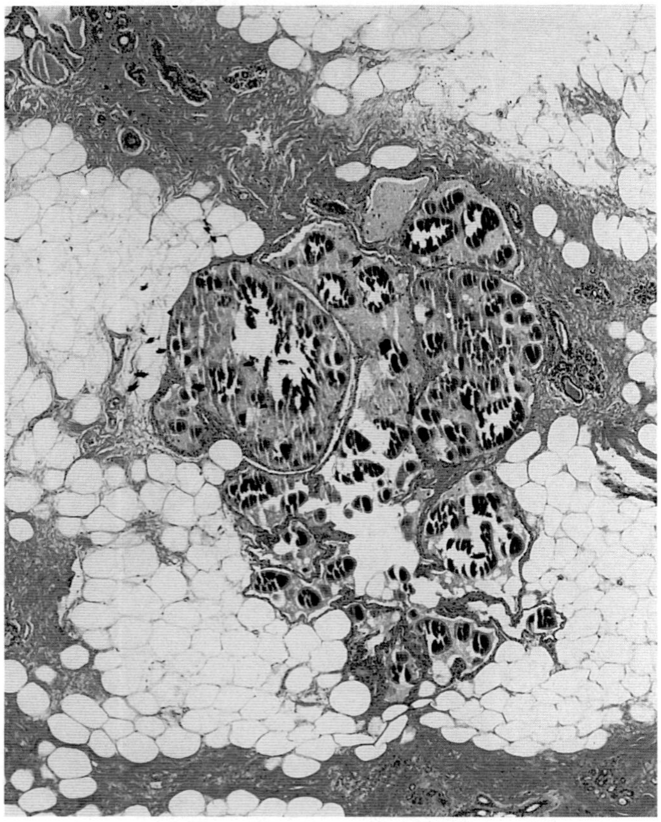

**Figure 4.23** Liesegang rings. (a&b) Numerous laminated inclusions probably reflecting complex proteins are sometimes present in cysts or spaces within the stroma. (H&E, (a) X40; (b) X240)

other elements including aluminum, potassium, sulfur, silicone, and titanium. An unusual combination of calcium, iron (hemosiderin), silicone, and sulfur form laminated inclusions referred to as Liesegang ring within some cysts; these are often mistaken for parasites (313) (Fig. 4.23). Furthermore, particles containing no calcium, but an admixture of other elements such as aluminum, magnesium, copper, nickel, lead, gold, chlorine, iodine, molybdenum, silicone, and titanium are also found within breast biopsies (280).

The biochemical makeup of the calcification has been correlated with the major background lesion in several studies (272,276,278,279,289,311,312). These studies have shown that calcium phosphate can be detected in either benign or malignant lesions. Calcium oxalate, on the other hand, has been identified mainly in benign lesions. Calcium oxalate occurs as the only form of calcification in approximately 11.5% of breast samples (300). While reports have also noted the presence of calcium oxalate in biopsies containing lobular carcinoma in situ (272,277,285), the intimate association of the crystals with the lobular carcinoma in situ can be confirmed in only one case (272). When it has been identified in carcinomas (one infiltrating duct and one intraductal carcinoma), its location has been specified as within the lumina of benign dilated ducts (311), or not specified at all (276).

Calcifications are present in a variety of benign and malignant lesions of the breast. Among benign lesions, they are observed with a high frequency approaching 50% in sclerosing adenosis. As mentioned before, about 40% to 50% of carcinomas have microcalcifications, but the range is from 30% to 75% (271); some investigators have found that the incidence of microcalcification in carcinomas is lower than in fibrocystic changes (268). Among carcinomas, they are seen frequently in intraductal comedocarcinomas and infiltrating duct carcinomas (297), while infiltrating lobular carcinomas are rarely calcified (271). In many studies regarding calcification in breast carcinomas, it is not specified whether the calcifications are within the carcinoma itself, or in adjacent ducts lacking a malignant proliferation.

Furthermore, regardless of their chemical composition and crystalline structure, it has not been settled whether microcalcifications reflect a degenerative process or a product of an active living cell. The amorphous types of calcification appear to reflect a dystrophic or degenerative type of process

B

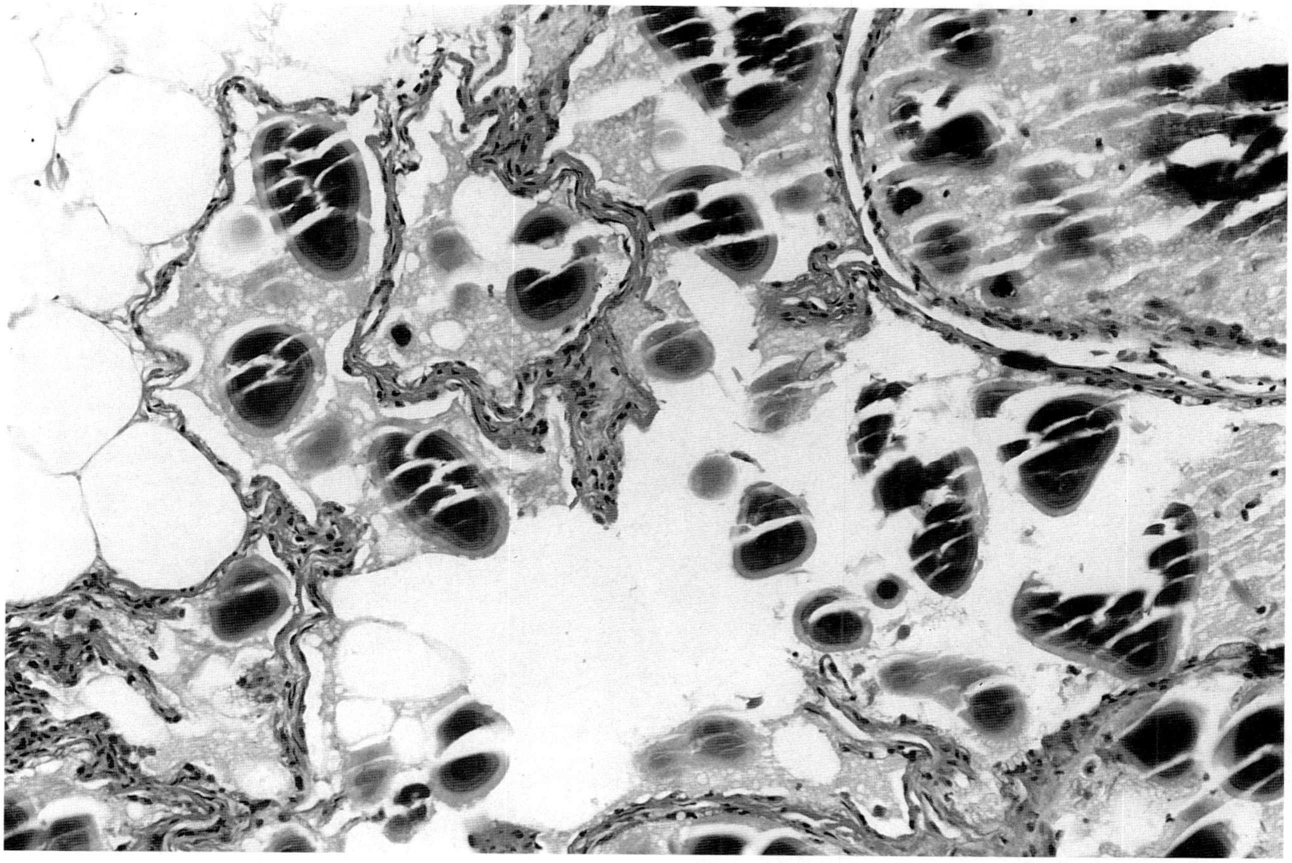

**Figure 4.23(b)** Legend on opposite page.

(272). It has been suggested that calcium apatite may also be degenerative or dystrophic in nature because of the possible existence of a gel phase in the beginning of its deposition (272). Calcium oxalate, however, may be the product of a living cell (308).

Mammographically-detected calcifications remain a valuable indication for biopsy in patients who have been treated by breast conserving surgery and radiation therapy for breast carcinoma. Approximately 58% of postirradiation biopsies performed because of such microcalcifications show either in situ or invasive carcinoma (306).

## INTRANUCLEAR HELIOID INCLUSIONS

This term was proposed by Ghadially et al (283) for inclusions identified during the course of an ultrastructural analysis of a breast adenoma removed from a 63-year-old woman. Subsequently, intranuclear inclusions resembling viral particles, which proved to be helioid inclusions (Fig. 4.24) at the ultrastructural level, were identified in eight cases of mammary intraductal hyperplasia (seven ordinary and one atypical hyperplasia) (310). The affected cells did not show any evidence of secretory activity in the cytoplasm.

Helioid intranuclear inclusions are single-membrane-bound rounded structures containing a laminated or homogeneously electron-dense core with a corona of radiating filaments resembling sun rays (hence the name, from Helios, the Greek god of the sun). Because of the similarity of the laminated structures to psammoma bodies, the possibility that these structures serve as a nidus for the development of microcalcifications was considered, but there was no evidence of any pattern of calcification within the affected or nearby ducts.

The most plausible mechanism of formation of these structures appears to be through intranuclear sequestration of secretory content of perinuclear cisternae or rough endoplasmic reticulum and the sub-

A

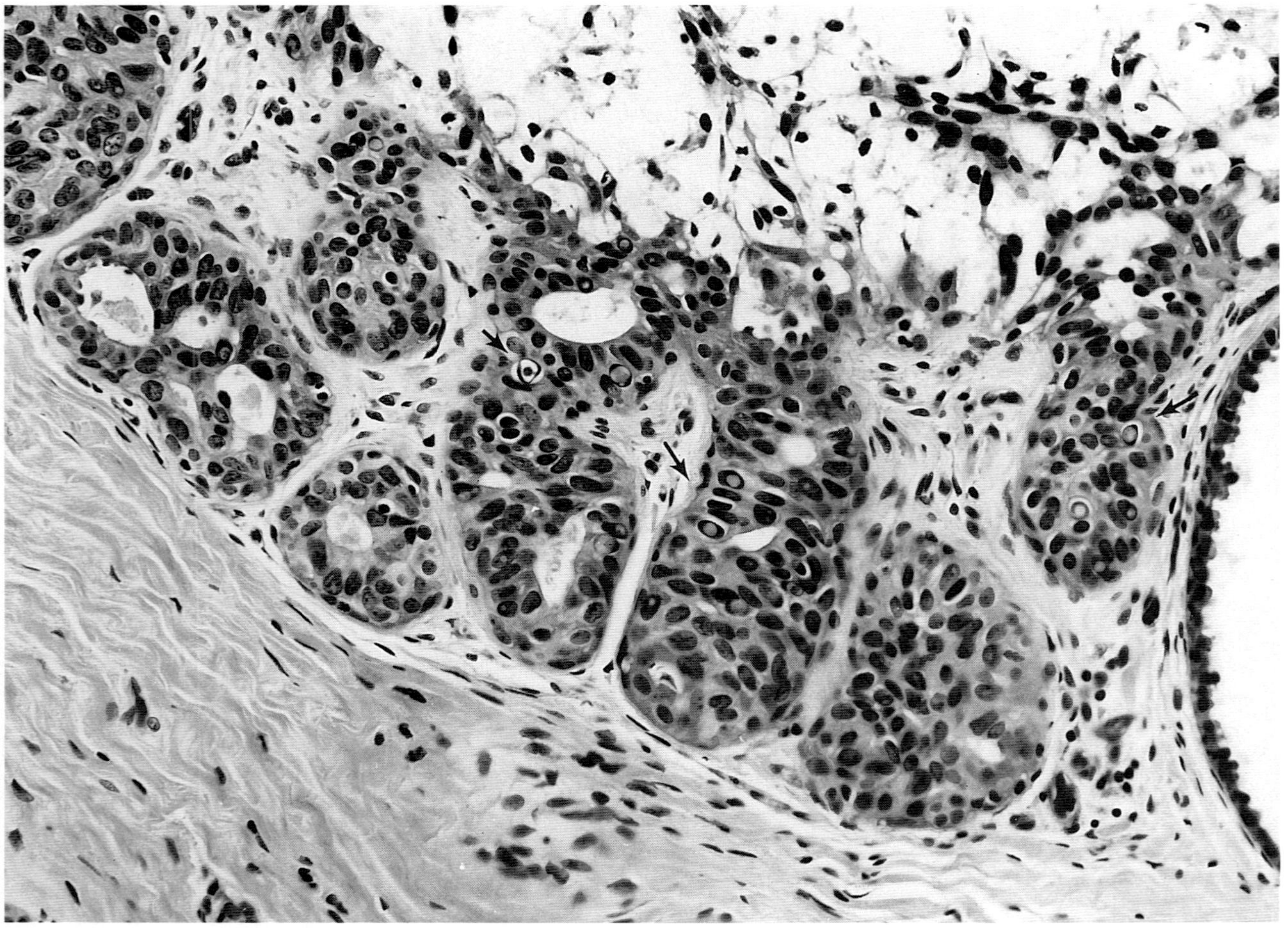

**Figure 4.24(a)** Helioid intranuclear inclusions. Several ducts with IDH show cells with intranuclear inclusions. (H&E, X400)

sequent transformation of the material into helioid bodies within the nucleus (283,284,310).

Similar inclusions have also been identified at light and electron microscopic levels within immature (nonsecreting) mucous cells of human labial salivary glands (309).

## COLLAGENOUS SPHERULOSIS

An incidental microscopic finding involving ductules, collagenous spherulosis, consists of intraluminal clusters of eosinophilic spherules measuring approximately 20 to 100 microns in diameter surrounded by epithelial and myoepithelial cell hyperplasia (Fig. 4.25). It occurs in women between 32 to 63 years of age. These spherules are generally found within secondary spaces of intraductal hyperplasia and papillomas. They vary somewhat in appearance from laminated fibrillar bodies, to more loosely-formed structures within a thick cuticle, and less frequently even a star-shaped pattern occurs (274). The spherules are rich in collagen, but also contain variable amounts of PAS-positive basement-membrane-like material, elastin (demonstrated as punctate black granules within the spherules by Wiegert van Gieson stain), and acidic mucin. The cells immediately surrounding these spherules are myoepithelial in nature at the ultrastructural level (287) and demonstrate a positive reaction with actin (287,296); it is this cell population that appears to be producing these spherules (296).

Collagenous spherulosis is a completely benign lesion which may be present within a solitary ductule or multiple, often adjacent, ductules. Its recognition is important to prevent misinterpretation as adenoid cystic carcinoma or intraductal signet-ring cell carcinoma. Adenoid cystic carcinoma is generally a clinically palpable lesion and an invasive process micro-

B

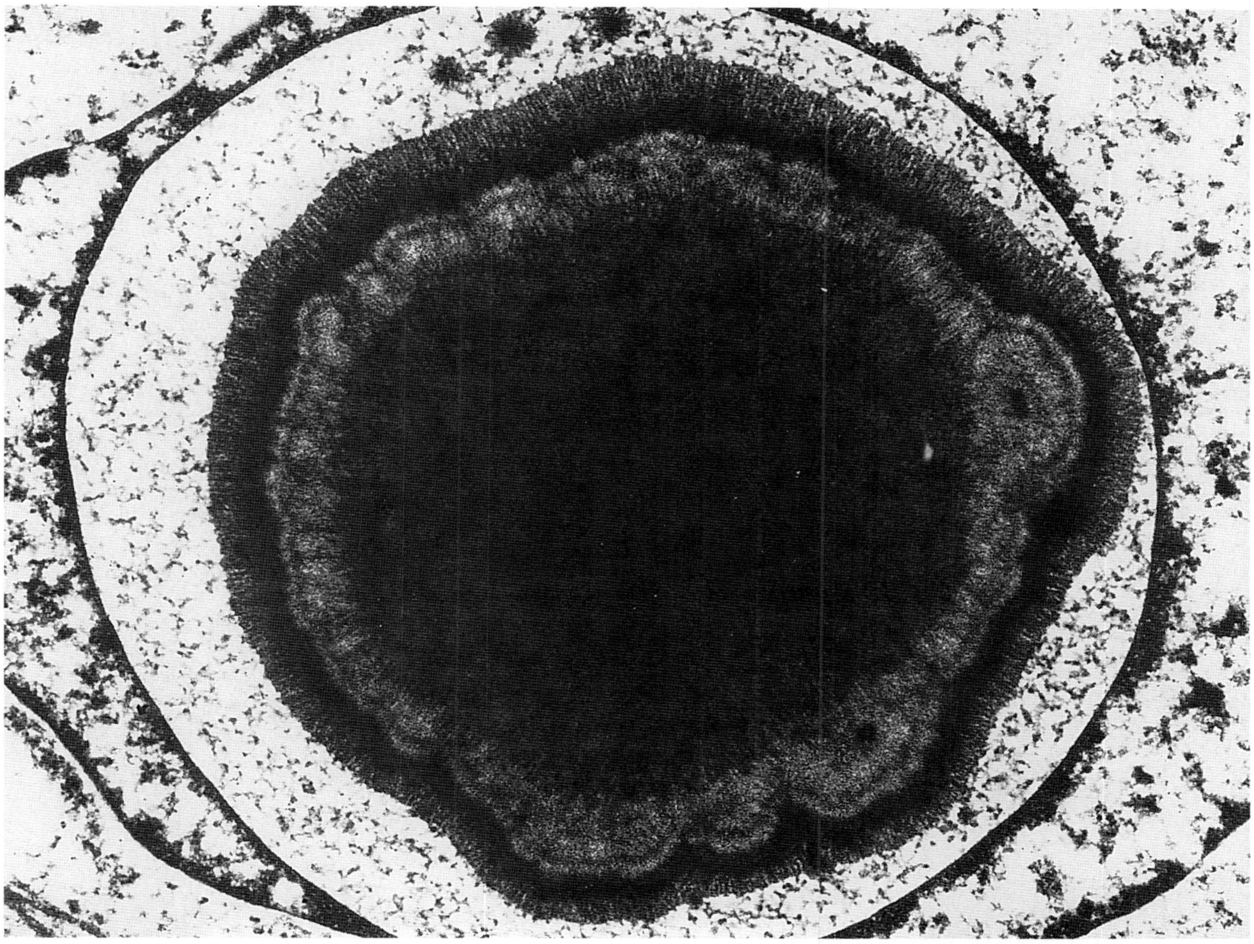

**Figure 4.24(b)** Helioid intranuclear inclusions. At the ultrastructural level, the inclusions display a laminated core, along with rigid rays of uniform length emanating from the core. (Uranyl acetate-lead citrate, X7,800) (Figure 4.24(b) reprinted from Tavassoli FA, et al: *Ultrastructural Pathol* 1991;15:267–279, with permission.)

scopically, in contrast to the incidental microscopic detection of collagenous spherulosis which is confined to ductules. Intraductal signet-ring cell carcinoma, aside from being quite rare, shows intracytoplasmic-mucin-positive, collagen-negative secretory content. Furthermore, there are no myoepithelial cells admixed with the signet-ring cells.

## SILICONE GRANULOMAS

The most extensive experience with silicone gel mammary prosthesis has been in the area of augmentation mammoplasty and correction of unilateral hypoplasia, though it is being used with increasing frequency for reconstruction of the breast following prophylactic and therapeutic subcutaneous mastectomy. The former account for approximately 80% of silicone implants utilized, while the latter account for around 20% of the usage.

The implants have two basic components, the silicone elastomere dispersion used for making the outer shell and the compliant silicone gel within the shell. In reality, however, the implant is a heterogeneous combination of polymers, mineral fillers, catalysts, and solvent residuals; about 14 chemical precursors are used to manufacture the final product (324).

Injected silicone, the use of which for breast augmentation has been forbidden (316,317), or silicone leaking through an envelope can cause a variety of complications. The human response to a gel prosthesis varies depending on the design of the prosthesis, extent of silicone bleed, the polymeric composition, the mechanical forces within the site, and the

A

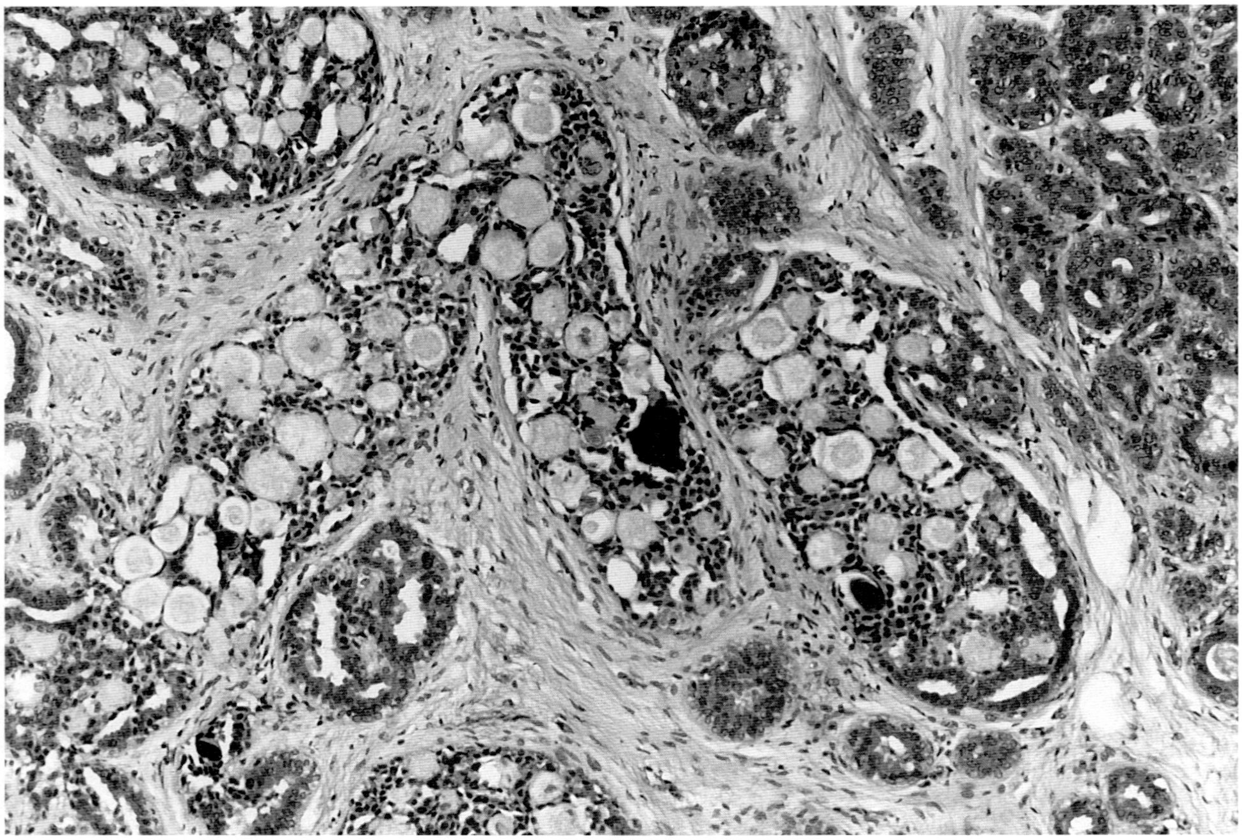

B

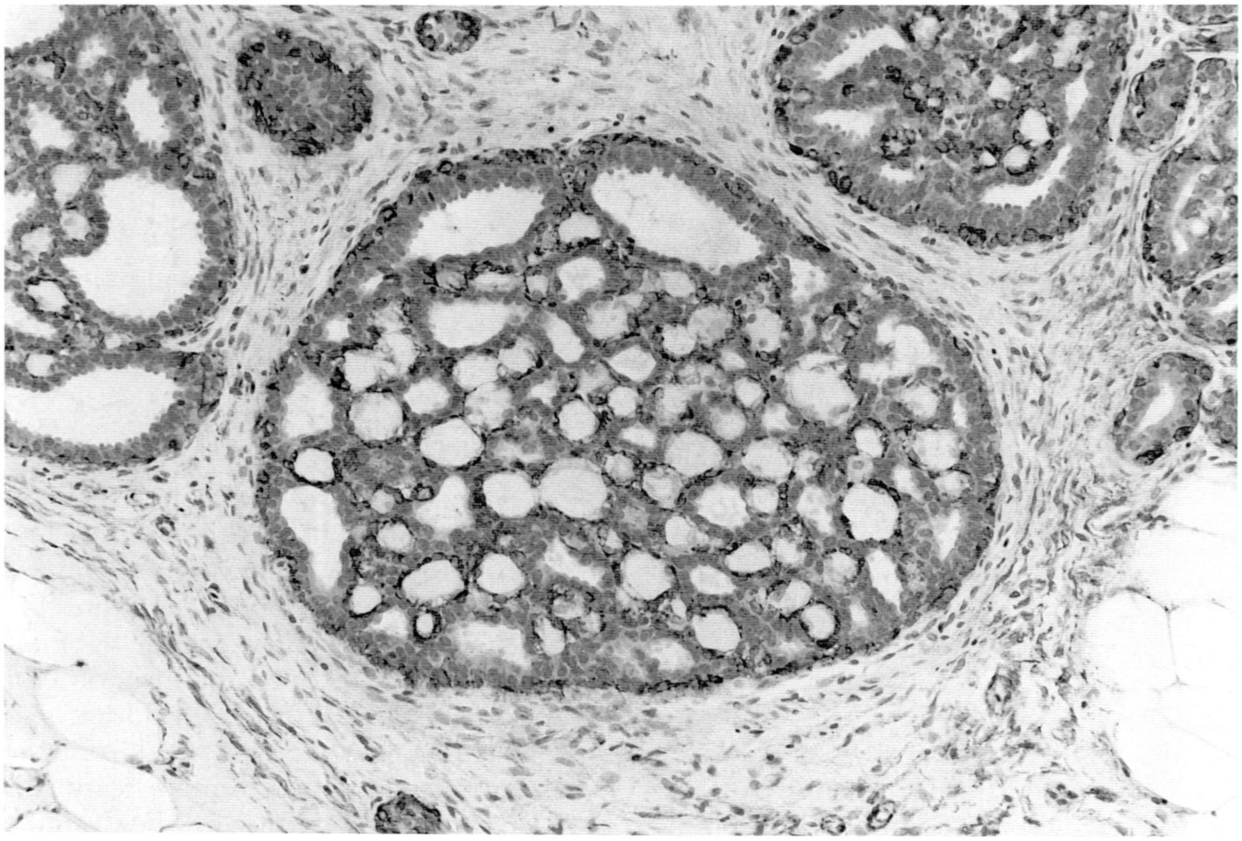

**Figure 4.25** Collageneous spherulosis. (a) Multiple typically discrete spherules within an area of epithelial hyperplasia. (H&E, X150) (b) Immunostain for actin decorates the myoepithelial cells surrounding the spherules. (X240)

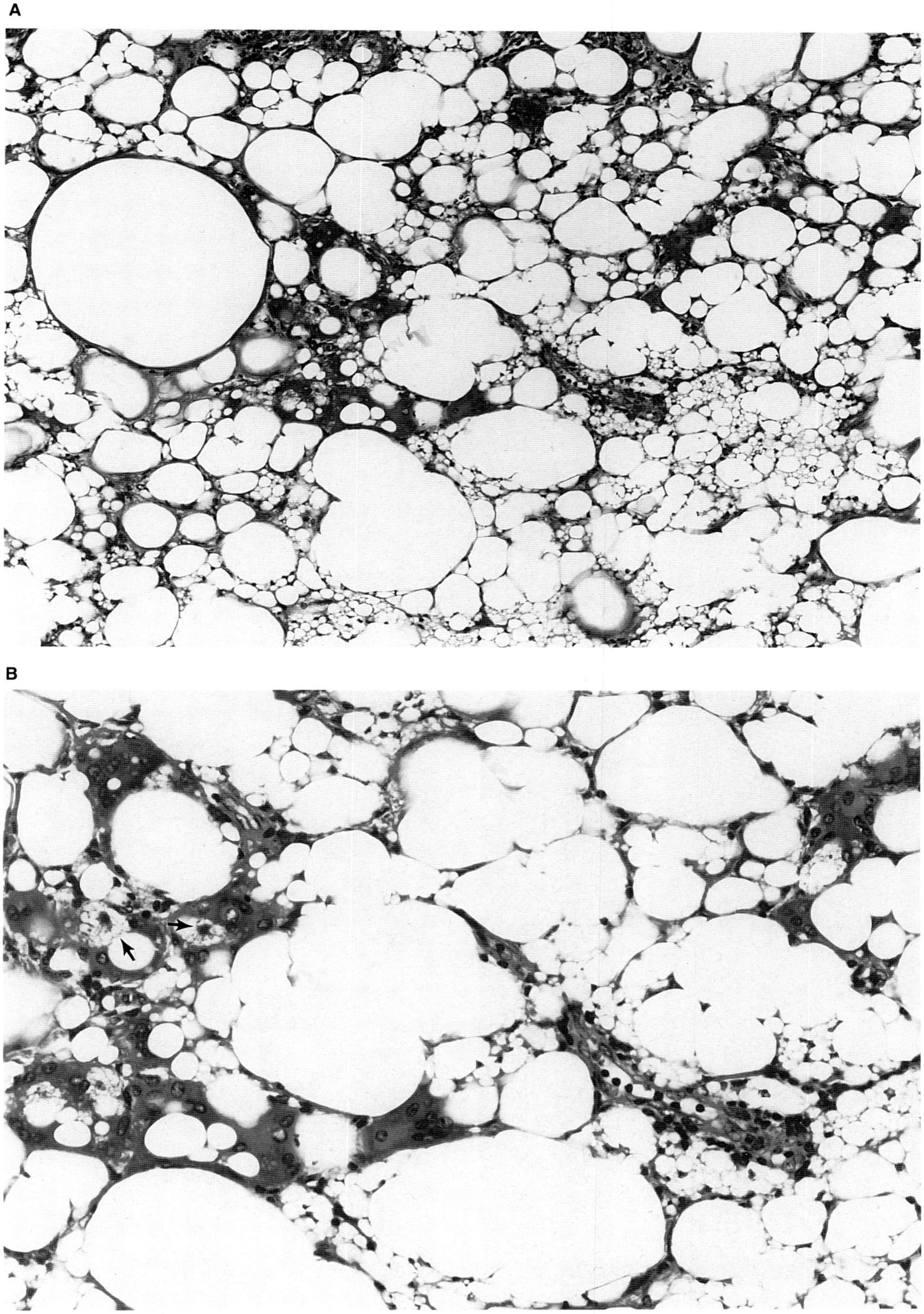


**Figure 4.26** Silicone granuloma. (a) Rounded spaces of highly variable size with numerous clusters of small vacuoles are typical. The spaces are often empty or lined by a thin eosinophilic band. (H&E, X200) (b) Giant cells may contain asteroid bodies. (H&E, X300)

C

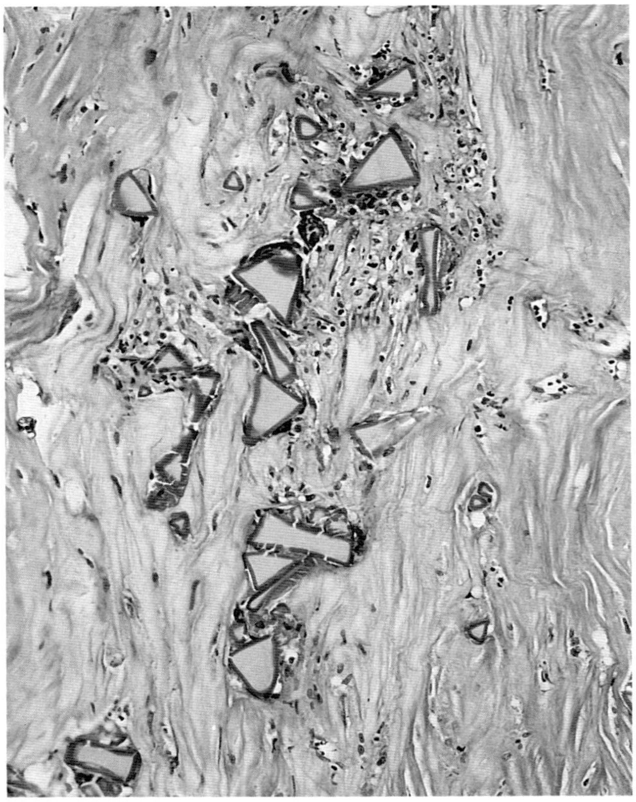

D

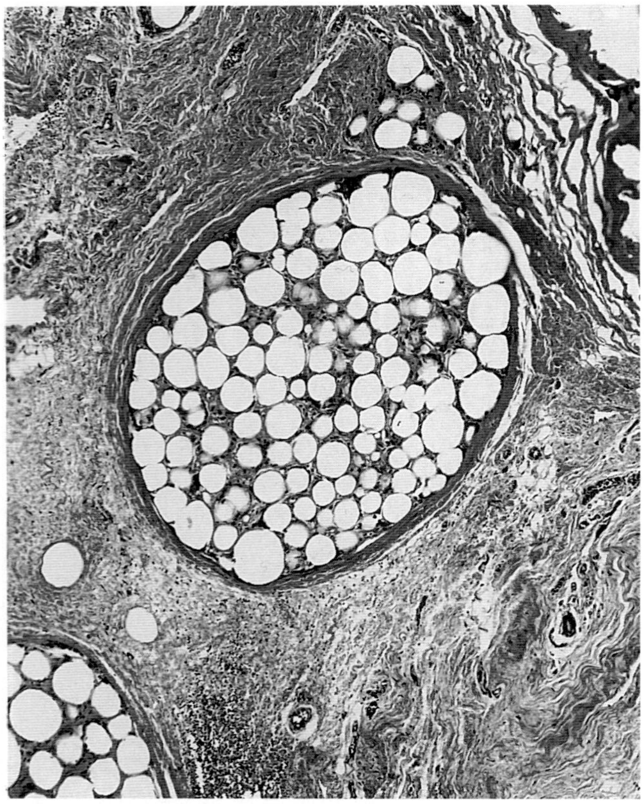

E

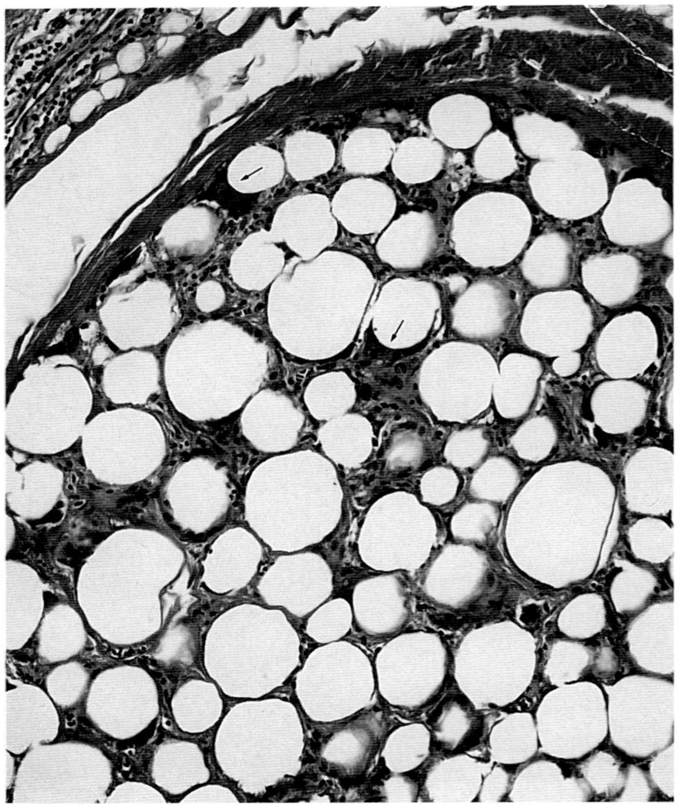

**Figure 4.26(c,d,e)** Silicone implant. (c) Unusually-shaped polyurethane crystals are rarely found in the fibrous capsule around the implant. (Oil-red-O, X75) (d) For comparison, paraffinoma in the breast is characterized by spaces of relatively uniform size clustered together and surrounded by a fibrous capsule. (H&E, X150) (e) A few foreign-body giant cells are present around some vacuoles (arrows). (H&E, X450)

individual's immune system (324). The most common complication reflects local reactive changes associated with the formation of numerous microcysts alternating with coalescent, rounded spaces of various sizes that may be empty or lined by a thick eosinophilic film (Fig. 4.26). Numerous histiocytes and foreign-body-type giant cells are also abundant. When the empty spaces dominate, the appearances simulate fat necrosis.

The literature contains conflicting reports regarding the type of localized soft tissue reaction to silicone. Some have reported little to no reaction to silicone in man or experimental animals (316,317, 325); others have noted the induction of a definite reaction, but without foreign-body-type response (318,320). Some investigators have actually observed a lipogranulomatous or foreign-body-type granulomatous response (321,323,326,328). In their pure form, the highly viscous silicone fluids—Dimethicone 350, an organosilicone polymer with the chemical formula of $[O\ Si\ (CH_3)_2]n$—are thought to reflect chemically and physically inert, nonallergenic substances that induce minimal tissue reaction and often no foreign-body-type reaction (316,317). It has been suggested that the granulomatous reaction to the leaking silicone may be in response to additives or adulterants in the silicone preparations, rather than to the silicone itself (319). The purpose of the additives, which often consist of vegetable oils and fatty acids, is to induce fibrosis and to ascertain firmness and immobilization.

Silicone fluid is capable of migrating relatively long distances from the breast to the inguinal region (321) and can induce a similar granulomatous reaction wherever it lodges. When it migrates to the bone marrow, it may be confused with a mucinous carcinoma. Silicone gel also gets carried to the axillary nodes where a similar foreign-body-type granulomatous reaction may ensue (322,327).

The long-term effects of silicone implants and possible development of systemic reactions to silicone leakage need to be studied in greater depth. There appears to be an increasing demand for implants in reconstruction procedures following breast cancer surgery particularly since smaller carcinomas are being detected in younger women who may not be candidates for conservative surgical treatment. Therefore, there is an unquestionable need for the availability of implants with a minimum of risk and complications.

## REFERENCES

### Fibrocystic Changes and Epithelial Metaplasias


1. Abrams AA: Use of vitamin E in chronic cystic mastitis. *N Engl J Med* 1965;272:1080–1081.
* 2. Ahmed A: Apocrine metaplasia in cystic hyperplastic mastopathy. Histochemical and ultrastructural observations. *J Pathol* 1975;115:211–214.
3. Anastassiades OTH, Tsakraklides E, Gogas J: The histology of fibrocystic disease of the female breast. *Path Res Pract* 1981;172:109–129.
4. Andersen AN, Larsen JF, Steenstrup OR, et al: Effect of bromocriptine on the premenstrual syndrome. A double blind clinical trial. *Br J Obstet Gynaecol* 1977;84:370–374.
5. Arias-Stella J: A topographic study of uterine epithelial atypia associated with chorionic tissue. *Cancer* 1959;12:782–790.
6. Archer F, Omar M: The fine structure of fibroadenoma of the human breast. *J Pathol* 1969;99:113–117.
7. Ariel IM: Enovid therapy (norethynodrel with mestranol) for fibrocystic disease. *Am J Obstet Gynecol* 1973;117:453–468.
8. Atkins HJB: The effect of endocrines on fibroadenosis. *Br Med J* 1949;1:750–752.
* 9. Azzopardi JG: *Problems in Breast Pathology*. London, WB Saunders, 1979, pp 57–72.
10. Barbieri RL, Ryan KJ: Danazol: Endocrine pharmacology and therapeutic applications. *Am J Obstet Gynecol* 1981;141: 453–463.
11. Bartow SA, Black WC, Waeckerlin RW, et al: Fibrocystic disease: A continuing enigma. *Pathol Annu* 1982;17:93–111.
* 12. Barwick KW, Kashgarian M, Rosen PP: Clear cell change within duct and lobular epithelium of the human breast. *Pathol Annu* 1982;17:319–328.
* 13. Bassler R: *Pathologie der Brustdruse*. Berlin, Springer-Verlag, 1978.
14. Birkett J: *The Diseases of the Breast*. London, Longman & Co, 1850.
15. Blackmore WP: Danazol in the treatment of benign breast disease. *J Int Med Res* 1977;5:101–108.
16. Blichert-Toft M, Anderson AN, Henriksen OB, et al: Treatment of mastalgia with bromocriptine: A double-blind crossover study. *Br Med J* 1979;1:237.
* 17. Bloodgood JC: The pathology of chronic cystic mastitis of the female breast with special consideration of the blue-domed cysts. *Arch Surg* 1921;3:445–542.
* 18. Bonser GM, Dossett JA, Jull JW: *Human and Experimental Breast Cancer*. London, Pitman Medical, 1961.
19. Bradlow HL, Skidmore FD, Schwartz MK, et al: Cation levels in human breast cyst fluids. *Clin Oncol* 1981;7:388–390.
20. Bradlow HL, Schwartz MK, Fleisher M, et al: Hormone levels in human breast cyst fluids, in: Angeli A, Bradlow HL, Dogliotti L (eds): *Endocrinology of Cystic Breast Disease*. New York, Raven Press, 1983, pp 59–75.

21. Brinton LA, Vessey MP, Flavel R, et al: Risk factors for benign breast disease. *Am J Epidemiol* 1981;113:203–214.
22. Brodie B: Lectures on sero-cystic tumors of the breast. *London Medical Gazette* 1846;25:808.
23. Bryant T: *The Diseases of the Breast*. London, Cassel & Co, 1887.
24. Bundred NJ, Miller WR, Walker RA: An immunohistochemical study of the tissue distribution of the breast cyst fluid protein, Zn-alpha$_2$ glycoprotein. *Histopathology* 1987; 11:603–610.
* 25. Cheatle GL, Cutler M: *Tumors of the Breast*. London, Edward Arnold & Co, 1931.
* 26. Ciatto S, Biggeri A, Rosselli Del Turco M, et al: Risk of breast cancer subsequent to proven gross cystic disease. *Eur J Cancer* 1990;26:555–557.
27. Colin C, Gaspard U, Lambotte R: Relationship of mastodynia with its endocrine environment and treatment in a double blind trial with lynestrenol. *Arch Gynaekol* 1978; 225(1):7–13.
* 28. Cowan DF, Herbert TA: Involution of the breast in women aged 50 to 104 years: A histopathologic study of 102 cases. *Surg Pathol* 1989;2:323–333.
29. Davis HH, Simons M, Davis JB: Cystic disease of the breast: Relationship to carcinoma. *Cancer* 1964;17:957–978.
30. Dawson EK: Sweat gland carcinoma of the breast. A morpho-histological study. *Edinburgh Med J* 1932;39:409–438.
31. Dennerstein L, Spencer-Gardner C, Gotts G, et al: Progesterone and the premenstrual syndrome; A double blind crossover trial. *Br Med J* 1985;290:1617–1621.
32. Devitt JE: Fibrocystic disease of the breast is not premalignant. *Surg Gynecol Obstet* 1972;134:803–806.
33. Dilley WG, Haagensen DE Jr, Leight GS, et al: Fluoxymetesterone stimulation of tumor marker secretion in patients with breast carcinomas. *Breast Cancer Res Treat* 1986;8:205–215.
* 34. Dixon JM: Cystic disease and fibroadenoma of the breast: Natural history and relation to breast cancer risk. *Br Med Bull* 1991;47:258–271.
* 35. Dixon JM, Scott WN, Miller WR: Natural history of cystic disease: the importance of cyst type. *Br J Surg* 1985;72:190–192.
* 36. Dixon JM, Miller WR, Scott WN, et al: The morphological basis of human breast cyst populations. *Br J Surg* 1983;70: 604–606.
37. Doberl A, Tobiassen T, Rasmussen T: Treatment of recurrent cyclical mastodynia in patients with fibrocystic disease. *Acta Obstet Gynecol Scand* (Suppl) 1984;123:177–184.
38. Dogliotti L, Mussa A, Sandrucci S: Prolactin and benign breast disease with special emphasis on bromocriptine therapy, in: Angeli A, Bradlow HL, Dogliotti L (eds): *Endocrinology of Cystic Breast Disease*. New York, Raven Press, 1983. pp 273–284.
* 39. Dupont WD, Page DL: Risk factors for breast cancer in women with proliferative disease. *N Engl J Med* 1985;312: 146–151.
40. Dupont WD, Page DL: Relative risk of breast cancer varies with time since diagnosis of atypical hyperplasia. *Hum Pathol* 1989;20:723–725.
41. Durning P, Sellwood RA: Bromocriptine in severe cyclical breast pain. *Br J Surg* 1982;69:248–249.
42. Eldar S, Meguid MM, Beatty JD: Cancer of the breast after prophylactic subcutaneous mastectomy. *Am J Surg* 1984; 148:692–693.
43. Erb H, Kallenberger A: The action of an oral high-dosed oestrogen-progestogen combination on the human breast. *Acta Endocrinol* 1972;70:143–155.
44. Ernster VL, Goodson WH, Hunt TK, et al: Vitamin E and benign breast "disease": A double-blind randomized clinical trial. *Surgery* 1985;97:490–494.
45. Estes NC: Mastodynia due to fibrocystic disease of the breast controlled with thyroid hormone. *Am J Surg* 1981; 142:764–766.
* 46. Foote FW, Stewart FW: Comparative studies of cancerous versus noncancerous breast. *Ann Surg* 1945;121:197–222.
* 47. Frantz VK, Pickren JW, Melcher GE, et al: Incidence of chronic cystic disease in so-called "normal breasts." A study based on 225 postmortem examinations. *Cancer* 1951; 4:762–783.
* 48. Geschikter CF: *Diseases of the Breast. Diagnosis–Pathology–Treatment*, ed 2. Philadelphia, JB Lippincott, 1945, pp 219–234; 723–732.
49. Goldman LD, Goldwyn RM: Some anatomical considerations of subcutaneous mastectomy. *Plast Reconstr Surg* 1973;51:501–505.
50. Golinger RC: Hormones and the pathophysiology of fibrocystic mastopathy. *Surg Gynecol Obstet* 1978;146:273–281.
* 51. Goodnight JE, Quagliana JM, Morton DL: Failure of subcutaneous mastectomy to prevent the development of breast cancer. *J Surg Oncol* 1984;26:198–201.
52. Greenblatt RB, Dmowski WP, Mahesh VB, et al: Clinical studies with an antigonadotropin—danazol. *Fertil Steril* 1971;22:102–112.
* 53. Haagensen CD: *Disease of the Breast*, ed 3. Philadelphia, WB Saunders, 1986, pp 250–266.
* 54. Haagensen CD: The relationship of gross cystic disease of the breast and carcinoma. *Surgery* 1977;185:375–376.
* 55. Haagensen DE Jr: Is cystic disease related to cancer? *Am J Surg Pathol* 1991;15:687–694.
56. Haagensen DE Jr, Mazoujian G: Biochemistry and immunohistochemistry of gross cystic disease fluid proteins of the breast, in: Haagensen CD: *Diseases of the Breast*, ed. 3. Philadelphia, WB Saunders, 1986, pp 474–500.
* 57. Haagensen DE Jr, Mazoujian GM, Dilley WG, et al: Breast gross cystic disease fluid analysis. I. Isolation and radioimmunoassay for a major component protein. *Surg Forum* 1981;32:413–414.
58. Haagensen DE Jr, Silva JS, Leight GS, et al: Fluoxymesterone stimulates plasma concentrations of gross cystic disease fluid protein in patients with metastatic breast carcinoma. *Surg Forum* 1981;32:413–414.

59. Harrington E, Lesnick G: The association between gross cysts of the breast and breast cancer. *Breast* 1980;7:13–17.

60. Hayward JL, Parks AG: Alterations in the microanatomy of the breast as a result of changes in the hormonal environment, in: Currie AR (ed): *Endocrine Aspects of Breast Cancer; Proceeding of a Conference at University of Glasgow*. Edinburgh, Livingstone, 1958, pp 133–134.

61. Hooper JH Jr, Welch VC, Shackelford RT: Abnormal lactation associated with tranquilizing drug therapy. *JAMA* 1961;178:506–507.

62. Humphrey LJ: Subcutaneous mastectomy is not a prophylaxis against carcinoma of the breast: Opinion or knowledge? *Am J Surg* 1983;145:311–312.

63. Huseby RA, Thomas LB: Histological and histochemical alterations in the normal breast tissues of patients with advanced breast cancer being treated with estrogenic hormones. *Cancer* 1954;7:54–74.

64. Hutchinson WB, Thomas DB, Hamlin WB, et al: Risk of breast cancer in women with benign breast disease. *J Natl Cancer Inst* 1980;65:13–20.

* 65. Hutter RVP: Consensus meeting: Cancer Committee of the College of American Pathologists: Is "fibrocystic disease" of the breast precancerous? *Arch Pathol Lab Med* 1986;110: 171–173.

66. Izuo M, Okagaki T, Richart RM, et al: DNA content in "apocrine metaplasia" of fibrocystic disease of the breast. *Cancer* 1971;27:643–650.

67. Jones BM, Bradbeber JW: The presentation and progress of macroscopic breast cysts. *Br J Surg* 1980;67:669–671.

* 68. Kiaer HW, Andersen JA: Focal pregnancy-like changes in the breast. *Acta Path Microbiol Scand A* 1977;85:931–947.

69. Kier LC, Kickey RC, Keettel WC, et al: Endocrine relationships in benign lesions of the breast. *Ann Surg* 1952;135: 782–790.

70. Kodlin D, Winger EE, Morgenstern NL, et al: Chronic mastopathy and breast cancer. *Cancer* 1977;39:2603–2607.

71. Lafaye C, Aubert B: Action de la progesterone locale dans les mastopathies benignes. *J Gynecol Obstet Biol Reprod* (Paris) 1978;7:1123–1139.

72. Lauersen NH, Wilson KH: The effect of danazol in the treatment of chronic cystic mastitis. *Obstet Gynecol* 1976;48: 93–98.

73. Leis HP Jr: Breast cancer patients at risk, in: Niebergs HE (ed): *Cancer Detection and Prevention*. New York, Marcel Dekker Inc, 1977.

74. Leis HP Jr: *Diagnosis and Treatment of Breast Lesions*. Flushing, New York, Medical Examinations Publishing Co, 1970.

75. Leis HP Jr: Fibrocystic disease of the breast. *J Med Assoc State Ala* 1962;32:97–104.

76. Leis HP, Kwon CS: Fibrocystic disease of the breast. *J Reprod Med* 1979;22:291–296.

77. Lendrum AC: On the "pink" epithelium of the cystic breast and the staining of its granules. *J Pathol Bacteriol* 1945;57:267–270.

78. London RS, Solomon DM, London ED, et al: Mammary dysplasia: clinical response and urinary excretion of 11-deoxy-17-ketosteroids and pregnanediol following alpha-tocopherol therapy. *Breast* 1978;4:19–22.

79. London RS, Sundaram GS, Goldstein PJ: Medical management of mammary dysplasia. *Obstet Gynecol* 1982;59:519–523.

80. London RS, Sundaram GS, Murphy L, et al: The effect of vitamin E on mammary dysplasia: A double-blind study. *Obstet Gynecol* 1985;65:104–106.

* 81. Love SM, Gelman RS, Silen W: Fibrocystic "disease" of the breast—a non-disease. *N Engl J Med* 1982;307:1010–1014.

82. Mansel RE, Hughes LE: The clinical and hormonal effects of treating mastalgia with danazol, in: Angeli A, Bradlow HL, Dogliotti L (eds): *Endocrinology of Cystic Breast Disease*. New York, Raven Press, 1983.

83. Mansel RE, Preece PE, Hughes LE: A double blind trial of the prolactin inhibitor bromocriptine in painful benign breast disease. *Br J Surg* 1978;65:724–727.

84. Marzetti L, Framarino dei Malatesta ML, Aaragona C: Prolactin and benign breast diseases, in: Angeli A, Bradlow HL, Dogliotti L (eds): *Endocrinology of Cystic Breast Disease*. New York, Raven Press, 1983.

85. Mauvais-Jarvis P, Sterkers N, Kuttenn F, et al: Traitement des mastopathies benignes par la progesterone, et les progestatifs. *J Gynecol Obstet Biol Reprod* (Paris) 1978;7:477–484.

* 86. Mazoujian G, Haagensen DE Jr: The immunopathology of gross cystic disease fluid proteins. *NY Acad Sci* 1990;586: 188–187.

* 87. Mazoujian G, Pinkus GS, Davis S, et al: Immunohistochemistry of a breast gross cystic disease fluid protein (GCDFP-15) in breast epithelium. *Am J Pathol* 1984;116:305–310.

88. Mills SE, Fechner RE: Focal pregnancy-like change of the breast. *Diagn Gynecol Obstet* 1980;2:67–70.

89. Minkowitz S, Hedayati H, Miller S, et al: Fibrous mastopathy. A clinical histopathologic study. *Cancer* 1973;32:913–916.

90. Minton JP, Poecking MK, Webster DJT, et al: Response of fibrocystic disease to caffeine withdrawal and correlation of cyclic nucleotides with breast disease. *Am J Obstet Gynecol* 1979;135:157–158.

91. Mongeau CJ, Madarnas P, Majem LS, et al: Risk of invasive breast carcinoma in patients with fibrocystic disease. Pathological and epidemiological study. *Path Res Pract* 1987;182:528.

92. Morandi G, Marchesoni M, Valdagni C: Chorionic gonadotropins in the therapy of fibrocystic mastosis. *Minerva Ginec* 1969;21:1655–1661.

93. Murad TM, von Haam E: The ultrastructure of fibrocystic disease of the breast. *Cancer* 1968;22:587–600.

* 94. Neilsen M, Thomsen JL, Primdahl S, et al: Breast cancer atypia among middle-aged women: A study of 110 medicolegal autopsies. *Br J Cancer* 1987;56:814–819.

* 95. Page DL: Cancer risk assessment in benign breast biopsies. *Hum Pathol* 1986;17:871–874.

* 96. Page DL, Vander Zwag R, Rogers LW, et al: Relation

between component parts of fibrocystic disease complex and breast cancer. *J Natl Cancer Inst* 1978;61:1055–1063.

* 97. Pastides H, Kelsey JL, LiVolsi VA, et al: Oral contraceptive use and fibrocystic breast disease with special reference to its histopathology. *J Natl Cancer Inst* 1983;71:5–9.

* 98. Patey DH: Two common non-malignant conditions of the breast. *Br Med J* 1949;1:96–99.

99. Pennisi VR: Subcutaneous mastectomy and fibrocystic disease of the breast. *Clin Plast Surg* 1976;3:205–216.

100. Pier WJ, Garancis JC, Kuzma JF: The ultrastructure of apocrine cells in intracytic papilloma and fibrocystic disease of the breast. *Archiv Pathol* 1970;89:446–452.

101. Pye JK, Mansel RE, Hughes SE: Clinical experience of drug treatments for mastalgia. *Lancet* 1985;2:373–376.

* 102. Reclus P: La maladie kystique des mammelles. *Bull Soc Anat* (Paris) 1883;68:428.

103. Renieri N, Stavropoulos C, Kappelou X, et al: Fibrocystic disease of the breast and HLA antigens. *Path Res Pract* 1984;179:59–60.

104. Ricciardi I, Ianniruberto A: Tamoxifen-induced regression of benign breast lesions. *Obstet Gynecol* 1979;54:80–84.

105. Roberts MM, Jones V, Elton RA, et al: Risk of breast cancer in women with a history of benign disease of the breast. *Br Med J* 1984;288:275–278.

* 106. Sandison AT: An autopsy study of the adult human breast: With special reference to proliferative epithelial changes of importance, in: *Pathology of the Breast*. Bethesda, National Cancer Institute Monograph 8, 1962, pp 55, 57–59.

* 107. Schimmelbusch C: Uber das Cystadenom der weiblichen Milchdruse. *Vbl Deutsch Gesell Chir* 1890;19:116.

* 108. Semb C: Pathologico-anatomical and clinical investigations of fibroadenosis cystica mammae and its relation to other pathological conditions in mammae, especially cancer. *Acta Chir Scand* 1928;64(Suppl):1–484.

109. Shaaban MM, Morad F, Hassan A: Treatment of fibrocystic mastopathy by an antiestrogen, tamoxifen. *Int J Gynaecol Obstet* 1980;18:348–350.

* 110. Silverberg SG, Chitale AR, Levitt SH: Prognostic implications of fibrocystic dysplasia in breasts removed for mammary carcinoma. *Cancer* 1972;29:574–580.

111. Sitruk-Ware R, Sterkers N, Mauvais-Jarvis P: Benign breast disease I: Hormonal investigation. *Obstet Gynecol* 1979;53: 457–460.

112. Sloss PT, Bennett WA, Clagett OT: Incidence in normal breasts of features associated with chronic cystic mastitis. *Am J Pathol* 1957;33:1181–1191.

113. Sundaram GS, London R, Manimekalai S, et al: Alpha-tocopherol and serum lipoproteins. *Lipids* 1981;16:223–227.

* 114. Tavassoli FA, Yeh I-T: Lactational and clear cell changes of the breast in non-lactating, nonpregnant women. *Am J Clin Pathol* 1987;87:23–29.

* 115. Tavassoli FA, Norris HJ: A comparison of the results of long-term follow-up for atypical intraductal hyperplasia and intraductal hyperplasia of the breast. *Cancer* 1990;65: 518–529.

* 116. Temple WJ, Lindsay RL, Magi E, et al: Technical considerations for prophylactic mastectomy in patients at high risk for breast cancer. *Am J Surg* 1991;161:413–415.

117. Tobiassen T, Rasmussen T, Doberl A, et al: Danazol treatment of severely symptomatic fibrocystic breast disease and longterm follow-up—the Hjorring project. *Acta Obstet Gynecol Scand* (Suppl) 1984;123:159–176.

* 118. Trapido EJ, Brinton LA, Schairer C, et al: Estrogen replacement therapy and benign breast disease. *J Natl Cancer Inst* 1984;73:1101–1105.

119. Vassar PS, Culling CFA: Fibrosis of the breast. *Arch Pathol* 1959;67:128–133.

* 120. Velpeau A: *A Treatise on Diseases of the Breast and Mammary Region*. Mitchell H (trans), London, Sydenham Society, 1856.

121. Veronesi V, Pizzocaro G: Breast cancer in women subsequent to cystic disease of the breast. *Surg Gynecol Obstet* 1968;126:529–534.

122. Vilanova JR, Simon R, Alvarez J, et al: Early apocrine change in hyperplastic cystic disease. *Histopathology* 1983; 7:693–698.

123. Vina M, Wells CA: Clear cell metaplasia of the breast: A lesion showing eccrine differentiation. *Histopathology* 1989; 15:85–92.

* 124. Vorherr H: Fibrocystic breast disease: Pathophysiology, pathomorphology, clinical picture, and management. *Am J Obstet Gynecol* 1986;154:161–179.

* 125. Warren S: Relation of "chronic mastitis" to carcinoma of breast. *Surg Gynec Obstet* 1940;71:257–273.

* 126. Wellings SR, Alpers CE: Apocrine cystic metaplasia: Subgross pathology and prevalence in cancer-associated versus random autopsy breasts. *Hum Pathol* 1987;18:381–386.

* 127. Wellings SR, Jensen HM, Marcum RG: An atlas of subgross pathology of the human breast with special reference to possible precancerous lesions. *J Natl Cancer Inst* 1975;55: 231–273.

128. Ylostalo P: Cycle of continuous treatment of premenstrual syndrome (PMS) with bromocriptine. *Eur J Obstet Gynecol Reprod Biol* 1984;17:337–343.

### Adenosis, Sclerosing, Nodular, Microglandular

* 129. Azzopardi JG: *Problems in Breast Pathology*. Philadelphia, WB Saunders, 1979, pp 168–174.

* 130. Bassler R: *Pathologie der Brustdruse*. Berlin. Springer-Verlag, 1978.

* 131. Bonser GM, Dossett JA, Jull JW: *Human and Experimental Breast Cancer*. London, Pittman Medical, 1961, pp 269–283.

* 132. Carter DJ, Rosen PP: Atypical apocrine metaplasia in sclerosing lesions of the breast: A study of 51 patients. *Modern Pathol* 1991;4:1–5.

* 133. Chan JCK, Ng WF: Sclerosing adenosis cancerized by intraductal carcinoma. *Pathology* 1987;19:425–428.

* 134. Clement PB, Azzopardi JG: Microglandular adenosis of the breast—a lesion simulating tubular carcinoma. *Histopathology* 1983;7:169–180.

135. Davies JD: Neural invasion in benign mammary dysplasia. *J Pathol* 1973;109:225–231.

136. Dawson EK: Fibrosing adenosis: A little recognized mammary picture. *Edinb Med J* 1954;61:391–401.

137. Diaz NM, McDivitt RW, Wick MR: Microglandular adenosis of the breast. An immunohistochemical comparison with tubular carcinoma. *Arch Pathol Lab Med* 1991;115:578–582.

*138. Fechner RE: Lobular carcinoma in situ in sclerosing adenosis, a potential source of confusion with invasive carcinoma. *Am J Surg Pathol* 1981;5:233–239.

139. Gould VE, Rogers DR, Sommers SC: Epithelial-nerve intermingling in benign breast lesions. *Arch Pathol* 1975;99:596–598.

140. Haagensen CD: *Diseases of the Breast*. ed 3. Philadelphia, WB Saunders, 1986, pp 106–117.

*141. Haagensen CD, Lane CD, Lattes R: Neoplastic proliferation of the mammary lobules. Adenosis, lobular neoplasia, and small cell carcinoma. *Surg Clin N Amer* 1972;52:497–524.

142. Heller EL, Fleming JC: Fibrosing adenomatosis of the breast. *Am J Clin Pathol* 1950;20:141–146.

*143. Jensen RA, Page DL, Dupont WD, et al: Invasive breast cancer risk in women with sclerosing adenosis. *Cancer* 1989;64:1977–1983.

144. Kay S: Microglandular adenosis of the female mammary gland: Study of a case with ultrastructural observations. *Hum Pathol* 1985;16:637–640.

145. MacErlean DP, Nathan BE: Calcification in sclerosing adenosis simulating malignant breast calcification. *Br J Radiol* 1972;45:944–945.

*146. McDivitt RW, Rubin GL, Stevens JA, et al: Benign breast disease histology and the risk of breast cancer (abstr). *Lab Invest* 1988;50:62.

147. McDivitt R, Stewart F, Berg J: *Tumors of the Breast*, Fasc 2. Atlas of Tumor Pathology, second series, Washington DC, Armed Forces Institute of Pathology, 1968.

*148. Nielsen BB: Adenosis tumor of the breast: A clinicopathological investigation of 27 cases. *Histopathology* 1987;11:1259–1275.

149. Peremans J: Sclerosing adenosis. *Belg T Geneesk* 1961;17:1120–1132.

150. Rosai J: Breast, in: Rosai J (ed): *Ackerman's Surgical Pathology*, ed 6. St Louis, CV Mosby, 1981, vol 2, pp 1087–1149.

*151. Rosen PP: Microglandular adenosis: A benign lesion simulating invasive mammary carcinoma. *Am J Surg Pathol* 1983;7:137–144.

*152. Rosenblum MK, Purrazella R, Rosen PP: Is microglandular adenosis a precancerous disease? A study of carcinoma arising therein. *Am J Surg Pathol* 1986;10:237–245.

153. Sandison AT: An autopsy study of the adult human breast: With special reference to proliferative epithelial changes of importance in the pathology of the breast, in: *Pathology of the Breast*. Bethesda, National Cancer Institute Monograph 8, 1962, pp 16–30.

*154. Sandison AT: A study of surgically removed specimens of breast, with special reference to sclerosing adenosis. *J Clin Pathol* 1958;11:101–109.

*155. Simpson JF, Page DL, Dupont WD: Apocrine adenosis—a mimic of mammary carcinoma. *Surg Pathol* 1990;3:289–299.

156. Symmers WSC: The breasts, in: Symmers WSC (ed): *Systemic Pathology*, ed 2. Edinburgh, Churchill Livingstone, 1978, vol 4, pp 1791–1796.

*157. Tanaka Y, Oota K: A stereomicroscopic study of the mastopathic human breast. I. Three dimensional structures of abnormal duct evolution and their histologic entity. *Virchows Arch A* 1970;349:195–214.

*158. Tavassoli FA, Norris HJ: Microglandular adenosis of the breast: A clinicopathologic study of 11 cases with ultrastructural observations. *Am J Surg Pathol* 1983;7:731–737.

*159. Taylor HB, Norris HJ: Epithelial invasion of nerves in benign diseases of the breast. *Cancer* 1967;20:2245–2249.

*160. Urban JA, Adair FE: Sclerosing adenosis. *Cancer* 1949;2:625–634.

### Radial Scar

*161. Andersen JA, Carter D, Linell F: A symposium on sclerosing duct lesions of the breast. *Pathol Annu* 1986;21(part 2):145–179.

*162. Andersen JA, Gram JB: Radial scar in the female breast: A long-term follow-up study of 32 cases. *Cancer* 1984;53:2557–2560.

*163. Anderson TJ, Battersby S: Radial scars of benign and malignant breast: Comparative features and significance. *J Pathol* 1985;147:23–32.

164. Azzopardi JG: *Problems in Breast Pathology*. Philadelphia, WB Saunders, 1979, pp 174–187.

*165. D'Amore E, Montes E, Le MG, et al: Le centre de proliferation d'Aschoff. *Ann Pathol* 1985;5:173–182.

166. Eusebi V, Grassigli A, Grosso F: Lesioni focali scleroelastiche mammarie simulanti carcinoma infiltrante. *Pathologica* 1976;68:507–518.

*167. Fenoglio C, Lattes R: Sclerosing papillary proliferations in the female breast. A benign lesion often mistaken for carcinoma. *Cancer* 1974;33:691–700.

168. Fisher ER, Palekar AS, Kotwal N, et al: A non-encapsulated sclerosing lesion of the breast. *Am J Clin Pathol* 1979;71:240–246.

*169. Hamperl H: Strahlige Narben und obliterierende Mastopathie. Beitrage zur pathologischen Histologie der Mamma XI. *Virch Arch* (A) 1975;369:55–68.

*170. Linell F, Ljungberg O, Andersson I: Breast carcinoma: Aspects of early stages, progression and related problems. *Acta Pathol Scand* (sect A) 1980 (suppl); 272:1–233.

*171. Nielsen M, Christensen L, Andersen J: Radial scars in women with breast cancer. *Cancer* 1987;59:1019–1025.

*172. Nielsen M, Jensen J, Andersen JA: An autopsy study of radial scar in the female breast. *Histopathology* 1985;9:287–295.

173. Rickert RR, Kalisher L, Hutter RVP: Indurative mastopathy: A benign sclerosing lesion of breast with elastosis which may simulate carcinoma. *Cancer* 1981;47:561–571.

174. Semb C: Fibroadenomatosis cystica mammae. *Acta Chir Scand* (Suppl) 1928;10:1–484.

175. Tremblay G, Buell RH, Seemayer TA: Elastosis in benign sclerosing ductal proliferation of the female breast. *Am J Surg Pathol* 1977;1:155–159.

* 176. Wellings SR, Alpers CE: Subgross pathologic features and incidence of radial scars in the breast. *Hum Pathol* 1984;15: 475–479.

### Mammary Duct Ectasia

* 177. Abramson DJ: Mammary duct ectasia, mammilary fistula and subareolar sinuses. *Ann Surg* 1969;169:217–226.

* 178. Adair FE: Plasma cell mastitis—a lesion simulating mammary carcinoma: A clinical and pathologic study with a report of 10 cases. *Arch Surg* 1933;26:735–749.

* 179. Azzopardi JG: *Problems in Breast Pathology*. Philadelphia, WB Saunders, 1979, pp 72–87.

* 180. Bloodgood JC: The clinical picture of dilated ducts beneath the nipple frequently to be palpated as a doughy worm-like mass—the varicocele tumor of the breast. *Surg Gynecol & Obstet* 1923;36:486–495.

* 181. Bonser GM, Dossett JA, Jull JW: *Human and Experimental Breast Cancer*. London, Pitman Medical, 1961, pp 237–265.

* 182. Cromar CDL, Dockerty MB: Plasma-cell mastitis. *Proc Staff Meet Mayo Clin* 1941;16:775–783.

* 183. Cutler M: Benign lesions of the female breast simulating cancer. *JAMA* 1933;101:1217–1222.

184. Davies JD: Inflammatory damage to ducts in mammary dysplasia: A cause of duct obliteration. *J Pathol* 1975;117: 47–54.

185. Davies JD: Pigmented periductal cells (ochrocytes) in mammary dysplasia: Their nature and significance. *J Pathol* 1974;114:205–216.

* 186. Dixon JM, Anderson TJ, Lumsden AB, et al: Mammary duct ectasia. *Br J Surg* 1983;70:601–603.

* 187. Franz VK, Pickren JW, Melcher GW, et al: Incidence of chronic cystic disease in so-called "normal breast." A study on 225 postmortem examinations. *Cancer* 1951;4:762–783.

188. Haagensen CD: *Diseases of the Breast*, ed 3. Philadelphia, WB Saunders, 1986, pp 357–368.

* 189. Haagensen CD: Mammary duct ectasia—a disease that may simulate carcinoma. *Cancer* 1951;4:749–761.

* 190. Ingier A: Uber obliterierende Mastitis. *Virch Arch Pathol Anat Physiol Klin Med* 1909;198:338–345.

* 191. Payne RL, Straus AF, Glasser RD: Mastitis obliterans. *Surgery* 1943;14:719–727.

192. Rees BI, Gravelle H, Hughes LE: Nipple retraction in duct ectasia. *Br J Surg* 1977;64:577–580.

193. Sandison AT, Walker JC: Inflammatory mastitis, mammary duct ectasia, and mammillary fistula. *Br J Surg* 1962;50:57–64.

194. Tedeschi LG, McCarthy PE: Involutional mammary duct ectasia and periductal mastitis in a male. *Hum Pathol* 1974;5:232–236.

* 195. Thomas WG, Williams RCN, Davies JD, et al: The clinical syndrome of mammary duct ectasia. *Br J Surg* 1982;69:423–425.

* 196. Tice GE, Dockerty MB, Harrington SW: Comedomastitis. A clinical and pathologic study of data in 172 cases. *Surg Gynecol Obstet* 1948;51:350–355.

* 197. Walker JC, Sandison AT: Mammary duct ectasia. A clinical study. *Br J Surg* 1964;512:350–355.

198. Young GB: Mammography in carcinoma of the breast. *J Royal Col Surg Edinbg* 1968;13:12–33.

### Adenomas

199. Azzopardi JG: *Problems in Breast Pathology*. Philadelphia, WB Saunders, 1979, pp 52–54.

* 200. Azzopardi JG, Salm R: Ductal adenoma of the breast: A lesion which can mimic carcinoma. *J Pathol* 1984;144:15–23.

* 201. Baker EM: Simple adenoma of the breast. *Va Med Mon* 1947;74:505–508.

202. Balance WA, Ro JY, El-Naggar AK, et al: Pleomorphic adenoma (benign mixed tumor) of the breast. An immunohistochemical, flow cytometric, and ultrastructural study and review of the literature. *Am J Clin Pathol* 1990; 93:795–801.

203. Carney JA, Toorkey BC: Ductal adenoma of the breast with tubular features. A probable component of the complex of myxomas, spotty pigmentation, endocrine overactivity, and Schwannomas. *Am J Surg Pathol* 1991;15:722–731.

* 204. Chen KTK: Pleomorphic adenoma of the breast. *Am J Clin Pathol* 1990;93:792–794.

205. Costa A: Una variante non conosciuta di adenoma puro della ghiandola mammaria: L'adenoma pura a cellule apocrine. *Arch de Vecchi Anat Patol* 1974;60:393–401.

206. Cuadros CL, Ryan SS, Miller RE: Benign mixed tumor (pleomorphic adenoma) of the breast: Ultrastructural study and review of the literature. *J Surg Oncol* 1987;34:1003–1005.

207. Diaz NM, McDivitt RW, Wick MR: Pleomorphic adenoma of the breast: A clinicopathologic and immunohistochemical study of 10 cases. *Hum Pathol* 1991;22:1206–1214.

208. Draheim JH, Neubecker RD, Spirinz H: An unusual tumor of the breast resembling eccrine spiradenoma. *Amer J Clin Path* 1959;31:511–516.

209. Finck FM, Schwinn CP, Keasbey LE: Clear cell hydradenoma of the breast. *Cancer* 1968;22:125–135.

* 210. Geschickter CG, Lewis D: Pregnancy and lactation changes in fibroadenoma of the breast. *Br Med J* 1938;1:499–504.

211. Giao T, Bianchi AE: Tumor mixto de la glandula mamaria en la hombre. *Semana Medica* 1930;2:1193–1198.

* 212. Gill AJ, Stirman JA, Gordon CE: Lactating adenomas of breast. *Tex Med J* 1953;49:231–234.

213. Gusterson BA, Sloane JP, Middwood C, et al: Ductal adenoma of the breast—a lesion exhibiting a myoepithelial/epithelial phenotype. *Histopathology* 1987;11:903–908.

* 214. Hertel BF, Zaloudek C, Kempson RL: Breast adenomas. *Cancer* 1976;37:2891–2905.

* 215. Hill RP, Miller FN: Adenomas of the breast. *Cancer* 1954;7: 318–324.

216. Hirst E, Rawle RM: The lactating nodule. *Austr N Z J Surg* 1961;31:17–24.

217. Jakimowicz JJ, Gramata S: Three cases of rare tumors of the mammary gland. *Arch Chir Neerl* 1977;29:203–208.

*218. Kermarec J, Plouvier S, Duplay H, et al: Tumeur mammaire a cellules myo-epitheliales. Etudes ultrastructurale. *Arch Anat Cytol Pathol* 1973;21:225–231.

*219. Lammie GA, Millis RR. Ductal adenoma of the breast—a review of fifteen cases. *Hum Pathol* 1989;20:903–908.

*220. Le Gal Y: Adenomas of the breast: Relationship of adenofibromas to pregnancy and lactation. *Am Surgeon* 1961;27: 14–22.

221. Makek M, Kochstetter AR: Pleomorphic adenoma of the human breast. *J Surg Oncol* 1980;14:281–286.

222. McClure J, Smith PS, Jamieson GG: "Mixed" salivary type adenoma of the human female breast. *Arch Pathol Lab Med* 1982;106:615–619.

223. Medina A, Uehlinger K: Das pleomorphe adenom der Mamma. *Hel Chir Acta* 1980;47:205–208.

224. Moran CA, Suster S, Carter D: Benign mixed tumours (pleomorphic adenomas) of the breast. *Am J Surg Pathol* 1990;14:913–921.

225. Morris JA, Kelly JF: Multiple bilateral breast adenomata in identical adolescent Negro twins. *Histopathology* 1982;6: 539–547.

*226. Nabert C, Kermanach G, Saout J: Epithelioma a stroma remanie ou tumeur mixte du sein: A propos d'une observation. *J Sci Med Lille* 1968;86:507–510.

227. Nanavati MP, Mandoli RC, Kanvinde MS: Pure adenoma of the breast. *Indian J Med Sci* 1969;23:257–258.

228. O'Hara MF, Page DL: Adenomas of the breast and ectopic breast under lactational influences. *Hum Pathol* 1985;16: 707–712.

229. Paikova LV: Smeshannaia opukhol' molochnyk zhelez. *Arkh Pathol* 1972;34:59–61.

230. Petrelli M: Pleomorphic adenomas of the breast. *N Y State J Med* 1986;86:232–233.

231. Poluektov IA, Shestakova LM: Smeshannaia opukhol molochnoi (odo nabliudenie). *Vopr Onkol* 1969;15:99–101.

*232. Persaud V, Talerman A, Jordon R: Pure adenoma of the breast. *Arch Pathol* 1968;86:481–483.

*233. Rottino A, Willson K: Osseous, cartilaginous, and mixed tumors of the human breast. A review of the literature. *Arch Surg* 1945;50:184–193.

234. Segan JC, Foo M, Richer S: Pleomorphic adenoma of the breast with positive estrogen receptors. *N Y State J Med* 1986;86:265–266.

235. Sheth MJ, Hathway D, Petrelli M: Pleomorphic adenoma ("mixed tumors") of human female breast mimicking carcinoma clinicoradiologically. *Cancer* 1978;41:659–665.

236. Smith BH, Taylor HB: The occurrence of bone and cartilage in mammary tumors. *Am J Clin Pathol* 1968;51:610–618.

*237. Soreide JA, Anda O, Erikson L, et al: Pleomorphic adenoma of the human breast with local recurrence. *Cancer* 1988;61:997–1001.

238. Stead RH, Qizilbach AH, Kontozoglov T, et al: An immunohistochemical study of pleomorphic adenoma of the salivary gland: Glial fibrillary acidic protein-like immunoreactivity identifies a major myoepithelial component. *Hum Pathol* 1988;19:32–40.

239. Tesluk H, Amott T, Goodnight JE: Apocrine adenoma of the breast. *Arch Pathol Lab Med* 1986;110:351–352.

240. van der Walt J, Rohlova B: Pleomorphic adenoma of the human breast. A report of a benign tumour closely mimicking a carcinoma clinically. *Clin Oncol* 1982;8:361–365.

241. Willen R, Uvelius B, Cameron R: Pleomorphic adenoma of the breast of a human female. *Acta Chir Scand* 1986;152:709–713.

242. Williams RW, Leach WB: Mixed tumor of the female breast of unusual duration and size. *South Med J* 1975;68:97–100.

243. Zawirska B, Cisek T, Markuszewka-Bernarz J: An unusual tumor of the female breast: Combined eccrine and apocrine adenoma. *Pat Pol* 1983;34;1:125–128.

### Hamartoma

*244. Arrigoni MG, Dockerty MB, Judd ES: The identification and treatment of mammary hamartoma. *Surg Gynecol Obstet* 1971;133:577–582.

245. Goussot JF, Coindre JM, Dilhuydy MH, et al: Hamartomes mammaires. A propos de onze cas. Revue de la litterature. *Sem Hop Paris* 1984;60:767–770.

*246. Hessler C, Schnyder P, Ozzello L: Hamartoma of the breast: Diagnostic observations of 16 cases. *Radiology* 1978; 126:95–98.

247. Hogeman KE, Ostberg G: Three cases of post lactational breast tumour of a peculiar type. *Acta Path Microbiol Scand* 1968;73:169–176.

248. Jones MW, Norris HJ, Wargotz ES: Hamartomas of the breast. *Surg Gynecol Obstet* 1991;173:54–56.

*249. Linnel F, Ostberg G, Soderstrom J, et al: Breast hamartomas. An important entity in mammary pathology. *Virch Arch Pathol Anat Histol* 1979;383:253–264.

250. Metcalf JS, Ellis B: Choristoma of the breast. *Hum Pathol* 1985;16:739–740.

251. Oberman HA: Hamartomas and hamartoma variants of the breast. *Semin Pathol* 1989;6:135–145.

252. Petrik PK: Mammary hamartoma. *Am J Surg Pathol* 1987; 11:234–235.

253. Skaane P: Das Fibro-adeno-lipom (Hamartom) der Mamma. *Fortschr Rontgenstr* 1981;135:747–748.

### Juvenile Hypertrophy

254. Azzopardi JG: *Problems in Breast Pathology*. Philadelphia, WB Saunders, 1979, p 77.

255. Barreto U: Juvenile mammary hypertrophy. *Plast Reconstr Surg* 1991;87:583–584.

256. Cardoso de Castro C, Aboudib JH, Salema R, et al: Massive breast hypertrophy in a young girl. *Ann Plast Surg* 1990;25: 497–501.

*257. Farrow JH, Ashikari H: Breast lesions in young girls. *Surg Clin N Am* 1969;49:261–269.

*258. Fechner RE: Fibroadenoma and related lesions, in: Page DL, Anderson TJ (eds): *Diagnostic Histopathology of the*

*Breast*. New York, Churchill Livingstone, 1987, Chapt 7, pp 72–85.

259. Fisher W, Smith JW: Macromastia during puberty. *Plast Reconstr Surg* 1971;47:445–451.

*260. Geschikter CF: *Diseases of the Breast. Diagnosis–Pathology–Treatment*, ed 2. Philadelphia, JB Lippincott, 1945, pp 97–132.

261. Griffith JR: Virginal breast hypertrophy. *J Adolesc Health Care* 1989;10:423–432.

*262. Haagensen CD: *Diseases of the Breast*, ed 3. Philadelphia, WB Saunders, 1986, pp 59–62.

263. Hines JR, Geurkink RE: Giant breast tumors in the adolescent female. *Am J Surg* 1965;109:810–813.

*264. Lewis D, Geschikter CF: Gynecomastia, virginal hypertrophy, and fibroadenoma of the breast. *Ann Surg* 1934;100: 779–795.

*265. Oberman HA: Breast lesions in the adolescent female. *Pathol Annu* 1979;14(part 1):175–201.

266. Sagot P, Mainguene C, Berriere P, et al: Virginal breast hypertrophy at puberty: A case report. *Eur J Obstet Gynecol Reprod Biol* 1990;34:289–292.

## Calcifications, Crystals, Inclusions

267. Ahmed A: Calcifications in human breast carcinomas: Ultrastructural observations. *J Pathol* 1975;117:247–251.

*268. Anastassiades TH, Bouropoulou V, Kontogeorgos G, et al: Microcalcifications in benign breast diseases. A histological and histochemical study. *Path Res Pract* 1984;178:237–242.

269. Barth V, Franz ED, Scholl A: Microcalcifications in mammary glands. *Natuwissenschaften* 1977;64:278–279.

270. Black WJ, Young B: A radiologic and pathological study of the incidence of calcification in diseases of the breast and neoplasms of other tissues. *Br J Radiol* 1965;38:596–598.

*271. Bouropoulou V, Anastassiades TH, Kontogeorgos G, et al: Microcalcifications in breast carcinomas. A histological and histochemical study. *Path Res Pract* 1984;179:51–58.

*272. Busing CM, Keppler U, Menges V: Differences in microcalcifications in breast tumors. *Virchows Arch* (B) 1981;393: 307–313.

273. Cheek HJ: Experience with breast biopsies from mammographic findings. *Breast* 1978;4:4–9.

*274. Clement PB, Young RH, Azzopardi JG: Collagenous spherulosis of the breast. *Am J Surg Pathol* 1987;11:411–417.

275. Contesso G, Masselot J, Pettit JY, et al: Microcalcifications en pathologie (TO). Le point de vue de l'anatomopathologiste. *Rev Fr Gynecol Obstet* 1991;86:20.

*276. Fandos-Morera A, Prats-Esteve M, Tura-Soteras JM, et al: Breast tumors: composition of microcalcifications. *Radiology* 1988;169:325–327.

277. Fisher ER, Dow AW, Posada H: Correlations between specimen roentgenograms (mammograms) and pathologic findings in breast disease. *Pathol Annu* 1973;8:453–471.

*278. Frappart L, Boudeulle M, Boumendil J, et al: Structure and composition of microcalcifications in benign and malignant lesions of the breast: Study by light microscopy, transmission and scanning electron microscopy, microprobe analysis, and X-ray diffraction. *Hum Pathol* 1984;15:880–889.

*279. Frappart L, Remy I, Lin HC, et al: Different types of microcalcifications observed in breast pathology. Correlations with histopathological diagnosis and radiological examination of operative specimen. *Virchows Arch A* 1986; 410:179–187.

*280. Galkin BM, Feig SA, Frasca P, et al: Noncalcified breast particles. A possible marker for breast cancer. *Invest Radiol* 1982;17:119–128.

281. Galkin BM, Feiz SA, Frasca P, et al: Photomicrographs of breast calcifications: Correlation with histopathologic diagnosis. *Radiographics* 1983;3:450–417.

282. Gerschon-Cohen J, Berger SM, Curcio BM: Breast cancer and microcalcifications: Diagnostic difficulties. *Radiology* 1966;87:613–622.

283. Ghadially FN, Stinson JC, Payne CM, et al: Intranuclear helioid inclusions. *J Submicrosc Cytol* 1985;17:469–475.

284. Ghadially FN (ed): *Ultrastructural Pathology of the Cell and Matrix*, ed 3. Boston, Butterworths, 1988, pp 86–89.

*285. Going JJ, Anderson TJ, Crocker PR, et al: Weddellite calcification in the breast: Eighteen cases with implications for breast cancer screening. *Histopathology* 1990;16:119–124.

*286. Gonzalez JEG, Caldwell RG, Valaitis J: Calcium oxalate crystals in the breast. Pathology and significance. *Am J Surg Pathol* 1991;15:586–591.

*287. Grignon DJ, Ro JY, Mackey BN, et al: Collagenous spherulosis of the breast. Immunohistochemical and ultrastructural studies. *Am J Clin Pathol* 1989;91:386–392.

288. Gump FE, Jicha DL, Ozella L: Ductal carcinoma in situ (DCIS): A revised concept. *Surgery* 1987;102:790–795.

289. Hassler O: Microradiographic investigation of calcifications of the female breast. *Cancer* 1969;23:1103–1109.

290. Keppler U, Nitsche D: Mikrokalke aus degeneriertem Gewebe der weiblichen Brust. *Natuwissenschaften* 1979;66: 214.

*291. Koehl RH, Snyder RE, Hutter RVP, et al: The incidence and significance of calcification within operative breast specimens. *Am J Clin Path* 1970;53:3–14.

292. Lagios MD, Westdahl PR, Margolin FR, et al: Duct carcinoma in situ. Relationship of extent of noninvasive disease to the frequency of occult invasion, multicentricity, lymph node metastases, and short term treatment failure. *Cancer* 1982;50:1309–1314.

293. Lang NP, Talbert GE, Shewmake KB, et al: The current evaluation of non-palpable breast lesions. *Arch Surg* 1987; 122:1389–1391.

*294. Leborgne R: Diagnostics de la tumores de la mamma por la radiographic simple. *Bol Soc Cirurgia Uruguay* 1949;20:407–422.

295. Levitan LH, Witten DM, Harrison EG: Calcification in breast disease: Mammographic pathologic correlation. *Am J Roentg* 1964;92:29–39.

296. Michal M, Skalova A: Collagenous spherulosis. A comment on its histogenesis. *Path Res Pract* 1990;186:365–370.

*297. Millis RR, Davis R, Stacey AJ: The detection and significance of calcifications in the breast: A radiological and pathological study. *Br J Radiol* 1976;49:12–26.

* 298. Millis RR: Mammography, in: Azzopardi JG (ed): *Problems in Breast Pathology*. Philadelphia, WB Saunders, 1979, pp 437–459.

299. Murphy WA, Deschryver-Kecskemeti K: Isolated clustered microcalcifications in the breast: Radiologic-pathologic correlation. *Radiology* 1978;127:335–341.

300. Radi MJ: Calcium oxalate crystals in breast biopsies: An overlooked form of microcalcification associated with benign breast disease. *Arch Pathol Lab Med* 1989;113:1376–1379.

301. Reid JD, Choi C, Oldroyd O: Calcium oxalate crystals in the thyroid: Their identification, prevalence, origin, and possible significance. *Am J Clin Pathol* 1987;87:443–454.

302. Salomon A: Beitrage zur Pathologie und Klinik der Mammakarzinome. *Arch Klin Chir* 1913;101:573–668.

303. Sandison AT: An autopsy study of the adult human breast: With special reference to proliferative epithelial changes of importance, in: *Pathology of the Breast*. Bethesda, National Cancer Institute Monograph 8, 1962, p 61.

304. Sickles EA: Breast calcifications: Mammographic evaluation. *Radiology* 1986;160:289–293.

305. Shepard IJ, Crile G Jr, Strittmatter WC: Roentgenographic evaluation of calcifications seen in paraffin block specimens of mammary tumors. *Radiology* 1962;78:967–968.

306. Solin LJ, Fowble BL, Troupin RH, et al: Biopsy results of new calcifications in the postirradiated breast. *Cancer* 1989; 63:1956–1961.

307. Snyder RE, Rosen PP: Radiography of breast specimens. *Cancer* 1971;28:1608–1611.

* 308. Stegner HE, Pape C: Beitrag zur Feinstruktur der sogenannten Mikrokalzifikation in Mammatumoren. *Zentralbl Allg Path* 1972;115:106–112.

309. Tandler B, Denning CR, Mandel ID, et al: Ultrastructure of human labial salivary glands. II. Intranuclear inclusions in the acinar secretory cells. *Z Zellforsch* 1969;94:555–564.

* 310. Tavassoli FA, Majeste RM, Snyder RC: Intranuclear helioid inclusions in mammary intraductal hyperplasias. *Ultrastruct Pathol* 1991;15:267–279.

311. Torell JA, Knight JP, Marcus PB: Intraluminal calcium hydroxyapatite crystals in breast carcinoma: An ultrastructural study. *Ultrstruct Pathol* 1984;6:9–14.

* 312. Tornos C, Silva EG, El-Naggar A, et al: Calcium oxalate crystals in breast biopsies: The missing microcalcifications. *Am J Surg Pathol* 1990;14:961–968.

* 313. Tuur SM, Nelson AM, Gibson DW, et al: Liesegang rings in tissue. How to distinguish Liesegang rings from the giant kidney worm, Dioctophyma renale. *Am J Surg Pathol* 1987;11:598–605.

* 314. Warren SL: A roentgenologic study of the breast. *Am J Roentgenol Radium Ther Nucl Med* 1930;24:113–124.

315. Yasue T: Histochemical identification of calcium oxalate. *Acta Histochem Cytochem* 1969;2:83–94.

### Reaction to Silicone Implants

316. Ashley FL, Braley S, McNall EG: The current status of silicone injection therapy. *Surg Clin North Am* 1971;51:501–509.

317. Ashley FL, Braley S, Rees TD, et al: The recent status of silicone fluid in soft tissue augmentation. *Plast Reconstr Surg* 1967;39:411–420.

318. Ben-Hur N, Neuman Z: Siliconoma—another cutaneous response to dimethylpolysiloxane: Experimental study in mice. *Plast Reconstr Surg* 1965;36:629–631.

319. Berger RA: Dermatologic experience with liquid silicones. *NY State J Med* 1966;66:2523–2526.

320. Brody GL, Frey CF: Peritoneal response to silicone fluid: A histologic study. *Arch Surg* 1968;96:237–245.

* 321. Delage C, Shane JJ, Johnson FB: Mammary silicone granulomas. Migration of silicone fluid to abdominal wall and inguinal region. *Arch Dermatol* 1973;108:104–107.

322. Hausner RJ, Schoen FJ, Pierson KK: Foreign body reaction to silicone gel in axillary lymph nodes after an augmentation mammoplasty. *Plast Reconstr Surg* 1978;62:381–384.

323. Nosanchuk JS: Silicone granuloma in breast. *Arch Surg* 1968;97:583–585.

* 324. Picha GJ, Goldstein JA: Analysis of soft-tissue response to components used in the manufacture of breast implants: Rat animal model. *Plast Reconstr Surg* 1991;87:490–500.

325. Rees TD, Vallantyne DL Jr, Seidman I, et al: Visceral response to subcutaneous and intraperitoneal injections of silicone in mice. *Plast Reconstr Surg* 1967;39:402–410.

326. Symmers W St C: Silicone mastitis in "topless" waitresses and some other varieties of foreign body mastitis. *Br Med J* 1968;3:19–22.

* 327. Tabatowski K, Elson CE, Johnston WW: Silicone lymphadenopathy in a patient with a mammary prosthesis. Fine needle aspiration cytology, histology and analytical electron microscopy. *Acta Cytol* 1990;34:10–14.

* 328. Winer LH, Sternberg TH, Lehman R, et al: Tissue reactions to injected silicone liquids. *Arch Dermatol* 1964;90:588–593.

# 5

# Intraductal Hyperplasias, Ordinary and Atypical



In search of a morphologic factor that would identify a woman at risk for the development of invasive breast carcinoma, pathologists have considered many lesions over the past several decades. After evaluation of a variety of lesions, it has become apparent that epithelial hyperplasias within ducts and lobules constitute an important risk factor (6,10–12,22,23,32). Among these hyperplastic changes, those that more closely resemble one of the recognized variants of in situ carcinoma are the most worrisome and have been designated as atypical hyperplasia. The atypical intraductal proliferations are worrisome because they have attained some or all features that are typically identified in intraductal carcinomas, yet they fall short of an intraductal carcinoma either by having retained some of the characteristics of ordinary hyperplasias, or because of their very limited quantity.

In our practice as consultants in breast pathology at AFIP, we have witnessed a tremendous surge in all variants of intraductal proliferative lesions for which a second opinion has been sought over the past ten years. This is in part due to increased patient awareness and to the detection of early proliferative lesions by technically advanced mammographic procedures. Another important factor is that general pathologists have been overwhelmed by the variety of early proliferative changes picked up by advanced screening procedures for which neither a precise definition nor any standardized criteria has been available. There is a dire need for a standardized approach to the classification, interpretation, and management of the ordinary and atypical proliferative lesions confined to the duct system. Furthermore, well-organized multicenter, national prospective programs are needed to evaluate the long-term significance of these changes. It is also important to educate women that their participation in these programs is necessary and an important factor in how much we may learn from these studies which will ultimately benefit them.

The terminology, diagnostic criteria, clinical significance, and management of patients with ordinary and atypical intraductal epithelial proliferations are presented in this chapter. Lobular neoplasia is discussed in Chapter 8. Once again, it is emphasized that it is not the site of origin of what is generally designated as a ductal or lobular type of proliferation that distinguishes the two, but rather the pattern of

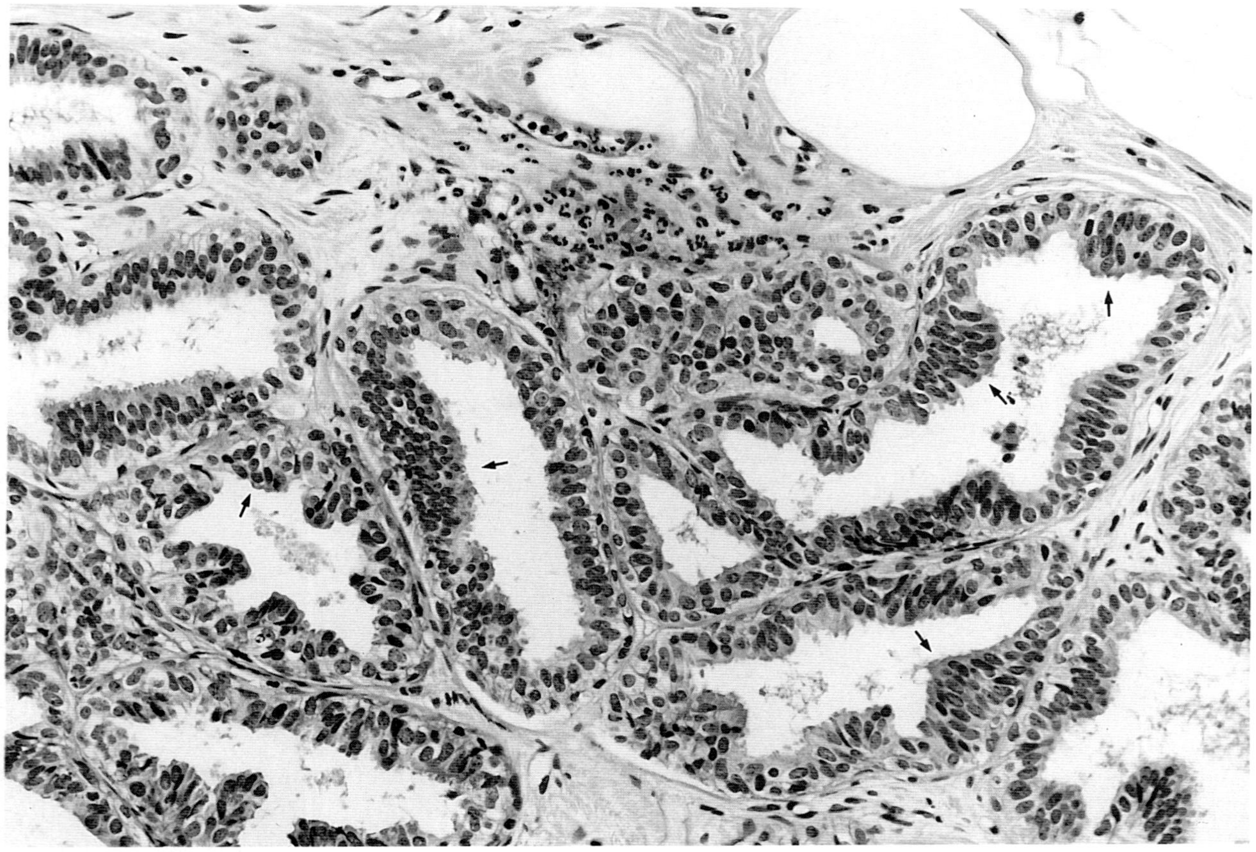

**Figure 5.1** Intraductal hyperplasia, mild. The ductules in this field show focal heaping up of the cells and tufting of three to four cells thick (arrows). (H&E, X160)

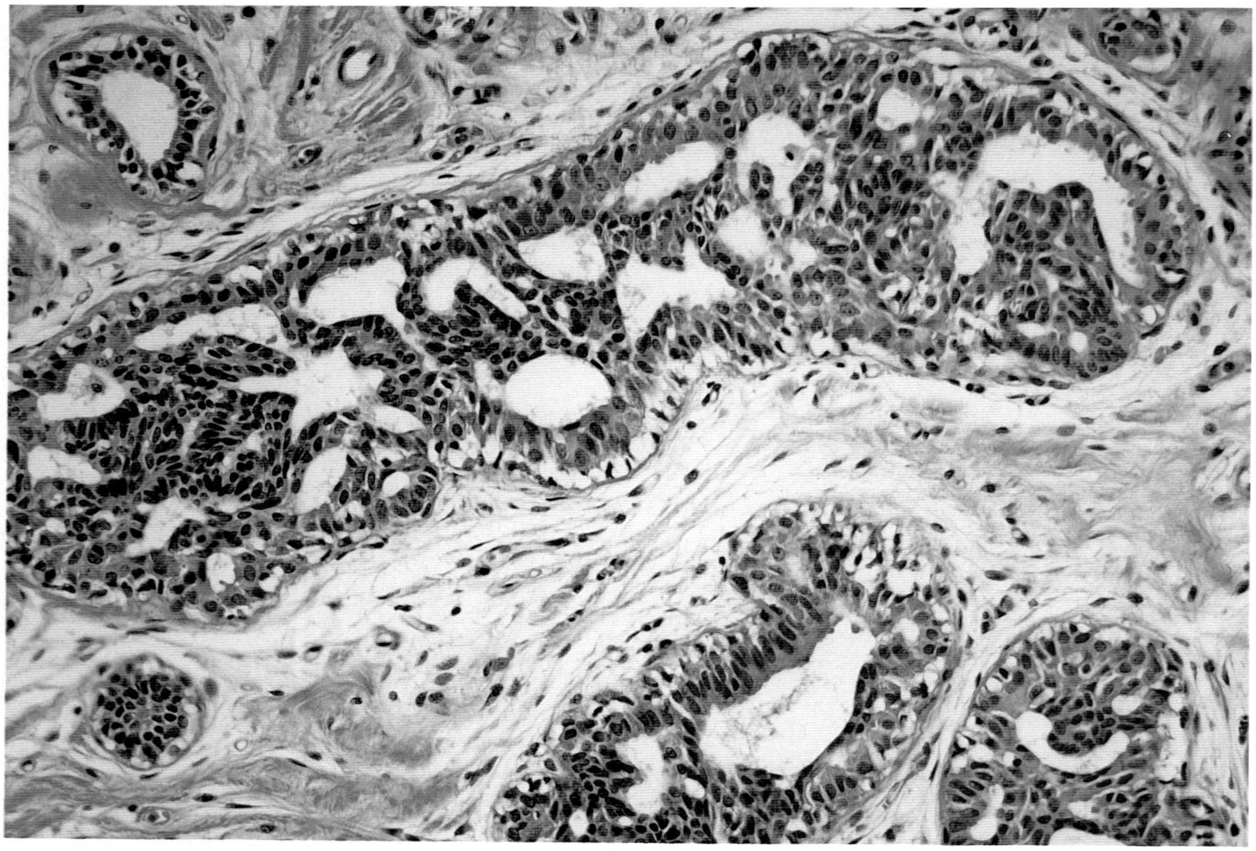

**Figure 5.2** Intraductal hyperplasia, moderate. The tips of the epithelial tufts meet and appear to or occasionally actually bridge across the lumen. (H&E, X320)

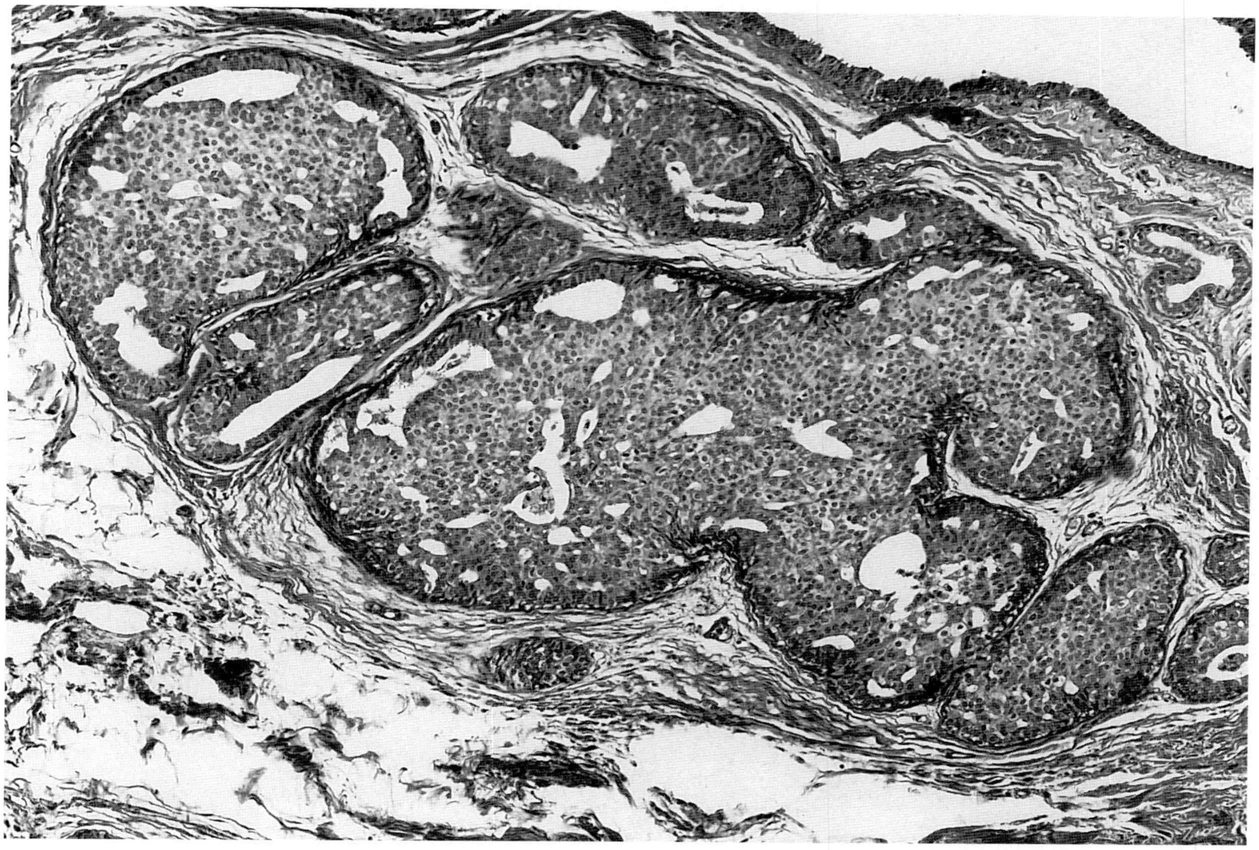

**Figure 5.3** Intraductal hyperplasia, severe. The ductal spaces are distended by solid and fenestrated clusters of hyperplastic cells, with formation of multiple secondary lumens (H&E, X200)

proliferation. There are intraductal proliferative lesions that develop in the major and lactiferous ducts, but whether ductal or lobular in their growth pattern, a majority of proliferative lesions in the breast begin in the terminal duct-lobular unit (TDLU) (32).

## TERMINOLOGY

Without qualification, the term hyperplasia could refer to epithelial proliferations that are perpendicular to the basement membrane, to an increase in the number of epithelial and myoepithelial cells resulting from a lateral expansion of lobules or increased branching of the duct system as observed during gestation, or to an increase in the number of unit structures (see Chapter 1) as in various patterns of adenosis and adenoma. It is the pattern of proliferation perpendicular to the basement membrane that is the subject of this chapter. This is referred to as intraductal hyperplasia (ordinary or atypical) to distinguish it from the type of hyperplasia that is observed during gestation or in adenosis.

Intraductal hyperplasia is present any time the number of cell layers lining a duct exceeds the two layers—a continuous layer of luminal epithelial cells surrounded by an interrupted layer of myoepithelial cells—typical of the normal unit structure. The designation of intraductal hyperplasia is preferred to epitheliosis (2) and papillomatosis (8,9,16) which are used by some pathologists for the same changes. The term epitheliosis is not commonly used in the United States, and it does not convey any information regarding the ductal growth pattern of these lesions; papillomatosis is also inaccurate considering the requirement of a fibrovascular supportive core for a papillary process.

Prior to the extensive use of mammography, about 25% of women who had breast biopsies were found to have intraductal hyperplasia (IDH), while about 2% to 5% of the women during the same period and subsequently have had atypical intraductal hyperplasia (AIDH) in their biopsies (15,17,21). These

A

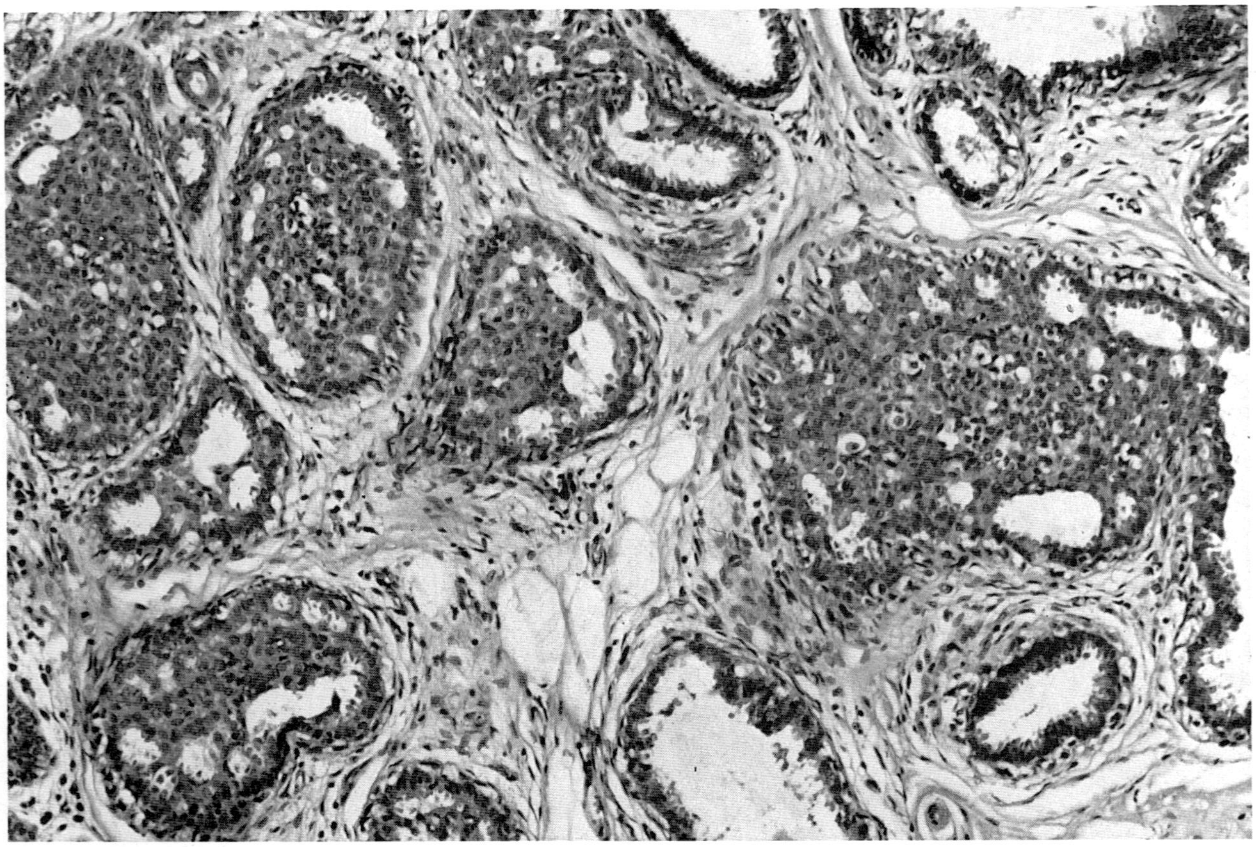

B

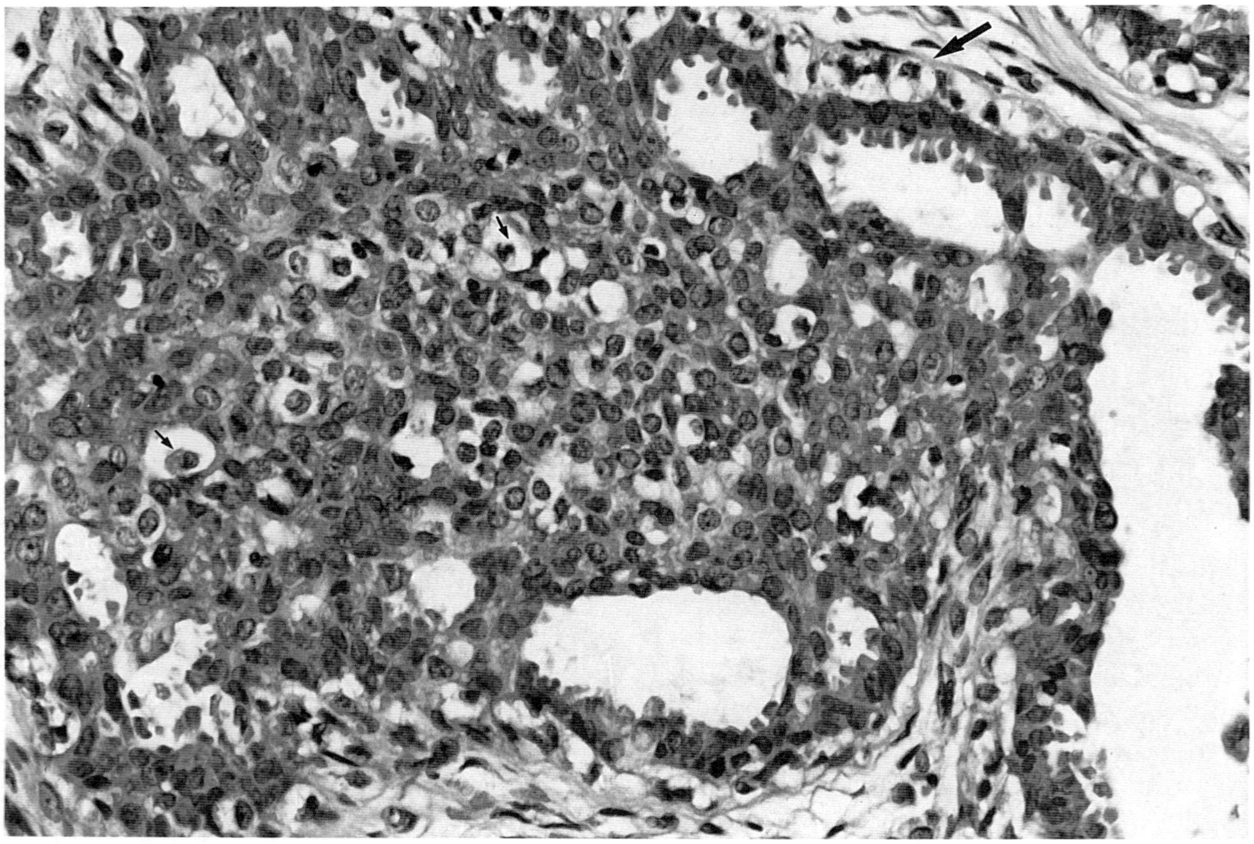

**Figure 5.4** Intraductal hyperplasia. (a) Multiple ducts are involved by the IDH. They all display predominance of peripheral fenestrations and a relatively solid area of central epithelial proliferation. (H&E, X200) (b) The epithelial proliferation is composed of epithelial and myoepithelial cells. Note the similarity of the naked nuclear appearance of the myoepithelial cells (short arrows) proliferating along with the epithelial cells to those in the normal myoepithelial cell layer at the periphery of the duct (long arrow). (H&E, X480)

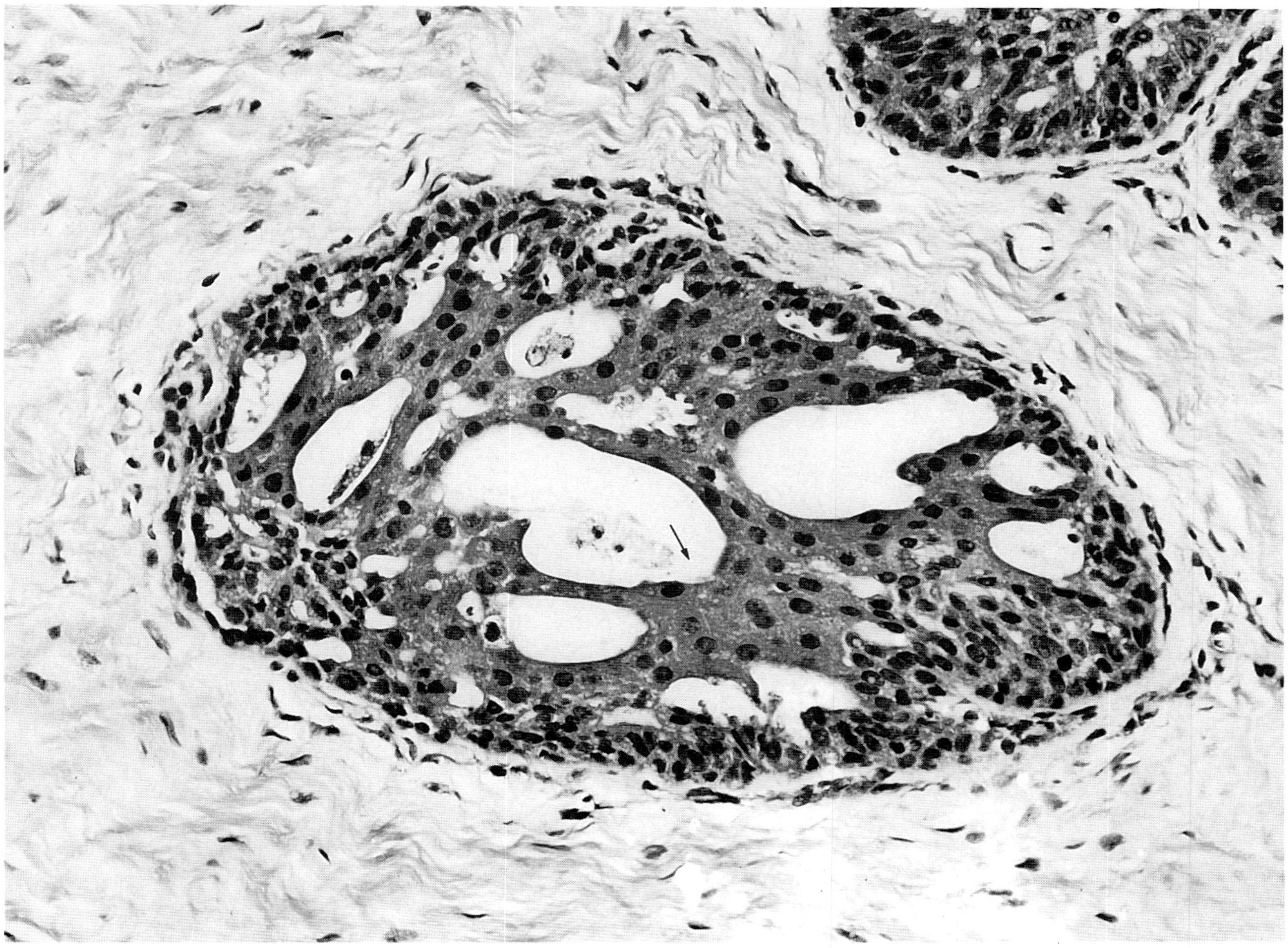

**Figure 5.5** Intraductal hyperplasia showing an admixture of epithelial and metaplastic apocrine cells (arrow). (H&E, X150)

changes are observed more frequently among mammographically directed biopsies (28).

The proliferating cells may display various forms of pleomorphism, or they may be quite uniform and even small, similar to those of lobular neoplasia. They may be composed purely of epithelial cells, or they may reflect an admixture of epithelial, metaplastic apocrine and/or myoepithelial cells.

The extent, quantity, and growth pattern of IDH are highly variable. The hyperplasia in the duct system may be focal or widespread. A hyperplastic duct may be partially or totally involved. The proliferating cells may assume a stratified appearance, show tufting, formation of epithelial bridges, a solid or fenestrated growth pattern. Furthermore, intraductal hyperplasia may be mild (3 to 4 cell layers above basement membrane), moderate (tufting and a tendency to cross lumens), or severe (formation of epithelial bridges across the lumen, or filling and distension of the duct), (Figs. 5.1–5.3). The degree of distension of a duct is not directly related to the amount of epithelial proliferation protruding into the lumen; ductal spaces may become cystically dilated even when there is minimal epithelial tufting.

Based on a combination of cellular and architectural characteristics, the intraductal proliferation is interpreted as either ordinary intraductal hyperplasia (IDH), atypical intraductal hyperplasia (AIDH), or intraductal carcinoma (IDCA) (29). Two previously proposed classifications for the intraductal hyperplasias regarded the changes as a spectrum and subdivided the spectrum into different categories morphologically (4,32). While both studies noted an increased association of the higher grade lesions (those comparable to AIDH and IDCA) with invasive carcinoma, they did not study the significance of the various categories within the system. I do not believe that IDH is within the same spectrum as AIDH and IDCA. The cytologic features observed in AIDH and IDCA are not present in IDH. The latter may also

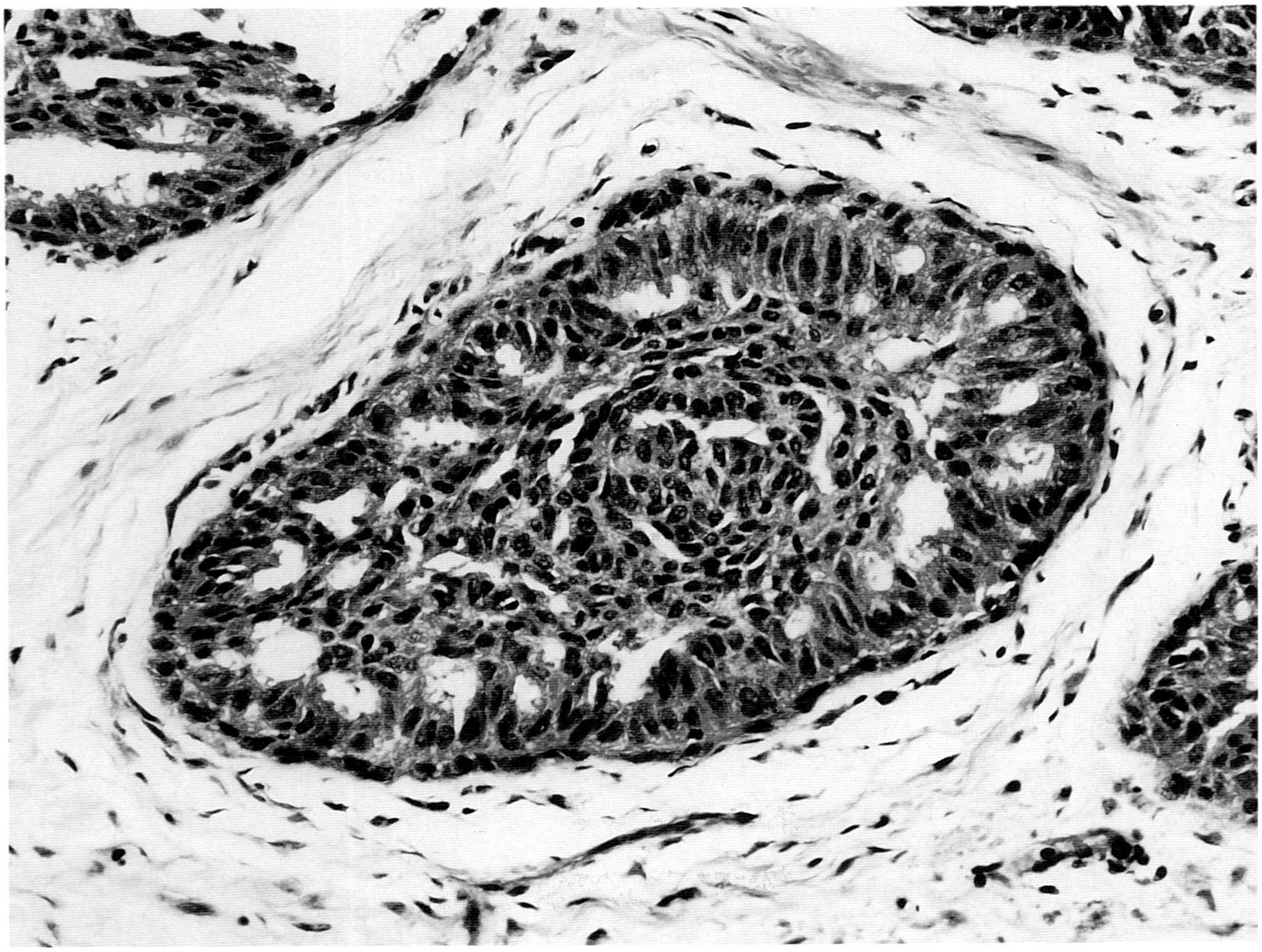

**Figure 5.6** Intraductal hyperplasia showing spindling and streaming of the cells. (H&E, X240)

show an admixture of cell types (epithelial, myoepithelial and metaplastic apocrine cells), in contrast to the uniformity of the proliferating cells observed in AIDH and the non-necrotic variants of IDCA. Azzopardi (2) used the designation of atypical intraductal hyperplasia reluctantly for a borderline group of lesions that showed a ductal pattern of proliferation within lobules. While I agree that what he illustrated in his Fig. 10.22 would qualify as AIDH by our criteria, he did not specify how the lesion he designated as AIDH differed from ordinary hyperplasia or why it did not qualify as intraductal carcinoma. Neither did Ashikari et al (1) specify the criteria for diagnosing AIDH in their study. Instead, they noted that the changes are difficult to characterize. During the 1980s, we learned more about IDH and AIDH through a number of reports from different centers (19–23,24–26,29). The following definitions and discussions are based on the AFIP experience and criteria (29), Tables 5.1 & 5.2.

## INTRADUCTAL HYPERPLASIA

### Definition of IDH

Intraductal hyperplasia is characterized by the proliferation of a heterogeneous cell population which may be purely epithelial or may have an admixture of epithelial, myoepithelial, and metaplastic apocrine cells (Figs. 5.4–5.5). The cells are irregular in outline with indistinct cell margins that frequently overlap; streaming of the cells may be present (Figs. 5.6–5.7). The nuclei are variable in appearance and lack a uniform, round contour. The proliferation is often fenestrated, but the secondary lumens are irregular in size and shape, angulated, slit-like, and sometimes peripheral in location (Figs. 5.8–5.11). The original duct lumen may persist as a crescent at one side of the duct. Epithelial bridges may form, but they are

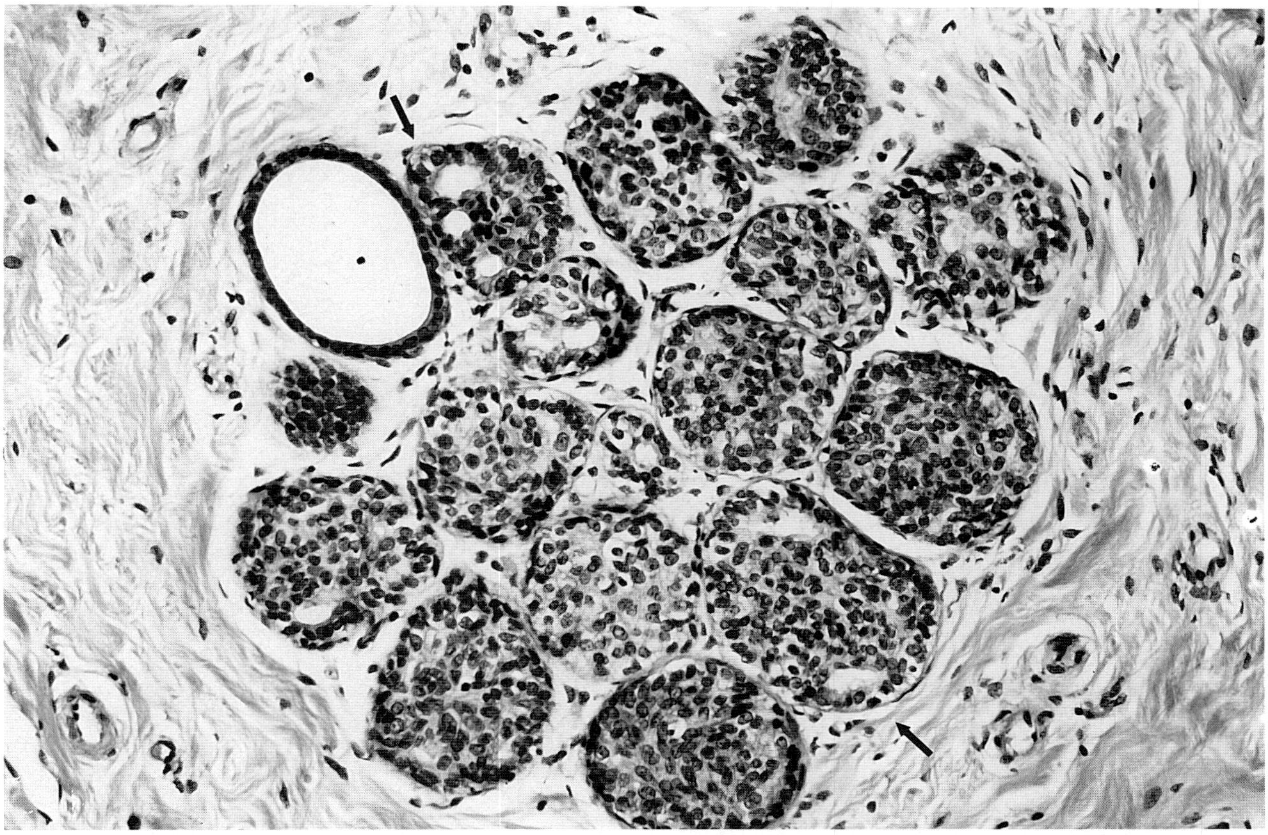

**Figure 5.7** Intraductal hyperplasia within TDLU. The more solid growth pattern mimics lobular neoplasia. The presence of two or more luminal spaces and epithelial bridging (arrows) within some ductules indicates a ductal growth pattern. The nuclei are variably shaped, irregularly distributed and show overlap; these features distinguish it from atypical hyperplasia. (H&E, X200) (Reproduced from Tavassoli FA, Norris HJ: *Cancer* 1990;65:518–529, with permission.)

stretched with elongation of the cells (Fig. 5.12). Sometimes the proliferation assumes the pattern observed in the hyperplastic ducts of gynecomastia (Fig. 5.13). This pattern may sometimes develop atypia (30); if and when it does, it would then qualify as AIDH. Foam cells may be present in the lumen of the hyperplastic ducts. Mitotic figures are observed only rarely, and their presence does not influence the ultimate diagnosis. Necrotic debris is also seen on rare occasions in the lumen (Fig. 5.14). It should be emphasized that the presence of luminal necrosis is not diagnostic of IDCA, and the lesion should be interpreted on the basis of the proliferating cell type.

Intraductal hyperplasia may be quite florid or of limited extent and degree. Mild intraductal hyperpla-

**Table 5.1** Morphologic Features of IDH

| |
|---|
| Cytologic features |
| Admixture of cell types (variably appearing epithelial cells, with or without myoepithelial, and/or metaplastic apocrine cells) |
| Variation in the appearance of epithelial cells displaying indistinct cell margins and deviation from round contour |
| Variation in the appearance of nuclei (angulated, spindled, oval, round) |
| Architectural Features |
| Irregular and slit-like fenestrations |
| Peripheral distribution of fenestrations |
| Stretched epithelial bridges |
| Streaming or spindling of cells |
| Uneven distribution of nuclei |

**Table 5.2** Morphologic Features of Nonapocrine AIDH

| |
|---|
| Cytologic features |
| Uniform, rounded cell population (or a tendency toward this appearance) |
| Subtle increase in nuclear/cytoplasmic ratio |
| Equidistant or rosette-like nuclear distribution |
| Rounded nuclei |
| Architectural features |
| Any of the patterns typical of IDH |
| Cribriform or micropapillary pattern involving anywhere from part of a single duct to multiple ducts or ductules, the aggregate cross-sectional diameter of which does not exceed 2 mm |

A

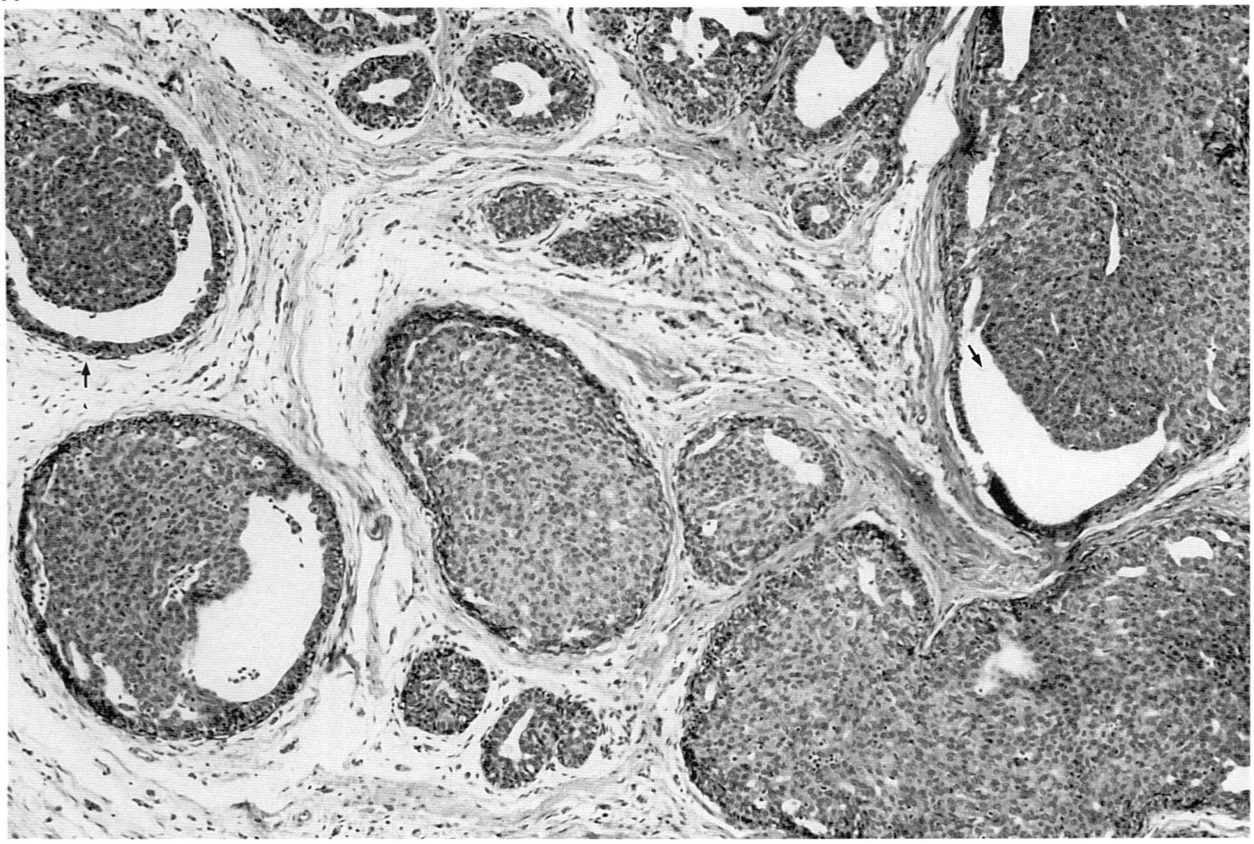

B

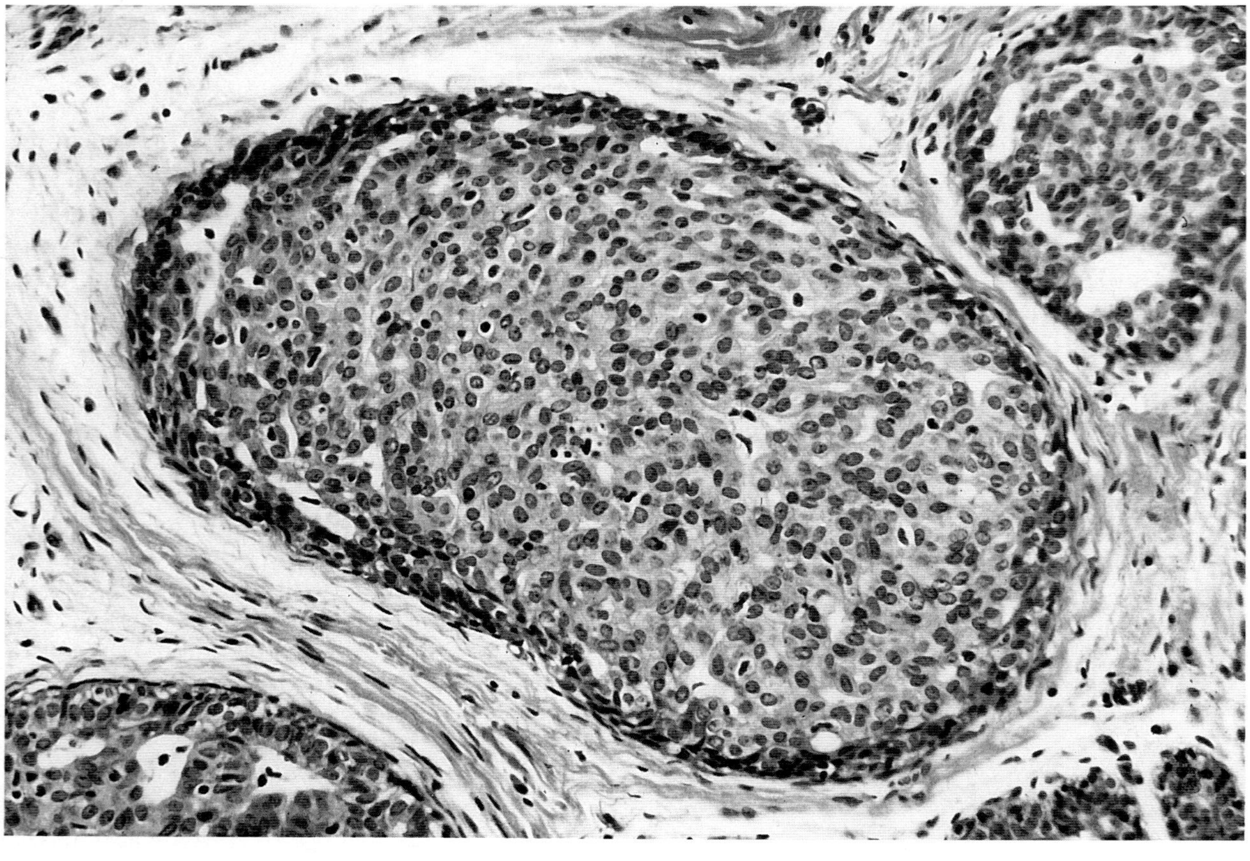

**Figure 5.8** Intraductal hyperplasia. (a) Several ducts show florid hyperplasia. Note crescents of residual lumen (arrows). (b) Small fenestrations are evident in the periphery. (H&E, (a) X75; (b) X240)

A

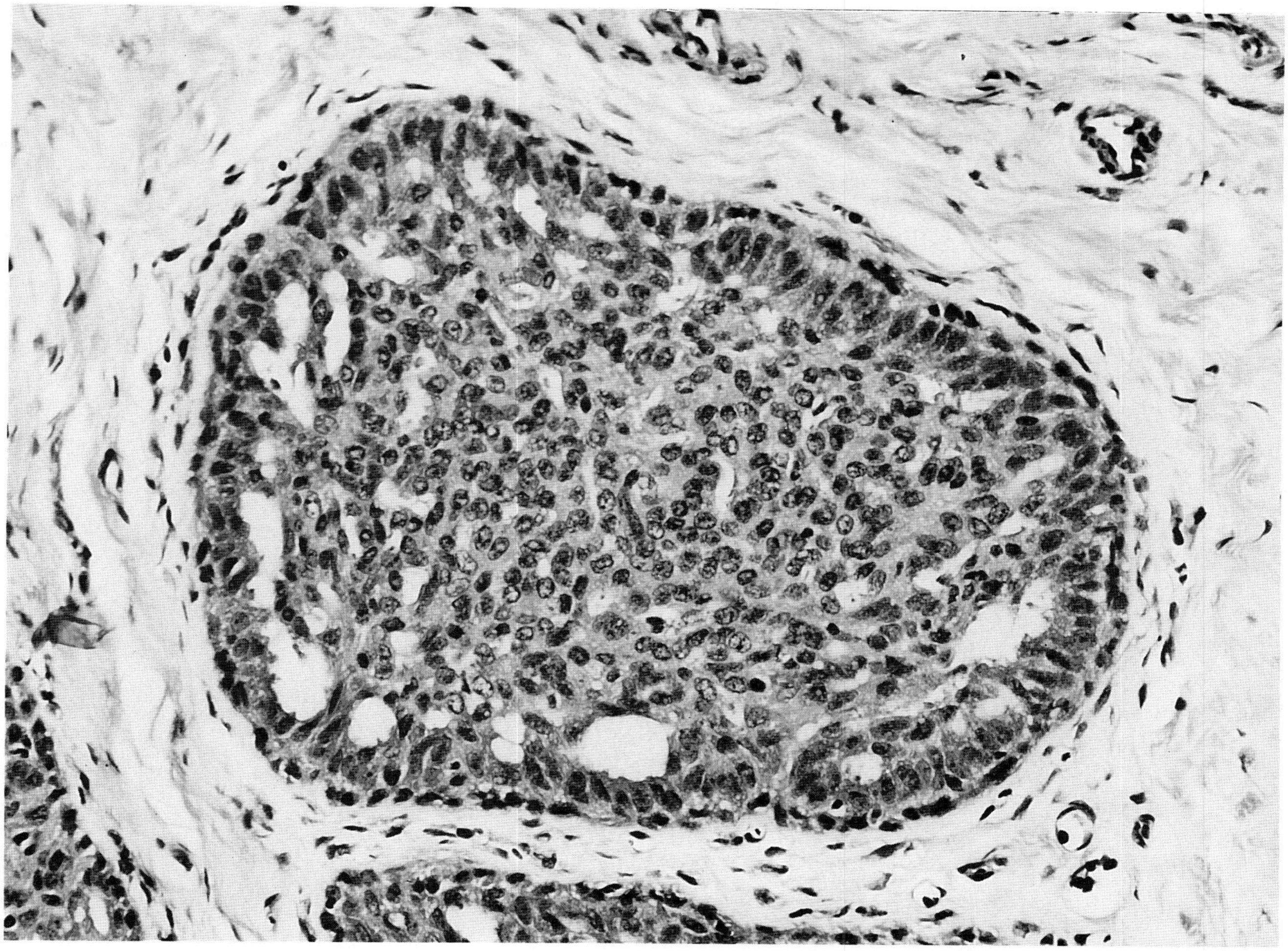

**Figure 5.9(a)** Intraductal hyperplasia. Fenestrations or the secondary lumens are variable in size and shape and predominantly peripheral in location. (H&E, X250)

sia is so common and relatively inconsequential that it was not included in the AFIP study that compared the follow-up of 117 women with IDH to that of 82 women with AIDH (30). Also excluded were proliferations composed purely of apocrine cells.

## Clinical Features and Significance of IDH

Women with IDH present with either a palpable mass, areas of induration, or mammographically suspicious areas. They range in age from 15 to 75 years with a median age of 45 years.

Women with IDH have a relative risk (see explanation of relative risk in Chapter 2, General Considerations and Chapter 7, Intraductal Carcinoma) for subsequent development of breast carcinoma that is one and a half to two times that of the general population (21). Of the 117 women with IDH in Tavassoli and Norris's series (29), three women (2.6%) developed subsequent invasive ductal carcinoma. The degree and/or extent of hyperplasia did not influence the outcome. The subsequent carcinomas developed 11.8, 14, and 17.5 years after the diagnosis of IDH; two of these were ductal, while one was lobular in type. They all developed in the same breast; two in the same quadrant, and the third in a quadrant below the almost completely excised quadrant harboring the IDH.

## Management of Patients with IDH

Because of the slight magnitude of the risk for development of subsequent invasive carcinoma associated with IDH, follow-up of the patient in the form of

B

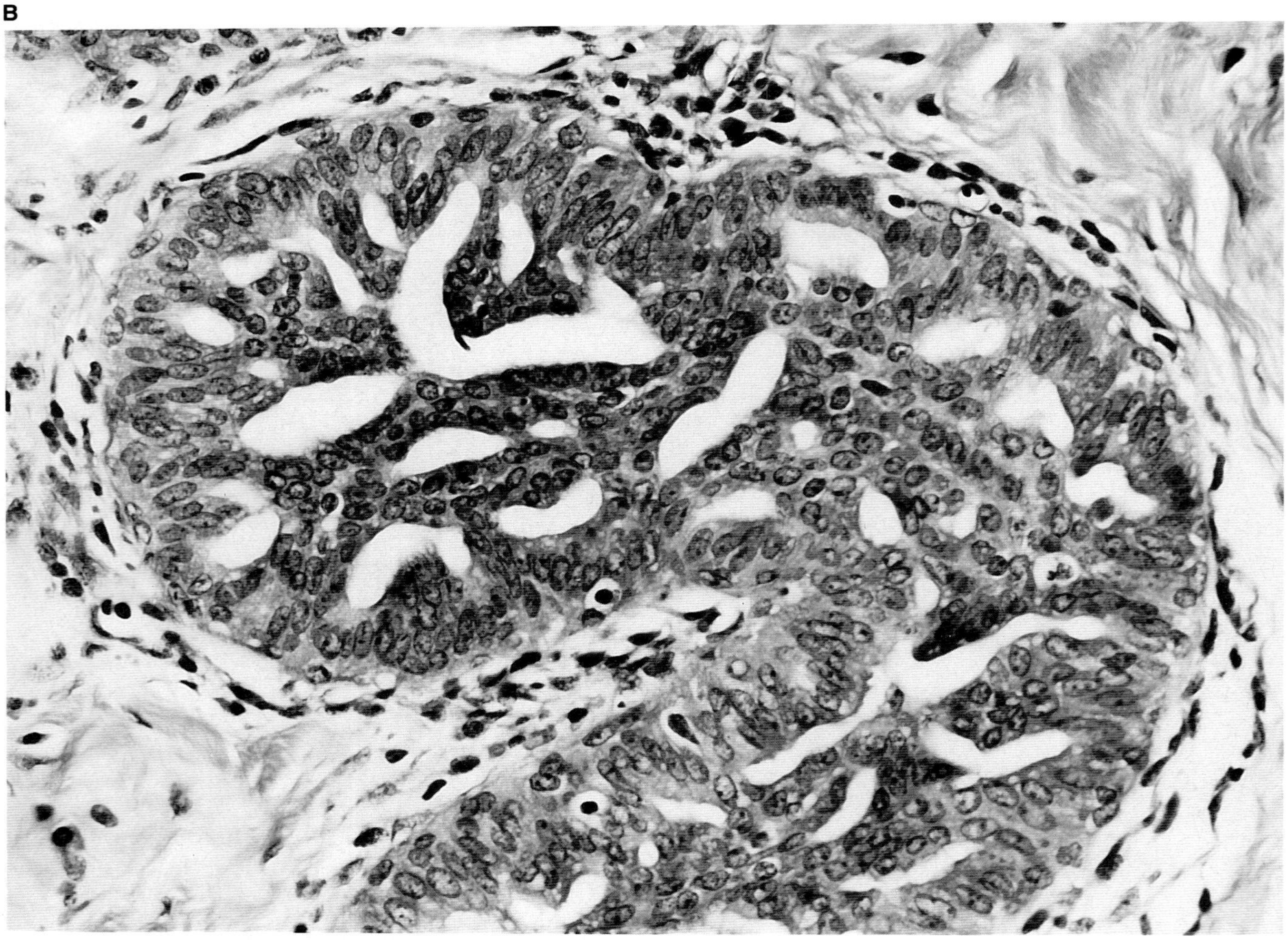

**Figure 5.9(b)** Intraductal hyperplasia. Note the angulated and variable size of the secondary lumens. (H&E, X250)

annual or biannual examination of the breasts by a physician is generally recommended. Patients need to become aware of the problem and learn breast self-examination. In the absence of other risk factors, mammography every one or two years for patients between 40 and 49 years of age would be prudent. Annual mammography is advised for women 50 years of age or older. Recent studies have shown that mammography, in addition to detecting small non-palpable invasive carcinomas, can identify IDH, AIDH, and IDCA (16).

## Juvenile Papillomatosis

First publicized by Rosen et al (24–26) as a distinctive clinicopathologic entity, a few previous reports had noted the occurrence of severe papillomatosis in young women (14,31). Juvenile papillomatosis (JP) is a localized lesion characterized by cystically dilated ducts and various degrees of intraductal proliferations that occurs in women less than 30 years of age. Two thirds of the patients with JP are less than 20 years of age, and it is rarely encountered after age 35. About 33% to 58% of women with JP have a positive family history of breast carcinoma (26).

Clinically, the lesion may present as a firm and discrete mass that is difficult to distinguish from a fibroadenoma, or it may present as a poorly defined dense area with cystic changes.

The presence of cysts of various sizes is characteristic of the gross specimen, and the basis for the designation of JP as "Swiss cheese hyperplasia." Microscopically, it is characterized by florid intraductal hyperplasia associated with fibrocystic changes

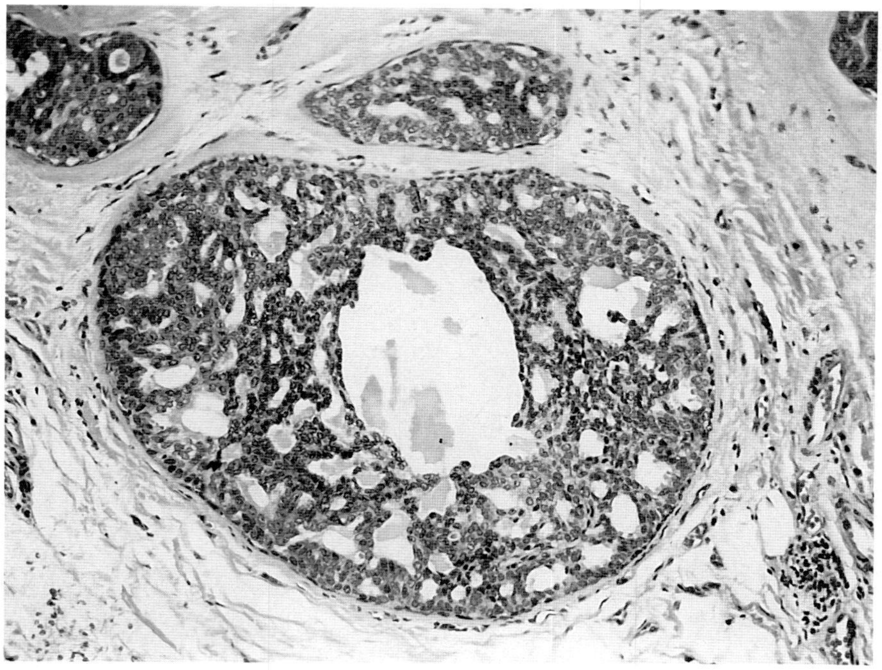

**Figure 5.10** Intraductal hyperplasia. Note the highly irregular shapes and the variable sizes of the secondary lumens; the original lumen persists at the center. (H&E, X160)

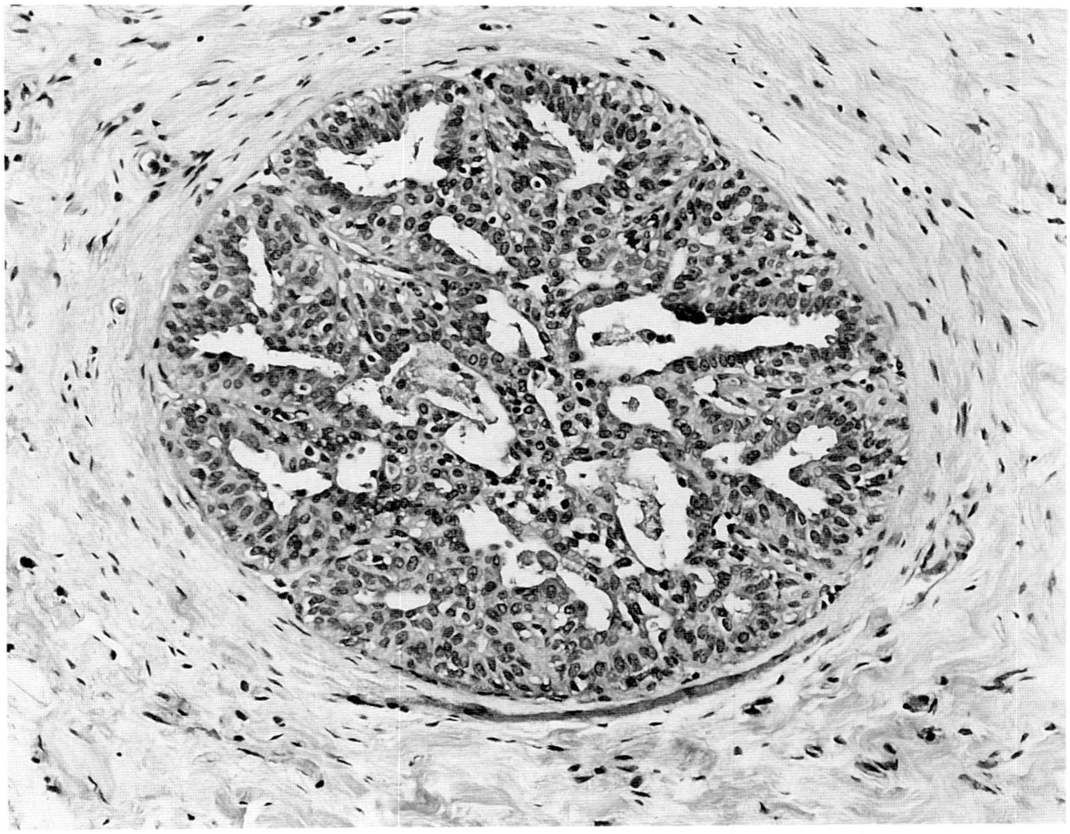

**Figure 5.11** This duct shows a combination of papillary and pure epithelial hyperplasia. In the papillary areas, the presence of a myoepithelial cell layer confirms their benign nature and the irregularly shaped, angulated secondary lumens reflect another feature of a benign hyperplasia. Furthermore, the cells lack the rounded nuclei and even spacing typical of atypicality. (H&E, X200)

A

B

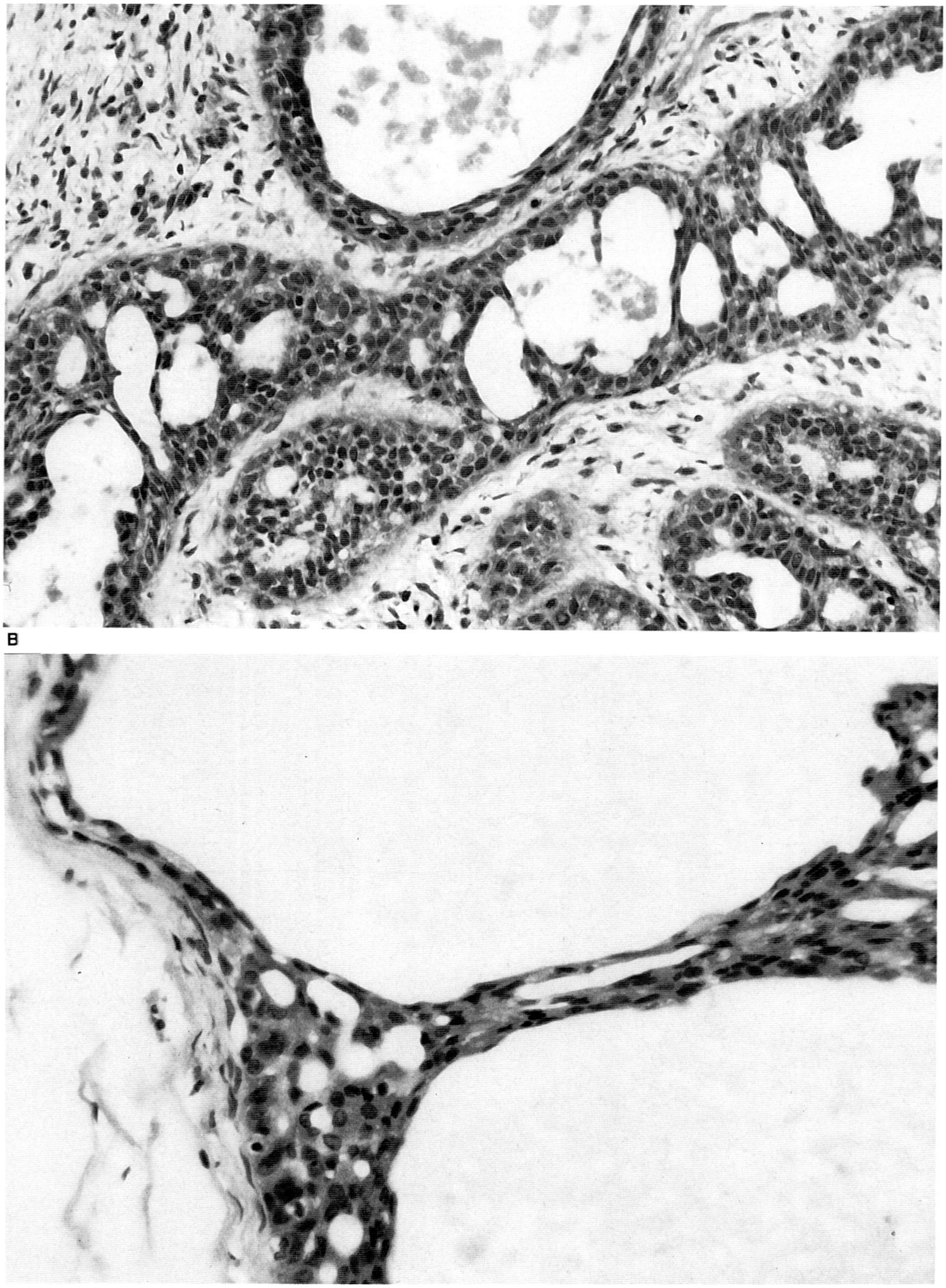

**Figure 5.12** Intraductal hyperplasia. (a, b) Epithelial bridges are thin and fragile, in contrast to the rigid nature of the bridges formed by cancer cells (c). (H&E, (a) X480; (b) X300) (Figure 5.12(b) reprinted from Tavassoli FA, Norris HJ: *Cancer* 1990;65:518–529, with permission).

c

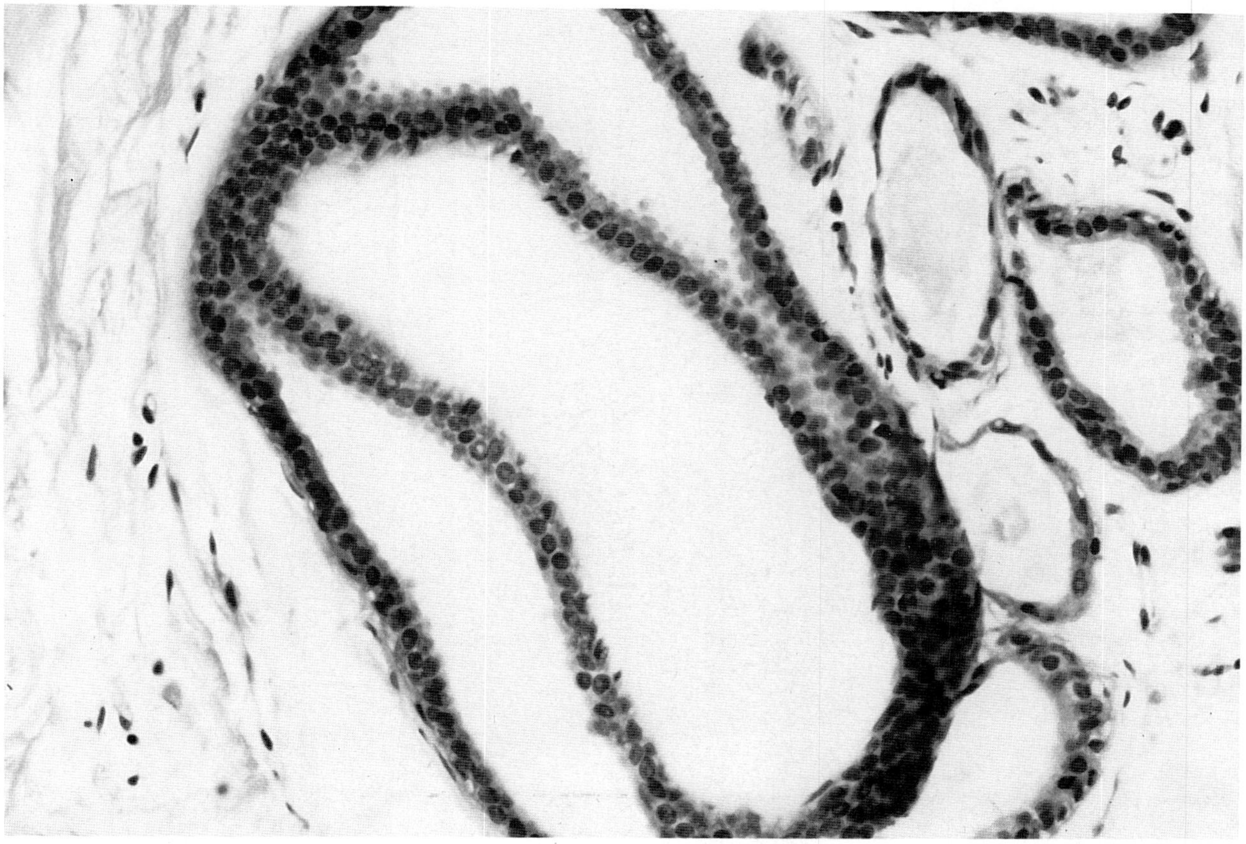

**Figure 5.12(c)** Rigid epithelial bridges formed by cancer cells. (H&E, X240)

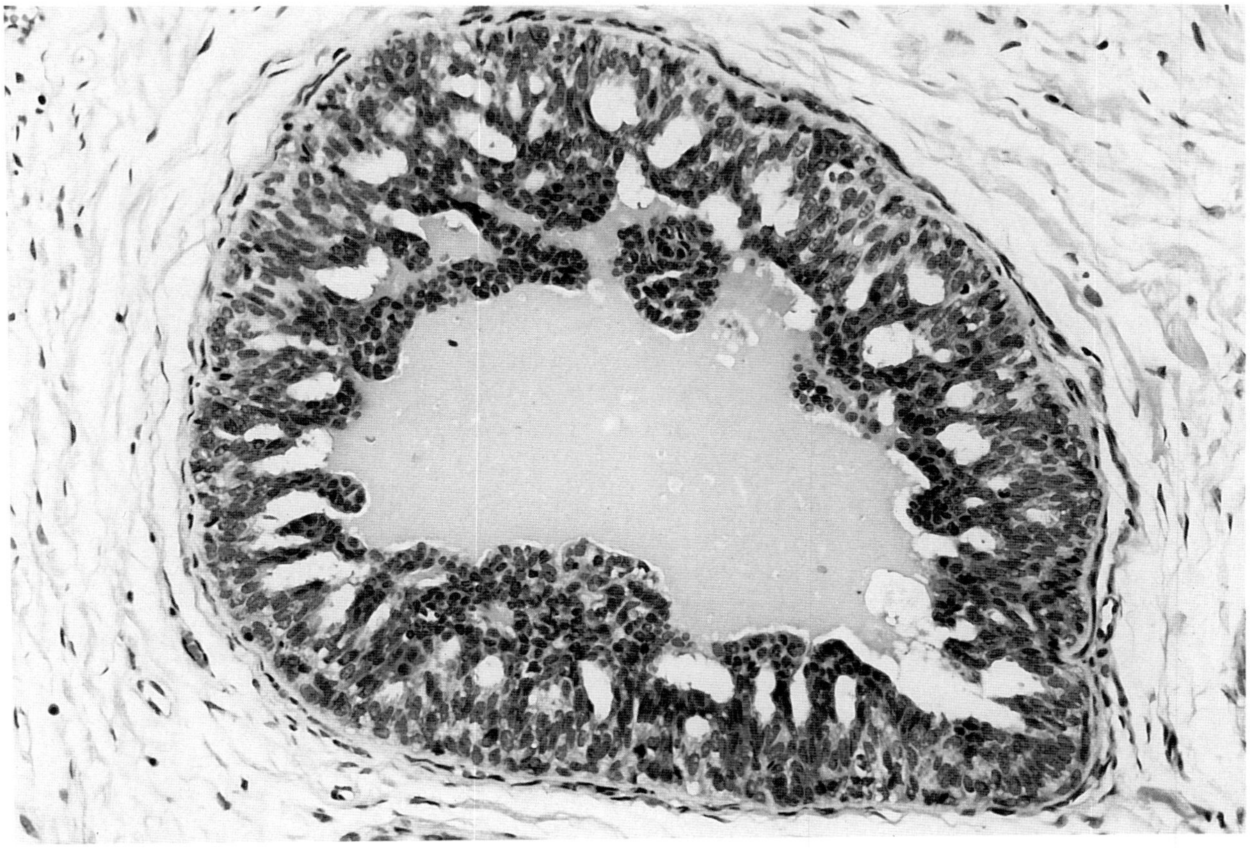

**Figure 5.13** Intraductal hyperplasia. This pattern resembles the type of proliferation often seen in the male breast in association with gynecomastia; It is distinguished from micropapillary IDCA by the presence of a combination or overlap of stratification and tufting, and lack of the rounded, evenly distributed nuclei. (H&E, X320)

A

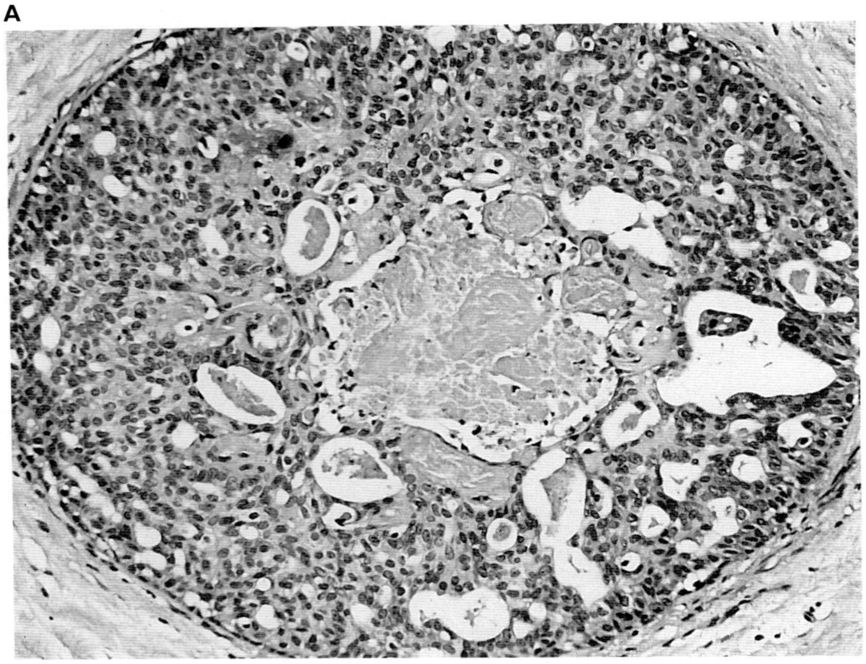

**Figure 5.14** (a&b) Intraductal hyperplasia with central necrosis; the cell type and growth pattern of the proliferating cells indicate the benign nature of this process. (H&E, (a) X160; (b) X300) (Figure 5.14(b) reprinted from Tavassoli FA, Norris HJ: *Cancer* 1990;65:518–529, with permission).

B

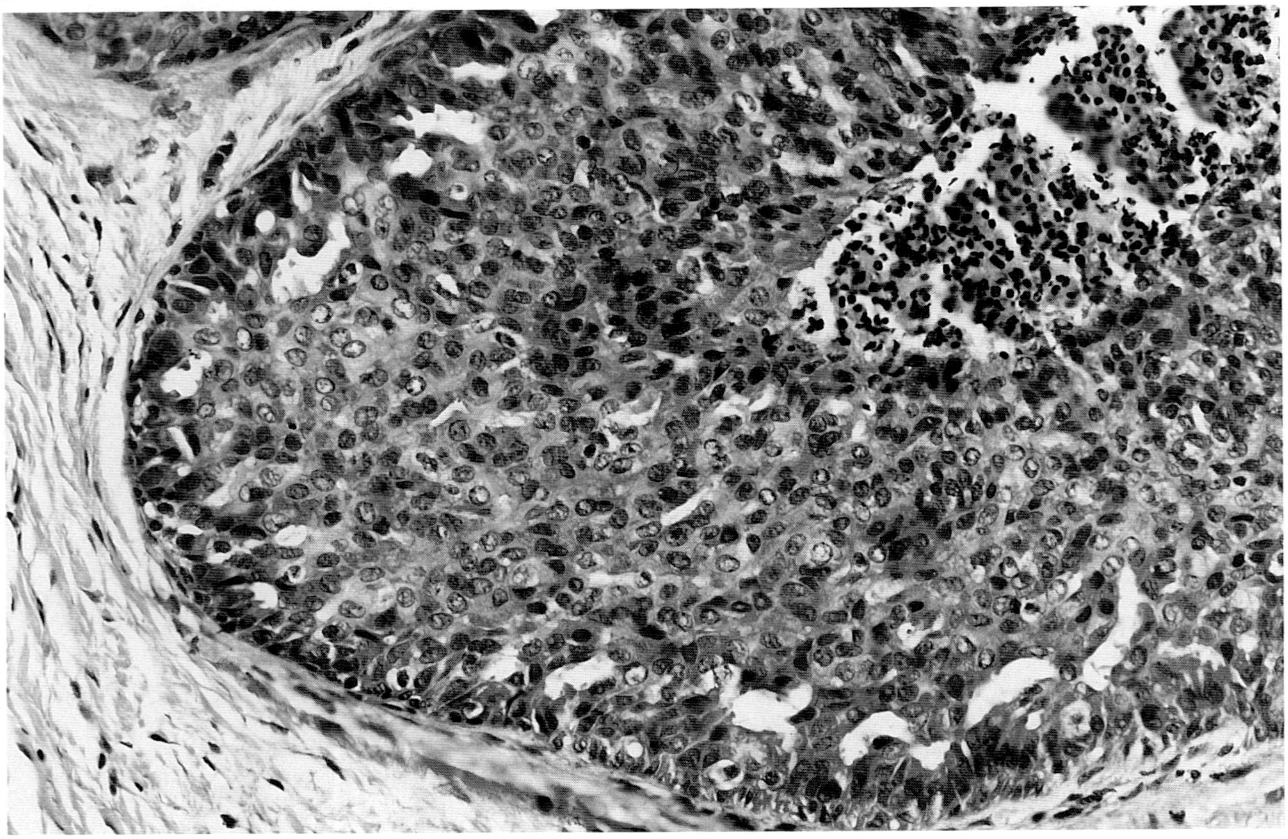

A

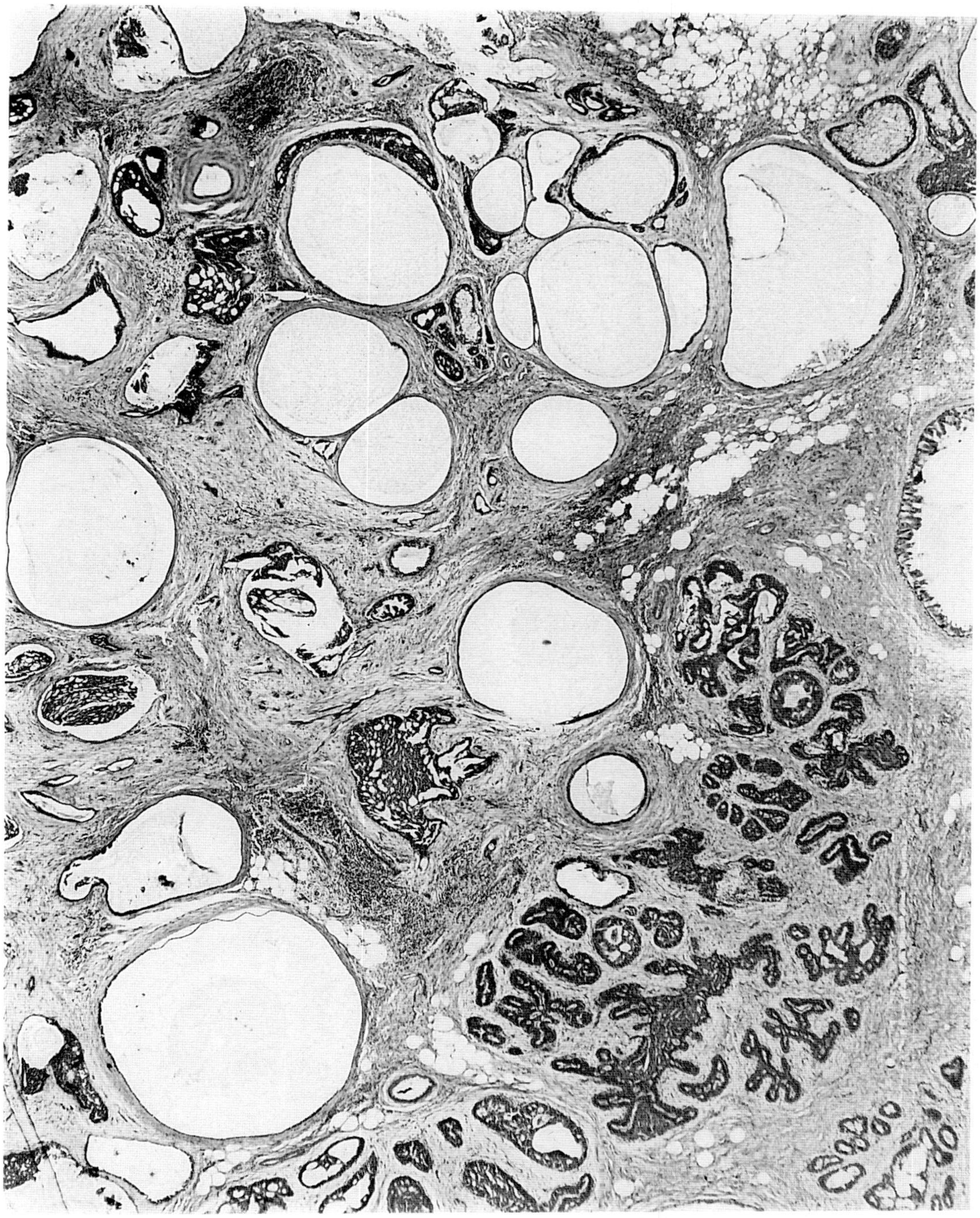

**Figure 5.15(a)** Juvenile papillomatosis. A 15-year-old girl presented with an area of irregular density in her breast. The lesion consisted of numerous cystically dilated ducts and intraductal hyperplasia. (H&E, X40)

(Fig. 5.15). Not infrequently, atypia is present in the hyperplastic epithelium. Intraductal carcinoma coexisting with JP has rarely been reported, but based on the criteria presented here, the intraductal carcinoma illustrated by Bazzocchi et al (3) would qualify as AIDH. Two cases of secretory carcinoma coexisting with or subsequent to JP have also been reported (7,26).

### *Risk of Breast Carcinoma in Patients with JP*

With a median follow-up of 14 years, breast carcinoma was identified in five (12%) of the 41 women reported by Rosen et al (26). All of these five patients had either bilateral, recurrent, or multifocal disease. All five patients had a positive family history of breast carcinoma, three in the mother, and two in either

B

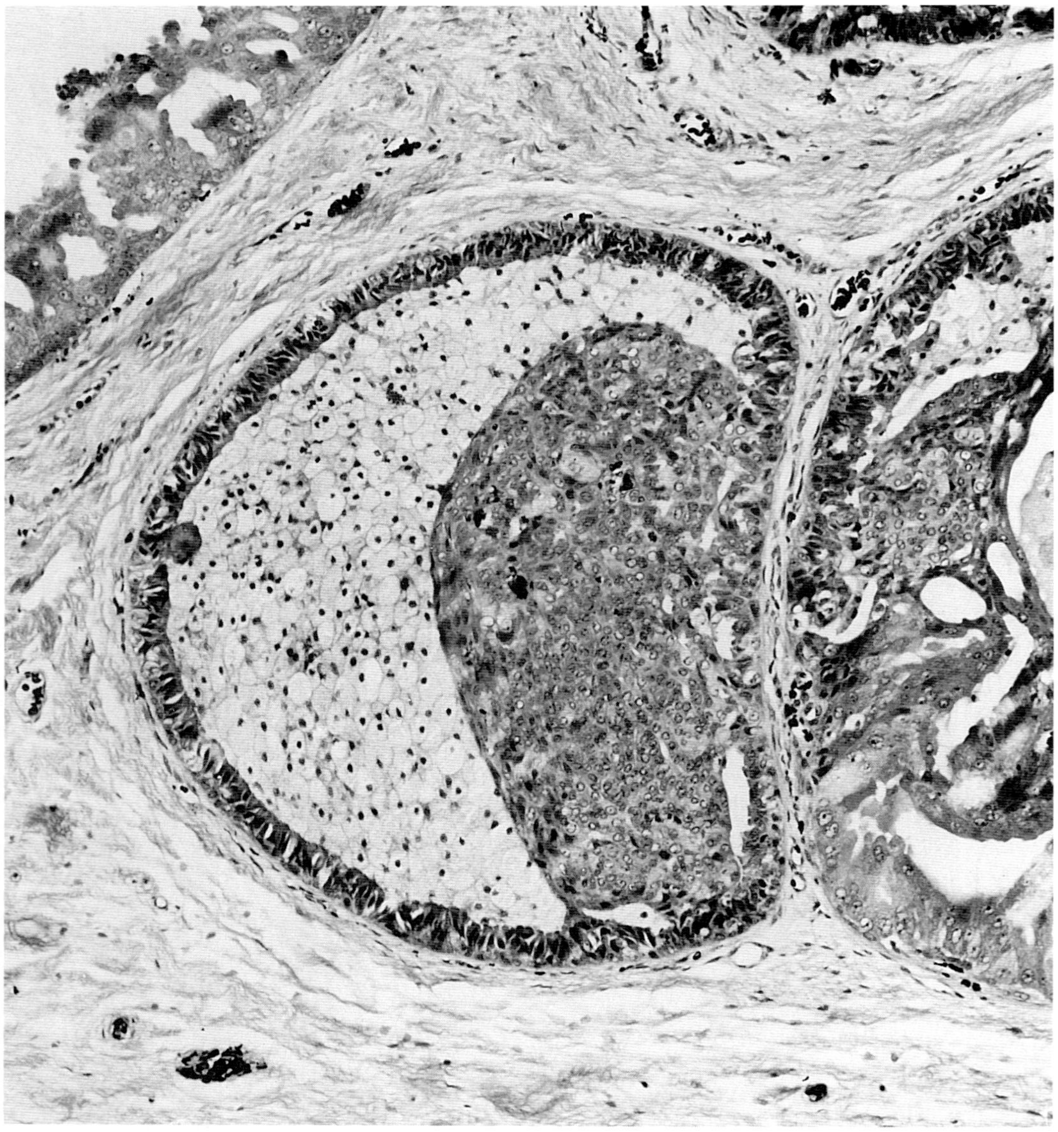

**Figure 5.15(b)** Juvenile papillomatosis. The areas of IDH, though florid, lacked atypia (H&E, X240)

paternal or maternal aunts. Fourteen of the 117 women with IDH in Tavassoli and Norris's study (29) were 30 years of age or younger. Morphologically, the findings in these 14 women with IDH and fibrocystic changes were identical to JP. None of these women developed a subsequent invasive carcinoma with follow-up ranging from 7 to 18.5 years; only two patients had less than ten years of follow-up. Considering the young age of these women, however, much longer follow-up would be necessary to accurately assess the course of the lesion.

### *Management of Patients with JP*

Excisional biopsy is adequate treatment. The patient should learn breast self-examination. Regular follow-up examinations should be scheduled annually. Those patients with bilateral, recurrent, or multifocal disease require closer follow-up, particularly if they also have a positive family history of breast carcinoma. Annual mammography is not routinely indicated for patients less than 40 years of age.

A

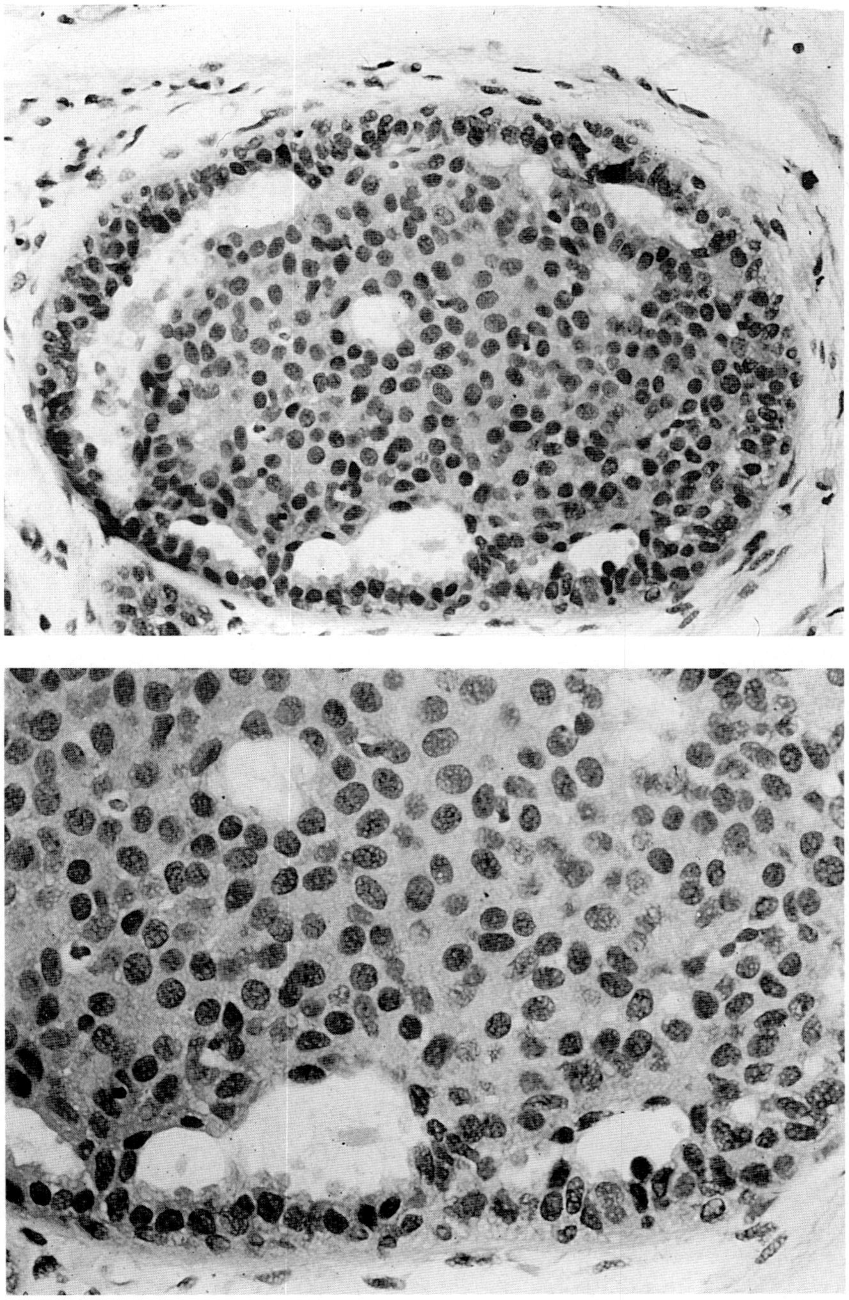

**Figure 5.16** Atypical intraductal hyperplasia. The architecture with the peripheral fenestrations is that of IDH (a), but the cells display a tendency toward nuclear rounding and uniformity (b). (H&E, (a) X160; (b) X250)

## ATYPICAL INTRADUCTAL HYPERPLASIA

### Definition of Atypical Intraductal Hyperplasia

Until recently, atypical intraductal hyperplasia (AIDH) was defined as a lesion that has some but not all features of an intraductal carcinoma. There was no attempt to specify the criteria that would separate atypical hyperplasia from intraductal carcinoma. What has been ignored in such definitions is that one of the major reasons an AIDH does not qualify as an IDCA is that AIDH has retained some of the features of an ordinary hyperplasia. In other words, certain features commonly associated with ordinary hyperplasia (IDH) have persisted in AIDH. In order to recognize AIDH, one should be thoroughly familiar not only with the many varieties, as well as the

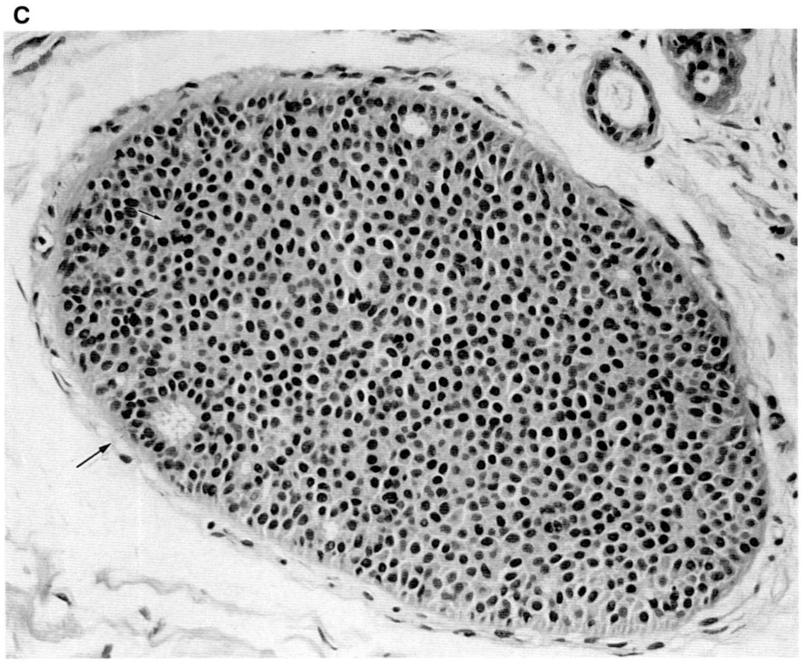

Figure 5.16(c) Atypical intraductal hyperplasia. A relatively solid proliferation with focal rosette-like arrangements of nuclei (arrows), and a trend toward uniformity in a duct less than 2 mm. (H&E, X250)

minimal requirement for a diagnosis of intraductal carcinoma, but also with the highly heterogeneous group of IDH. To define what is atypical, and to distinguish atypical intraductal hyperplasia from intraductal carcinoma, a precise definition of the minimal requirements for a diagnosis of intraductal carcinoma is needed. At the same time, to separate atypical intraductal hyperplasia from the ordinary intraductal hyperplasia, it is necessary to be familiar with the features of ordinary intraductal hyperplasia.

In 1990, Tavassoli and Norris (29) emphasized the cytologic appearance as the most important feature in separating atypical hyperplasias (AIDH) from the ordinary hyperplasias (IDH); it is the cytologic aspect of atypical hyperplasia that simulates intraductal carcinoma even when the architecture is clearly not that of any of the recognized variants of intraductal carcinoma. Their criteria (Table 5.2) specifically excluded apocrine proliferations. An atypical intraductal hyperplasia generally displays a cytologic monotony and uniformity that is characteristic of the

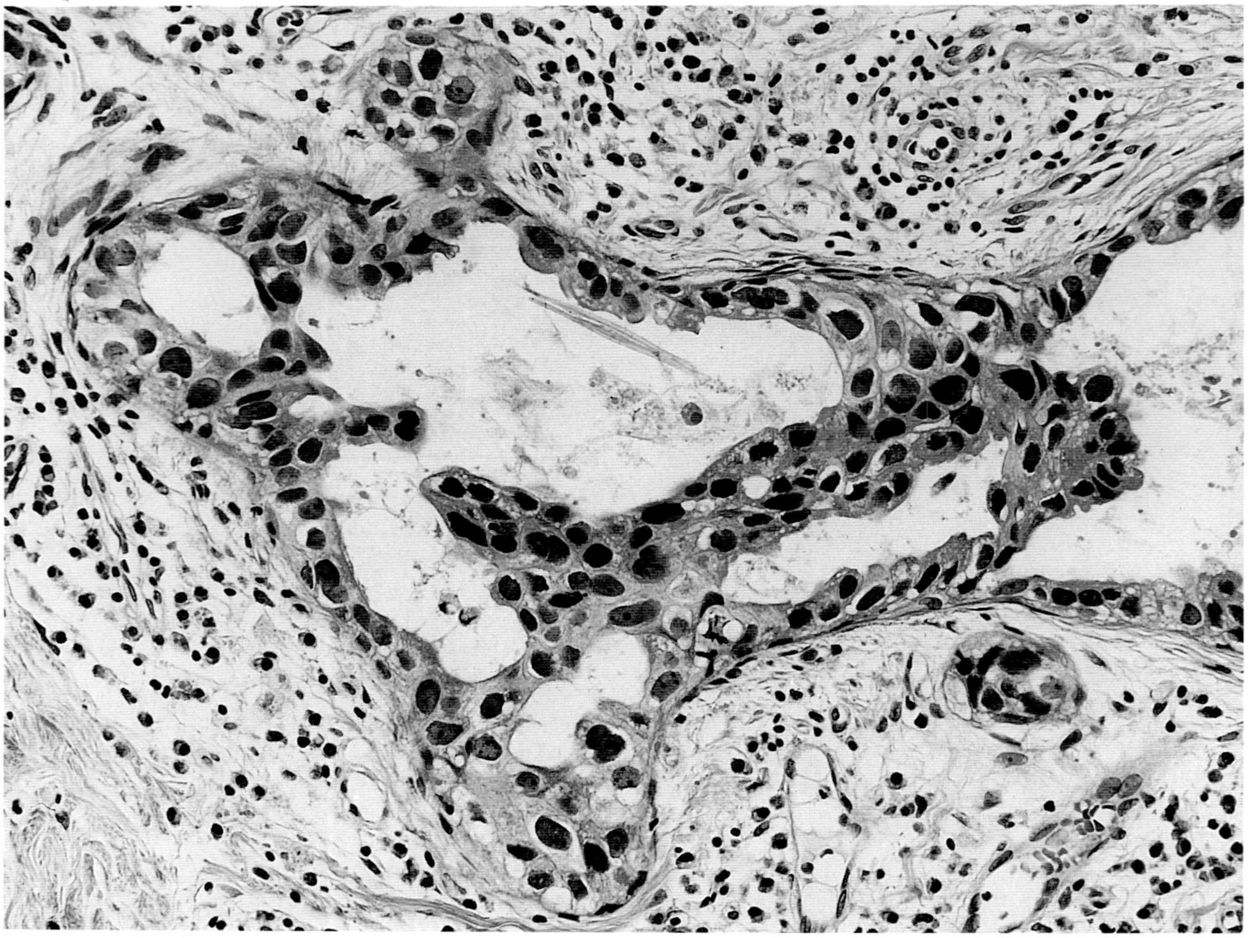

Figure 5.17 Atypical intraductal hyperplasia. The fenestrations or secondary lumens vary in size and shape as in IDH, but the cells are clearly atypical partially involving a duct. (H&E, X1,000)

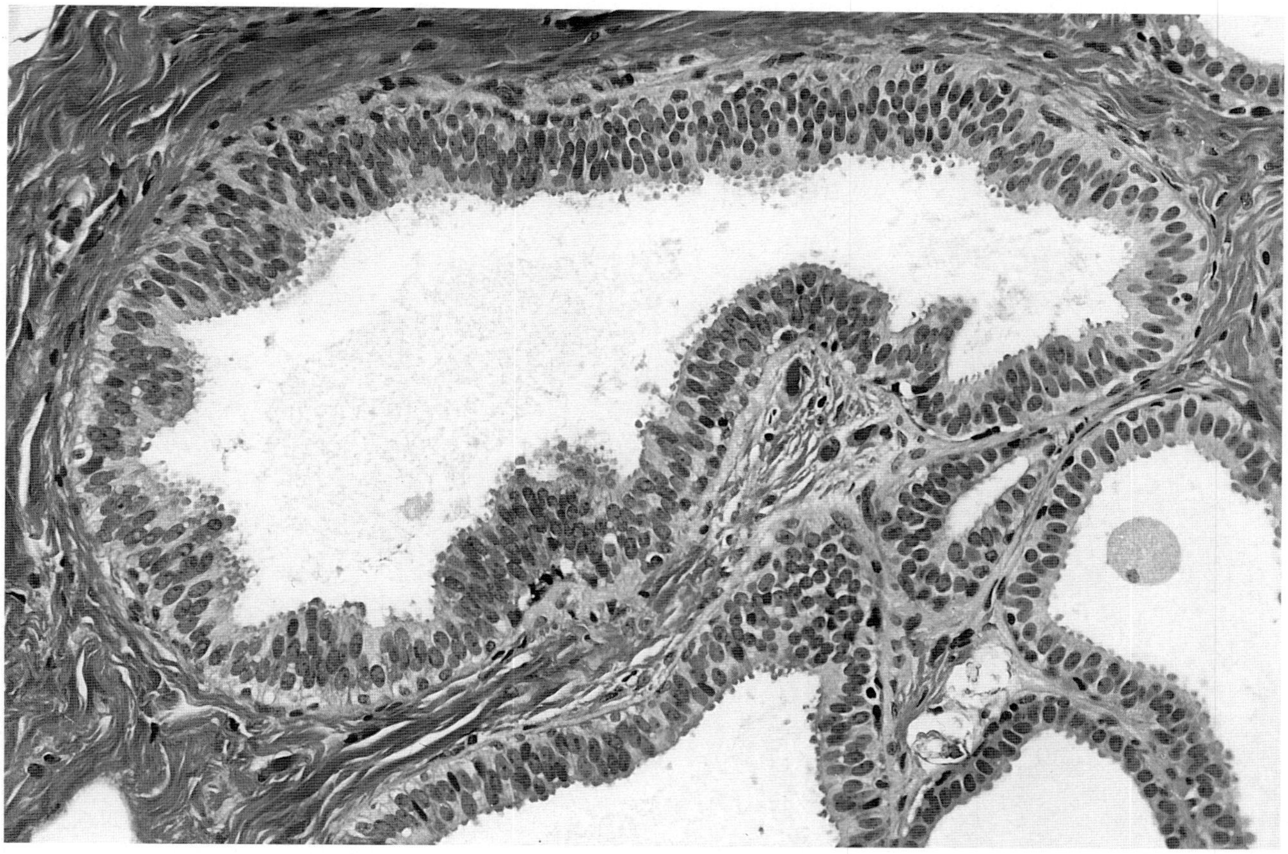

**Figure 5.18** Atypical intraductal hyperplasia. Rarely, distended ducts are lined by a population of uniform ovoid to spindle cells showing a pattern of stratification similar to that typical of the stratified spindle cells variant of intraductal papillary carcinoma. This pattern is often observed in association with intraductal carcinomas. (H&E, X400)

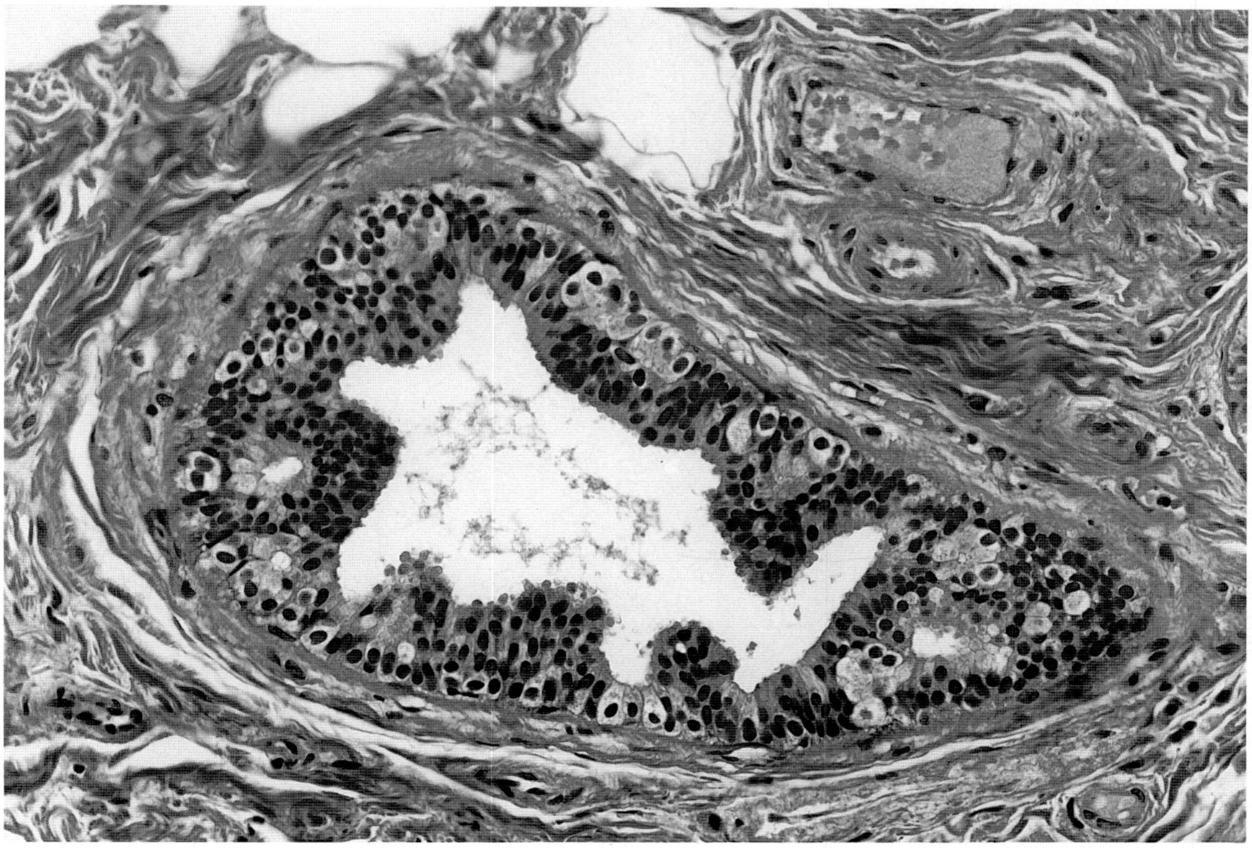

**Figure 5.19** Atypical intraductal hyperplasia displaying tufts and epithelial arches formed by two atypical cell types. (H&E, X400)

A

B

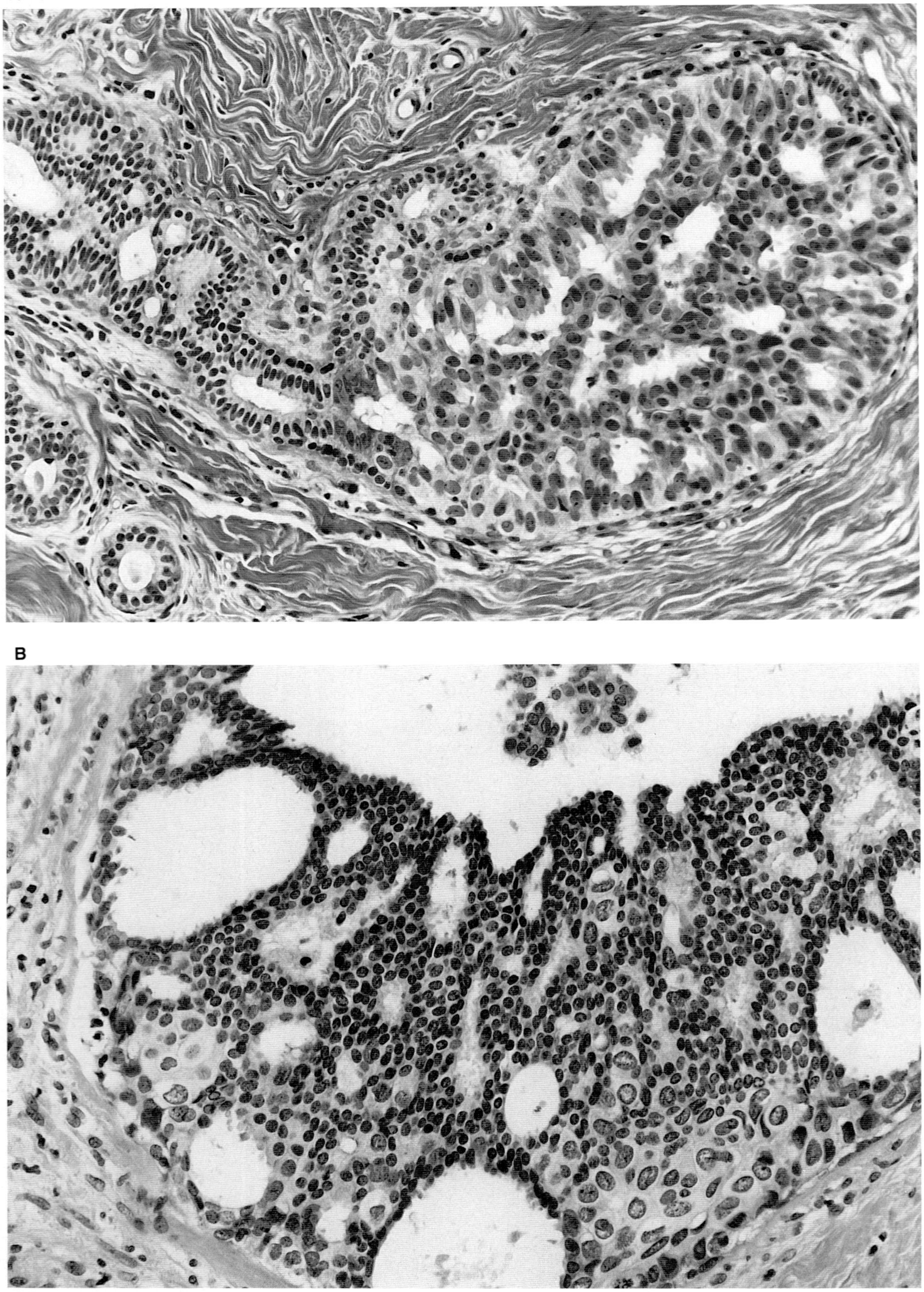

**Figure 5.20** Atypical intraductal hyperplasia. (a) The proliferation is composed of two cell types. While the small cells are quite uniform and the larger ones also display a tendency toward uniformity, neither one forms a recognizable pattern of intraductal carcinoma. (b) Another case showing proliferation of two cell populations within a single duct. (H&E, (a&b) X480)

A

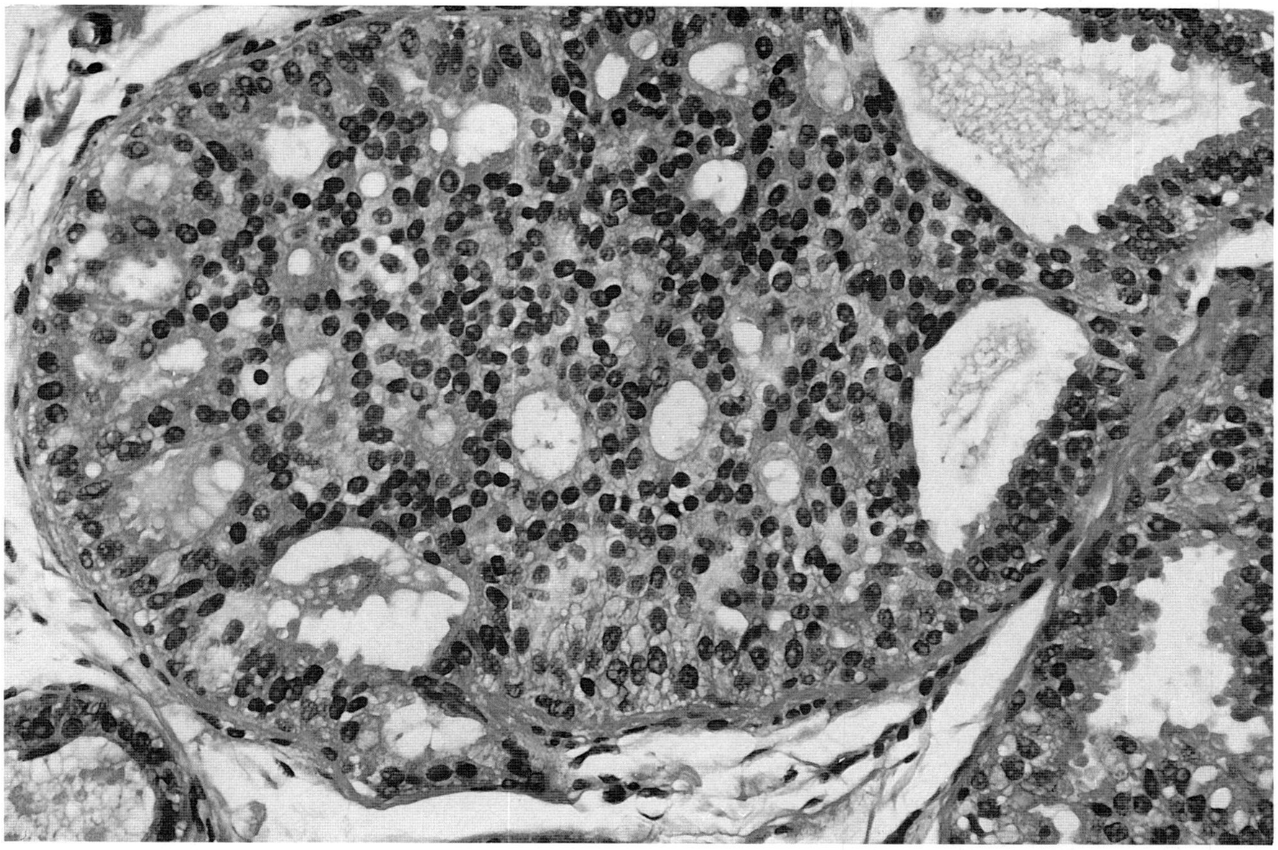

B

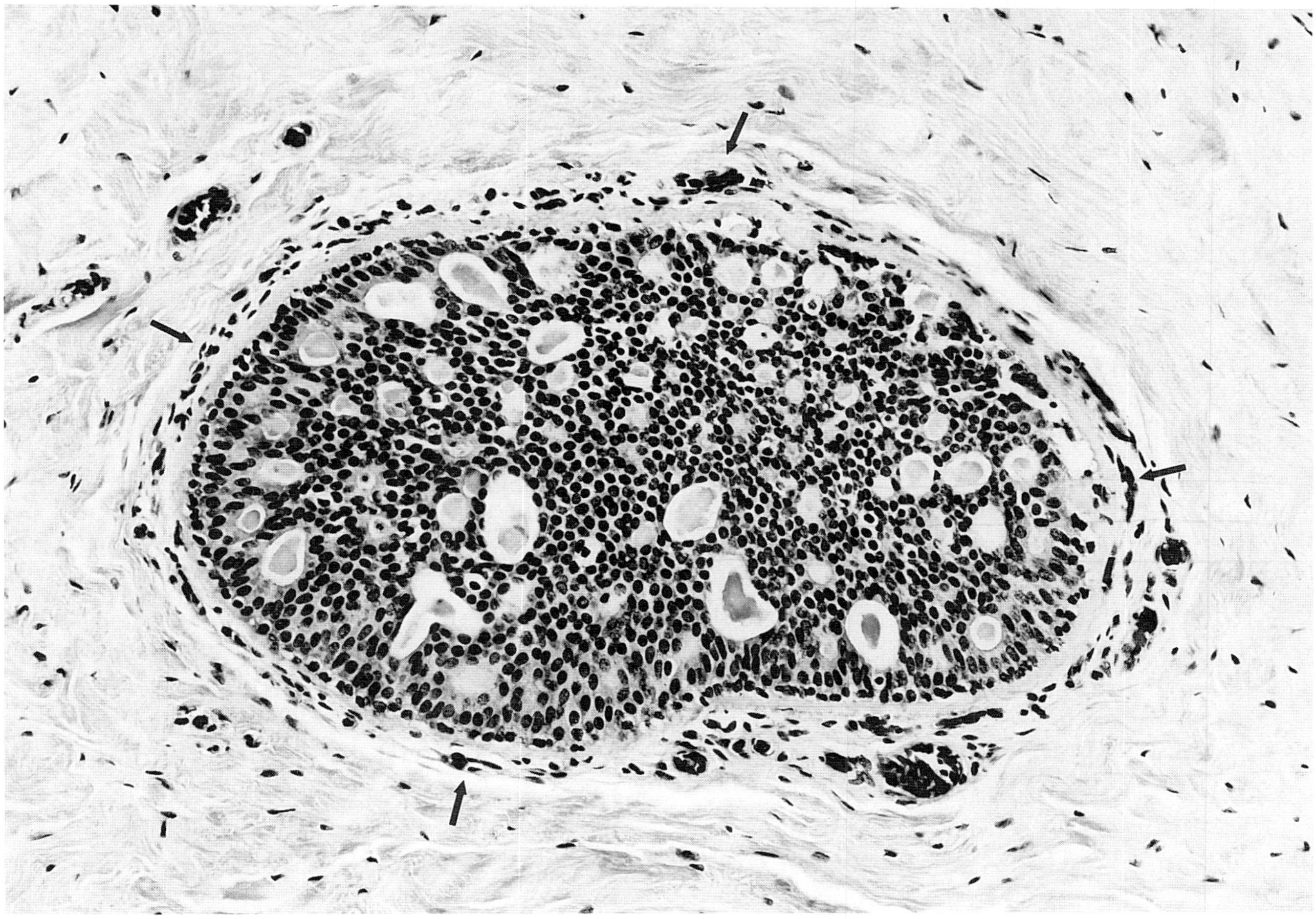

**Figure 5.21** Atypical intraductal hyperplasia. (a) The cell type and architecture of cribriform intraductal carcinoma partially involve a duct that is less than 2 mm in cross-sectional diameter. (b) A monotonous population of round cells with a cribriform pattern involves a duct less than 2 mm in cross-sectional diameter; note the layer of small vascular spaces all around the duct (arrows). (H&E, (a) X800; (b) X700)

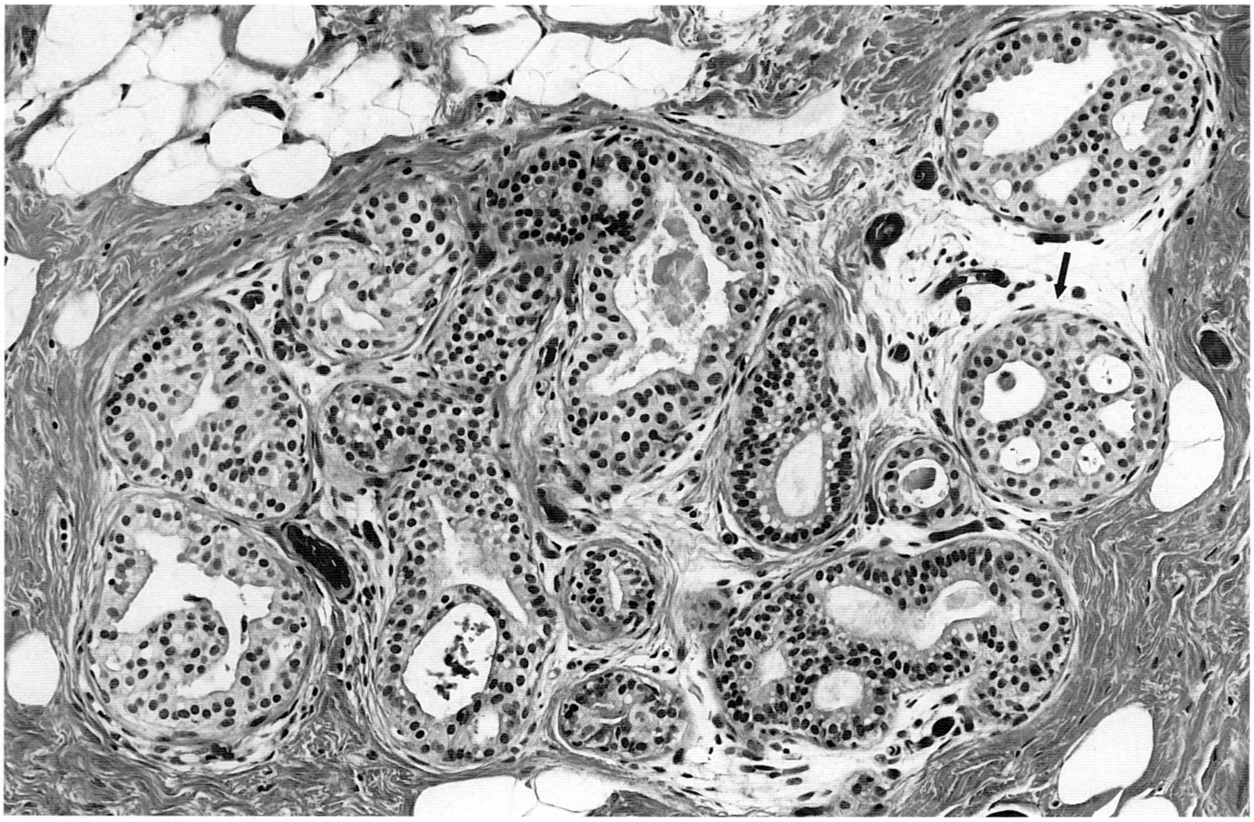

**Figure 5.22** Atypical intraductal hyperplasia in a TDLU. A uniform cell population is proliferating in a majority of the ductules forming epithelial tufts and bridges. Only one of the ductules (arrow) shows a fully-developed cribriform arrangement and it is less than 2 mm in its cross-sectional diameter; this duct is qualitatively identical to the cribriform variant of intraductal carcinoma, but quantitatively insufficient to warrant a diagnosis of IDCA. All other ductules show partial features of the cribriform pattern of IDCA.

non-necrotic variants of intraductal carcinoma. It is the presence of this cell type that distinguishes AIDH from IDH. An ordinary hyperplasia has neither the cytologic, nor the architectural, features of an intraductal carcinoma. The atypical cytology may involve an area of hyperplasia either partially or totally. When the cytologic features of IDCA are present in the hyperplasia, but the architecture is that of a classic IDH, then the lesion is diagnosed as AIDH (Figs. 5.16–5.19). Also, if both the cytologic and architectural features of IDCA are present partially within one or more ducts (Figs. 5.20–5.21), or completely involve one or more ducts that do not exceed 2 mm in aggregate cross-sectional diameter, the lesion qualifies as AIDH (Figs. 5.22–5.25). The latter group is qualitatively identical to an intraductal carcinoma, but quantitatively, it is insufficient to warrant a diagnosis of carcinoma. The 2 mm aggregate diameter was introduced arbitrarily after noting that it was at the level of one or more small ducts or ductules measuring around 2 mm in aggregate cross-sectional diameter that most pathologists felt hesitant in diagnosing a lesion as an intraductal carcinoma. In Tavassoli and Norris's study (29), those patients with the latter type of atypical intraductal hyperplasia were not more prone to developing subsequent invasive carcinomas compared to women whose atypical hyperplasias lacked the architectural features of intraductal carcinoma. The AIDH gradually and eventually unfolds the lobule (Figs. 5.26–5.27), causing a ductal transformation of the involved lobule.

The method of measurement of the ductules is illustrated in Figures 5.28–5.31. On occasions, I have been asked what should be done if we have a longitudinal section of the duct rather than a cross section. It should be kept in mind that these lesions begin in the TDLU where the ductules or acini are more or less spherical in shape. If the proliferative activity distorts the cross section to an ovoid or irregular shape, then the maximum length of the structure is measured. When the IDCA actually involves larger ducts, it is often advanced enough that problems in diagnosis are very limited and there is no need to resort to this quantitative approach.

A

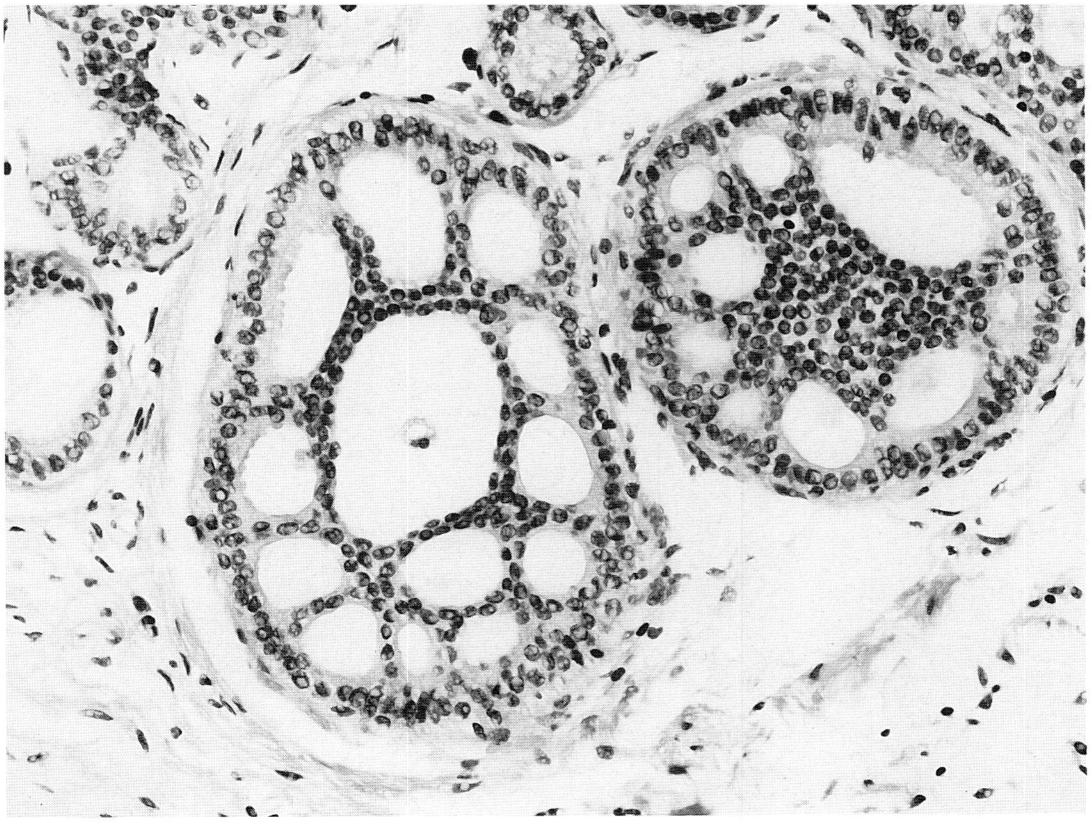

B

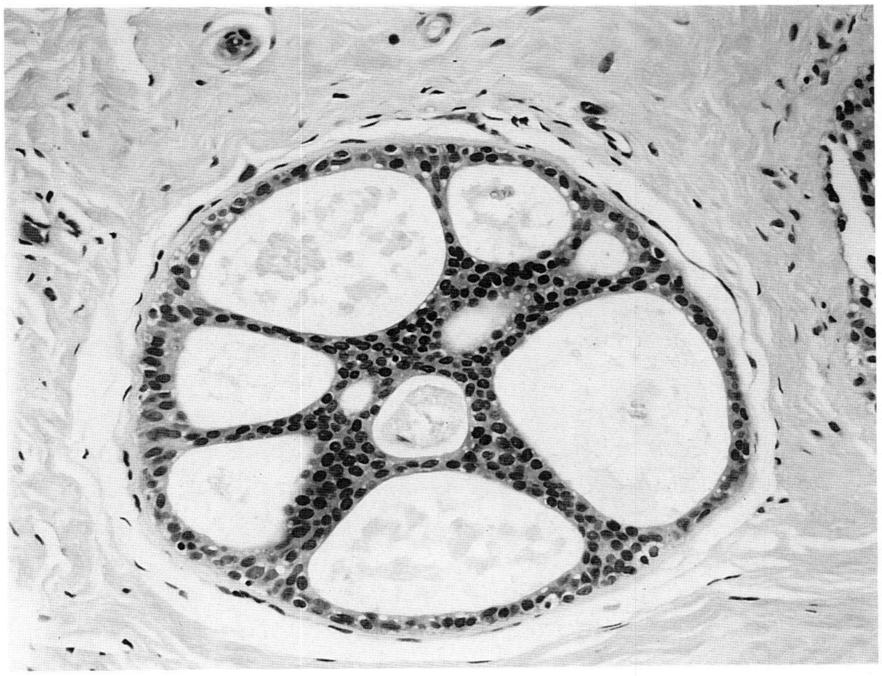

**Figure 5.23** Atypical intraductal hyperplasia. The larger duct in (a) and the one in (b) are qualitatively identical to the cribriform variant of intraductal carcinoma, but quantitatively insufficient to qualify as IDCA because each is smaller than 2 mm in its cross-sectional diameter. (H&E, (a) X250; (b) X250) (Figure 5.23(a) reprinted from Tavassoli FA, Norris HJ: *Cancer* 1990;65:518–529, with permission).

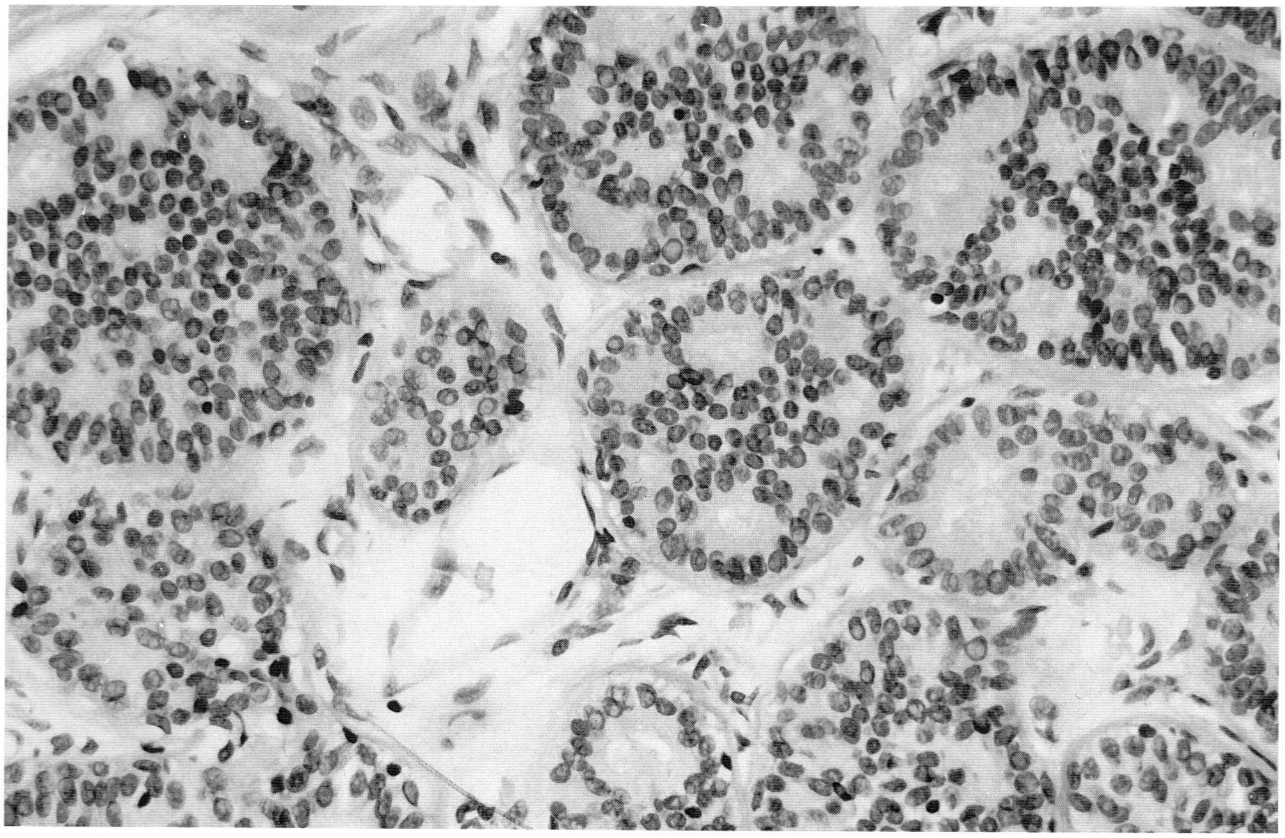

**Figure 5.24** Atypical intraductal hyperplasia. Several ductules in a TDLU show both the architectural and cytologic features of cribriform intraductal carcinoma. While at this high magnification it may hard to appreciate, the aggregate cross-sectional diameter of these ductules is less than 2 mm and the changes do not qualify as IDCA. (H&E, X800)

Also, it is noteworthy that persistence of a myoepithelial cell layer around the duct wall does not influence the diagnosis of the proliferative lesion (IDH, AIDH, or IDCA) within the duct; it is the admixture of cell types within the areas of proliferation that is significant since even comedocarcinomas can have a myoepithelial cell layer around the duct that harbors the carcinoma (Fig. 5.32).

Both IDH and IDCA are frequently rather florid and quite widespread throughout a biopsy. In comparison, AIDH is almost always focal in nature and of limited extent; it is found either in a background of florid IDH, or it is present as an isolated lesion. This finding suggests that whatever induces proliferation of the epithelial cells in the ducts may either induce a malignant or atypical cell population from the onset, or cause a benign cellular proliferation. The continuous proliferative activity and cell division of the benign cells, however, provides additional opportunities for a malignant clone to develop at some point. If such a cell type develops, it can progressively displace or replace the benign cell population. Some of these may proceed to the eventual development of a recognizable carcinoma and invasion, unless the progression is interrupted by a biopsy. I have observed rare cases of extensive (present almost diffusely in every section of 5 to 8 cm biopsies) cribriform intraductal carcinoma—treated by biopsy alone because of patient's refusal to undergo additional surgery—that have recurred after 15 to 17 years in a more limited extent and persisted in an in situ phase. These cases suggest that progression to an invasive carcinoma is by no means inevitable or universal (see also Chapter 7 on IDCA). Apparently, while some cancer cells have or quickly develop the potential to invade, not all cancer cells have this capability, or they attain it over such a long period of time that it may be considered inconsequential for an elderly patient.

## Unusual Atypical Intraductal Hyperplasias

Occasionally, a rather bizarre proliferating cell population is identified which is characterized by enlarged

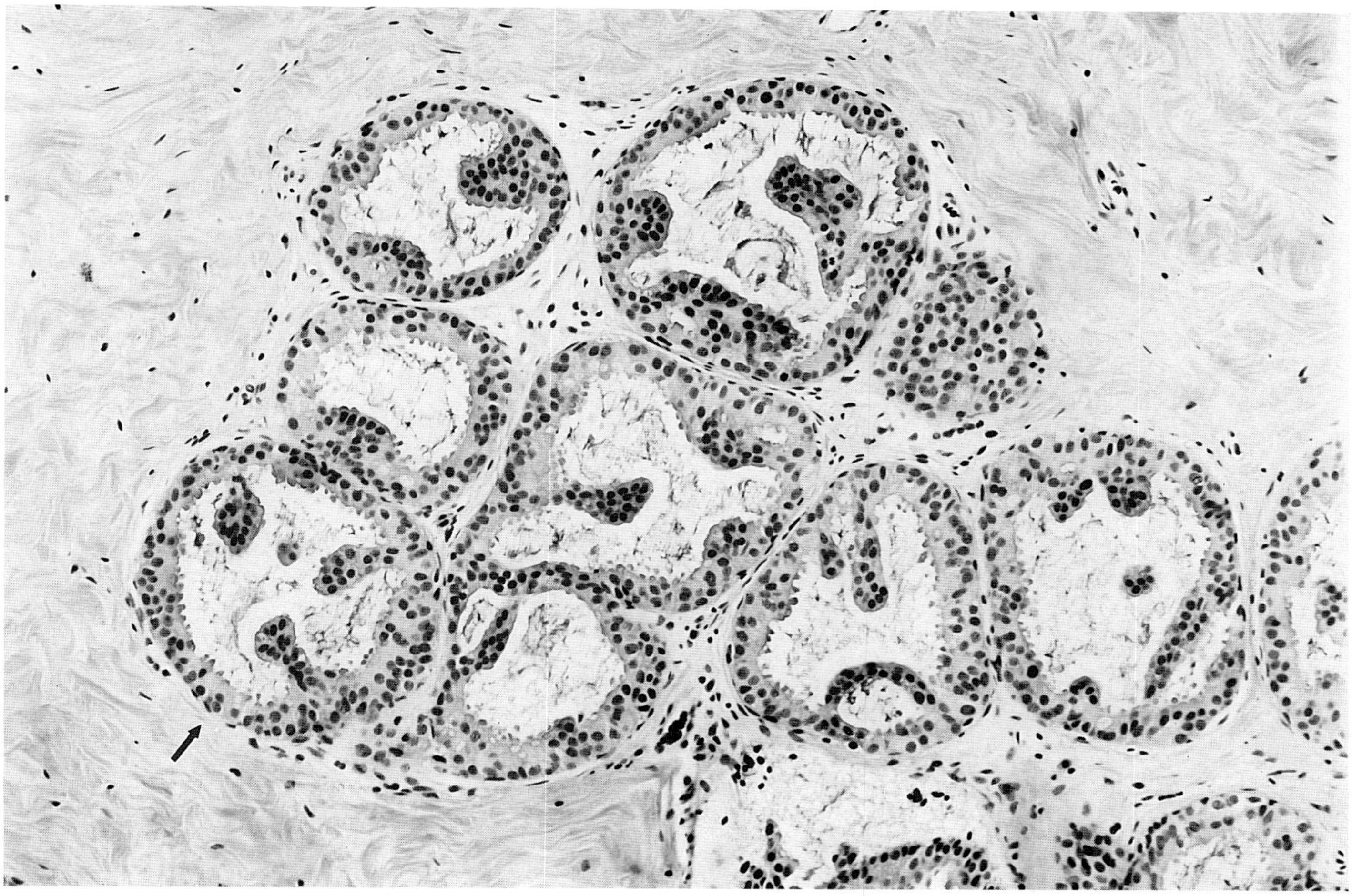

**Figure 5.25** Atypical intraductal hyperplasia. All ductules within this lobule or TDLU show proliferation of a monotonous cell population forming epithelial tufts similar to those of micropapillary intraductal carcinoma. The fully-developed micropapillary pattern is evident in one ductule only (arrow); the cross-sectional diameter of this ductule is less than 2 mm. The remaining ductules show partial formation of the classic pattern. (H&E, X250)

and sometimes multilobulated nuclei. Nucleoli may appear quite prominent. The hyperplastic cells may be rather limited in their distribution, or they may be quite abundant (Fig. 5.33). The cytologic features of the atypical cells are reminiscent of viral alterations, and to a lesser degree simulate radiation-induced atypia.

The three lesions in our files with this morphology were all incidental findings in breast biopsies from women in their twenties with no history of prior radiation therapy. Ultrastructural evaluation of one of these cases showed enlarged cells with abundant fine fibrillar and granular material within the cytoplasm and lobulated nuclei (Fig. 5.34). Viral inclusions were not identified in the sampled specimen. We have designated these changes as atypical hyperplasia as well. While these alterations may reflect early stages in the development of comedocarcinoma, I am not absolutely convinced that they are not an unusual reactive change of a viral type.

## Clinical Significance of AIDH

The clinical presentation of women with AIDH is similar to that of patients with IDH. The median age of these women is 50 years with a range of 15 to 78 years. This median age is five years older than the median for women with IDH. The risk for subsequent development of invasive carcinoma associated with AIDH is four to five times that of the general population (23). Of 82 women with AIDH in our study (29), eight (9.8%) subsequently developed invasive carcinomas within an average of 8.2 years. Six of these carcinomas developed within 6.1 years of the diagnosis of AIDH. Six of the subsequent carcinomas developed within the same breast, four of which were in the same quadrant; five of the carcinomas were invasive ductal, while one was an invasive lobular in type. None of the patients had any evi-

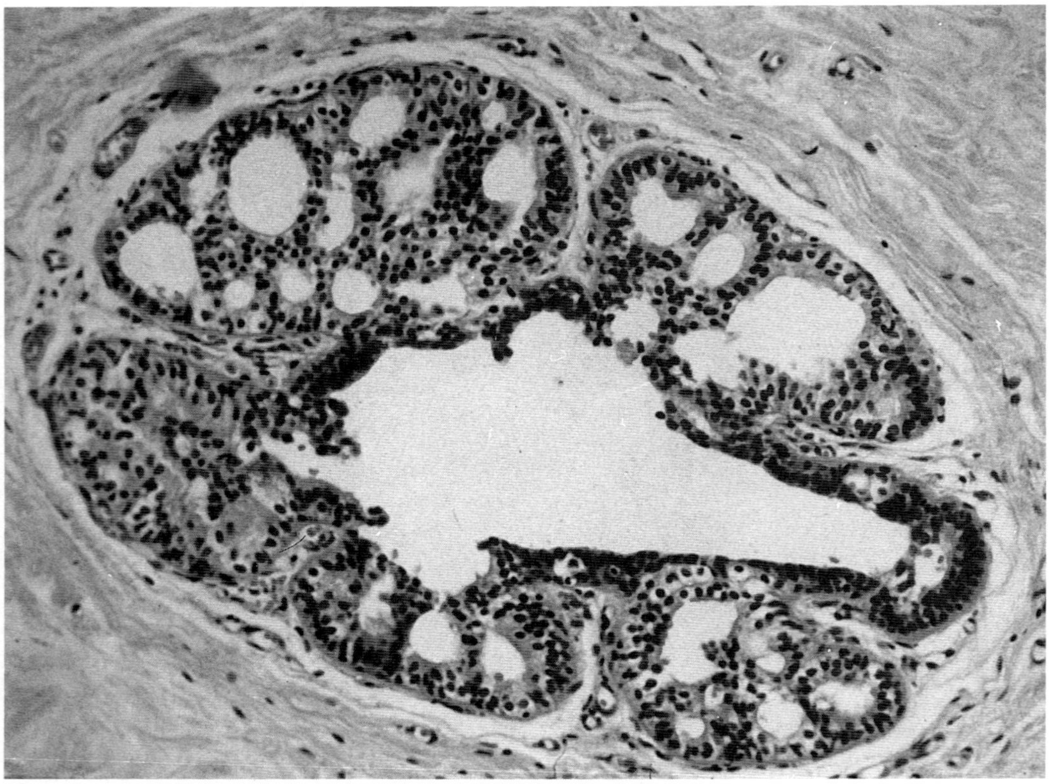

**Figure 5.26** Atypical intraductal hyperplasia unfolding the TDLU. The central dilated area reflects the intralobular segment of the terminal duct leading to the cluster of ductules within the lobule. The ductules are all either partially or totally involved by a proliferation similar to the cribriform pattern of IDCA. The changes are qualitatively similar to IDCA, but are quantitatively insufficient. (H&E, X400)

dence of lobular disease in their previous biopsies, however. The remaining two women developed invasive ductal carcinomas 16.9 and 20 years later in the contralateral breast. In Page et al's series (23) 12% of women with AIDH developed subsequent invasive carcinomas, also within an average of 8.2 years. Of the subsequent carcinomas, 55% were in the ipsilateral breast.

Therefore, patients with AIDH are not only at greater risk for development of invasive carcinoma, but when they do develop subsequent invasive carcinoma, they do so within a shorter period of time (average interval of 8.3 years) compared to patients with IDH (average interval of 14.3 years).

## Influence of Family History of Breast Carcinoma

The presence of a family history of breast carcinoma in a sister, mother, or daughter of a patient with either IDH or AIDH doubles the risk in either group (23). In effect, a woman with AIDH and a family history of breast carcinoma has the same risk as one with intraductal carcinoma.

## Management of Patients with AIDH

In view of the moderately increased risk for development of subsequent carcinoma associated with AIDH, and the shorter interval to the development of subsequent carcinoma compared to IDH (8.2 years versus 14.4 years), women with AIDH require closer follow-up. The follow-up regimen recommended includes three to four examinations of both breasts by a physician each year, along with annual mammograms for those over 40 years of age.

While the presence of multiple risk factors may not be indicative of the invariable development of a subsequent invasive carcinoma, it does contribute to increased patient and physician anxiety regard-

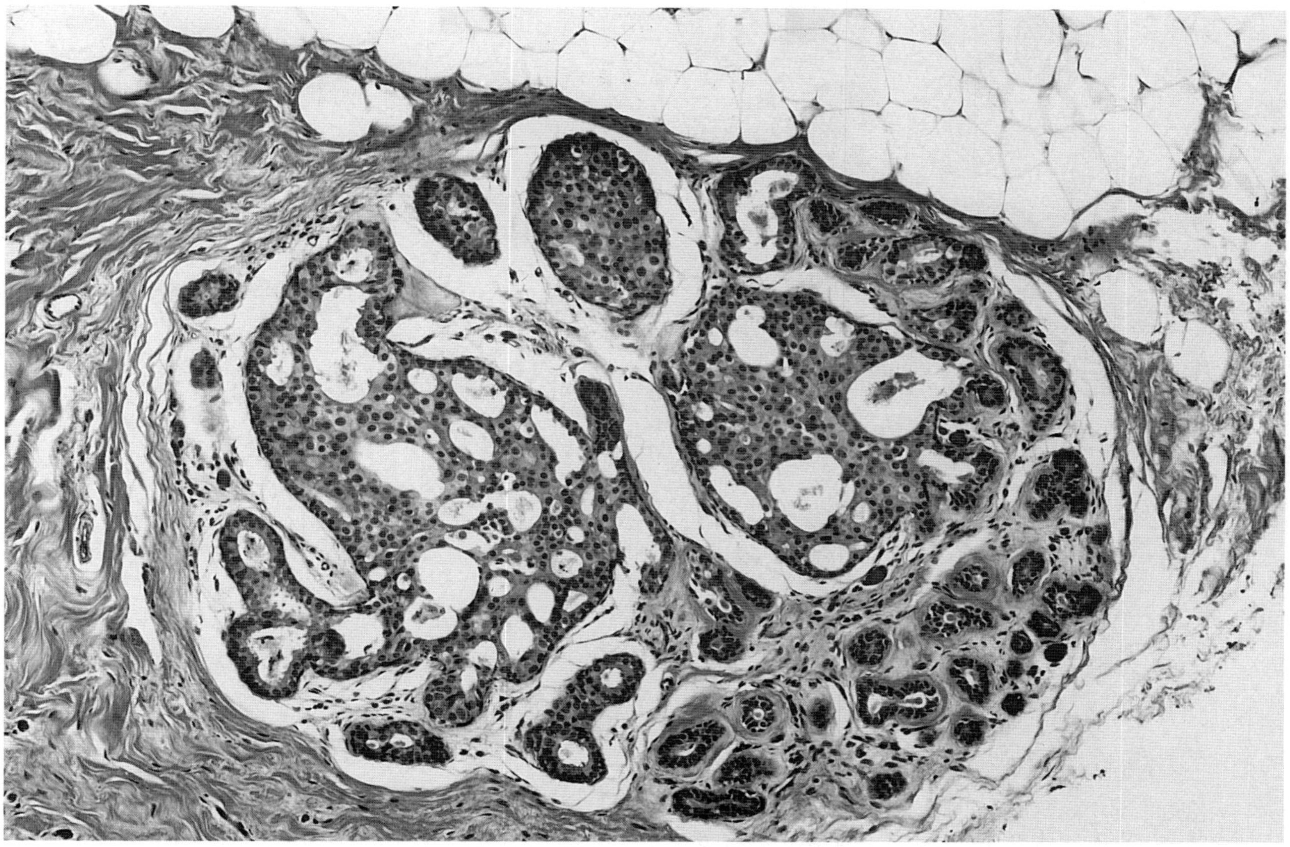

**Figure 5.27** Atypical intraductal hyperplasia unfolding the TDLU. The more peripheral ductules are not yet involved, and the lobular location of the process is readily recognized. (H&E, X400)

ing the course of the disease. This anxiety is heightened when proper mammographic screening or monitoring is hampered by the density of breast tissue. In practice, the final therapeutic decision is often determined not only based on the magnitude of the risk involved, but also by assessing the patient's level of understanding of this risk, her reliability in adhering to the follow-up regimen, and her level of anxiety.

A successful program for management of patients at high risk for the development of invasive breast carcinoma or those with invasive breast carcinoma in a medical center that attends to a large number of patients should include a pathologist(s) with special training in breast pathology and a thorough understanding of the implications of the presence of IDH, AIDH, and IDCA in a breast biopsy. It is only through a team effort that we may some day succeed in controlling or altering the course of the development of breast cancer.

## Special Studies

At present, there are no special studies or antibodies that could help distinguish AIDH from either IDH or IDCA, though some cases of AIDH may express certain tumor-associated antigens such as DF3 (18).

## Differential Diagnosis

As mentioned earlier AIDH should be distinguished from IDH and IDCA. Occasionally, a relatively solid pattern of AIDH may be confused with lobular neoplasia since both originate in the TDLU, and both may be composed of a small uniform cell population. The morphologic features of IDH and features that help distinguish IDH from AIDH have been dis-

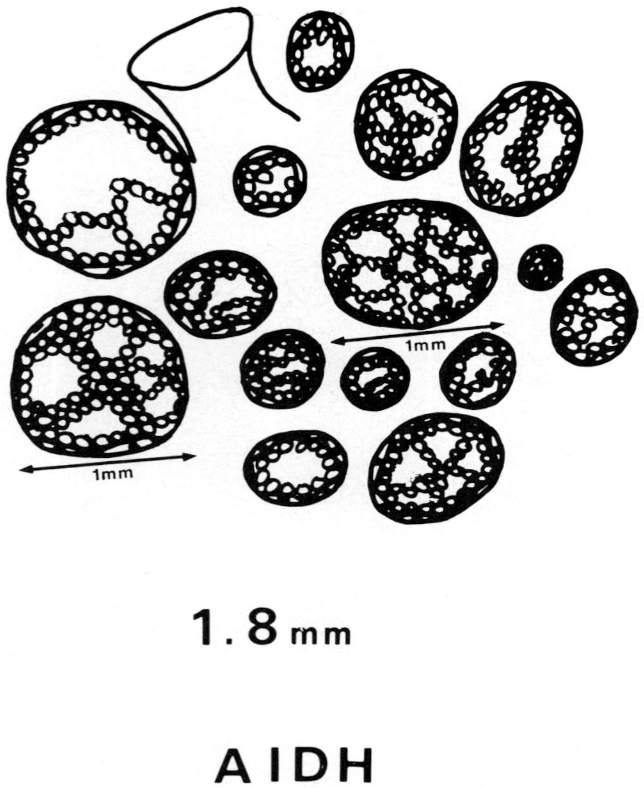


Figure 5.28 Two ductules in this TDLU show a complete cribriform arrangement. Together, they measure 1.8 mm; this is less than the required 2 mm aggregate diameter for a diagnosis of IDCA. Therefore, the proliferation qualifies as AIDH.

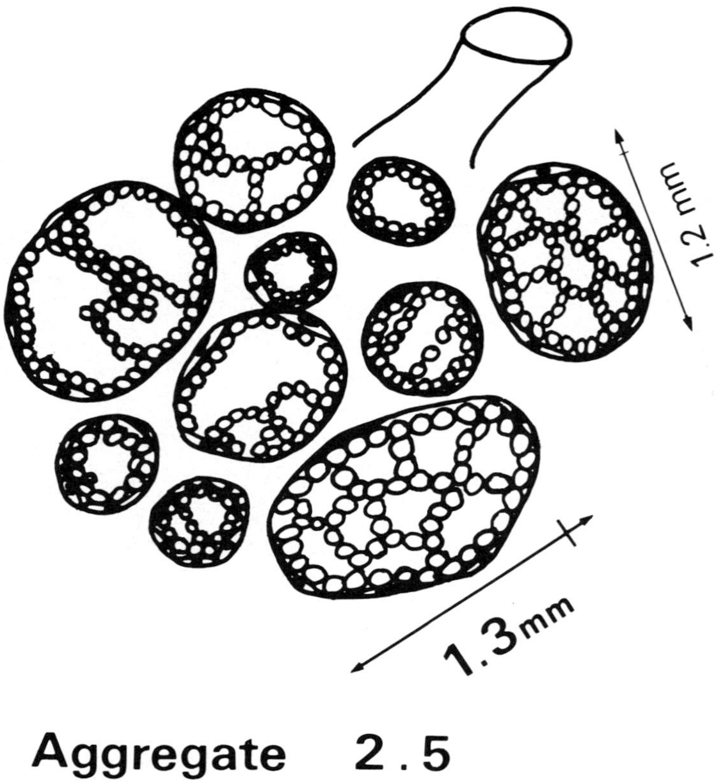


Figure 5.29 The two involved ductules here exceed 2 mm in aggregate measurement. Therefore, the changes qualify as IDCA.

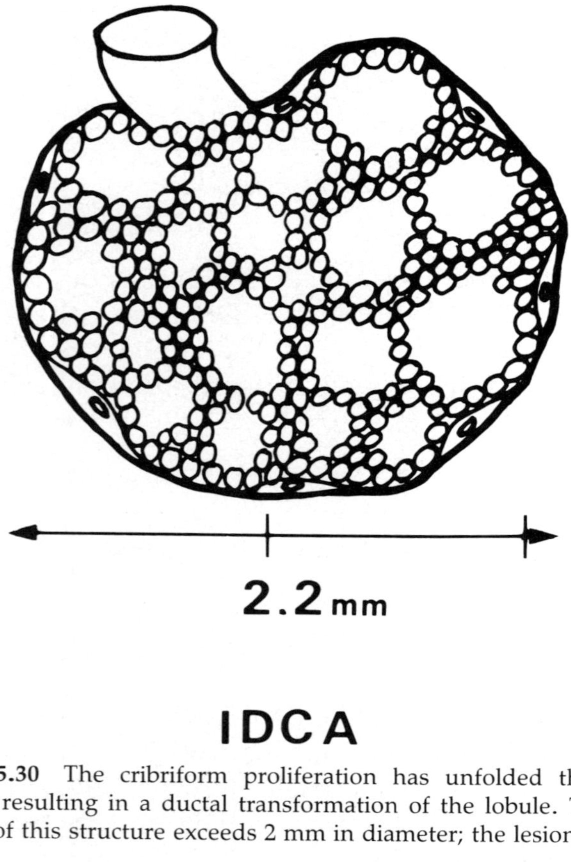


Figure 5.30 The cribriform proliferation has unfolded the TDLU (lobule) resulting in a ductal transformation of the lobule. The cross section of this structure exceeds 2 mm in diameter; the lesion qualifies as IDCA.

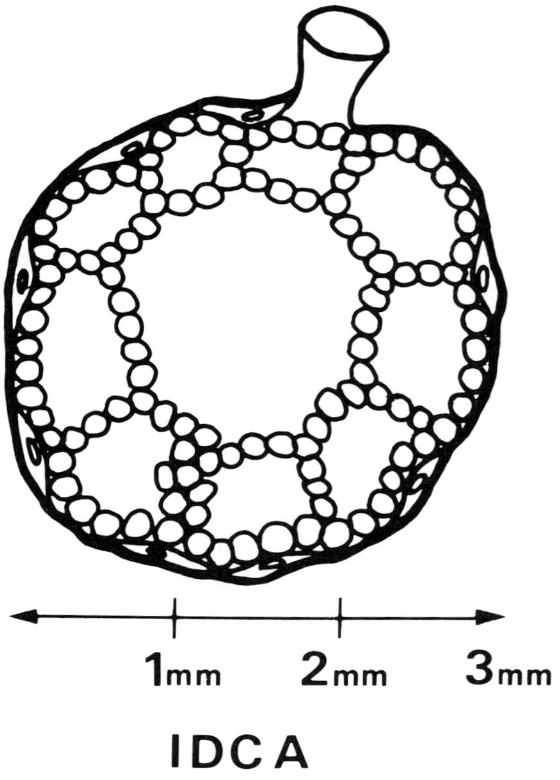


Figure 5.31 Another TDLU unfolded by the proliferation of a uniform population of cells forming epithelial bridges. The cross-sectional diameter of this structure is over 2 mm and the lesion qualifies as IDCA.

cussed earlier. To differentiate AIDH from IDCA, it is important to be familiar with the many varieties of IDCA as well as the minimal requirements for a diagnosis of IDCA.

## Morphologic Criteria for Diagnosis of Intraductal Carcinoma

There are several varieties of intraductal carcinoma. The most readily recognizable one is comedocarcinoma which is characterized by the proliferation of an atypical, sometimes anaplastic, cell population in a relatively solid manner with persistence of a central lumen which contains necrotic debris. This type of IDCA and other variants with central necrosis are not a problem in the differential diagnosis of AIDH. It is the non-necrotic variant, characterized by the proliferation of a uniform cell population, with either a micropapillary or cribriform pattern, that is a source of diagnostic problems.

What is the minimal requirement for a diagnosis of intraductal carcinoma of the cribriform or micropapillary types? Page et al (23) defined intraductal carcinoma as an intraductal proliferation of evenly-spaced, round, cuboidal, or polygonal cells with monotonous, hyperchromatic, round or oval nuclei forming regular and smooth, round spaces, rigid, geometric configuration and bridges lacking attenuation, or micropapillae with narrow bases and no swirls or streaming. They demanded that all features of intraductal carcinoma be uniformly present throughout two separate spaces before IDCA is diagnosed. They did not specify what they meant by two spaces, however. Neither did they provide criteria for separating AIDH from IDH. Anything less than the definition of IDCA qualified as atypical intraductal hyperplasia if some features of carcinoma in situ were present.

A shortcoming of this definition is the vagueness of the two-space requirement. Afterall, most pathologists would not hesitate to call a lesion an intraductal carcinoma if a single 2 cm or 1 cm duct is completely involved by the cribriform growth pattern of IDCA. Even in subsequent elaboration of the criteria (20), there is no mention of what is meant by two spaces, or how large a space they are referring to. Furthermore, identification of nuclear hyperchromasia is very much influenced by the technical aspects of tissue preparation; pyknotic and compressed nuclei may be confused with hyperchromasia. Elston (6) deleted this feature from the criteria for grading infiltrating duct carcinoma; it should be deleted from the criteria for intraductal carcinoma as well for the same reasons.

In order to further refine the available criteria and elaborate on the features that help distinguish regular intraductal hyperplasia (IDH) from AIDH, and AIDH from IDCA, Tavassoli and Norris (29) introduced a new set of criteria incorporating cytologic, architectural, and precise quantitative features. Proliferations composed purely of metaplastic apocrine cells were excluded from the study. These criteria are listed in Tables 5.1 and 5.2.

## Distinction from Lobular Neoplasia

Some ductal proliferations are also composed of a uniform, small cell population similar to those of lobular neoplasia, while some lobular neoplasias show a cell population larger than those of the typical lesion. Since both lobular and ductal lesions originate in the TDLU, occasionally, the early, solid phase of proliferation of the ductal process may be confused with lobular neoplasia. A distinction can be made only when the more advanced areas of the proliferation within the same TDLU show recognizable ductal patterns, such as a rosette-like arrangement of the nuclei or formation of multiple secondary lumens (Fig. 5.35 a–c). With one exception, the cell type is not as helpful because of the variety of accepted cell populations for both ductal and lobular lesions. The presence of intracytoplasmic lumens within the proliferating cells would favor a lobular type of proliferation.

Lobular neoplasia may also present primarily within the ducts (22). In this setting distinctions from atypical ductal hyperplasia is facilitated by the distinctive nature of the lobular neoplasia cells and their pagetoid growth pattern within the involved ducts.

In our consultation practice at AFIP, ductal hyperplasias and lobular neoplasia coexist in around 10% of the biopsies. The cells forming the two patterns may be identical in appearance, or they may differ morphologically.

A

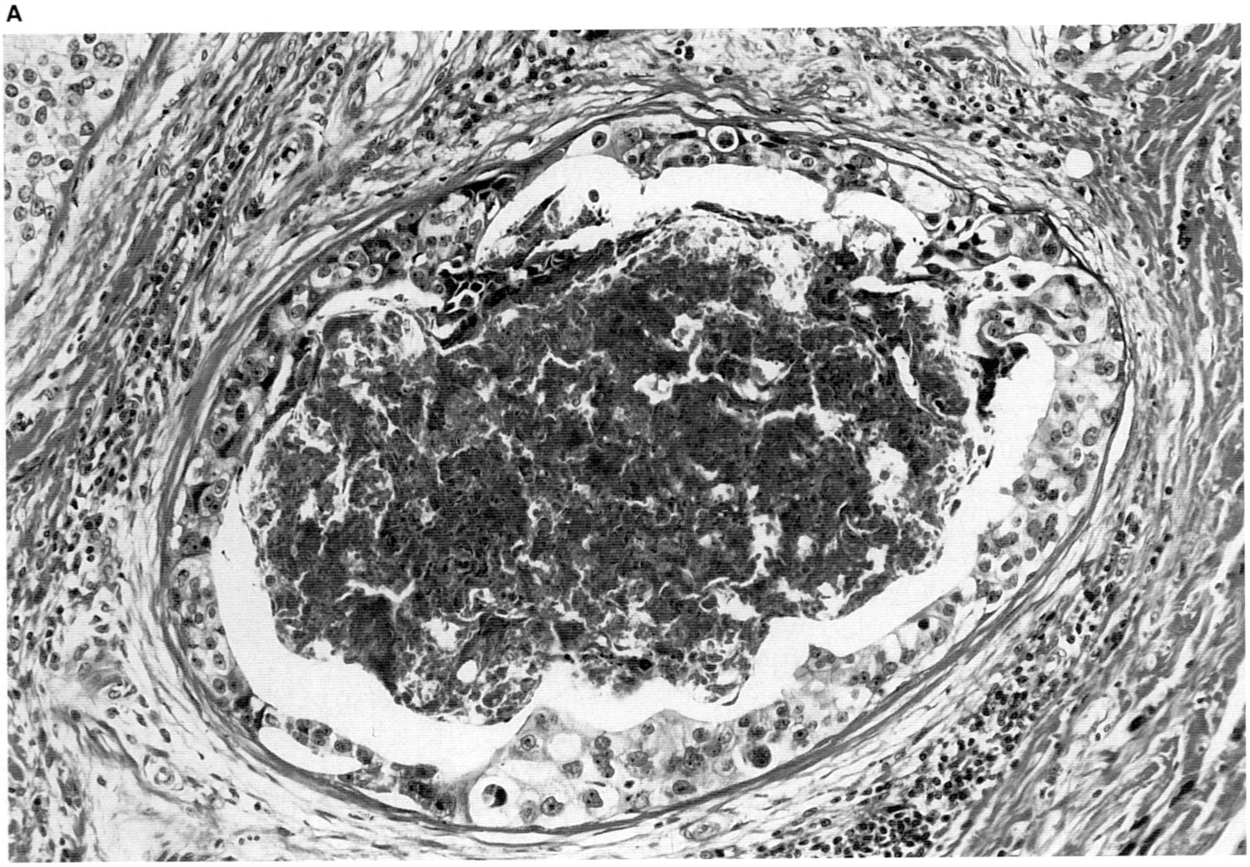

B

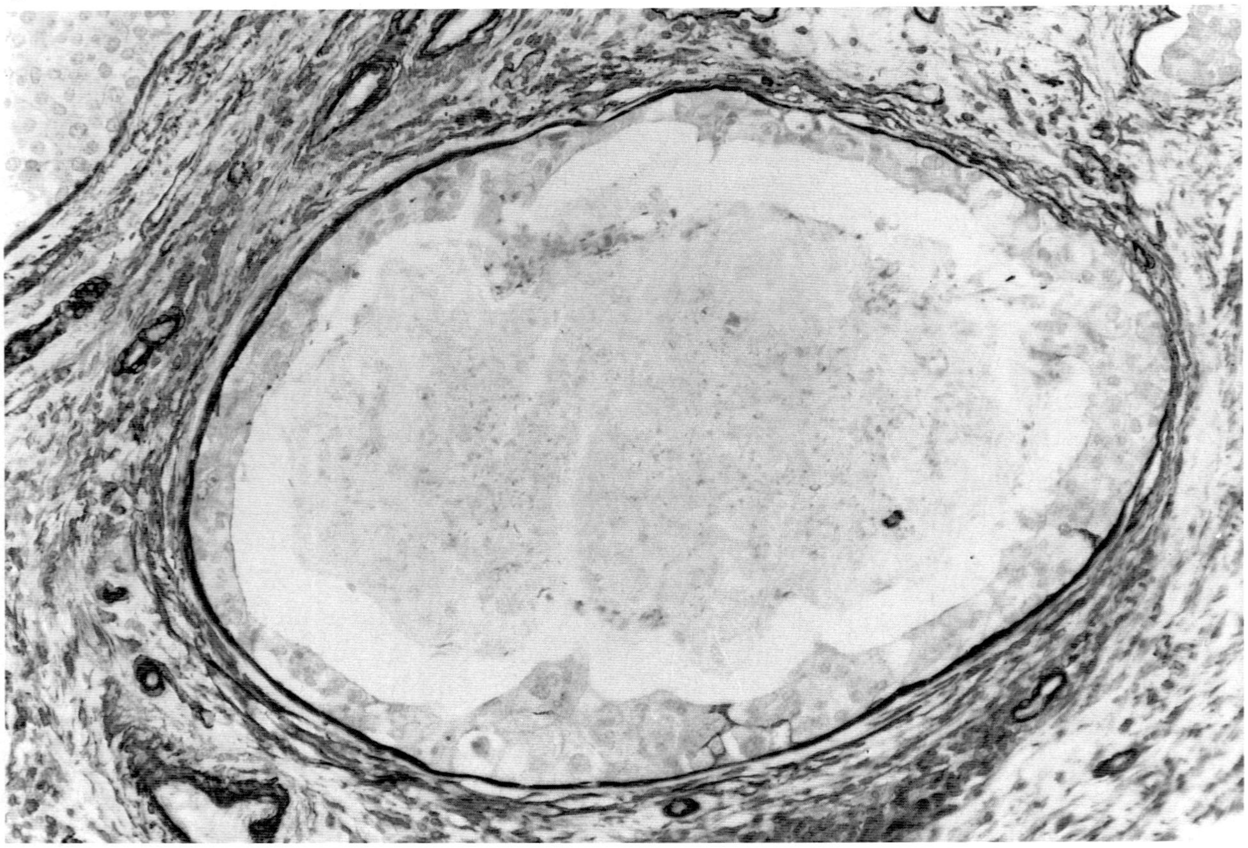

**Figure 5.32** Intraductal carcinoma with central necrosis (a), showing persistence of myoepithelial cell layer confirmed by immunostain for actin (b). (H&E, (a) X75; Immunostain for actin, (b) X150)

A

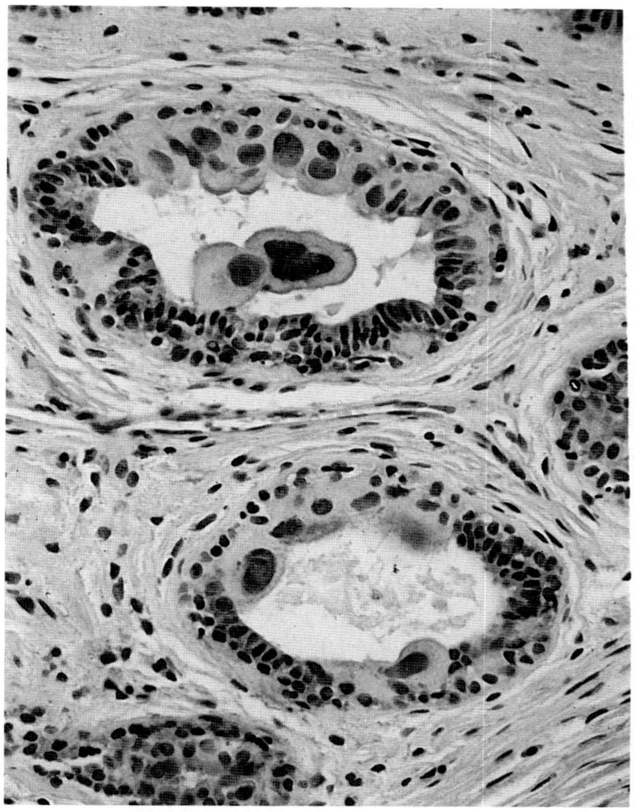

**Figure 5.33** Unusual atypical intraductal hyperplasia showing large cells with lobulated nuclei partially replacing the normal duct epithelium (a), and with prominent intranuclear inclusion (arrow) (b). (H&E, (a) X160; (b) X240)

B

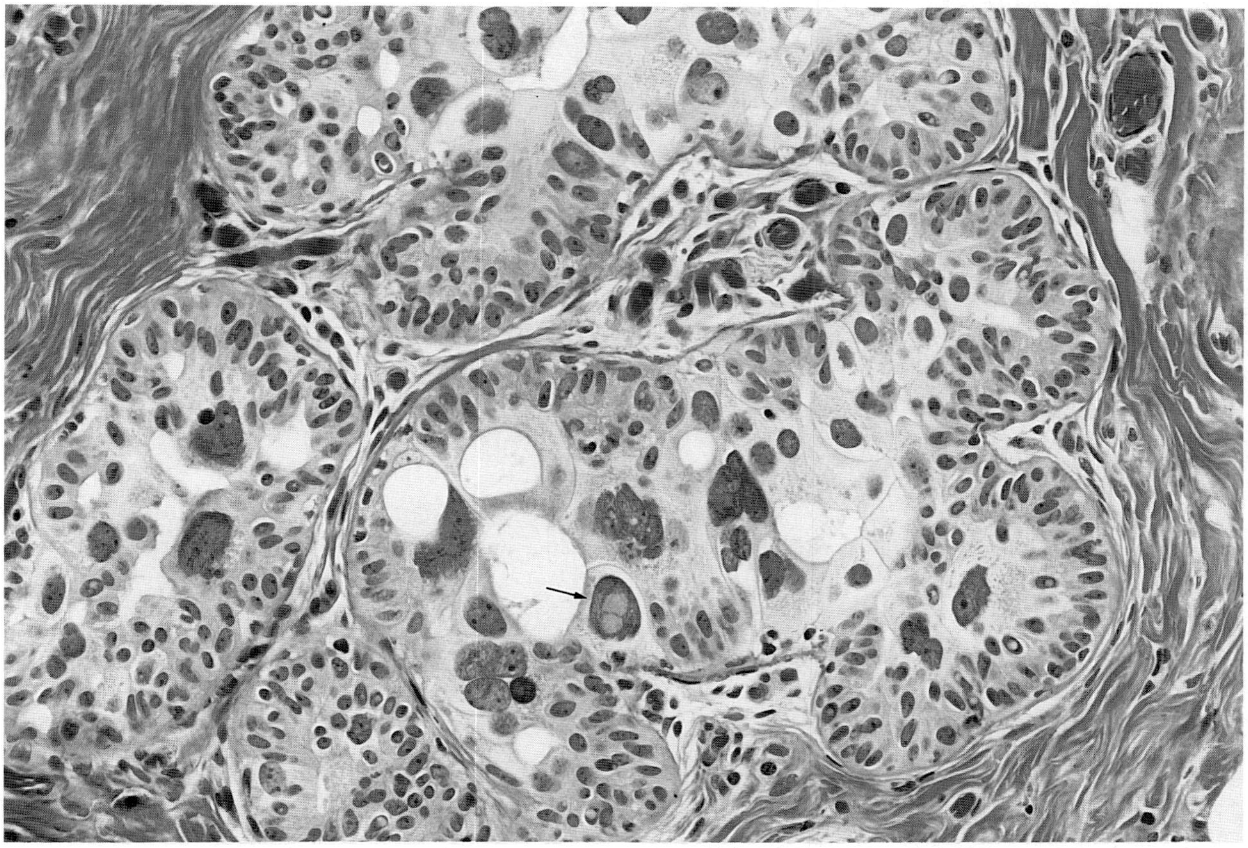

A

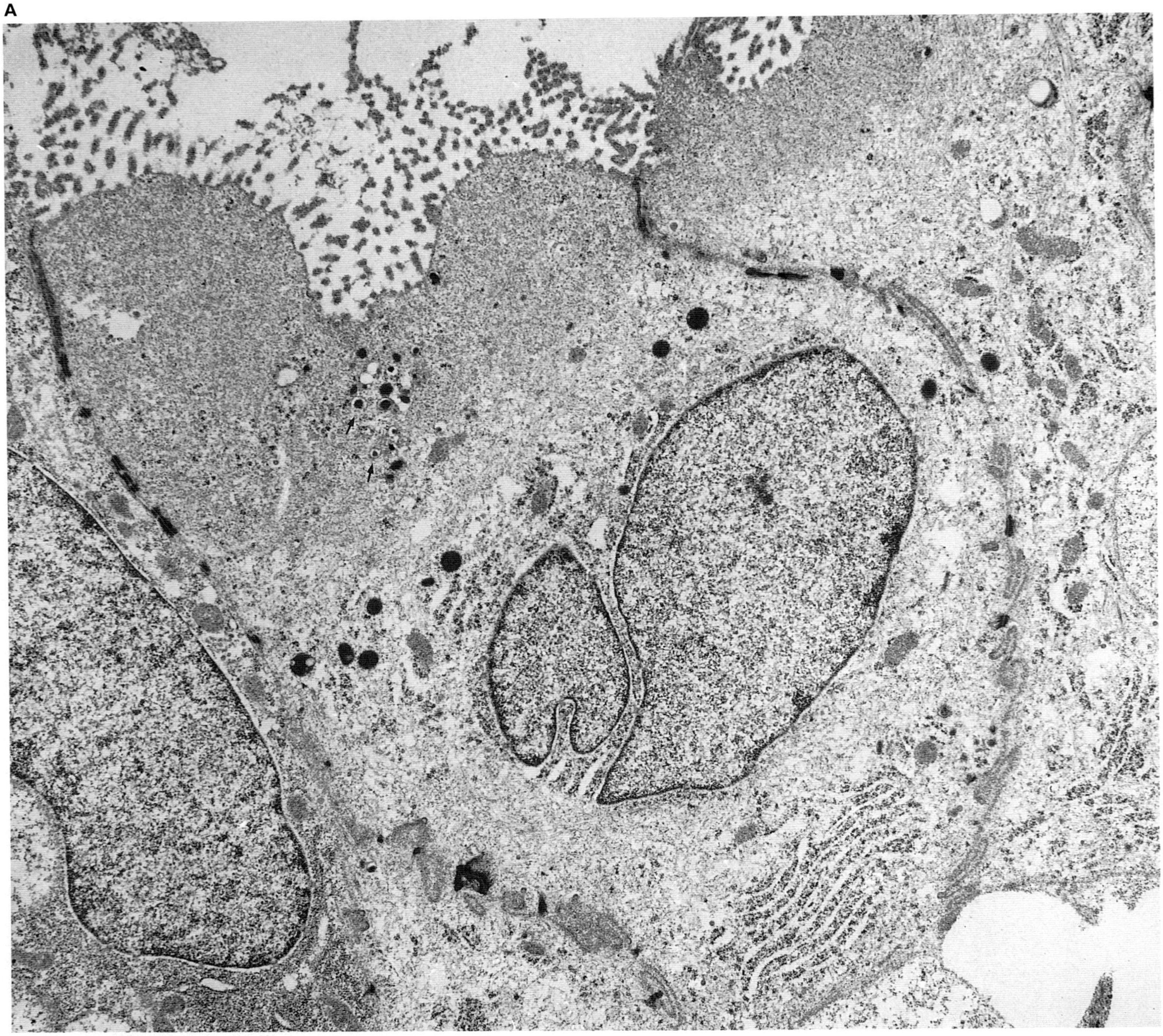

**Figure 5.34(a)** At the ultrastructural level, the atypical cells illustrated in Figure 5.32 stand out as conspicuously large with abundant cytoplasm containing granular to fine fibrillar material as well as clusters of small membrane bound dense bodies (arrows). (Uranyl acetate-lead citrate, X5,700)

## INTRODUCTION OF NEW TERMINOLOGY

The issue of using the term ductal mammary intraepithelial neoplasia (DMIN) for "borderline" ductal lesions of the breast has been raised in a recent report (27). Although I prefer to use the term lobular neoplasia rather than dividing the spectrum into atypical hyperplasia and lobular carcinoma in situ, application of this concept to ductal proliferations is more difficult. One important reason is that the variety of ductal proliferations are not part of a morphologic spectrum, even though the ascending magnitude of the risk associated with IDH, AIDH, and IDCA may suggest otherwise. Notably, ordinary hyperplasia is

B

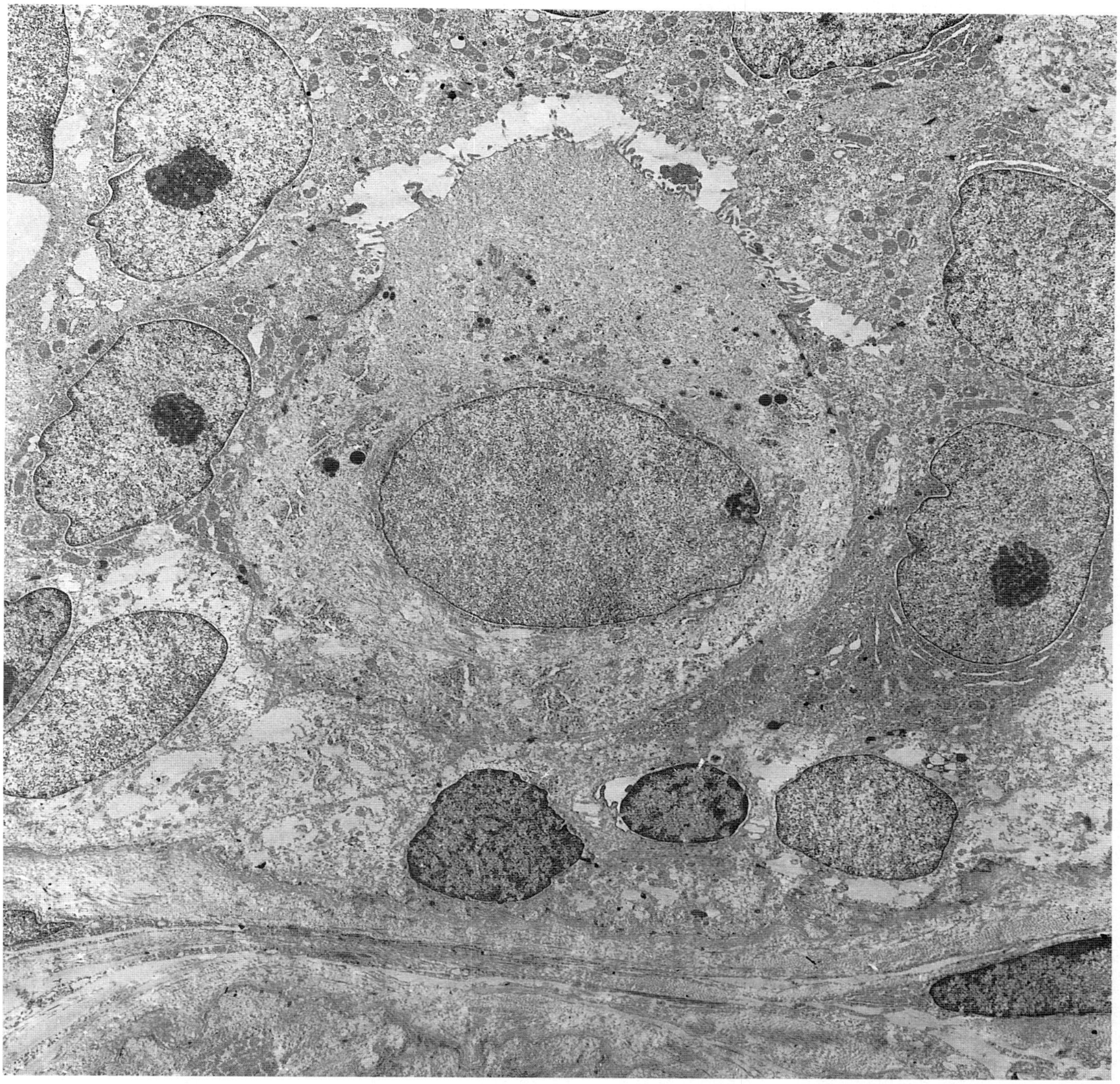

**Figure 5.34(b)** Even the smallest atypical cells were at least twice the size of adjacent normal cells. (Uranyl acetate-lead citrate, X5,700)

not in the same league (or spectrum) with atypical intraductal hyperplasia and IDCA. The cell population in IDH is totally different from those in AIDH and IDCA. Intraductal hyperplasia is characterized by the proliferation of a heterogeneous cell population; sometimes, there is an admixture of epithelial, myoepithelial, and/or metaplastic apocrine cells. When only the epithelial cell population proliferates, it is cytologically different from the cells proliferating in AIDH or IDCA, lacking a trend toward, or actual uniformity and monotony of, the cells characteristically found proliferating in AIDH. In lobular neoplasia, a distinctive cell population proliferates and either displaces or replaces the native epithelial cells, sometimes even dislodging the myoepithelial cells. The spectrum of lobular neoplasia refers to the various extents or degrees of proliferation of this distinctive cell population within the lobules. There is no

A

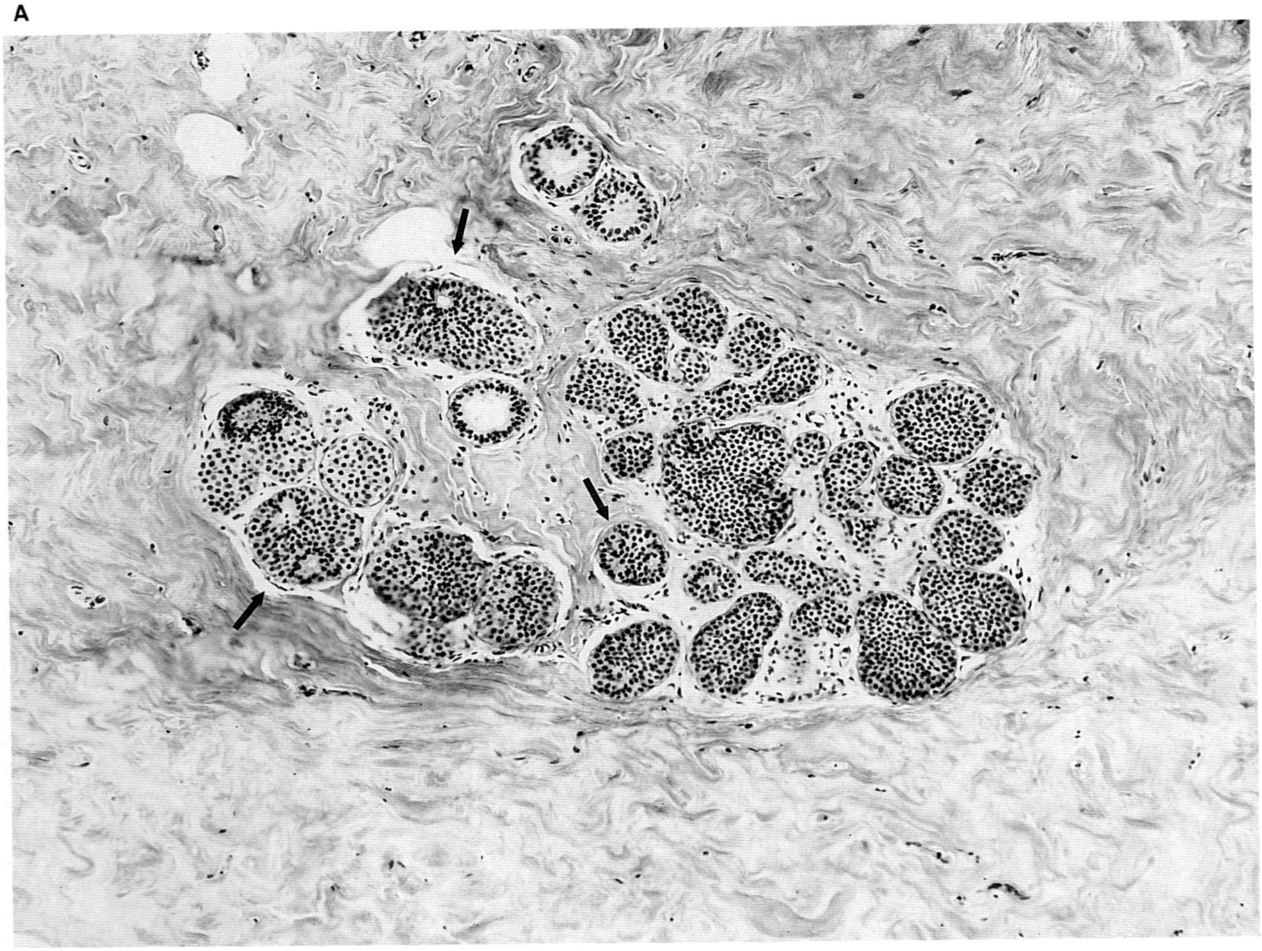

**Figure 5.35** (a–c) Atypical ductal proliferations within TDLU simulating lobular neoplasia. Three examples of the solid variant of ductal proliferation which show either rosette-like arrangement of the proliferating cells or multiple secondary lumen formation (arrow) in a few more advanced areas of proliferation within the TDLU. (H&E, X150)

counterpart for IDH within the spectrum of lobular neoplasia. Therefore, if the term DMIN were to be applied to the ductal proliferations, it should be exclusive of IDH since there is no justification to include IDH in the same spectrum just because morphologically it also reflects a proliferative process.

The cells in AIDH do resemble the cells of IDCA, however. Therefore, if we were to grade DMIN, the atypical intraductal hyperplasias characterized by proliferation of a cell population with a trend toward monotony and rounding of nuclei, or those actually simulating the cells of IDCA, but with the architecture of regular IDH could be designated as DMIN 1. Those lesions which are both cytologically and architecturally (qualitatively) identical to IDCA, but quantitatively too limited (less than 2 mm in aggregate cross-sectional diameter) to warrant a diagnosis of IDCA, could be regarded as DMIN 2. Finally, all proliferations that meet both the qualitative and quantitative criteria for the non-necrotic cribriform or micropapillary variants of IDCA would be designated as DMIN 3. But is there an advantage to this approach? Currently, DMIN 1 and 2 are lumped together as AIDH by the AFIP criteria. Those pathologists who already have problems separating this "spectrum" into two groups (AIDH and IDCA) will have even more problems separating them into three groups (DMIN 1, 2, and 3).

Furthermore, the AFIP study (29) has shown that lesions morphologically identical to the non-necrotic cribriform or the micropapillary variants of IDCA, but involving one or more ducts which are less than 2 mm in aggregate cross-sectional diameter do not behave any differently from atypical proliferations that exhibit the cytologic features of intraductal carcinoma but retain the architecture of ordinary hyperplasia. About 10% of the 82 women with AIDH developed subsequent invasive carcinoma with an

B

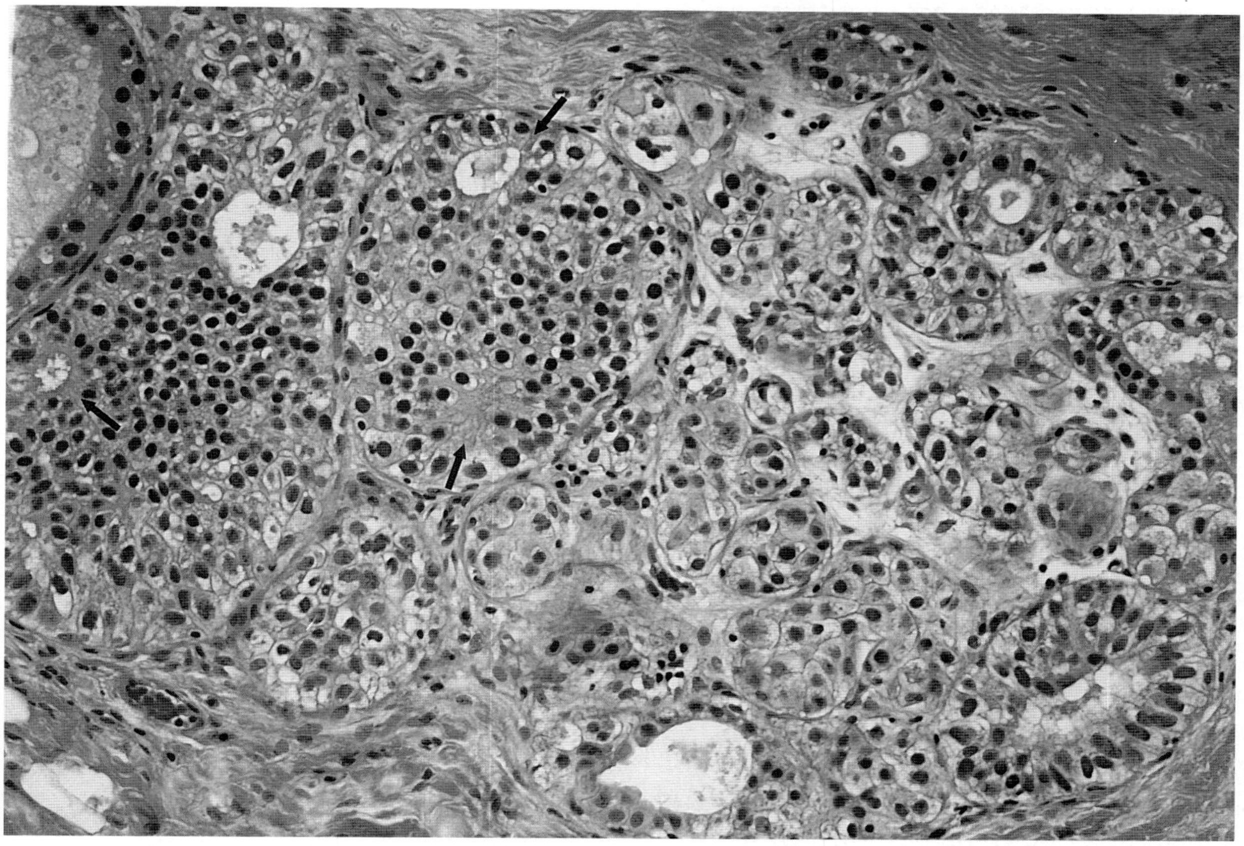

C

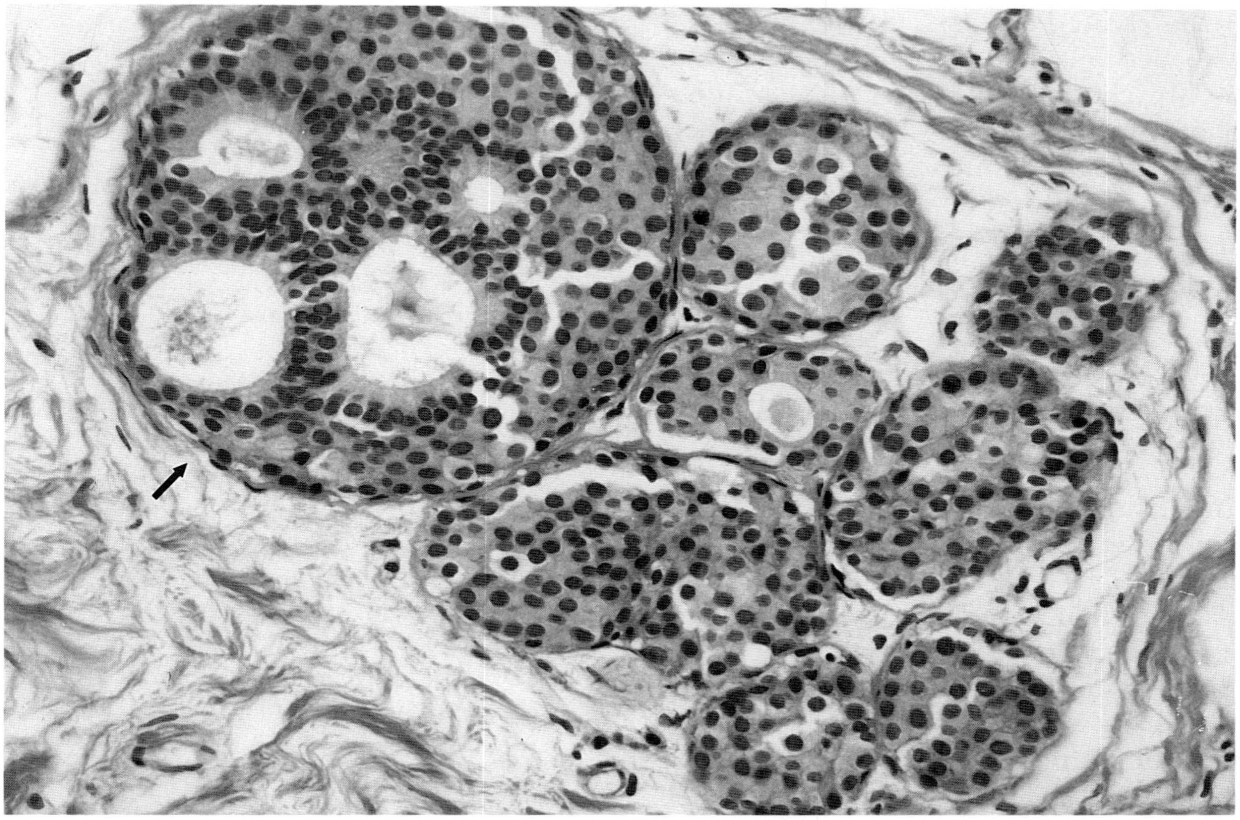

**Figure 5.35(b,c)** AIDH in TDLU. Note distinct cell margins in (b) and multiple secondary lumens (arrows) in (b) and (c). (H&E, (b&c) X800)

average follow-up of 12.4 years. In comparison, over a ten-year period, anywhere from 25% to 50% of women with IDCA of all types will eventually develop invasive carcinoma.

It seems inappropriate to introduce a new terminology of questionable value when we have just begun to define, enumerate criteria for, and better understand atypical ductal hyperplasias. It should be expected that pathologists would disagree on the interpretation of a given lesion when using different criteria, but this does not justify changing the present terminology and introducing a new one. Rather, an effort should be made to standardize criteria for the diagnosis of IDH and AIDH. Pathologists should be given time to learn and become familiar with the criteria for the diagnosis of AIDH before they are introduced to a new system of terminology. If there remains a significant difference of opinion among pathologists using the standardized criteria, then attempts can be made to modify the criteria.

It is noteworthy that differences of opinion have always existed and will continue to exist not only among pathologists but also among clinicians. We have all witnessed the different approaches to treatment for the same diagnosis, as well as different diagnoses based on the same clinical signs and symptoms, by our clinical colleagues. These differences should prompt us to study more vigorously the various approaches to arrive at a consensus rather than give up altogether or use umbrella designations.

## APPLICATIONS OF NEW TECHNIQUES

The value of morphometric and immunohistochemical studies as an aid in the diagnostic process remains to be determined.

There is a lot of information available in the literature that may be of interest as a reflection of the amount of effort committed to this area of proliferative disease. There are also accomplishments in areas of investigation not yet proven to assist our diagnostic problems or management decisions. Some of these are confirmations or continuations of works quoted in this chapter. A small sample of these references is listed (33–46) for those who may wish to utilize them.

## REFERENCES


* 1. Ashikari R, Huvos AG, Snyder RE, et al: A clinicopathologic study of atypical lesions of the breast. *Cancer* 1977;33:310–317.

2. Azzopardi JG: *Problems in Breast Pathology*. Philadelphia, WB Saunders, 1979, pp 213–214.

3. Bazzocchi F, Santini D, Marinelli G, et al: Juvenile papillomatosis (epitheliosis) of the breast. A clinical and pathologic study of 13 cases. *Am J Clin Pathol* 1986;86:745–748.

* 4. Black MM, Chabon AB: In situ carcinoma of the breast. *Pathol Annu* 1969;4:185–210.

* 5. Dupont WD, Page DL: Risk factors for breast cancer in women with proliferative breast disease. *N Engl J Med* 1985;312:146–151.

6. Elston CW: Grading of invasive carcinoma of the breast, in: Page DL, Anderson TJ (eds): *Diagnostic Histopathology of the Breast*. Edinburgh, Churchill Livingstone, 1988, pp 300–311.

7. Ferguson BT, McCarty KS Jr, Filston HC: Juvenile secretory carcinoma and juvenile papillomatosis: Diagnosis and treatment. *J Pediatr Surg* 1987;22:637–639.

8. Foote FW, Stewart FW: Comparative studies of cancerous versus non-cancerous breasts. *Ann Surg* 1945;121:6–53.

9. Haagensen CD: *Diseases of the Breast*, ed 3. Philadelphia, WB Saunders, 1986, pp 118–124.

10. Hutter RVP, et al: Consensus meeting. Is "fibrocystic disease" of the breast precancerous? *Arch Pathol Lab Med* 1986;110:171–173.

11. Jensen RA, Page DL, Dupont WD, et al: Invasive breast cancer risk in women with sclerosing adenosis. *Cancer* 1989;64:1977–1983.

12. Jensen RA, Rice JR, Wellings SR: Preneoplastic lesions in the human breast. *Science* 1976;191:295–297.

13. Ketcham AS, Moffatt FL: Vexed surgeons, perplexed patients and breast cancers which may not be cancer. *Cancer* 1990;65:387–393.

14. Kiaer HW, Kiaer WW, Linell F, et al: Extreme duct papillomatosis in the juvenile breast. *Acta Pathol Microbiol Scand* 1979;87(A):353–359.

15. Kodlin D, Winger EE, Morgenstern RG: Chronic mastopathy and breast cancer: A follow-up study. *Cancer* 1977;39:2603–2607.

16. McDivitt RW, Stewart FW, Berg JW: *Tumors of the Breast*, Fasc 2. Atlas of Tumor Pathology, Second Series. Washington, Armed Forces Institute of Pathology, 1968.

17. Nielsen M, Thomsen JL, Primdahl S, et al: Breast cancer and atypia among young and middle-aged women: A study of 110 medicolegal autopsies. *Br J Cancer* 1987;56:814–819.

18. Ohuchi N, Page DL, Merino MJ, et al: Expression of tumor-associated antigen (DF3) in atypical hyperplasias and in situ carcinomas of the human breast. *JNCI* 1987;79:109–117.

19. Page DL: Cancer risk assessment in benign breast biopsies. *Hum Pathol* 1986;17:871–874.

*20. Page DL, Anderson TJ, Rogers LW: Epithelial hyperplasia, in: Page DL, Anderson TJ (Eds): *Diagnostic Histopathology of* *the Breast*. Edinburgh, Churchill Livingstone, 1988, pp 120–156.

21. Page DL, Dupont WD: Anatomic markers of human premalignancy and risk of breast cancer. *Cancer* 1990;66:1326–1335.
22. Page DL, Dupont WD, Rogers LW: Ductal involvement by cells of atypical lobular hyperplasia in the breast: A long-term follow-up study of the cancer risk. *Hum Pathol* 1988;19:201–207.
*23. Page DL, Dupont WD, Rogers LW, et al: Atypical hyperplastic lesions of the female breast: A long-term follow-up study. *Cancer* 1985;55:2698–2708.
24. Rosen PP, Cantrell B, Mullen DL, et al: Juvenile papillomatosis (Swiss cheese disease) of the breast. *Am J Surg Pathol* 1980;4:3–12.
25. Rosen PP, Holmes G, Lesser ML, et al: Juvenile papillomatosis and breast carcinoma. *Cancer* 1985;55:1345–1352.
*26. Rosen PP, Kimmel M: Juvenile papillomatosis of the breast. A follow-up study of 41 patients having biopsies before 1979. *Am J Clin Pathol* 1990;95:599–603.
27. Rosai J: Borderline epithelial lesions of the breast. *Am J Surg Pathol* 1991;15:209–221.
28. Rubin E, Alexander RW, Visscher DW, et al: Proliferative disease and atypia in biopsies performed for mammographically detected nonpalpable lesions. *Cancer* 1988;61:2077–2082.
*29. Tavassoli FA, Norris HJ: A comparison of the results of long-term follow-up for atypical intraductal hyperplasia and intraductal hyperplasia of the breast. *Cancer* 1990;65:518–529.
30. Tham K-T, Dupont WD, Page DL, et al: Micro-papillary hyperplasia with atypical features in female breasts, resembling gynecomastia. *Progress in Surgical Pathology* 1989;X:101–109.
31. Uriburu JV, Mosta AM, Gomez MA: Displasia proliferative juvenil focalizada. *Pren Med Argentina* 1975;62:172–176.
*32. Wellings SR, Jensen HM, Marcum RG: An atlas of subgross pathology of the human breast with special reference to possible precancerous lesions. *J Natl Cancer Inst* 1975;55:231–273.

### Additional Reading

33. Bhattacharjee DK, Harris M, Faragher EB: Nuclear morphometry of epitheliosis and intraduct carcinoma of the breast. *Histopathology* 1985;9:511–516.
34. Black MM, Kwon S: Precancerous mastopathie: Structural and biological considerations. *Path Res Pract* 1980;166:491–514.
35. Cardiff RD, Wellings SR, Faulkin LJ: Biology of breast preneoplasia. *Cancer* 1977;39:2734–2746.
36. Cook MG, Rohan TE: The patho-epidemiology of benign proliferative epithelial disorders of the female breast. *J Pathol* 1985;146:1–15.
37. Ferguson DJP: Ultrastructural characterisation of the proliferative (stem?) cells within the parenchyma of the normal "resting" breast. *Virchows Arch* (*Pathol Anat*) 1985;407:379–385.
38. Goldenberg VE, Goldenberg NS, Sommers SC: Comparative ultrastructure of atypical ductal hyperplasia, intraductal carcinoma, and infiltrating ductal carcinoma of the breast. *Cancer* 1969;24:1152–1167.
39. Humphrey LJ, Swerdlow MA: Large duct epithelial hyperplasia and carcinoma of the breast. *Arch Surg* 1968;97:592–594.
40. Jarasch E-D, Nagle RB, Kaufmann M, et al: Differential diagnosis of benign epithelial proliferations and carcinomas of the breast using antibodies to cytokeratins. *Hum Pathol* 1988;19:276–289.
41. Joshi K, Smith JA, Perusinghe N, et al: Cell proliferation in the human mammary epithelium. Differential contribution by epithelial and myoepithelial cells. *Am J Pathol* 1986;124:199–206.
42. Kramer WM, Rush BF: Mammary duct proliferation in the elderly. A histopathologic study. *Cancer* 1973;31:130–137.
43. Schuerch C, Rosen PP, Hirota T, et al: A pathologic study of benign breast diseases in Tokyo and New York. *Cancer* 1982;50:1899–1903.
44. Simpson HW, Mutch F, Halberg F, et al: Bimodal age-frequency distribution of epitheliosis in cancer mastectomies. Relevance to preneoplasia. *Cancer* 1982;50:2417–2422.
45. Squartini F, Sarnelli R: Structure, functional changes, and proliferative pathology of the human mammary lobule in cancerous breasts. *JNCI* 1981;67:33–46.
46. Wells S, Hasleton PS: A dilutional immunoperoxidase study of proliferative ductal lesions and carcinomata of the breast. *Histopathology* 1981;5:517–526.

# 6

# Papillary Lesions



## GENERAL COMMENTS

Included among papillary lesions of the breast are papilloma, papillomatosis, sclerosing papilloma, atypical papilloma, carcinoma arising in a papilloma, intraductal papillary carcinoma, and invasive papillary carcinoma. Haagensen et al (19) divided papillary lesions into solitary papilloma, multiple papillomas and papillary carcinoma. Judging from recent studies, multiplicity itself is not a factor that should influence the classification of papillary lesions. Rather, it is their location or their site of origin—central versus peripheral (origin in the TDLU)—that is associated with differences in clinical behavior (25,26).

As emphasized by Azzopardi (1), the term papilloma should be applied strictly to lesions with a papillary, arborescent growth pattern supported by a fibrovascular stalk. Therefore, juvenile papillomatosis—as defined by Rosen and characterized by an intraductal epithelial proliferation, not supported by a fibrovascular stalk—is excluded from this chapter. Furthermore, intraductal hyperplasia (epitheliosis) of the solid and fenestrated types, as well as those intraductal carcinomas forming micropapillae or tufts not supported by a fibrovascular connective tissue stalk are, by definition, excluded from the category of papillary lesions. In this chapter, "papilloma" will be used for the central and often solitary lesions, and "papillomatosis" for the peripheral, multifocal papillomas originating in the TDLU with or without extension to adjacent terminal and major ducts. The designations of "papilloma" and "papillomatosis" are preferred to the terms "central papilloma" and "peripheral papilloma," as proposed by Ohuchi et al (25,26). Papillary carcinomas also may be either solitary and centrally located, or multifocal and peripherally located (within TDLUs); the latter would be the malignant counterpart of papillomatosis. A majority of papillary carcinomas are intraductal and noninvasive accounting for their excellent prognosis. When invasion is present, it should be noted in the diagnosis as an invasive papillary carcinoma.

The most crucial task of a pathologist in assessing a papillary lesion is to determine whether it is benign or malignant. The single most important feature that distinguishes a benign papilloma from a papillary carcinoma is the presence of a relatively uniform myoepithelial (ME) cell layer in the proliferating, papillary intraluminal component of the lesion. It is important to emphasize that a myoepithelial cell layer is often present in the lining of the duct wall into which the papillary carcinoma proliferates, and the presence of this layer does not exclude the diag-

A

B

C

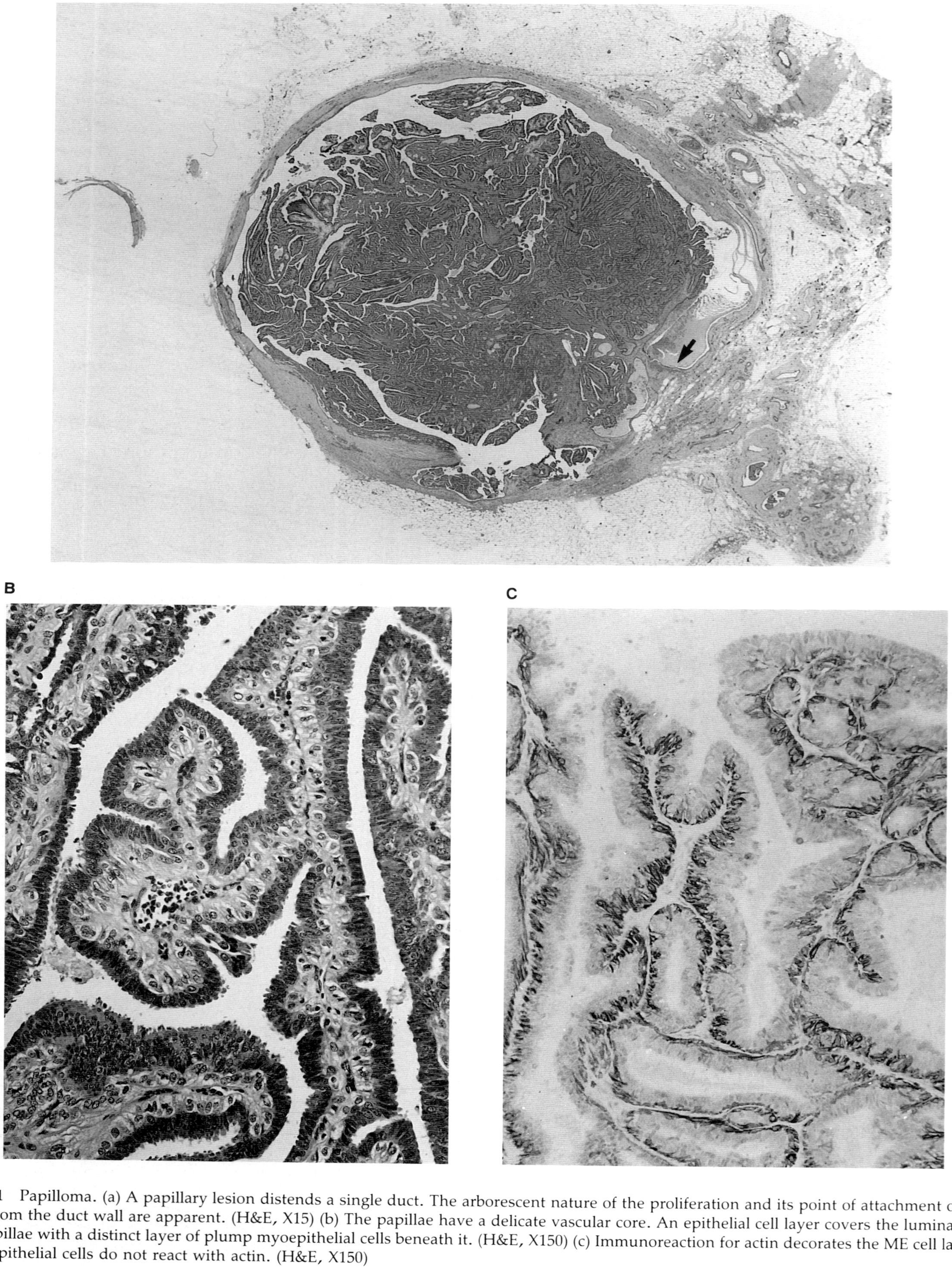

**Figure 6.1** Papilloma. (a) A papillary lesion distends a single duct. The arborescent nature of the proliferation and its point of attachment or origin (arrow) from the duct wall are apparent. (H&E, X15) (b) The papillae have a delicate vascular core. An epithelial cell layer covers the luminal aspect of the papillae with a distinct layer of plump myoepithelial cells beneath it. (H&E, X150) (c) Immunoreaction for actin decorates the ME cell layer; the luminal epithelial cells do not react with actin. (H&E, X150)

nosis of papillary carcinoma. The myoepithelial cell layer surrounding the duct is not a component of the neoplastic papillary proliferation.

Since identification of the ME cell layer is the most important feature in the accurate interpretation of papillary lesions, it is important to refrain from freezing papillary lesions. Freezing diminishes the tinctorial differences between the epithelial and ME cells, making their distinction difficult even on permanent sections.

Some of the numerous publications on the subject of papillomas, papillomatosis, and papillary carcinoma will not be discussed in detail because of the confusion in the use of the term papillomatosis and the fact that they make no reference to the significance of the myoepithelial cell layer in separating the benign papillary proliferations from the malignant ones. The failure to note the significance of the ME cells stemmed from a general lack of familiarity with this cell type until recently. Kraus and Neubecker (4) listed and illustrated the presence of a single cell type as one of the features of papillary carcinoma in an excellent and often-quoted study. They emphasized the presence of a double cell layer (luminal and basal cells), in some areas at least, as a hallmark of a papilloma. Apparently, the authors did not recognize that the "basal cell layer" is the ME cell layer. They further stated, "A third cell type, the myoepithelial cell, is inconspicuous and is usually not recognized in routine sections. To our knowledge, it is not involved in papillary epithelial proliferative lesions." It is important to emphasize that a complete absence of the myoepithelial cell layer in a papillary lesion displaying a proliferation of ordinary (nonmetaplastic) epithelial cells always identifies a papillary carcinoma.

Occasionally, two tinctorially different variants of epithelial cells may be present in papillary carcinomas with one proliferating underneath the other in a pagetoid fashion, simulating a proliferating ME cell layer. In contrast to myoepithelial cells, these cells do not react with either actin or S-100 protein, however.

Rarely, papillary carcinomas can and do have sporadic myoepithelial cells (7,8,36). It is the accurate separation of these papillary carcinomas from papillomas, and the determination of the point at which the amount of myoepithelial cells exceeds that acceptable for a carcinoma that is most difficult. Papotti et al (8) have illustrated what they refer to as a papillary carcinoma with persistent ME cells. It is not clear, however, what proportion of the papillary processes in the papillary carcinoma illustrated in Figs. 11a–b of their paper contained a ME cell layer. According to Papotti et al, other carcinoma areas in the same slide were completely devoid of a ME cell layer. It is doubtful that Papotti et al would have designated the papillary areas illustrated in Figs. 11a–b of their 1983 paper as carcinoma in the absence of the other areas of fully-developed carcinoma, however. By the criteria that will be discussed in this chapter, the lesion they have illustrated and discussed reflects either an atypical papilloma or a carcinoma arising in a papilloma. Based on available data, the significance of a papillary lesion which only partially displays the morphologic features of carcinoma (complete absence of a ME cell layer in some papillae, or cribriform growth patterns identical to cribriform intraductal carcinoma overlying the ME cell layer) is not known. Since there are no absolute rules established on this issue, arbitrary guidelines are provided in this chapter for separating benign papilloma, atypical papilloma, carcinoma arising in a papilloma, and papillary carcinoma based mainly on the presence or absence of the ME cell layer, the proliferating cell types, and their quantity within each lesion. Immunoreactions for actin and/or S-100 protein are often useful and sometimes necessary for making a distinction between the varieties of papillary lesion.

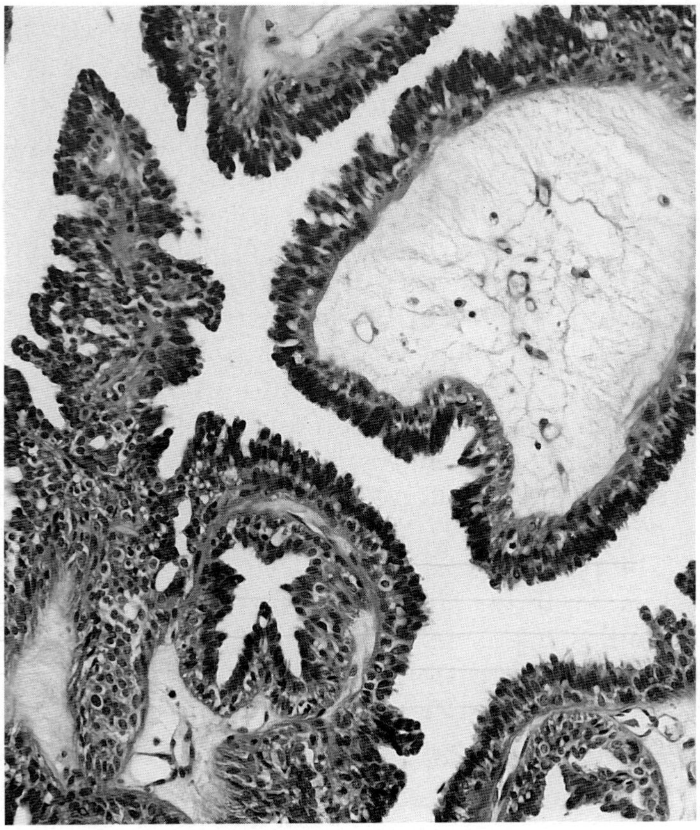

**Figure 6.2** Papilloma. The papillary stalk shows an edematous stroma and a distinct ME cell layer. (H&E, X50)

Focal apocrine metaplasia, as a minor component, is often observed in benign papillomas, but is invariably absent in classic papillary carcinomas. Some papillary lesions show a complete replacement of the epithelial cell layer by metaplastic apocrine cells. In this setting, the recognition of the ME cell layer may become difficult particularly when the apocrine cells display hyperplasia with formation of epithelial bridges and cribriform arrangements. Immunostain for actin is helpful in unmasking the myoepithelial cell layer in this situation and confirming the benign, albeit atypical in some instances, nature of the papillary process. There are also exceptionally rare, atypical, and mitotically active papillary lesions that are composed exclusively of apocrine cells and display complete absence of a myoepithelial cell layer and regular epithelial cells. Even though a diagnosis of papillary apocrine carcinoma would seem appropriate based on the presence of a single, atypical cell type proliferating in the lesion, the degree of aggressiveness of this rare lesion has not been established.

## PAPILLOMA

Papillomas are generally solitary and located in the subareolar region or major ducts and involve a single duct or a number of contiguous ducts without any significant sclerosis or hyalinization. Serous or serosanguinous nipple discharge is present in up to 87% of women (1,2,6,9,12,15,16,21,34), and is frequently the major presenting symptom (9,12,34). Papillomas manifest most often during the fifth and sixth decade of life (1,20,29). While a case of intraductal papilloma has been reported in a seven-month-old infant (32), this lesion is rare in children and adolescent females (31) and occurs most frequently in women over 50 years of age. Papillomas occur in both male and female.

The possible role of papillomas lacking atypia as a risk factor in the subsequent development of breast carcinomas needs further evaluation, but currently, the general impression is that solitary, central papillomas are not associated with a significant risk for subsequent development of invasive breast carcinoma (30).

The evolution of our understanding of papillomas and gradual acceptance of these lesions as benign despite their large size and association with nipple discharge is well illustrated by three studies from a single institution. A total of 109 papillomas have been reported from the Johns Hopkins Hospital over a period of 72 years (2,3,5). With a follow-up of up to 25 years, 16% of the patients developed recurrences and 6% developed subsequent carcinomas. It is interesting that 78% of the first group of 95 patients seen between 1895 to 1924 were treated by either simple or radical mastectomy (3). Nine of these women developed recurrences, but none of them developed a subsequent carcinoma. The second study involved 32 women during the period of 1925 to 1941 (5). Simple or radical mastectomy was performed on 28% of these patients; two developed recurrences, but none developed a carcinoma during the period of follow-up of up to 25 years. The third study (2) covered the period of 1949 to 1967 and included 64 women with 5 to 17 years of follow-up; all of these women were treated by local excision alone. Six developed recurrences and six developed subsequent carcinomas; only four of the carcinomas were invasive.

Three other studies from different institutions and with a total of 235 cases also reported a relatively high 8% incidence of subsequent carcinomas during up to 16 years of follow-up (11,22,23). If some of the Hopkins' studies are grouped differently with others, however, from a total of 427 patients with papillomas in five separate studies (3,4,5,19,21), only two (0.4%) of the women developed subsequent carcinomas during the follow-up periods ranging from 1 to 22 years. Many of the patients in some of the older studies had been treated by mastectomies, however. The real frequency of subsequent carcinoma is probably somewhere in between 0.4% and 8%, and its development is undoubtedly influenced by the presence of other proliferative lesions which frequently coexist in the same breast.

### Microscopic Features

Microscopically, papillomas are characterized by formation of epithelial fronds supported by a fibrovascular stroma. Epithelial cells line the luminal aspect of the papillae and a myoepithelial cell layer is invariably present between the epithelial cells and the basement membrane (Figs. 6.1–6.3). Metaplastic apo-

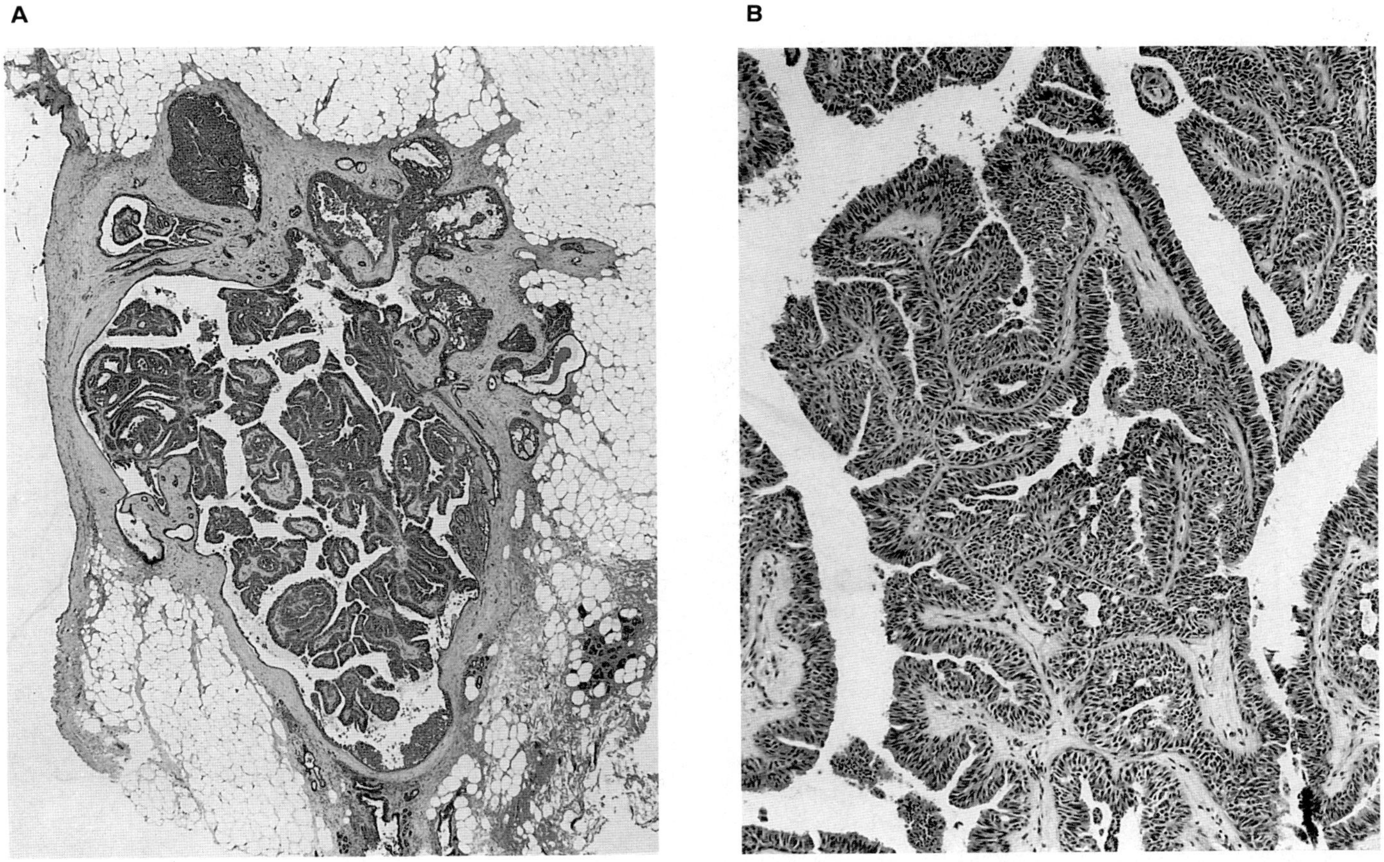


**Figure 6.3** Papilloma. (a) The papillary proliferation involves a major duct and extends into the adjacent branches. (H&E, X20) (b) The epithelial cells show stratification and hyperplasia but the persistence of the ME cell layer identifies this lesion as a benign papilloma. (H&E, X100)

crine cells are readily identifiable in 20% of papillomas (Fig. 6.4). Solid and fenestrated epithelial hyperplasia as well as stratification of the epithelial cells without cytologic atypia is present focally or diffusely in approximately 30% of papillomas. The involved duct is always dilated and sometimes cystic.

Hemorrhagic infarction secondary to the torsion of some of the fronds or the entire papilloma occurs occasionally (Fig. 6.5). When the entire papillary lesion is infarcted, it is best to regard the process as an infarcted papilloma since it is impossible to identify any evidence of malignancy or confirm the absence of a myoepithelial cell layer in an infarcted lesion. Sometimes, a few peripheral papillae remain viable and show the double cell layer typical of a benign papilloma, however, (Fig. 6.6). Partially or completely infarcted papillomas are not rare among the consultation cases reviewed at AFIP, indicating the dilemma faced by a pathologist when dealing with an infarcted papilloma. As a rule, a diagnosis of papillary carcinoma should not be made unless there is unequivocal and recognizable evidence of malignancy which requires the presence of viable tissue.

Squamous metaplasia is seen occasionally within papillomas, particularly in the vicinity of areas of infarction (Fig. 6.7). Three of the six infarcted papillomas reported by Flint and Oberman (14) had squamous metaplasia. Mucinous (Fig. 6.8), clear cell and sebaceous metaplasia also occur in papillomas but at a much lower frequency than squamous metaplasia.

## PAPILLOMATOSIS

Papillomatosis is defined here as a proliferation of papillary fronds, supported by fibrovascular stalks within multiple TDLUs with or without extension into the adjacent terminal ducts of the duct system (Figs. 6.9–6.10). Also referred to as "multiple papillomas," papillomatosis may present as a palpable lesion or it may be a microscopic lesion that is detected either mammographically, if associated with calcification or significant structural alterations, or

A B

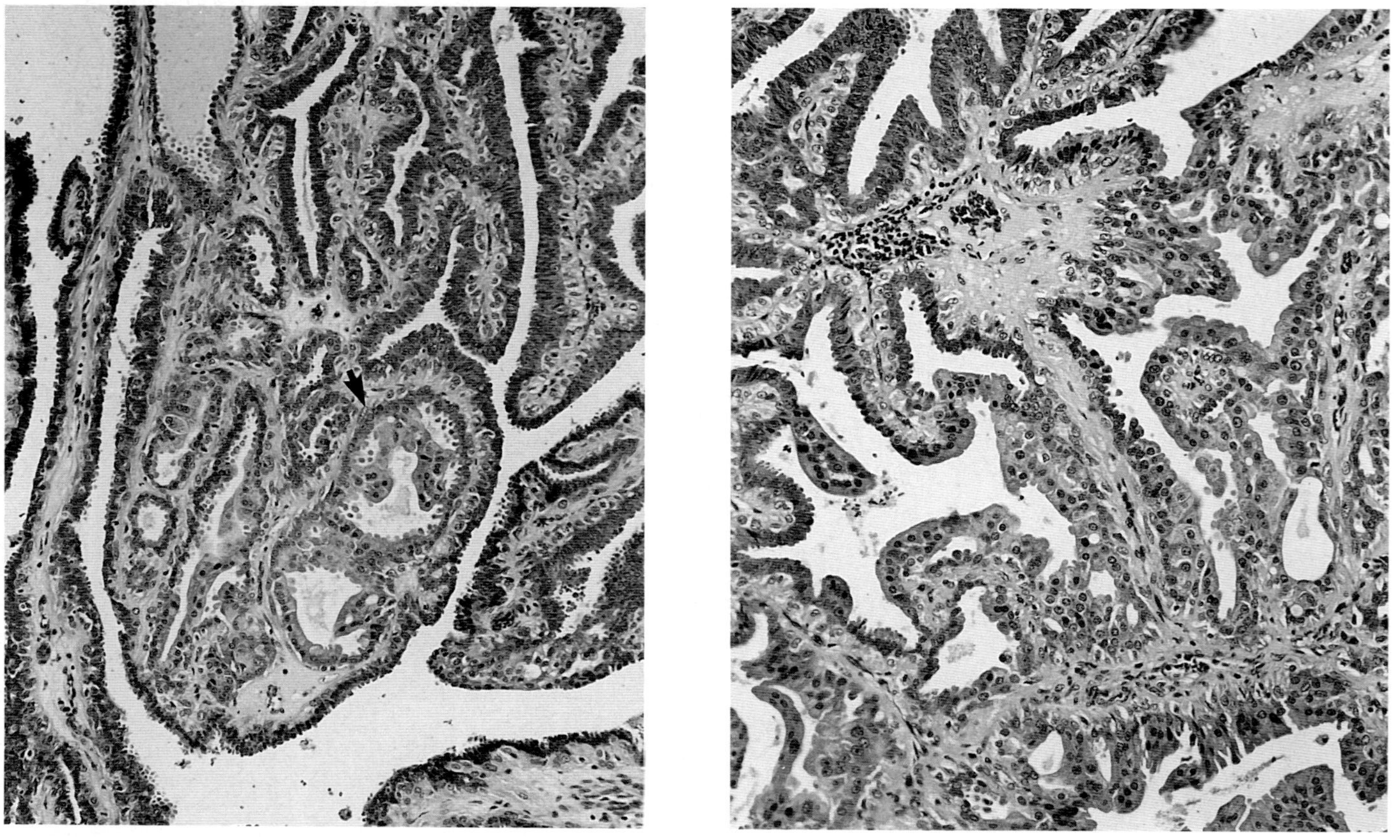

**Figure 6.4** Papilloma. (a) In addition to the epithelial and myoepithelial cell layers, there are metaplastic apocrine cells (arrow) in the papilloma. (H&E, X120) (b) Notice that the myoepithelial cell layer has become less distinctive in areas lined by metaplastic apocrine cells. (H&E, X200)

incidentally in biopsies removed for other reasons. Patients with papillomatosis are generally younger than those with either solitary, central papillomas or papillary carcinoma. Patients with "multiple papillomas" average 11 years younger than patients with papillary carcinoma; their median age is 39 years with occasional patients less than 20 years of age (7). Nipple discharge is present in about one third of the patients. Since both Murad et al (7) and Haagensen's series (19) of multiple papillomas included lesions central and peripheral in location, about 25% of the cases (those centrally located) in either series would not qualify as papillomatosis according to the definition used here.

## Microscopic Features

Microscopically—in contrast to a papilloma which is frequently attached to the duct wall in one or, at most, a few foci—papillomatosis is often characterized by a simultaneous proliferation and protrusion of multiple papillae into the duct lumen (Figs. 6.11–6.12). This variant of papillomatosis may be confused with micropapillary intraductal carcinoma if the presence of a ME cell layer is missed. A majority of the papillae in papillomatosis start as simple, nonbranching structures which become more complex as the lesion progresses. Each of these papillary processes has both an epithelial and a myoepithelial cell layer overlying a distinct fibrovascular stromal support. Atypia may develop in papillomatosis. Atypia is manifested by a proliferation of stratified spindle cells or by the focal loss of the myoepithelial cell layer in some of the papillary fronds. In general, the atypical papillomatosis appears more complex and cellular with the papillary processes often filling the lumen of the involved ducts. These can be difficult to diagnose accurately on H&E sections. Immunoreactions for actin often show the absence of a myoepithelial cell layer in a minority of the papillae.

The risk of carcinoma developing subsequent to, or in the presence of, papillary disease has been a

A

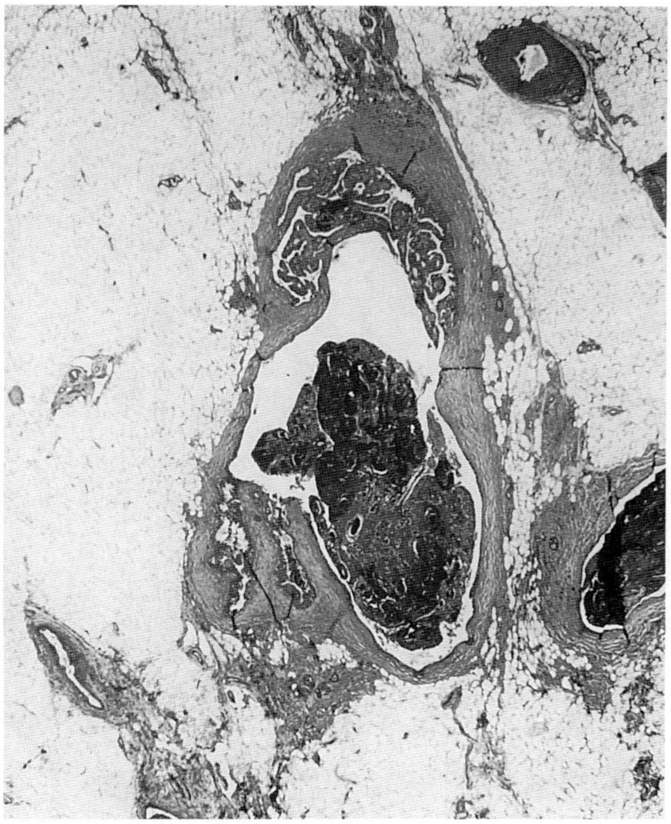

B

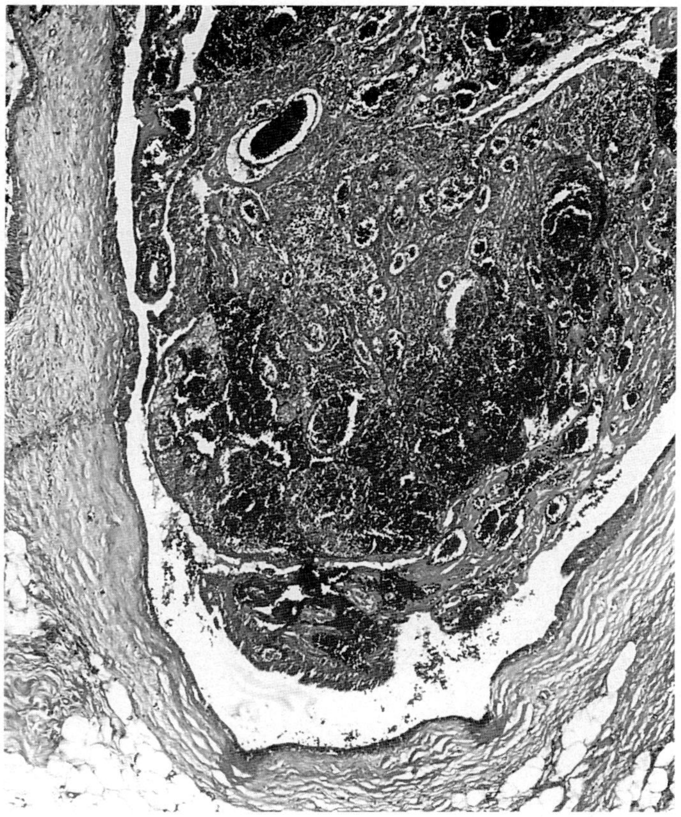

C

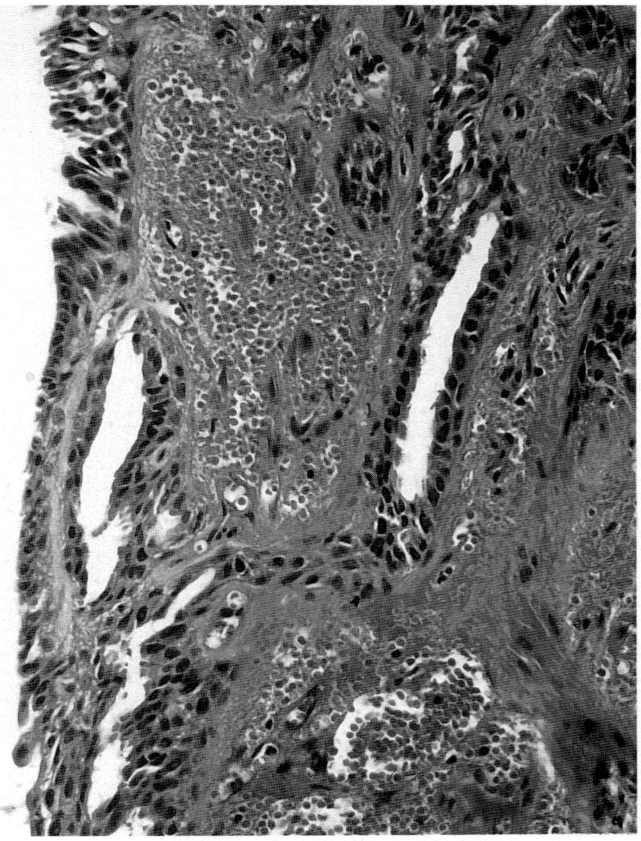

**Figure 6.5** Papilloma with hemorrhagic infarction. (a) The darker papillary process reflects the presence of significant hemorrhage. (b) Much cf the papillae shows congested vessels and extravasated red cells without viable epithelial cells. (c) At the periphery, some residual epithelial and ME cells are apparent. (H&E, (a) X15; (b) X60; (c) X250)

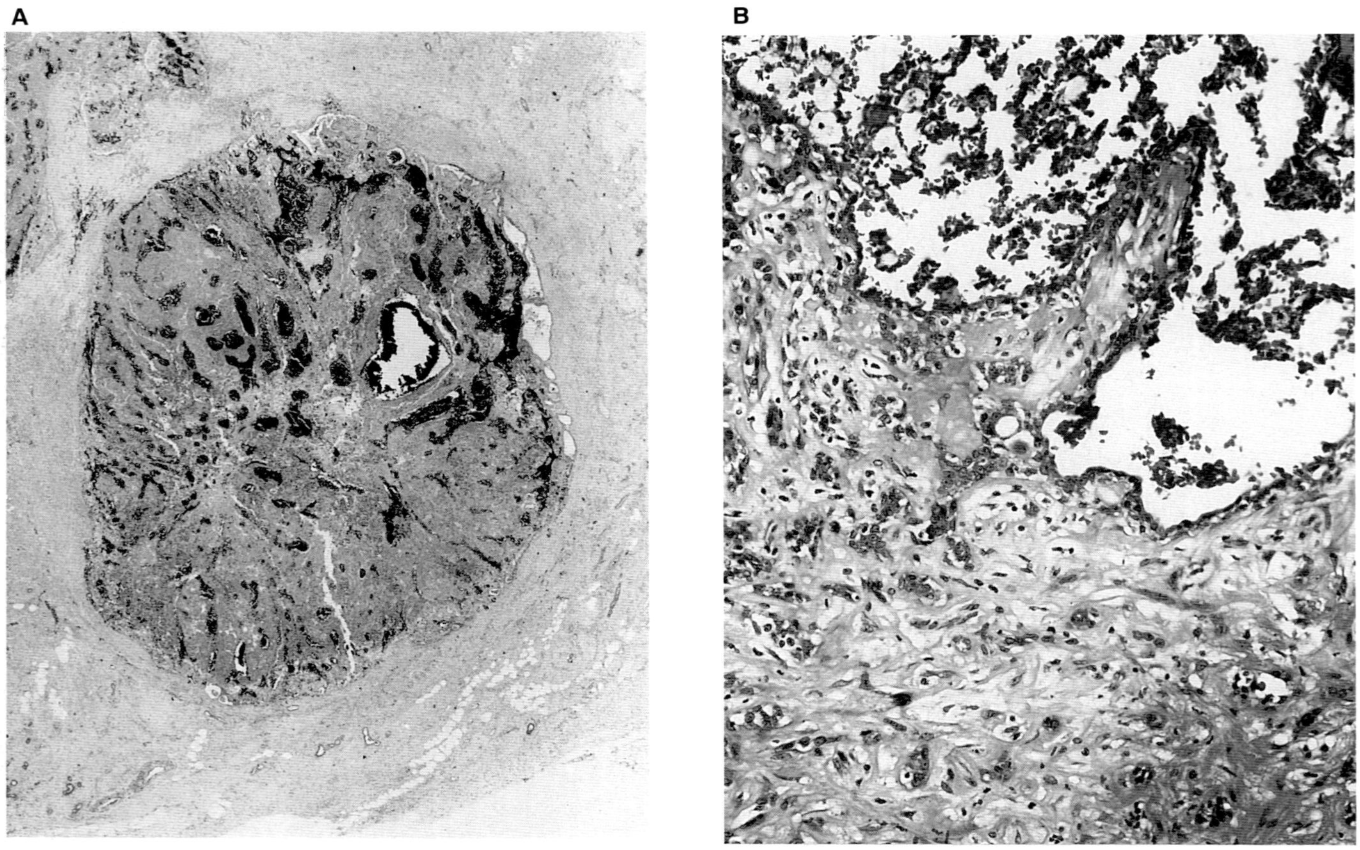

**Figure 6.6** Infarcted papilloma. (a) This papilloma is almost entirely infarcted. (b) Small areas of viable epithelial and ME cells are apparent in the periphery. (H&E, (a) X12; (b) X150)

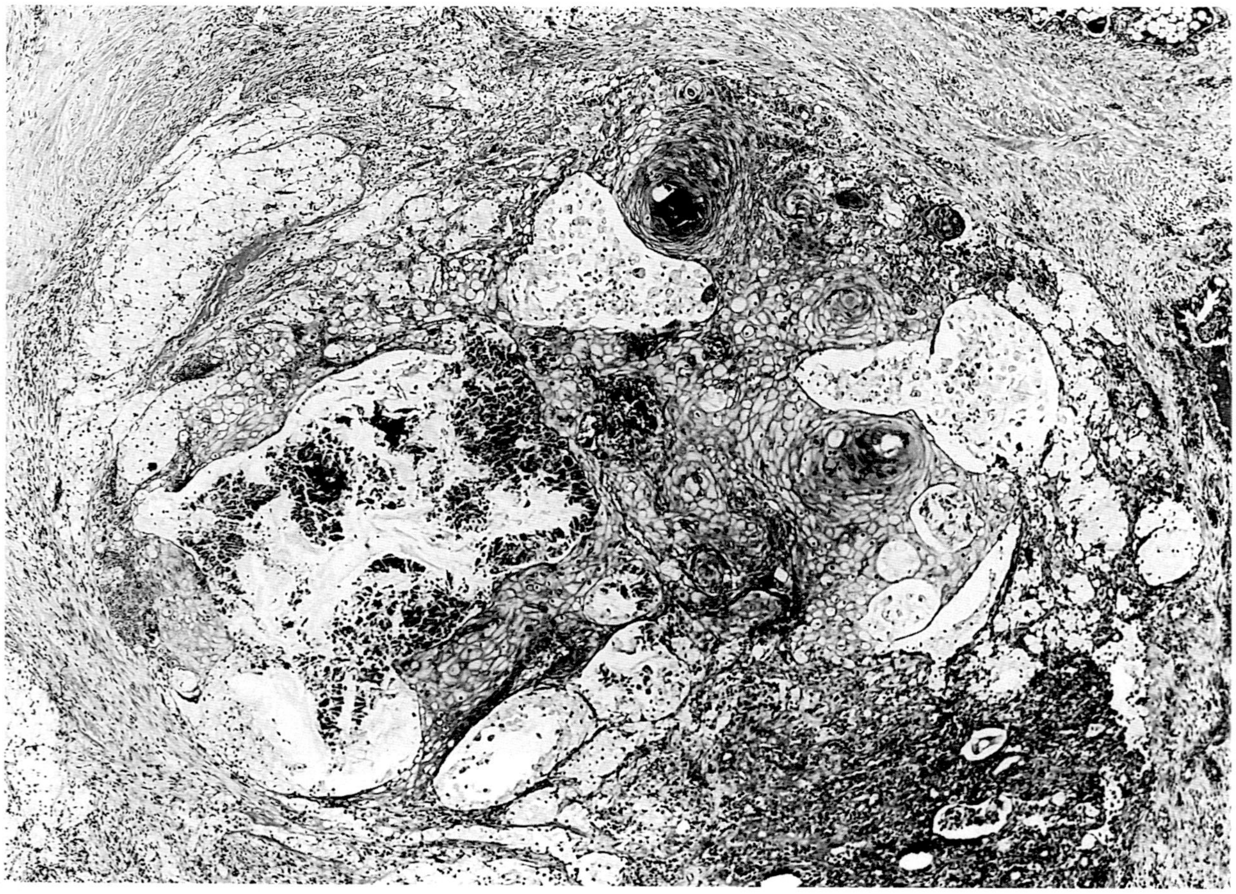

**Figure 6.7** Papilloma with extensive squamous metaplasia. (H&E, X240)

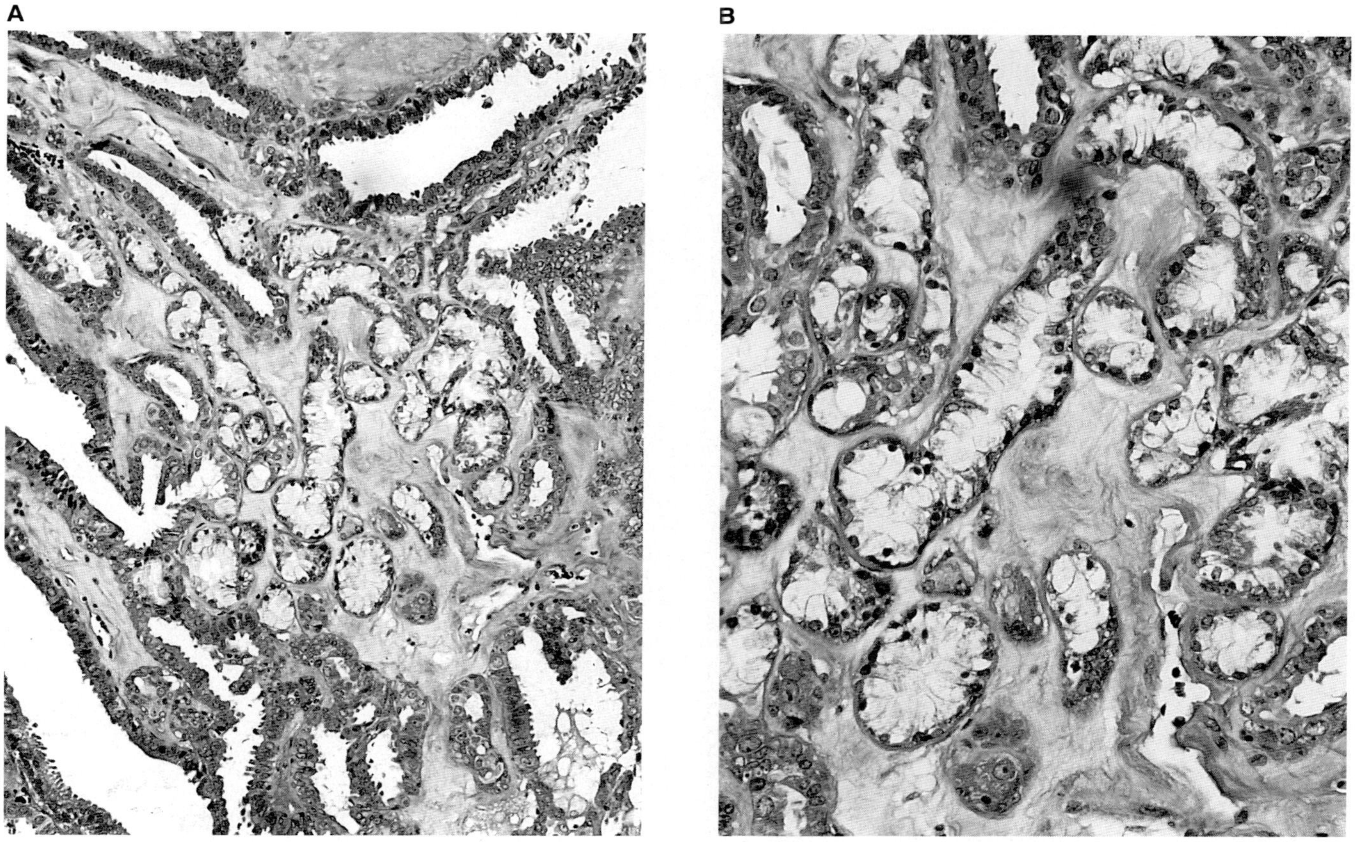


**Figure 6.8** (a&b) Papilloma with a small focus of mucinous metaplasia. In addition to apocrine and squamous metaplasia, mucinous metaplasia also occurs in papillomas but with a far lower frequency. (H&E, (a) X160; (b) X250)

subject of interest for a long time (22,27). Papillomatosis is often present simultaneously with intraductal epithelial hyperplasia (Fig. 6.9c) with or without atypia, as well as with intraductal carcinoma (Fig. 6.13). Papillomatosis is associated with a malignant lesion in 20% to 39% of cases (6,20). The malignant process may be an intraductal carcinoma or an invasive carcinoma. The frequent association of papillomatosis with various patterns of "intraductal" epithelial proliferation (IDH, AIDH, and IDCA) is understandable since all of these lesions generally originate in the TDLU, leading to eventual unfolding of this unit or its transformation into a duct-like structure. Once the TDLU is stimulated to proliferate, the proliferation may assume any of the variety of patterns ranging from ordinary intraductal hyperplasia to multifocal, peripheral papillary carcinoma. Occasionally, the lumen may contain both fenestrated intraductal hyperplasia and a few papillary processes.

## SCLEROSING PAPILLOMA

Papillomas (solitary or multiple, grossly visible or microscopically identified) may undergo extensive sclerosis leading to prominent areas of hyalinization, distortion and pseudoinvasive patterns that are easily mistaken for carcinoma. None of the 30 sclerosing papillomas reported by Fenoglio and Lattes (13) developed recurrences after a median follow-up of six years.

### Clinical Features

Patients range in age from 11 to 67 with a median age of 45 years. While a majority present with a lump, in

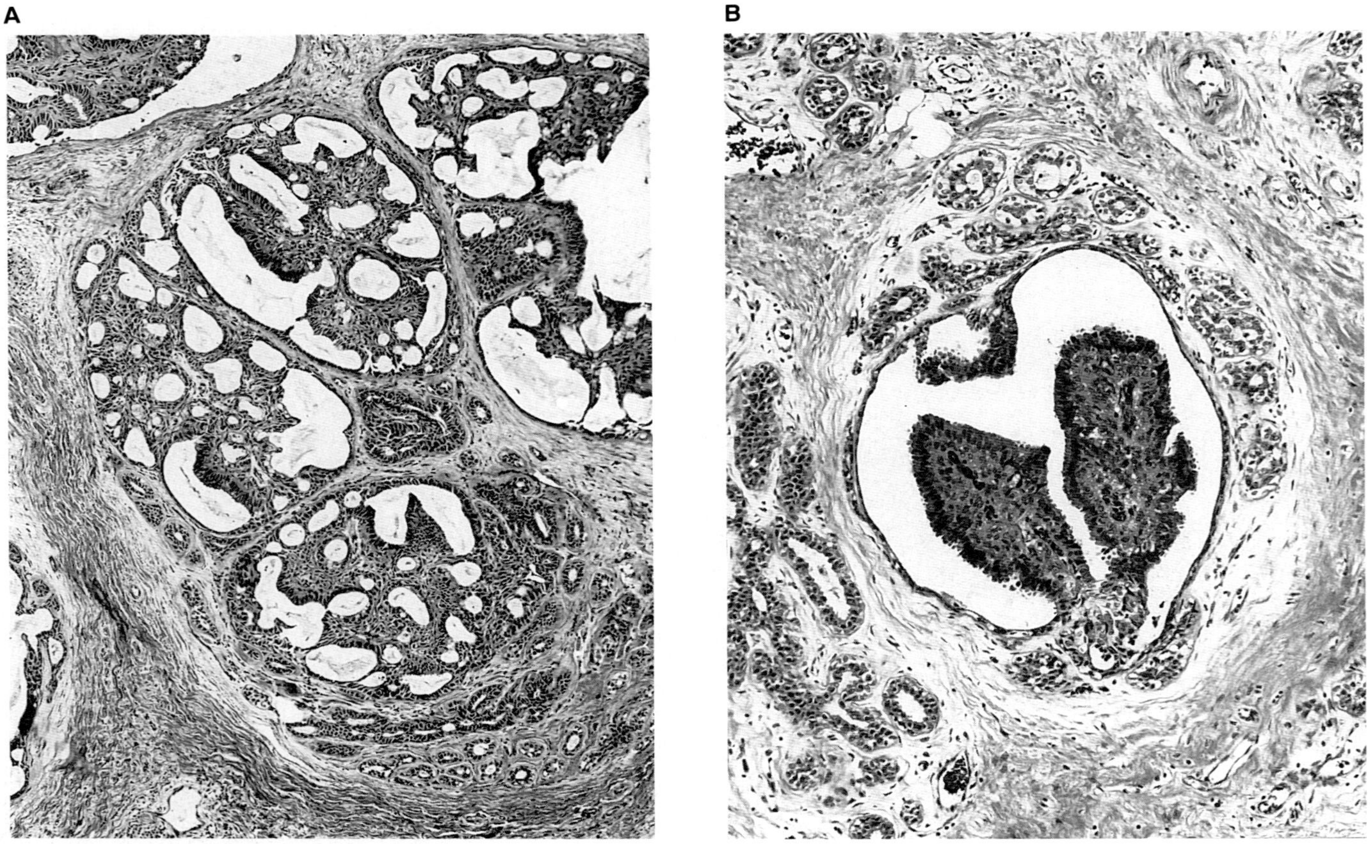


**Figure 6.9** Papillomatosis. (a,b) Several papillary lesions at different stages of development are evident in multiple TDLUs. (H&E, (a) X75; (b) X120)

some cases, the lump is caused by either cystic disease, adenosis, or a combination of both. On rare occasions, the patient may complain of pain or nipple discharge. The lesion may be fixed to the overlying skin.

## Macroscopic Features

Only rarely does sclerosing papilloma appear as an intracystic mass. It varies in size from micrcscopic to a grossly visible lesion of 3.5 cm diameter.

## Microscopic Features

At low magnification, the papillary and intraductal nature of these lesions is readily apparent in many cases (Figs. 6.14–6.16). The sclerotic changes may be focal or diffuse. Sometimes there is a stellate pattern of central fibrosis simulating a radial scar. The sclerotic areas generally display distorted, entrapped tubules imitating an invasive carcinoma. At higher magnification, the persistence of myoepithelial cells in any residual papillary process and the entrapped ductules and tubules in the sclerotic areas of the lesions affirms their benign nature. The duct wall is often prominently thickened. In some cases, the entire duct is surrounded by a band of florid sclerosing adenosis. In some planes of section, some of these lesions may appear as solid, intraductal proliferations of sclerosing tubules, for which a diagnosis of ductal adenoma (10,17,18) would seem appropriate (Fig. 6.17). Deeper levels of these solid growths often show a few papillary processes. The sclerosis may be diffuse, transforming the involved duct into a hyalinized nodule peppered by a few distorted ductules (Fig. 6.18), or it may be focal in an otherwise typical papilloma. Occasionally sclerosing papillomas develop extensive squamous metaplasia (Fig. 6.19).

c

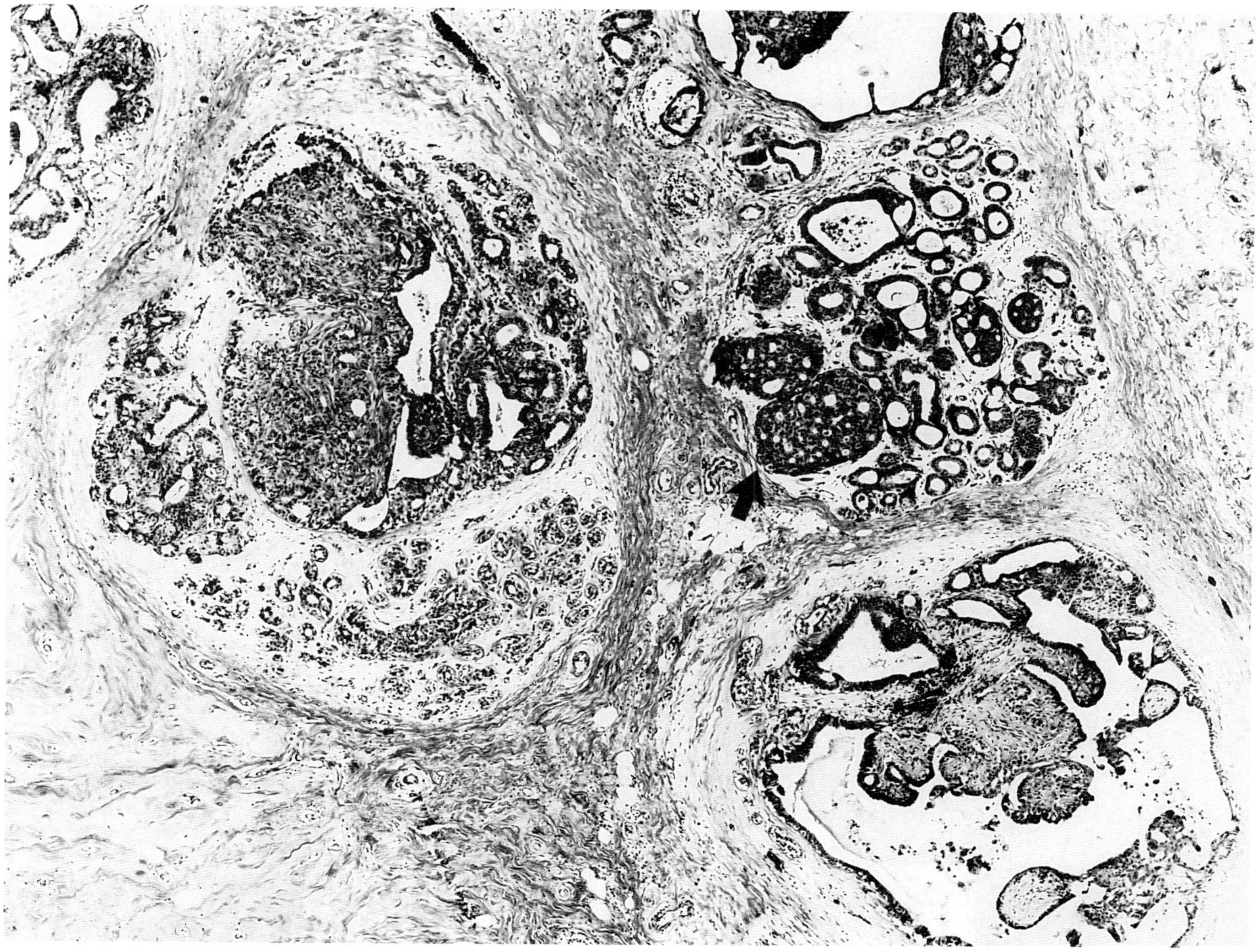

**Figure 6.9(c)** Papillomatosis. Note simultaneous papillomatosis and AIDH (arrow) in adjacent TDLU's. (H&E, X160)

Some sclerosing papillomas reflect extension of sclerosing adenosis into the duct lumen along with florid sclerosing adenosis around the duct (Fig. 6.20); see also sclerosing adenosis in Chapter 4.

## ATYPICAL PAPILLOMAS AND CARCINOMA ARISING IN A PAPILLOMA

Atypical papilloma (Figs. 6.21–6.23) displays focal areas within the papillary processes with proliferation of a monotonous cell population similar to that observed in atypical intraductal hyperplasia. Areas identical to the cribriform or other variants of nonnecrotic intraductal carcinoma characterized by a monomorphic cell population are sometimes present within a papilloma. Such areas may be interpreted as carcinoma arising in a papilloma when they occupy at least a third of the lesion in the cross section of the duct under evaluation. If less than a third of the lesion in a ductal cross section shows these changes, the designation of atypical papilloma would be appropriate (Fig. 6.23). Rarely, a highly atypical cell population with or without abundant mitotic activity proliferates in a solid or cribriform pattern over a persistent ME cell layer; the designation of carcinoma arising in a papilloma would also be appropriate in this setting. Sometimes the papillary processes may show stratification of atypical spindled epithelial cells but with a distinctive ME cell layer persisting throughout the lesions; such a lesion would qualify as atypical papilloma (Fig. 6.24). The same pattern

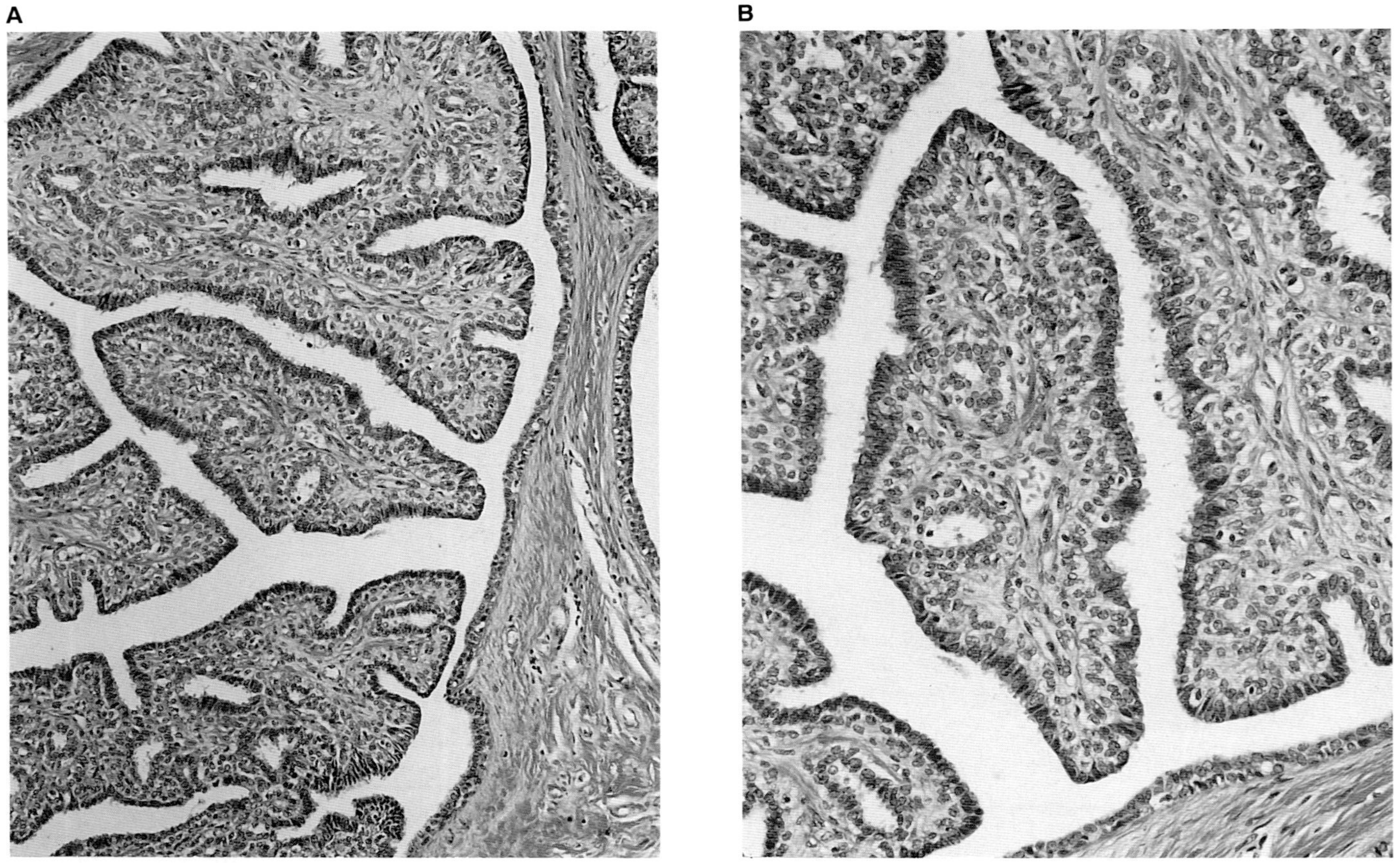


**Figure 6.10** Papillomatosis. (a) The papillary processes are broad, and the stroma appears cellular. (b) The cellularity is due to myoepithelial cell layer is prominence and hyperplasia. (H&E, (a) X120; (b) X200)

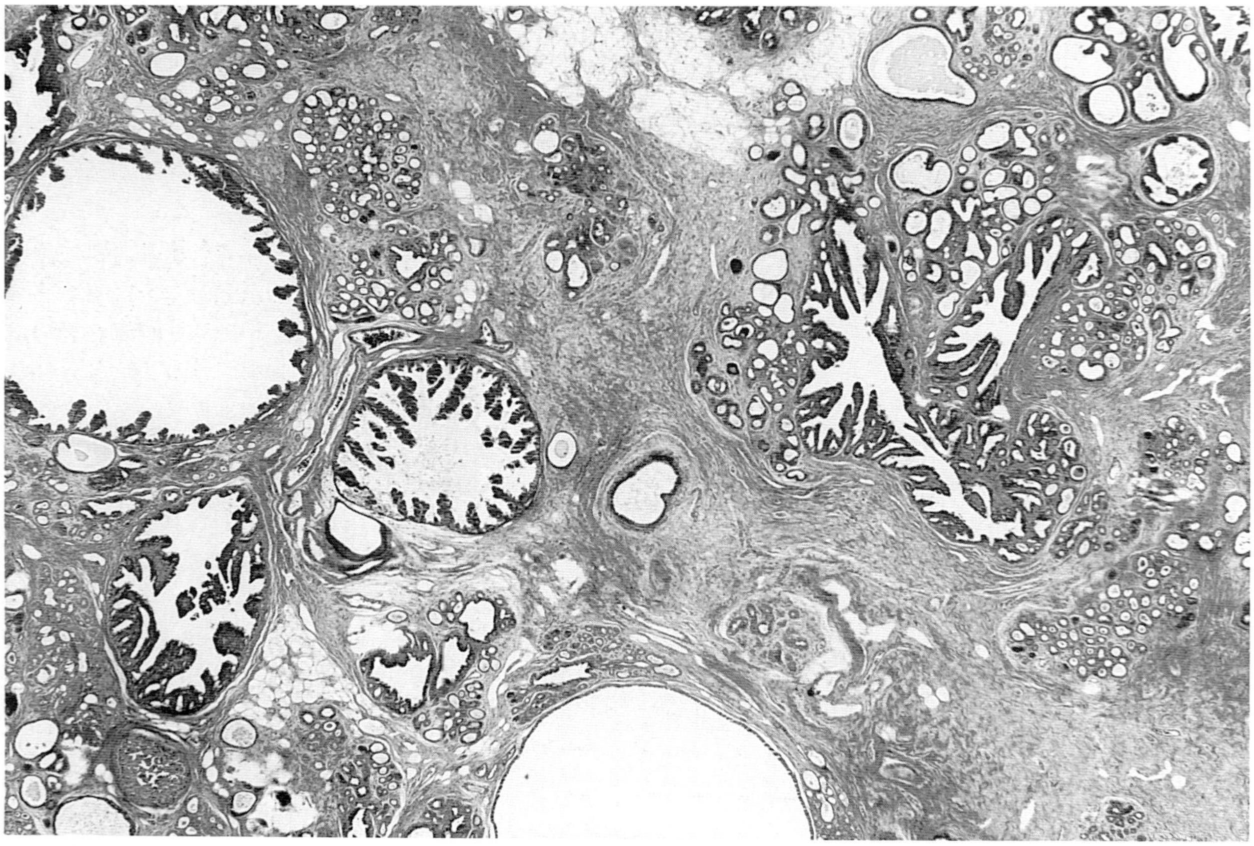

**Figure 6.11** Papillomatosis. Multiple peripheral ducts display various patterns of papillary intraluminal proliferation. (H&E, X30)

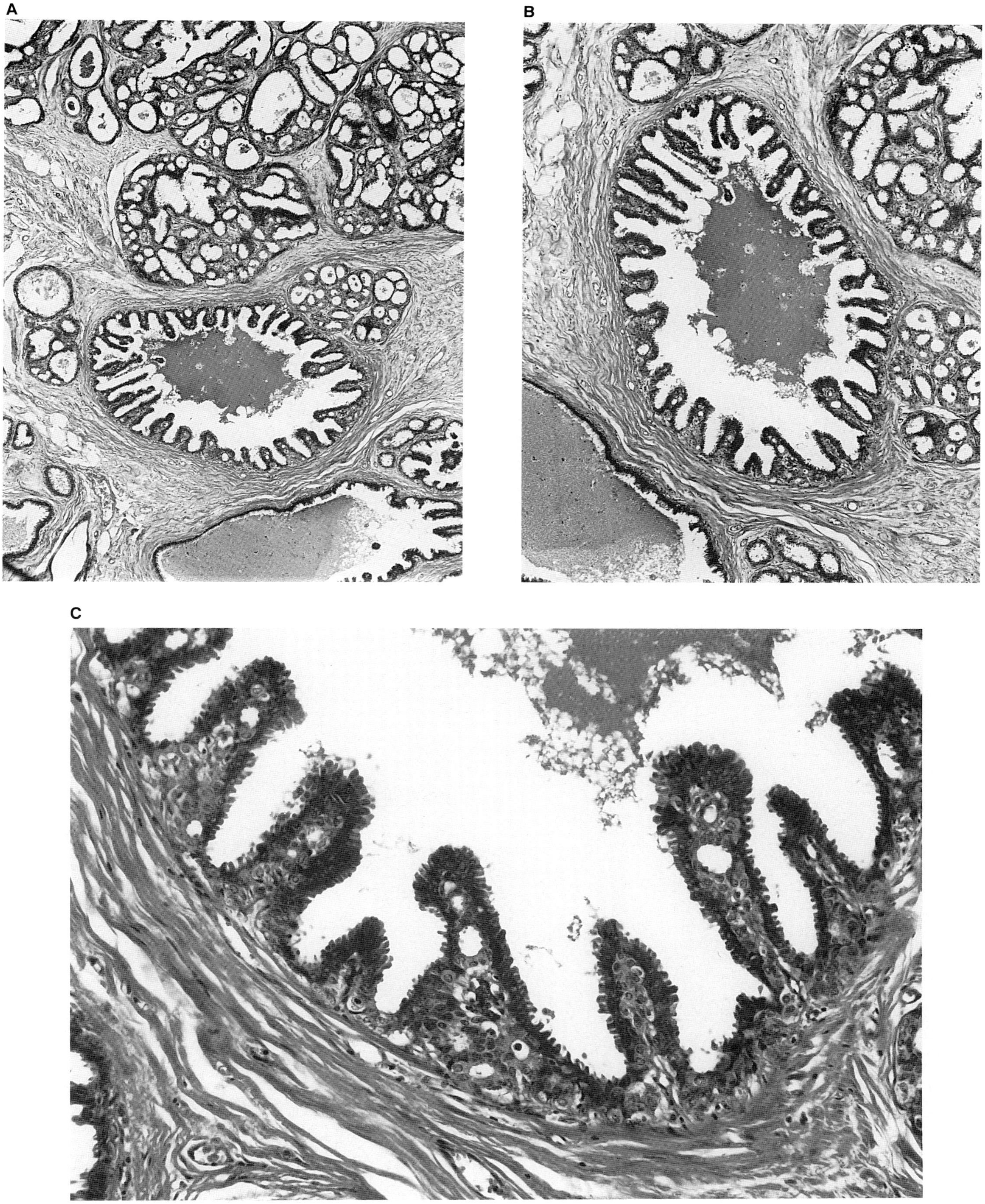

**Figure 6.12** Papillomatosis. (a) Multiple patterns of proliferation in the peripheral ducts. (b) Note the small papillary processes distributed all around this duct mimicking micropapillary carcinoma. (c) The papillary processes have epithelial and myoepithelial cell layers; the epithelial cells display prominent apical snouts. (H&E, (a) X40; (b) X60; (c) X150)

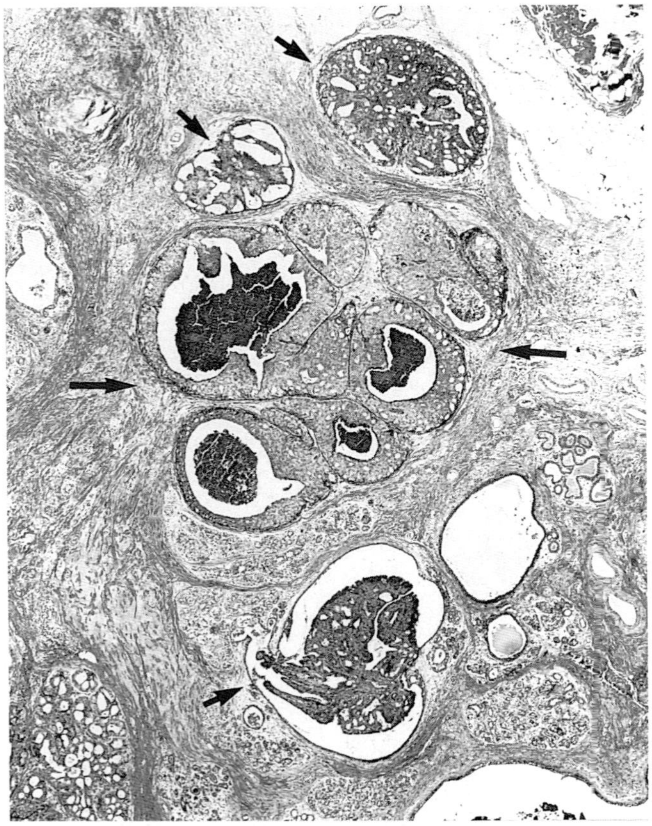

**Figure 6.13** Simultaneous papillomatosis and intraductal carcinoma. Several ducts between the two long arrows show intraductal carcinoma with central necrosis; papillomatosis is evident in the surrounding ducts (short arrows). (H&E, X15)

present as multiple lesions in the TDLU would qualify as atypical papillomatosis (Fig. 6.25). Alternatively, a small proportion of the papillary fronds in an otherwise benign papilloma will show stratification of the epithelial cells with loss of the ME cell layer. At least a third of the papillary fronds in a given section of a ductal space should show absence of the ME cell layer for the lesion to qualify as carcinoma arising in a papilloma. Otherwise, a designation of atypical papilloma would be appropriate.

The clinical significance of carcinoma arising in a papilloma has not been established, however. It is possible that when only a third of a papillary lesion is replaced by intraductal carcinoma, it would have a different behavior compared to one in which close to 90% of the lesion displays features of a carcinoma. Until data becomes available on the significance of carcinoma arising in a papilloma, it is proposed that when less than a third of a papillary lesion within a given cross section of a ductal space displays a proliferation morphologically indistinguishable from carcinoma, it should be regarded as atypical papilloma. Those with at least a third, but less than 90%, of the lesion displaying such areas, should be designated as carcinomas arising in a papilloma, with a

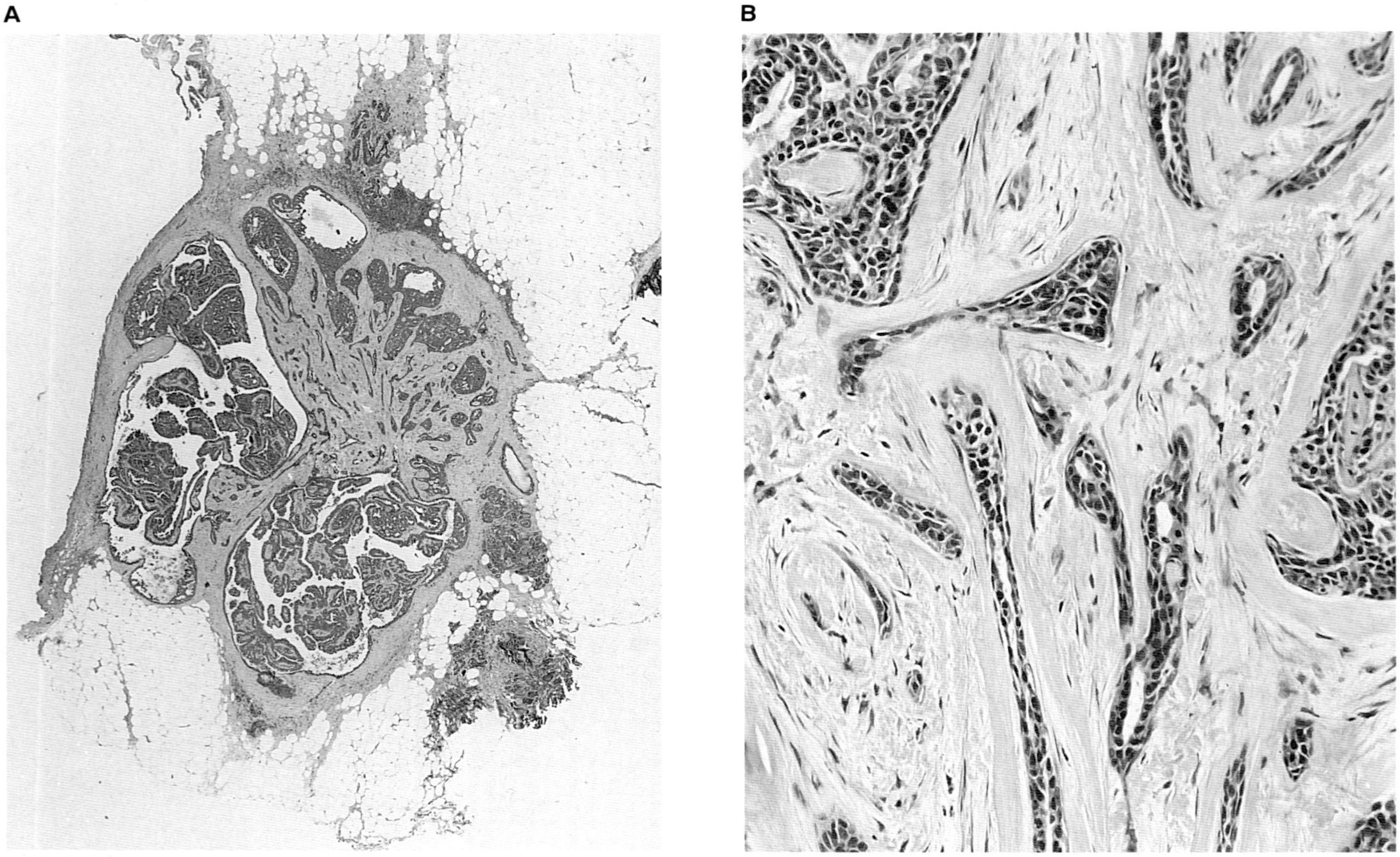


**Figure 6.14** Sclerosing papilloma. (a) About a third of this lesion appears relatively solid at low magnification. (b) The more solid area shows distorted, compressed tubules within a dense, sclerotic stroma; the ME cell layer, though attenuated, is recognizable (arrow). (H&E, (a) X15; (b) X200)

A

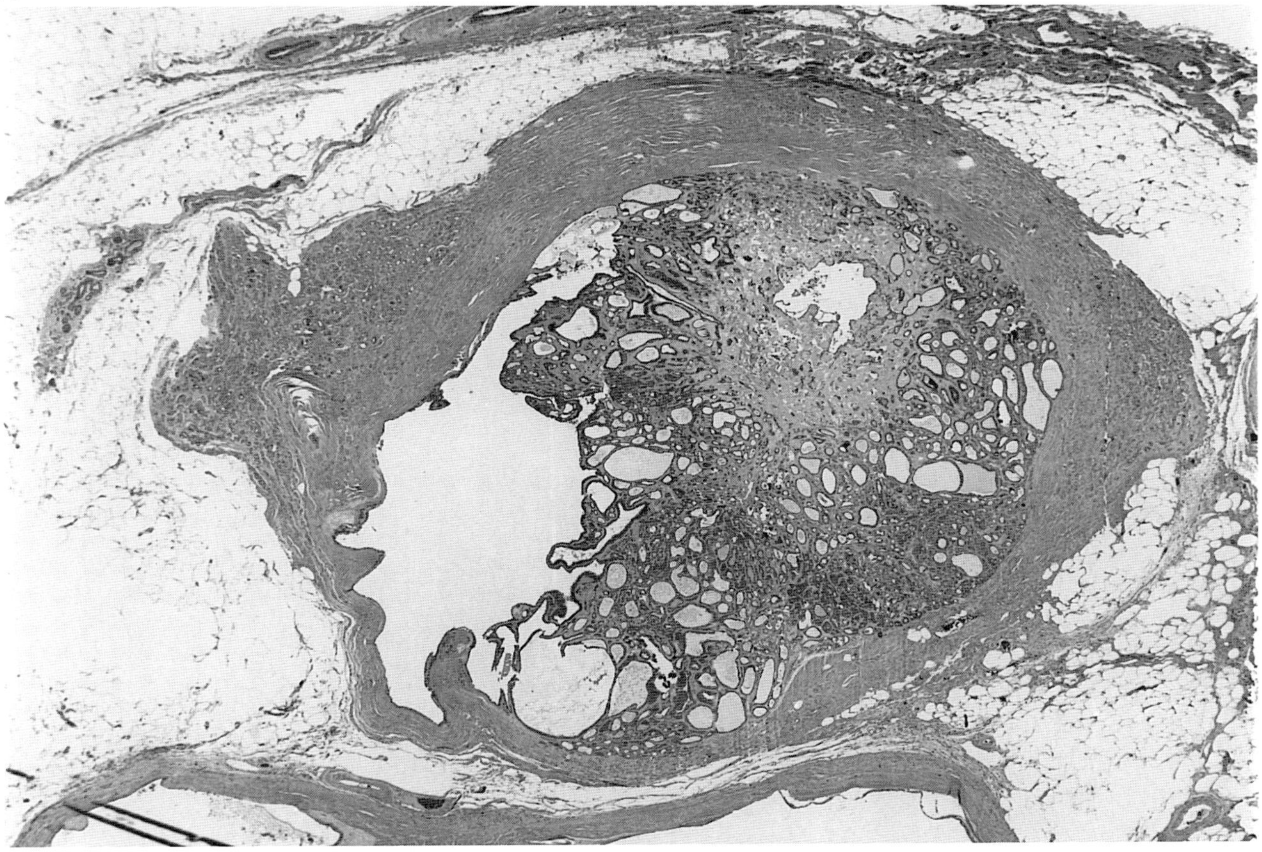

B

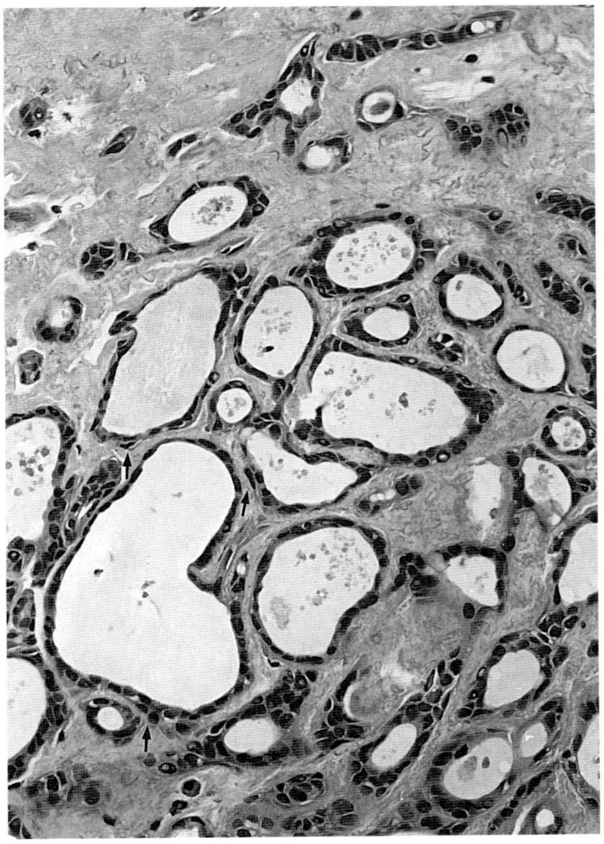

**Figure 6.15** Sclerosing papilloma. (a) A relatively solid, but fenestrated and sclerosing process with a minor papillary component (arrows) proliferates in a thick walled duct. (b) The sclerotic area shows numerous irregularly shaped tubules. All tubules are lined by an epithelial and a ME cell layer identifying them as benign. (H&E, (a) X15; (b) X240)

A

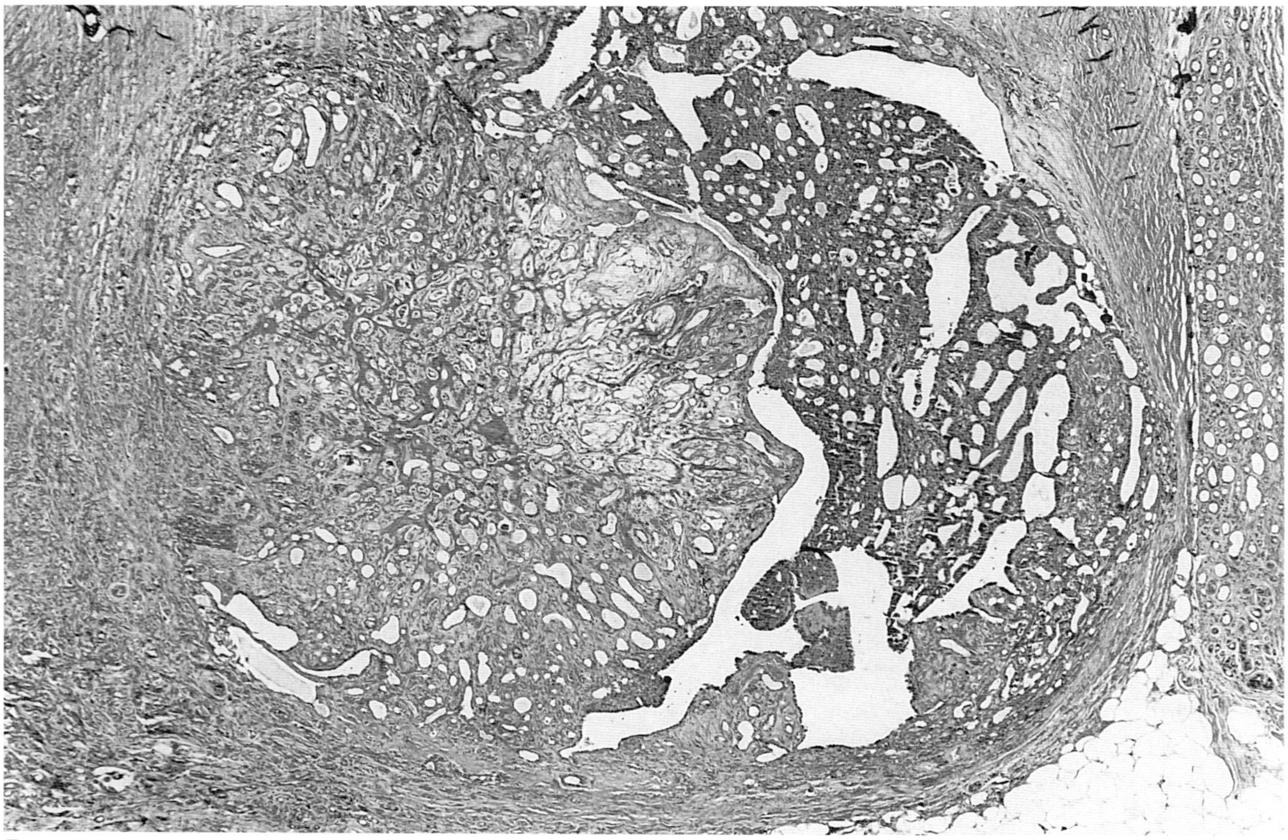

B

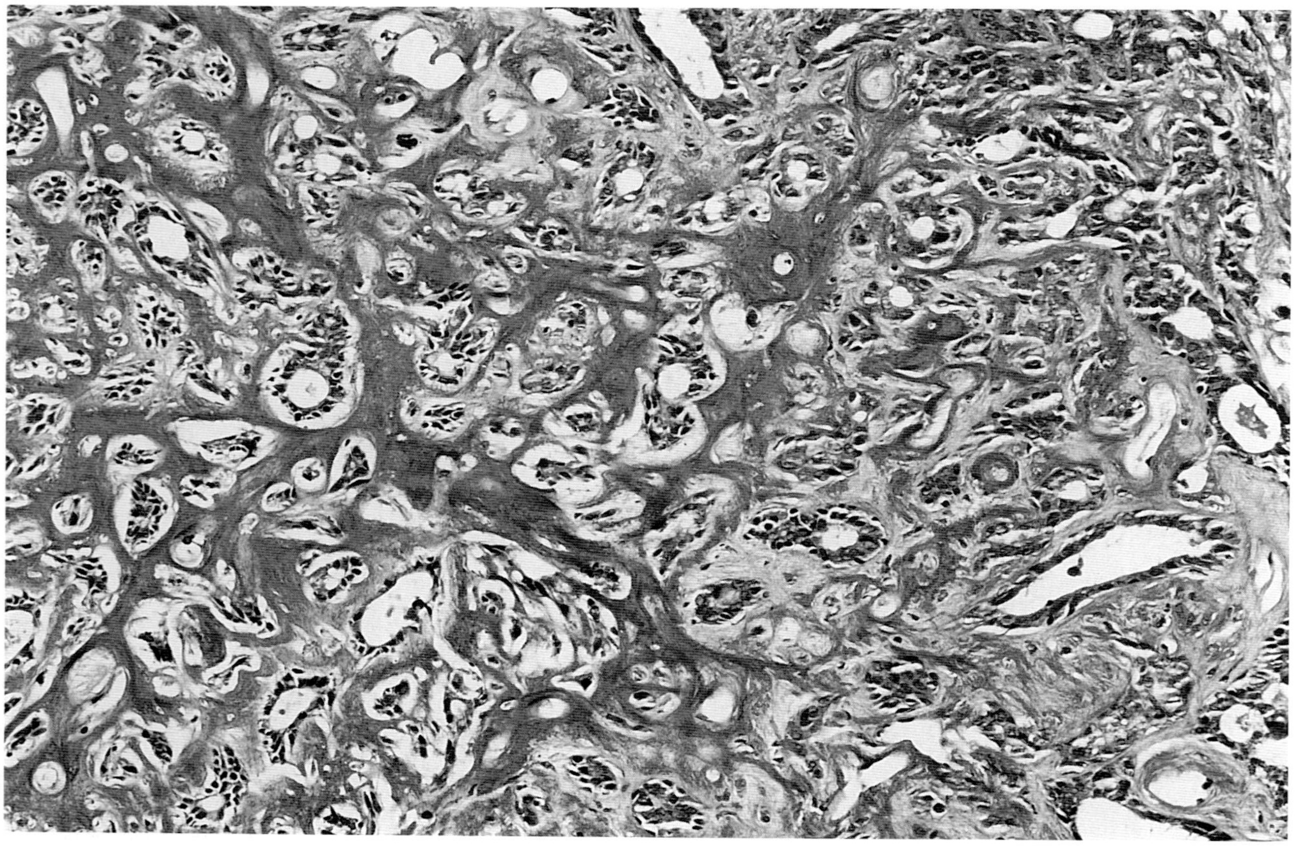

**Figure 6.16** Sclerosing papilloma. (a) A combination of intraluminal papillary and nodular sclerosing growth. (b) Despite the sclerosis, the myoepithelial cell layer around the entrapped tubules is apparent. (H&E, (a) X50; (b) X240)

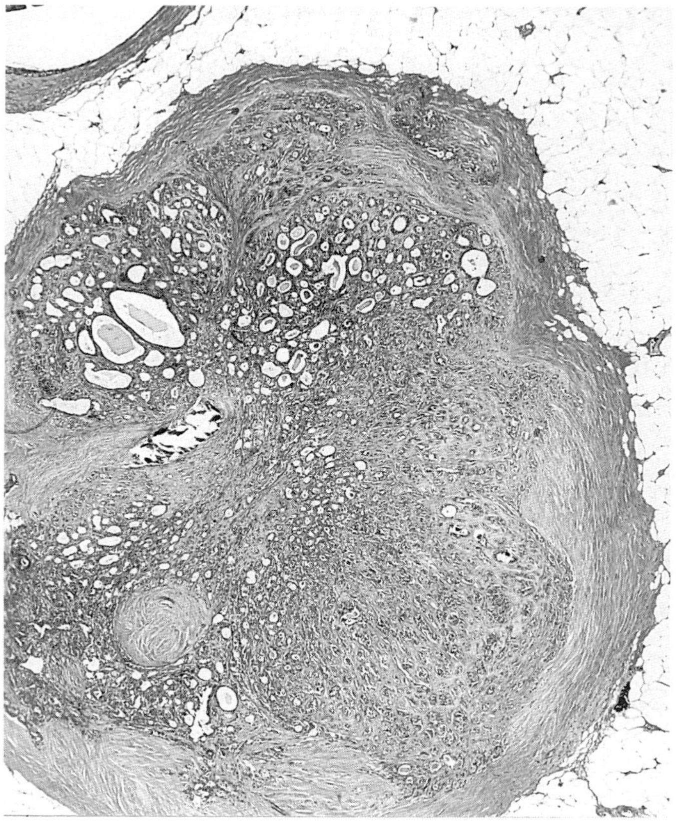

**Figure 6.17** Sclerosing papilloma (ductal adenoma). This variant is characterized by an occlusive, adenosis growth pattern within the duct lumen. The thick, fibrotic duct wall distinguishes this intraductal lesion from nodular sclerosing adenosis. The designation of ductal adenoma has been used for this lesion. (X30)

proviso added that these may be less aggressive than a fully-developed papillary carcinoma. The low degree of aggressiveness displayed by a classic, noninvasive papillary carcinoma, in general, justifies this conservative approach.

This quantitative criterion is completely arbitrary, but it is provided to serve as a guideline in categorizing these lesions until we have a large enough population and a long enough follow-up on such cases to determine the efficacy of these guidelines. Considering the fact that a fully-developed or classic papillary carcinoma is an intraductal lesion and not highly aggressive, it may be possible to eventually lump atypical papillomas and carcinoma arising in a papilloma together, facilitating future classification.

It is particularly important to distinguish central papillary carcinomas from the multifocal peripheral variety since the frequency of multifocality in the latter would necessitate a different therapeutic approach depending on the extent of the lesion. The peripheral multifocal papillary carcinoma is considered a variant of intraductal carcinoma since its origin in the TDLU and its distribution parallel that of intraductal carcinoma and would justify a similar management.

## Treatment

Total excision of atypical papilloma and carcinoma arising in a papilloma, with a rim of uninvolved breast tissue for the latter, is advised. Careful evaluation of the surrounding breast tissue is necessary to exclude the presence of intraductal carcinoma elsewhere in the more peripheral duct system. A clinicopathologic study of these lesions with at least 10 to 15 years of follow-up is necessary to establish their mode of behavior.

# PAPILLARY CARCINOMA

## Clinical Features

Papillary carcinoma accounts for approximately 2% of all breast carcinomas (39). The patients range in age from 25 to 89 years, with a majority being in the fifth and sixth decades of life (2,37,39,40). While most occur in women, papillary carcinomas also develop in the male breast (44). Nipple discharge occurs in 22% to 26% of patients (35,39), and in a majority the discharge is blood-tinged at least on some occasions. A palpable tumor is present in up to 90% of the patients; more than half of the tumors are centrally located. Occasionally, the lesion causes a protuberance with reddening of the overlying skin which may eventually ulcerate. Skin dimpling, nipple retraction, or deviation occurs in 28% of the patients. In some reports, the term papillary carcinoma has been used for the solitary, centrally located lesions excluding the microscopic, multifocal lesions that are located more peripherally in the duct system. In contrast to solitary, centrally-located papillary carcinomas which often present with a lump or nipple discharge, the multifocal, peripheral papillary carcinomas may not be palpable and actually present as microscopic lesions in up to 50% of cases.

Papillary carcinoma is a variant of intraductal carcinoma but unequivocal stromal invasion occurs in

A B

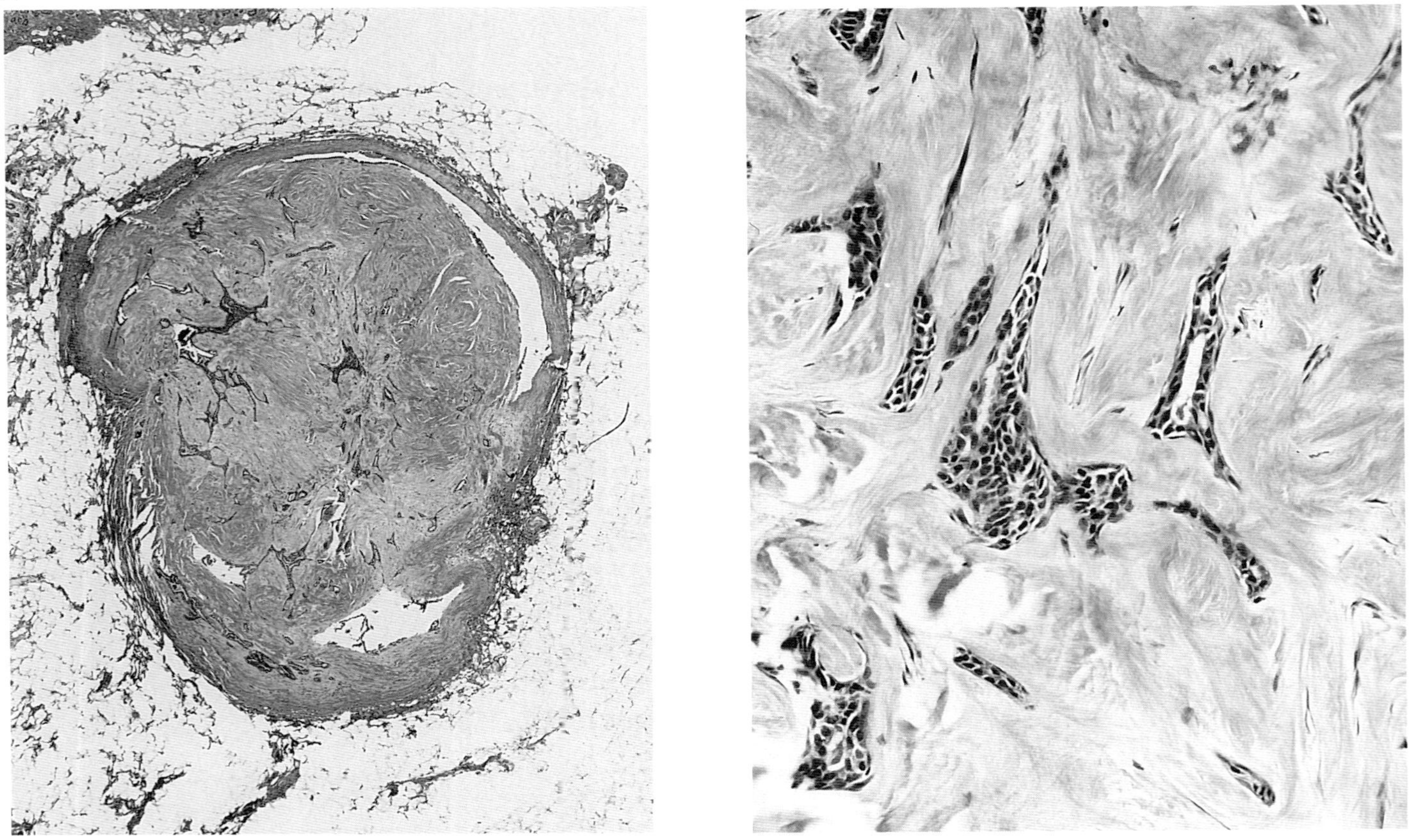

**Figure 6.18** Sclerosing papilloma. (a) An almost end stage sclerosing papilloma with a crescent of the residual duct lumen apparent at the top. (X20) (b) Despite the distortion, an attenuated layer of spindle ME cells is apparent around most of these tubules. (X200)

A B

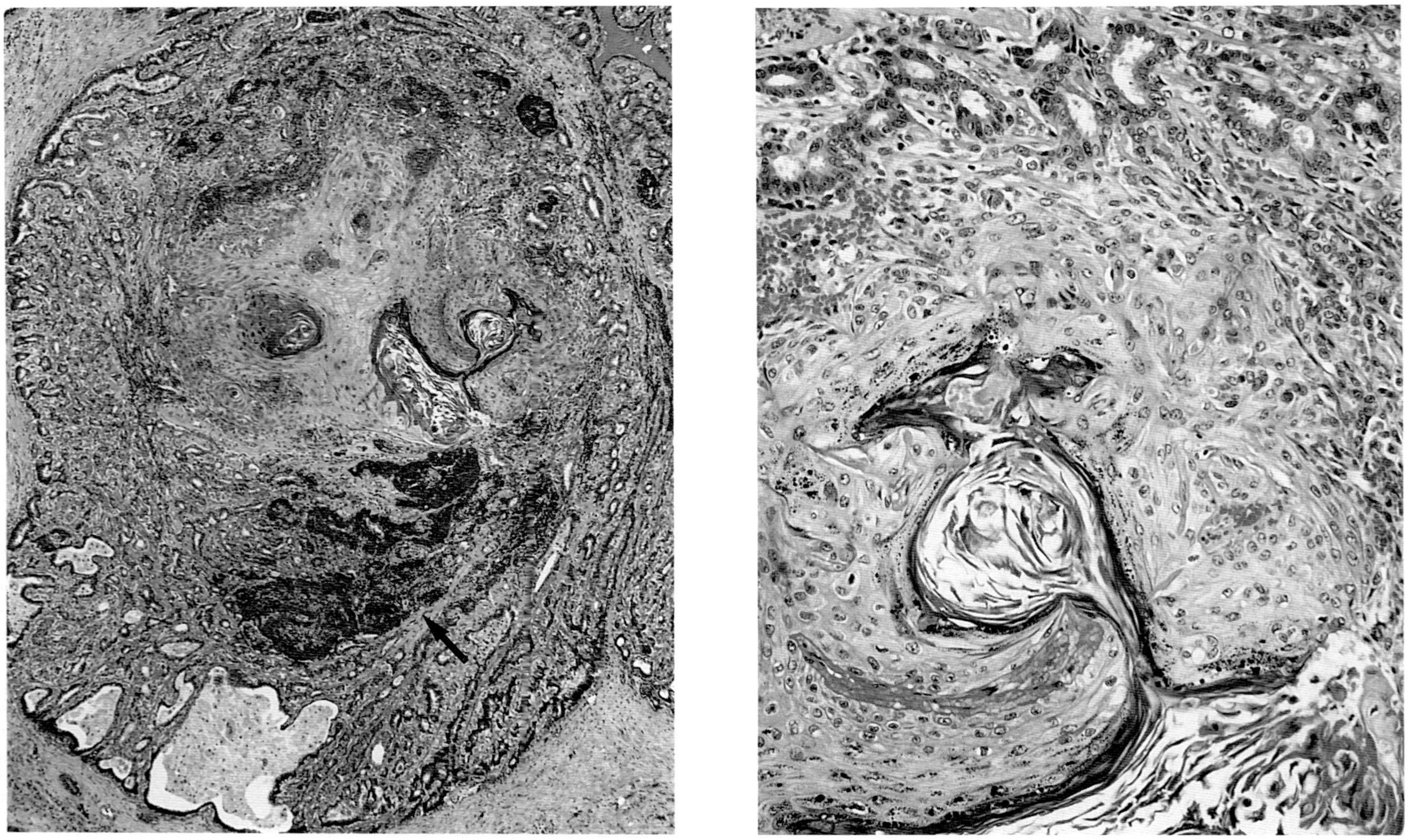

**Figure 6.19(a&b)** Sclerosing papilloma with extensive squamous metaplasia. (H&E, (a) X60; (b) X160)

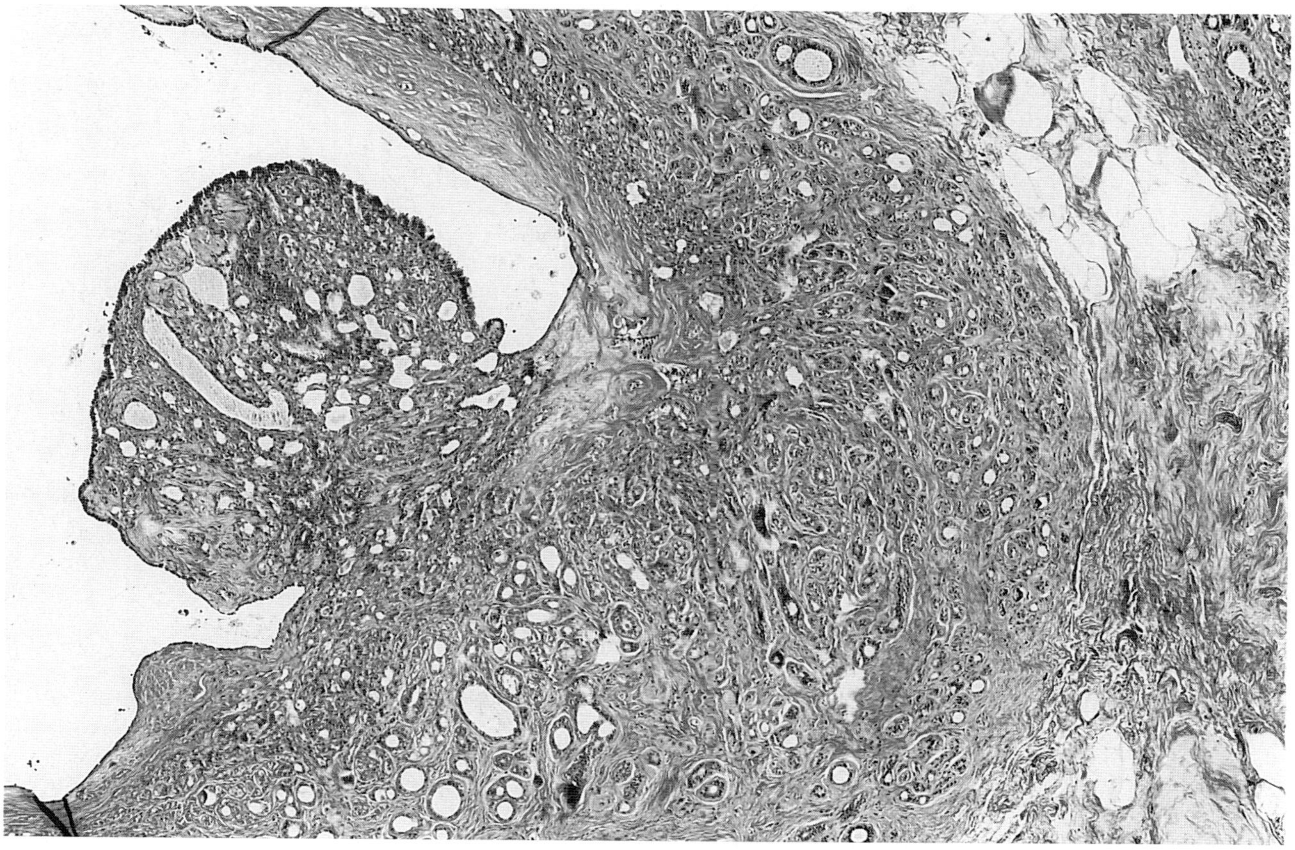

**Figure 6.20** Sclerosing papilloma. In this lesion, there is extensive sclerosing adenosis proliferating around and into the duct lumen. (H&E, X50)

a small minority (38). Many papers on papillary carcinomas have not specified the proportion of cases with stromal invasion. In the absence of stromal or vascular invasion, these tumors basically reflect a variant of in situ or intraductal carcinoma localized to a single duct. Therefore, the absence of axillary node metastases and the excellent survival rates are not at all surprising. With follow-up of up to 15 years (2), there is no report of a woman having died from papillary carcinoma. Obviously, those tumors associated with invasion are expected to behave more aggressively. The five-year survival rate for invasive papillary carcinoma in Murad et al's (6) series was 93.4% with 79.8% of the patients remaining disease free at five years.

## Macroscopic Features

The grossly visible, centrally located, papillary carcinoma grows either within a dilated duct that simply expands to accommodate the proliferating lesion or one that becomes cystically dilated. In my opinion, the term intracystic papillary carcinoma should be restricted to those associated with a grossly visible cyst (Fig. 6.26). Otherwise, all papillary carcinomas are in effect located within a dilated, cystic duct and the term would serve no distinctive purpose. Papillary carcinoma may appear actually papillary, or it may be nodular with a somewhat shaggy or rough surface. Hemorrhage is not uncommon because either some or all of the papillary structures may undergo torsion and hemorrhagic infarction. The tumors are generally about 2.5 to 3 cm in size, soft and friable.

## Microscopic Features

The quintessential morphologic feature of papillary carcinoma is the absence of a ME cell layer in the papillary processes proliferating into the distended duct lumen (Fig. 6.27). Generally, an experienced pathologist, familiar with the range of appearances of ME cells, can readily determine the presence or absence of a myoepithelial cell layer. If difficulty is

A B

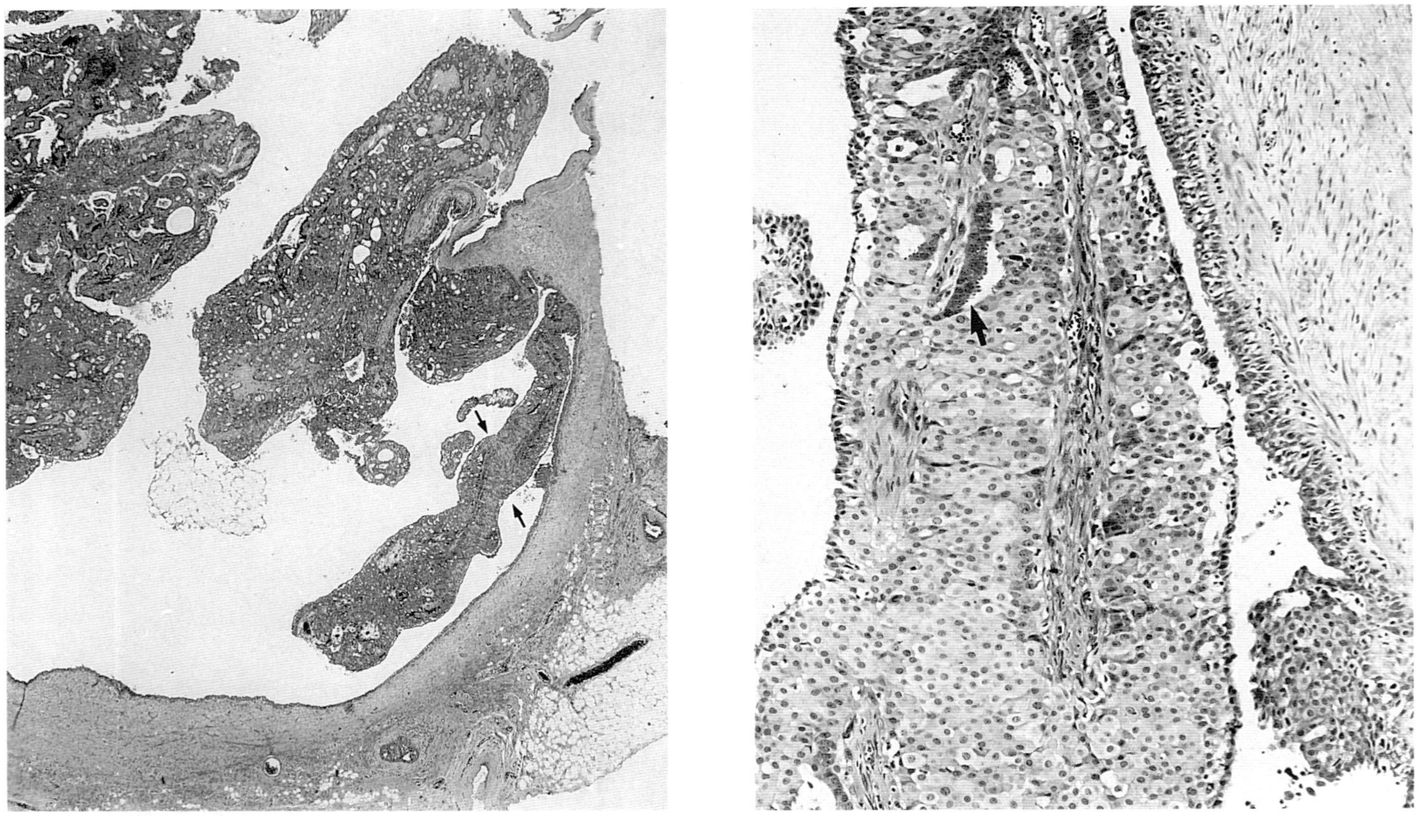

**Figure 6.21** Atypical papilloma. (a) A cystically-dilated duct shows several papillary processes, one of which displays a sheet-like cellular proliferation (arrows). (b) The proliferating cells are uniform in appearance and replace the original epithelial cell layer (arrow) in some areas and extend under the adjacent epithelial cell layer elsewhere. This area reflects atypical hyperplasia. (H&E, (a) X30; (b) X120)

A B

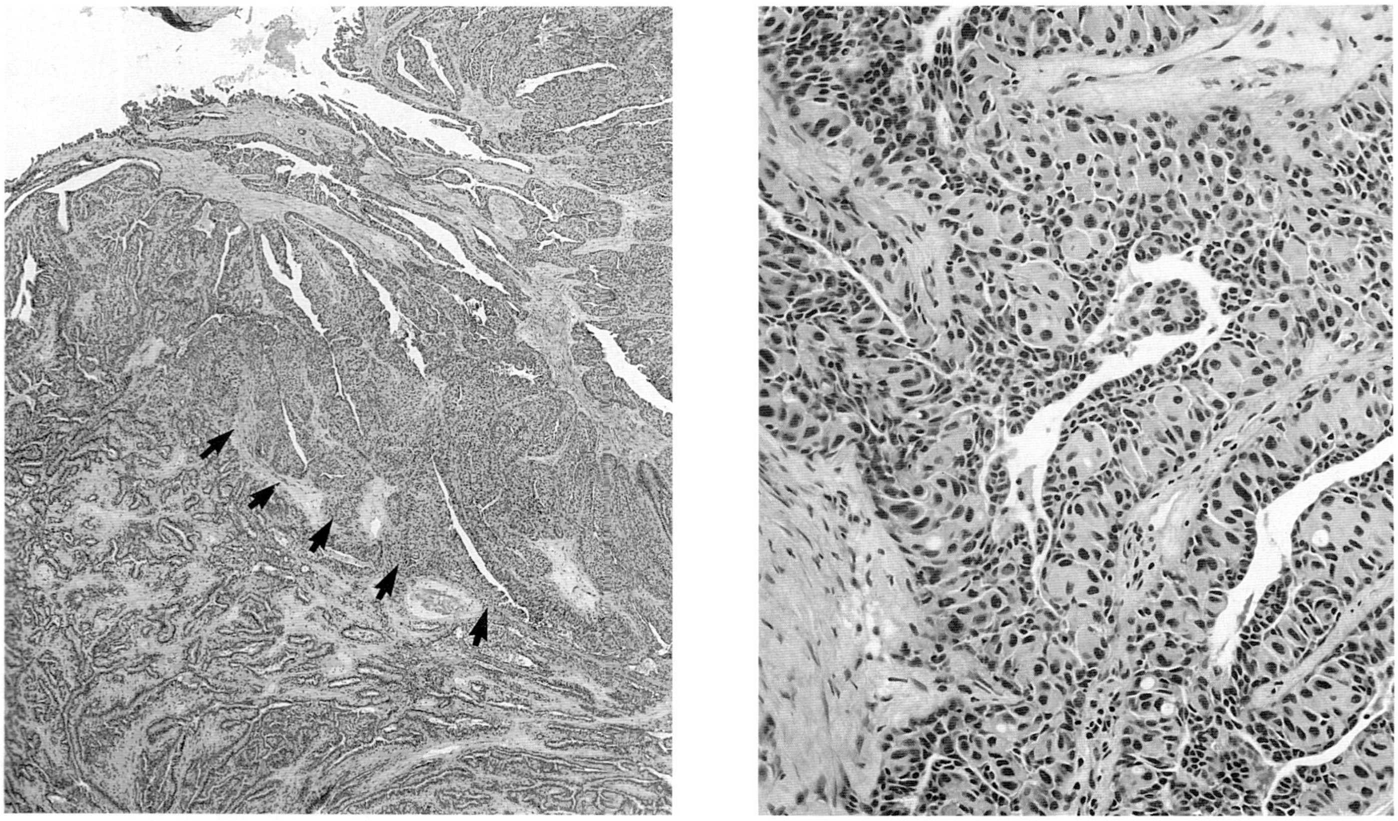

**Figure 6.22** Atypical papilloma (Lobular neoplasia involving a papilloma). (a) A portion of the papilloma (arrows) appears more cellular than the rest of the lesion. (b) These cells are proliferating in a pagetoid fashion between the epithelial and ME cell layers and, despite their large size, suggest lobular neoplasia involving the papilloma. (H&E, (a) X30; (b) X200)

A

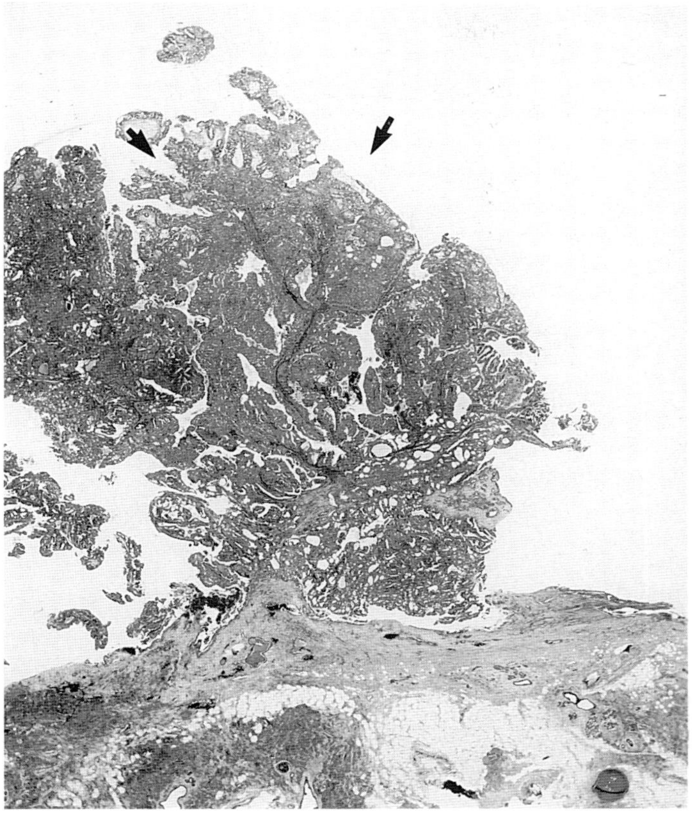

B

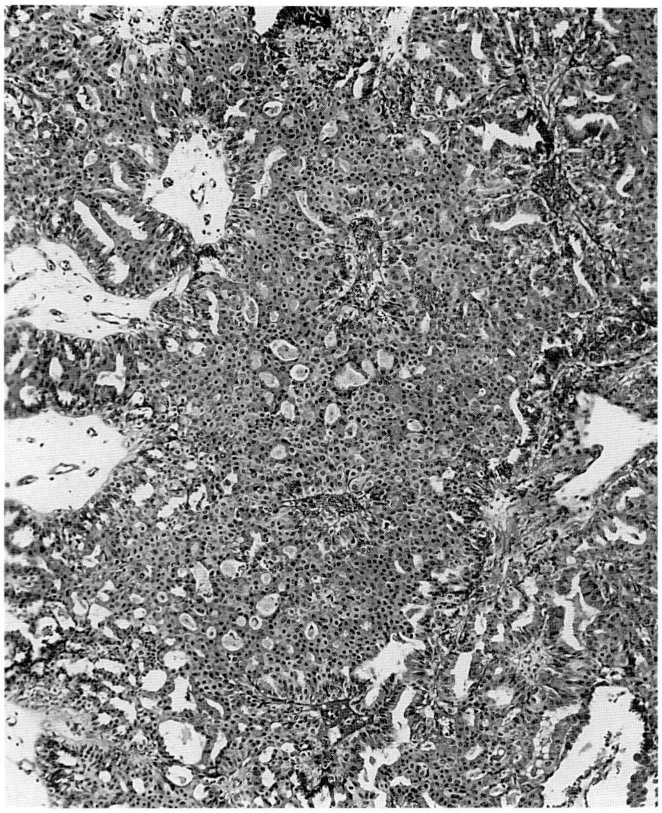

C

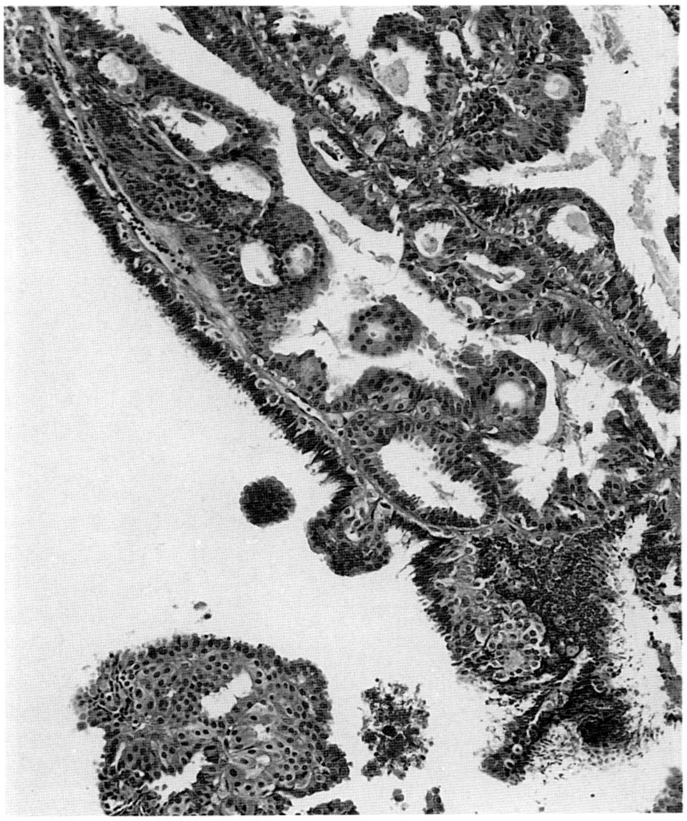

**Figure 6.23** Atypical papilloma. (a) Some of the papillary processes appear broader and more cellular (arrows). (X7.5) (b) The atypical cellular area constitutes less than a third of the lesion and is composed of a fenestrated proliferation of a uniform cell population similar to the cribriform variant of intraductal carcinoma. (X75) (c) Elsewhere, typical benign papillary processes lined by epithelial and ME cells abound. (X120)

A

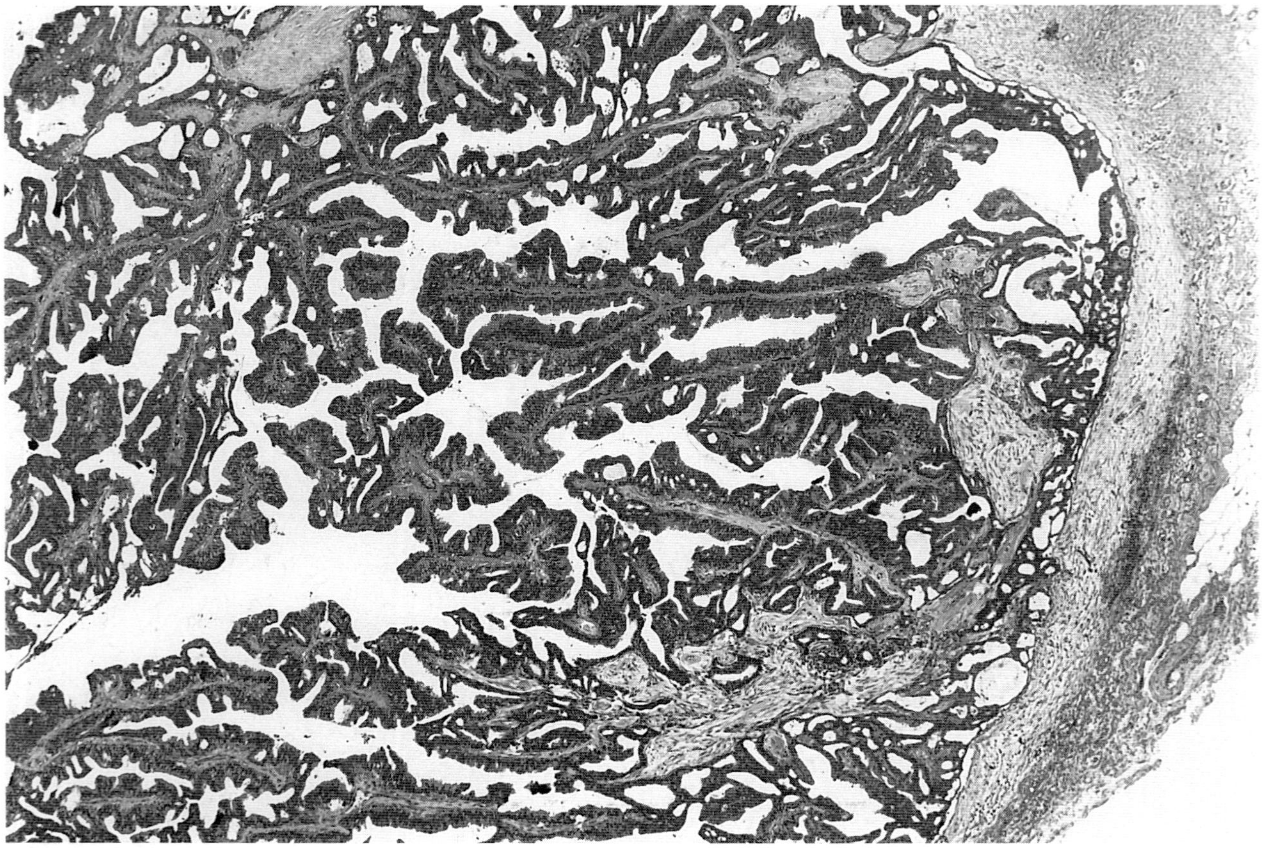

B

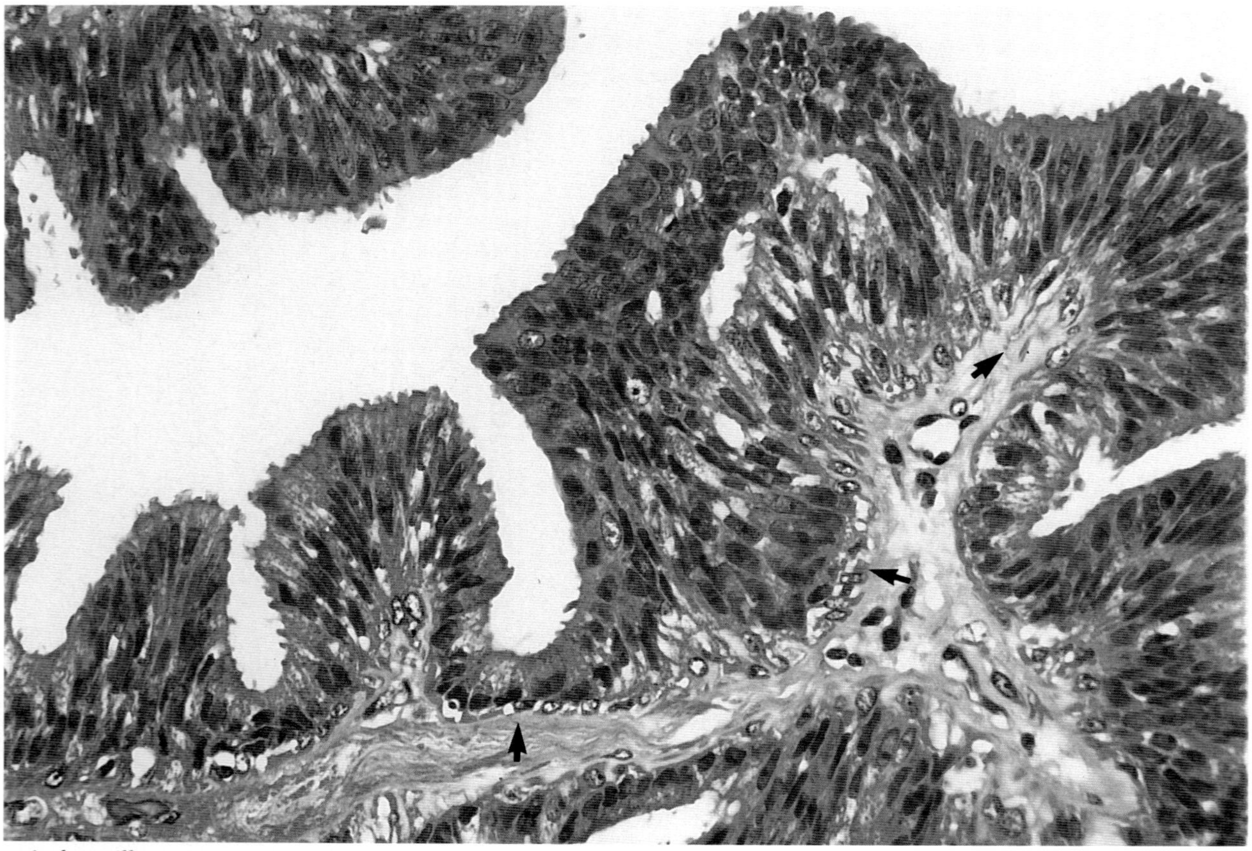

**Figure 6.24** Atypical papilloma. (a) At low magnification, papillary processes with delicate fibrovascular stalks are evident. The stratified spindle cell appearance of the proliferating epithelial cells suggest a papillary carcinoma. (X60) (b) At higher magnification, the epithelial cells appear spindled and stratified, but a distinct myoepithelial cell layer is apparent (arrows) throughout the lesion, excluding the diagnosis of carcinoma and qualifying the lesion as an atypical papilloma. (X300)

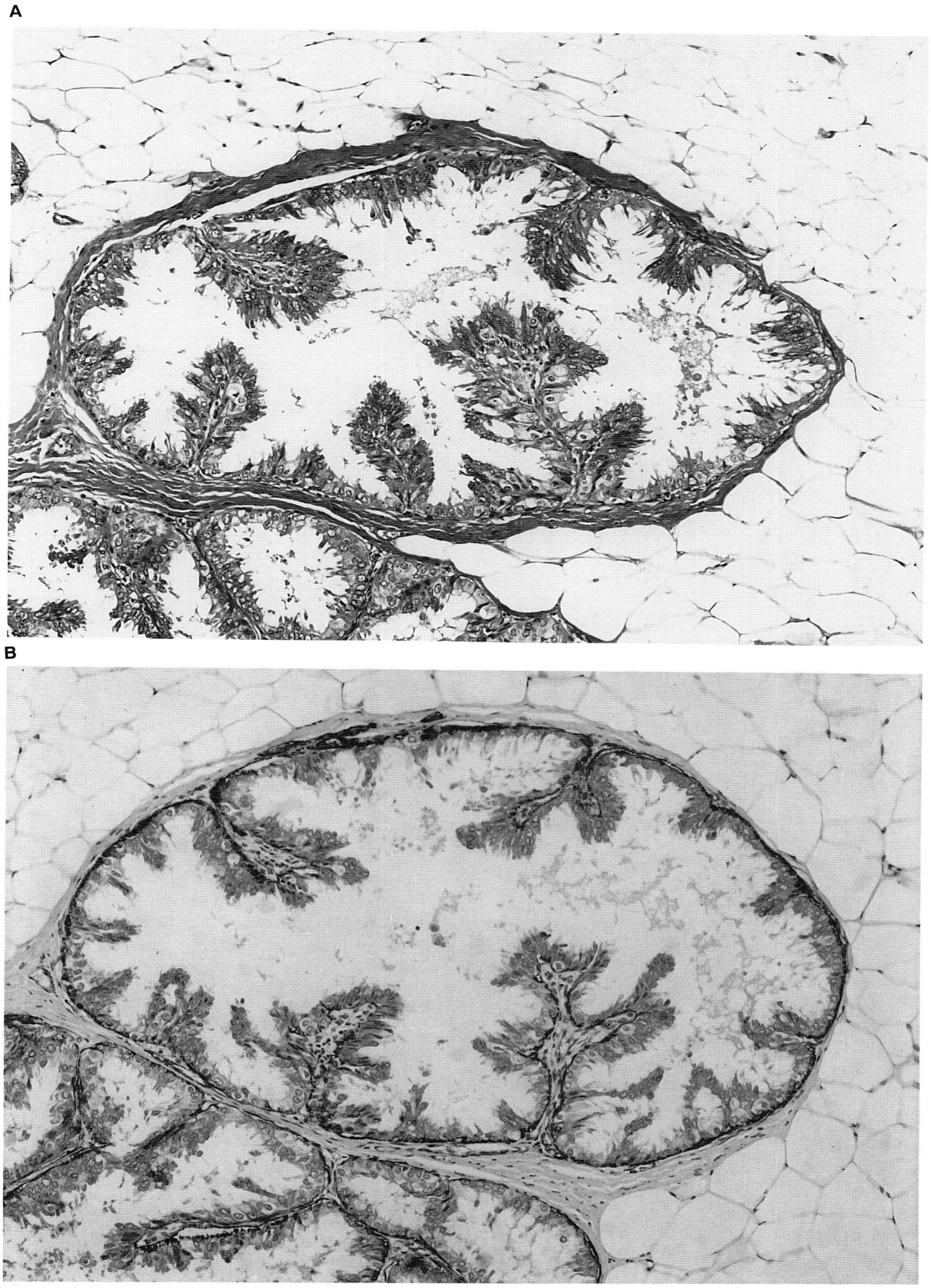


**Figure 6.25** Atypical papillomatosis. (a) Papillary processes in a peripheral duct show stratified spindle cells. (b) Immunostain for actin decorates the ME cell layer in the papillae and around the entire duct. (H&E, (a) X120; Immunostain for actin, (b) X120)

C

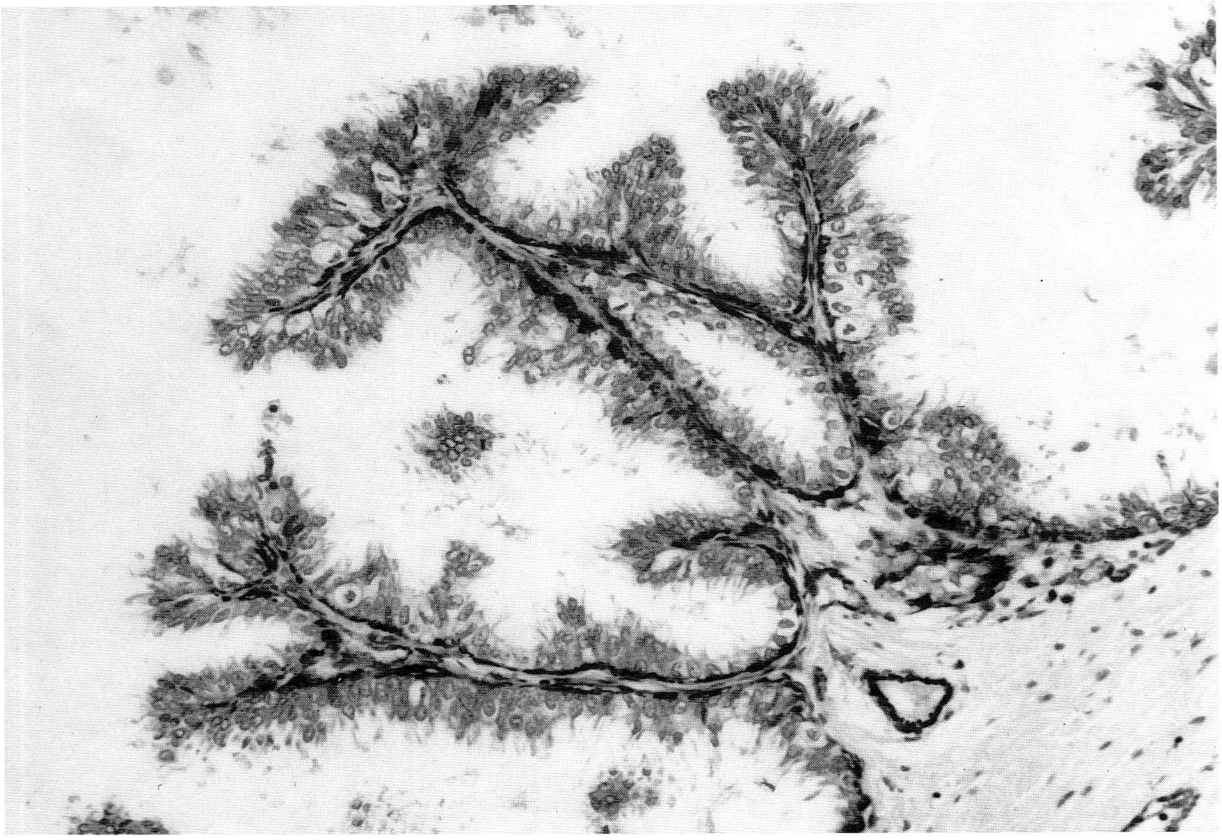

**Figure 6.25(c)** Atypical papillomatosis. The plump cells (arrows) are not myoepithelial cells, but a second epithelial cell population. (Immunostain for actin, X240)

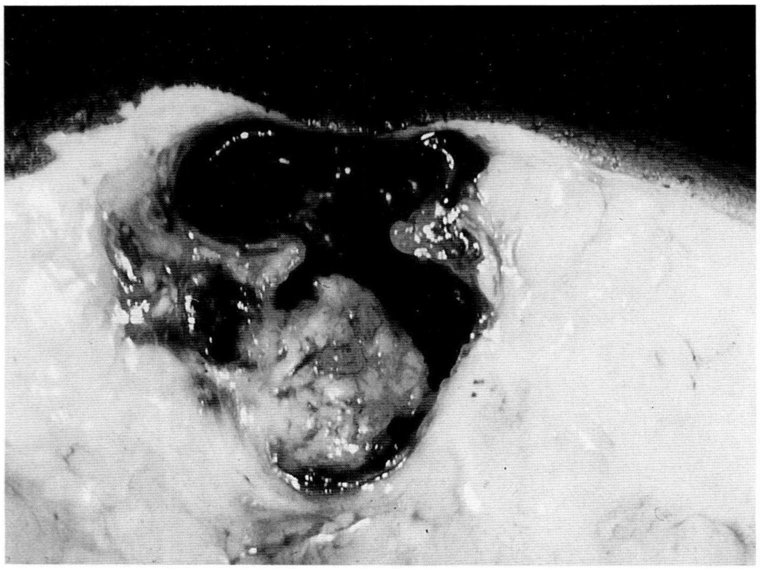

**Figure 6.26** Intracystic papillary carcinoma. A grossly visible cyst qualifies this lesion as an intracystic papillary lesion.

A B C

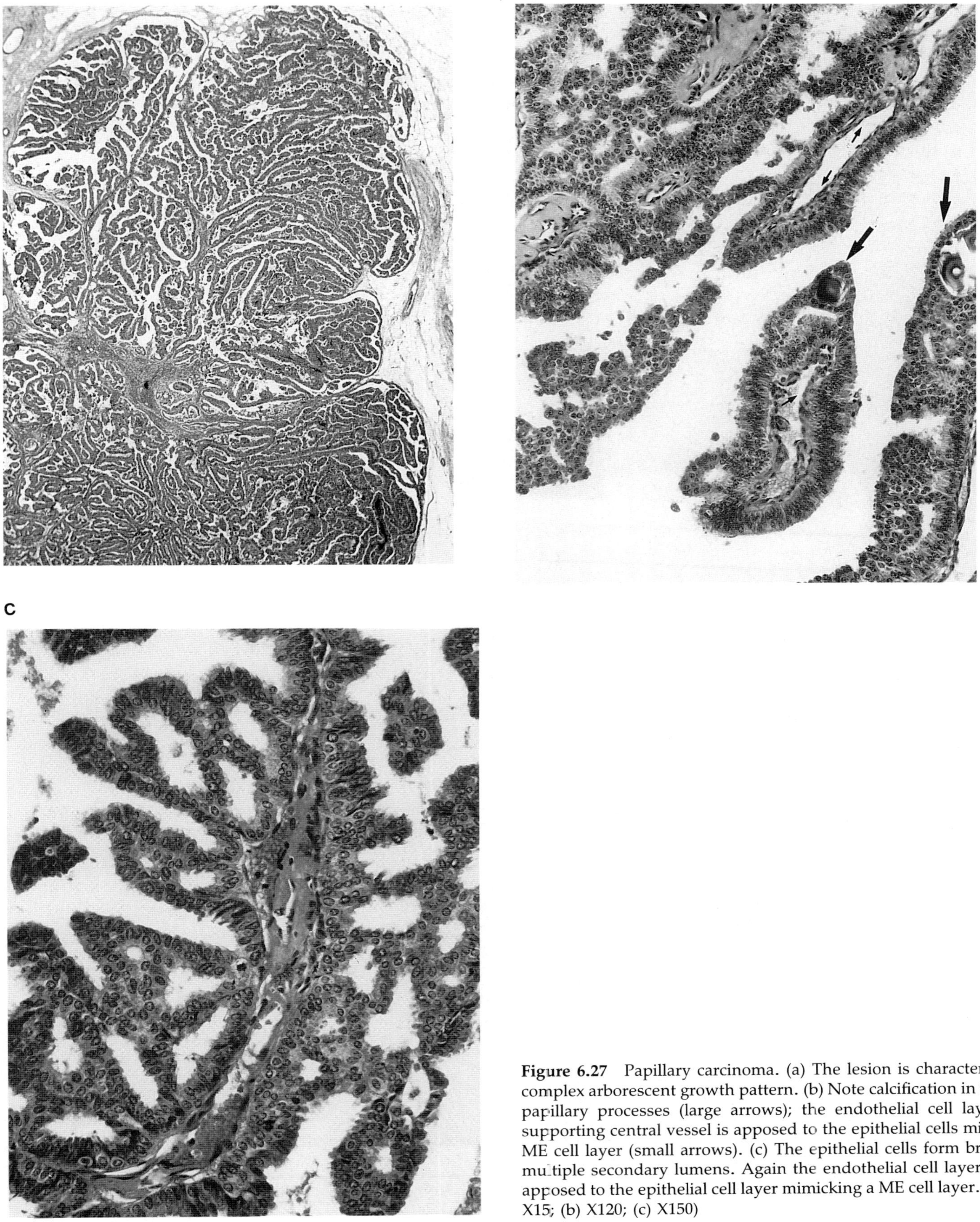

**Figure 6.27** Papillary carcinoma. (a) The lesion is characterized by a complex arborescent growth pattern. (b) Note calcification in two of the papillary processes (large arrows); the endothelial cell layer of the supporting central vessel is apposed to the epithelial cells mimicking a ME cell layer (small arrows). (c) The epithelial cells form bridges and multiple secondary lumens. Again the endothelial cell layer is closely apposed to the epithelial cell layer mimicking a ME cell layer. (H&E, (a) X15; (b) X120; (c) X150)

A

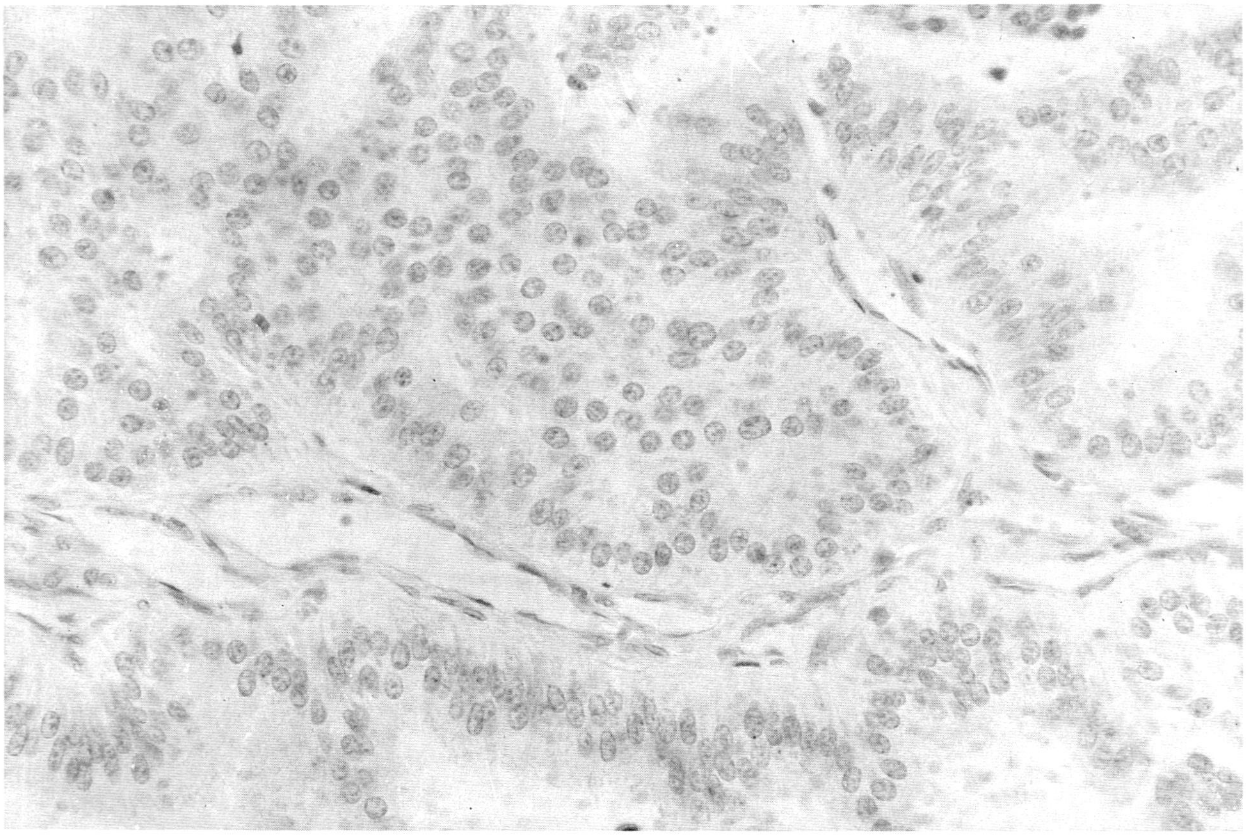

B

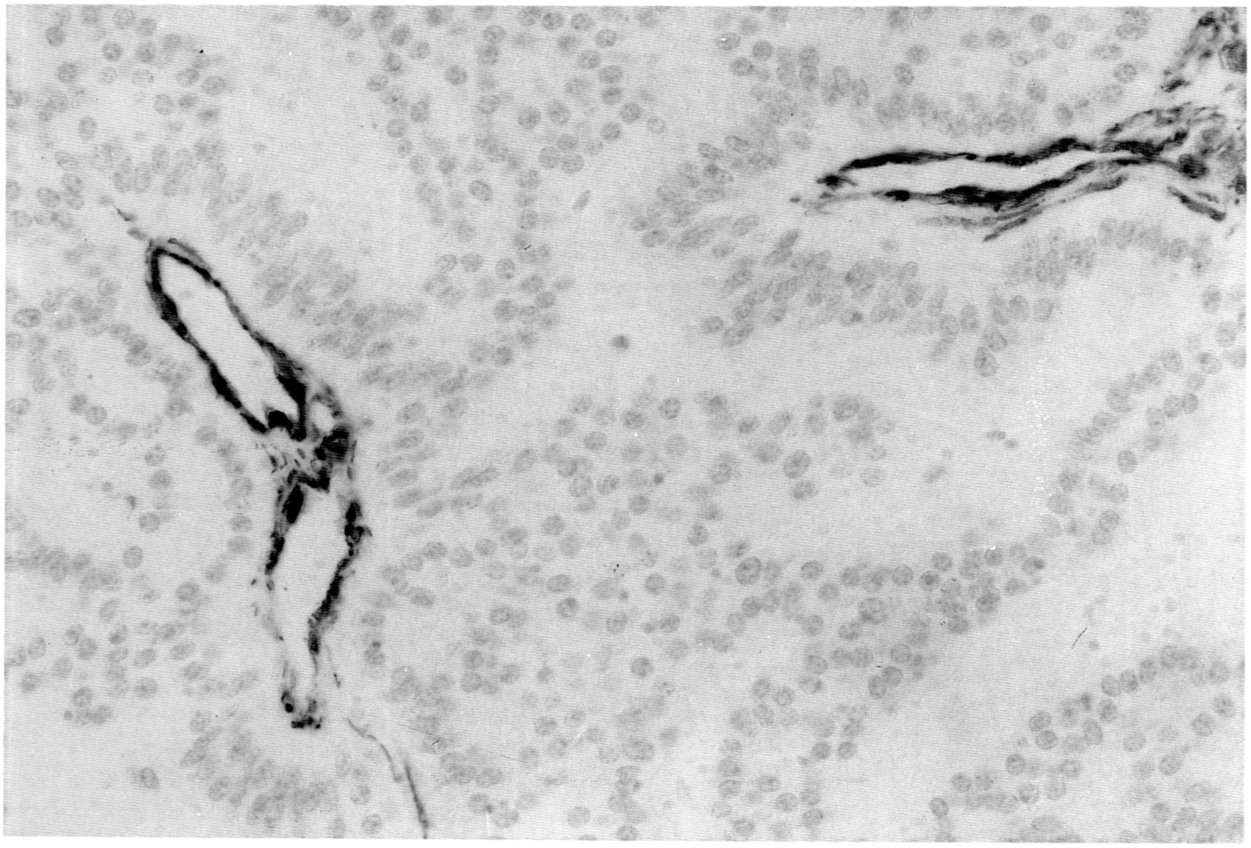

**Figure 6.28** (a) Immunostain for S-100 protein shows no evidence of a ME cell layer. (X600) (b) Immunostain for actin does decorate the vascular spaces and should not be misinterpreted as reflecting the presence of a ME cell layer. (X600)

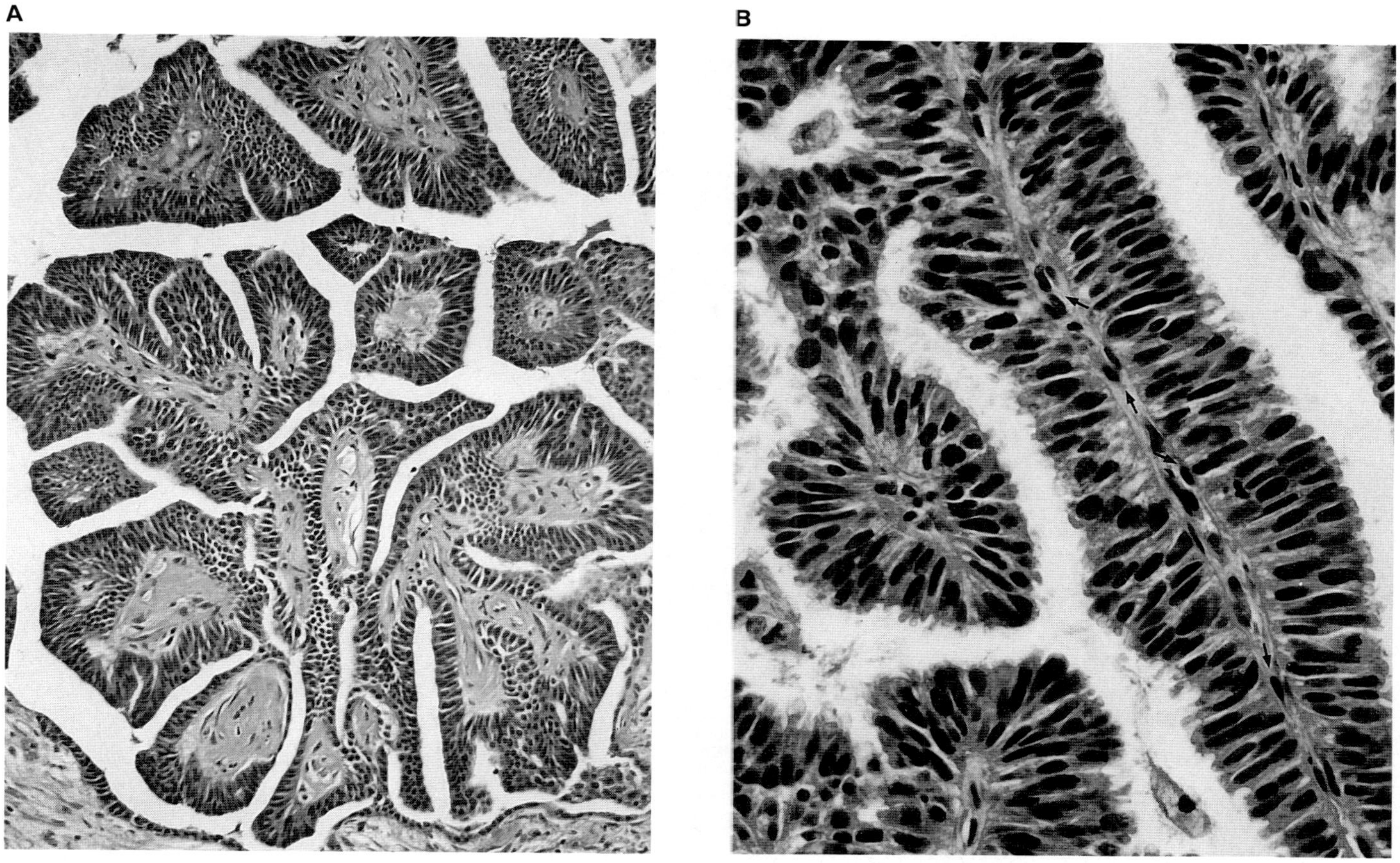


**Figure 6.29** Papillary carcinoma, stratified spindle cell variant. The spindle cells are more atypical than usual and the ME cell layer is absent, but the delicate endothelial-lined vascular spaces may be confused with a ME cell layer. (X75) (b) Elsewhere in the same lesion, the absence of the ME cell layer is more readily appreciated. (X400)

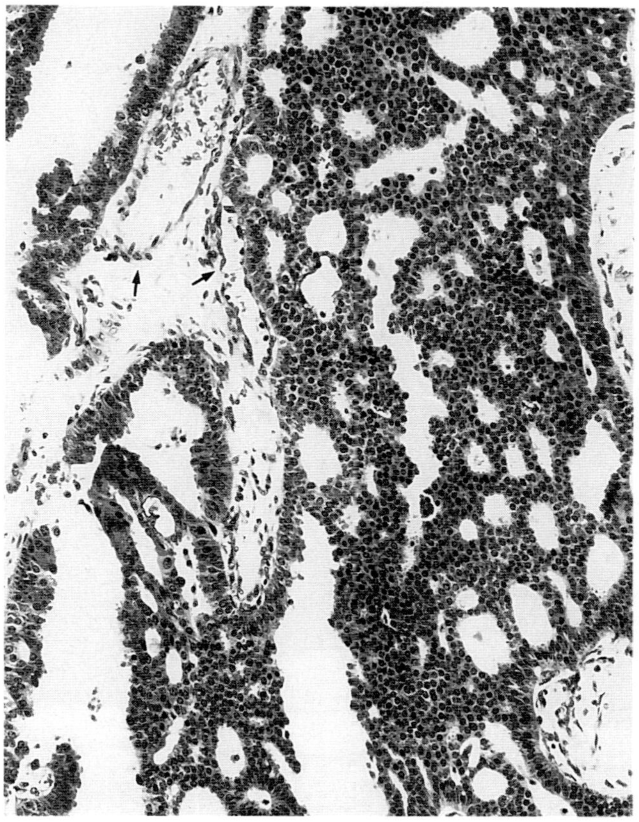

**Figure 6.30** Papillary carcinoma. The epithelial cells show a cribriform pattern of proliferation overlying the fibrovascular stalks. There is no ME cell layer. The endothelial-lined vascular spaces (arrows) should not be mistaken for a ME cell layer. (X100)

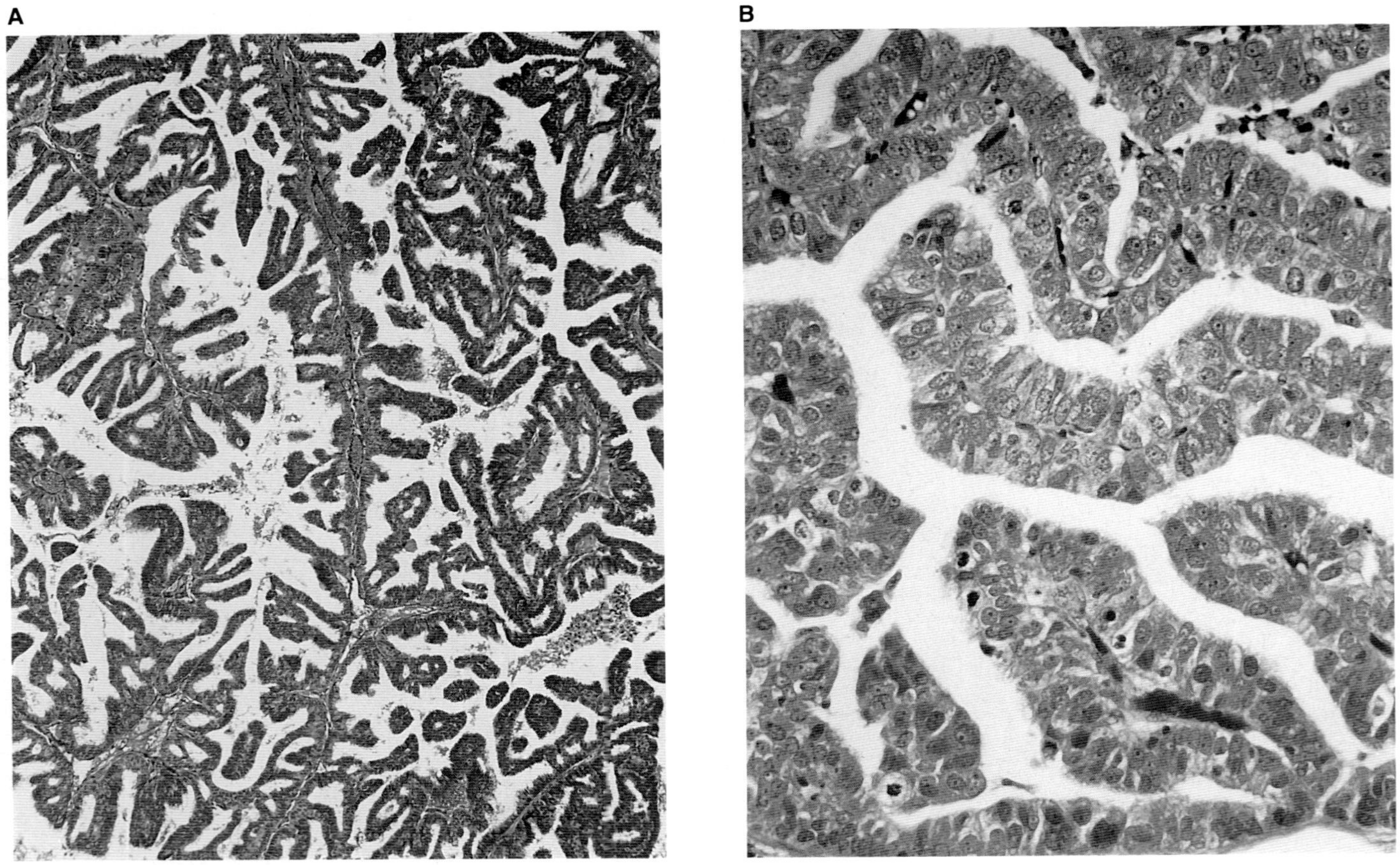


**Figure 6.31** Papillary carcinoma. (a) The delicate main papillary processes show epithelial proliferation in the form of tufts. (X60) (b) The smaller papillary processes have a delicate vascular core; the epithelial cells are atypical and the ME cell layer is absent. (X250)

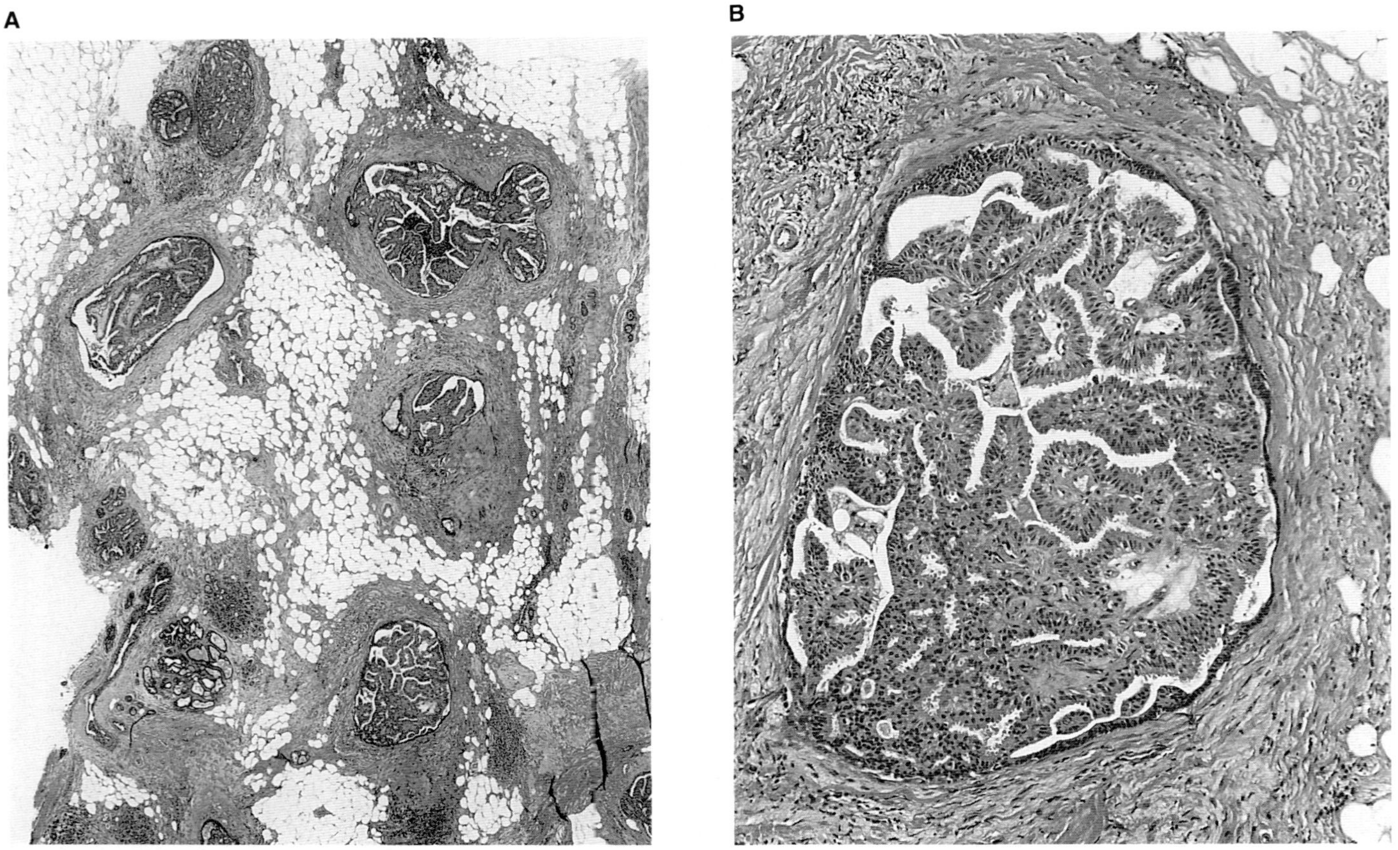


**Figure 6.32** Multifocal peripheral papillary carcinoma (Intraductal carcinoma, stratified spindle cell papillary variant). (a) In contrast to the centrally-located solitary papillary carcinomas, this lesion is multifocal, located in the TDLU, and often shows an admixture with benign papillomatosis. (X12) (b) The absence of a ME cell layer qualifies this papillary proliferation as malignant. (X120)

A

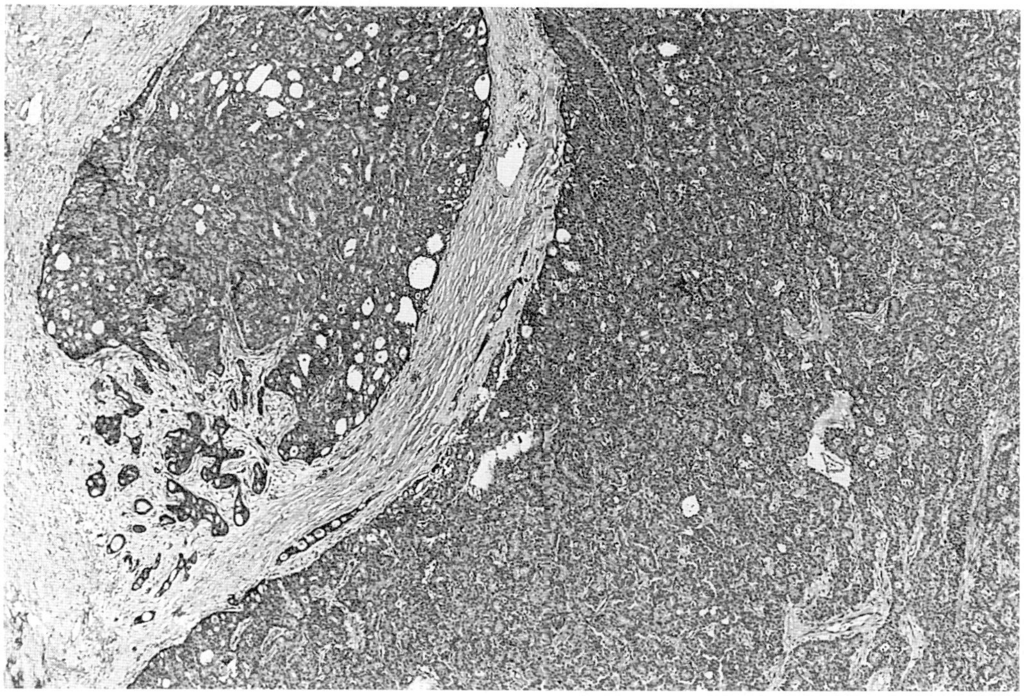

B

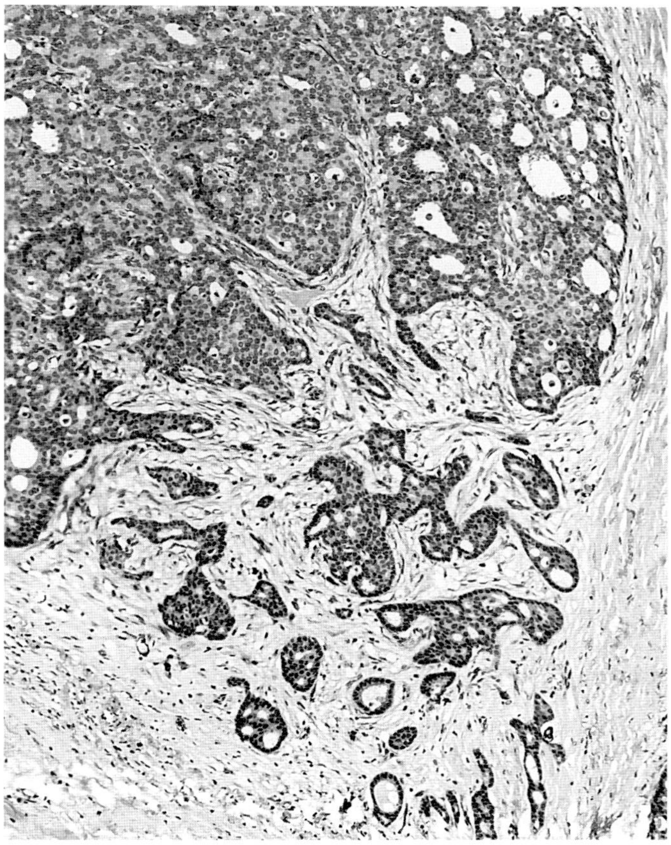

**Figure 6.33** Invasive papillary carcinoma. (a) The relatively solid appearance is due to the cribriform proliferation of the epithelial cells overlying the papillary processes. There is a cluster of irregular tubules (arrow) adjacent to the intraductal lesion. (X60) (b) Higher magnification of the irregular tubules confirms their invasive nature. (X120)

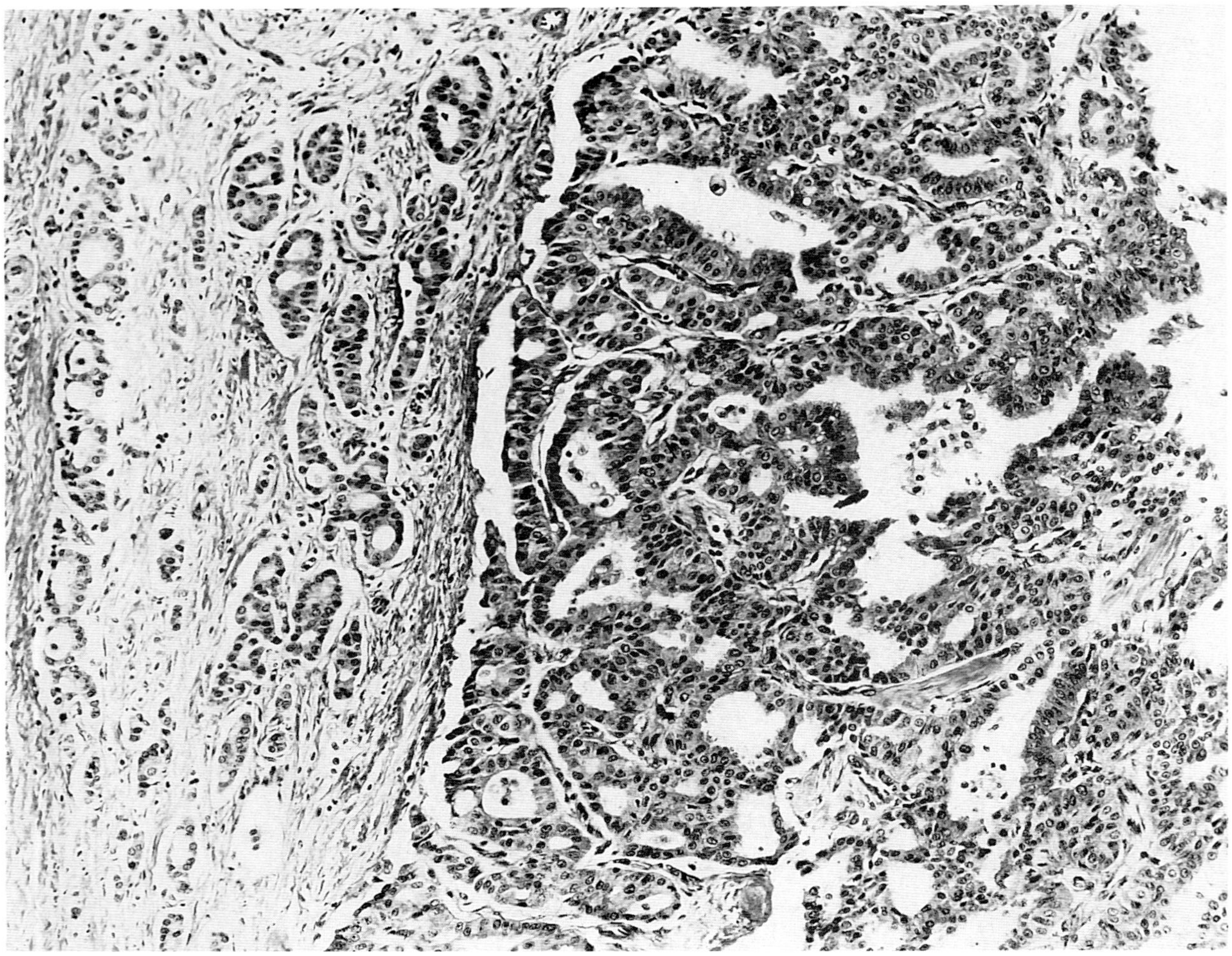

**Figure 6.34** Invasive papillary carcinoma. The invasive area assumes the pattern of a well-differentiated ordinary duct carcinoma. (H&E, X240)

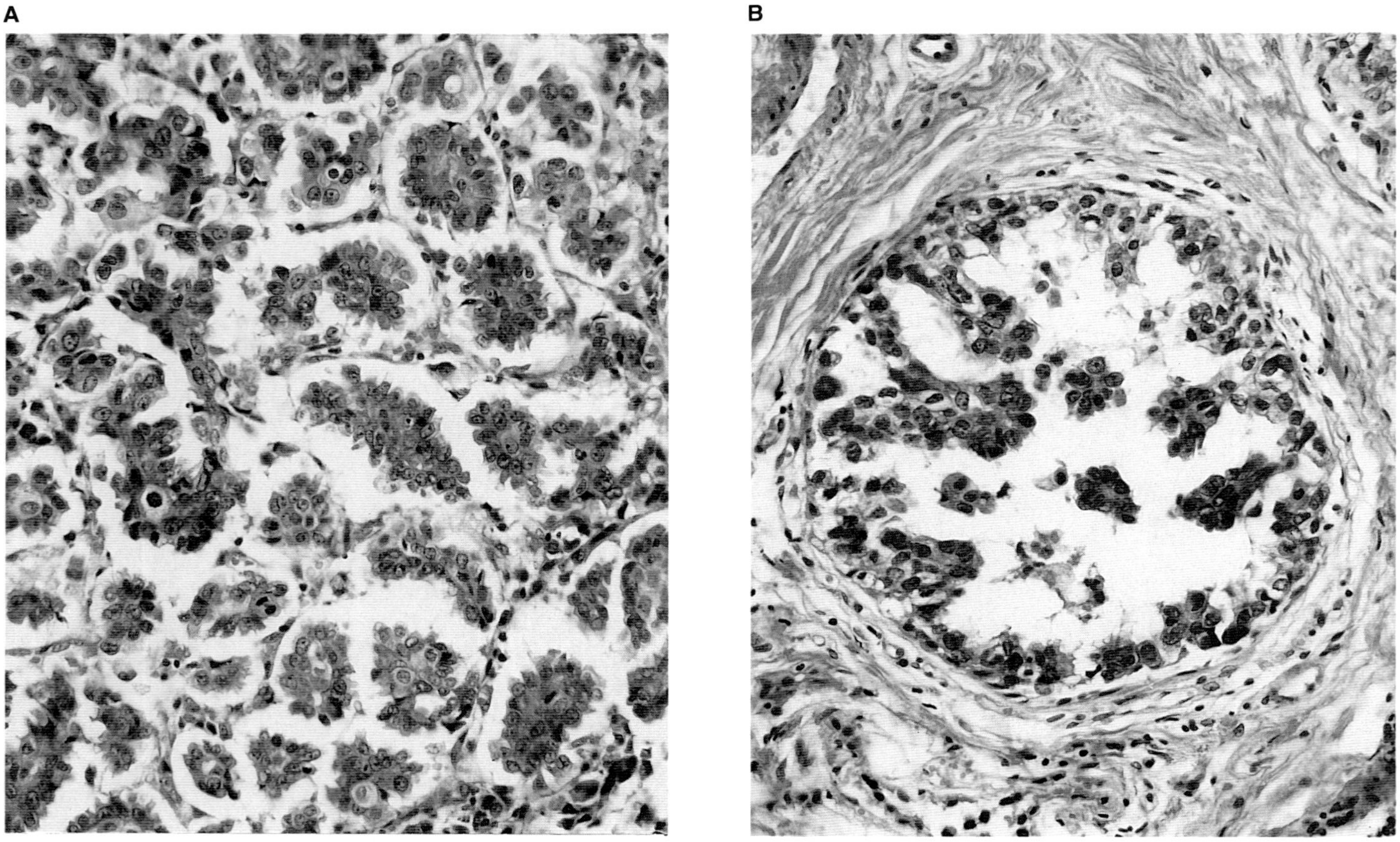


**Figure 6.35** Invasive micropapillary carcinoma. (a) There are numerous papillary cell clusters within stromal spaces; these spaces lack an endothelial lining. (b) The associated intraductal carcinoma is a micropapillary carcinoma; the epithelial tufts are identical to those invading the stroma. (H&E, (a&b) X250)

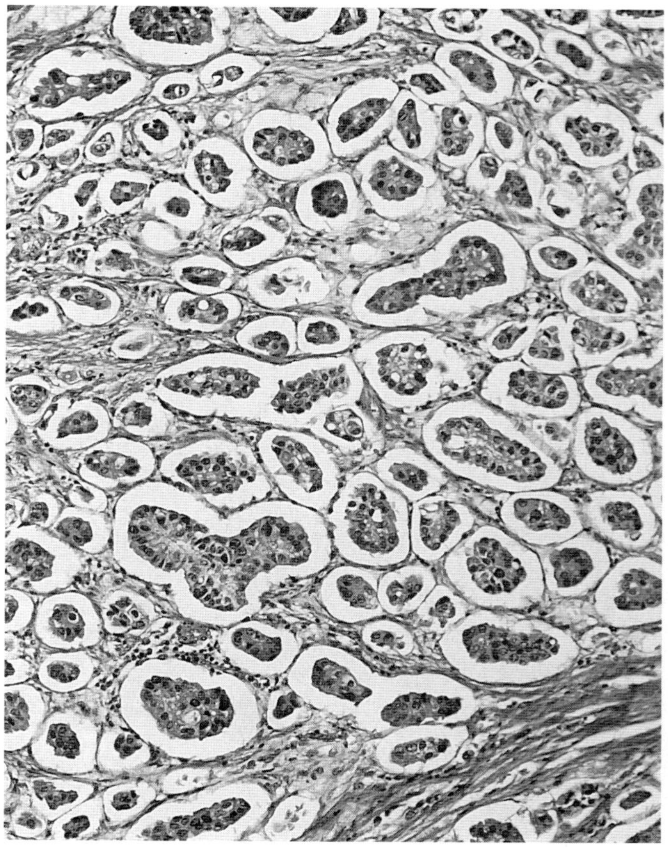


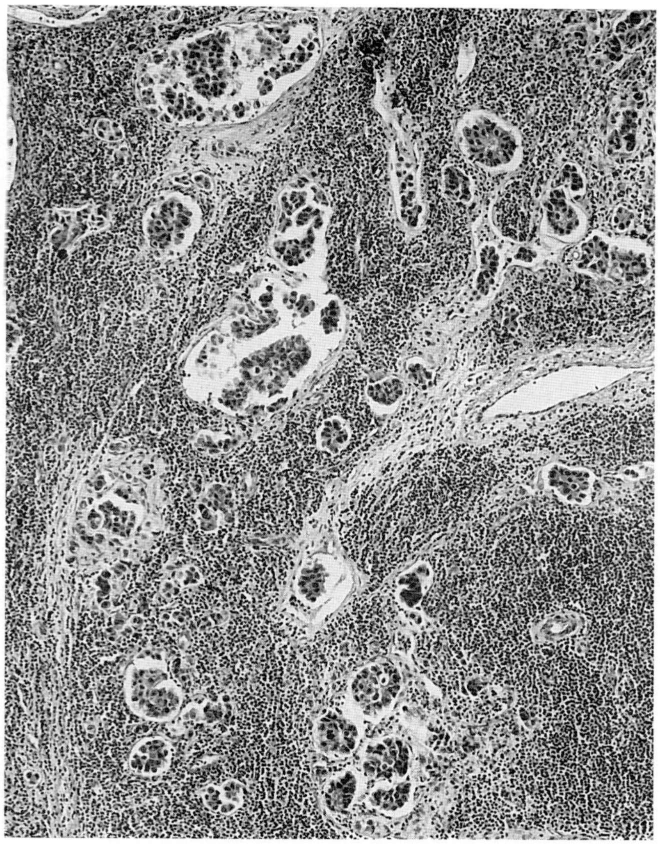


**Figure 6.36** Invasive micropapillary carcinoma with axillary node metastases. (a) Numerous papillary cell clusters are dispersed within vascular-like spaces in the breast. These spaces are surrounded by stromal cells, however. (b) The metastatic tumor in the axillary node has retained its papillary configuration and the spaces around the cell clusters. (H&E, (a) X120; (b) X100)

encountered in confirming the presence of this important cell layer, then immunostains for actin can be utilized for identifying these cells. The efficacy of immunoreactivity of ME cells for actin as a feature distinguishing papillary carcinoma from benign papillomas has been discussed by Papotti et al (42). One characteristic of actin that could cause a problem is that it also decorates the vessel walls in the fibrovascular core of the papillary stalks. At times, these endothelial-lined vascular spaces become closely apposed to the epithelial cells and, associated with a positive reaction with actin, they could be misinterpreted as a ME cell layer (Fig. 6.28a). Simultaneous use of immunoreaction for S-100 protein is helpful in these cases. At least some of the ME cells, if present, should react with S-100 protein, but there will be no reaction with the endothelial cells lining the vessel walls (Fig. 28b). The exclusive use of S-100 protein has several drawbacks, also, however. S-100 protein does not react uniformly with the ME cells in some laboratories. Furthermore, it may also react with epithelial cells in a patchy fashion causing confusion. The epithelial cells in papillary carcinoma show a positive reaction for carcinoembryonic antigen (CEA) in 85% of the cases in contrast to none in the benign papillomas (42).

As long as the limitations of the various antibodies are kept in mind, immunostains for actin and S-100 protein can be used judiciously to assist in the interpretation of difficult papillary lesions.

The type or amount of stroma in the papillary stalks, nuclear/cytoplasmic ratio, nuclear appearance, or pattern of epithelial proliferation are secondary and relatively insignificant features for separating benign and malignant papillary lesions. While there is no absolute feature separating benign from malignant papillary lesions, the complete absence of a myoepithelial cell layer is the one feature that invariably identifies a papillary carcinoma. In 15 cases of classic papillary carcinoma immunostained with actin and S-100 protein that I personally reviewed recently, a myoepithelial cell layer was not present in a single

A

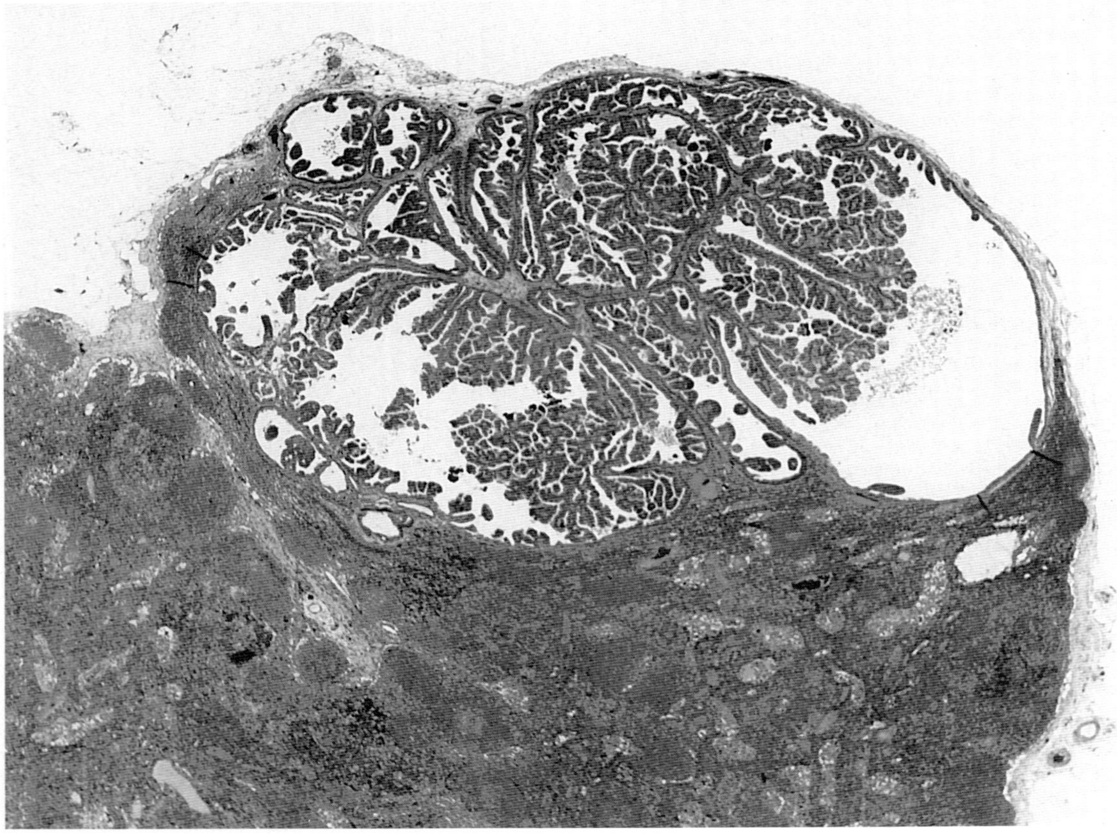

B

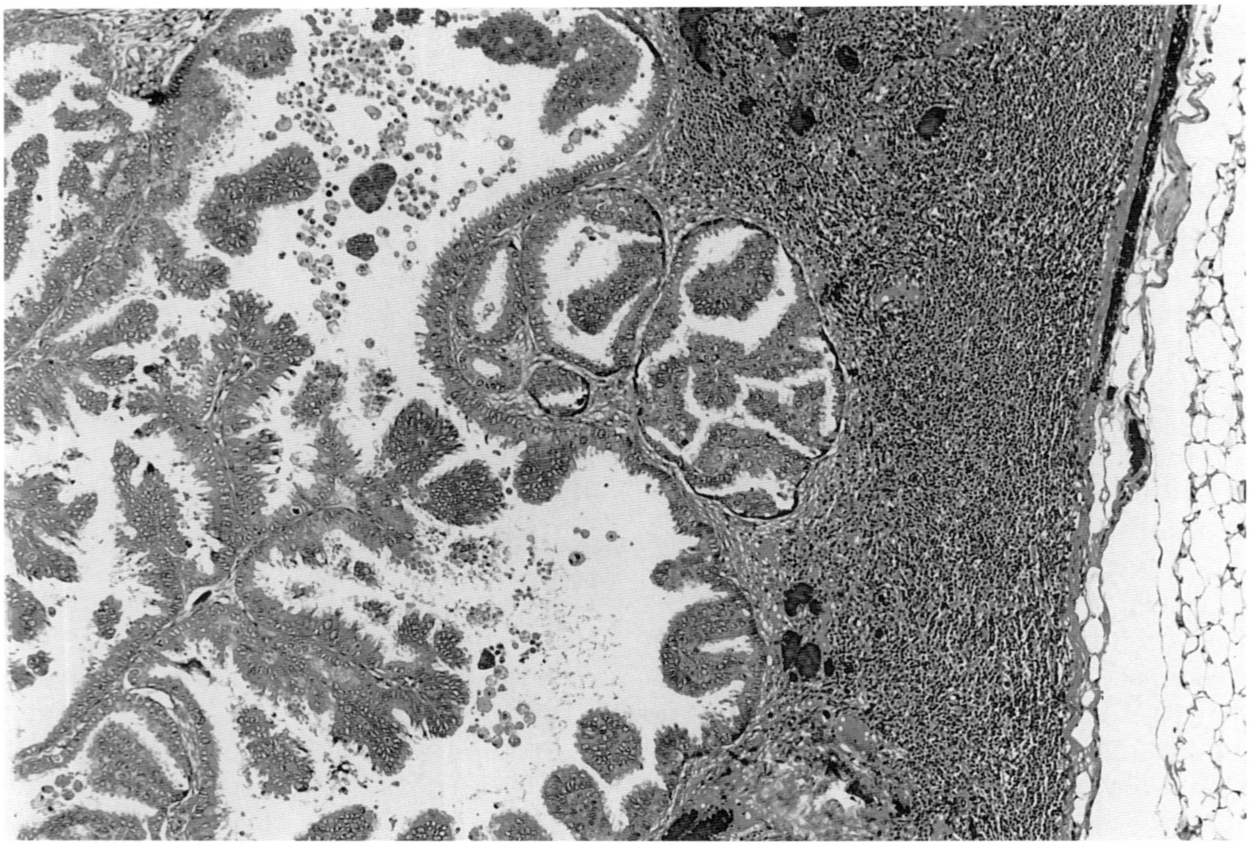

**Figure 6.37** Lymph node with metastatic papillary carcinoma. (a–c) The papillary pattern is well retained. (c) The papillae lack a myoepithelial cell layer. The possibility of origin from intranodal ectopic breast tissue should be excluded in all such cases. This patient had two nodes showing the papillary pattern as well as a recent carcinoma diagnosed in the breast. (H&E, (a) X20; (b) X120; (c) X300)

c

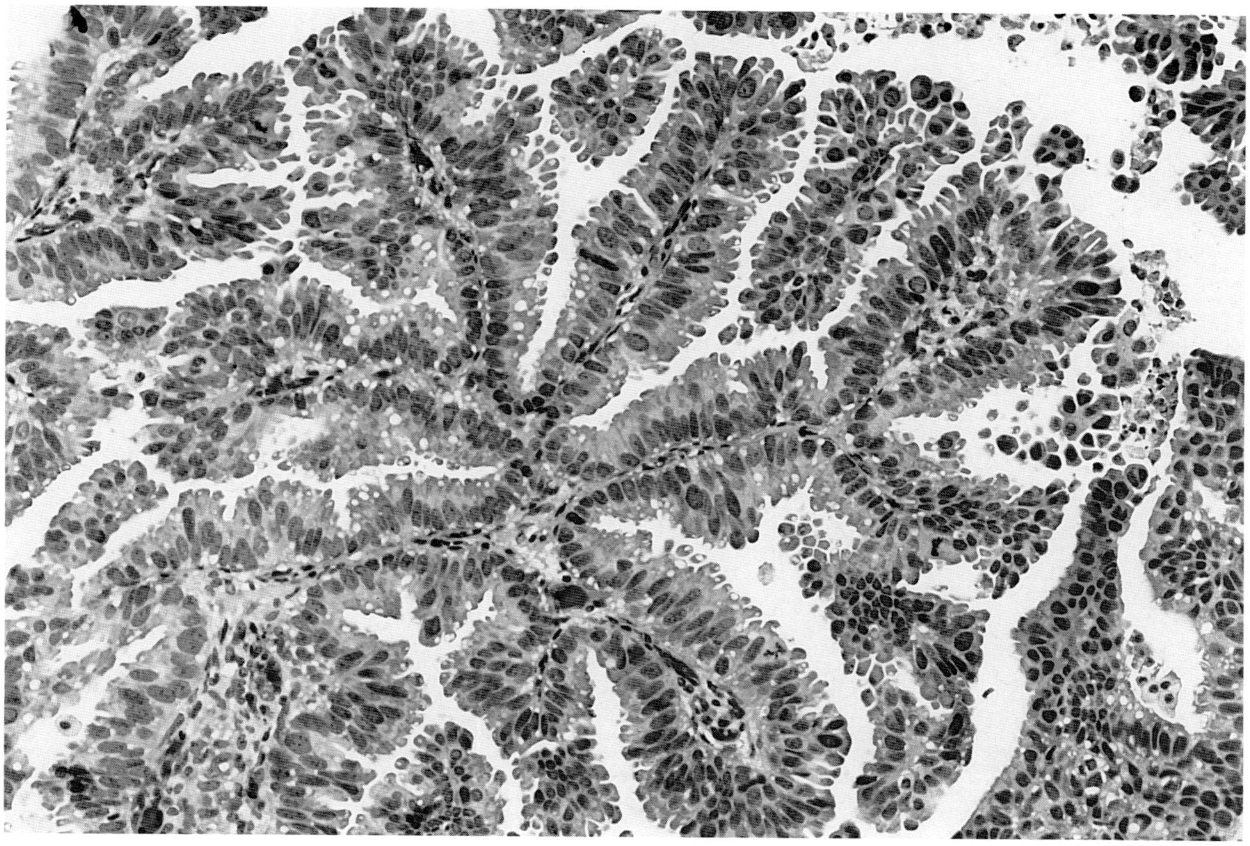

**Figure 6.37(c)** Legend on opposite page.

case. As noted before, however, it is possible that an occasional, sporadic ME cell may be present in some large papillary carcinomas; according to the guidelines described, these ME cells should be confined to less than 10% of the papillary processes in an otherwise typical papillary carcinoma.

The epithelial cells supported by the fibrovascular stalk assume a variety of proliferative patterns (7). Some papillary carcinomas simply display stratification of spindled epithelial cells (Fig. 6.29), while others show tufting (micropapillae), sieve-like or rosette-forming, cribriform growth of the neoplastic epithelial cells (Fig. 6.30). Sometimes, the neoplastic cells exhibit atypia (Fig. 6.31) and abundant mitotic activity, but more often, the cells are characterized by a notoriously deceptive uniformity and monotonous appearance. Rarely, the cells may even develop neuroendocrine granules (44).

Papillary carcinoma of the stratified spindle cell variant may also present as a multifocal microscopic lesion involving the TDLUs (Fig. 6.32). This variant can be particularly difficult to diagnose accurately because benign papillomatosis may be present simultaneously in adjacent ducts. Again, immunostains for actin can be extremely helpful in distinguishing the benign areas from the malignant ones.

Many papillary carcinomas appear deceptively bland because of the absence of anaplastic pleomorphism. The neoplastic epithelial cells may have apical snouts or display apocrine features, but true metaplastic apocrine cells are absent as a second cell population in papillary carcinomas. The presence of intraductal carcinoma of any type in the same biopsy is irrelevant to the diagnosis of a given papillary lesion. Benign papillomas and papillary carcinoma can and do coexist in biopsies with or without other benign or malignant intraductal proliferations.

## INVASIVE PAPILLARY CARCINOMA

A small proportion of papillary carcinomas have an associated focus of unequivocal stromal invasion

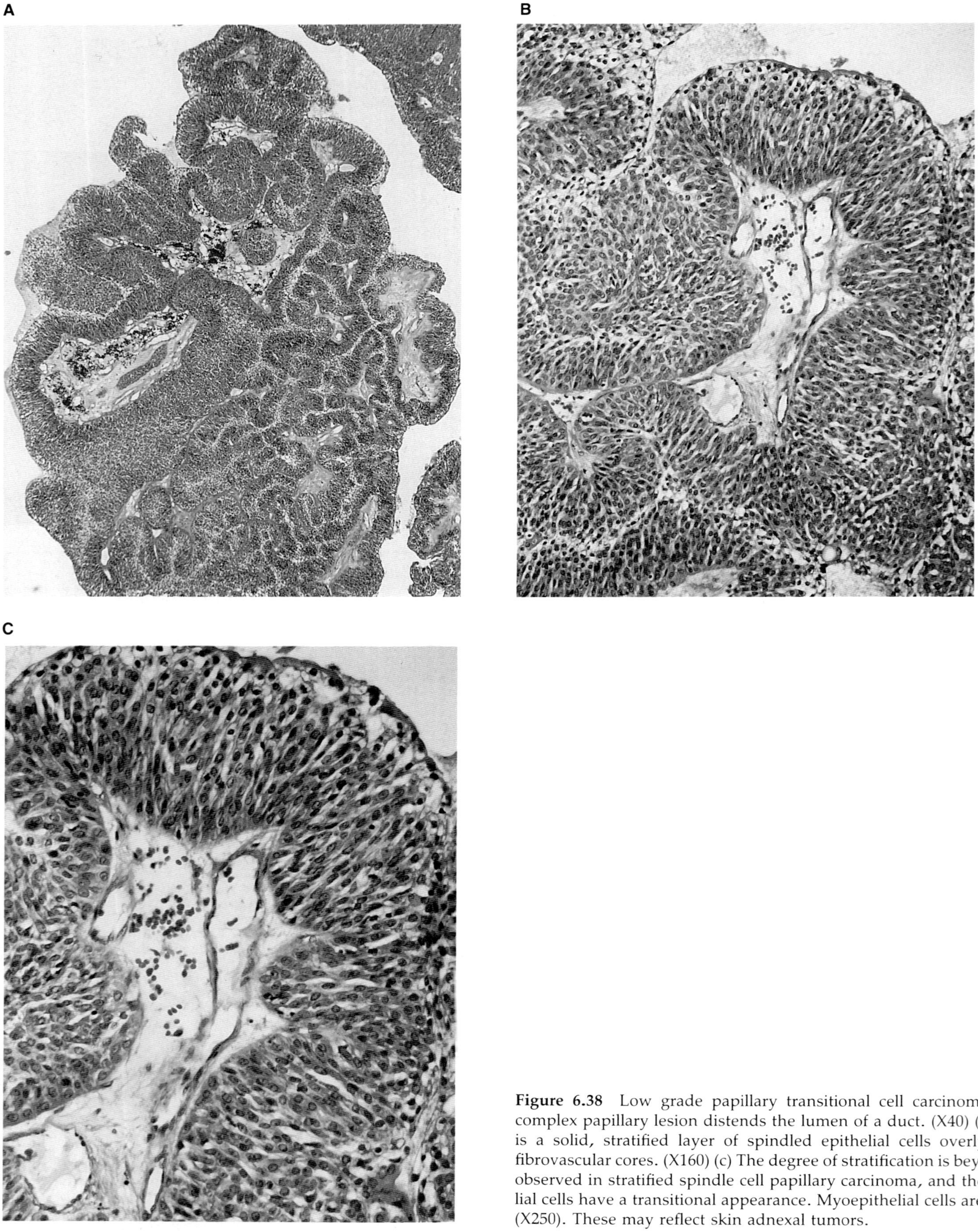


**Figure 6.38** Low grade papillary transitional cell carcinoma. (a) A complex papillary lesion distends the lumen of a duct. (X40) (b) There is a solid, stratified layer of spindled epithelial cells overlying the fibrovascular cores. (X160) (c) The degree of stratification is beyond that observed in stratified spindle cell papillary carcinoma, and the epithelial cells have a transitional appearance. Myoepithelial cells are absent. (X250). These may reflect skin adnexal tumors.

(Figs. 6.33–6.34), accounting for 1.5% to 2.5% of all invasive mammary carcinomas (38,41). The morphology of the associated invasion varies from tubular carcinoma to regular infiltrating duct carcinoma. Rarely, the invasive carcinoma displays a micropapillary appearance (43) which persists even in metastatic foci (Figs. 6.35–6.36). This invasive pattern is seen in association with a grade II intraductal carcinoma of the micropapillary type, or without an in situ component. In all such cases, the possibility of a metastasis from an ovarian serous carcinoma should be carefully investigated. The invasive papillae are often surrounded by a space simulating extensive vascular invasion. Immunostains for Factor VIII fail to show an endothelial cell lining around these spaces, however. As pointed out by Fisher et al (38), aside from Carter (2) who refers to the intraductal nature of the papillary carcinomas in his study, and McDivitt et al (41) who based their comments on an unknown number of cases but a definite group of invasive papillary carcinomas, the issue of the presence or absence of invasion is not addressed properly in many reports.

Among 1,603 invasive breast carcinomas, Fisher et al (38) found only 35 invasive papillary carcinomas accounting for 2.5% of all cancers examined in National Surgical Adjuvant Breast Project, protocol #4. Invasive papillary carcinoma occurs with a significantly higher frequency among postmenopausal and non-caucasian women.

While many patients are clinically judged to have regional node metastases, nodal involvement is not commonly found. A high proportion of the palpable lymph nodes show sinus histiocytosis accounting for the erroneous clinical observation. When present, nodal metastases are limited to fewer than four nodes, with only 9% of the patients having four or more positive nodes. The nodal metastases generally display an ordinary invasive ductal carcinoma pattern. On very rare occasions, however, the papillary pattern is retained in the nodal metastases (Fig. 6.37). Even less frequently, papillary carcinomas may arise from ectopic breast tissue in an axillary node (46).

Only three of the 35 patients in Fisher et al's series experienced treatment failure after five years, while only one patient died from papillary carcinoma. Consequently, Fisher et al (38) concluded that invasive papillary carcinoma is associated with a favorable prognosis.

## Treatment

Since most papillary carcinomas are noninvasive intraductal carcinomas, they should be treated as such. A solitary intraductal papillary carcinoma located centrally would be a good candidate for conservative treatment particularly in light of the findings that patients treated by lumpectomy did not develop subsequent recurrences unless another variant of intraductal carcinoma was also evident (35). Microscopic intraductal papillary carcinomas which are generally found in the peripheral ducts and the TDLU are often multifocal and require a more cautious determination of their extent if conservative therapy, in the form of lumpectomy, is considered.

## UNUSUAL PAPILLARY LESIONS

Rarely, the proliferating cells within centrally located, intraductal papillary lesions assume a transitional-squamoid appearance (Fig. 6.38). Myoepithelial cells are absent in these papillary processes and a designation of a low grade, transitional cell, papillary carcinoma seems appropriate for these tumors. These lesions probably reflect a skin adnexal tumor, however.

A case of an oncocytic papilloma has also been reported by Nielsen (24). This lesion probably reflects a papillary adenomyoepithelioma judging from the distribution of the oncocytic cells and the presence of actin-like filaments at the ultrastructural level.

## REFERENCES

### General


* 1. Azzopardi JG: Papilloma and papillary carcinoma, in *Problems in Breast Pathology*. Philadelphia, WB Saunders, 1979, pp 150–166.

* 2. Carter D: Intraductal papillary tumors of the breast. A study of 78 cases. *Cancer* 1977;39:1689–1692.

* 3. Hart D: Intracystic papillomatous tumors of the breast, benign and malignant. *Arch Surg* 1927;14:793–835.

* 4. Kraus FT, Neubecker RD: The differential diagnosis of papillary tumors of the breast. *Cancer* 1962;15:444–455.

* 5. Lewison EF, Lyons JG Jr: Relationship between benign breast disease and cancer. *Arch Surg* 1953;66:94–114.

* 6. Murad TM, Contesso G, Mouriesse H: Papillary tumors of large lactiferous ducts. *Cancer* 1981;48:122–133.

7. Murad TM, Swaid S, Pritchett P: Malignant and benign papillary lesions of the breast. *Hum Pathol* 1977;8:379–390.

8. Papotti M, Gugliotta P, Ghiringhello B, et al: Association of breast carcinoma and multiple intraductal papillomas: An histological and immunohistochemical investigation. *Histopathology* 1984;8:963–975.


### Papilloma, Sclerosing Papilloma, Papillomatosis


9. Andersen A, Koudal G: Papillome intracanaliculaire du sein. *Acta Chir Scand (Suppl)* 1965;343:37–41.

10. Azzopardi JG, Salm R: Ductal adenoma of the breast: A lesion which can mimic carcinoma. *J Pathol* 1984;144:11–23.

* 11. Buhl-Jorgensen SE, Fischermann K, Johansen H, et al: Cancer risk in intraductal papilloma and papillomatosis. *Surg Gynecol Obstet* 1968;127:1307–1312.

12. Estes AC, Phillips C: Papilloma of lacteal duct. *Surg Gynecol Obstet* 1949;89:345–348.

* 13. Fenoglio C, Lattes R: Sclerosing papillary proliferations in the female breast. *Cancer* 1974;33:691–700.

* 14. Flint A, Oberman HA: Infarction and squamous metaplasia of intraductal papilloma. A benign breast lesion that may simulate carcinoma. *Hum Pathol* 1984;15:764–767.

15. Forrest H: Intraductal papilloma of the breast. *Br J Surg* 1966;53:1028–1032.

16. Gray HK, Wood GA: Significance of mammary discharge in cases of papilloma of the breast. *Arch Surg* 1941;42:203–208.

17. Gusterson BA, Sloane JP, Middwood C, et al: Ductal adenoma of the breast—A lesion exhibiting a myoepithelial/epithelial phenotype. *Histopathology* 1987;11:103–110.

* 18. Lammie GA, Millis RR: Ductal adenoma of the breast—A review of fifteen cases. *Hum Pathol* 1989;20:903–908.

* 19. Haagensen CD, Stout AP, Philips JS: The papillary neoplasms of the breast. I. Benign intraductal papilloma. *Ann Surg* 1951;133:18–36.

* 20. Haagensen CD: *Diseases of the Breast*, ed 3. Philadelphia, WB Saunders, 1986, pp 136–174.

21. Hendrick JW: Intraductal papilloma of the breast. *Surg Gynecol Obstet* 1957;105:215–223.

22. Kilgore AR, Fleming R, Ramos MD: The incidence of cancer with nipple discharge and the risk of cancer in the presence of papillary disease of the breast. *Surg Gynecol Obstet* 1953;96:649–660.

23. Moore SW, Pearce J, Ring E: Intraductal papilloma of the breast. *Surg Gynecol Obstet* 1961;112:153–158.

24. Neilsen BB: Oncocytic breast papilloma. *Virchows Archiv (Pathol Anat)* 1981;393:345–351.

* 25. Ohuchi N, Abe R, Kasai M: Possible cancerous change of intraductal papillomas of the breast. A 3-D reconstruction study of 25 cases. *Cancer* 1984;54:605–611.

* 26. Ohuchi N, Abe R, Takahashi T, et al: Origin and extension of intraductal papillomas of the breast: A 3-D reconstruction study. *Breast Cancer Res Treat* 1984;4:117–128.

27. Page DL, Zwang RV, Rogers LW, et al: Relation between component parts of fibrocystic disease complex and breast cancer. *J Natl Cancer Inst* 1978;61:1055–1063.

* 28. Page DL, Andersen TJ: *Diagnostic Histopathology of the Breast*. New York, Churchill Livingstone, 1987, pp 104–119;186–190.

29. Pellettiere EV II: The clinical and pathologic aspects of papillomatous disease of the beast: A follow-up study of 97 patients treated by local excision. *Am J Clin Pathol* 1971;55:740–748.

* 30. Rosen PP: A. P. Stout and papilloma of the breast. Comments on the occasion of his 100th birthday. *Am J Surg Pathol* 1986;10(Suppl 1):100–107.

* 31. Rosen PP: Papillary duct hyperplasia of the breast in children and young adults. *Cancer* 1985;56:1611–1617.

32. Simpson JS, Barson AJ: Breast tumours in infants and children. *Can Med Assoc J* 1969;101:100–102.

33. Snyder WH, Chaffin L: Main duct papilloma of breast. *Arch Surg* 1955;70:685–688.

34. Tailhefer A, Pilleron JP: 130 cas de mamelle saignante. *Med Acad Chir* 1956;82:612–617.


### Papillary carcinoma


* 35. Carter D, Orr SL, Merino MJ: Intracystic papillary carcinoma of the breast. After mastectomy, radiotherapy or excisional biopsy alone. *Cancer* 1983;52:14–19.

36. Chan JKC, Saw D: One or two cell types in papillary carcinoma of the breast. *Pathology* 1986;18:479–481.

37. Czernobilsky B: Intracystic carcinoma of the female breast. *Surg Gynecol Obstet* 1967;124:93–98.

* 38. Fisher ER, Palekar AS, Redmond C, et al: Pathologic findings from the National Surgical Adjuvant Breast Project (Protocol No. 4). VI. Invasive papillary carcinoma. *Am J Clin Pathol* 1980;73:313–320.

* 39. Haagensen CD: *Diseases of the Breast*, ed 3. Philadelphia, WB Saunders, 1986, pp 729–757.

40. Hunter CE Jr, Sawyers JL: Intracystic papillary carcinoma of the breast. *South Med J* 1980;73:1484–1486.

41. McDivitt RW, Holleb AI, Foote FW: Prior breast disease in patients treated for papillary carcinoma. *Arch Pathol* 1968;85:117–124.

* 42. Papotti M, Gugliotta P, Eusebi V, et al: Immunohistochemical analysis of benign and malignant papillary lesions of the breast. *Am J Surg Pathol* 1983;7:451–461.

43. Pettinato G, Manival JC, Panico L, et al: Pseudopapillary (serous-like) carcinoma of the breast. An aggressive variant of ductal carcinoma. *Mod Pathol* 1991;4:13A.

44. Ramos CV, Boeshart C, Restrapo GL: Intracystic papillary carcinoma of the male breast. *Arch Pathol Lab Med* 1985;109:858–861.

45. Veronesi U, Giarrusso A, Guarino M: Il carcinoma papillefero della mammella. *Tumori* 1964;50:421–430.

* 46. Walker AN, Fechner RE: Papillary carcinoma arising from ectopic breast tissue in an axillary lymph node. *Gynecol Obstet* 1982;4:141–145.

# 7

# Intraductal Carcinoma



Among the many carcinomas that originate in the terminal duct-lobular unit (TDLU), a majority assume patterns that we have come to recognize as ductal in type. In addition, there are carcinomas that actually originate in the extralobular ducts: papillary carcinomas and Paget's disease within the major lactiferous ducts are among this group.

While in 1941 the term lobular carcinoma in situ (LCIS) was introduced for a noninvasive, microscopic lesion not clinically or grossly detectable, the designation of intraductal carcinoma (IDCA) has been used to refer to a highly heterogeneous group of lesions ranging from microscopic to grossly detectable intraductal carcinomas as well as predominantly IDCA with areas of stromal invasion. Although IDCA is not considered at all uncommon in the current practice of surgical pathology, in 1960, Gillis et al (34) reported 36 cases of intraductal carcinoma particularly noting that it is rare in its pure form. In the late 1960s and early 1970s, the definition of IDCA was narrowed to a noninvasive tumor (53,71). This definition is by no means universally accepted, however. Haagensen (38) continued to follow Stout's classification, considering a breast carcinoma as intraductal when less than 50% of the lesion was invasive. Most, if not all, pathologists would now consider this to be an unacceptable definition. Subdivision of intraductal carcinomas into gross IDCA (lesions presenting as a palpable mass, Paget's disease, or nipple discharge) and microscopic IDCA (lesions detected mammographically or found incidentally at microscopic examination) has been used by one group (37). Others stratify intraductal carcinomas into microfocal, tumor forming, and diffuse forms (3). The term intraductal carcinoma, as used in this chapter, refers to a malignant epithelial proliferation confined within a "duct," with no evidence of stromal invasion apparent on routinely prepared sections. Several morphologic variants of intraductal carcinoma are recognized. For some variants, a minimal quantity of the changes are required before the lesion is designated as intraductal carcinoma. (See Chapter 5, page 182.)

## CLINICAL FEATURES

Prior to the widespread application of screening mammography, IDCA constituted 0.84% to 5.6% of breast carcinomas (25,45,48,71,77,83,87,103), and a majority of intraductal carcinomas were clinically obvious lesions that presented as a palpable mass, Paget's disease, nipple discharge, or a combination of these findings (5,90). During the two-year period of 1985–1986, IDCA represented 22% of all new breast cancers accessioned at the Children's Hospital of San Francisco, compared to 5% prior to the introduction of mammography (48). Elsewhere, among mammographically-screened patients, 15% to 33% manifest this type of carcinoma (7,57,64,78,80,96), and 20% to 40% of occult tumors are IDCA (10,79,82,84). Among biopsies performed due to mammographically-detected microcalcifications, about 10% to 77% are noninvasive carcinomas; and of these, a majority are ductal rather than lobular (65,79).

When mammography is interpreted as "suspicious calcifications," a carcinoma of predominantly the intraductal type is identified in 25% of the specimen (76). In two separate studies, one of which was nationwide (7), 58% and 59% of IDCA were detected by mammographic calcification (7,81). A high proportion of lesions that are currently biopsied based on mammographic abnormalities are minuscule lesions, the biologic and clinical significance of which has never been established. Other patients, however, continue to present with either areas of irregularity or lumpiness in the breast that have been discovered on self-examination by the patient or during routine check-up by a clinician. Among 83 consecutive, unselected female autopsies, and after excluding six women with prior diagnosis of invasive breast carcinoma, 14 (18%) of the remaining 77 women had in situ carcinoma (59). Eleven of these women (14.3%) had IDCA, while six had lobular carcinoma in situ (LCIS); obviously some women had both lesions simultaneously. The multicentricity and bilaterality of IDCA was 33.3% and 9.1% respectively; the corresponding figures for LCIS were 42.9% and 16.7% (59).

Patients with IDCA range in age from 16 to 85 years with an average age of 55 years. Compared to patients with infiltrating duct carcinoma, some studies have found no significant difference in the mean age of the patients (83). Others, however, have reported a lower mean age of about three years for patients with IDCA (102).

## THE SITE OF ORIGIN OF INTRADUCTAL CARCINOMA

The study of Wellings et al (101) has demonstrated that a majority of carcinomas originate within the terminal duct-lobular unit. Depending on the pattern of proliferation, the lesion is designated as either ductal or lobular. Furthermore, some of the structures that we recognize as a duct basically reflect an unfolded or a transformed lobule. Sometimes, the same proliferating small cell population may manifest a ductal growth pattern in half of a lobule and a lobular pattern in the other half. The reason we continue to separate the "ductal" lesions from the "lobular" ones is that the latter pattern is associated with clinically distinct features.

## GROSS PATHOLOGIC FEATURES

When comedocarcinoma is extensive and there is abundant necrotic debris in the duct lumens, these areas may be apparent to the naked eye. As a rule, other variants of intraductal carcinoma are not grossly detectable. In a high proportion of cases, even when a patient presents with a palpable lesion, the mass is generally not a cancer, but rather some form of benign pathology with only microscopic foci of IDCA. Neither is the presence of a serous or bloody nipple discharge indicative of carcinoma in situ. Intraoperative frozen section diagnosis is discouraged since it does not always allow accurate morphologic interpretation (95). Furthermore, the tissue alterations induced by freezing may render the lesion permanently uninterpretable on subsequent paraffin embedded sections.

A

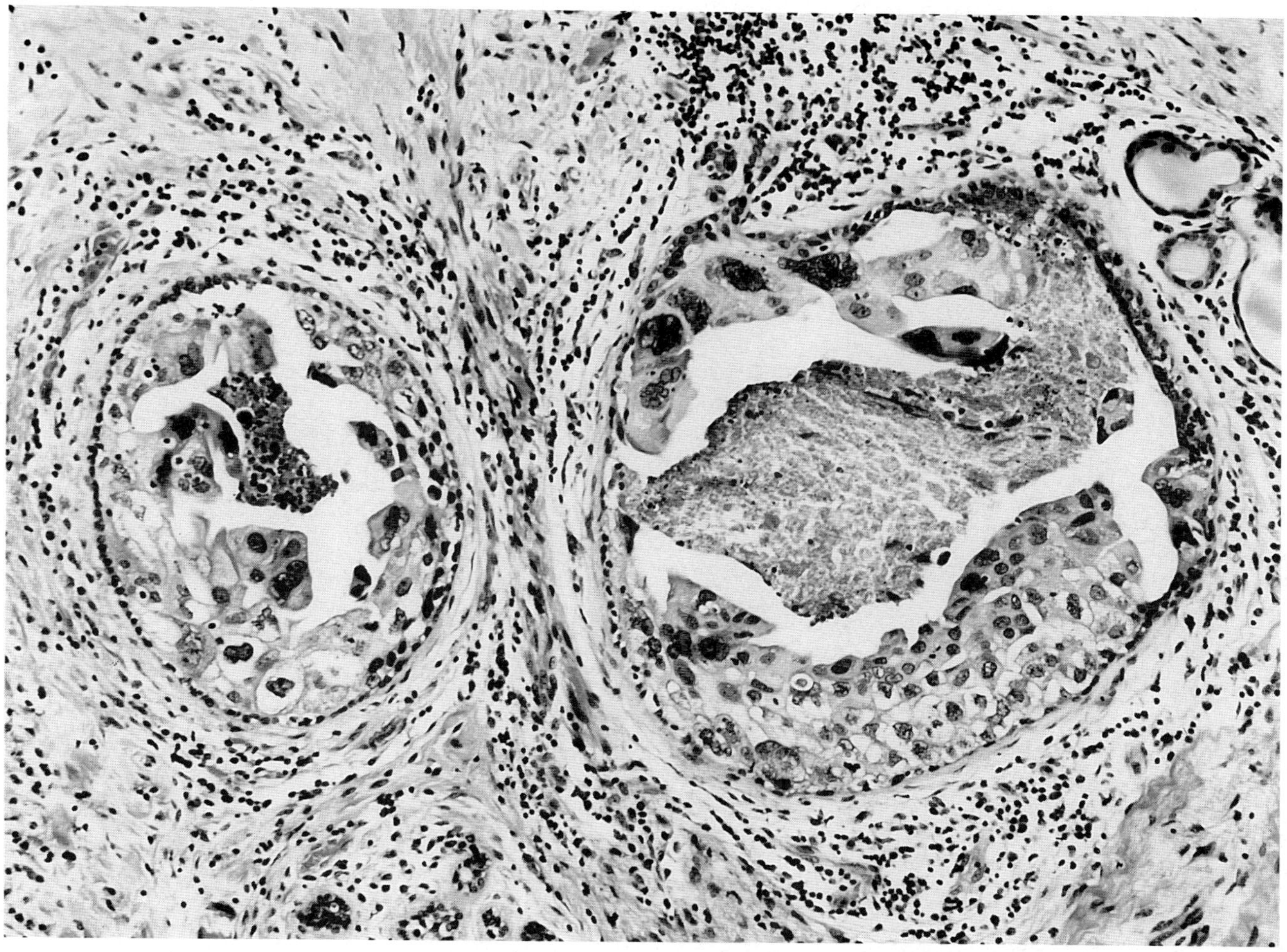

**Figure 7.1(a)** Comedocarcinoma (high grade IDCA). Two ducts show a highly atypical cellular proliferation and central necrosis. (H&E, X300)

## MICROSCOPIC VARIANTS

There are several morphologic variants of IDCA. The most readily recognizable pattern is comedocarcinoma. Also relatively well-known are the papillary, cribriform and micropapillary variants. The latter two have come to constitute a high proportion of intraductal carcinomas since the use of mammography. There are a variety of additional patterns including intraductal apocrine, clear cell, clinging and signet ring-cell carcinomas. In addition, some of the rare special types of carcinoma (secretory, spindle cell, carcinoma with neuroendocrine granules, lipid-rich, etc) also have an in situ counterpart; these are discussed in sections addressing each of these special types of carcinoma. Intraductal papillary carcinoma is discussed in Chapter 6, Papillary Lesions.

The histologic features and criteria for the diagnosis of each variant are presented separately. Generally, two or more of these patterns coexist. Among the different variants, comedocarcinoma most frequently presents as the sole pattern in a biopsy.

### Comedocarcinoma

Comedocarcinoma is characterized by the presence of necrosis, cytologic atypia, and often loosely cohesive cells (Figs. 7.1–7.2). Mitotic figures are abundant in some cases and few in others. A diagnosis of comedocarcinoma is warranted even if a single small duct shows these classic features. Some of the most extensive intraductal carcinomas are of this type showing the involvement of practically every TDLU in a generous (larger than 5 cm) breast biopsy. The myoepithelial cell layer may be well retained around the

B

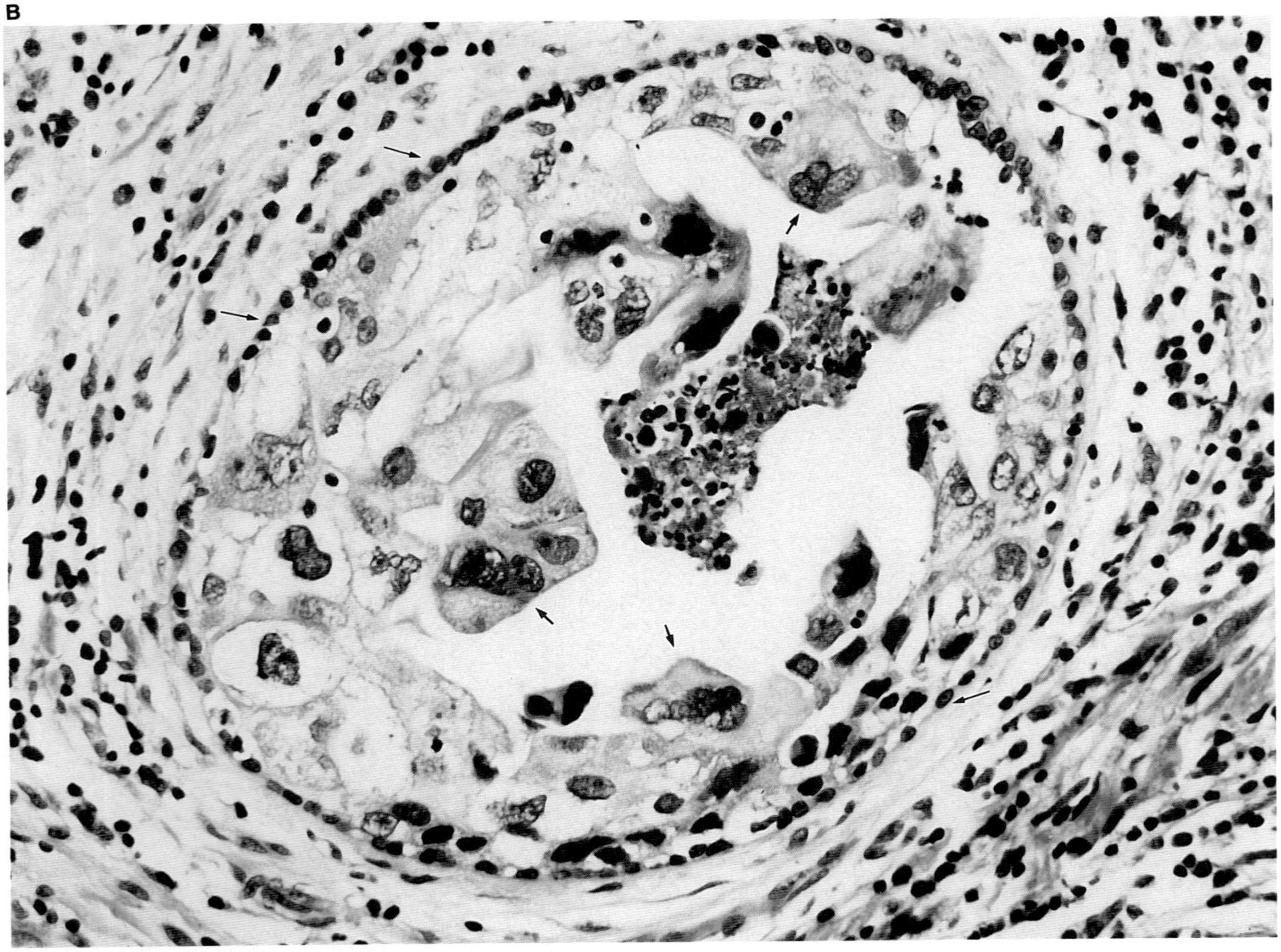

**Figure 7.1(b)** Comedocarcinoma (high grade IDCA). Higher magnification of the smaller duct shows some multinucleated cells and cells with lobulation of the nuclei (small arrows). The myoepithelial cell layer is well retained (large arrows). A prominent lymphocytic infiltrate surrounds the ducts. (H&E, X800)

ducts in some cases and barely apparent due to attenuation, or absent in others. It is noteworthy that breaks in the basement membrane, even if present, are not detectable on H&E stained sections. Sometimes the stroma surrounding the ducts displays a reactive or desmoplastic appearance, and occasionally a prominent lymphoplasmacytic infiltrate surrounds the ducts.

## Non-necrotic Cribriform Variant

The cribriform pattern is characterized by proliferation of a uniform population of cells forming a sieve-like arrangement (Fig. 7.3). The secondary lumens are generally rounded and often surrounded by low columnar cells with basally located nuclei. The epithelial bridges are rigid. The nuclei are round to ovoid and evenly distributed with minimal, if any, nuclear overlap. Mitotic figures are only rarely observed. Calcification can be prominent within the secondary lumens. This variant itself has a tremendous range of appearances. The growth pattern sometimes assumes a spokewheel appearance, with a central nest of cells connected to the duct wall by numerous epithelial bridges. Occasionally, the central part of the lumen is empty and the cellular proliferation forms a single or multi-tiered arcade(s) or "Roman bridges," (Fig. 7.4). A relatively solid variant, with rosette-like arrangement of the nuclei as the only sign of early secondary lumen formation, also occurs. Cytologically, some

A

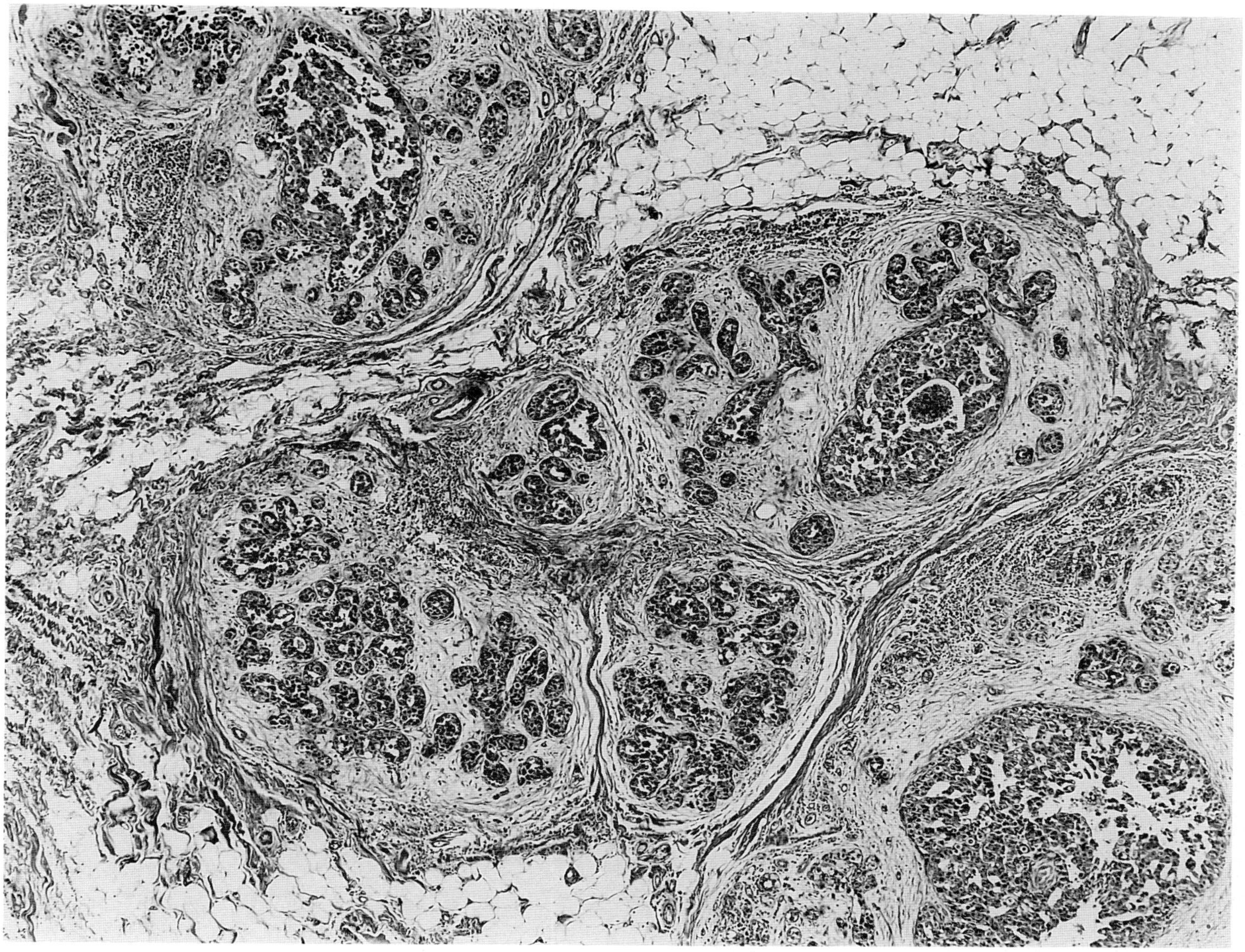

**Figure 7.2(a)** Comedocarcinoma involving the TDLU. There is expansion of the intralobular segment of the terminal duct with extension of the malignant cells to replace the native epithelium of all ductules within the TDLUs. Note the stromal alteration around the involved TDLUs. (H&E, X120)

lesions are composed of small, uniform cells with rounded nuclei and sparse cytoplasm. Others are composed of a slightly more atypical cell population with some nuclear variation and small amounts of granular eosinophilic cytoplasm.

## Micropapillary Type

A uniform cell population similar to that described for the cribriform variant, but forming epithelial tufts projecting into the lumen, proliferates in the micropapillary type (Fig. 7.5). The tufts are often regularly distributed around the duct walls. In the interval between the epithelial tufts, two cell layers line the duct wall; the luminal epithelial cell layer may appear identical to those proliferating within the tufts or it may appear normal. The myoepithelial cell layer is generally unaltered. Occasionally, the neoplastic cells display atypia and even a hobnail appearance. This pattern has a deceptively bland appearance and is one of the most difficult ones to recognize as a carcinoma when present by itself.

There are frequent transitional forms of IDCA whereby, the micropapillary patterns appear to transform into the cribriform variety (Fig. 7.6). Either the cribriform or the micropapillary pattern may display cytologic atypia occasionally. Intraluminal necrosis may sometimes be observed in association with either

B

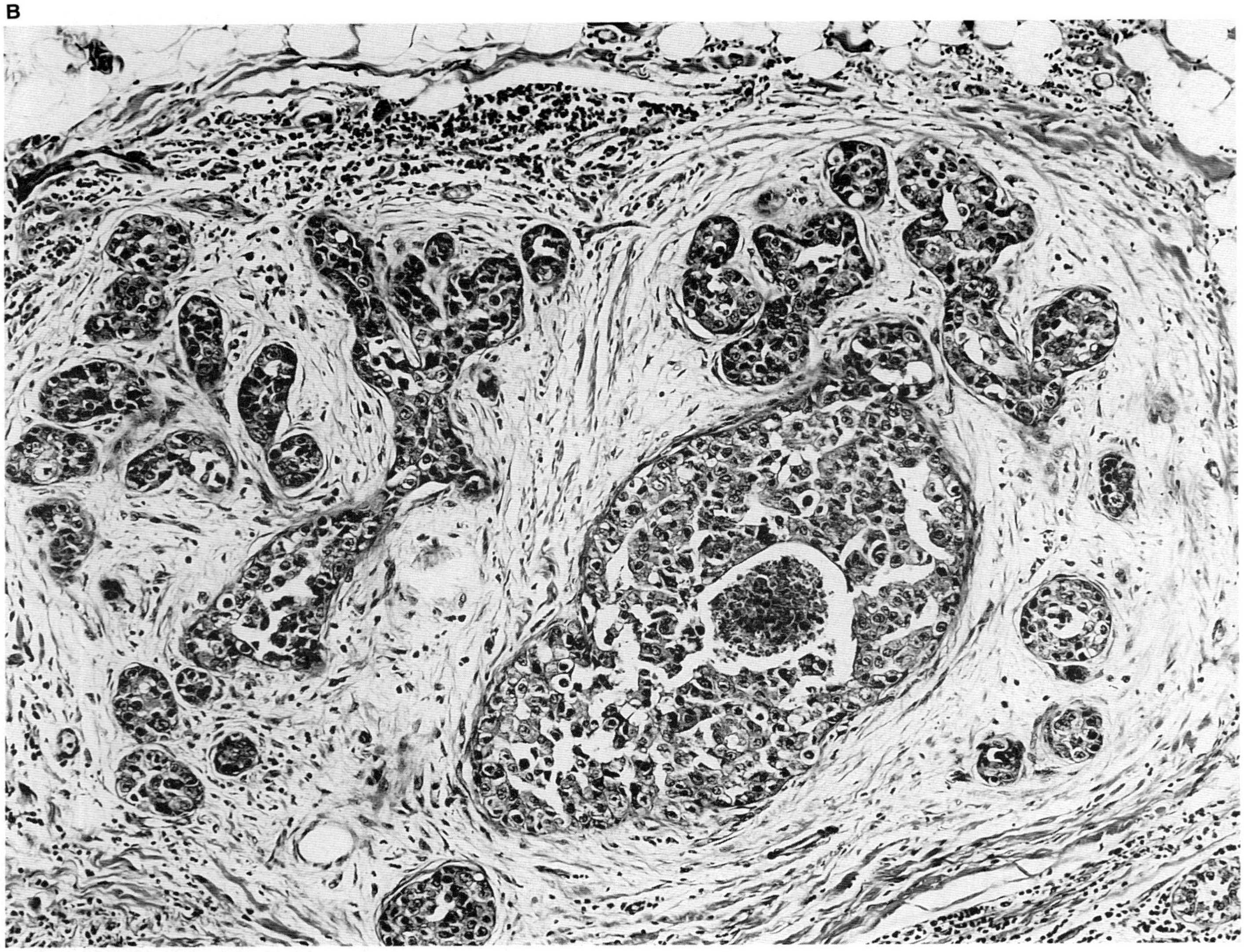

**Figure 7.2(b)** Comedocarcinoma involving the TDLU. The neoplastic cells are atypical and there is intraluminal necrosis. (H&E, X400)

pattern even in the absence of cytologic atypia. Occasionally, either pattern may show distension of the ducts or ductules with abundant intraluminal secretory material which has prompted the designation of cystic hypersecretory intraductal carcinoma (36,74); this designation would not be appropriate if the cystically dilated ducts lack one of the classic patterns of IDCA. I would prefer to classify the IDCA on the basis of its pattern and cytologic features regardless of the presence or absence of secretory material within the lumens. Actually, the malignant nature of some the lesions reported with this designations (20) has been questioned (43).

*To qualify as intraductal carcinoma either the cribriform or the micropapillary pattern should completely involve one or more ducts that measure 2 mm in their aggregate cross-sectional diameter* (see Figs. 5.28–5.31, Chapter 5). The involved ducts are generally present in close proximity within a single tissue section, but occasionally they may be identified in different sections.

## Papillary Intraductal Carcinoma, Peripheral Type

This variant is discussed in Chapter 6, Papillary Carcinomas.

A

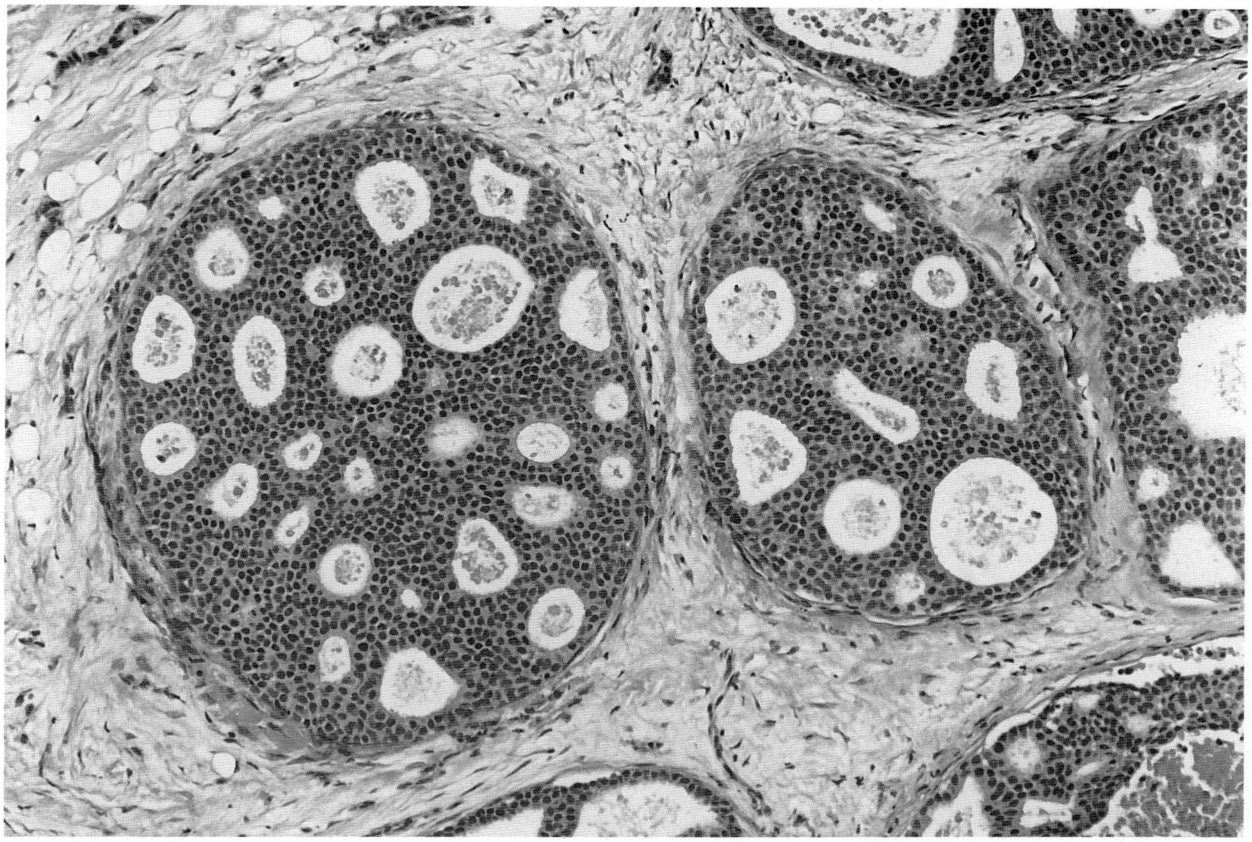

**Figure 7.3(a)** Intraductal carcinoma, cribriform variant. Two ducts show a classic cribriform growth pattern with a monotonous cell population forming rounded lumens and rigid epithelial bridges. (H&E, X240)

## Intraductal Apocrine Carcinoma

To qualify as intraductal apocrine carcinoma, the proliferating cells should display abundant granular, eosinophilic cytoplasm, moderate to severe atypia and central necrosis (Fig. 7.7). Some cells contain coarse intracytoplasmic, eosinophilic granules, while others show vacuolization. Apical cytoplasmic protrusions are not always evident. Alternately, there may be no definite necrosis, but the cells appear highly anaplastic (Fig. 7.7c), or they may display moderate atypia, but distinctive cell margins imparting a mosaic appearance to the cells that form a solid or cribriform growth pattern. Nucleoli are often present in either setting. When necrosis is present, involvement of even a single duct is sufficient for a diagnosis of carcinoma regardless of the duct size. When necrosis is absent, the same quantitative rule used for the cribriform and micropapillary patterns is applied. Because of the high frequency of apocrine metaplasia and hyperplasia in association with fibrocystic changes, it is important to be particularly cautious in the diagnosis of apocrine IDCA. Therefore, very stringent criteria are required to prevent misinterpretation of the common hyperplasia or metaplasia of apocrine cells as malignant and to avoid overdiagnosis of carcinoma. In this regard, prominent nucleoli are also observed in benign apocrine cells and, by themselves, do not indicate atypia or malignancy.

## Intraductal Clear-cell Carcinoma

Intraductal clear-cell carcinoma is characterized by a proliferation of cells with optically clear cytoplasm and distinct cell margins forming any of the variants of the cribriform pattern (Fig. 7.8). Central necrosis is not uncommon. A solid pattern is also seen within the terminal duct-lobular unit (TDLU), particularly in the earlier stages of its development. This pattern is often seen admixed with the usual cribriform variant.

B

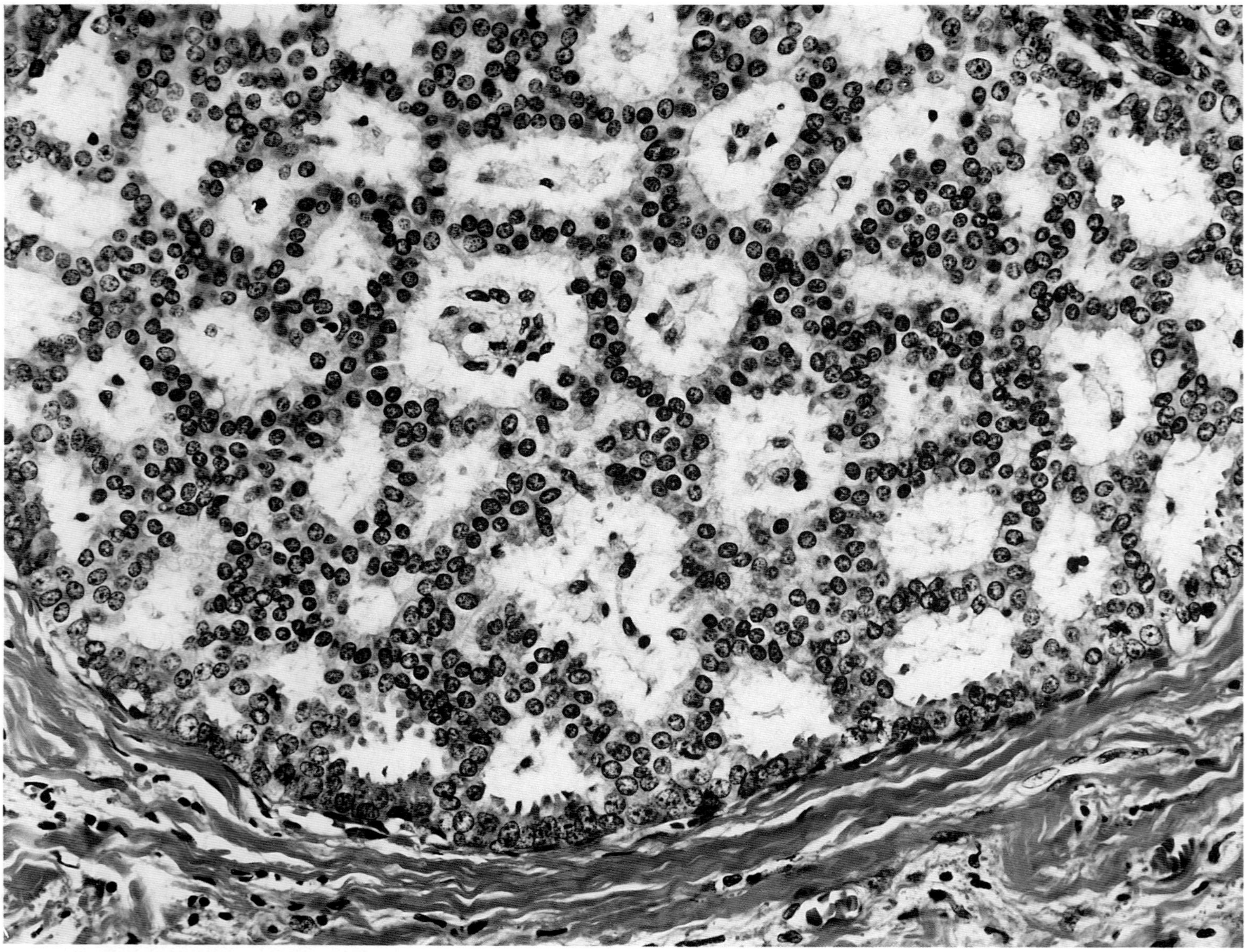

**Figure 7.3(b)** Intraductal carcinoma, cribriform variant. Another example showing a uniform population of cells with rounded nuclei forming rigid epithelial bridges and multiple rounded secondary lumens. Pyknotic nuclei are present within the lumens, but there is no necrosis. (H&E, X680)

Sometimes a single duct may show an admixture of clear cells and the uniform cells typical of the non-necrotic variants of IDCA. It is also seen in association with invasive clear-cell or "glycogen-rich" carcinomas.

## Clinging Carcinoma

This variant was described by Azzopardi (6), and consists of two subtypes (Fig. 7.9). One is similar to comedocarcinoma, but lacks the necrotic luminal debris. This variant shows ducts that are lined by several layers of highly atypical cells; the lumens are empty or contain granular secretory material. In the second type, there is no necrosis, and the native epithelial cell lining of the duct or ductules is replaced by a single layer of atypical cells. Whether these cells reflect an in situ cellular transformation or replacement of the native epithelial cell layer by proliferating neoplastic cells from adjacent foci is difficult to establish. While at AFIP we accept the first subtype of clinging carcinoma and simply designate it as intra-

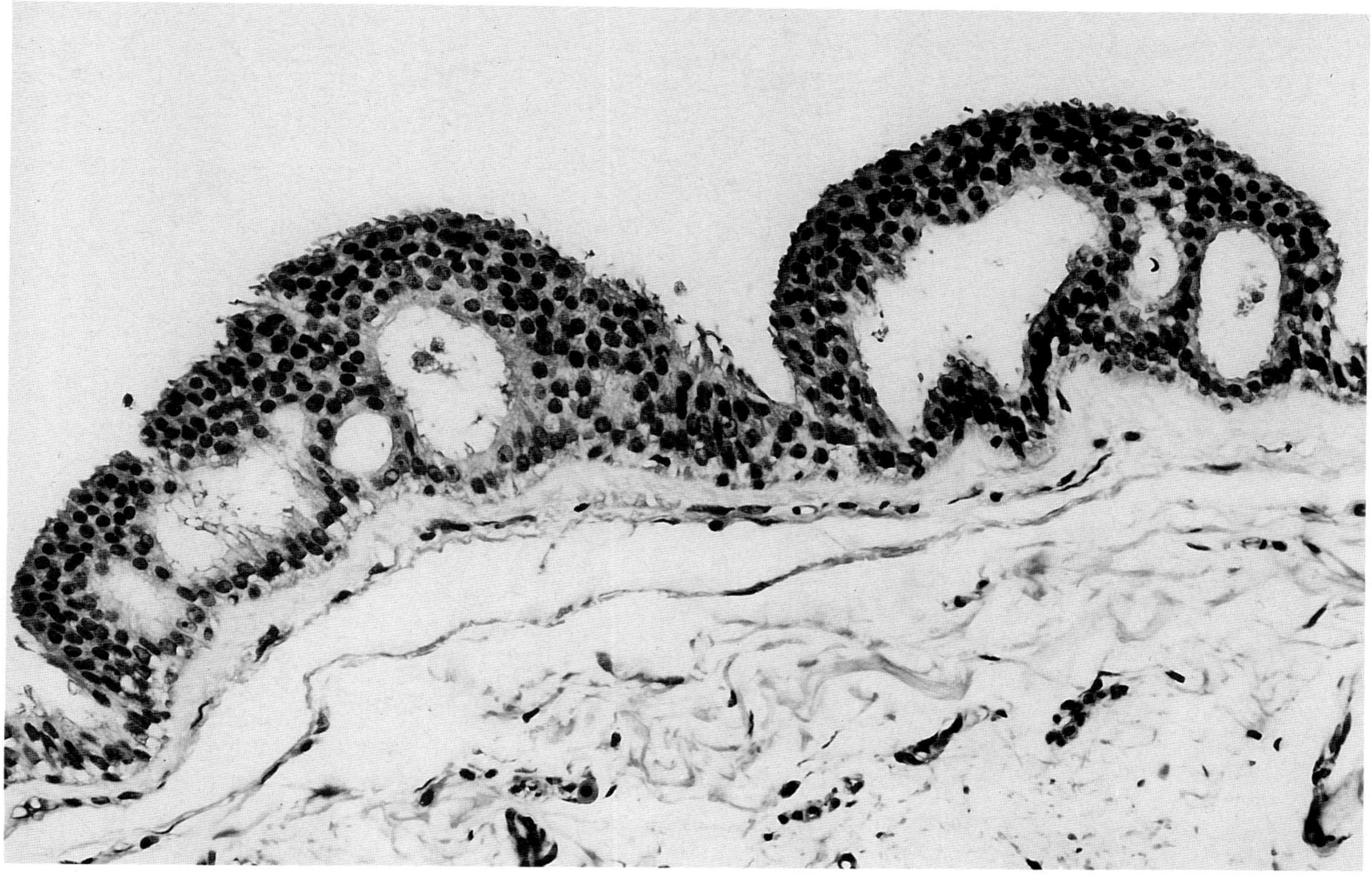

**Figure 7.4** Epithelial arcades are one of the variety of growth patterns observed in the cribriform variant. (H&E, X480)

ductal carcinoma, we are much more reluctant to accept the second subtype. When the native epithelial cell layer is replaced by an atypical cell population, we would carefully and exhaustively evaluate all of the biopsy sample to exclude the presence of a more typical and recognizable intraductal carcinoma. If there is no other lesion, the changes are interpreted as atypical hyperplasia. When the degree of cytologic anaplasia in these cells is great, we have invariably identified necrosis on deeper levels of the block, precluding a designation of clinging carcinoma.

The lesions illustrated by Azzopardi (6) in his Figs. 10.1, 10.4, 10.5, 10.6, and 10.7 would not qualify as carcinoma by the criteria utilized at AFIP. With a few exceptions, most of the changes illustrated as examples of clinging carcinoma by Azzopardi would qualify as atypical intraductal hyperplasia by the AFIP criteria. I have seen lesions similar to those illustrated by Azzopardi in his Figs. 10.2 and 10.3 transformed to typical comedocarcinomas on deeper levels. The example of clinging carcinoma illustrated by Eusebi et al (24) shows some necrosis and significant cytologic anaplasia, and I would designate it as a variant of comedocarcinoma.

## Intraductal Signet-ring Cell Carcinoma

This very rare variant of IDCA is characterized by the proliferation of signet ring cells in solid or papillary growth patterns (see invasive signet ring cell carcinoma). I have seen only two convincing examples of this variant of in situ carcinoma in the absence of an invasive component. Several of the illustrations by Fisher et al (28) in their report on this type of intraductal carcinoma are not convincing and appear to reflect collagenous spherulosis (see Chapter 4).

A

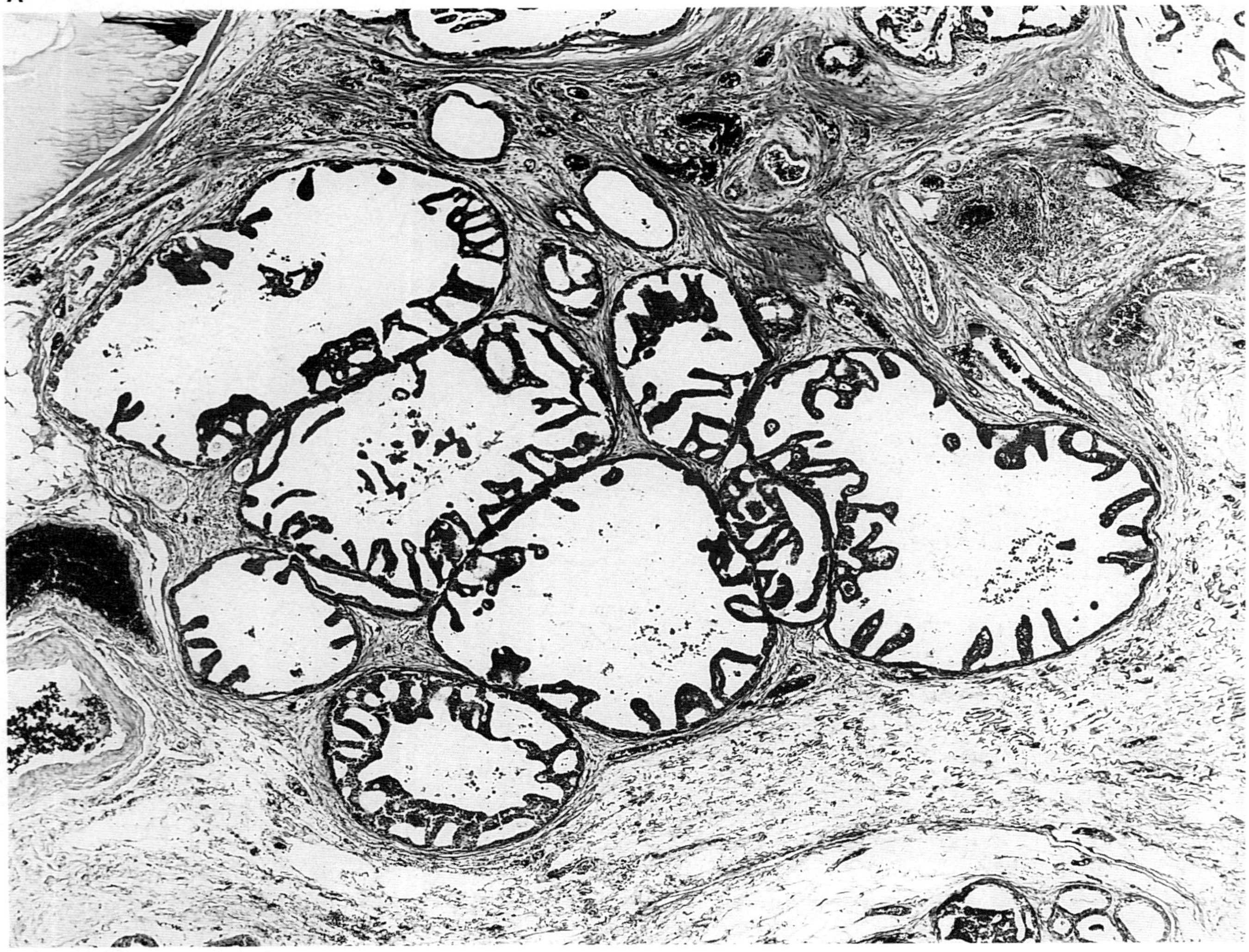

**Figure 7.5** Intraductal carcinoma, micropapillary variant (low grade IDCA). (a&b) A monomorphic cell population forms epithelial tufts around the duct. (H&E, (a) X240; (b) X800).

## Combined Patterns and Rare Types

Frequently, more than a single pattern or cell type is evident in a given biopsy. The different cell types and patterns sometimes display gradual transition (Fig. 7.10), or they may collide (Fig. 7.11) and result in unusual appearances. A solid, "mosaic" pattern of intraductal carcinoma is also observed composed of large round to polygonal cells with distinct cell margins (Fig. 7.12). The intraductal spindle cell carcinoma is one of the most difficult patterns to recognize. I have only made this diagnosis when the intraductal lesion was associated with an invasive spindle cell carcinoma or when other patterns of unequivocal intraductal carcinoma merge with it (see carcinoma with neuroendocrine granules). The possibility of myoepitheliosis should be excluded in these rare cases using immunostain for actin and cytokeratin. The intraductal spindle cell carcinoma is actin negative, but cytokeratin positive (see also adenocarcinoma with spindle cell metaplasia).

## GRADING OF IDCA

There has long been a general suspicion that the comedo variant of intraductal carcinoma is associated with a worse prognosis. This suspicion has been confirmed by the rare available studies correlating the type of intraductal carcinoma with clinical behavior in conservatively treated patients. Lagios et al (48)

B

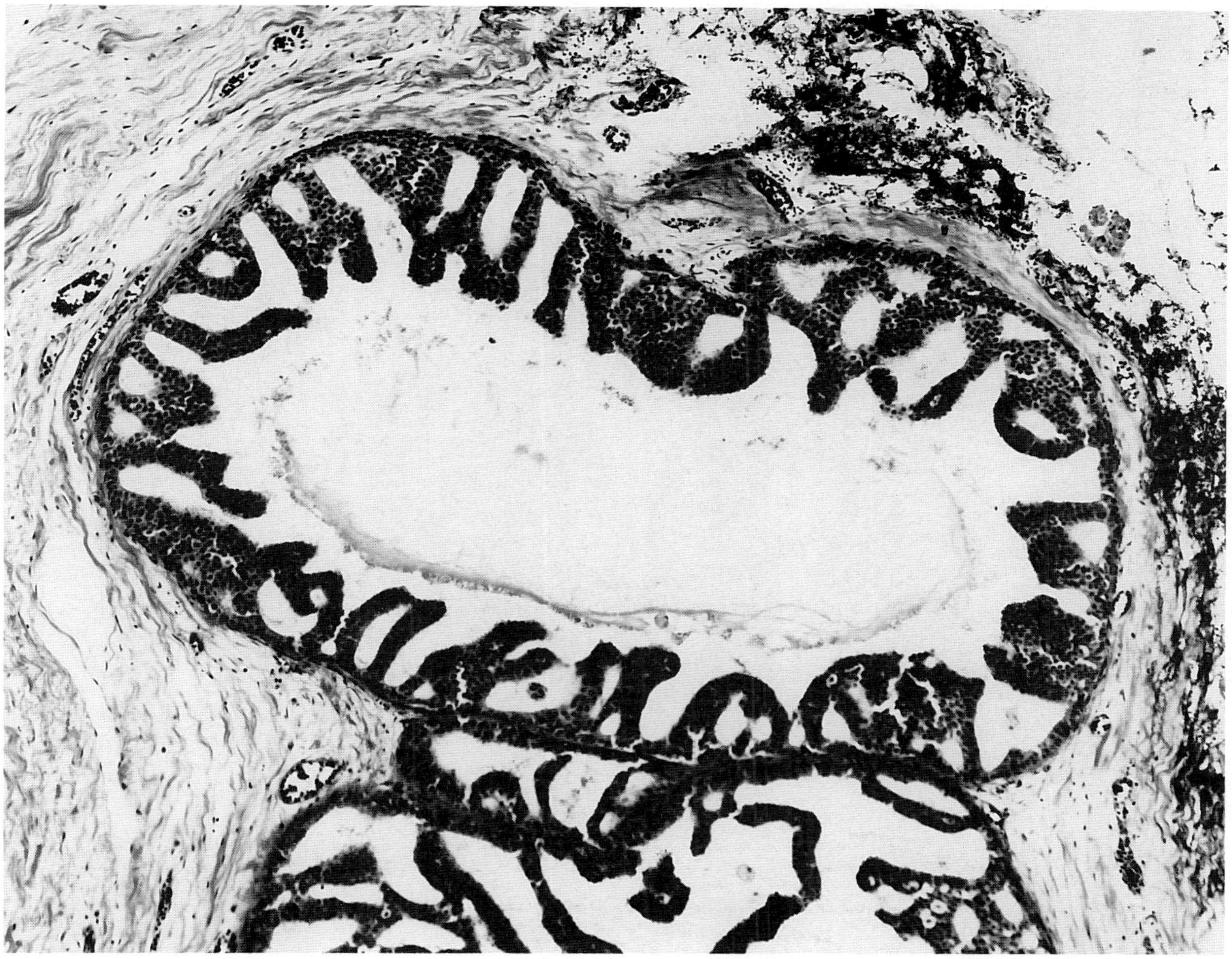

**Figure 7.5(b)** Intraductal carcinoma, micropapillary varient (low grade IDCA). Legend on opposite page.

found a greater number of recurrences among patients with the comedo pattern of IDCA. Their findings suggested that grading of the intraductal carcinoma may be useful as a prognostic factor. Lagios et al subdivided the intraductal carcinomas into comedo, cribriform with necrosis, cribriform with anaplasia, and micropapillary based on nuclear features. I prefer a slight modification to their approach and grade them as high grade, intermediate grade, and low grade based mainly on the presence of necrosis and atypia but also considering cell types.

*High Grade:* Intraductal carcinomas displaying both cytologic atypia and necrosis and those composed purely of classic signet ring cells qualify as high grade lesions (Fig. 7.1). All comedocarcinomas and many intraductal apocrine carcinomas fall into this category. The designation of the signet ring cell variant of IDCA as high grade is purely judgmental and based on the aggressiveness manifested by invasive carcinomas having a signet-ring cell component.

*Moderate Grade:* Three groups of intraductal carcinoma are interpreted as moderately differentiated. In the first group, the proliferating cells lack atypia and may form solid, cribriform or micropapillary patterns with central necrosis; these do not display the cytologic anaplasia characteristic of comedocarcinoma (Fig. 7.13). The second group consists of cribriform, micropapillary or solid patterns with cytologic atypia, but no necrosis (Fig. 7.5c,d). The third group consists of the rare variants (clear cell) and other variants showing an admixture of two uniform cell types (Fig. 7.11), with or without necrosis.

*Low Grade:* Cribriform and micropapillary patterns of intraductal carcinoma composed of a uniform population of cells lacking necrosis or atypia would qualify as low grade (Figs. 7.4, 7.5a,b).

C

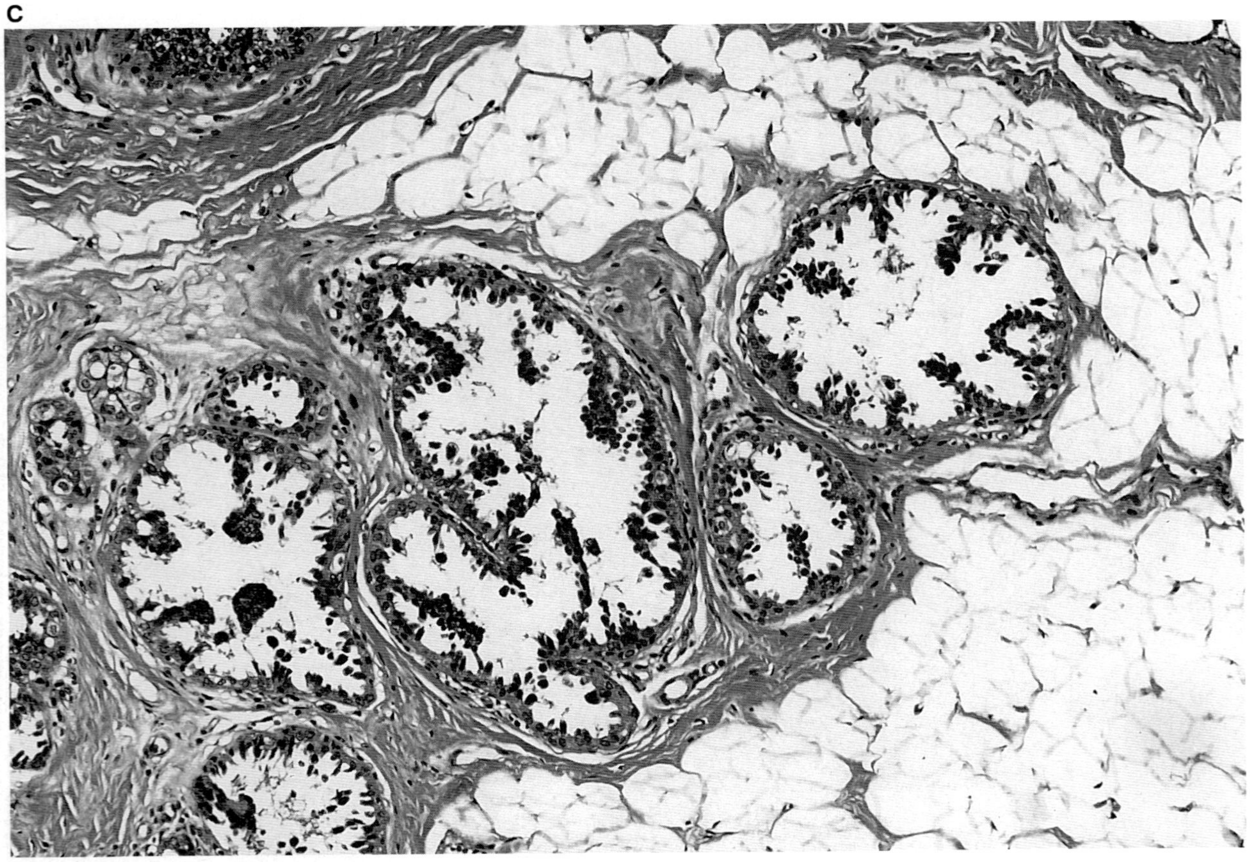

D

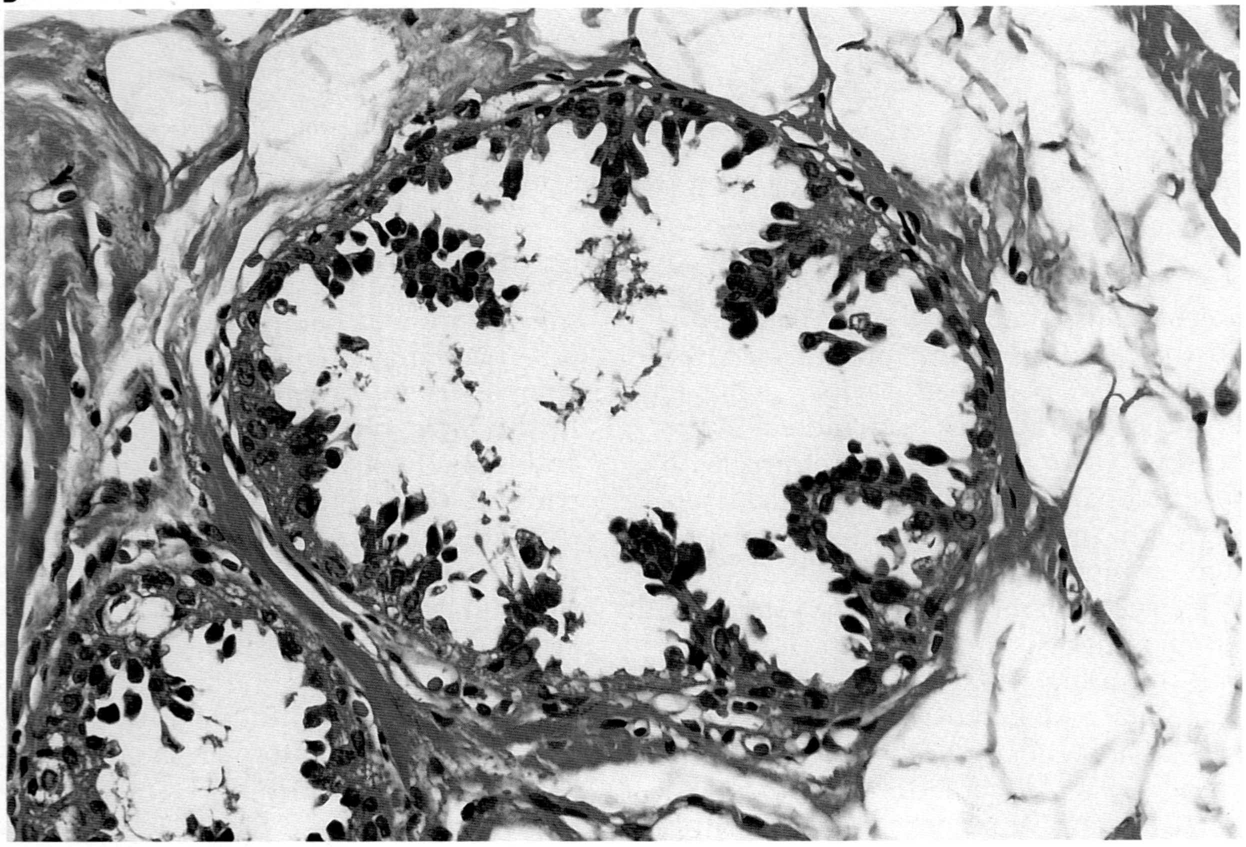

**Figure 7.5(c,d)** Intraductal carcinoma, micropapillary variant. Another tumor composed of a slightly more atypical cell population and somewhat more disorderly micropapillary formations. (H&E, (c) X80; (d) X400)

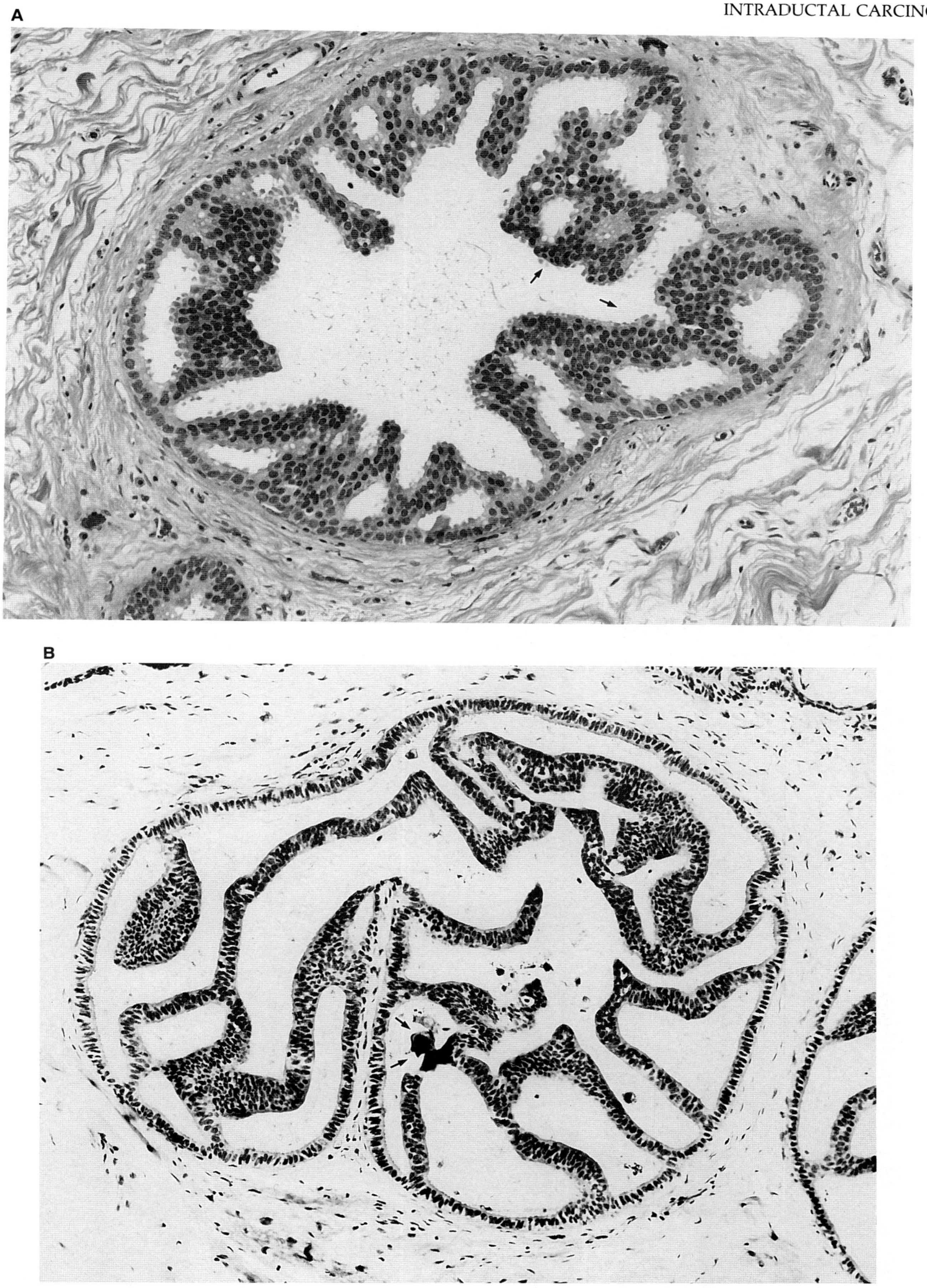


**Figure 7.6** Transitional forms of low grade IDCA. These forms show features of the micropapillary IDCA transforming into the cribriform variant. (a) The tips of the micropapillae merge forming single and double-tiered arcades (arrows). (b) Arcades and a few transluminal bridges have formed, and there is microcalcification (arrows). (H&E, (a) X300; (b) X300)

A

B

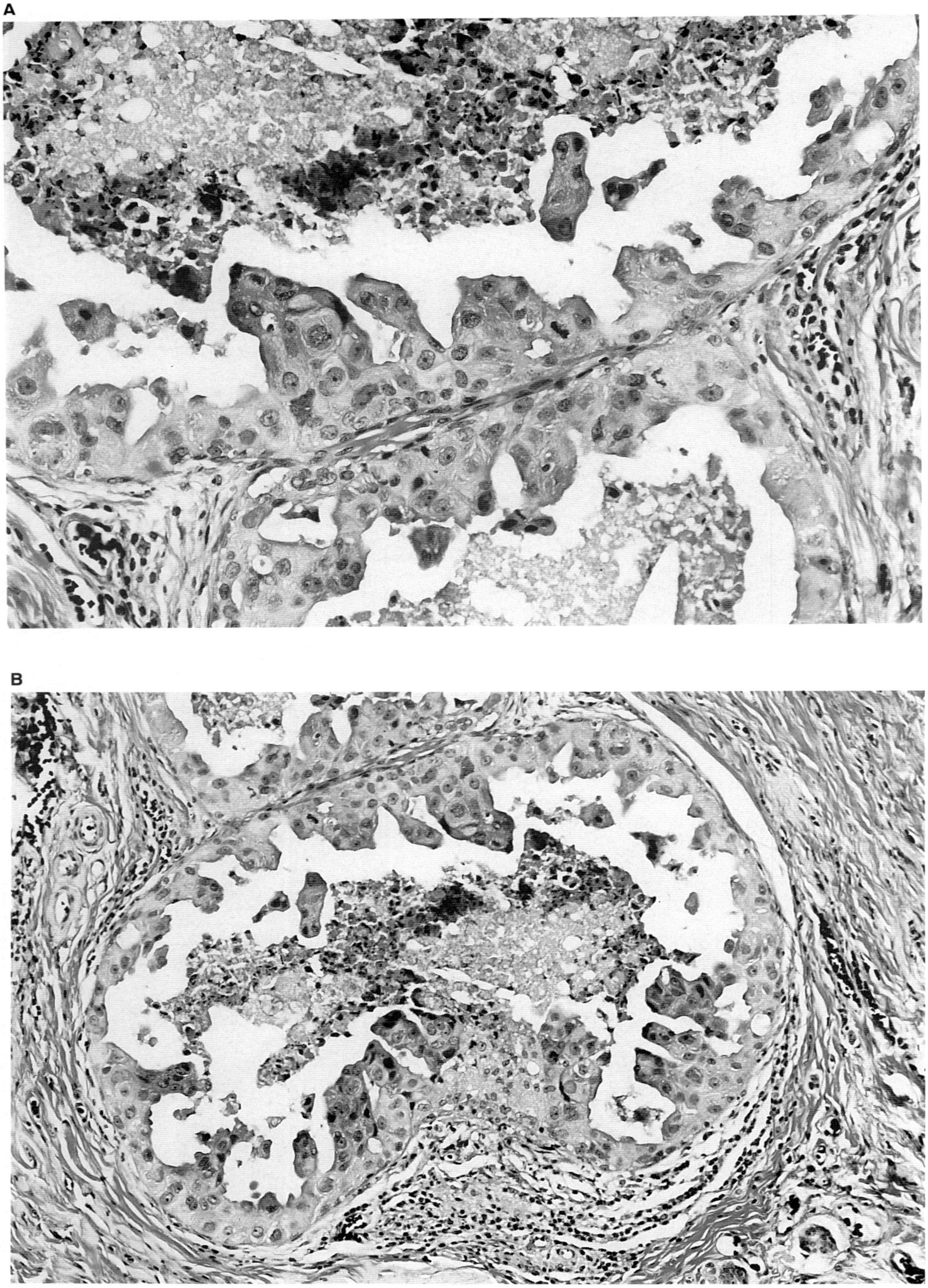

**Figure 7.7(a,b)** Apocrine IDCA. (a) Moderately atypical cells with abundant proliferate in a duct with central necrosis. (b) Higher magnification showing prominent nucleoli and a mitotic figure. (H&E, (a) X320; (b) X480)

C

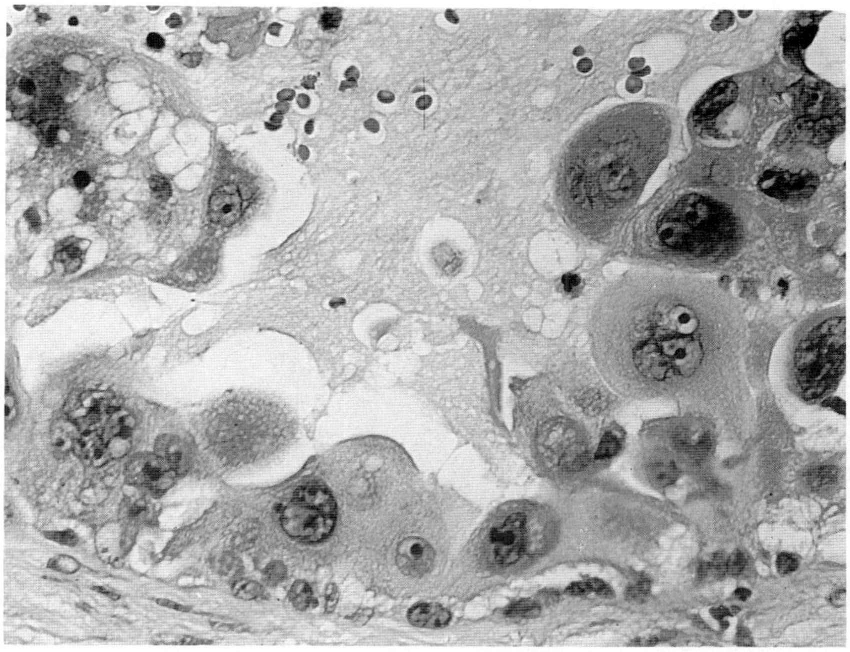

D

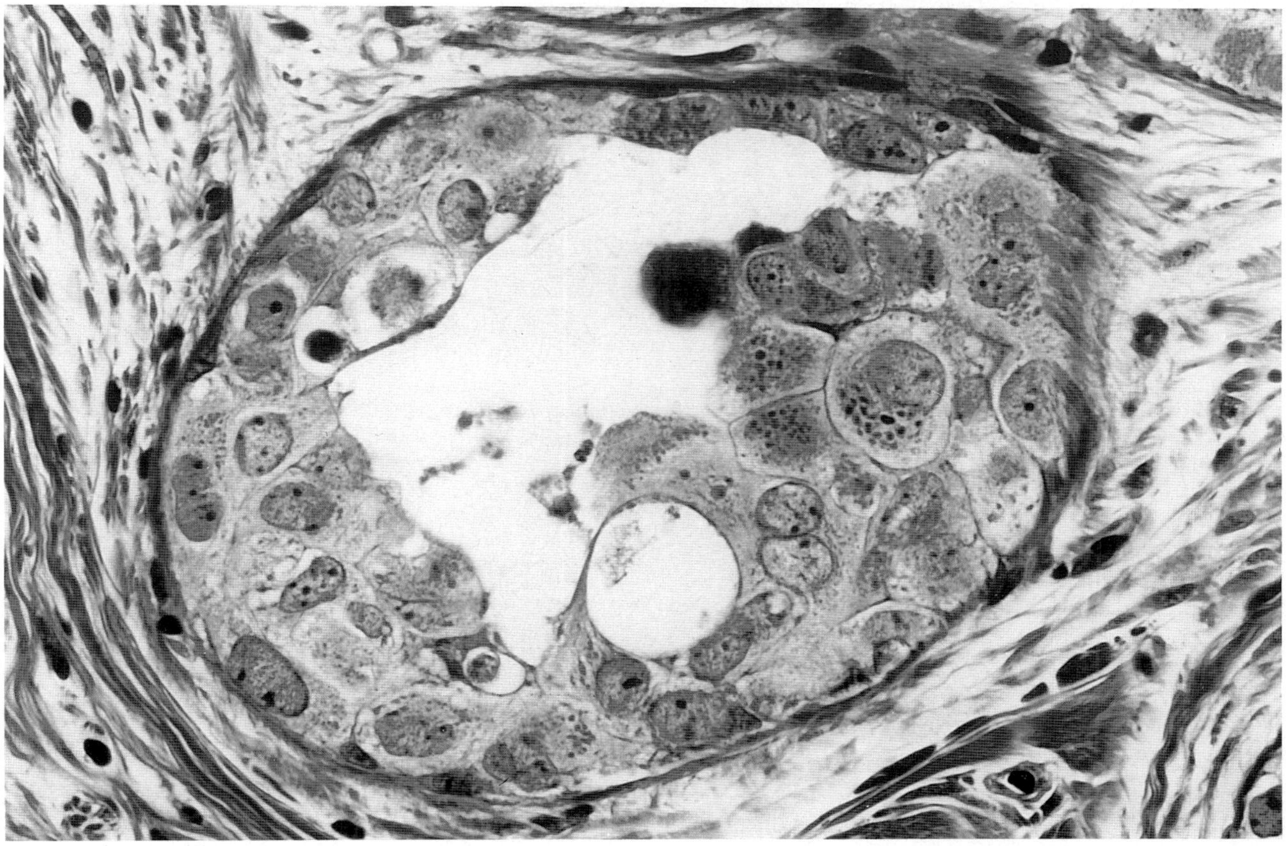

**Figure 7.7(c,d)** Apocrine IDCA. (c) The cells are bizarre with multinucleated cells displaying prominent nucleoli, but no unequivocal central necrosis. (d) Some of the neoplastic cells contain course intracytoplasmic granules. (H&E. (c) X240; (d) X500)

A

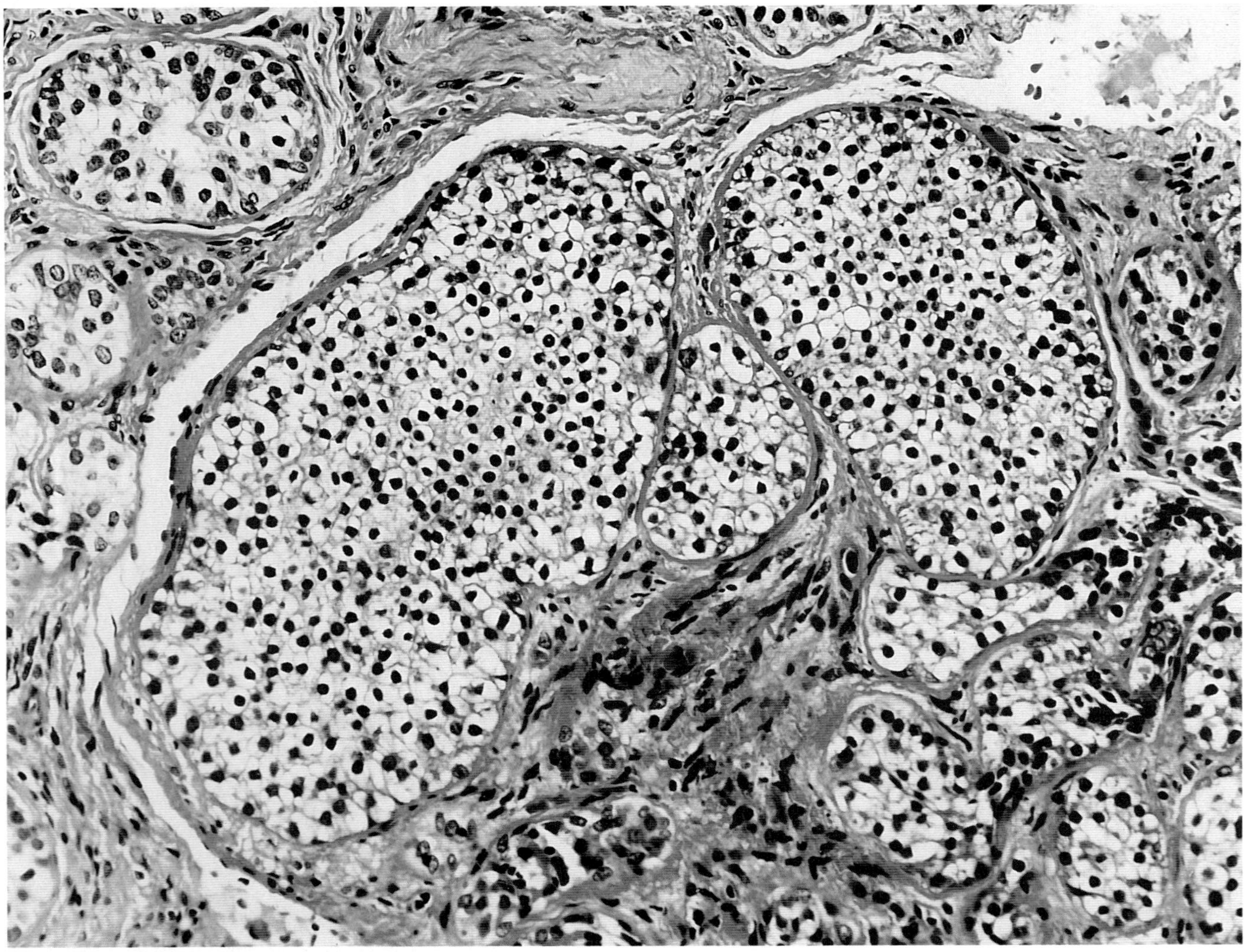

**Figure 7.8** Intraductal clear cell carcinoma. (a) The clear cells may form a solid growth pattern with distinctive cell margins, (b) they may display intraluminal calcification and necrosis, or (c) they may form multiple secondary lumens. Several patterns generally coexist within a biopsy. (H&E, (a) X640; (b) X150; (c) X320)

## DIFFERENTIAL DIAGNOSIS

In many cases, the diagnosis of intraductal carcinoma is simple and straightforward. Sometimes, however, the distinction from AIDH can be quite troublesome. This topic is discussed in detail in Chapter 5. As a rule, in borderline cases and when there is uncertainty, it is best to make the more benign or conservative diagnosis.

Intraductal carcinoma involving lobules (26) or sclerosing adenosis sometimes poses as a diagnostic problem, and it may be misinterpreted as lobular neoplasia or an invasive carcinoma. The cells of ductal carcinoma involving lobules are generally more pleomorphic and larger than the cells of lobular neoplasia. Even when the cells are small and uniform, the formation of rosette-like arrangement of the nuclei, multiple secondary lumen formation, and distinct, cohesive cell margins support a ductal type of proliferation. The presence of a well-defined PAS-positive basement membrane and myoepithelial cells around the proliferating tubules helps distinguish IDCA involving sclerosing adenosis from invasive carcinoma (23). Immunostain for actin may be required to unmask and enhance the myoepithelial cell layer.

Sometimes it is difficult to determine if there is stromal invasion, particularly in cases of extensive comedocarcinoma. Often the areas of early invasion are characterized by blurring of the normally sharp epithelial-stromal interface and altered stroma ap-

B

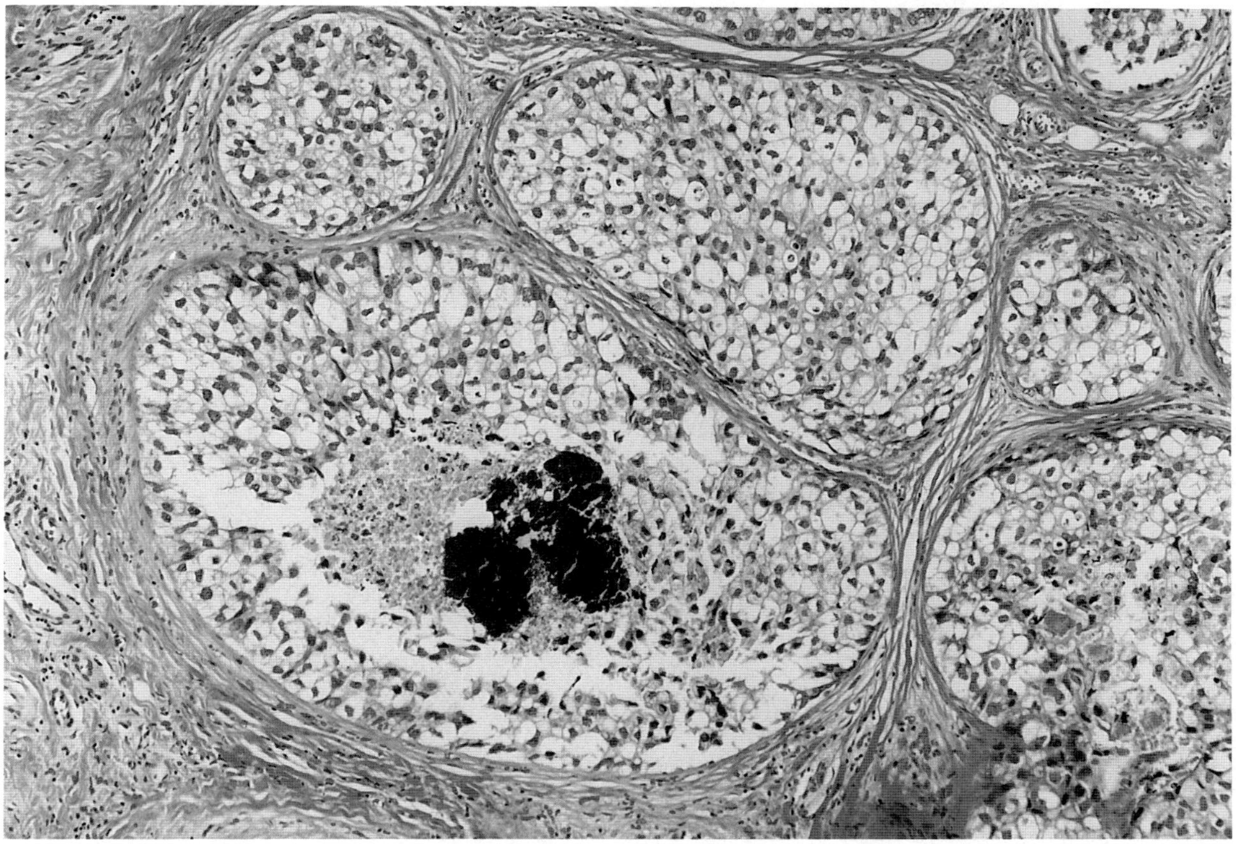

C

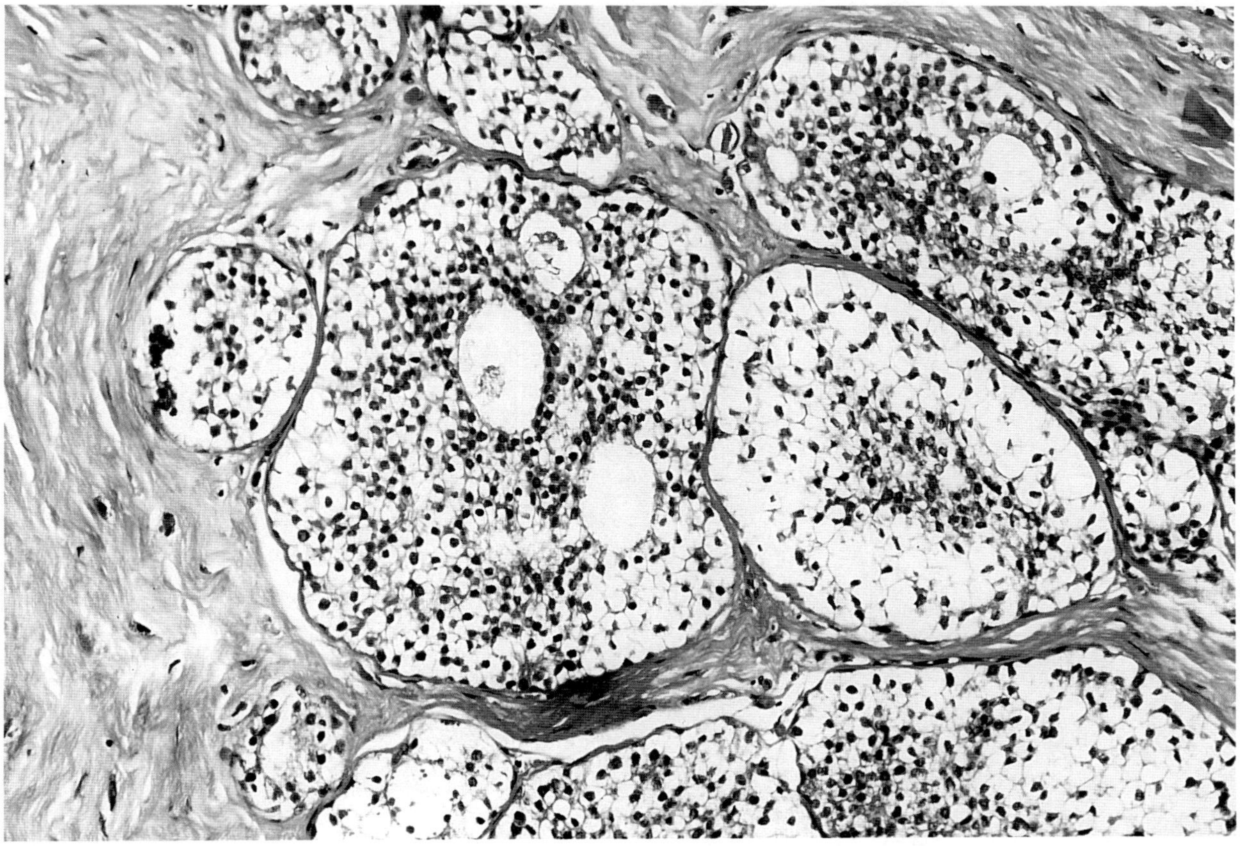

**Figure 7.8(b,c)** Intraductal clear cell carcinoma. Legend on opposite page.

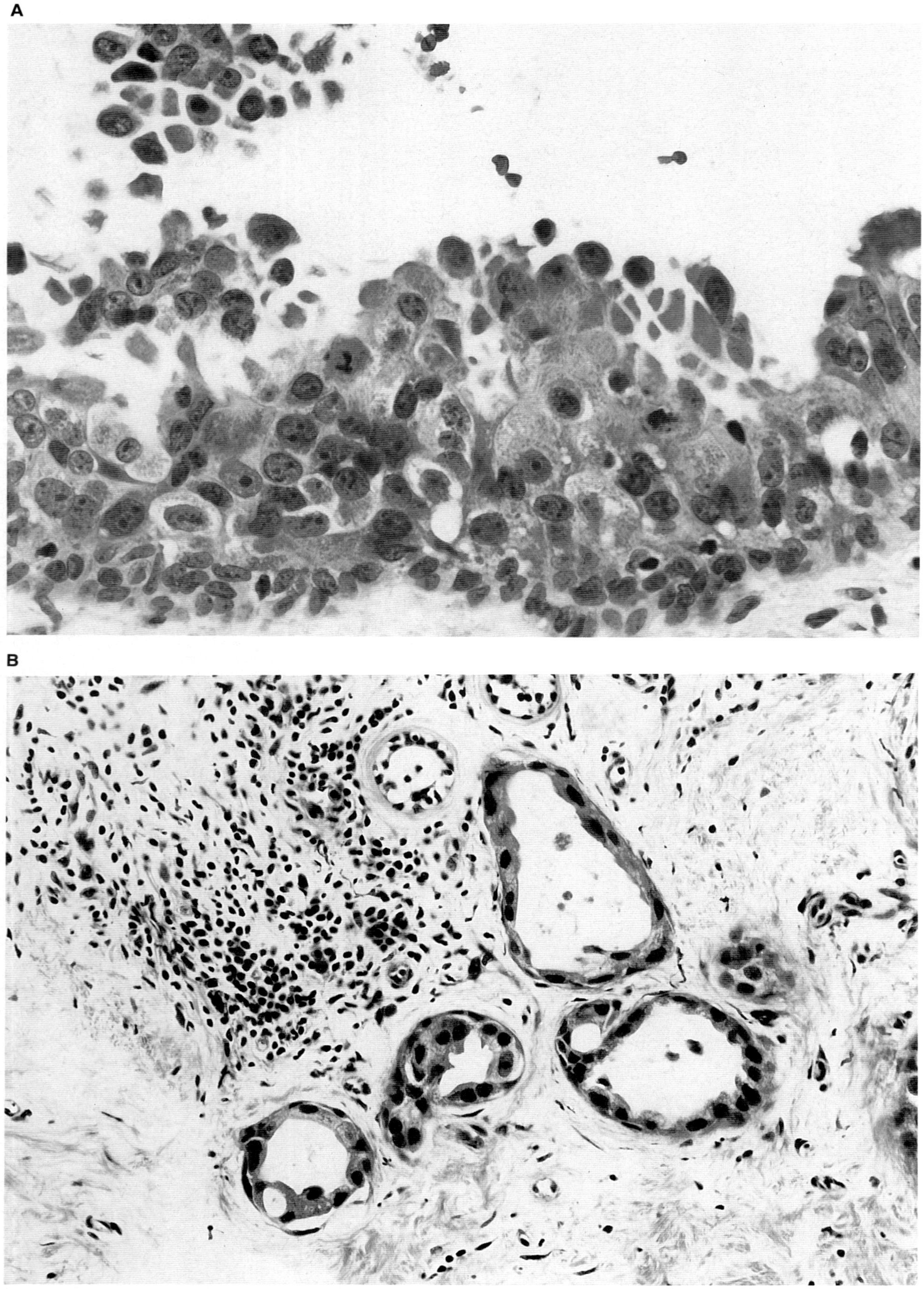


**Figure 7.9** Intraductal clinging carcinoma. (a) The subtype acceptable as a carcinoma is characterized by proliferation of pleomorphic, atypical cells, but there is no central necrosis; the lumen contains granular secretory material and histiocytes. (b) The subtype that I would designate as atypical intraductal hyperplasia shows replacement of the normal epithelial cell layer by a single layer of atypical cells, but no necrosis. This finding requires thorough evaluations of the biopsy to exclude the presence of recognizable IDCA. (H&E, (a) X400; (b) X480)

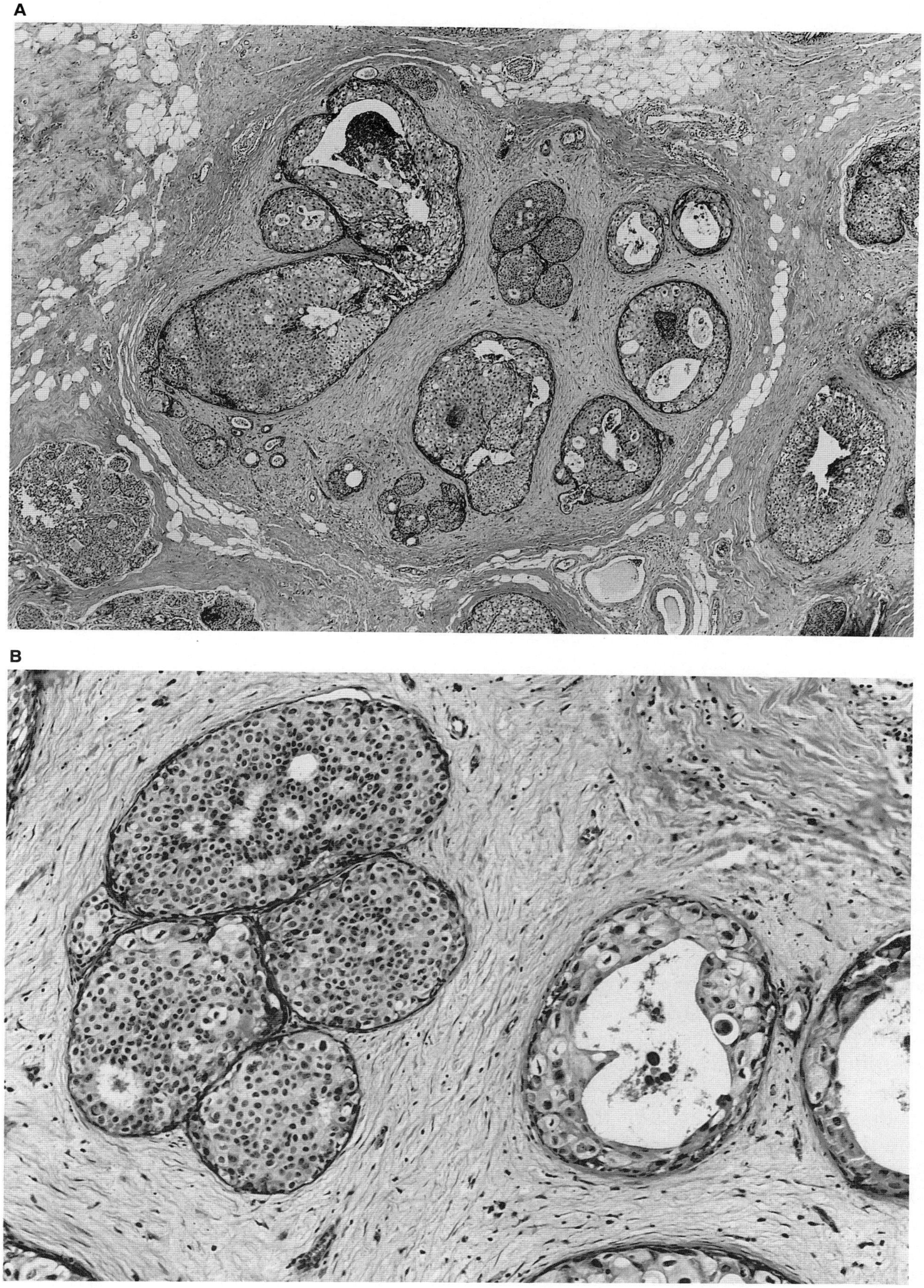


**Figure 7.10** Intraductal carcinoma showing proliferation of several patterns and cell types (a&b). (H&E, (a) X60; (b) X240)

A

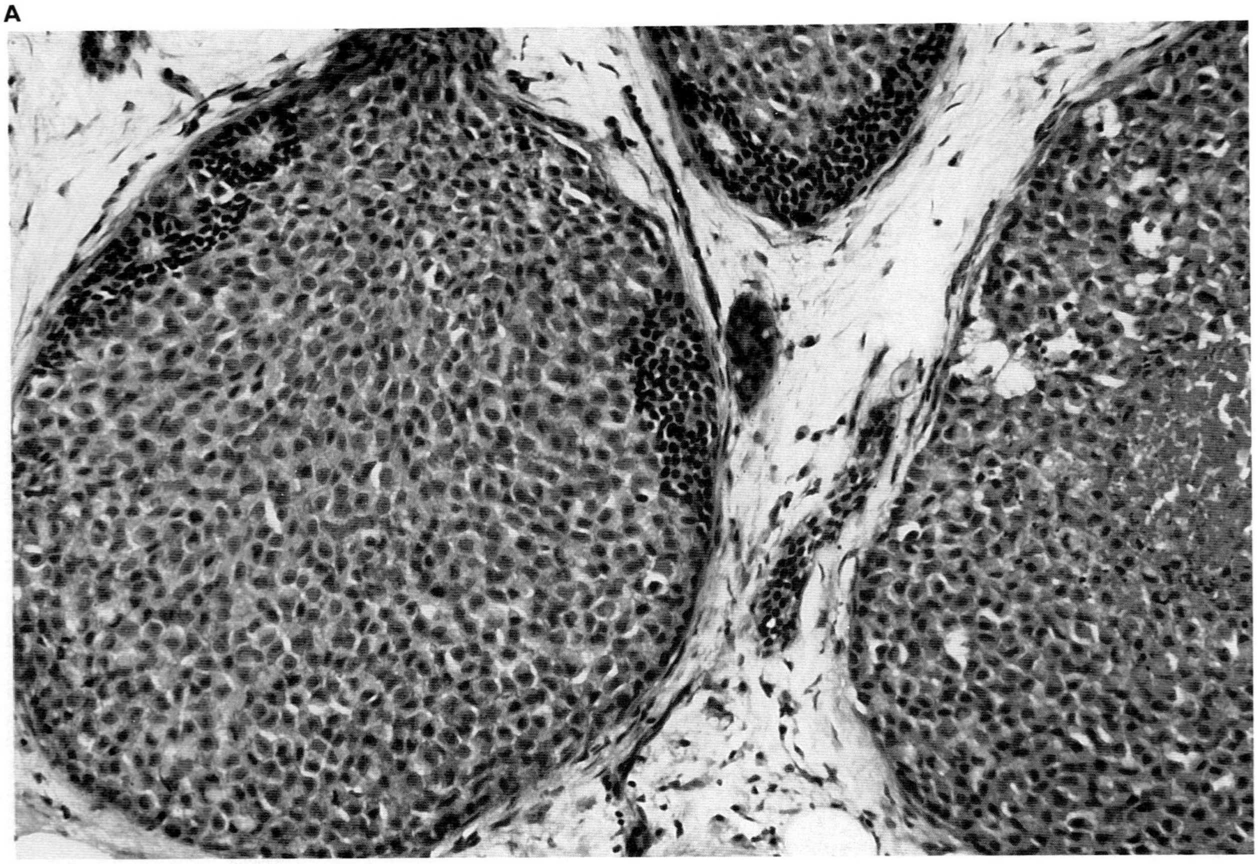

**Figure 7.11** Collision of two types of IDCA. (a) One of the ducts shows larger cells with central necrosis, the other shows rosette-like arrangement of cells with hyperchromatic nuclei and sparse cytoplasm focally around the larger cells. (H&E, X400) (b) More of the smaller cells with rosette-like arrangement of the nuclei are apparent in the periphery of the duct. Elsewhere in the biopsy some ducts had a pure proliferation of the hyperchromatic cells, while others displayed a pure proliferation of the larger cells with central necrosis. (H&E, X240) (c) Two adjacent ducts, one showing a predominance of the cribriform pattern with hyperchromic cell, the other a predominance of the solid growth pattern. (H&E, X240)

pearance (more edematous or more reactive desmoplasia, occasionally containing a few inflammatory cells) compared to the periductal stroma elsewhere (see also the section on microinvasive carcinoma in Chapter 9). Since our routine diagnosis is based on evaluation of H&E sections, unless there is unequivocal evidence of invasion, it is best to designate the lesion as in situ. Such lesions deserve careful evaluation of sometimes numerous levels of the areas of concern before designating the changes as either in situ or invasive carcinoma. In this regard, it is worth noting that frequently patterns identical to those we recognize as intraductal carcinomas are seen in metastatic foci within lymph nodes. It is unlikely that these reflect true in situ carcinomas. Apparently, invasive carcinomas can sometimes assume patterns indistinguishable from an intraductal carcinoma. Therefore, some of the foci that we interpret as intraductal carcinoma may actually reflect patterns of invasive carcinoma. It is not surprising, then, that 1% to 2% of women with IDCA have axillary node metastases at the time of diagnosis (6). Ultrastructural and immunohistochemical evaluation of the integrity of basement membrane (BM), using BM proteins such as laminin and type IV collagen, may be useful in identifying areas of invasion (8,61), but the practical value of these techniques has not been established. In my personal experience with immunostains using laminin and type IV collagen, there are sufficient problems associated with the technique and interpretation of the results that I would not recommend absolute reliance on the presence of breaks in the basement membrane identified by these methods as an indicator of invasion.

B

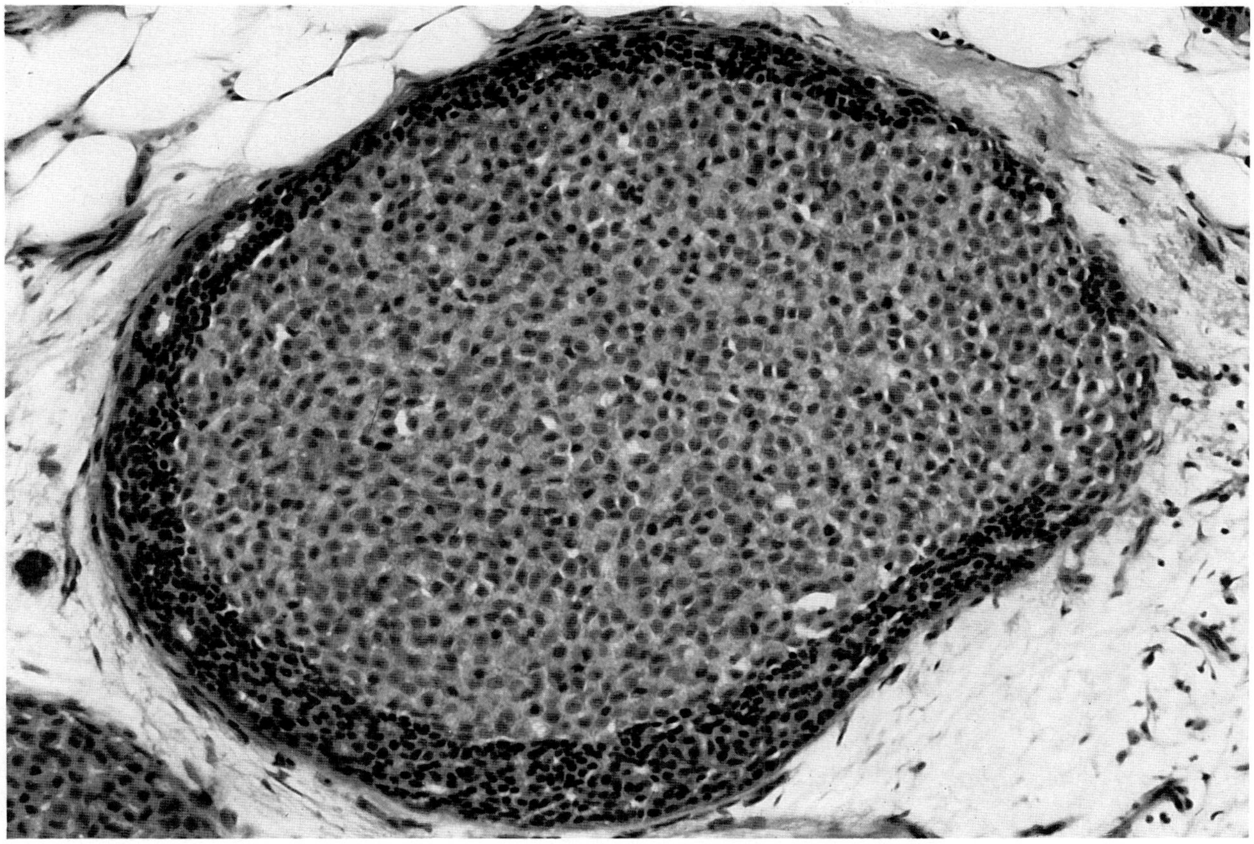

C

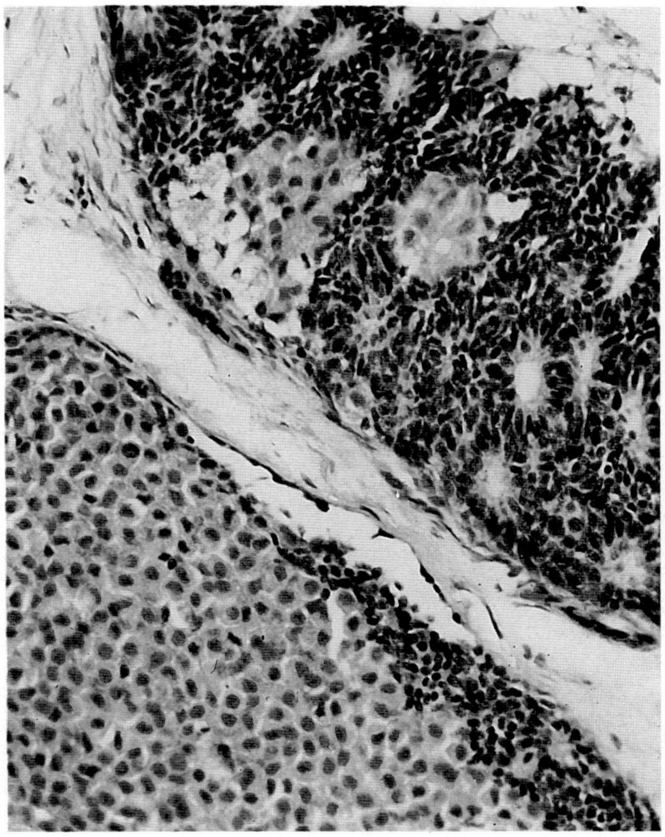

**Figure 7.11(b,c)** Collision of two types of IDCA. Legend on opposite page.

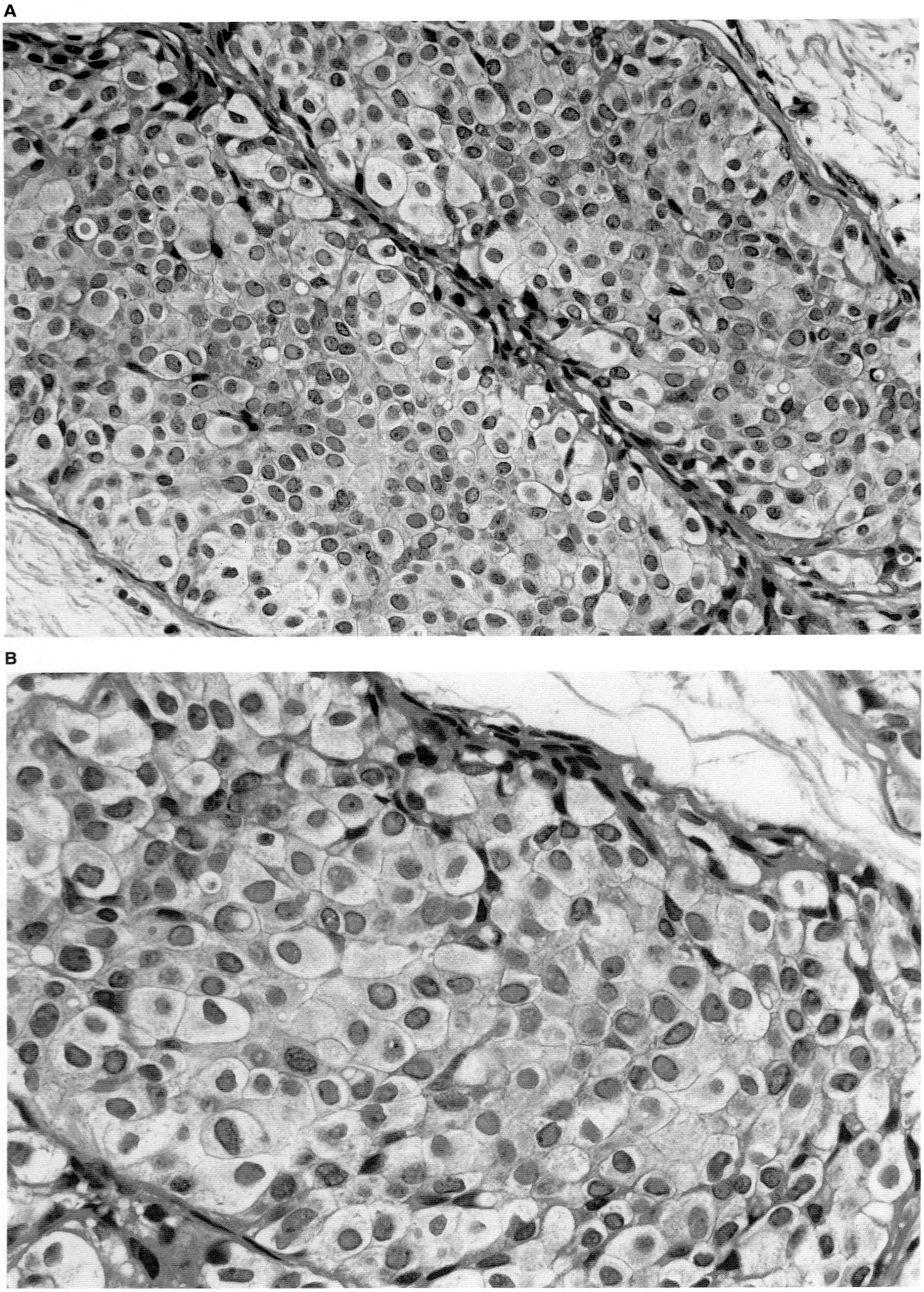

**Figure 7.12** Solid "mosaic" variant of intraductal carcinoma. (a&b) The atypical proliferating cells are round to polygonal, with distinctive cell margins imparting a mosaic appearance to the lesion, grow in a solid fashion, and occlude the lumens. (H&E, (a) X600; (b) X800)

A

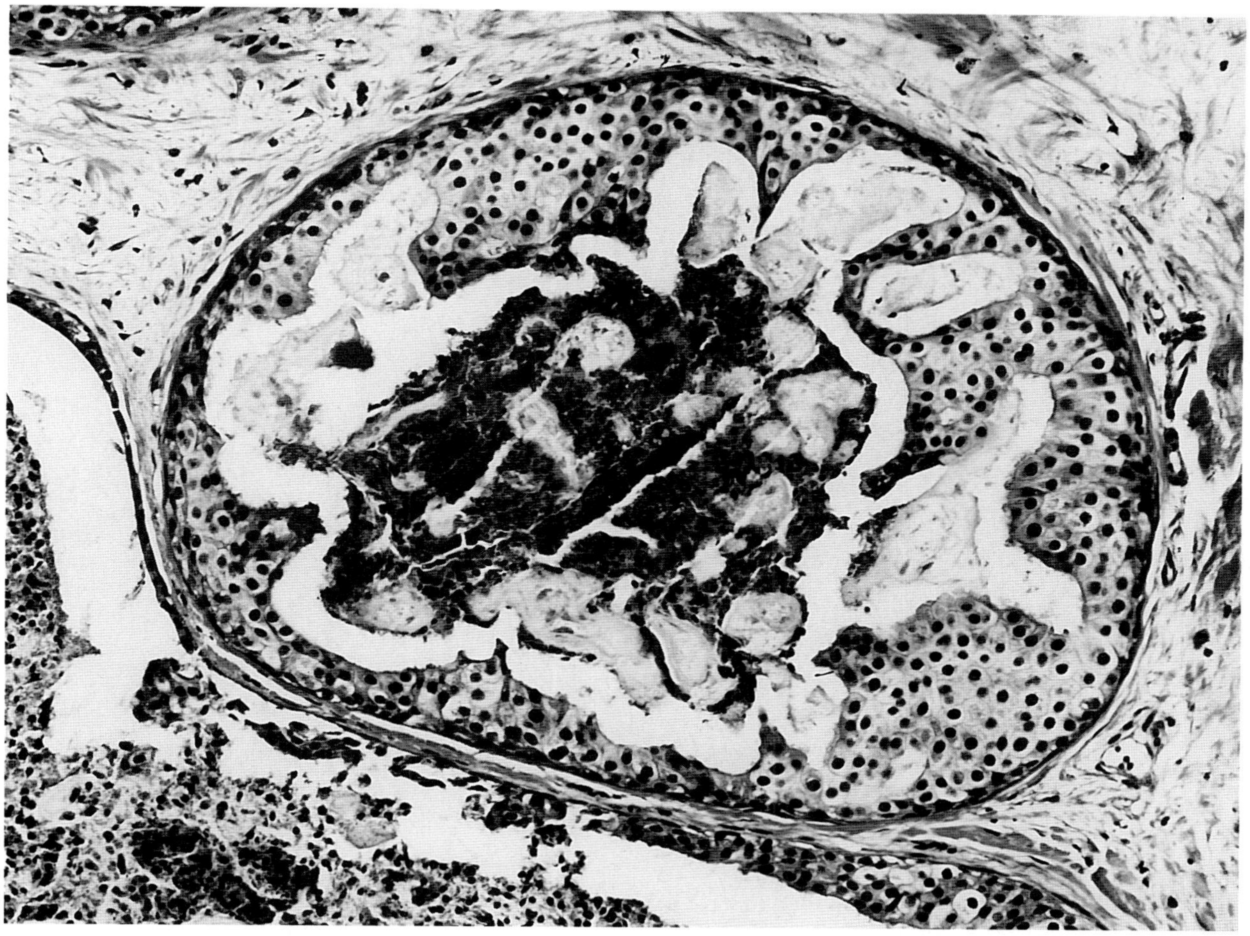

**Figure 7.13(a)** Intraductal carcinoma, intermediate grade. There is central necrosis, but the proliferating cells are uniform, lacking pleomorphism. (H&E, X300)

## SPECIAL STUDIES, HORMONE RECEPTORS, AND ULTRASTRUCTURAL ANALYSIS

Obviously, there are several morphologic variants of IDCA. Some of these variants may have a significant proliferative, but negligible invasive, potential. Whether or not these are all precursors of invasive carcinoma has not been established—some of the low-grade, non-necrotic variants may prove to be biologically inactive. The high frequency of intraductal carcinoma in autopsy series of asymptomatic women (58), and in the contralateral breast of 13% of the women with invasive breast cancer (93) suggests that not all IDCAs become invasive. Unfortunately, we have no reliable means of predicting which lesions may progress to invasive carcinoma. To unravel the mysteries surrounding the biologic significance of the proliferating cells, attention has been focused on a variety of special approaches including biomarkers that may help the pathologists in assessing the aggressive potential of a given lesion.

One of the biomarkers utilized extensively in a number of studies on a variety of breast carcinomas is c-erbB-2 or neu-protein. Neu-protein overexpression was detected immunohistochemically in nearly all specimens showing IDCA with large nuclear size, poor cytonuclear differentiation, high mitotic rate, and in none of the small-cell IDCA tested (93). Neu-protein has membrane receptor characteristics and is homologous with the epidermal growth factor. Its presence in large-cell IDCA (comedocarcinoma) has been interpreted as an expression of rapid growth (93). It appears that basically neu-protein has confirmed the more aggressive potential of the comedo variant of IDCA which had been suspected on the

B

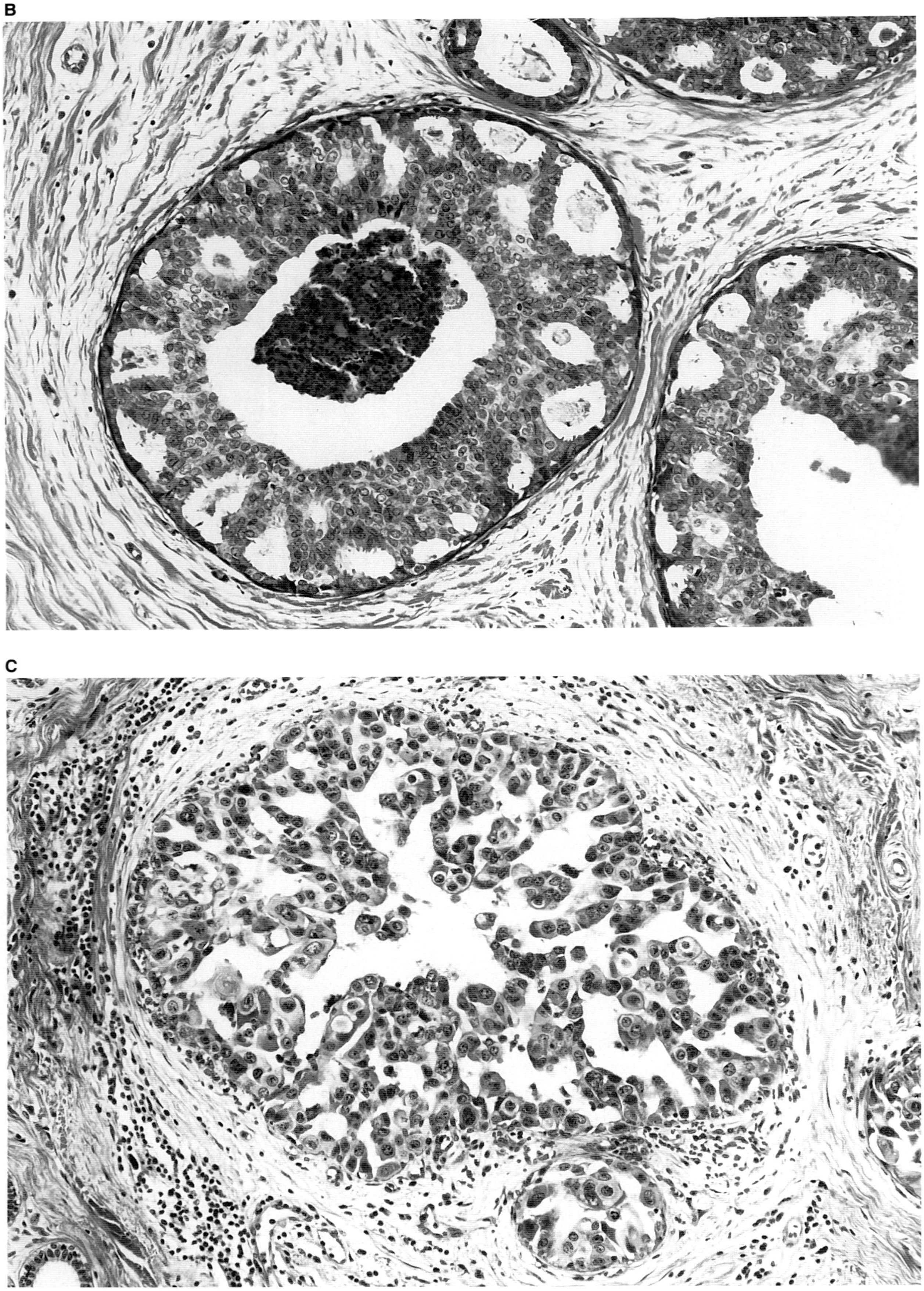

C

**Figure 7.13(b,c)** Intraductal carcinoma, intermediate grade. (b) A relatively uniform cell population proliferates in a cribriform pattern, but with central necrosis. (H&E, X300) (c) There is no necrosis, but the cells are more atypical than those of classic micropapillary IDCA. (H&E, X300)

basis of its histomorphology and confirmed in clinical follow-up studies (48).

Ploidy is another feature of malignancies that often correlates with their behavior. An aneuploid DNA content in IDCA seems to be related to early recurrence after excisional biopsy (18). About 30% of IDCA and atypical intraductal hyperplasias have displayed aneuploidy. Among 26 cases of IDCA associated with invasive carcinoma, 22 (88.4%) displayed aneuploid cells. Of 16 cases of concurrent IDCA and invasive carcinoma, both phases of the carcinoma were aneuploid in 11 cases, both were diploid in one, and in four cases the IDCA was aneuploid, whereas, the invasive component was diploid.

Another aspect of the different variants of IDCA that has been evaluated and compared is their proliferative rate. The growth rate of comedocarcinoma is more rapid than that of other types of intraductal carcinoma. Comedocarcinomas are composed of a more anaplastic cell population which displays a higher proliferative rate as determined by thymidine labeling index (TLI) compared to other types of IDCA (54). The utility of TLI as a prognostic factor and its value in determining the optimal therapeutic regimen for an individual patient with IDCA has not been defined, however.

Morphometric studies have shown that the mean diameter of ducts containing IDCA with necrosis is 470 $\mu$m compared to a mean diameter of 192 $\mu$m for IDCA without necrosis (52). Furthermore, necrosis is found in 94% of ducts larger than 180 $\mu$m in radius, compared to 34% of ducts less than 180 $\mu$m in size. These findings have been noted as providing indirect evidence for the existence of a hypoxic compartment in IDCA that could explain the higher local failure rate after conservative surgery and irradiation in cases of comedocarcinoma.

Estrogen receptor proteins have been reported in ICDA (72). They have been observed in less than 20% of comedocarcinomas and over 50% of the cribriform, papillary and solid variants (35). These findings provide additional support for the more poorly differentiated nature of the cells in comedocarcinoma.

Ozzello (61) has shown that a high proportion of lesions interpreted as intraductal carcinoma histologically show evidence of basement membrane irregularity and foci of early invasion at the ultrastructural level. It is neither practical, nor proven efficacious, however, to evaluate IDCA at the ultrastructural level for the determination of early stromal invasion.

## BILATERALITY AND MULTICENTRICITY

The incidence of bilaterality for IDCA varies from 2.2% to 10% (26,49,55,81,86,102). Of the 28 women reported by Millis and Thynne (55), two had bilateral IDCA. In a study by Alpers and Wellings (1), intraductal carcinoma was found in 48% of breasts contralateral to the one harboring an invasive cancer, yet in a prospective study of 1,458 women with invasive breast carcinoma, 94 new primaries developed in the contralateral breast 20 years following the diagnosis of the initial cancer (69), or a cumulative risk of 12.5% after 20 years. On the other hand, four of 116 (3.4%) patients with IDCA developed subsequent breast cancer in the contralateral breast within an average of nine years (100). The incidence of previous, concurrent, and subsequent invasive carcinoma in the contralateral breast ranges from 4.7% (102) to 10% (11). In one study based on 112 patients, however, 32 (29%) of the women had prior, simultaneous, or subsequent carcinoma (in situ or invasive) in the contralateral breast (4). This is a rather high frequency of contralateral breast carcinoma and comparable to the 36.5% noted for LCIS in the same study (4). Unfortunately, the diagnostic criteria for IDCA are not clearly stated.

The frequency of multicentricity ranges from 12% to 45.5%, but has been noted to be as high as 64% to 76% (19,49,75,79) in patients with IDCA treated by mastectomy. The definition of multicentricity is not uniform in various studies, however, and this may account for the wide range noted. Some use the terms "multifocal" and "multicentric" interchangeably; I use them to express two different extents of distribution (see Chapter 2, General Considerations). A majority of IDCA are multifocal, but a much smaller number are multicentric.

## TREATMENT

The management of patients with IDCA must be tempered by the available data regarding its multicentricity, bilaterality, and the lack of information regarding its bioclinical progression if left behind. Until recently, mastectomy was the treatment of choice for intraductal carcinoma. Two recent devel-

**Table 7.1** Results of Treatment of Ductal Carcinoma In Situ

| No. of Patients | Therapeutic Method, (Ref.) | Presentation | Follow-up | Local Recurrence | Salvage of Patients with Local Recurrence* | Overall Survival (%) |
|---|---|---|---|---|---|---|
| 74 | MastX, (5) | Palpable Mass | 11 yr | 0 | N/A | 100 |
| 68 | MastX, (90) | Palpable Mass | 10 yr (min) | 0 | N/A | 95 |
| 181 | MastX, (25) | Palpable Mass | 5–20 yr** | 2 | N/A | 98 |
| 40 | CS&RT, (68) | Palpable Mass | 44 mo (med) | 4 | 4 | 100 |
| 54 | CS&RT, (104) | Palpable Mass | 55 mo (med) | 3 | 2 | 98 |
| 56 | CS&RT, (56) | Palpable Mass | 60 yr (med) | 2 | 1 | 98 |
| 29 | CS&RT, (31) | Palpable Mass | 24 mo (mean) | 2 | 1 | 100 |
| 259 | CS&RT, (89) | 40% Mammographic | 78 mo (med) | 28 | 24 | 94 |
| 71 | CS, (48) | 100% Mammographic | 43 mo (mean) | 6 | 6 | 100 |
| 22 | CS, (31) | Palpable Mass | 39 mo (mean) | 5 | 5 | 100 |
| 96 | RT, (84) | 70% Mammographic | 42 mo (med) | 7 | 6 | N/A |

*Abbreviations:* No. = number; ref. = reference; MastX. = mastectomy; CS = conservative surgery; RT = radiation therapy; min = minimum; N/A = not available; * Salvage is defined as freedom from further recurrence after treatment of the local recurrence; ** range of follow-up, median not reported.

Modified with permission from Schnitt SJ, et al: *N Engl J Med* 1988;318:898–903.

opments have raised questions regarding the efficacy of this approach, and have prompted a reassessment of the management of patients with ICDA. As a result, two conservative options have been offered on a limited basis to patients with IDCA over the past ten years: complete excision, or complete excision followed by external radiotherapy (31,47,56,68,104) (see Table 7.1)

One of the developments that has resulted in the more conservative options is increased patient awareness coupled with widespread use of screening mammography and improved mammographic techniques. Together, these have led to the detection of lower grade IDCA and IDCA of very limited extent—some less than a few millimeters in size and confined to a small cluster of ductules. The biologic significance of these early morphologic carcinomas is not known. Some pathologists have already started categorizing those intraductal proliferations morphologically identical to the cribriform or micropapillary variants of IDCA, but involving less than two separate spaces (63), or those involving one or more ducts measuring less than 2 mm in aggregate cross-sectional diameter (91), as AIDH. One of the major reasons for separating the smaller lesions and categorizing them as AIDH has been to prevent the drastic measure of mastectomy which until recently, was the only treatment for IDCA, and remains the basic approach to the treatment of intraductal carcinomas in many hospitals in the United States regardless of the type and amount of the IDCA.

Another factor that has refocused our attention on the management of IDCA is that lumpectomy and radiation therapy are now offered as the equivalent of mastectomy to many patients with invasive carcinomas less than 2 cm in size that have not metastasized to axillary nodes ($T_2N_0$) (2,16,27,38,40,56,58,97). This current shift to a more conservative treatment for invasive carcinomas makes it difficult to justify mastectomy for in situ carcinomas in order to prevent the development of an invasive carcinoma which could be treated by lumpectomy.

Let us examine the results of the various available options.

## Mastectomy

Mastectomy has been the most successful form of treatment in preventing recurrences and providing a cure for patients with IDCA. But even mastectomy is not an absolute curative measure, since failures due to chest wall recurrences occur even among patients so treated (32,86,90). The type of surgery performed on patients with IDCA varies from subcutaneous mastectomy to radical mastectomy; the use of the latter procedure has declined gradually, but significantly, over the past two decades. Prophylactic subcutaneous mastectomy, which is sometimes performed for early IDCA or borderline lesions in high risk patients, leaves behind a substantial amount of breast tissue. It has been estimated that 5% of the breast tissue left behind is in the regions of the tail of the breast, beneath the nipple, and in the thick skin flaps after subcutaneous mastectomy (92). Based on anecdotal reports, this procedure is associated with an incidence subsequent breast carcinoma of about 1% (92). It is noteworthy that even a standard total mastectomy performed for breast cancer frequently leaves breast tissue within the superficial pectoralis major muscle, and the lower skin flap (92). According to Temple et al (92), if total glandular extirpation of the breast is intended, then mastectomy must be extended to include a layer of the pectoralis major fascia as well as the lower-level axilla, and the lower skin flaps must be made very thin.

Farrow (25) reported the result of mastectomy (ranging from simple to radical) performed on 181 patients with clinically palpable IDCA. The follow-up period ranged from 5 to 20 years. Two patients (1.1%) having the comedo type of IDCA developed local recurrences.

In Ashikari's (5) group of 78 women with palpable IDCA followed for a maximum of 11 years, none developed any recurrences following mastectomy, but specific criteria for diagnosis of IDCA are not provided and there are no illustrations of the morphology either. Neither did any of the 68 patients with clinically palpable IDCA and a minimum of ten years of follow-up reported by Sunshine et al (90) develop recurrent lesions.

Ninety-seven of the 208 patients with IDCA in Silverstein et al's (86) group were treated with mastectomy. The maximum follow-up was ten years. Two patients developed recurrences. One of them developed a chest wall nodule 25 months after the initial diagnosis which proved to be an invasive carcinoma. The other patient developed metastatic carcinoma within 62 months. Her initial tumor had an area of microinvasion. Included among the 208 patients in Silverstein et al's study were 28 women who had IDCA with microinvasion. The precise distribution of these 28 women among the three treatment categories is not clear.

In summary, local recurrences develop in 0% to 2% of women treated by mastectomy, and the overall survival rates are nearly 100% (5,27,32,45,92).

## Breast Conserving Treatment

In general, the trials for conservative treatment of IDCA involve a relatively small number of cases, suffer from inconsistency of tissue processing (sampling technique and evaluation of margins), and inclusion of a heterogeneous group of IDCA's (palpable, nonpalpable, mammographically-detected, extensive, focal, comedo, non-necrotic), as well as short follow-up periods. As a rule, there has been a higher incidence of recurrences in patients treated conservatively compared to those treated by mastectomy. It is uncertain, however, what effect local recurrences would have on the ultimate patient survival (27,29, 41). Therefore, every attempt should be made to maintain a low rate of local recurrence and to carefully monitor patients managed by lumpectomy for early and prompt detection of recurrences. In order to reduce the recurrence rate due to residual disease, attempts have been made to ascertain an uninvolved margin of excision. This approach might require excision of a large amount of tissue judging from Holland et al's (42) finding that 40% of IDCAs are larger than 5 cm with a mean size of 9 cm. They found that the clinical and mammographic assessment of the lesion size does not correlate with the pathologic extent. Therefore, they defined size as the microscopically assessed area within which foci of IDCA were distributed. Based on these findings and in reference to conservative therapy, they stated that even quadrantectomy would not remove all foci of IDCA.

Clearly, we need to learn more about the biologic significance of the different variants of IDCA in order to better determine the extent of the surgical excision for a patient. Until then, patients who select conservative therapy require a rigorous follow-up regimen to include physical examination three to four times a year and annual or biannual mammography (78,91). The results of available trials should be viewed cautiously and as preliminary until results of better planned prospective studies provide more definitive answers to some of our questions.

### *Treatment by Biopsy Alone*

There have been no controlled studies to assess the natural history of in situ ductal carcinoma interrupted by biopsy alone. There are only a few retrospective studies of such cases, and it is difficult to compare the results of these studies because of the highly variable definitions used, inclusion of an admixture of clinically and mammographically detected lesions, as well as either inclusion of several morphologic variants of IDCA, or lack of information regarding the variants of IDCA included in the study. It should be kept in mind that a high proportion of the patients in these studies were not put on a regular follow-up regimen.

In 1938, Lewis and Geschikter (50) reported the follow-up on eight women who had been previously diagnosed and reported to have "intraductal comedocarcinoma" by Bloodgood (11) and treated by local excision only. Six of the eight patients developed local recurrence within a four-year period. Three of these women were found to have axillary node metastases when radical mastectomy was performed for the recurrent disease.

Betsil et al (9) collected a group of 25 women with "low grade papillary" IDCA treated by biopsy only. Of ten women in this group for whom long-term follow-up was available, six (60%) developed subsequent invasive carcinoma after an average interval of 9.7 years (9); another patient developed subsequent IDCA. Two of the seven patients who subsequently developed carcinoma also had lobular neoplasia in their biopsy. Rosen et al (73) subsequently added five additional patients to this group. Of these 15 women, all with the micropapillary variant of IDCA, eight (53%) developed subsequent invasive carcinoma. Two other patients developed recurrent IDCA.

Farrow (25) reported 25 patients with IDCA treated by biopsy alone. The histologic types were not specified. Five (20%) of these women developed subsequent carcinomas within one to eight years after the initial diagnosis.

Page et al (62) published a similar study of 28 women with IDCA treated by biopsy alone; these were carcinomas that were incidental histologic findings and had been missed on the initial review of the biopsies. Invasive carcinoma developed in seven of the 25 (28%) women who had at least three years of follow-up. With the exception of classic comedocarcinoma, the entire morphologic spectrum of IDCA appears to have been included in the study.

Fisher et al (31) reported on a group of 78 women with IDCA, 22 of whom were treated by lumpectomy alone. The median follow-up was 24 months. Recurrence developed in five of the 22 (23%) women treated by lumpectomy at or close to the site of the original biopsy within an average of 39 months. Only one of the 78 women in this study had a clinically occult lesion detected by mammography.

Lagios et al (48) evaluated the frequency of local recurrence and subsequent invasive carcinoma in 79 women with mammographically-detected foci of ductal carcinoma in situ with histologically-confirmed extents of 25 mm of less treated by tylectomy without radiation or axillary node dissection. The median follow-up was 44 months. Eight patients (10%) developed recurrences in the immediate vicinity of the previous biopsy. Four women developed recurrent in situ carcinoma detected mammographically. The other four patients developed subsequent invasive carcinoma, two of which were detected mammographically. Lagios et al (48) subdivided the IDCA into high grade, intermediate grade and low grade based on nuclear morphology. Among high grade IDCA (comedocarcinoma and carcinomas with high grade nuclear morphology), 19% developed local recurrences within an average interval of 26 months. Only one of ten (10%) women with the intermediate grade IDCA developed local recurrence at 87 months. None of the 33 women with the low grade IDCA (micropapillary/non-necrotic cribriform type) developed local recurrences.

Price et al (66) had a group of 37 women treated conservatively along with patients who had other types of treatment. The median follow-up for the entire series was seven years. Of those treated by lumpectomy, 54% developed subsequent recurrences.

Carpenter et al (17) had 28 patients treated by lumpectomy, with a mean follow-up of 38 months. Five patients (18%) developed recurrences.

Gallagher et al (33) treated 13 women with IDCA by lumpectomy. The median follow-up was 100 months. Five patients (38%) developed recurrences.

### *Lumpectomy and Radiotherapy*

Bornstein et al (12) reported a group of 38 women with IDCA treated by local excision (without evaluation of resection margins) and radiation therapy. This study included 20 of the women previously reported by Recht et al (68). The median follow-up was 81 months. Eight patients (21%) developed recurrences; seven at or near the site of the primary lesion. The recurrences developed 17 to 104 months following initial treatment. Five of the recurrent carcinomas were invasive, whereas the remaining were in situ carcinomas.

Silverstein et al (86) had 96 cases (including cases with microinvasion) of IDCA treated by excision and radiotherapy, and seven developed recurrences. The median follow-up was 42 months. Six of the seven recurrences occurred in women whose initial tumor was a comedocarcinoma, the other recurrence was a cribriform carcinoma. Two of the recurrent tumors were invasive, five were IDCA. The recurrences developed 26 to 63 months after the initial biopsy. One of the original lesions was IDCA with microinvasion; the recurrence was IDCA. All recurrences were treated by mastectomy. One of the two patients who subsequently developed invasive carcinoma died from her tumor.

Fisher et al (31) reported the results of lumpectomy and radiotherapy for 29 women with IDCA. The median follow-up was 24 months. Two patients developed recurrences; one was an in situ carcinoma, the other was an invasive carcinoma. The local recurrence rate for excision plus radiation therapy was 7%, compared with 23% in the excision-only group.

Zafrani et al (104) had 54 patients treated by conservative surgery and radiotherapy. With a median follow-up of 55 months, two patients developed recurrent in situ carcinoma, and one developed invasive carcinoma.

Recht et al (68) reported their results following conservative surgery and irradiation on 40 cases. The median follow-up was 44 months. Four patients developed recurrent tumor; two were invasive and two were in situ.

Montague et al (56) treated 56 women with IDCA with conservative surgery and radiotherapy. With a median follow-up of 60+ months, one woman developed in situ, and another an invasive carcinoma.

Kurtz et al (46) had 47 patients so treated (the group included three women who also had LCIS). The median follow-up was 61 months. Six percent of the patients developed recurrences.

Fowble et al (32) reported on 46 women (including 20 patients previously reported by Recht et al). The median follow-up was 35 months and 4% developed recurrences.

DeLouche et al (22) had 22 patients with a median follow-up of 132 months and 5% recurrence.

Stotter et al (88) had 44 patients with a median follow-up of 92 months and 7% recurrence.

The largest series included 259 women from nine institutions in Europe and the United States (89). All patients had complete gross excision of the lesion and definitive radiotherapy. Forty percent of the IDCA's were detected mammographically. With a median follow up of 78 months (range 11 to 197 months), 28 women developed recurrences; 50% of these were invasive carcinoma, the other 50% were intraductal carcinomas. The median time to recurrence was 50 months. Of these 28 women, 24 were salvaged and four developed distance metastases. An additional two women developed distant metastases, but no local recurrences. The ten-year actuarial failure rate was 16%. The ten-year actuarial survival was 94%, and the ten-year cause-specific survival rate was 97%. The status of the surgical margin was not known in 46% of the cases. Unfortunately, there is no information provided regarding the type of intraductal carcinomas. It would have been important to find out if the recurrences correlated with the type of intraductal carcinoma (ie, the high grade lesions, or the more extensive ones).

In summary, the recurrence rate for patients treated by biopsy alone varies from 10% to 60% (17,31,31,48). Breast conservative treatment with radiation is associated with 3.5% to 23% recurrence rates (12,22,31,32,46,68,78,86,88,89,104). Radiation therapy appears to reduce the rate of local relapse (31). When excision is followed by radiation therapy, the recurrence rate drops to around 2% to 11% (95).

Whether conservative surgery is justifiable for IDCA remains controversial. Randomized clinical trials are needed to determine whether lumpectomy with or without postoperative radiotherapy is effective in the treatment of IDCA. These studies should utilize a uniform approach to sampling of the biopsy, a standardized manner of measuring the microscopic size of the intraductal carcinoma, and a grading system to stratify the intraductal carcinomas according to the morphologic subtype. It is noteworthy that about 50% of women with IDCA will not develop a significant invasive carcinoma during their lifetime following treatment by biopsy alone (9,63).

## OCCULT INVASIVE CARCINOMA AND AXILLARY NODE METASTASES IN IDCA

The frequency of occult invasive carcinoma in the mastectomy specimen of women with IDCA ranges from 6% to 21% in different reports (19,49,73,75,98).

The axillary nodes show metastatic carcinoma in 1% to 4.5% of women with in situ (ductal or lobular) carcinomas (34,45,70). Contesso & Petit (20) had one axillary node recurrence among 41 women treated by mastectomy for IDCA. Lagios et al (49) reported 2% nodal involvement in their series. Von Reuden et al (98) had 0% nodal involvement in the group of patients treated with modified radical mastectomy after excisional biopsy. It is assumed that these nodal metastases are due to the presence of areas of invasion that escape detection by the routine methods of specimen evaluation.

Silverstein et al (85) removed the axillary lymph nodes from 100 patients with IDCA treated by either mastectomy (49 patients) or lumpectomy and radiotherapy (51 patients). The average number of axillary nodes removed was 16; none of the women had evidence of nodal metastases. They concluded that IDCA has little potential for axillary node metastases.

## CONCLUSIONS

In conclusion, we have no accurate data regarding the percentage of women with minimal foci of the non-necrotic variants of IDCA, which constitute a large proportion of the mammographically detected lesions, or even the proportion of women with the comedo variant of IDCA, who will develop subsequent invasive carcinoma if treated by lumpectomy alone. We do not know if subsequent carcinomas that develop in patients so treated and followed by regular palpation and mammography, would be at early enough stages so that the hazard of the lesion would be minimal compared to those that clinically manifest themselves as a palpable mass in the absence of close clinical follow-up. The length of follow-up on currently available studies is too short to provide a response to these uncertainties. The study by Lagios et al (48) is important because it only deals with mammographically-detected lesions and stratifies the lesions according to the grade of the IDCA; none of the low grade IDCA in this study recurred. The highest recurrence rates have been associated with comedocarcinoma (48,90). The presence of IDCA in 14.3% of 77 asymptomatic women at autopsy (59) raises additional questions regarding the biologic significance of at least some variants of IDCA.

Obviously we need to learn a lot more about the biologic significance of these lesions. Even if some foci of IDCA are left behind by a lumpectomy, would the actual percentage of women who develop subsequent invasive carcinoma justify mastectomy for the remaining group?

Whether a positive family history of breast carcinoma should influence the management of patients with IDCA has not been established, either. Cady (15) estimated that the incidence of subsequent invasive carcinoma in patients with IDCA and a negative family history of breast carcinoma is 2% annually and 40% after 20 years. For women with a positive family history of breast carcinoma, he estimated a 4% annual incidence of subsequent invasive breast carcinoma and an incidence of 60% at 15 years. This is an issue that should be carefully evaluated as it may help determine the optimum management of the woman with IDCA.

Currently, three treatment options are available to the patient: mastectomy, lumpectomy, and lumpectomy with radiotherapy. Due to the rarity of axillary node metastases, a watch policy for the axilla has been considered safe (95). The optimal management of the contralateral breast in patients with IDCA has not been established, but some form of follow-up would be prudent.

There are many ongoing studies in the process of accumulating data to resolve these questions. Meanwhile, my personal preference would be to follow patients with mammographically-detected, localized, low grade, non-necrotic variants of micropapillary and cribriform IDCA after the diagnostic biopsy; patients with mammographically-detected diffuse microcalcifications or disease in multiple quadrants are not considered ideal subjects for conservative treatment and follow-up (89). The follow-up should be life-long and include careful palpation of the breasts by an experienced clinician two to four times a year, along with annual mammography. For extensive high grade intraductal carcinomas (ie, comedo type), a mastectomy seems more appropriate regardless of the manner of presentation or detection. Treatment for other variants of IDCA could be more individualized after considering the extent of the disease in the biopsy, family history of breast carcinoma, and the patient's level of anxiety.

### REFERENCES

1. Alpers CE, Wellings SR: The prevalence of carcinoma in situ in normal and cancer-associated breast. *Hum Pathol* 1985;16:796–807.
* 2. Amalric R, Santamaria F, Robert F, et al: Radiation therapy with or without limited surgery for operable breast cancer: A 20-year experience at the Marseille Center Institute. *Cancer* 1982;49:30–34.
* 3. Andersen J, Blichert-Toft M, Dyreborg U: In situ carcinomas of the breast. Types, growth pattern, diagnosis, and treatment. *Eur J Surg Oncol* 1987;13:105–111.
4. Ashikari R, Hajdu SI, Robbins GF: Intraductal carcinoma of the breast (1960–1969). *Cancer* 1971;28:1182–1187.

5. Ashikari R, Huvos AG, Snyder RE: Prospective study of non-infiltrating carcinoma of the breast. *Cancer* 1977;39: 435–439.

6. Azzopardi JG: *Problems in Breast Pathology*. London, WB Saunders Co, 1979, pp 266–273.

7. Baker LH: Breast Cancer Detection Demonstration Project: five-year summary report. *CA* 1982;32:194–225.

8. Barsky SH, Siegal GP, Jannotta F, et al: Loss of basement membrane component by invasive tumors but not by their benign counterparts. *Lab Invest* 1983;49:140–147.

* 9. Betsill WL, Rosen PP, Lieberman PH, et al: Intraductal carcinoma. Long-term follow-up after treatment by biopsy alone. *JAMA* 1978;239:1863–1867.

10. Bigelow R, Smith R, Goodman PA, et al: Needle localization of nonpalpable breast masses. *Arch Surg* 1985;120:565–663.

11. Bloodgood JC: Comedocarcinoma (or comedo-adenoma) of the female breast. *Am J Cancer* 1934;22:842–849.

* 12. Bornstein BA, Recht A, Connoly JL, et al: Results of treating ductal carcinomas in situ of the breast with conservative surgery and radiation therapy. *Cancer* 1991;67:7–13.

13. Brown PW, Silverman J, Owens E, et al: Intraductal "non-infiltrating" carcinoma of the breast. *Arch Surg* 1976;111: 1063–1067.

* 14. Bussolati G, Botta G, Gugliotta P: Actin-rich (myoepithelial) cells in ductal carcinoma-in-situ of the breast. *Virchows Arch (B) Cell Path* 1980;34:251–259.

15. Cady B: New diagnostic, staging, and therapeutic aspects of early breast cancer. *Cancer* 1990;65:634–647.

* 16. Calle R, Pilleron JP, Schlienger P, et al: Conservative management of operable breast cancer: Ten years' experience at the Foundation Curie. *Cancer* 1978;42:2045–2053.

* 17. Carpenter R, Boulter PS, Cooke T, et al: Management of screen detected ductal carcinoma in situ of the female breast. *Br J Surg* 1989;76:564–567.

18. Carpenter R, Gibbst N, Matthews J, et al: Importance of cellular DNA content in pre-malignant breast disease and pre-invasive carcinoma of the female breast. *Br J Surg* 1987;74:905–906.

19. Carter D, Smith RL: Carcinoma in situ of the breast. *Cancer* 1977;40:1189–1193.

20. Collandrea JM, Schmookler BM, O'Dowd GJ, et al: Cystic hypersecretory duct carcinoma of the breast. Report of a case with fine-needle aspiration. *Arch Pathol Lab Med* 1988; 112:560–563.

* 21. Contesso G, Petit JY: Les adenocarcinomes intracanalaires non infiltrants du sein. *Bull Cancer* (Paris) 1979;66:1–8.

* 22. Delouche G, Bachelot F, Premont M, et al: Conservation treatment of early breast cancer: Long term results and complications. *Int J Radiat Oncol Biol Phys* 1987;13:29–34.

23. Eusebi V, Collina G, Bussolati G: Carcinoma in situ in sclerosing adenosis of the breast: An immunocytochemical study. *Sem Diagn Pathol* 1989;6:146–152.

24. Eusebi V, Foschini MP, Cook MG, et al: Long-term follow-up of in situ carcinoma of the breast with special emphasis on clinging carcinoma. *Sem Diagn Pathol* 1989;6: 165–173.

25. Farrow JH: Current concepts in the detection and treatment of the earliest of the early breast cancers. *Cancer* 1970;25:468–477.

* 26. Fechner RE: Ductal carcinoma involving the lobule of the breast. A source of confusion with lobular carcinoma in situ. *Cancer* 1971;28:274–281.

27. Fisher B: Breast-cancer management: alternatives to radical mastectomy. *N Engl J Med* 1979;301:326–328.

28. Fisher ER, Brown R: Intraductal signet ring carcinoma. A hitherto undescribed form of intraductal carcinoma of the breast. *Cancer* 1985;55:2533–2537.

* 29. Fisher B, Redmond C, Fisher ER, et al: Ten-year results of randomized clinical trial comparing radical mastectomy and total mastectomy with or without radiation. *N Engl J Med* 1985;312:674–681.

* 30. Fisher B, Redmond C, Poisson R, et al: Eight-year results of randomized clinical trial comparing radical mastectomy and lumpectomy with or without radiation in the treatment of breast cancer. *N Engl J Med* 1989;320:822–828.

* 31. Fisher ER, Sass R, Fisher B, et al: Pathologic findings from the National Surgical Adjuvant Breast Project (Protocol 6) I. Intraductal carcinoma. *Cancer* 1986;57:197–208.

32. Fowble BL, Solin LJ, Goodman RL: Results of conservative surgery and radiation for intraductal noninvasive breast cancer (abstr). Proceedings of the American Radium Society. *Am J Clin Oncol* 1987;10:110–111.

* 33. Gallagher WJ, Koerner FC, Wood WC: Treatment of intraductal carcinoma with limited surgery: Long-term follow-up. *J Clin Oncol* 1989;7:376–380.

34. Gillis DA, Dockerly MB, Clagett OT: Preinvasive intraductal carcinoma of the breast. *Surg Gynecol Obstet* 1960;110: 555–562.

35. Giri DD, Dundas SAC, Nottingham JF, et al: Oestrogen receptors in benign epithelial lesions and intraduct carcinomas of the breast: an immunohistochemical study. *Histopathology* 1989;15:575–584.

36. Guerry P, Erlandson RA, Rosen PP: Cystic hypersecretory hyperplasia and cystic hypersecretory duct carcinoma of the breast. Pathology, therapy, and follow-up of 39 patients. *Cancer* 1988;61:1611–1620.

* 37. Gump FE, Jicha DL, Ozzello L: Ductal carcinoma in situ (DCIS): A revised concept. *Surgery* 1987;164:285–301.

38. Haagensen CD: *Diseases of the Breast*, 3 ed. Philadelphia, WB Saunders, 1986, pp 782–789.

39. Haffty BG, Kornguth P, Fischer D, et al: Mammographically detected breast cancer: Results with conservative surgery and radiation therapy. *Cancer* 1991;67:2801–2804.

* 40. Harris JR, Hellman S, Kinne DW: Limited surgery and radiotherapy for early breast cancer. *N Engl J Med* 1985;313: 1365–1368.

41. Hellman S, Harris JR: The appropriate breast cancer paradigm. *Cancer Res* 1987;47:339–342.

* 42. Holland R, Veling SHJ, Mravunac M, et al: Histologic multifocality of Tis, T1-2 breast carcinomas: Implications

for clinical trials of breast-conserving surgery. *Cancer* 1985; 56:979–990.

43. Jensen RA, Page DL: Cystic hypersecretory carcinoma: What's in a name? *Arch Pathol Lab Med* 1988;112:1179.

44. Kinne DW, Petrek JA, Osborne MP, et al: Breast carcinoma in situ. *Arch Surg* 1989;124:22–36.

* 45. Kouchoukos NT, Ackerman LV, Butcher HR Jr: Prediction of axillary nodal metastases from the morphology of primary mammary carcinomas. *Cancer* 1967;20:948–960.

* 46. Kurtz JM, Jacquemier J, Torhorst J, et al: Conservation therapy for breast cancers other than infiltrating duct carcinoma. *Cancer* 1989;18:283–287.

47. Lagios MD: Human breast precancer: Current status. *Cancer Surv* 1983;2:383–402.

* 48. Lagios MD, Margolin FR, Westdahl PR, et al: Mammographically detected duct carcinoma in situ. Frequency of local recurrence following tylectomy and prognostic effect of nuclear grade on local recurrence. *Cancer* 1989;63:618–624.

49. Lagios MD, Westdahl PR, Margolin FR, et al: Duct carcinoma in situ: Relationship of extent of noninvasive disease to the frequency of occult invasion, multicentricity, lymph node metastases, and short-term treatment failures. *Cancer* 1982;50:1309–1314.

50. Lewis D, Geschickter CF: Comedocarcinoma of the breast. *Arch Surg* 1938;36:225–244.

51. Margolin FR, Lagios MD: Mammographic detection of early breast cancer: Ten years' experience in a community hospital. *West J Med* 1986;144:46–48.

52. Mayr NA, Staples JJ, Robinson RA, et al: Morphometric studies in intraductal breast carcinoma using computerized image analysis. *Cancer* 1991;67:2805–2812.

* 53. McDivitt RW, Stewart FW, Berg JW: *Tumors of the Breast*, Fasc 2. Atlas of Tumor Pathology, second series, Washington DC, Armed Forces Institute of Pathology, 1968, pp 29–49.

54. Meyer JS: Cell kinetics of histologic variants of in situ breast carcinoma. *Breast Cancer Res Treat* 1986;7:171–180.

* 55. Millis RR, Thynne GSJ: In situ intraduct carcinoma of the breast: A long term follow-up study. *Br J Surg* 1975;62:957–962.

* 56. Montague ED: Conservation surgery and radiation therapy in the treatment of operable breast cancer. *Cancer* 1984; 53(suppl 3):700–704.

* 57. Moskowitz M, Russell P, Fidler J, et al: Breast cancer screening. Preliminary report of 207 biopsies performed in 4,128 volunteer screeners. *Cancer* 1975;36:2245–2250.

* 58. Nielsen M, Thomsen JL, Primdahl S, et al: Breast cancer and atypia among young and middle-aged women: A study of 110 medicolegal autopsies. *Br J Cancer* 1987;56: 814–819.

* 59. Nielsen M, Jensen J, Andersen J: Precancerous and cancerous breast lesions during lifetime and at autopsy. A study of 83 women. *Cancer* 1984;54:612–615.

* 60. NIH Consensus Conference. Treatment of early stage breast cancer. *JAMA* 1991;265(3):391–395.

61. Ozzello L: Ultrastructure of intraepithelial carcinoma of the breast. *Cancer* 1971;28:1508–1515.

* 62. Page DL, Dupont WD, Rogers LW, et al: Intraductal carcinoma of the breast. Follow-up after biopsy only. *Cancer* 1982;49:751–758.

* 63. Page DL, Dupont WD, Rogers LW, et al: Atypical hyperplastic lesions of the female breast: A long-term follow-up study. *Cancer* 1985;55:2698–2708.

64. Patchefsky AS, Schwartz GF, Finklestein SD, et al: Heterogeneity of intraductal carcinoma of the breast. *Cancer* 1989;63:731–741.

* 65. Powell RW, McSweeney MD, Wilson C: X-ray calcifications as the only basis for breast biopsy. *Ann Surg* 1983;197:555–559.

66. Price P, Walsh G, A'Hern RP, et al: Predictors of local recurrence and progression in patients treated by surgery alone for in situ breast carcinoma (abstr). *Br J Cancer* 1988;58:522.

67. Recht A, Connolly JL, Schnitt SJ, et al: Conservative surgery and radiation therapy for early breast cancer: Results, controversies, and unsolved problems. *Sem Oncol* 1986;13:434–449.

* 68. Recht A, Danoff BS, Solin LJ, et al: Intraductal carcinoma of the breast: Results of treatment with excisional biopsy and irradiation. *J Clin Oncol* 1985;3:1339–1343.

* 69. Robbins GF, Berg JW: Bilateral primary breast cancers: A prospective clinicopathological study. *Cancer* 1964;17:1501–1527.

* 70. Rosen PP: Axillary lymph node metastases in patients with occult noninvasive breast carcinoma. *Cancer* 1980;46:1298–1306.

71. Rosen PP: The pathological classification of human mammary carcinoma: Past, present and future. *Ann Clin Lab Sci* 1979;9:144–156.

72. Rosen PP: The pathology of breast carcinoma, in: Harris JR, Hellman S, Henderson IC, et al (eds): *Breast Diseases*. Philadelphia, JB Lippincott, 1987, p 149.

* 73. Rosen PP, Brown DW, Kinne DE: The clinical significance of preinvasive breast carcinoma. *Cancer* 1980;46:919–925.

74. Rosen PP, Scott M: Cystic hypersecretory duct carcinoma of the breast. *Am J Surg Pathol* 1984;8:31–41.

* 75. Rosen PP, Senie R, Schottenfeld D, et al: Noninvasive breast carcinoma. Frequency of unsuspected invasion and implications for treatment. *Ann Surg* 1979;189:377–382.

76. Rosen PP, Snyder RE, Robbins G: Specimen radiography for nonpalpable breast lesions found by mammography: Procedures and results. *Cancer* 1974;34:2028–2033.

* 77. Rosner D, Bedwani RN, Vana J, et al: Noninvasive breast carcinoma. Results of a national survey by the American College of Surgeons. *Ann Surg* 1980;192:139–147.

* 78. Schnitt SJ, Silen W, Sadowsky NL, et al: Current concepts: Ductal carcinoma in situ (intraductal carcinoma of the breast). *N Engl J Med* 1988;318:898–903.

79. Schwartz GF, Patchefsky AS, Feig SA, et al: Clinically occult breast cancer: multicentricity and implications for treatment. *Ann Surg* 1980;191:8–12.

80. Schwartz GF, Feig SA, Patchefsky A: Significance and staging of nonpalpable carcinomas of the breast. *Surg Gynecol Obstet* 1988;166:6–10.

81. Schwartz GF, Patchefsky AS, Finklestein SD, et al: Nonpalpable in situ carcinoma of the breast. *Arch Surg* 1989; 124:29–32.

82. Sickles EA: Mammographic features of 300 consecutive nonpalpable breast cancers. *Am J Radiol* 1986;146:661–663.

83. Silverberg SG, Chitale AR: Assessment of significance of proportions of intraductal and infiltrating tumor growth in ductal carcinoma of the breast. *Cancer* 1973;32:830–837.

* 84. Silverstein MJ, Gamagami P, Colburn WJ, et al: Nonpalpable breast lesions: Diagnosis with slightly overpenetrated screen-film mammography and hook wire-directed breast biopsy in 1,014 cases. *Radiology* 1989;171:633–638.

* 85. Silverstein MJ, Rosser RJ, Gierson ED, et al: Axillary lymph node dissection for intraductal carcinoma: Is it indicated? *Cancer* 1988;59:1819–1824.

* 86. Silverstein MJ, Waisman JR, Gamagami P, et al: Intraductal carcinoma of the breast (208 cases). Clinical factors influencing treatment choice. *Cancer* 1990;66:102–108.

87. Smart CR, Myers MH, Gloeckler LA: Implications from SEER data on breast cancer management. *Cancer* 1978;41: 787–789.

88. Stotter RT, McNeese M, Oswald MJ, et al: The role of limited surgery with radiation in primary treatment of ductal in situ breast cancer. *Int J Radiat Biol Phys* 1990;18: 283–287.

* 89. Solin LJ, Recht A, Fourquet A, et al: Ten-year results of breast-conserving surgery and definitive irradiation for intraductal carcinoma (ductal carcinoma in situ) of the breast. *Cancer* 1991;68:2337–2344.

* 90. Sunshine JA, Moseley HS, Fletcher WS, et al: Breast carcinoma in situ: A retrospective review of 112 cases with a minimum 10-year follow-up. *Am J Surg* 1985;150:44–51.

* 91. Tavassoli FA, Norris HJ: A comparison of the results of long-term follow-up for atypical intraductal hyperplasia and intraductal hyperplasia of the breast. *Cancer* 1990;65: 518–529.

* 92. Temple WJ: Technical considerations for prophylactic mastectomy in patients at high risk for breast cancer. *Am J Surg* 1991;161:413–415.

93. Tuluson AH, Ronay G, Egger H, et al: A contribution to the natural history of breast cancer. V. Bilateral primary breast cancer: Incidence, risks and diagnosis of simultaneous primary cancer in the opposite breast. *Arch Gynecol* 1985; 237:85–91.

94. Van De Vijver MJ, Peterse JL, Mool WJ, et al: Neu-protein overexpression in breast cancer. Association with comedo-type ductal carcinoma in situ and limited prognostic value in stage II breast cancer. *N Engl J Med* 1988;319:1239–1245.

* 95. Van Dongen JA, Fentiman IS, Harris JR, et al: In situ breast cancer: The EORTC consensus meeting. *Lancet* 1989;2:25–27.

* 96. Verbeek ALM, Hendriks JHCL, Holland R, et al: Reduction of breast cancer mortality through mass screening with modern mammography: First results of the Nijmegen Project, 1975–1981. *Lancet* 1984;1:1222–1224.

97. Veronesi U, Saccozzi R, DelVecchio M, et al: Comparing radical mastectomy with quadrantectomy, axillary dissection, and radiotherapy in patients with small cancers of the breast. *N Engl J Med* 1981;305:6–11.

98. Von Rueden DG, Wilson RE: Intraductal carcinoma of the breast. *Surg Gynecol Obstet* 1984;158:105–111.

99. Wecksell A, Altkiss MD, Shahamatpour M: Recurrent intraductal breast carcinoma following radiation therapy: A case report. *Breast* 1982;8:13–15.

* 100. Webber BL, Heise H, Neifeld JP, et al: Risk of subsequent contralateral breast carcinoma in a population of patients with in-situ carcinoma. *Cancer* 1981;47:2928–2932.

* 101. Wellings SR, Jensen HM, Marcum RG: An atlas of subgross pathology of the human breast with special reference to possible precancerous lesions. *J Natl Cancer Inst* 1975;55: 231–273.

102. Westbrook KC, Gallager HS: Intraductal carcinoma of the breast. A comparative study. *Am J Surg* 1975;130:667–670.

103. Wulsin JH, Schreiber JT: Improved prognosis in certain patterns of carcinoma of the breast: Colloid, medullary with lymphoid stroma, and intraductal. *Arch Surg* 1962;85: 791–800.

* 104. Zafrani B, Fourquet A, Vilcoq JR, et al: Conservative management of intraductal breast carcinoma with tumorectomy and radiation therapy. *Cancer* 1986;57:1299–1301.

# 8

# Lobular Neoplasia (Lobular Carcinoma In Situ)



In 1941, two designations were offered for a histologically distinct proliferation within one or more terminal duct-lobular units (TDLU), characterized by a uniform population of generally small and loosely cohesive cells growing in a solid, occlusive fashion with or without distension of the affected acini. Foote and Stewart (31) used the term lobular carcinoma in situ (LCIS) for this change, while Muir (56) referred to it as intra-acinus carcinoma. Among lesions designated as intra-acinus carcinomas, Muir also included cribriform variants of intraductal carcinoma originating in the TDLU. It appears that Muir had a broader concept of intra-acinus carcinoma which was inclusive of various patterns of proliferation besides the solid, occlusive growth typical of LCIS. Prior to general understanding of the concept of noninvasive carcinoma and introduction of the term "in situ carcinoma," the same lesion had been illustrated as an example of a precancerous change by Ewing in 1919 (27). An undeniable example of this lesion, surrounded by an invasive carcinoma, and also designated as acinar carcinoma by Cornil (21), was recorded as early as 1908. Broder (17) in 1932 illustrated five examples of carcinoma in situ in various parts of the body; one of these was from the breast and is clearly an example of LCIS. This lesion obviously was not totally unfamiliar to pathologists even prior to the 1940s.

Foote and Stewart (31), who are rightfully credited for drawing attention to this lesion as a distinct entity, observed this lobular alteration occurring alone in two of a series of 300 patients treated by radical mastectomy for breast carcinoma. They also found 12 additional cases in which the same noninvasive lesion was associated with infiltrating carcinoma. The cells confined to the lobules were identical to those infiltrating the stroma, which was considered an important justification for designating the former lesion as the in situ phase of the invasive carcinoma, or lobular carcinoma in situ (LCIS).

The term lobular carcinoma in situ was immediately adopted by most pathologists even though no scientific evidence of its malignant nature had been offered. Regardless of the appropriateness of the term, the listing of some of the major characteristics of LCIS by Foote and Stewart (31) remains the most significant contribution of their report. They noted that LCIS is always an incidental finding that does not form a palpable mass and cannot be recognized grossly. Microscopically, aside from the lobular changes described earlier, there is often a pagetoid involvement of the extralobular ducts, while Paget's disease of the nipple is notably absent. Foote and Stewart noted that "there is a type of carcinoma which apparently takes its origin in smaller ducts and which begins in cells of pagetoid type, identical with those seen in lobular carcinoma in situ, and this type of cancer may occur in the non-lobule-containing atrophic breast." This comment was made following a statement that existence of lobular carcinoma in situ presupposes the presence of lobules and that LCIS cannot be diagnosed in atrophic breast.

Furthermore, Foote and Stewart noted that LCIS is generally multifocal and has the potential to progress to an invasive small cell carcinoma. In support of the multicentric nature of LCIS, Warner (86), combining results from several reports, noted that residual foci of LCIS were described in up to 70% of mastectomy specimen removed after a biopsy diagnosis of LCIS. Because of the multicentricity and the possibility of progression to an invasive carcinoma, Foote and Stewart (31) recommended simple mastectomy as essential with additional procedures dependent on any subsequent findings.

Subsequent studies and reviews noted a high frequency of bilaterality (12,15,41,50,53,54,58,73,80, 84,85). The bilaterality may be synchronous or metachronous. Urban (84,85) noted concurrent carcinoma in the contralateral breast in 10 of 22 women who presented with LCIS in one breast; 90% of the contralateral carcinomas were LCIS.

It also became apparent that a high proportion of women with LCIS are premenopausal (2,4,50,61,74). Contrary to some earlier observations (41), however, LCIS (and infiltrating lobular carcinoma) have been recorded in postmenopausal women as well (29,42, 61,72); in my experience, the oldest woman with LCIS has been 89 years of age. Approximately 90% of the patients are premenopausal, however (42).

In about a decade after Foote & Stewart's paper it gradually became evident that while in some patients the disease progresses to invasive carcinoma, there are many patients who do not develop invasive carcinoma even after prolonged follow-up (12,15,37). In 1967, McDivitt et al (54) projected a 20-year cumulative risk of 35% for subsequent ipsilateral carcinoma and 25% for contralateral carcinoma after follow-up of women with LCIS who did not have a mastectomy. This report was the first to note that both breasts are at increased risk for subsequent development of carcinoma. Subsequent reports confirmed that the presence of LCIS in one breast requires careful observation of the contralateral breast as well (42,73,80).

## EVOLUTION OF ATYPICAL LOBULAR HYPERPLASIA (ALH)

In an attempt to resolve the mystery surrounding lesions that progress, attention was soon focused on the extent of lobular involvement as a feature that may be of prognostic value and helpful in predicting the course of the disease. In their original paper, Foote and Stewart (31) did not remark on the number of lobules involved, proportion of acini within a lobule displaying the proliferating cells, extent of acinar distension, or persistence of central lumens within the acini as a significant factor in the interpretation of the lesion. As a matter of fact, they specifically stated that ". . . these lobules may be within normal limits in size or even smaller than normal, etc," and their main illustrations show persistence of lumens in some of the involved acini.

Subsequently, however, pathologists started to use the designation of atypical hyperplasia for lesions in which there was either persistence of residual lumens in the acini, minimal distension of the acini, proliferation of the typical cells admixed with the native epithelial and myoepithelial cells, or involvement of only a single lobule. Wheeler et al (90) used the term "atypical lobular hyperplasia" (ALH) for terminal ductules that contained cells morphologically identical to LCIS cells, but in which a few normal epithelial or myoepithelial cells persisted. They noted that these atypical lobules are often closely associated with LCIS, but may be seen as an isolated lesion. They also included in the category of atypical lobular hyperplasia lesions that showed persistence of ductular (acinar) lumens and those that lacked ductular distension (10). Others (47,48) required involvement of two or three lobules for a diagnosis of LCIS, and subsequently McDivitt et al

(54) stated that a diagnosis of LCIS should not be made if only one lobule was involved. Consequently, along with a diagnosis of ALH, follow-up of the patient was advised. In contrast, a diagnosis of LCIS portended mastectomy.

In 1985, Page et al (66) specified the minimal requirement for a diagnosis of LCIS. They defined LCIS as a proliferation of evenly-spaced, round, cuboidal, or polygonal cells with usually round, monotonous, hyperchromatic nuclei completely filling, distorting, and distending one half—subsequently changed to more than half (69)—of the acini in a TDLU. Anything less would be atypical lobular hyperplasia (ALH). They offered no definition of what is distension in either their original paper or subsequent discussions of the topic (64–69).

Because of the lack of standardized criteria, the threshold for the diagnosis of LCIS varies among pathologists. A lesion that is interpreted as ALH by one pathologist may be designated as LCIS by another. Some pathologists diagnose LCIS rather frequently, while others rarely make this diagnosis. For example, Rosen et al (73) had diagnosed only 13 cases of ALH during the same period in which they collected 99 examples of LCIS. A comparison of the follow-up of a large number of women diagnosed as having ALH with those having LCIS based on one set of criteria is necessary to determine if an absolute subdivision into these two categories and different therapeutic approaches for the two groups is warranted.

Another important issue is that there is overlap in the appearance of early atypical intraductal hyperplasia and lobular neoplasia which may be variably interpreted by different pathologists. For example, if the ductules within a TDLU show an epithelial proliferation that occludes some ductules, leaves a residual lumen in others, and actually forms two secondary lumens in even one of the ductules, I would interpret the process as a ductal type of growth; the same type of proliferation has been designated as an atypical lobular hyperplasia by others (66, Fig. 4).

Obviously, many pathologists use a quantitative approach by requiring complete replacement of the native acinar epithelial cell population filling the lumens, complete involvement of the acini with or without distension, or involvement of more than one lobule. Curiously, no one has defined what is implied by distension. Recently, some breast pathologists have suggested that the presence of six to eight neoplastic cells across the occluded ductular (acinar) lumen is indicative of distention; others would consider a ductule as distended whenever it is larger than the "average" size of the normal lobules in a given biopsy. These definitions do not always overlap. For example, in elderly women with atrophic breasts, the presence of only four to five neoplastic cells across ductules displaying an occlusive growth often reflects distension compared to the surrounding atrophic acini, but would not qualify as such if the presence of six to eight cells were required. I prefer to compare the involved acini to the appearance of the largest of surrounding normal acini for determination of distension. It is noteworthy that the proliferating cell population is the same in both ALH and LCIS. Therefore, implicit in the mere division of this spectrum into ALH and LCIS is the introduction of a quantitative parameter. Interestingly, Wheeler & Enterline (89), who themselves clearly introduced a quantitative parameter by separating ALH from LCIS, objected to Hutter et al's (49) requirement of involvement of at least two or three lobules for a diagnosis of LCIS on the grounds that introduction of a quantitative element is unwarranted in the diagnosis of cancer.

## INTRODUCTION OF THE TERM "LOBULAR NEOPLASIA"

As follow-up information became available on women with LCIS who for some reason or other had not had mastectomy, some investigators began to question whether or not the lesion warranted a designation of carcinoma, and hence, a mastectomy (22). Haagensen was the only individual, however, who objected seriously enough to the designation of LCIS and the pursuant mastectomy that he changed the terminology to lobular neoplasia. This term includes the entire spectrum of lobular disease from those showing only partial lobular involvement to those showing massive distension of acini in numerous lobules.

My personal preference also is to use the designation of lobular neoplasia for the entire spectrum of changes within the lobules, rather than splitting the spectrum into LCIS and ALH on the basis of features of questionable therapeutic and absolute prognostic value.

## CLINICAL FEATURES

Lobular neoplasia (LN) [or lobular carcinoma in situ (LCIS)] is identified in 0.3% to 3.8% of all breast biopsies (11,35,39,51,90), or about 1.5% of all biopsies performed for benign breast lesions (2,51). Wheeler and Enterline (89) noted that ALH accounted for 0.4% of all biopsies in their practice, while LCIS accounted for 0.8%, or a total of 1.2% when the two are grouped together. Variations in the reported frequency of the disease are due to differences in criteria, extent of sampling, and the thoroughness of the microscopic evaluation. Patients with LN range in age from 15 to the late 80s. A majority of the patients are premenopausal (52), with 80% (76) to 89% (40) of the lesions presenting in women less than 54 years of age. The average age of women with LCIS is between 44 and 46 (71), which is ten years younger than the average age of patients with infiltrating duct carcinoma and 15 years younger than that of infiltrating lobular carcinoma. Lobular neoplasia is less common in blacks (10).

Additional important characteristics of LN that were noted by Foote and Stewart and subsequent investigators are summarized below.

1) Lobular neoplasia is predominantly a pathologic diagnosis; it does not produce a palpable mass, rather, it is generally an incidental finding in patients biopsied for other reasons.
2) The lesion is generally multifocal and multicentric, as well as frequently bilateral in 35% to 59% of cases (75,79,84).
3) With prolonged follow-up exceeding 20 years and based on autopsy findings, up to a third of the lesions will progress to an invasive carcinoma (62) of the small cell or some other histologic type.

Mammographically, an important finding noted in the mid 1960s was the presence of localized abnormality with minute calcific densities grouped in an irregular manner (79). The calcification is generally found in adjacent uninvolved lobules, rather than those affected by LN (79). With more advanced technology, mammography has been utilized effectively to pick up lesions at early stages of malignancy, as well as many atypical proliferation. In a study of 100 consecutive breast biopsies performed for nonpalpable lesions detected mammographically, Rubin et al (77) demonstrated that mammography can identify a high percentage of women with pathologic lesions associated with increased risk for subsequent development of invasive carcinoma. In addition to its ability to detect carcinomas in 20% of these women (55% of which were noninvasive), atypical hyperplasia was found in 10% of the biopsies, whereas ordinary hyperplasia was found in an additional 21% of the women.

## PATHOLOGIC FEATURES

As it is obvious from previous discussions, LN does not produce a grossly visible lesion.

Microscopically, the term lobular neoplasia (LN) refers to the entire spectrum of pathologic epithelial proliferations within the lobules characterized by a solid, occlusive proliferation of a relatively uniform population of loosely cohesive, and often small, round cells with sparse cytoplasm (Fig. 8.1). In about 30% to 40% of the cases, there is a pagetoid extension into adjacent terminal ducts. The morphologic appearances of the lesions within this spectrum vary depending upon the degree of acinar distension and the proportion of acini involved within a lobule. The cells in classic lobular neoplasia are often small and uniform, with rather indistinct cell margins, and sparse cytoplasm. Frequently, however, the cells deviate from this "classic appearance." The cell may display minor variations in size, and occasionally develop abundant granular, eosinophilic cytoplasm with apocrine-like features (Fig. 8.2). Sometimes, the cells show secretory differentiation (8,13,26,33). Intracytoplasmic lumens (Fig. 8.3), mucous globules (8), and a signet-ring-cell appearance have also been observed; intracytoplasmic lumens and mucous globules are a relatively common finding. The nuclei of LN cells are generally round and uniform, but occasionally display variation in size and shape. When the cells assume an apocrine appearance, the nuclei may display prominent nucleoli. The proliferating cells may appear closely-packed and coherent, loosely cohesive, or completely loose and detached. It is extremely rare to observe distinct cell margins evident even among LN cells that appear coherent. The native epithelial cells in the TDLU are either completely replaced or simply displaced and lifted by the proliferating cells (Fig. 8.4). The neoplastic cells

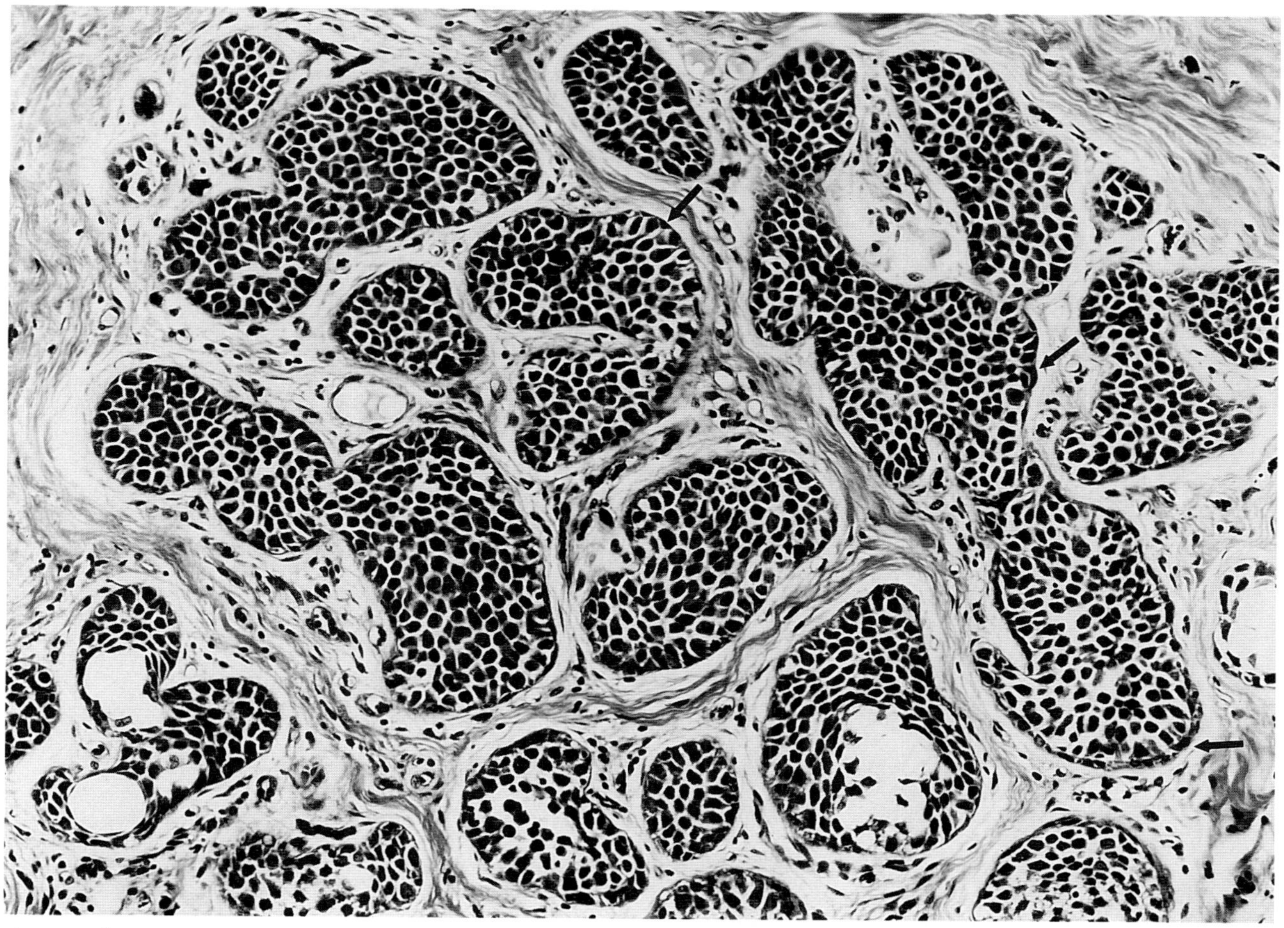

**Figure 8.1** Lobular neoplasia (LN2). The acini within this lobule are distended by a proliferation of a loosely cohesive, uniform cell population in a solid occlusive manner. The acinar outlines are distinct with intervening stroma. The ME cell layer (arrows) is identifiable around many of the acini. (H&E, X250)

may extend to adjacent terminal ducts in a pagetoid fashion (Fig. 8.5). Sometimes this pagetoid ductal involvement may be the only change evident in the biopsy (29,67).

If the pathologist wishes to convey the extent and degree of advancement of these lobular changes, the alterations can be graded as LN1 to LN3, based on the extent and degree of proliferation (Table 8.1). To qualify as LN1, there should be partial or complete replacement or displacement of the normal epithelial cells of acini within one or more lobules by a proliferation of LN cells which may fill the lumens, but without any evidence of distension of the acini (Fig. 8.6), when compared to adjacent uninvolved acini. LN2 should display more abundant proliferation of LN cells that fill and distend some or all acini, but the acinar outlines remain distinct and separate from one another with persistence of intervening stroma (Fig. 8.7); residual lumens may persist in some acini. To warrant a designation of LN3, either an occlusive epithelial proliferation distending the acini to the point that they appear almost confluent—macroacini of Haagensen et al (42)—or acinar distension by a population of signet ring cells proliferating in a solid occlusive manner within the acini should be present (Figs. 8.8–8.10); residual lumens are absent and generally there is involvement of multiple acini. In my experience, LN1 and LN3 are quite rare, while LN2 is the most common. I would like to emphasize that this grading system should be used to convey information regarding the extent of the disease only; whether or not this grading has any prognostic significance has not been established.

Judging from the illustrations in Page et al's paper (66), their Figs. 2, 3, and probably 6 would qualify as LN1. Figures 1 and 4 show at least two lumens per some acini in the illustrated TDLU, and I would interpret the changes as a ductal pattern of hyperplasia. In Fig. 5, there is simply compression of the ductules and, in my opinion, no evidence of hyperplasia. They designated all of these as atypical lobular hyperplasia. Obviously, the range of changes

A

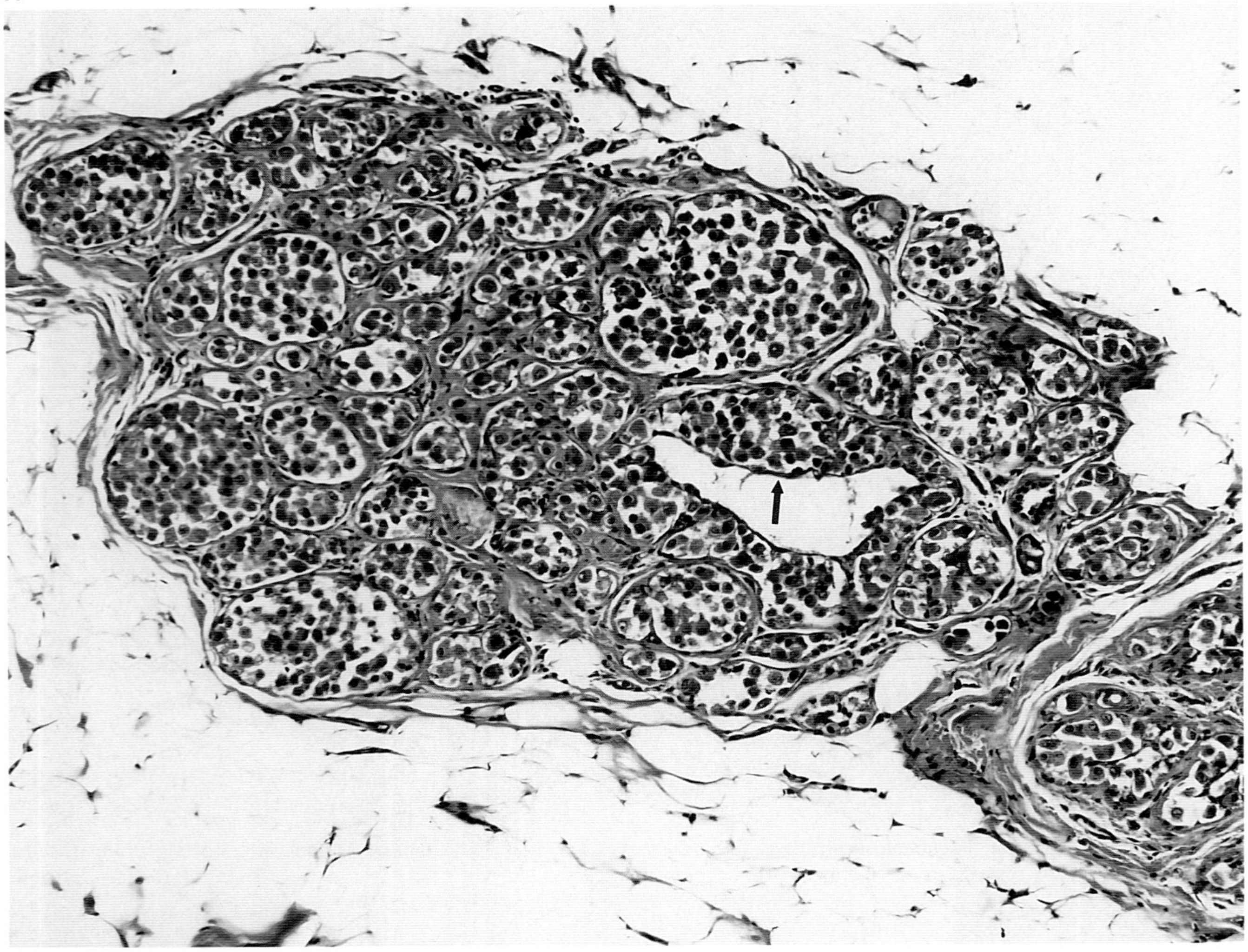

**Figure 8.2(a)** Lobular neoplasia (LN3). The cells are loosely cohesive and variable in size; note pagetoid growth pattern and attenuated native epithelial cell layer (arrow). (H&E, X300)

accepted as atypical lobular hyperplasia or LN1 varies depending on the rigidity of the criteria used.

*Necrosis and calcification* do rarely occur in lobular neoplasia and do not necessarily imply a ductal growth pattern. I have seen necrosis mainly in LN3 lesions (Fig. 8.11) that involved almost all lobules within a biopsy with such massive distension of the acini that a single acinus dwarfed a cluster of residual uninvolved lobules. While apparently necrosis is a reflection of a far advanced LN, calcification may be seen in LN1 and LN2 as well, albeit rarely.

The appearance of the myoepithelial cell layer is quite variable in LN (17,18,26). In some cases, it presents as a distinct layer in its original, normal location. In others, it is displaced and disrupted with some cells pushed or dislodged into the bolus of cellular proliferation. Finally, in a small number of LN3 lesions, it is hardly visible on H&E stained slides; immunostains for actin shows widening of the intermyoepithelial cell gaps.

The basement membrane (BM) around the acini is generally intact. Using special stains for reticulin or PAS, the basement membrane is not always present as a smooth band around the acini when closely inspected. Rather, it sometimes appears to have notches that protrude up in between the acinar lining cells; when these areas are cut tangentially, one may get the erroneous impression that there is a defect in the basement membrane. The presence of a few irregularities or breaks in the continuity of BM on

B

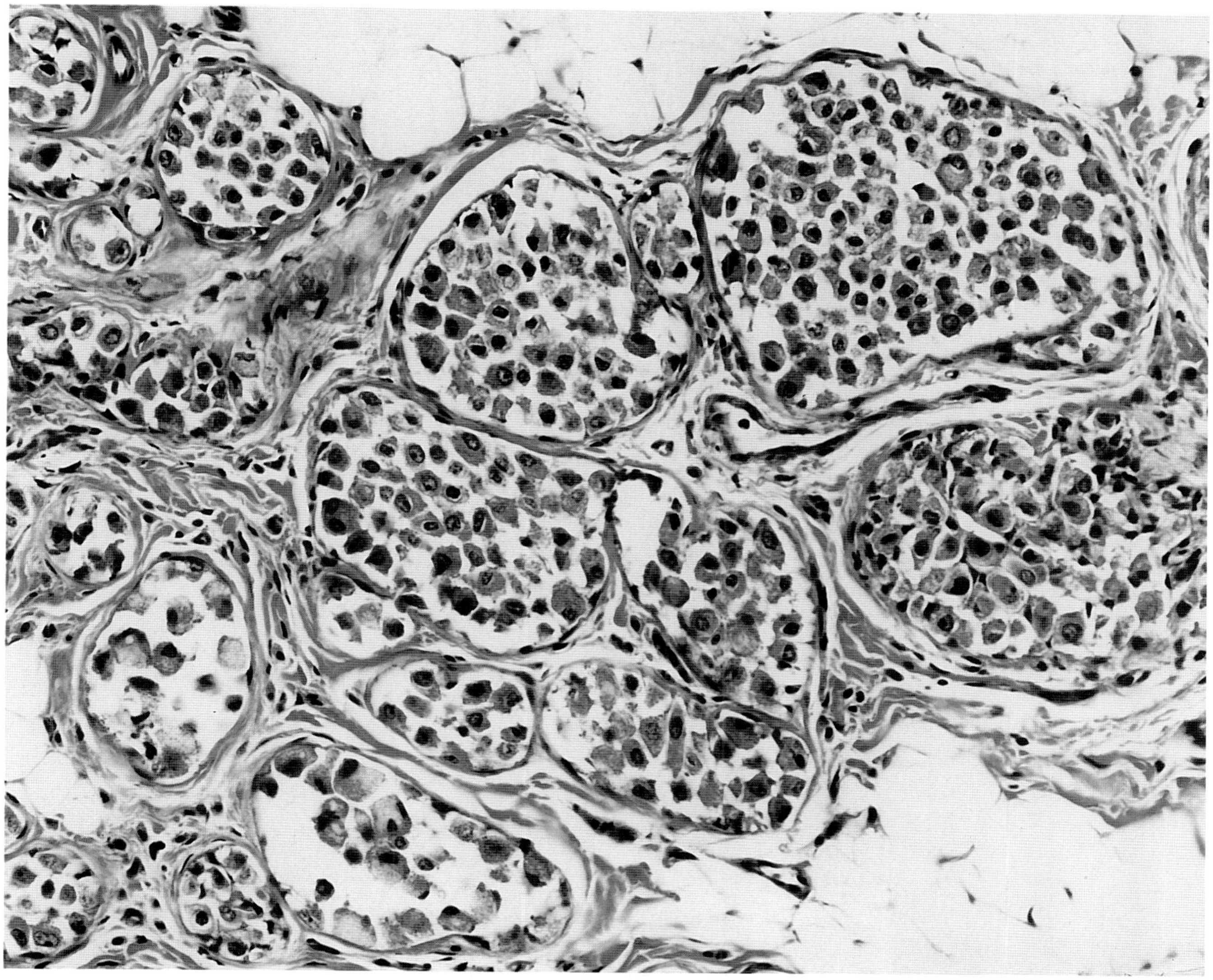

**Figure 8.2(b)** Lobular neoplasia (LN3). The cells have abundant eosinophilic cytoplasm, displaying apocrine-like features; the lesion is designated as LN3 because of the atypical cell population. (H&E, X600)

reticulin or PAS stains should not be considered as evidence of imminent invasion. Andersen (7) has shown that reticulin and PAS stains are not completely reliable in assessing the intact nature of the basement membrane since even normal lobules showed defects in up to half of their cases; I believe the major reason for this is the presence of convolutions and anatomic variation in the shape of the basement membrane. Even immunostains for type IV collagen and laminin used in our laboratories show similar flaws in adjacent normal lobules. These antibodies are very effective only when the basement membrane is thickened or multilayered as in microglandular adenosis (see Chapter 4).

Judging from two series published in 1978 (42,73), it appears that dividing this spectrum of lobular changes into ALH and LCIS has no prognostic significance. These studies conclude that a variety of qualitative and quantitative features generally used to subdivide the changes into LCIS and ALH are not of prognostic significance. The features evaluated by these studies as possible prognostic factors included the presence of cysts, perilobular lymphocytic infiltrate, persistence of central lumen, distension of acini, involvement of one or more lobules, macroacini, variation in cell type, loss of cell cohesion, closely-packed, hyperchromatic cells, and presence of an admixture of small and large cells. The only two features for which the subsequent risk was found to be higher than that for all other patients with LN were the presence of closely-packed, hyperchromatic cells (42), and an admixture of small and large cell

A

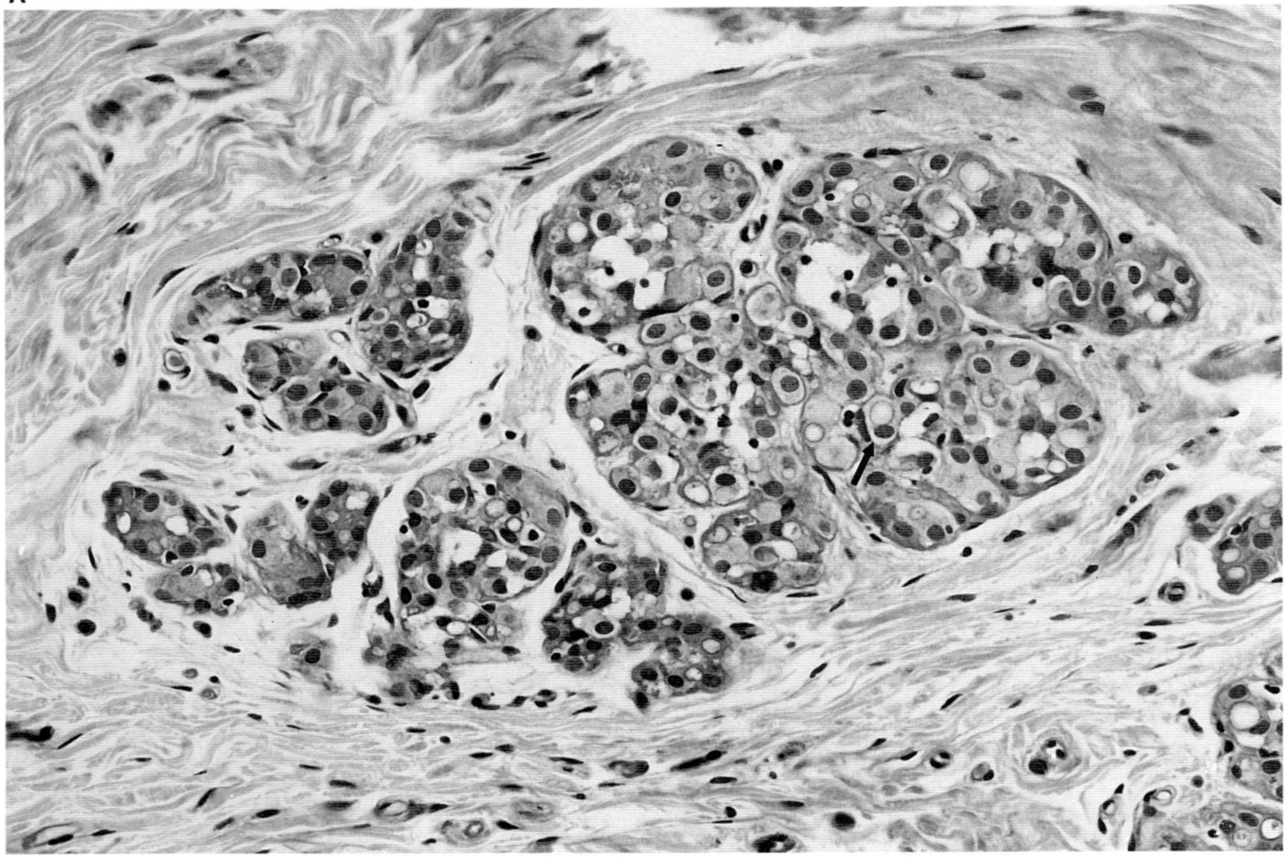

B

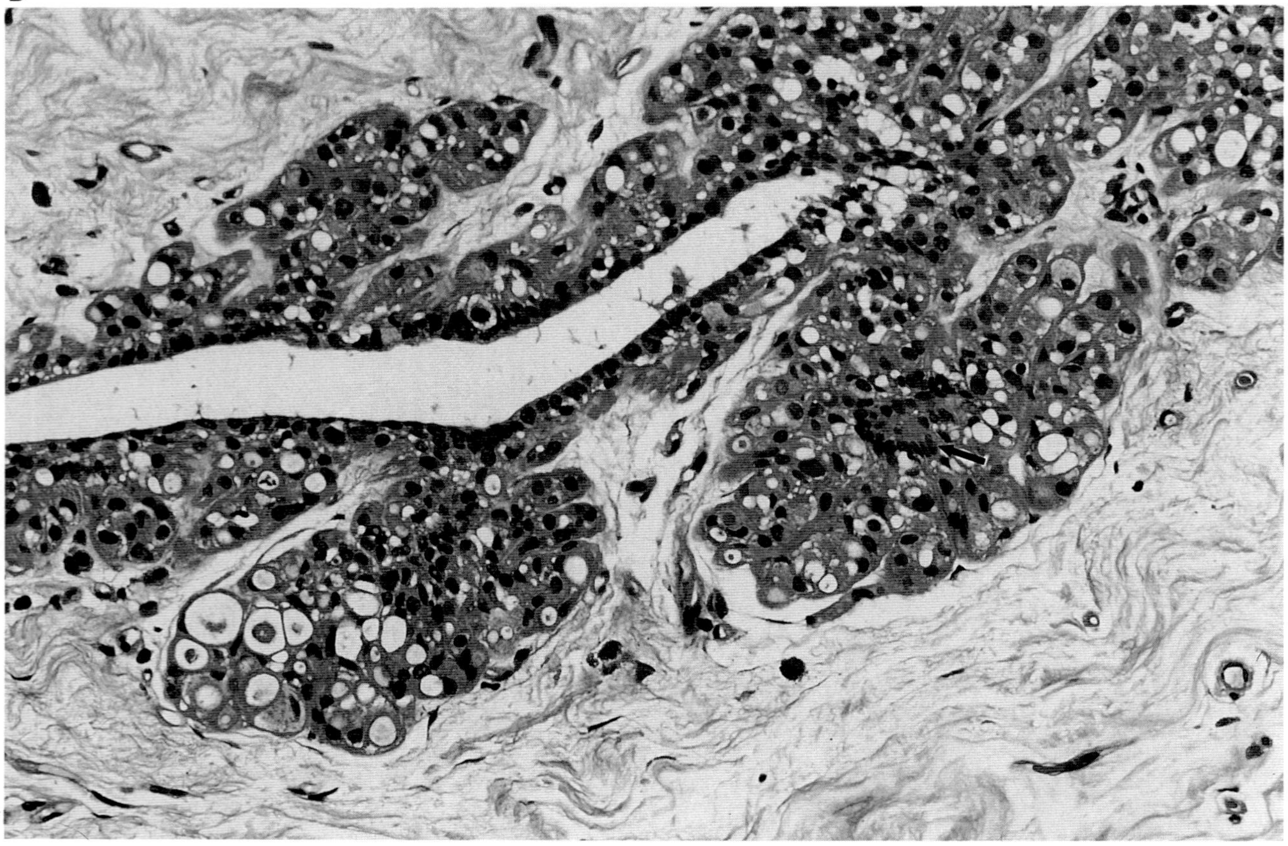

**Figure 8.3** Lobular neoplasia (LN2). The cells are larger with abundant cytoplasm. (a) Intracytoplasmic lumens of various sizes, some containing secretory droplets are evident in the neoplastic cells (arrow). (b) Residual epithelial cells are evident in one of the distorted acini (arrow). (H&E, (a&b) X400)

A

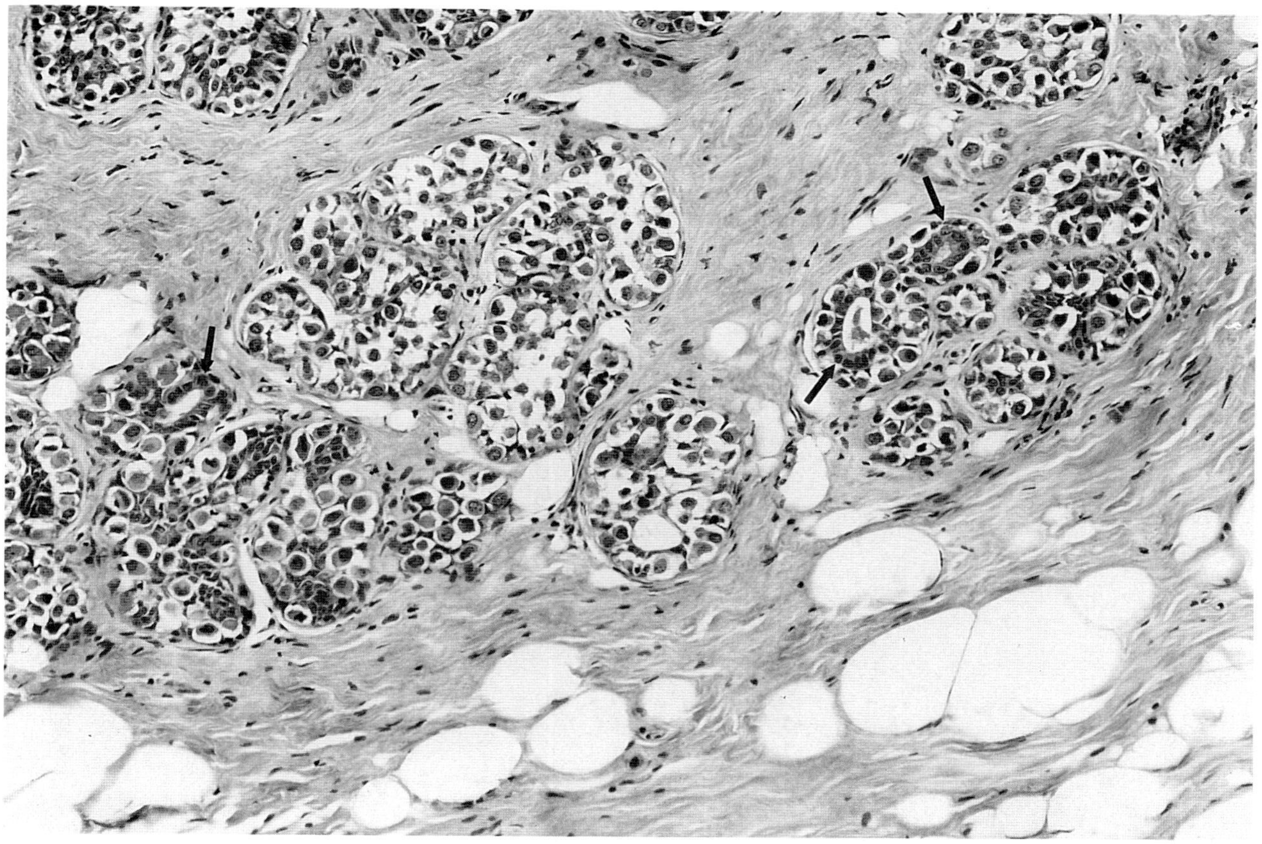

B

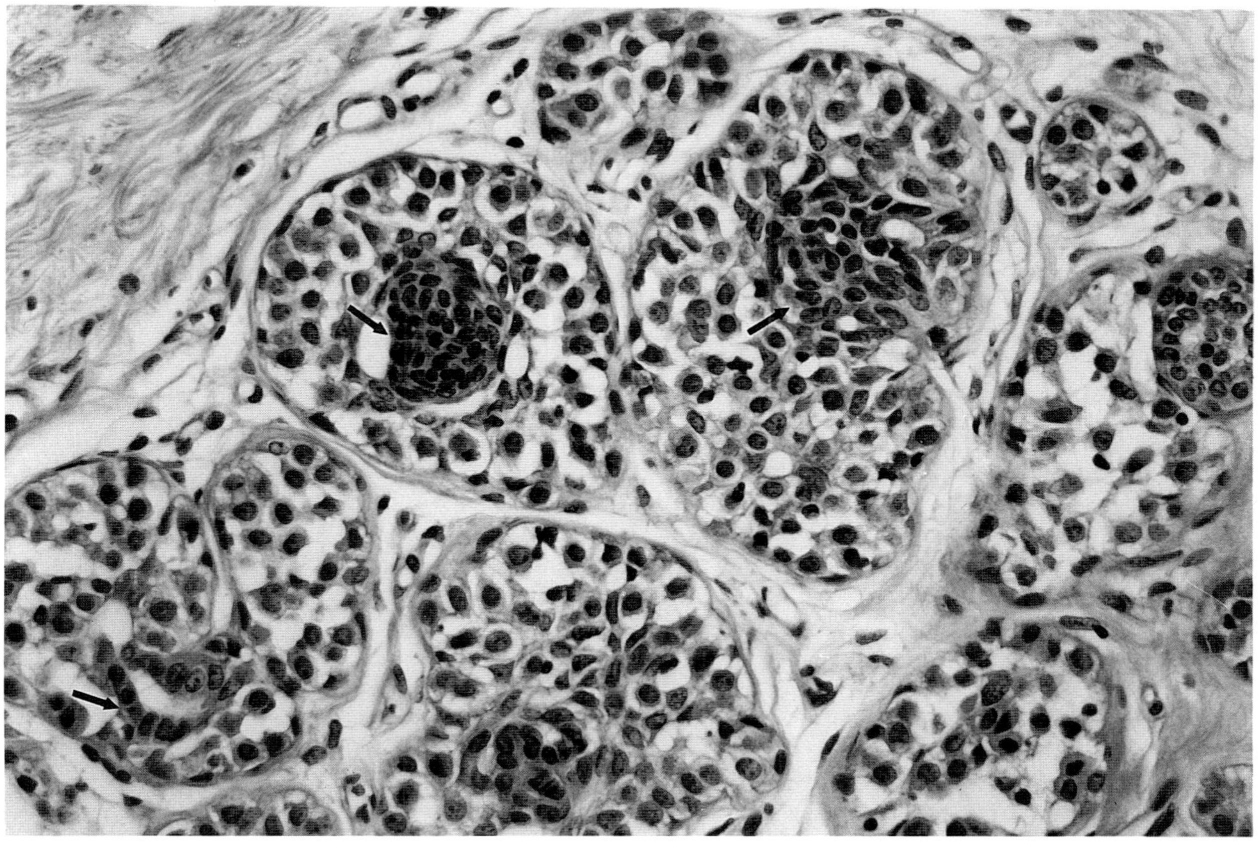

**Figure 8.4** Lobular neoplasia (LN2). (a) The native epithelial cells line displaced residual lumens (arrows). (b) The smaller native epithelial cells are compressed into solid clusters or line residual lumens (arrows). (H&E, (a) X200; (b) X500)

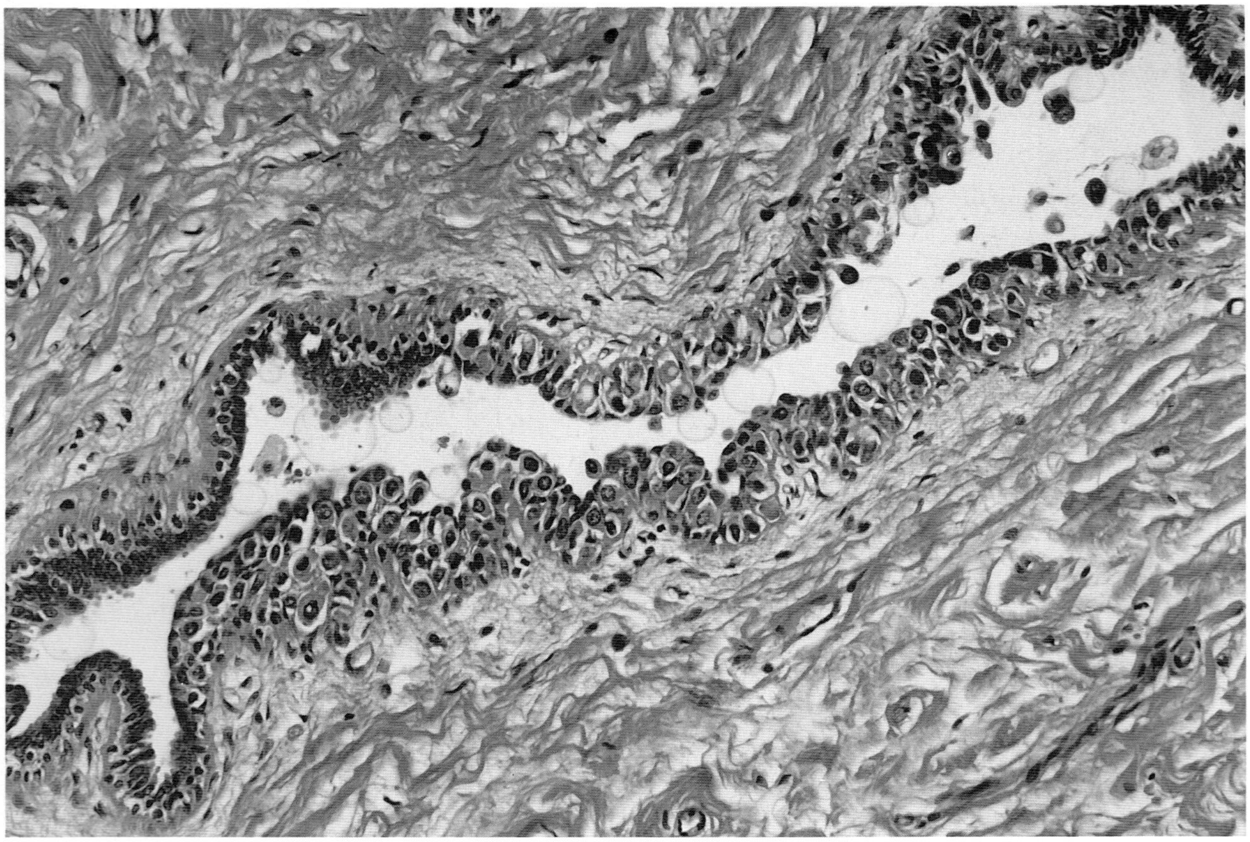

**Figure 8.5** Pagetoid involvement of a terminal duct by LN cells proliferating underneath the epithelial cell layer. (H&E, X100)

types (73). There were, however, only 12 patients with the former characteristic and 12 with the latter—too few to be considered significant.

Two subsequent studies (66,69) suggest that the lesions at the lowest end of the proliferative spectrum are associated with a lower risk for subsequent development of carcinoma. It is possible, however, that inclusion of cases such as illustrated in the Fig. 5 of one of the studies (66)—which in my opinion does not show lobular disease—may have diluted the effect of the presence of true lobular disease in their calculations. Furthermore, in a population of 10,542 women with otherwise benign breast biopsies, Page et al discovered 126 (66) cases of atypical lobular hyperplasia with proper follow-up and only 39 cases (0.5%) (69) of lobular carcinoma in situ with long-term follow-up. Obviously, Page et al are far more conservative in diagnosing LCIS compared to Rosen

**Table 8.1** Subclassification of LN Based on Extent of Lobular Involvement

LN1. There is partial or complete replacement or displacement of the normal epithelial cells of the acini within one or more lobules by a proliferation of generally uniform cells with poorly-defined margins which may fill, but do not distend, the acinar lumens (in comparison to adjacent uninvolved acini).

LN2. There is more abundant proliferation of similar cells as in LN1 that fill and actually distend some or all acini, but the acinar outlines remain distinct and separate from one another with persistence of intervening lobular stroma. Residual lumens may persist in some acini.

LN3. *Type 1.* There is proliferation of cells similar to those of LN1 and LN2, but occasionally a more atypical cell population dominates. An important feature is the massive degree of acinar distension to the point that the acini appear almost confluent. The interacinar stroma is barely evident.

*Type 2.* In this variant the proliferating cells are completely of the signet-ring cell type. This variant may not display significant acinar distension.

The myoepithelial cells may remain in their usual location or may be dislodged in any of these variants. In a small number of LN3 lesions, the myoepithelial cell layer is hardly visible on H&E stained slides; immunostain for actin shows widening of the intermyoepithelial cell gaps.

LN = Lobular neoplasia.

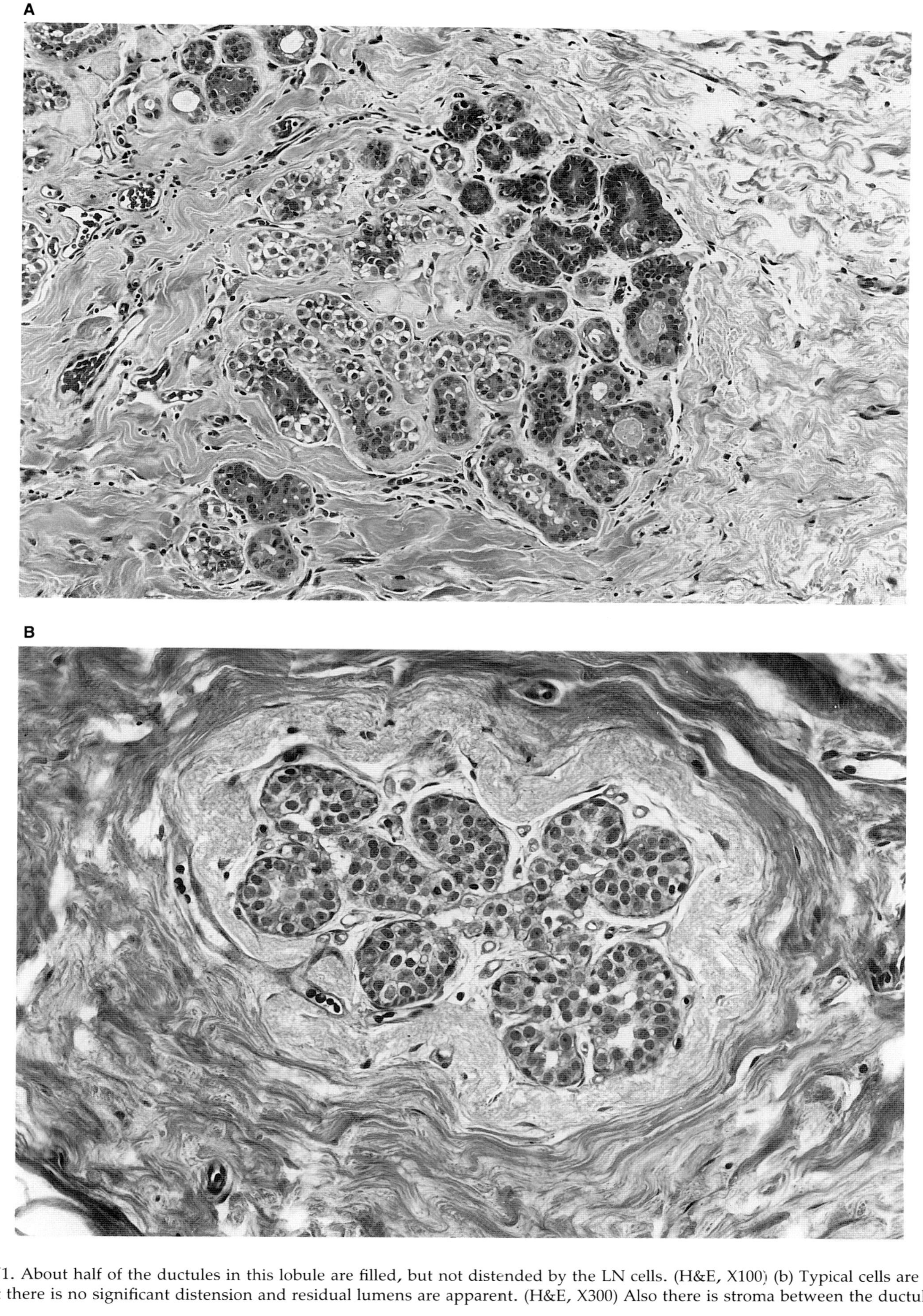


**Figure 8.6** LN1. About half of the ductules in this lobule are filled, but not distended by the LN cells. (H&E, X100) (b) Typical cells are present in all ductules but there is no significant distension and residual lumens are apparent. (H&E, X300) Also there is stroma between the ductules in both (a) and (b).

A

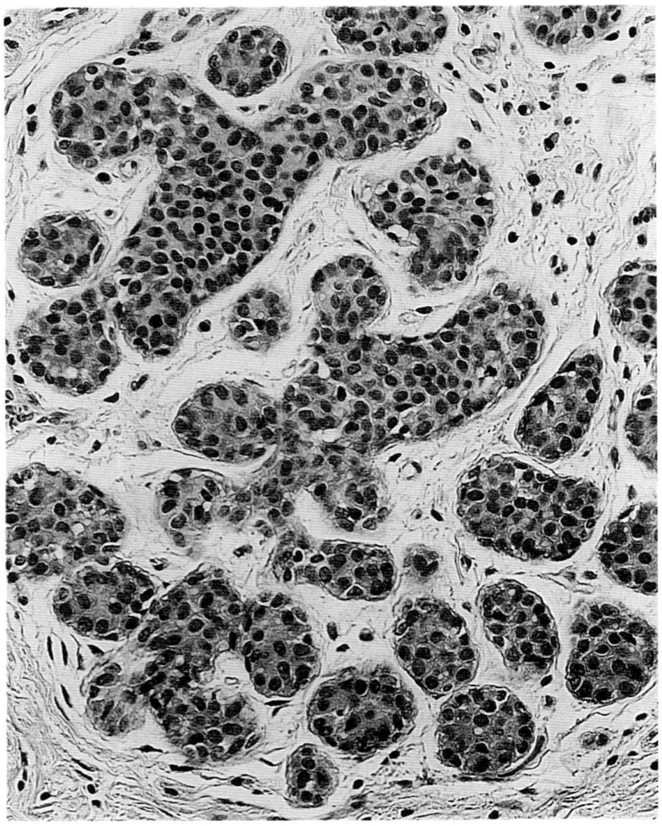

**Figure 8.7(a)** LN2. All ductules are involved, but are not very much expanded. There is stroma present between the ductules. (H&E, X120)

et al (71) who interpreted only 13 cases as ALH during the period when they diagnosed 99 cases (only 83 of which had proper follow-up evaluation) of LCIS (1.3%) among their breast biopsies. The fact that both Rosen et al (71) and Page et al (69) concluded that the relative risk for subsequent development of invasive carcinoma is 9.0 for women with LCIS while using different criteria and analytic approach indicates that the value of splitting this spectrum into two prognostically distinct groups has not been confirmed.

## DUCTAL INVOLVEMENT BY LOBULAR NEOPLASIA

Pagetoid involvement of ducts and its variants have been amply discussed by many investigators (5,29,32, 39,54,73,83,89). Haagensen (39) has stated that in some cases, the ducts are more extensively involved by LN than are the lobules. He illustrated what he refers to as the "clover-leaf" pattern of ductal involvement in Figures 14.13 to 14.15 of his book (39). I believe there is an overdiagnosis of ductal involvement by lobular neoplasia mainly due to a misperception of altered lobules as ducts. Just as the ductal type proliferations can unfold the lobules, the acini occluded by lobular neoplasia can sometimes alter the lobules by pulling away from the intralobular segment of the terminal duct creating the so-called "clover-leaf" pattern (Fig. 8.12). I find it difficult to accept that neoplastic cells would pattern themselves around a tubal structure in a clover-leaf fashion. It is physically much more likely for occluded acini to pull away from the intralobular segment of terminal duct located in their midst by the shear weight of the solid occlusive proliferation within them, creating the so-called "clover-leaf" pattern. Or, the proliferation may actually unfold the lobule, transforming it into a duct-like structure. The proliferation within such an altered lobule is recognized as a lobular process on the basis of formation of a complete collar by the LN cells (pagetoid appearance) throughout the unfolded TDLU, and retention of the luminal layer of native epithelial cells overlying the LN cells (Fig. 8.13); it does not reflect a pagetoid extension to an extralobular duct. I would accept ductal involvement by LN only when part of the duct wall retains its normal two-cell layer appearance while other areas show a pagetoid growth, or when the location of the duct adjacent to a lobule is such that it can be reasonably interpreted as an extralobular duct (Fig. 8.14). It is interesting that a flattening of the native epithelial cell layer of the ducts occurs even if involved by a small number of these "pagetoid cells."

## LOBULAR NEOPLASIA IN SCLEROSING ADENOSIS (SA)

Lobular neoplasia may extend into areas of sclerosing adenosis (30) (Fig. 8.15), or it may be evident only within areas of sclerosing adenosis. In this setting, it may be confused with an invasive carcinoma. Evaluation of the lesion at low magnification is crucial in its recognition since the nodular or lobulated outline and the presence of streaming, compressed ductules at the periphery of the lesion are best evident at low magnification. If doubts persist regarding the possibility of invasion, immunostains for actin can be used

B

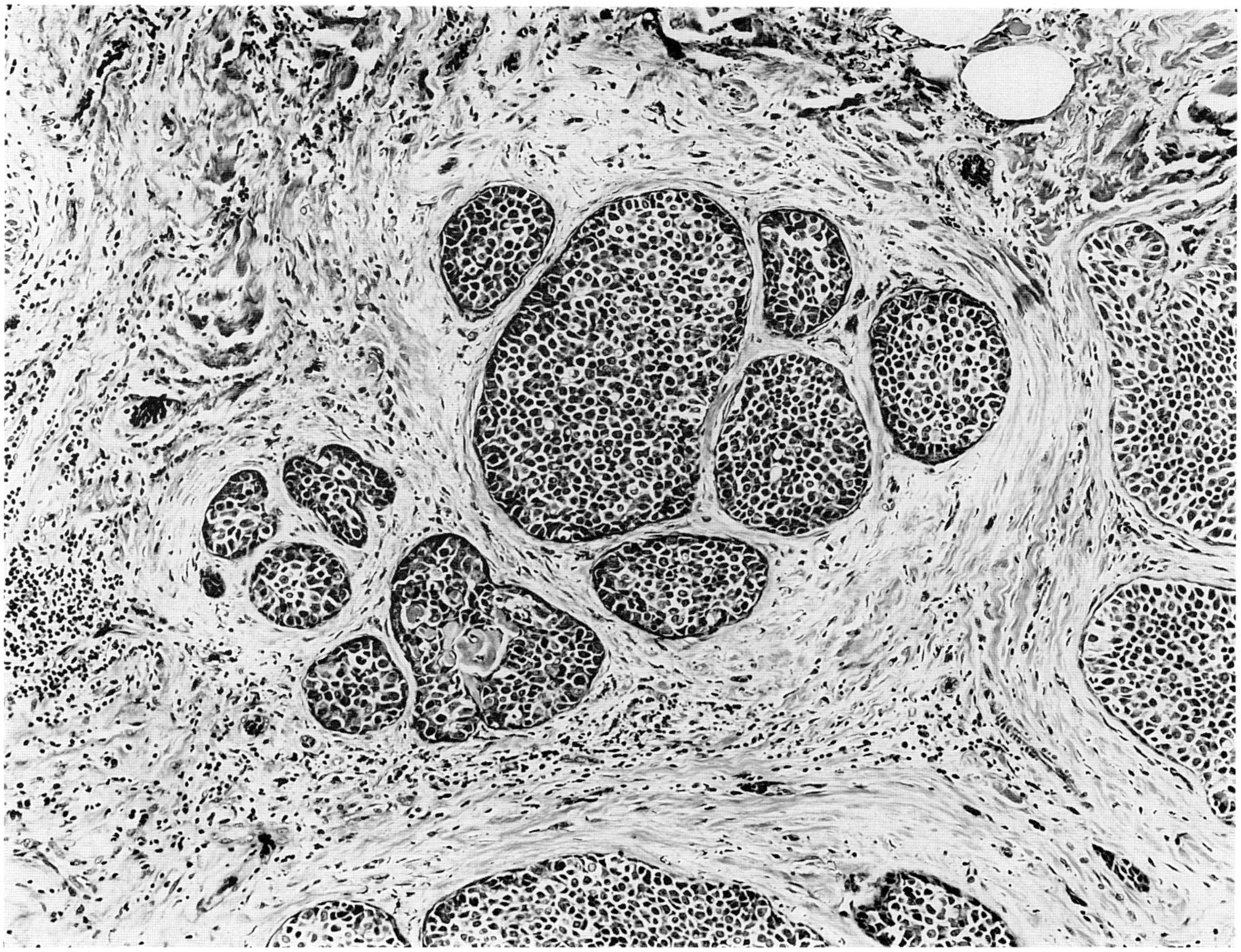

**Figure 8.7(b)** LN2. There is distension of these ductules, but they remain separated by intervening stroma. (H&E, X80)

to unmask the myoepithelial cell layer around the ductules of SA filled by LN cells, thereby resolving the problem.

## LN INVOLVING RADIAL SCARS AND FIBROADENOMA

These conditions are discussed under radial scars and fibroadenoma in Chapters 4 and 11, respectively.

## DISTINCTION FROM AIDH AND IDCA WITHIN THE TDLU

As mentioned in Chapter 5, Intraductal Hyperplasias, lesions with both ductal and lobular patterns originate in the TDLU (87). The frequent occurrence of carcinoma within the lobules was recognized by Dawson even in the early 1930s (23). Distinction of LN from ductal atypical hyperplasias and in situ carcinomas within the TDLU which have not yet unfolded the lobule can be difficult and a source of confusion (28). In general, IDCA will retain some of its classic features (11). Features that help identify the relatively solid variants of ductal growth patterns within the TDLU include formation of multiple—albeit minuscule—secondary lumens, rosette-like arrangement of the nuclei (Figs. 8.16 and 8.17), and distinctive cell margins bestowing a mosaic pattern upon the solid proliferation. The presence of large cells with abundant cytoplasm and pleomorphism associated with any of the features just mentioned would further support interpretation of the lesion as ductal rather than lobular.

Features that favor lobular neoplasia include

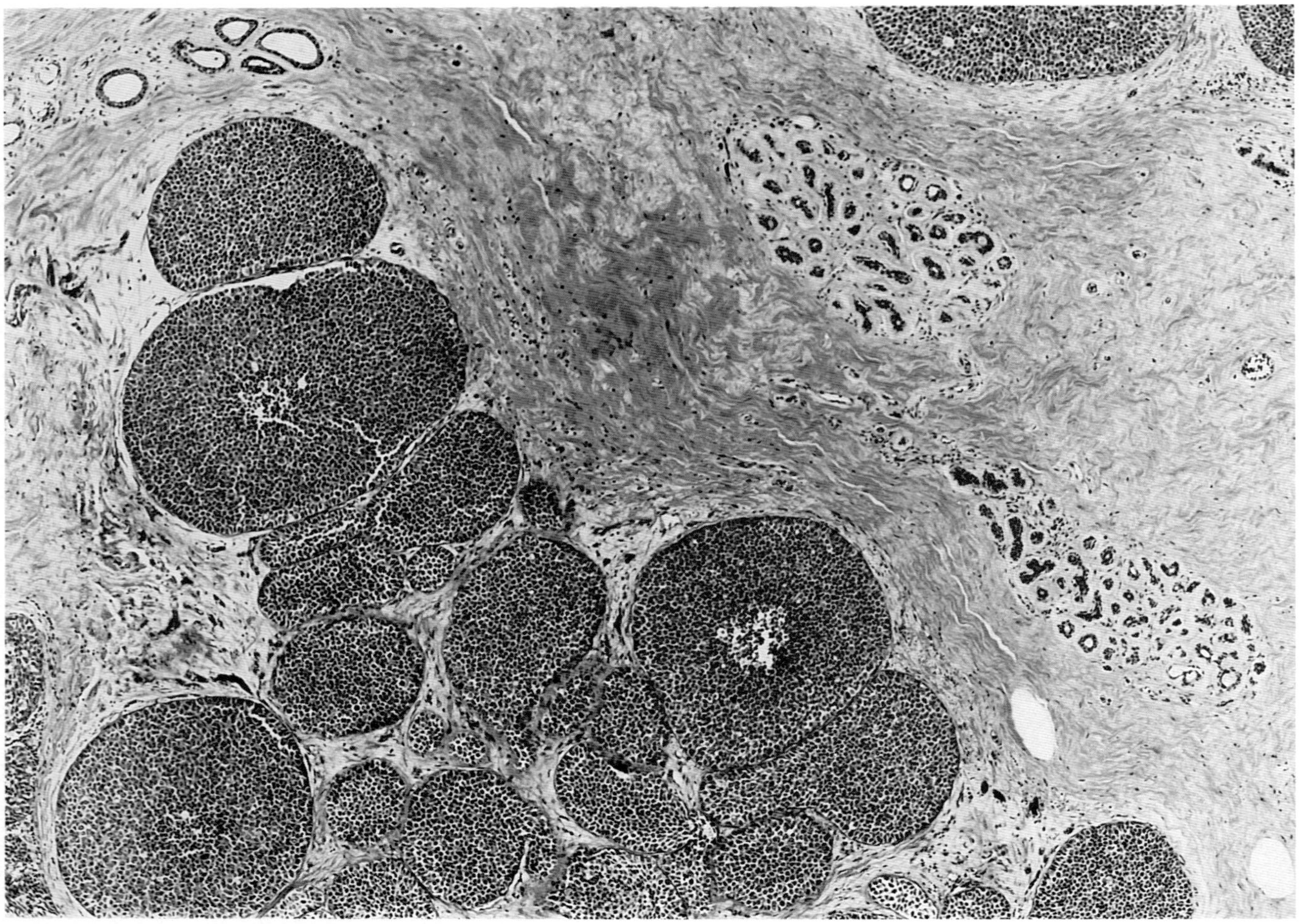

**Figure 8.8** LN3. There is massive distension of some ductules (acini), with minimal, if any, intervening stroma. Note the extent of acinar distension compared to the acini of adjacent normal lobules. (H&E, X80)

loosely cohesive cells and the presence of intracytoplasmic lumens (13) or secretory globules (8) and mucin positivity. The presence of intracellular sialomucin has been noted as another feature that may help distinguish LN from ductal carcinomas in the TDLU (33). Gad & Azzopardi (33) found that the mucosubstance in the LN cells is alcianophilic and periodic acid-Schiff (PAS) positive after diastase digestion.

Despite the variety of helpful features mentioned above, it is sometimes impossible to make such a distinction.

Regardless of whether a lesion forms epithelial bridges and multiple secondary lumens (ductal growth pattern), or a solid, occlusive proliferation (lobular growth pattern), it is noteworthy that some authors make no distinction between these different patterns of carcinoma when the lesion is composed of small cells (82). This approach would mask some of the distinctive qualities of LN enumerated by various investigators.

It is quite possible that the two distinctive patterns simply reflect versatility in the potential of a single neoplastic cell population. Nonetheless, the fact that the solid, lobular growth pattern has a significantly different clinical behavior compared to the fenestrated, ductal growth pattern implies that there is a morphologically inapparent factor, possibly as defects at the chromosomal level, that determines the ultimate architectural and clinical manifestation of these morphologically similar small cells.

## COEXISTENCE OF LOBULAR NEOPLASIA AND INTRADUCTAL CARCINOMA

Various investigators have commented on the simultaneous finding of LN and intraductal or inva-

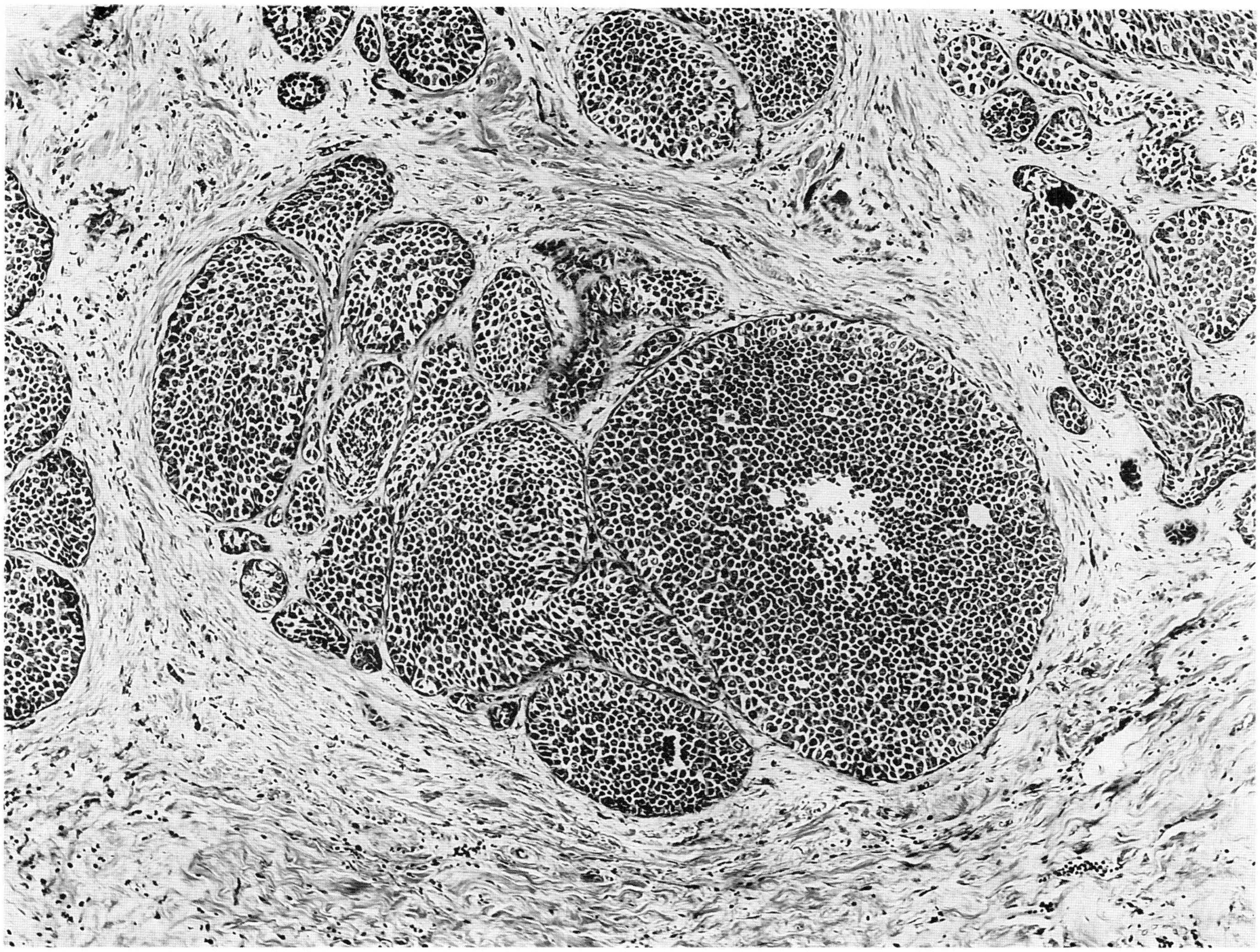

**Figure 8.9** LN3. The acini are distended and almost confluent. The cells are loosely cohesive. (H&E, X120)

sive ductal carcinoma within a biopsy (Fig. 8.18) as well as within a single terminal duct-lobular unit (39,40,70). The frequency of this coexistence has been noted to range from 12% to 16% (39,70). Haagensen et al (39) found that patients in whom LN occurred alone were generally younger than the group of patients having LN associated with other forms of breast carcinoma. Biopsies from the latter group displayed LN with loss of cell cohesion, macroacini, and maximal amounts of the lesion more frequently.

With the more extensive sampling of breast biopsy specimen in the current practice of surgical pathology, it is not surprising that we are observing an increase in the frequency of this association.

## DISTRIBUTION OF LN

Since the diagnosis of LN is mainly based on an evaluation of biopsies removed for other lesions, it is difficult to assess the distribution of LN in the breast. Only one study is available that addresses this issue. Lambird and Shelley (51) studied nine simple mastectomy specimen by first dividing them into quadrants, and incising the quadrants radially from the nipple to the periphery. The radial segments were cut circumferentially from the nipple to the periphery into 2.5 cm blocks. Eight of the breasts were totally blocked and embedded for evaluation. The ninth breast was quite large, weighing 2,600 grams; it was

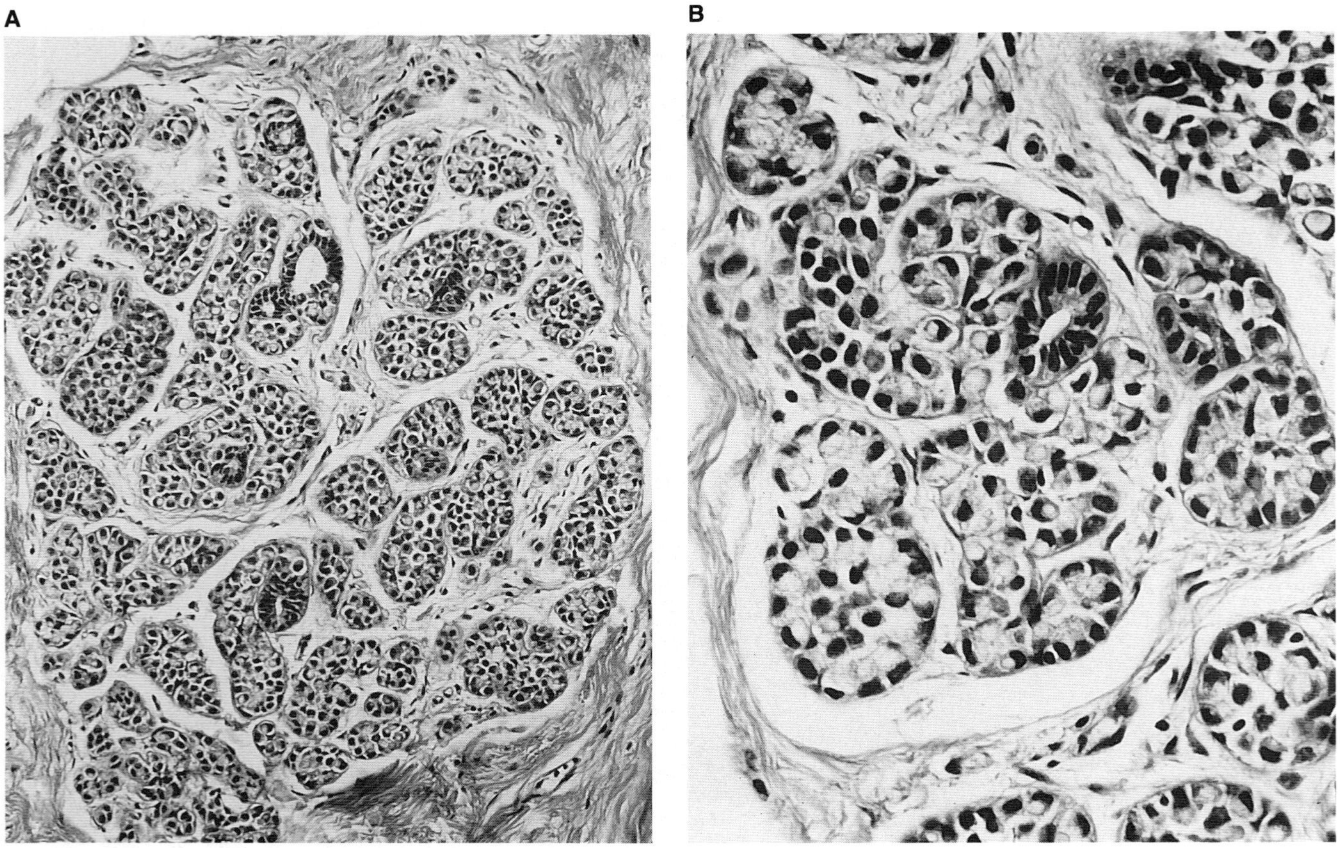


**Figure 8.10** LN3. (a) The acini are distended, but not massively so. There is even persistent lumen lined by native epithelial cells. The proliferating cells appear different even at this magnification, however. (b) All of the LN cells have a signet ring-like appearance. This patient had invasive carcinoma in her mastectomy specimen. (H&E, (a) X80; (b) X200)

step blocked and every third block was embedded. The sections were reviewed and they found LN most frequently in the upper outer quadrant (25%), then the upper inner quadrant (13.9%), the lower outer quadrant (7.2%), and finally, the lower inner quadrant (0.5%). From a circumferential view, LN was found most frequently in the subareolar and periareolar regions within 5 cm of the nipple. Of the sections from this central area, 20% contained the lesion, while 8.7% of the more peripheral sections showed the disease.

## DIAGNOSIS BY FINE-NEEDLE ASPIRATION (FNA)

The increasing utilization of FNA in the management of breast lesions mandates a brief remark regarding its application to the diagnosis of lobular neoplasia. Reports describing the features of LN on FNA are sparse (78) and have utilized the ALH/LCIS classification in evaluating only three patients. The findings indicate that the presence of loosely cohesive cell groups composed of uniform cells with frequent eccentric nuclei, minimal nuclear atypia, and occasional intracytoplasmic lumens are suggestive of ALH or LCIS; a distinction between the two is not possible on FNA. In contrast, the invasive lobular carcinomas are more cellular and have a higher proportion of noncohesive single cells, with increased nuclear atypia and pleopmorphism; also, intracytoplasmic lumens are observed with greater frequency in the invasive carcinomas (78).

It is important to keep in mind the limitations of FNA. A negative FNA does not exclude the possibility of LN. In most cases, a biopsy confirmation is obtained.

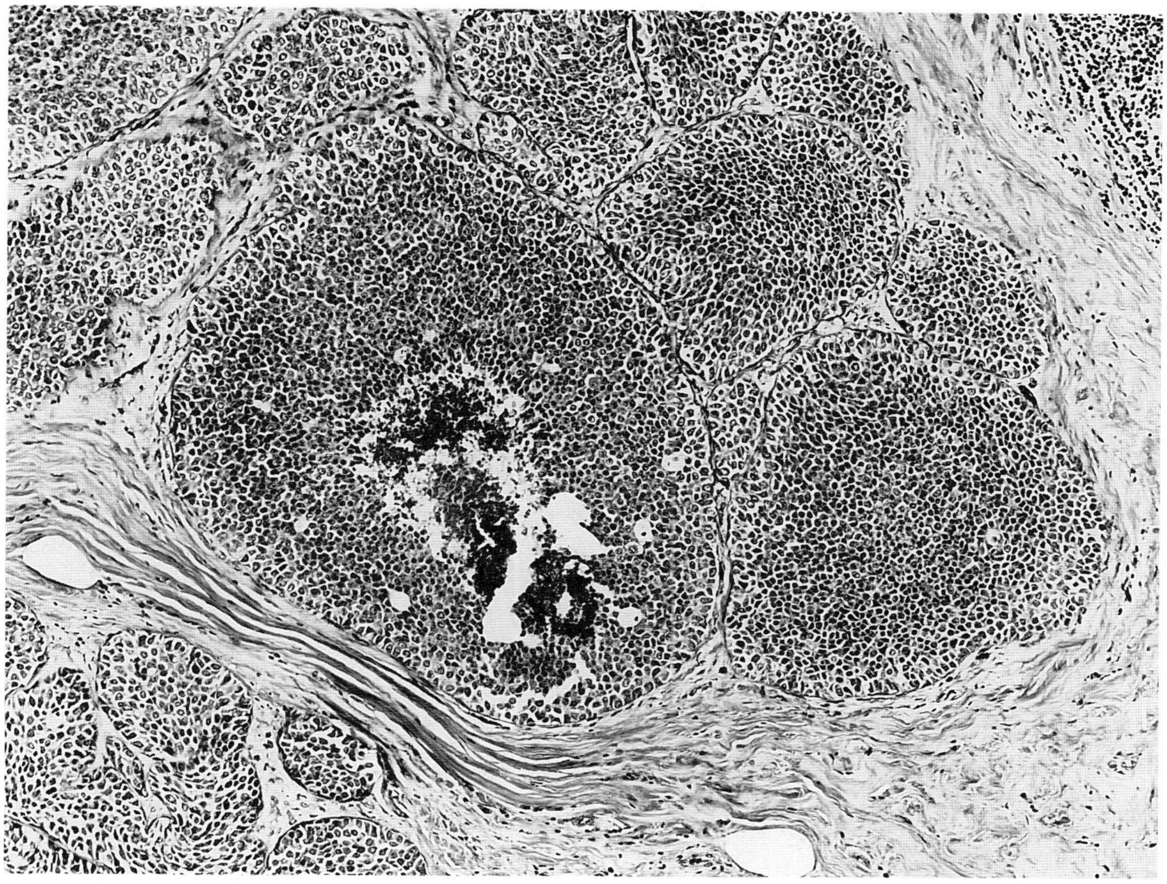

**Figure 8.11** LN3 with necrosis. An area of necrosis is evident in a massively enlarged acinus of this diffuse example of LN. (H&E, X100)

## ULTRASTRUCTURAL FEATURES

It appears as if in the early 1970s, the possibility of a myoepithelial (ME) cell origin for breast carcinomas had become popular among some investigators (44,45,56). Based on the light microscopic features or the finding of intracytoplasmic fibrils within the neoplastic cells, several investigators raised the possibility of a myoepithelial cell origin for LN (20,44,45). The finding of secretory activity as evidenced by the presence of intracytoplasmic lumens containing secretory droplets and identification of intracytoplasmic lumens with microvilli at the ultrastructural level (63), however, contradict a myoepithelial differentiation. Furthermore, the persistence of a uniform layer of normal ME cells around some classic examples of LN (18,19,59) without any transition to the neoplastic cells makes it difficult to explain origin from ME cells. It is important to realize that the mere presence of intracytoplasmic fibrils does not indicate a ME cell origin or differentiation. Intracytoplasmic fibrils are seen in a variety of epithelial cells. I have personally observed them in hyperplastic epithelial cells, atypical epithelial cells, and invasive ductal carcinomas. Others have also observed intracytoplasmic fibrils in infiltrating ductal carcinomas (88). One of the important diagnostic features of ME cells is the presence of pinocytotic vesicles; this has never been demonstrated in any of the ultrastructural reports on LN cells.

The LN cells may display a prominent Golgi apparatus (81). The neoplastic cells are attached to one another and to adjacent ME cells by well developed desmosomes. The ME cells are attached to the surrounding basement membrane by hemidesmosomes.

The basement membrane (BM) is generally intact (59), with intrusions between the ME cells and tortuosity as it follows the contour of the enclosed cells (81). Occasionally, gaps in the basement membrane are evident (63); these may serve as the points through which invasion of the stroma takes place. Nesland et al (59) stated that in infiltrating lobular carcinoma, the epithelial cells break through the ME cell layer and basal lamina, coming

A

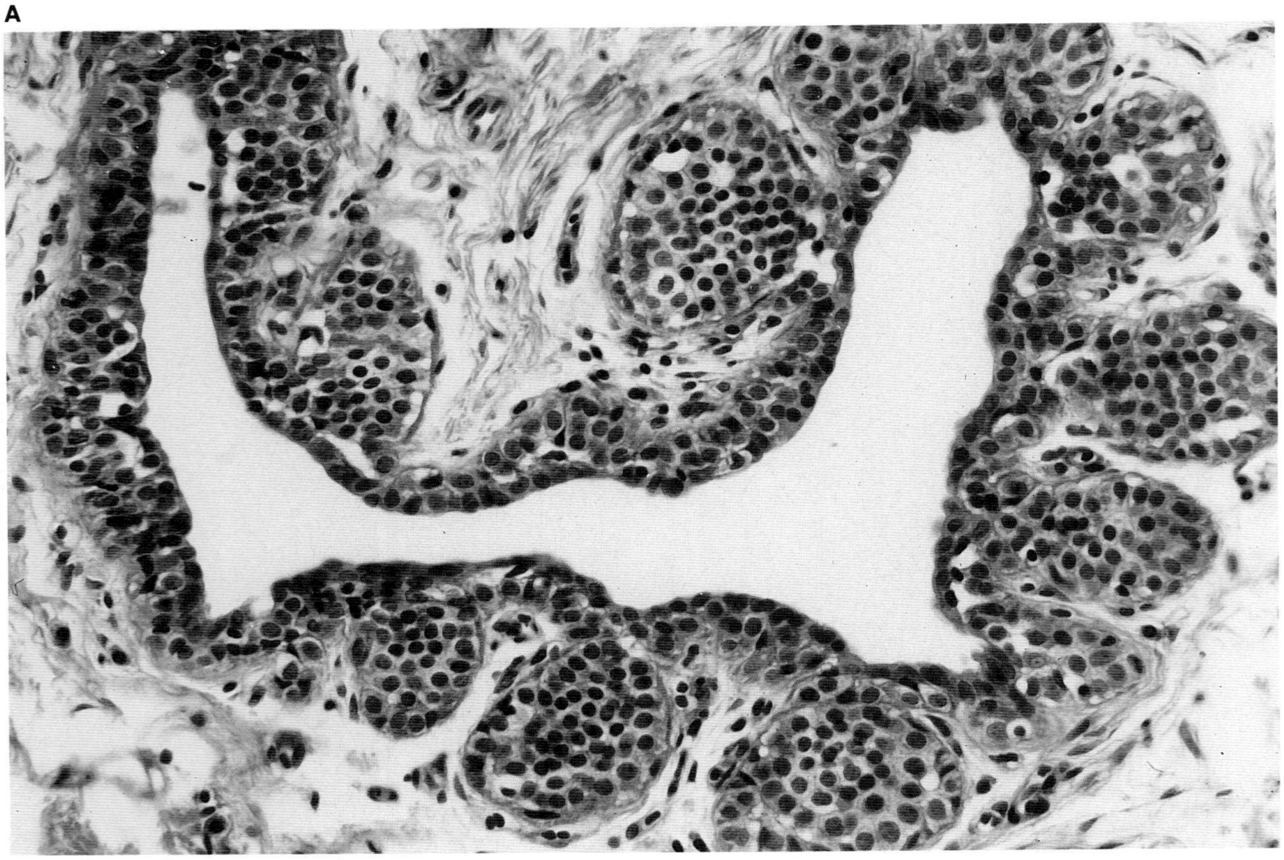

B

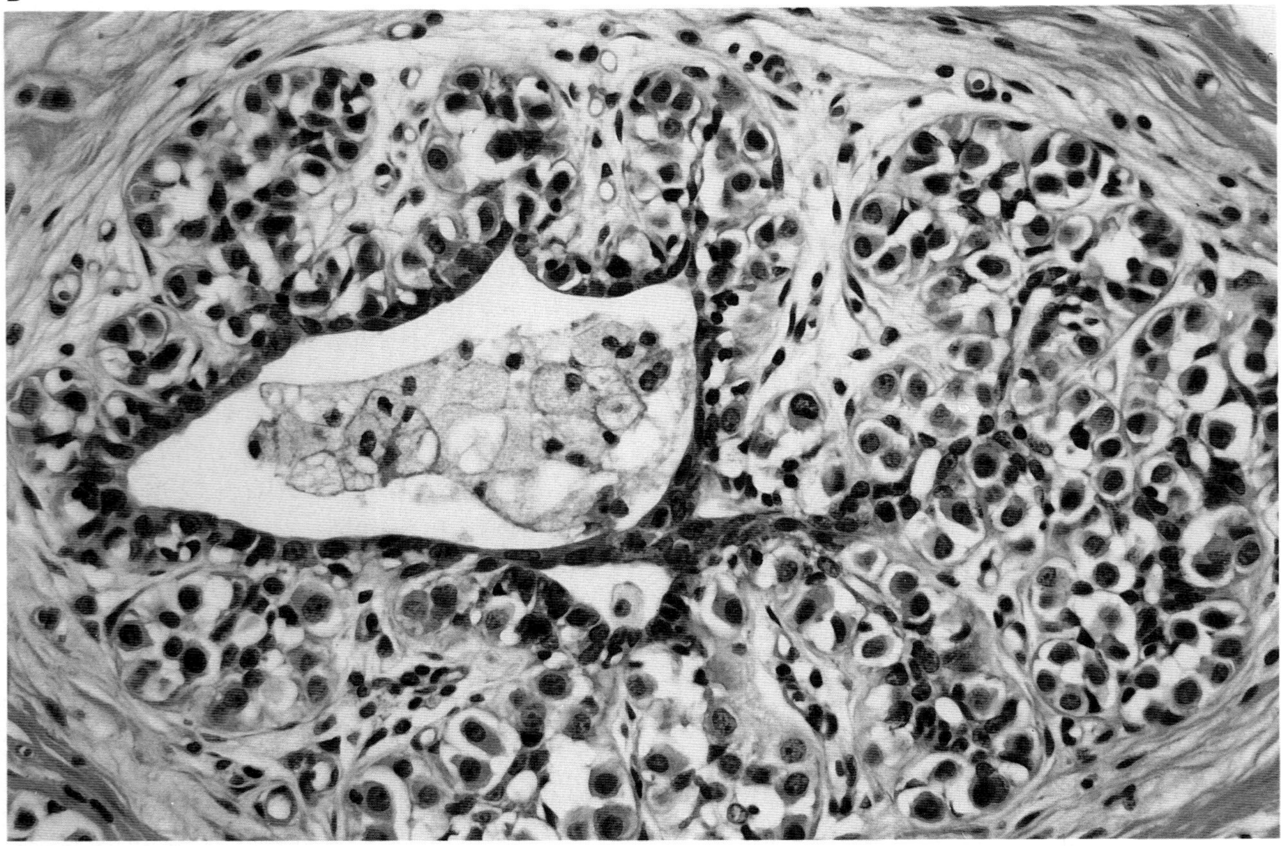

**Figure 8.12** LN, clover-leaf pattern. (a–c) Acini filled by LN cells of various appearances pull away from the intralobular segment of the terminal duct distending the latter. All of these structures reflect altered lobules or TDLUs; this pattern does not reflect pagetoid extension to an extralobular duct. (H&E, (a) X200; (b) X300; (c) X200)

c

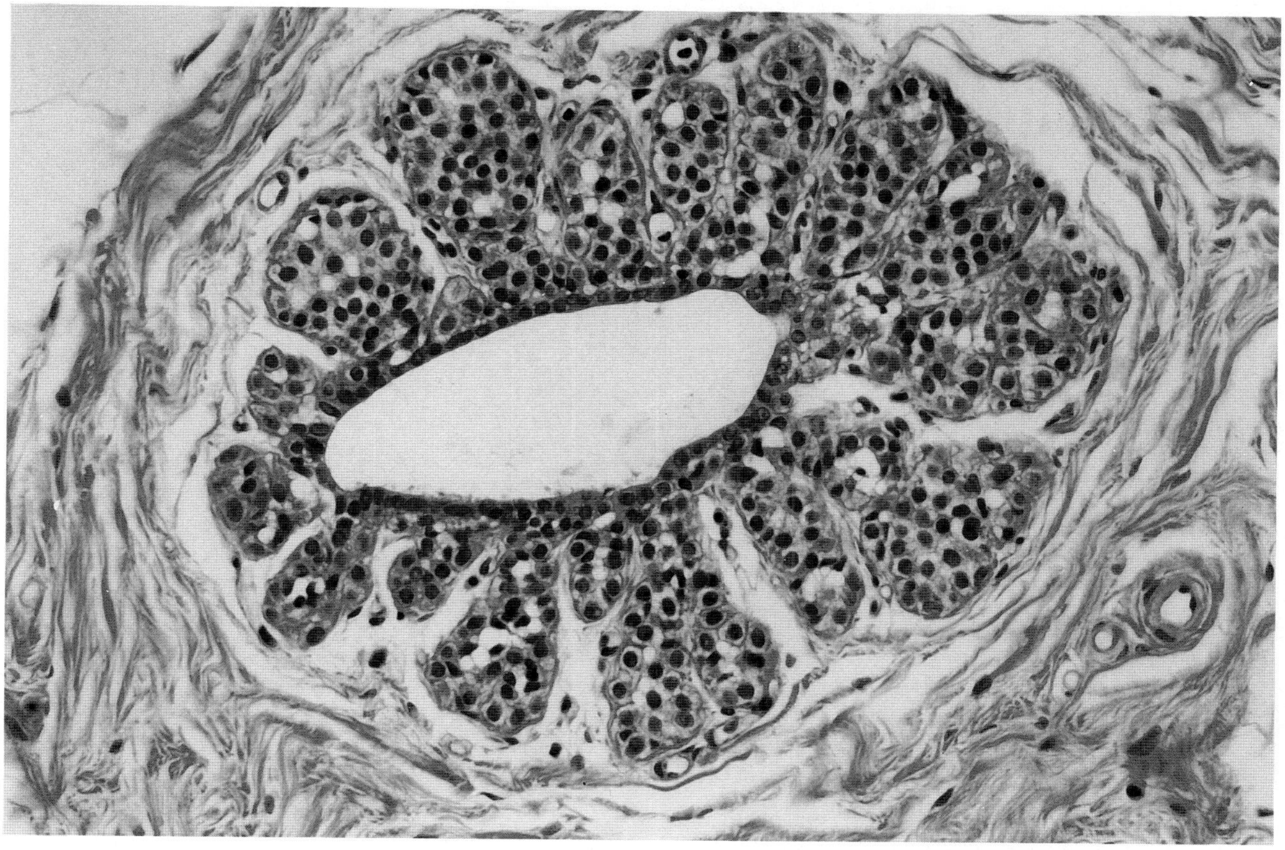

**Figure 8.12(c)** LN, clover-leaf pattern. Legend on opposite page.

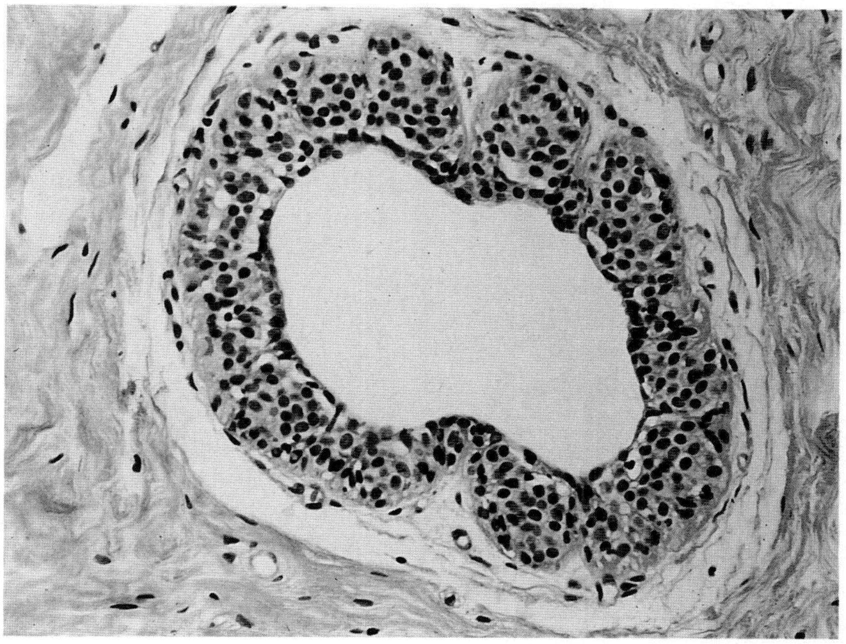

**Figure 8.13** An unfolded lobule with a collar of LN cells displaying a pagetoid appearance. The partial clover-leaf pattern is an important clue regarding the lobular location of the process. (H&E, X150)

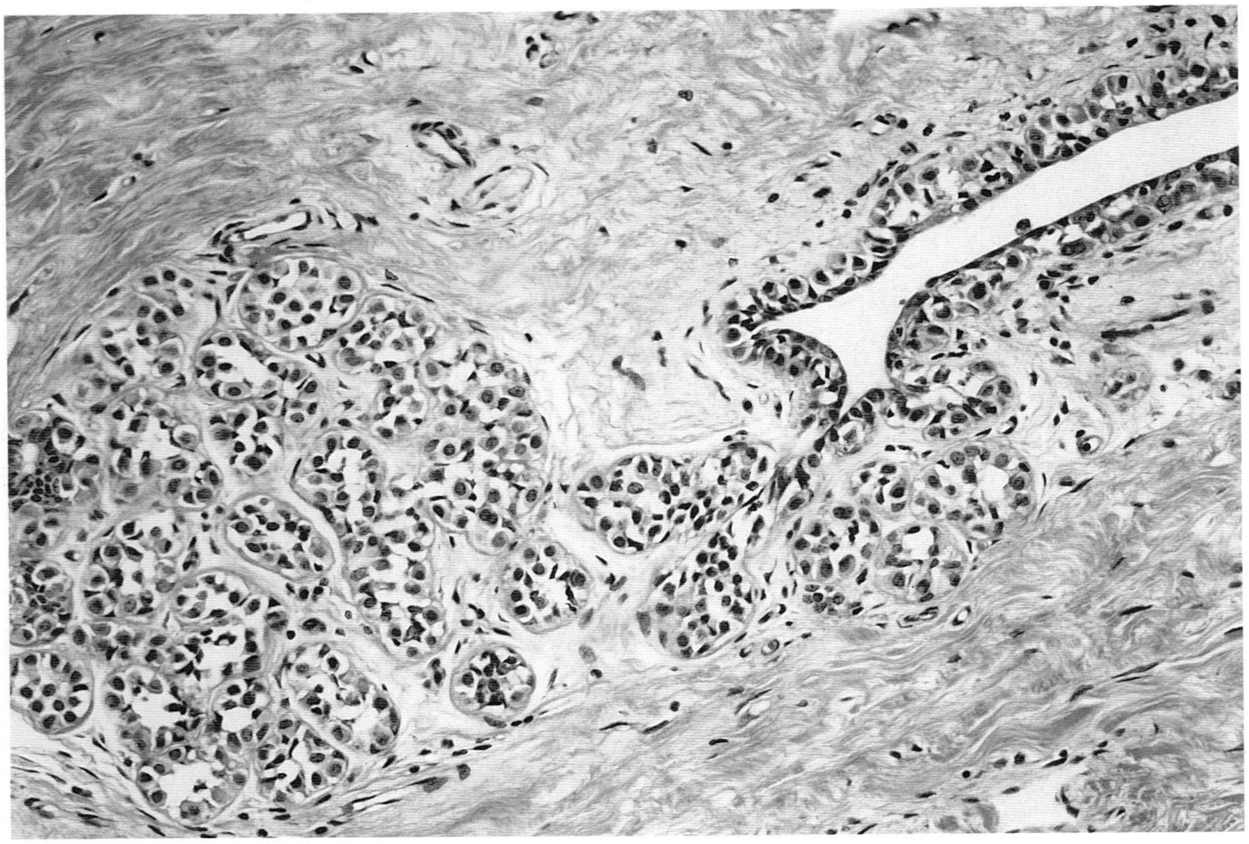

**Figure 8.14** Pagetoid involvement of an extralobule terminal duct. (H&E, X160)

into direct contact with the surrounding stroma. Their illustration of this process in their Fig. 6 is not convincing, however. An identical picture can be seen in normal lobules where the epithelial cells are in direct contact with the BM through the intermyoepithelial cell gap; the BM at these points may not stand out distinctively, giving the erroneous impression of a defect in the BM.

## HORMONE RECEPTORS AND TUMOR MARKERS

Using immunohistochemical staining, ten examples of LCIS were evaluated for estrogen receptor (ER) expression by Giri et al (36). Nine of the ten cases of LCIS showed variable expression of ER, and six of these (60%) displayed significant nuclear staining. Among a group of benign and malignant lesions evaluated by a panel of markers including c-erbB-2, collagen, type IV, B72.3, EP4, and progesterone receptors at AFIP, the only marker that displayed a consistently positive reaction in 14 examples of LN was type IV collagen. The positive reaction to type IV collagen was evident around the acini containing the neoplastic cells indicating persistence of the basal lamina. All 14 lesions were negative for c-erbB-2, only one showed positivity for B72.3, one for EP4, and five displayed nuclear positivity for progesterone receptor protein. Eleven of 14 intraductal carcinomas, in contrast, showed a positive reaction for EP4. The 14 invasive lobular carcinomas differed from LN mainly in their reaction to collagenase; 11 of the 14 cases displayed absolutely no positivity with collagen type IV. One example of LCIS evaluated by Nesland et al (59) displayed a positive reaction for CEA, prekeratin, and casein, but failed to react with lactalbumin.

Eusebi (26) found casein in the cytoplasm of five examples of LCIS and 21 of infiltrating lobular carcinoma. In addition, alpha lactalbumin and lactoferritin

A

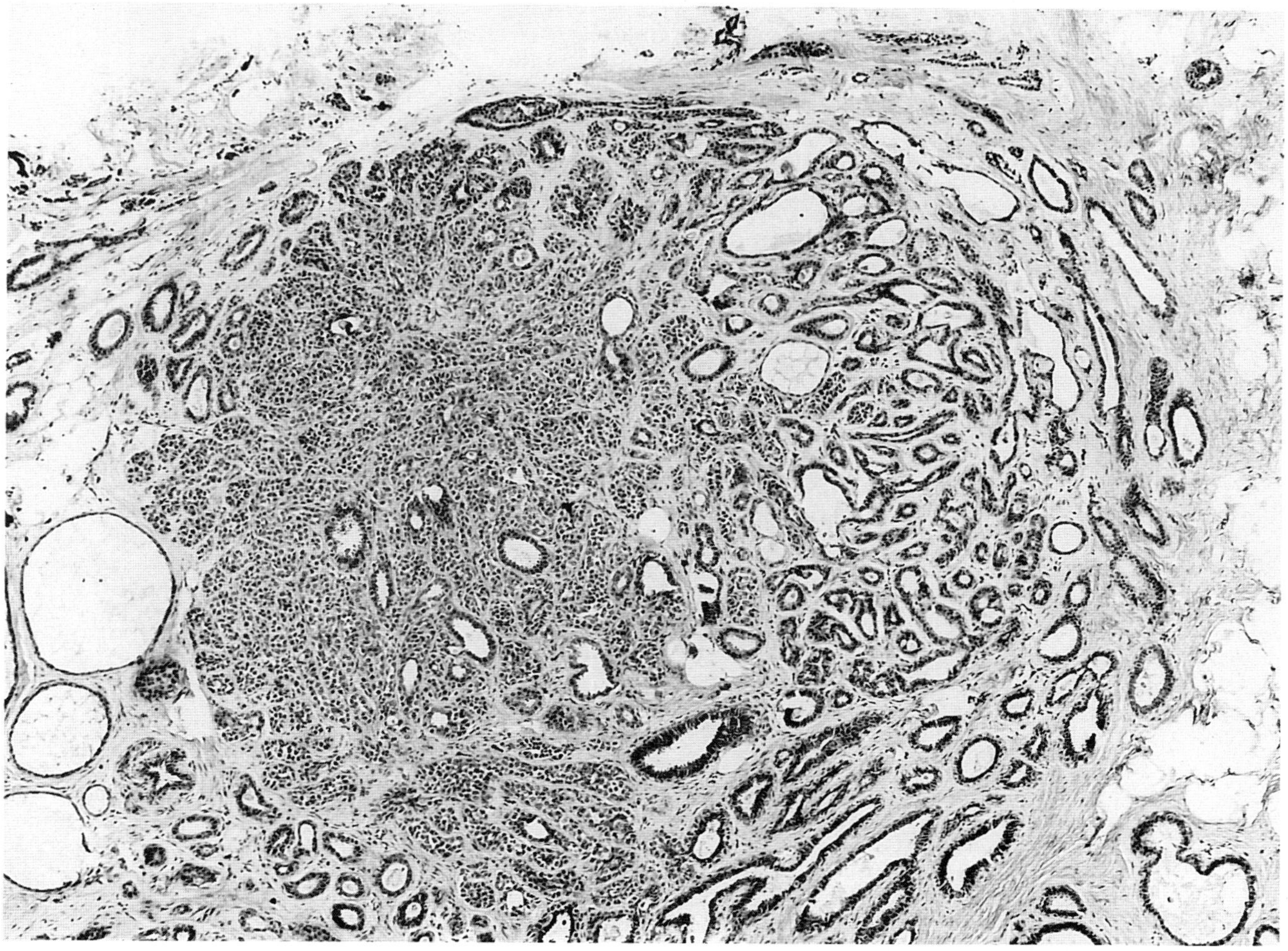

**Figure 8.15(a)** LN2 involving sclerosing adenosis (SA). The lobules on the left side of this area of SA are filled by a uniform cell population. (H&E, X100)

were identified in both infiltrating and in situ lobular carcinoma.

## LESIONS ASSOCIATED WITH LN

A variety of lesions are found in the biopsies associated with the incidental finding of LN. These include fibrocystic changes, adenosis, sclerosing adenosis, stromal fibrosis, fat necrosis, duct ectasia, hypertrophy, fibroadenoma, and cystosarcoma phyllodes (39,86). It would be of interest to determine the behavior of LN detected mammographically and unassociated with any other clinically palpable abnormalities.

## RESULTS OF LONG-TERM FOLLOW-UP AFTER DIAGNOSTIC BIOPSY ONLY

Comparison of the long-term follow-up results of different studies is difficult because of variations in the criteria used for the diagnosis of LCIS, as well as differences in the sampling and evaluation of the specimen. For example Andersen (2–4) and Wheeler et al (89) diagnosed LCIS even when only a single lobule showed the typical pattern of proliferation, whereas, Hutter and Foote (48) required involvement of at least two to three lobules for a diagnosis of LCIS. Haagensen et al's series (39) probably includes lesions that would qualify as ALH by the criteria utilized by a majority of other investigators. Rosen

B

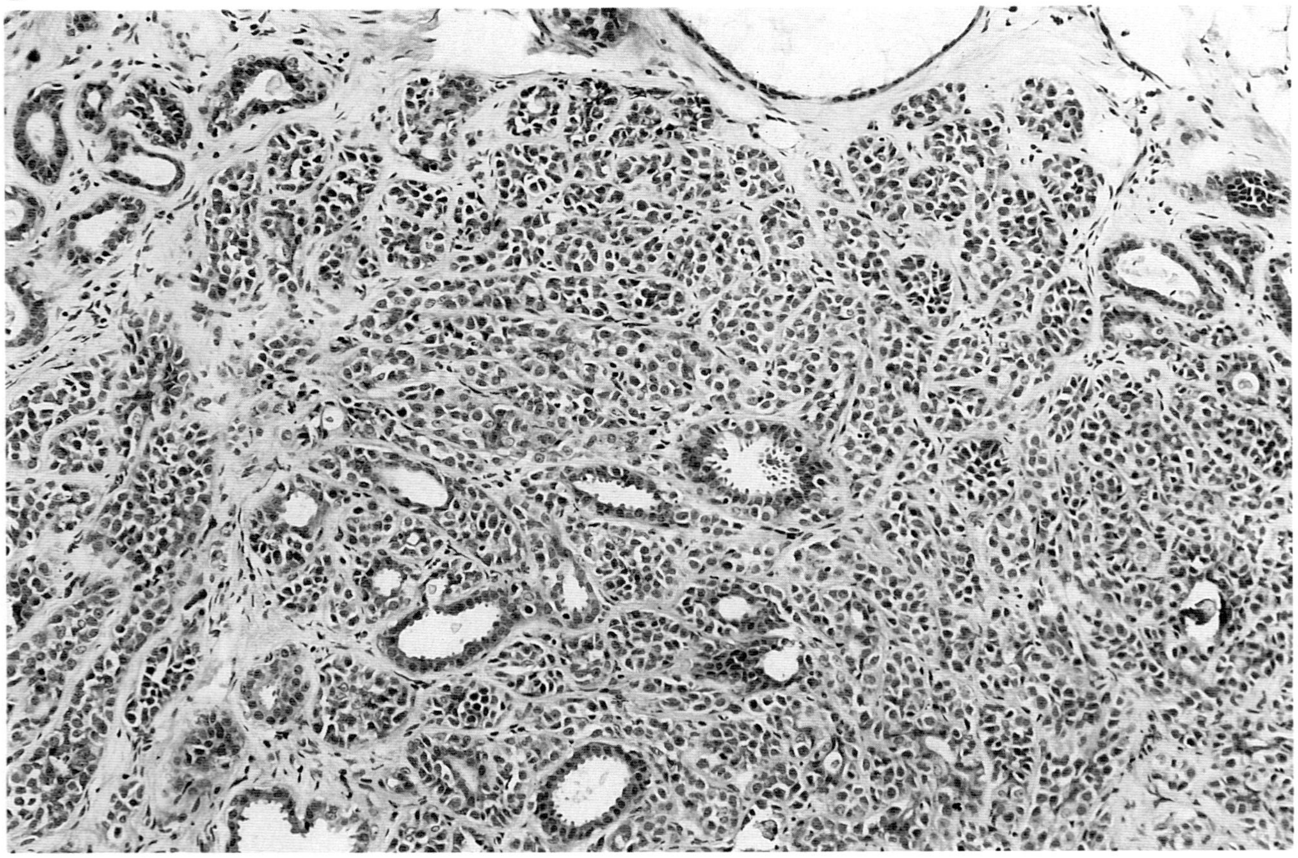

**Figure 8.15(b)** LN2 involving sclerosing adenosis (SA). At higher magnification, the solid occlusive growth of loosely cohesive cells confirms LN. Though the proliferation appears compact because of the background lesion, there is not much distension of each tubule. (H&E, X200)

(72) provided no firm criteria for separating the cases of ALH from LCIS. These studies have provided a large amount of information regarding the clinical significance of lobular neoplasia.

Women with ALH, as defined by Page et al (66), have a risk for subsequent development of invasive carcinoma that is 4 to 5.3 times that of the general population (25,64–66). Of 126 women with ALH in their study, 16 (13%) developed subsequent invasive carcinoma; they did so within an average of 11.9 years (66). Sixty-nine percent of the invasive carcinomas were in the ipsilateral breast (66).

Excluding Page et al's 1985 study (66) which specifically addresses ALH and subtracting patients with previous or current invasive breast carcinoma and those who had mastectomy within six months of the biopsy from the various published reports, from a total of 535 women in 11 separate studies (Table 8.2) on lesions diagnosed as either LCIS or LN, 130 (24.3%) eventually developed invasive carcinoma (2,3,15,35,39,42,49,69,72,73). Of these 535 women, 61 (13.3%) developed carcinoma in the ipsilateral breast, while 59 (11%) did so in the contralateral breast. Therefore, both breasts are at almost equal risk for the subsequent development of invasive carcinoma. Only 39 (7.3%) of the 535 women died of the subsequent invasive carcinoma. In all seven women who died of their subsequent invasive carcinoma in Haagensen et al's series (39), the LN had been missed on the original biopsy and they were not followed and examined systematically every four months. If these seven women are excluded, then 32 (5.9%) of the 535 women died from their invasive breast carcinomas. None of the patients who developed subsequent invasive carcinomas had axillary node metastases.

Andersen (2) calculated the risk for subsequent development of invasive carcinoma in patients with LCIS to be about 12 times that expected in comparable Danish women without LCIS. The calculated ratio of observed to expected carcinomas was 9:1 in Rosen et al's series (73) and Page et al's study (69), while in Haagensen et al's study (42), the ratio of observed to

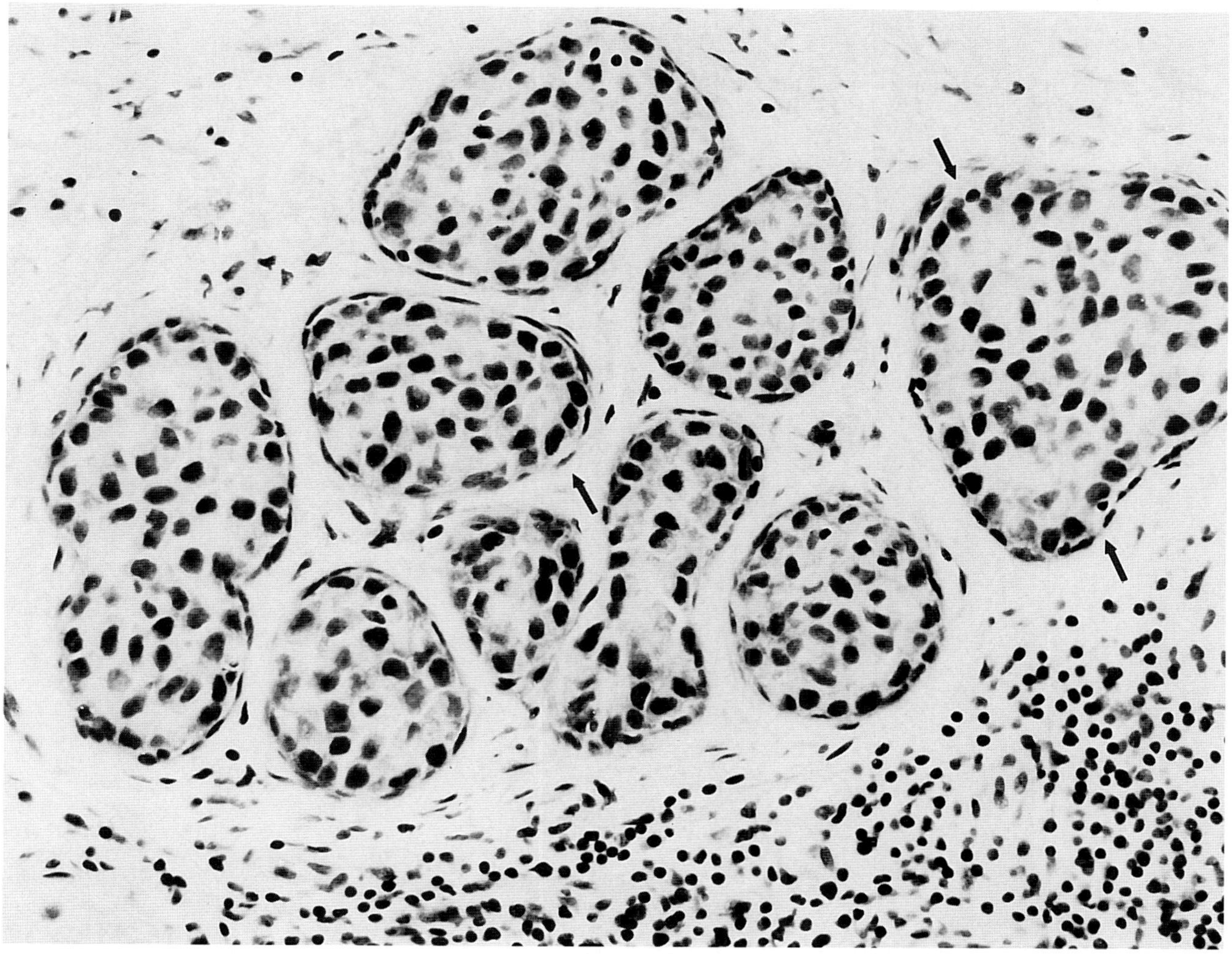

**Figure 8.16** AIDH in lobules. This ductal proliferation involving a lobule mimics LN1, but the presence of a rosette-like arrangement of the nuclei (arrows) discloses the ductal nature of the proliferation. Erroneous inclusion of such lesions among cases of LN (LCIS) may explain the high frequency of subsequent invasive ductal carcinomas in many previous studies on LN (LCIS). (H&E, X500)

expected carcinomas was 6.9:1. Haagensen's data are given for the study's time frame for developing subsequent carcinoma. Rosen et al found an increased "hazard rate" in later years.

Only a small proportion of the subsequent carcinomas develop within ten years of the diagnostic biopsy. Haagensen's data (39) indicates that the probability of the development of carcinoma in both breasts increases uniformly up to 25 years following treatment by biopsy alone. During the first ten years after a biopsy diagnosis of LCIS, only 17% of all subsequent invasive carcinomas in the ipsilateral breast, and about 20% of those intended to develop in the contralateral breast manifest themselves. In Page et al's series (69), the absolute risk of infiltrating breast carcinoma after LCIS was 17% at 15 years.

## INFLUENCE OF FAMILY HISTORY OF BREAST CARCINOMA

The presence of a family history of breast carcinoma in a sister, mother, or daughter of a patient with ALH doubles the risk from around 5.3 to 11 times that of women who have nonproliferating lesions without a family history of breast carcinoma (25,66). In effect, a woman with ALH and a family history of breast carcinoma has the same risk as one with intraductal carcinoma.

It is not well known if and how the presence of additional risk factors may alter the prognosis of patients with either a diagnosis of LN or LCIS. An increase in the risk has been noted by Haagensen et al

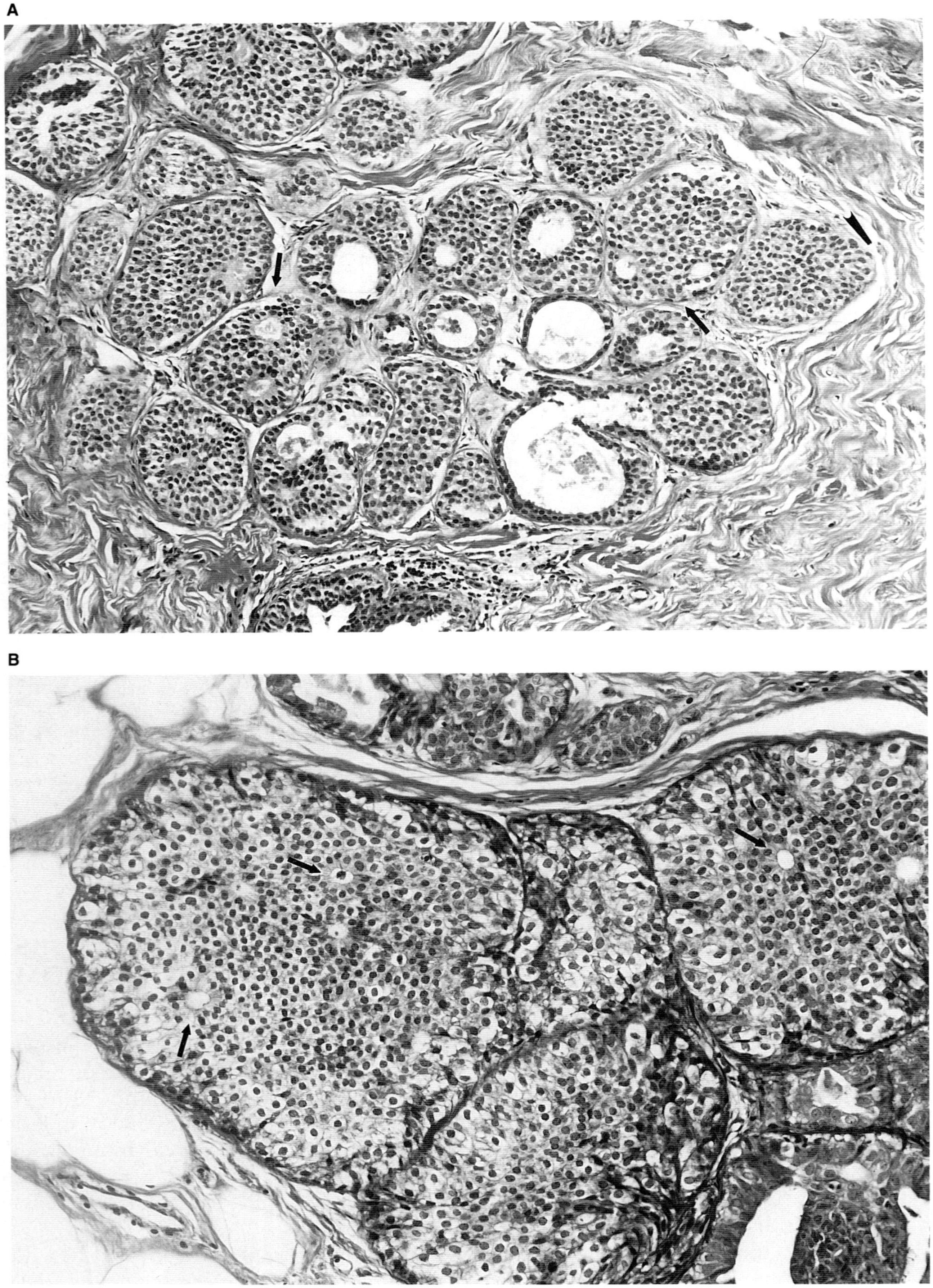

Figure 8.17 Atypical ductal hyperplasia within lobules. (a,b) Although the cells are uniform and small, the formation of rosette-like structures (arrows), indicates a ductal growth pattern. (H&E, (a) X100; (b) X200)

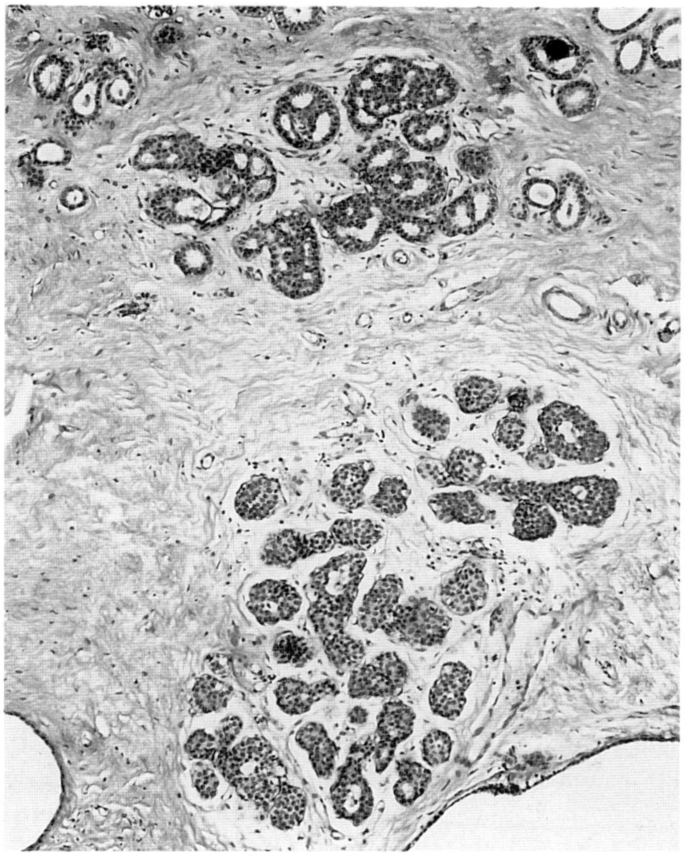

**Figure 8.18** Coexistence of LN and AIDH. Note adjacent lobules showing two different growth patterns. Elsewhere in the same biopsy, the patient had both LN2 and LCIS. (H&E, X200)

**Table 8.2** Number of Subsequent Carcinomas in Ipsilateral and Contralateral Breast in Women with LN/LCIS Treated by Biopsy Alone and No Previous or Concurrent Breast Carcinoma

| Reference | Number of Cases | Number of Subsequent Invasive CA in Ipsilateral Breast | Number of Subsequent Invasive CA in Contralateral Breast |
|---|---|---|---|
| Andersen (2–3) | 44 | 9 | 4 |
| Benfield (15) | 5 | 0 | 0 |
| Hutter (48) | 33 | 6 | 4 |
| Haagensen (41,42) | 263 | 27 | 24 |
| Herrman (46) | 5 | 0 | 0 |
| Giordano (35) | 19 | 2 | ? |
| Gaton (34) | 6 | 0 | 1 |
| Haefliger (43) | 13 | 3 | 2 |
| Page (69) | 39 | 5 (+1)* | 4 |
| Rosen (73) | 83 | 18 | 17 |
| Wheeler (90) | 25 | 1 | 3 |
| TOTAL | 535 | 71 | 59 |

* = One patient in this series developed subsequent invasive carcinomas in both breasts.

(41,42) in patients who have a family history of breast carcinoma and gross cystic disease in addition to lobular neoplasia; the ratio of observed to expected subsequent carcinomas rose from 7.2 for all women with LN but without a family history of breast carcinoma or gross cystic disease to 11.8 for those who also had a positive family history and gross cystic disease. In Rosen et al's study (73), 5 of 12 (42%) women with a family history of breast carcinoma subsequently developed invasive carcinoma, compared to 22 of 62 (36%) women without a positive family history. The difference between a positive and negative family history was not significant. Page et al (69) concluded that family history did not further affect the risk.

## LOCATION AND TYPE OF SUBSEQUENT INVASIVE CARCINOMAS

In patients who are treated by biopsy alone, the subsequent invasive carcinoma is of the small cell infiltrating (lobular) type in 43% of the patients (39). Haagensen categorized 90% of the subsequent invasive carcinomas detected through the course of close periodic follow-up in his series as well differentiated. Tulusan et al (83) observed that 46% of invasive carcinomas identified prior to, simultaneous with, or after a diagnosis of LCIS are of the invasive lobular, or the small cell type.

Rosen et al (75) tabulated the findings from three studies including their own whereby the mastectomy specimen performed for a biopsy diagnosis of LCIS were evaluated for the presence of residual LCIS and infiltrating carcinoma. They found that residual LCIS is present in 60% to 65% of the cases, and an invasive carcinoma is identified in 4% to 6% of the mastectomy specimen. The residual LCIS involved quadrants other than the biopsy site in 80% of the cases.

In Page et al's series (69), ten subsequent invasive carcinomas developed in nine patients. Seven of these were pure lobular or lobular variants, two were tubular, and one was ductal of no particular type.

As mentioned earlier, in the absence of other in situ or invasive lesions, LN has not been associated with axillary node metastases.

## MANAGEMENT OF PATIENTS WITH LOBULAR NEOPLASIA

The appropriate management of patients with lobular neoplasia (LN)/lobular carcinoma in situ (LCIS) has been an enigma, with divergent viewpoints expressed practically since the recognition of the lesion (3,9,16,35,38,39,47,81). Simple mastectomy was recommended by Foote and Stewart (31). This recommendation was followed by many as the treatment of choice (12,37,53). Some advised modified radical mastectomy (48,61). Because of the high incidence of bilaterality, Newman (60) suggested an ample biopsy of the contralateral breast which subsequently became common practice (15,49,61,84), while others went so far as to suggest bilateral mastectomy on prophylactic or therapeutic grounds (12,14,16). For many years mastectomy with or without contralateral breast biopsy (24,70–73) was the only treatment offered to patients with LN/LCIS. Fortunately, a few persistently questioned mastectomy as too radical and considered a more conservative approach of close observation after the biopsy (1,3,22,41,42,82, 90).

Wheeler et al (90) and Haagensen (42) were among the first to argue against mastectomy as the treatment for patients with LN/LCIS and actually proposed the alternative approach of life-long, periodic follow-up for patients whose biopsies showed lobular neoplasia.

Currently, there is general agreement that when either LN, LCIS or ALH occurs, the breasts should be regarded as a single organ. Therefore, since both breasts are at an almost equal risk for subsequent development of invasive carcinoma, there appear to be two alternative approaches to treatment: bilateral mastectomy or periodic follow-up for the remainder of the patient's life.

Based on the relatively young age of many patients with lobular neoplasia, the relatively long interval between detection of lobular disease and the development of a majority of subsequent invasive carcinomas, the low mortality from breast carcinoma within a ten-year follow-up (3) and our inability to predict which breast will manifest the subsequent invasive carcinoma, periodic follow-up seems more justifiable. The follow-up should include examination of both breasts by a physician four times a year. The follow-up regimen should also include annual mammography for patients over 40 years of age if the breast tissue density allows mammographic assessment.

When both LN and IDCA (non-necrotic variants) are present in a mammographically-directed biopsy, the issue becomes more complex. Haagensen et al (40) found that 92 (31%) of 282 carcinomas present in 237 women who had concurrent LN reflected a variety of intraductal carcinomas. Of these 92 patients, 32% had axillary node metastases; this is a high percentage considering the rarity of axillary node metastases associated with intraductal carcinoma alone, and the absence of any documented case of axillary node metastases associated with LN alone. In view of the current trend toward a more conservative approach to treatment, there is no good data available to help in the management of these patients.

It is important to ascertain that the patient and the physician are aware of the risks involved and the necessity of long-term follow-up over the remainder of the patient's life. The ideal approach would be to have a team composed of a mammographer, surgeon, pathologist and oncologist, preferably with an epidemiologist/statistician, to follow all these patients in a systematic manner.

Why some women develop subsequent invasive carcinoma, while others fail to do so, remains an unexplained aspect of this disease and an area that requires continued investigation.

## QUESTIONS RAISED BY THE CHANGING TRENDS IN TREATMENT OF BREAST CARCINOMA

Considering the recent recommendation of lumpectomy for invasive carcinomas that present as tumors less than 2 cm in size and with no evidence of lymph node metastases, one might question if the presence of concurrent LN in this group would in any way alter the prognosis or the management of the patient. There is very minimal amount of information available in the literature that might be of any help in this regard. Haagensen et al (40) compared the ratio of observed to expected carcinomas in the contralateral breast in three groups of women: 1) women with unilateral carcinoma and no prior LN treated by mastectomy; 2) patients with unilateral carcinoma and concurrent LN also treated by mastectomy; and

3) women with LN followed after biopsy who subsequently developed invasive carcinoma. The ratio of observed to expected carcinoma for the first group was 3 to 1; for the second group it was 8.3 to 1 and for the third group it was 9.4 to 1. Compared to all patients with carcinoma, the risk for a contralateral breast carcinoma was noted to be three times as high for postmenopausal and two times as high for premenopausal women with concurrent LN and carcinoma. Simultaneous breast carcinoma was five times more frequent in women who had concurrent LN and carcinoma compared to those with no prior lobular neoplasia. Ninety-one of the 282 carcinomas concurrent with LN were of the invasive small cell type; 45% of these cases had axillary node metastases. This was comparable to the 40.3% frequency of axillary node metastases found in women with cancer in general.

We also need to know how many and which varieties of lesions known to be risk factors and/or types of carcinomas (IDCA, ordinary infiltrating duct carcinoma, tubular carcinoma, colloid carcinoma, etc) are allowed to coexist in a biopsy before changing the treatment of a candidate for conservative management from lumpectomy to mastectomy.

## REFERENCES


1. Ackerman LV, Katzenstein AL: The concept of minimal breast cancer and the pathologist's role in the diagnosis of "early carcinoma." *Cancer* 1977;39(suppl):2755–2763.
* 2. Andersen JA: Lobular carcinoma in situ. A long-term follow-up in 52 cases. *Acta Pathol Microbiol Scand* (A) 1974;82: 519–533.
* 3. Andersen JA: Lobular carcinoma in situ of the breast. An approach to rational treatment. *Cancer* 1977;39:2597–2602.
* 4. Andersen JA: Lobular carcinoma in situ: A histologic study of 52 cases. *Acta Pathol Microbiol Scand* (A) 1974;82:735–741.
* 5. Andersen JA: Lobular carcinoma in situ of the breast with duct involvement: Frequency and possible influence on prognosis. *Acta Pathol Microbiol Scand* (A) 1974;82:655–662.
* 6. Andersen JA: Multicentric and bilateral appearance of lobular carcinoma in situ of the breast: A retrospective study. *Acta Pathol Microbiol Scand* (A) 1974;82:730–734.
7. Andersen JA: The basement membrane in lobular carcinoma in situ of the breast: A light microscopic study. *Acta Pathol Microbiol Scand* (A) 1975;83:245–250.
8. Andersen JA, Vendelboe ML: Cytoplasmic mucous globules in lobular carcinoma in situ. *Am J Surg Pathol* 1981;5:251–255.
9. Andersen JA, Fechner RE, Lattes R, et al: Lobular carcinoma in situ (lobular neoplasia) of the breast (a symposium). *Pathol Annu* 1980;21:193–223.
10. Ashikari R, Huvos AG, Snyder RE, et al: A clinicopathologic study of atypical lesions of the breast. *Cancer* 1974;33:310–317.
* 11. Azzopardi JG: *Problems in Breast Pathology*. Philadelphia, WB Saunders, 1979, pp 128–146; 192–233, 266–273.
12. Barnes JP: Bilateral lobular carcinoma in situ of the breast. *Texas State J Med* 1959;55:581–584.
13. Battifora H: Intracytoplasmic lumina in breast carcinoma. A helpful histopathologic feature. *Arch Pathol* 1975;99:614–617.
14. Benfield JR, Fingerhut AG, Warner NE: A multidisciplinary view of lobular breast carcinoma. *Am Surgeon* 1972;38:115–116.
15. Benfield JR, Jacobson M, Warner NE: In situ lobular carcinoma of the breast. *Arch Surg* 1965;91:130–135.
16. Benfield JR, Fingerhut AG, Warner NE: Lobular carcinoma of the breast—1969. A therapeutic proposal. *Arch Surg* 1969;99:129–131.
* 17. Broder AC: Carcinoma in situ contrasted with benign penetrating epithelium. *JAMA* 1932;99:1670–1674.
18. Bussolati G: Actin-rich (myoepithelial) cells in lobular carcinoma in situ of the breast. *Virchows Arch (Cell Pathol)* 1980;32:165–176.
19. Bussolati G, Botto-Micca F, Eusebi V, Betts CM: Myoepithelial cells in lobular carcinoma in situ of the breast: A parallel immunocytochemical and ultrastructural study. *Ultrastructural Pathol* 1981;2:219–230.
20. Carter D, Yardley JH, Shelley WM: Lobular carcinoma of the breast. An ultrastructural comparison with certain duct carcinomas and benign lesions. *Johns Hopkins Med J* 1969;125: 25–43.
* 21. Cornil V: *Les Tumeurs du Sein*. Paris, Librairie Germer Bailliere and Co, 1908.
22. Dall'Olmo CA, Ponka JL, Horn RC Jr, et al: Lobular carcinoma of the breast in situ. Are we too radical in its treatment? *Arch Surg* 1975;110:537–542.
23. Dawson EK: Carcinoma in the mammary lobule and its origin. *Edinb Med J* 1933;40:57–82.
24. Donegan WL, Perez-Mesa CM: Lobular carcinoma: An indication for elective biopsy of the second breast. *Ann Surg* 1972;176:178–187.
25. Dupont WD, Page DL: Risk factors for breast cancer in women with proliferative breast disease. *N Engl J Med* 1985;312:146–151.
26. Eusebi V, Pich A, Macchiorlatti E, et al: Morpho-functional differentiation in lobular carcinoma of the breast. *Histopathology* 1977;1:307–314.
27. Ewing J: *Neoplastic Diseases*, ed 1. Philadelphia, WB Saunders, 1919, pp 473–475.
28. Fechner RE: Ductal carcinoma involving the lobule of the breast: A source of confusion with lobular carcinoma in situ. *Cancer* 1971;28:274–281.
29. Fechner RE: Epithelial alterations in the extralobular ducts of breasts with lobular carcinoma. *Arch Pathol* 1972;93:164–171.

30. Fechner RE: Lobular carcinoma in situ in sclerosing adenosis. A potential source of confusion with invasive carcinoma. *Am J Surg Pathol* 1981;5:233–239.

31. Foote FW, Stewart FW: Lobular carcinoma in situ: A rare form of mammary cancer. *Am J Pathol* 1941;17:491–495.

32. Fisher ER, Fisher B: Lobular carcinoma of the breast: An overview. *Ann Surg* 1977;85:377–385.

33. Gad A, Azzopardi JG: Lobular carcinoma of the breast: A special variant of mucin-secreting carcinoma. *J Clin Path* 1975;28:711–716.

34. Gaton E, Czernobilsky B: Lobular carcinoma in situ of the breast. A retrospective study from a general hospital in Israel. *Isr J Med Sci* 1974;10:1106–1111.

35. Giordano JM, Klopp CT: Lobular carcinoma in situ: Incidence and treatment. *Cancer* 1973;31:105–109.

36. Giri DD, Dundas SAC; Nottingham JF, et al: Oestrogen receptors in benign epithelial lesions and intraduct carcinomas of the breast: An immunohistochemical study. *Histopathology* 1989;15:575–584.

37. Godwin JT: Chronology of lobular carcinoma in the breast. Report of a case. *Cancer* 1952;5:259–266.

38. Gump FE: Lobular carcinoma in situ. Pathology and treatment. Breast Cancer: Strategies for 1990's. *Surg Clin N Am* 1990;70:873–883.

*39. Haagensen CD: *Diseases of the Breast*, ed 3. Philadelphia, WB Saunders, 1986, pp 192–249.

40. Haagensen CD, Lane N, Bodian C: Coexisting lobular neoplasia and carcinoma of the breast. *Cancer* 1983;51:1468–1482.

*41. Haagensen CD, Lane N, Lattes R: Neoplastic proliferation of the epithelium of the mammary lobules: Adenosis, lobular neoplasia, and small cell carcinoma. *Surg Clin North Am* 1972;52:497–524.

*42. Haagensen CD, Lane N, Lattes R, et al: Lobular neoplasia (so-called lobular carcinoma in situ) of the breast. *Cancer* 42:737–769, 1978.

43. Haefliger J-M: Etude catamnestique de 18 cas de carcinome lobulaire de la glande mammaire. *Schweiz Med Wochenschr* 1974;104:229–234.

44. Hamperl H: Das lobulare carcinoma in situ der Mamma. *Deutsche Medizinische Wocheschrift* 1971;96:1585–1588.

45. Hamperl H: Zur Kenntnis des sog. Carcinoma lobulare in situ der Mamma. *Z Krebsforsch* 1972;77:231–246.

46. Hermann JB: Treatment of in situ mammary carcinoma. *Int Surg* 1972;57:127–129.

*47. Hutter RVP: The management of patients with lobular carcinoma in situ of the breast. *Cancer* 1984;53:798–802.

*48. Hutter RVP, Foote FW: Lobular carcinoma in situ: Long-term follow-up. *Cancer* 1969;24:1081–1085.

*49. Hutter RVP, Foote FW Jr, Farrow JW: In situ lobular carcinoma of the female breast 1939–1968, in: *Breast Cancer—Early and Late*. Chicago, Year Book, 1968, pp 201–226.

50. Kahn L, Webber B: Lobular carcinoma of the breast: A review. *South Afr J Surg* 1974;12:51–55.

51. Lambird PA, Shelley WM: The spatial distribution of lobular in situ mammary carcinoma. Implications for size and site of breast biopsy. *JAMA* 1969;210:689–693.

52. Lattes R: Lobular neoplasia (lobular carcinoma in situ) of the breast: A histological entity of controversial clinical significance (review article). *Path Res Prat* 1980;166:415–429.

53. Lewison EF, Finney GG Jr: Lobular carcinoma in situ of the breast. *Surg Gynec Obstet* 1968;126:1280–1286.

*54. McDivitt RW, Hutter RVP, Foote FW Jr, et al: In situ lobular carcinoma: A prospective follow-up study indicating cumulative patient risks. *JAMA* 1967;201:82–86.

*55. Muir R: The evolution of carcinoma of the mamma. *J Pathol Bacteriol* 1941;52:155–172.

56. Murad TM: A proposed histochemical and electron microscopic classification of human breast cancer according to cell of origin. *Cancer* 1971;27:288–299.

57. Murad TM: Ultrastructure of ductular carcinoma of the breast (in situ and infiltrating lobular carcinoma). *Cancer* 1971;27:18–28.

58. Nazari T, Benitez L, Robbins S, et al: In situ lobular cancer of the breast. *Int J Surg* 1967;47:140–143.

59. Nesland JM, Holm R, Johannessen JV: Ultrastructural and immunohistochemical features of lobular carcinoma of the breast. *J Pathol* 1985;145:39–52.

60. Newman W: In situ lobular carcinoma of the breast. Report of 26 women with 32 cancers. *Ann Surg* 1963;157: 591–599.

61. Newman W: Lobular carcinoma of the breast. Report of 73 cases. *Ann Surg* 1966;164:305–314.

62. Nielsen M, Jensen J, Andersen J: Precancerous and cancerous breast lesions during lifetime and autopsy. A study of 83 women. *Cancer* 1984;54:612–615.

63. Ozzello L: Ultrastructure of intra-epithelial carcinomas of the breast. *Cancer* 1971;25:1508–1515.

64. Page DL: Cancer risk assessment in benign breast biopsies. *Hum Pathol* 1986;17:871–874.

65. Page DL, Dupont WD: Anatomic markers of human premalignancy and risk of breast cancer. *Cancer* 1990;66: 1326–1335.

*66. Page DL, Dupont WD, Rogers LW, et al: Atypical hyperplastic lesions of the female breast: A long-term follow-up study. *Cancer* 1985;55:2698–2708.

*67. Page DL, Anderson TJ, Rogers LW: Epithelial hyperplasia, in: Page DL, Anderson TJ (eds): *Diagnostic Histopathology of the Breast*. Edinburgh, Churchill Livingstone, 1988, pp 145–156; 174–184.

68. Page DL, Dupont WD, Rogers LW: Ductal involvement by cells of atypical lobular hyperplasia in the breast: A long-term follow-up study of the cancer risk. *Hum Pathol* 1988;19: 201–207.

69. Page DL, Kidd TE, Dupont WD, et al: Lobular neoplasia of the breast: Higher risk for subsequent invasive cancer predicted by more extensive disease. *Hum Pathol* 1991;22:1232–1239.

*70. Rosen PP: Coexistent lobular carcinoma in situ and intraductal carcinoma in a single lobular-duct unit. *Am J Surg Pathol* 1980;4:241–246.

71. Rosen PP: Lobular carcinoma in situ: Recent clinicopathologic studies at Memorial Hospital. *Path Res Pract* 1980;166: 430–455.

*72. Rosen PP, Braun DW, Lyngholm B, et al: Lobular carcinoma in situ of the breast: Preliminary results of treatment by ipsilateral mastectomy and contralateral breast biopsy. *Cancer* 1981;47:813–819.

*73. Rosen PP, Lieberman PH, Braun DW Jr, et al: Lobular carcinoma in situ of the breast: Detailed analysis of 99 patients with average follow-up of 24 years. *Am J Surg Pathol* 1978;2:225–251.

74. Rosen PP, Seni RT, Farr GH, et al: Epidemiology of breast carcinoma: Age, menstrual status, and exogenous hormone usage in patients with lobular carcinoma in situ. *Surgery* 1979;85:219–224.

*75. Rosen PP, Senie R, Schottenfeld D, et al: Noninvasive breast carcinoma. Frequency of unsuspected invasion and implications for treatment. *Ann Surg* 1979;189:377–382.

76. Rosner D, Bedwani RN, Vana J, et al: Noninvasive breast carcinoma. Results of a national survey by the American College of Surgeons. *Ann Surg* 1980;192:139–147.

77. Rubin E, Alexander RW, Visscher DW, et al: Proliferative disease and atypia in biopsies performed for mammographically detected nonpalpable lesions. *Cancer* 1988;61:2077–2082.

78. Salhany KE, Page DL: Fine-needle aspiration of mammary lobular carcinoma in situ and atypical lobular hyperplasia. *Am J Clin Pathol* 1989;92:22–26.

79. Snyder RE: Mammography and lobular carcinoma in situ. *Surg Gynecol Obstet* 1966;122:255–260.

80. Tamura H: In situ and infiltrating lobular carcinoma of breast: Presence of lobular carcinoma in situ indicates careful observation of contralateral breast. *Rhode Island Med J* 1967;50:545–548.

81. Tobon H, Price HM: Lobular carcinoma in situ. *Cancer* 1972;30:1082–1091.

82. Toker C, Goldberg JD: The small cell lesion of mammary ducts and lobules. *Pathol Annu* 1971;12(1):217–249.

83. Tulusan AH, Egger H, Ober KG: Lobular carcinoma in situ and its relation to invasive breast cancer, in Zander J, Baltzer J (eds): *Early Breast Cancer. Histopathology, Diagnosis, and Treatment*. New York, Springer-Verlag, 1985, pp 48–51.

*84. Urban JA: Bilaterality of cancer of the breast: Biopsy of the opposite breast. *Cancer* 1967;20:1867–1870.

85. Urban JA: Biopsy of the "normal" breast in treating breast cancer. *Surg Clin N Amer* 1969;49:2291–2301.

86. Warner N: Lobular carcinoma of the breast. *Cancer* 1969;23: 840–846.

87. Wellings SR, Jensen HM, Marcum RG: An atlas of subgross pathology of the human breast with special reference to possible precancerous lesions. *J Natl Cancer Inst* 1975;55:231–273.

88. Wellings SR, Roberts P: Electron microscopy of sclerosing adenosis and infiltrating duct carcinoma of the human mammary gland. *J Nat Cancer Inst* 1963;30:269–287.

*89. Wheeler JE, Enterline HT: Lobular carcinoma of the breast, in situ and infiltrating. *Pathol Annu* 1976;11(2):161–188.

*90. Wheeler JE, Enterline HT, Roseman JM, et al: Lobular carcinoma in situ of the breast. Long-term follow-up. *Cancer* 1974;34:554–563.

# 9

# Infiltrating Carcinomas, Common and Familiar Special Types



This chapter will cover the common and major categories along with some of the more recognized special variants of invasive carcinoma. With due respect to our conventional approach, the division of breast carcinomas into ductal and lobular types on the basis of their presumed origin in ducts versus lobules is no longer a tenable concept since it has been well established that a majority of carcinomas originate in the terminal duct-lobular unit. It is also well known that about 50% of carcinomas developing following a diagnosis of lobular neoplasia are ductal in type. Furthermore, the so-called classic "Indian file" growth pattern of invasive carcinomas also occurs in association with and following classic examples of intraductal carcinoma. Based on these observations, it appears that once carcinoma cells invade they may assume any of the recognized patterns of invasion regardless of the pattern of the in situ phase. This would explain why almost 50% of subsequent infiltrating carcinomas observed following a diagnosis of lobular neoplasia display patterns recognized as ductal types. While certain invasive patterns are commonly associated with a given in situ pattern, there are enough deviations from these associations that the interpretation of the invasive tumor should be based only on its own morphologic pattern. Since one of the most distinctive characteristics of the in situ ductal carcinoma is the formation of secondary lumens and epithelial bridges in contrast to the solid growth pattern typical of lobular neoplasia, any infiltrating carcinoma that forms gland-like lumens and tubules in an attempt to form a duct-like structure should be designated as a variant of ductal carcinoma.

While a large proportion of invasive carcinomas reflect a pure subtype, combined patterns within a lesion, or two distinct patterns of infiltrating carcinoma within different regions of the breast occur in a substantial group of tumors (15). Though there are exceptions, as a rule, a carcinoma is designated according to the pattern dominating in 90% or more of the tumor. If the proportion of the minor component is larger, particularly when the minor component is a more aggressive variant, the diagnosis should always reflect its presence. According to Azzopardi (3), in about 3% to 4% of the cases, it is

**Table 9.1** Percent Distribution of Major Histologic Subtypes of Invasive Carcinoma in Different Populations

| | United States | | Denmark | Sweden | | Edinburgh | Japan |
|---|---|---|---|---|---|---|---|
| Type | Rosen (54) | Fisher (15) | Carstens (185) | Linnel (200) | Wallgren (74) | Page (51) | Sakamoto (61–63) |
| Ductal | 78.5 | 53 (NOS) | 74.4* | 56.2 | 64 (NST) | 70 (NST) | 47% (Common scirrhous) |
| Lobular | 8.8 | 5 | 8.9 | 12.9 | 14 | 10 (7% variants) | 2 |
| Tubular | 1.0 | 1 | 6.5 | 21 | 7 | 3 | |
| Colloid | 2.6 | 2 | 2.4 | 4.2 | | 2 | 4 |
| Medullary | 4.3 | 6 | 3.9 | 5.6 | 6 | 5 (3% variants) | 2 |
| Comedo | 4.6 | | 1.8 | | | 9% Cribriform or papillary | |
| | | 4 (papillary) | | | | 4 Cribriform | 22 Pappillotubular |
| | | 28 (combined) | | | | 2 Combined | 20 solid-tubular |

Abbreviations: NOS = not otherwise specified; NST = no special type; * After exclusion of pure tubular carcinoma.
From Fisher et al (15), Page et al (51), Rosen (54), Sakamoto (61–62), Sakamoto et al (63), Wallgren (74), Carstens et al (185), Linell and Ljungberg (200).

impossible to determine whether an invasive carcinoma is ductal or lobular in type; he has suggested that these should be designated as invasive carcinoma of uncertain type. My personal preference is to designate any invasive carcinoma that displays formation of one or more tubules or lumens (gland-like structures), as well as those composed of atypical cells displaying irregularly shaped, angulated, small or large clusters of generally cohesive cell clusters, as a ductal type of carcinoma regardless of the cell size unless it displays features of any one of the special types of carcinoma. Furthermore, any invasive carcinoma forming "Indian files" and composed of a uniform small cell population or larger cells containing intracytoplasmic lumens should be designated as infiltrating lobular carcinoma. Other types of invasive carcinoma can also form "Indian files," but generally not as an exclusive pattern throughout the lesion. Round, loosely-cohesive cells forming solid nests and islands, generally without significant intervening stroma, are also accepted as variants of infiltrating lobular carcinoma. If these basic rules are applied, the number of unclassifiable cases would be substantially reduced.

The classification used here is a modification of the WHO classification (78) which is based on that proposed by Foote and Stewart (17). As is evident in Table 9.1, there is no universally accepted terminology and classification. The classification that deviates most in its terminology and subdivision of the common types of infiltrating carcinoma from that used elsewhere throughout the world is the Japanese system (61–63). Not only is there a difference between the classification systems used in Japan and the United States, there are also differences in the frequencies of various types of carcinomas observed among Japanese and American women. The Japanese women have a higher frequency of colloid and medullary carcinomas, they have a higher proportion of circumscribed tumors, and their tumors are associated with more intense lymphoid infiltrate in and around the carcinoma (55). Infiltrating lobular carcinoma, however, is less common among Japanese women. American women show a higher frequency of intralymphatic tumor emboli. Joint studies by major American and Japanese cancer institutions have provided interesting data regarding these international variations. Because of the differences in the terminology, criteria, classification of the common carcinomas, and the diversity of the populations from an epidemiologic standpoint, however, it is difficult to compare results of studies published from different countries. These variations are partially reflected in the designations and percentages of different types of carcinoma in several countries (Table 9.1).

## INFILTRATING DUCT CARCINOMA

Infiltrating duct carcinoma accounts for the largest single category of mammary carcinomas (54). Also referred to as infiltrating carcinoma, not otherwise specified (NOS) (3,4), or infiltrating carcinoma of no special type (NST) (51), the diagnosis of this tumor is made on the basis of exclusion—a lesion that cannot be classified as any special type of breast carcinoma (78).

Infiltrating duct carcinoma accounts for 47% to 75% of all invasive breast carcinomas (15,18,51,54,61–63,74). The frequency varies in different countries depending on the diagnostic criteria used. The largest percentages are from the United States, while the lowest one is from Japan (Table 9.1). The diagnosis of infiltrating duct carcinoma is based on the growth pattern of the tumor regardless of the type, and the presence or absence of any associated intraductal carcinoma (3).

Though the possibility of myoepithelial origin was raised at one time (48), the epithelial origin of infiltrating duct carcinoma is now firmly established.

Women with infiltrating duct carcinoma are generally in the mid to late 50s. They present either with a mass detected by palpation or mammography. The tumor is generally about 2 to 3 cm in size on palpation, but may be massive and occupy a significant portion of the breast. Skin fixation, edema, "peau d'orange," nipple retraction and/or discharge, Paget's disease, and even ulceration of large tumors was seen more often prior to the 1980s. With the trend toward earlier detection of lesions, many of these changes, which basically reflect advanced disease, are now encountered less frequently in the United States.

Among the many varieties of infiltrating carcinoma, women with infiltrating duct pattern have a worse overall prognosis (16,60).

## Macroscopic Features

Infiltrating duct carcinoma appears either well circumscribed, stellate, or shows a combination of invasive and pushing margins. The stellate variant is associated with extensive fibrosis and is also referred to by the alternate designation of "scirrhous carcinoma," or "stellate carcinoma" (21). McDivitt et al (45) designated these as infiltrating ductal carcinoma with productive fibrosis in 1968. The stellate cancers have a central mass and radiate into the surrounding breast tissue. They often display yellowish, chalky streaks. The circumscribed or nodular tumor is well-delineated, rounded and lobulated. The stellate tumor is more common than the circumscribed variety, accounting for two thirds of the lesions. Necrosis is not uncommon in infiltrating carcinomas and is manifested as soft, chalky white areas. The hard gray to white areas correspond to a desmoplastic stromal response; these areas are the basis for the term "scirrhous" derived from the Greek word *skirhoss*, meaning hard. The yellow to white streaks often reflect elastosis. Cystic change is rare in either variety.

The size of the tumor is highly variable ranging from a few millimeters to more than 14 cm. Assessment of the size of the tumor is an important prognostic parameter. Ideally, the size should be expressed in three dimensions. Practically, however, the irregular shape of the tumor and the fragmentation of the tumor prior to its arrival to the surgical pathology laboratory may allow only an expression of the maximum dimensions of a specimen bisected to expose the largest flat cross section of the tumor. It is encouraging that this significant parameter is being recorded more frequently now compared to 20 years ago. In a review of 100 consecutive surgical pathology reports contributed by 100 different pathologists to AFIP in 1978, the maximum tumor diameter was expressed in centimeters or millimeters in 45% of the cases; an additional 12% provided a rather vague measurement. In 1990, a similar review yielded this information in approximately 86% of the reports. Although there is an obvious improvement in the recording of this important feature, this crucial prognostic information should be provided in 100% of cases.

## Microscopic Features

Microscopically, infiltrating duct carcinoma (NOS) is characterized by either a pushing or infiltrating margin (Fig. 9.1) and the presence of irregular or rounded, solid clusters of tumor admixed with single cells and cords of tumor cells lacking the morphologic features of any of the special types of invasive carcinoma. Poorly-formed tubules and glandular lumens may be evident. The appearance of these tumors is highly variable depending on the degree of cellularity, extent of stromal reaction and alterations, presence or absence of necrosis, as well as the presence and amount of inflammatory cell infiltrate. A dense lymphoplasmacytic infiltrate occurs in about 20% of infiltrating ductal carcinomas (15,59); the lymphocytic infiltrate is composed predominantly of T-lymphocytes of the cytotoxic-suppressor phenotype (23).

Based on the degree of tubule formation, nuclear appearance, and mitotic activity, the tumor should be graded (Figs. 9.2–9.3) for prognostic purposes (See grading in Chapter 2, General Considerations). Some

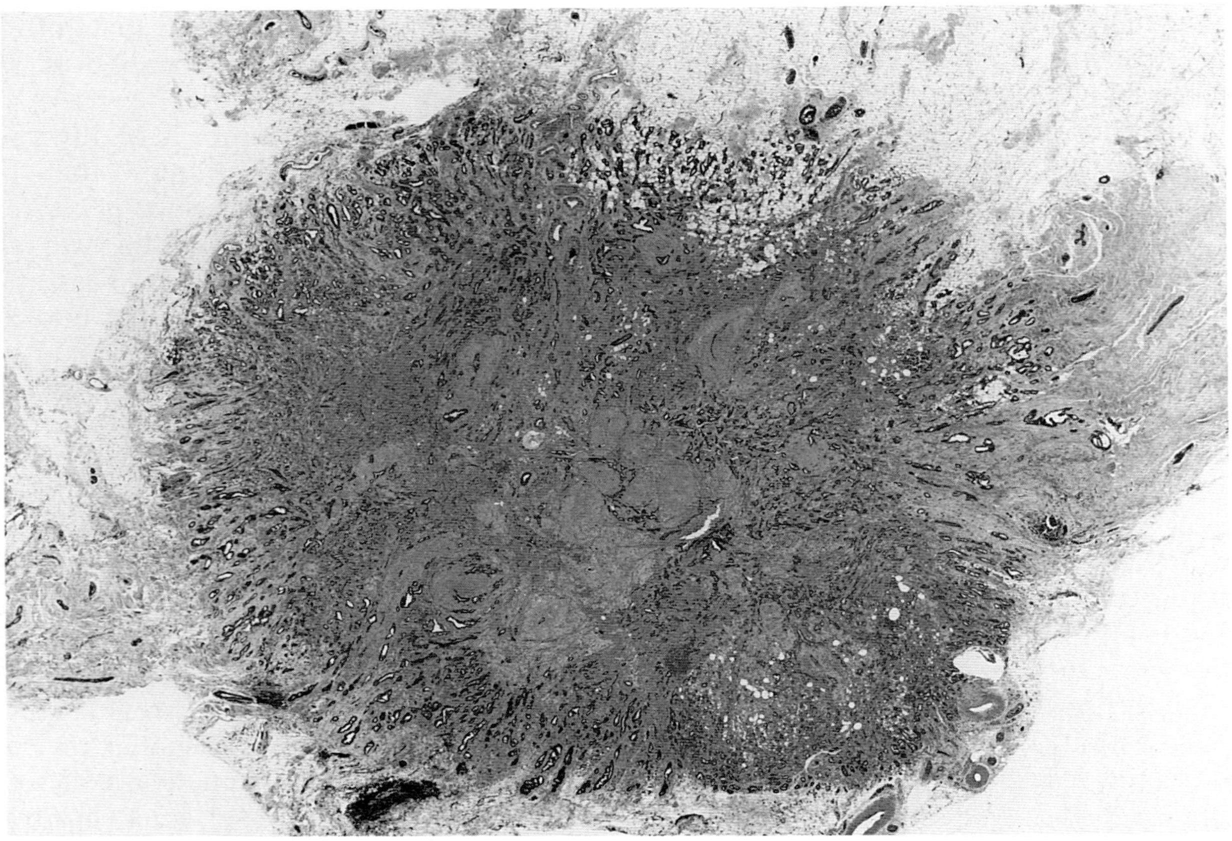

**Figure 9.1** Infiltrating duct carcinoma displaying a well-defined, but infiltrating margin and central, patchy elastosis. (H&E, X20)

poorly-differentiated carcinoma cells display phagocytic activity engulfing red and white blood cells as well as other tumor cells (Fig. 9.4). The stroma may be fibroblastic, collagenous, or elastotic (1). Occasionally, a granulomatous reaction is observed around the tumor or in the axillary nodes in association with infiltrating carcinomas (25,50,69).

In a majority of well-sampled cases, an in situ ductal carcinoma will be present. On the other hand, an in situ carcinoma is not identified despite exhaustive sampling in approximately 20% of the lesions (3). In some tumors, both ductal and lobular types of in situ carcinoma may be present. In a small proportion of cases, an invasive ductal carcinoma may be accompanied by an in situ lobular carcinoma in the absence of an apparent ductal in situ carcinoma.

## Infiltrating Duct Carcinoma with Extensive In Situ Component

The amount of the intraductal carcinoma (IDCA) associated with infiltrating duct carcinoma is highly variable, and the assessment of its extent or proportion is highly subjective. In approximately 72% of 972 carcinomas in one study, there was little or no IDCA, while 66% or more of the tumor was composed of IDCA in 11% of the tumors (15); the presence of abundant IDCA within the tumor was associated with a tendency to also have IDCA beyond the tumor margin and multicentric carcinoma. A better prognosis and a decreased frequency of nodal metastases has been noted for invasive tumors associated with a prominent intraductal carcinoma component (42,68). More recently, infiltrating duct carcinoma with extensive in situ component has been defined as an invasive tumor in which 25% of the overall area involved by the invasive carcinoma is composed of IDCA, and there is also IDCA beyond an imaginary line drawn around the area of invasive carcinoma (65). Identification of this extensive IDCA component seems to be important prognostically and assists the clinicians in determining the optimal therapeutic option for the patient. This finding generally contraindicates a conservative approach (lumpectomy with radiation therapy), because of its asso-

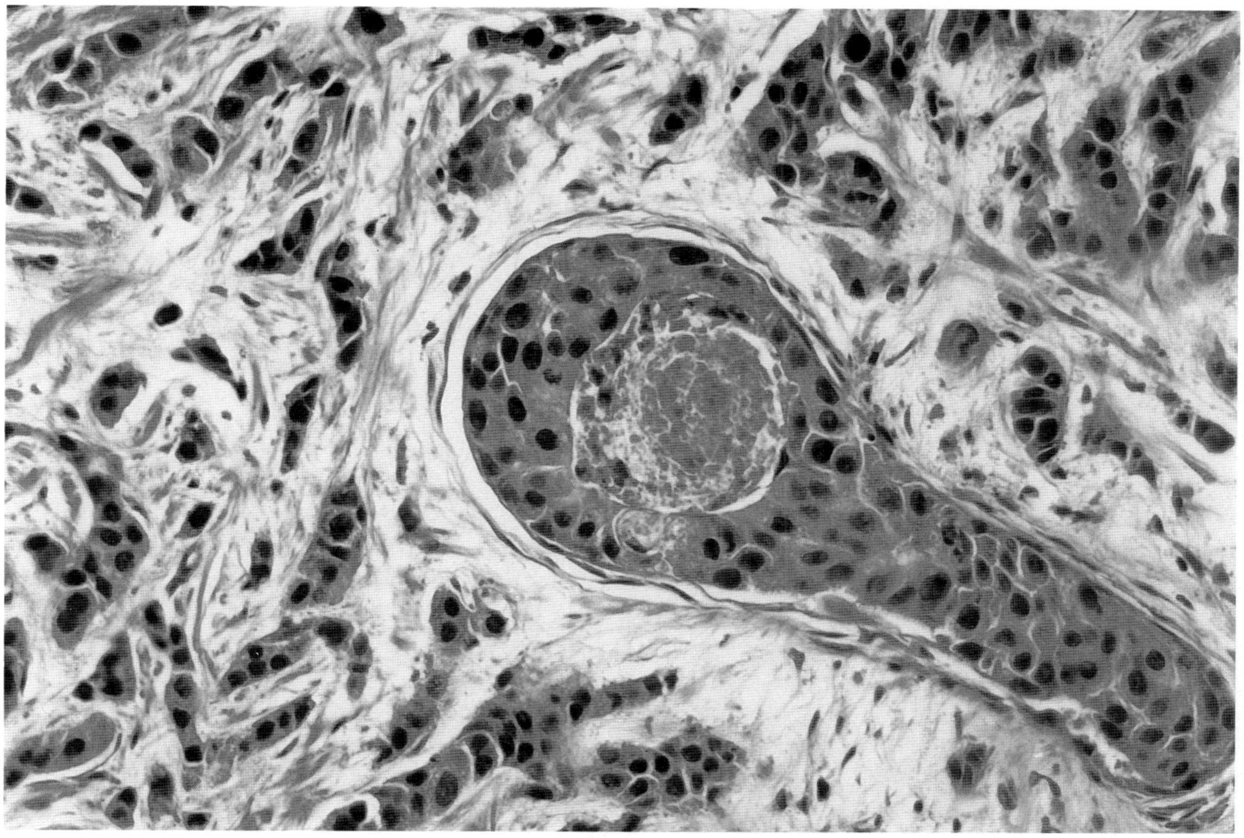

**Figure 9.2** Infiltrating duct carcinoma, moderately differentiated. The total grading score is 7 (tubule formation 3, mitotic figures 2, nuclei 2), qualifying the lesion as a moderately-differentiated carcinoma. (H&E, X420).

ciation with a higher rate of local recurrence and treatment failure (65).

## Minimal, Occult, and Early Breast Cancer

The term "minimal breast cancer" introduced and subsequently elaborated upon by Gallager and Martin (19–21), refers to a heterogeneous group of noninvasive carcinomas of either ductal or lobular type, as well as invasive carcinoma having a volume not greater than that of a sphere 0.5 cm in diameter (0.065 cm 3). The term "minimal carcinoma" was intended to reflect a stage in the progression between atypical hyperplasia and invasive carcinoma. Subsequently, McDivitt proposed that the term minimal breast carcinoma be restricted to infiltrating carcinomas less than 1.0 cm in diameter (45), while Hutter (32) expanded the concept to include the low grade variants of breast carcinoma which he enumerated as medullary, colloid, and tubular carcinoma regardless of their size, as well as unusual carcinomas such as those presenting in the axillary tail, arising in a fibroadenoma, and the noninfiltrating Paget's disease of the nipple. Shortly thereafter, this list was further expanded to include adenoid cystic and intracystic papillary carcinomas, as well as some cases of cystosarcoma phyllodes (76). Finally, as a result of a survey by the American College of Surgeons in 1981 (6), all invasive carcinomas less than or equal to 1 cm in diameter, lobular carcinoma in situ, and intraductal carcinomas were included in the definition of minimal breast carcinoma (8,30). Obviously, the term "minimal" has been used to refer to a highly heterogeneous group of neoplasms.

Minimal breast carcinoma should be distinguished from "occult" breast cancer; the latter refers to a nonpalpable, asymptomatic, and to some (67), not even mammographically demonstrable cancer. Minimal breast carcinoma would qualify as a subset of "early" breast carcinoma which encompasses all carcinomas confined to the breast, or a carcinoma of any size, but without axillary node metastases (33). Since the recent consensus recommendation that women with stage I and II breast

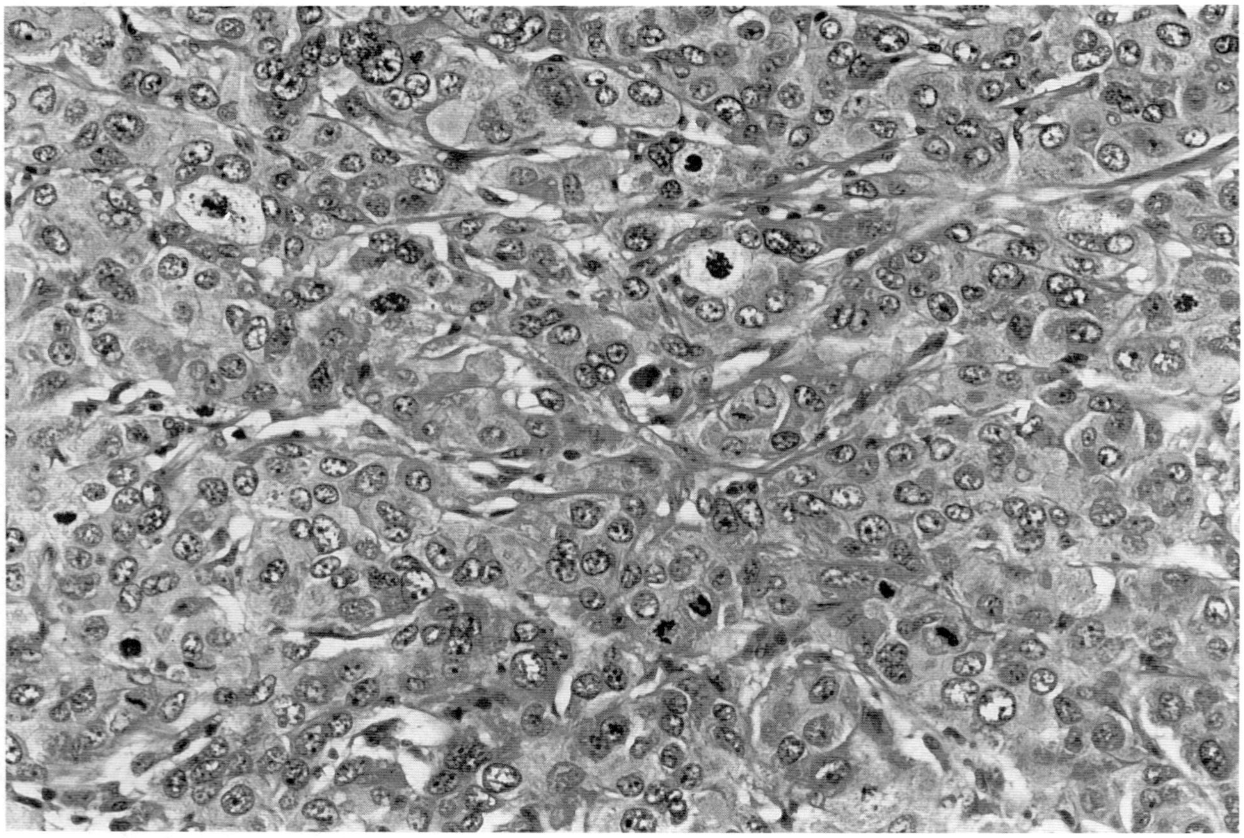

**Figure 9.3** Infiltrating duct carcinoma, poorly-differentiated. The total grading score is 8 (tubule formation 3, mitotic figure 3, nuclei 2), qualifying the lesion as a poorly-differentiated carcinoma. (H&E, X400)

carcinomas can be treated conservatively, and the availability of TNM classification which allows for various tumor sizes, there seems to be no point and justification in using the term "minimal" carcinoma, which has been so variably, vaguely, and broadly defined.

Survival and recurrence rates are better in patients with invasive carcinomas less than 1 cm in diameter and negative lymph nodes compared to those having tumors larger than 1 cm and negative nodes (6). Patients with tumors 1 cm or less in diameter and tumor emboli within lymphatic spaces do not experience a significant number of recurrences, but 43% of patients with similar finding in tumors between 1 to 2 cm in diameter develop recurrences (56).

## Microinvasive Carcinoma

In view of the vastly different and paradoxical treatment recommendations for intraductal and early stage infiltrating ductal carcinoma (frequently mastectomy for the former and lumpectomy with or without radiation for the latter), a small group of lesions require special attention. These are lesions that are predominantly intraductal carcinomas, but focally, the tumor cells have barely broken through the ductal boundaries, invading the stroma immediately adjacent to the defective portion of the duct wall. The invasion is sometimes no more than an overflow or tongue-like projection of cohesive cells that have not lost continuity with the intraductal component through a minor disruption of the basement membrane (Fig 9.5). Or, single and clusters of tumor cells, already dissociated from the intraductal component, infiltrate the stroma in the immediate vicinity of the defect in the basement membrane. The maximum diameter of the invasive area (inclusive of the intervening stroma separating the invasive cells) beyond the basement membrane rarely exceeds 1 mm, and I have set an arbitrary limit of 2 mm maximum diameter as the upper limit for these lesions. In general, such foci of microinvasion are identified after deeper levels of an initially suspicious

A

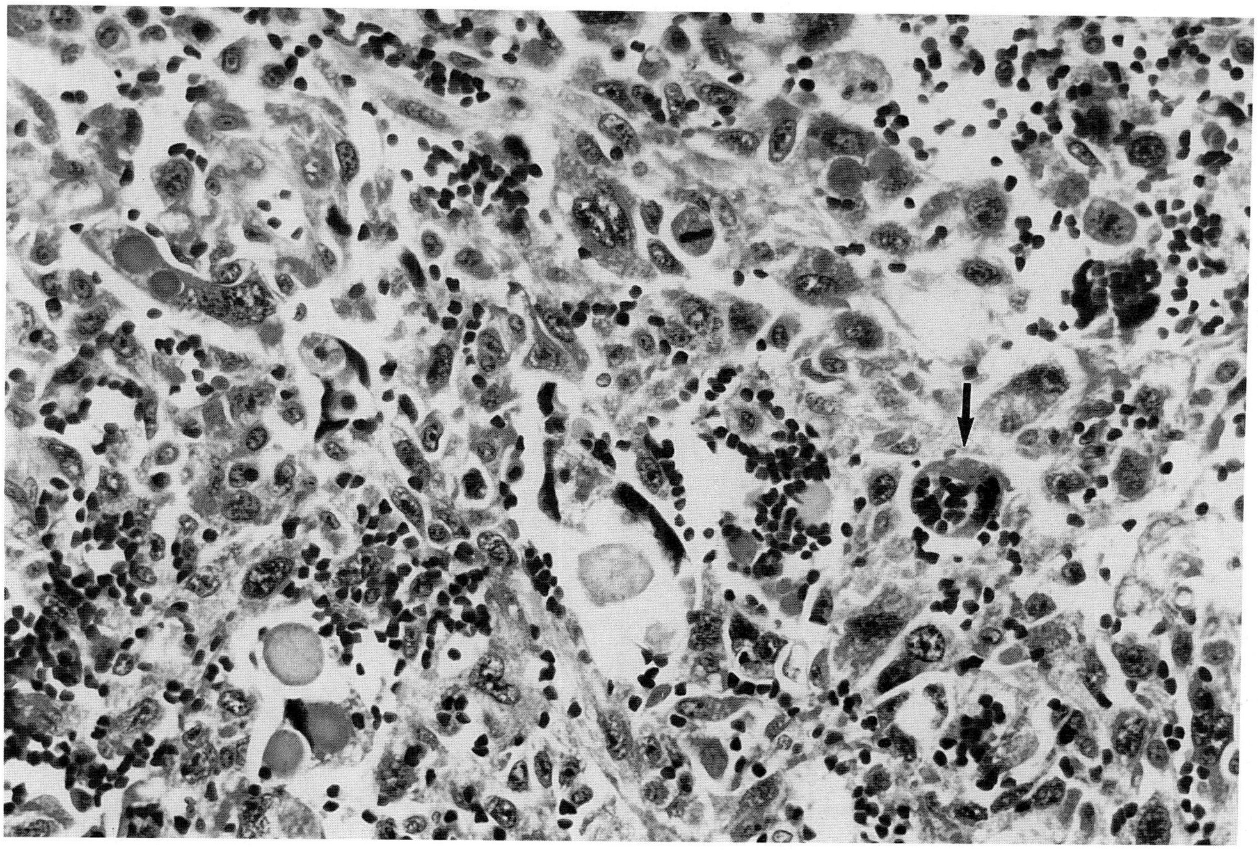

B

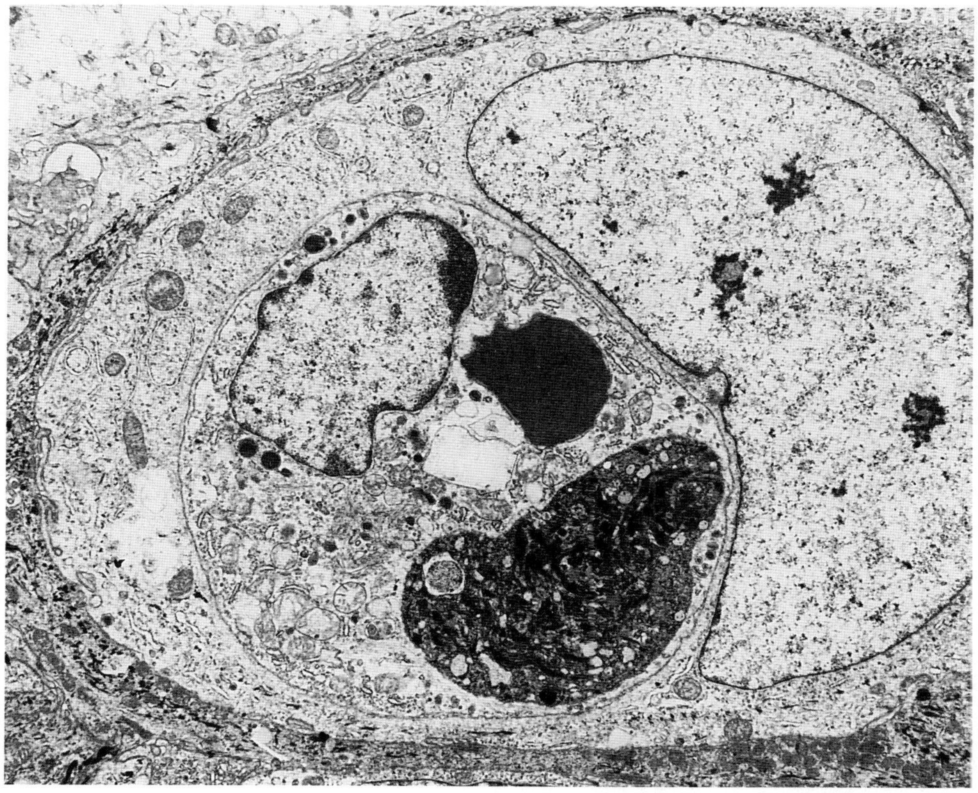

**Figure 9.4** (a) Poorly differentiated carcinoma cells displaying erythrophagocytosis (arrow). (H&E, X500) (b) A cancer cell phagocytizing another cells. (Uranyl acetate-lead citrate, X3,400)

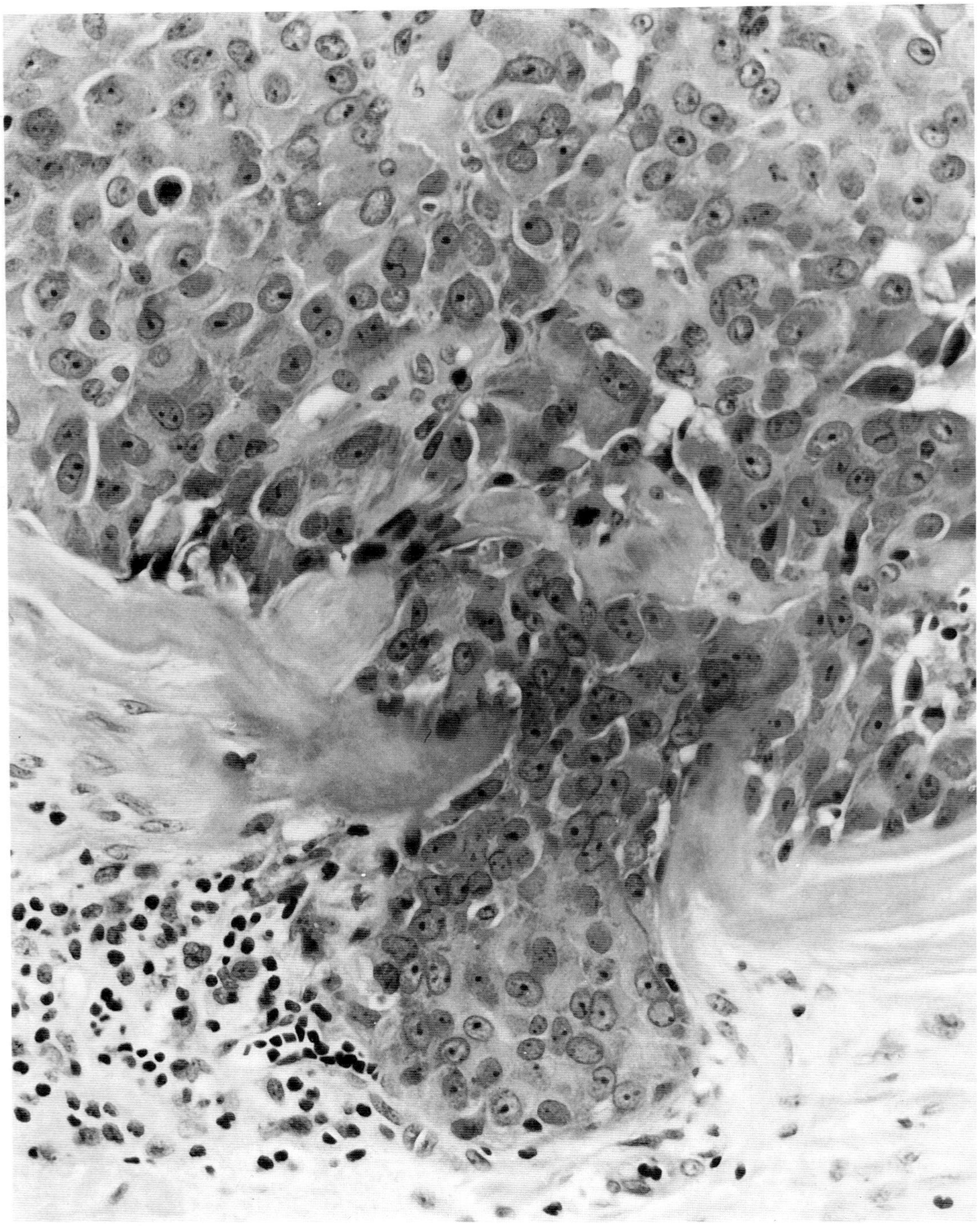

**Figure 9.5** Microinvasive carcinoma characterized by a small cluster of cells breaking through the basement membrane. (H&E, X980)

focus of irregularity in a duct wall are evaluated in a biopsy with extensive intraductal carcinoma.

Luminal necrosis may or may not be present in the affected or surrounding ducts. Whether these tumors should be managed according to the status of the associated and generally extensive IDCA, or as an invasive carcinoma needs to be addressed. I consider these lesions as examples of microinvasive breast carcinoma, and feel that they should be managed according to the type and extent of the intraductal carcinoma.

## Hormone Receptors and Tumor Markers

Infiltrating duct carcinomas are estrogen receptor (ER) positive in 55% to 72% of cases (2,29,39,43,46,

58,73). The ER positivity decreases in lower grade (more poorly-differentiated) carcinomas (58). The presence of abundant elastosis has been reported to be associated with estrogen receptor positivity (24,41,53). Progesterone receptor (PR) positivity is present in approximately 33% to 70% of infiltrating duct carcinomas; 33% of the poorly-differentiated carcinomas show positivity compared to 69% of the well-differentiated tumors (10). In about 15% of cases, the tumors are ER positive, but PR negative. It is believed that PR synthesis is controlled by estrogen and requires an intact ER pathway. Therefore, the presence of defective cytoplasmic ER proteins which prevent translocation of these receptors, as well as either defective or absent nuclear binding sites which are required for estrogen action could result in negative PR levels.

While a variety of other markers [CEA (22,34,38, 66,75), HCG (31,38,75), pregnancy specific beta-1 glycoprotein (31,38,75), human placental lactogen (31,38), casein (52), and alpha lactalbumin (5)] have been identified in infiltrating duct carcinomas, their significance as a prognostic factor remains controversial.

The finding of a positive reaction for S-100 protein in 45% of infiltrating ductal carcinomas is noteworthy (13). This could be a source of confusion since the differential diagnosis of metastatic breast carcinomas composed of large cells with prominent nucleoli (some of which present primarily as an axillary mass) includes malignant melanoma which also displays a positive reaction for S-100 protein. Aside from a mucicarmine stain, which if positive would establish a diagnosis of carcinoma, utilization of tumor markers including cytokeratin and HMB-45 will resolve the problem. Melanomas are negative for epithelial markers (cytokeratin and epithelial membrane antigen), while they display a positive reaction for HMB-45.

## Treatment

Until mid to late 1960's, radical mastectomy was the most common mode of treatment used for patients with infiltrating duct carcinoma. But even during that period, an occasional study recommended a more conservative approach for some of the low grade variants of breast carcinoma and consideration was given to local excision and irradiation as an alternative for treatment of early breast cancer (35,77). Subsequently, there was a gradual shift toward a less radical mastectomy procedure with increasing use of modified radical and simple or total mastectomy. Initially these more limited procedures were performed for some of the less aggressive variants of breast carcinoma. This was followed by a trend toward an even less extensive surgery with increasing use of partial mastectomy, quadrantectomy, and finally lumpectomy (9,14,36,37,64,71,72).

This section will be confined to a summary of the 1990 consensus recommendation (49) regarding the treatment of early stage carcinomas, and will not discuss the complex issue of treatment for all stages of breast carcinoma. For those interested in more detail on treatment of breast carcinoma, several excellent publications that address this topic in great depth are recommended (12,26,27,40).

The NIH Consensus Conference held in June 1990 (49) concluded that breast conservation treatment is appropriate as primary therapy for a majority of patients with stage I and II breast cancer, and "is preferable because it provides survival rates equivalent to those of total mastectomy and axillary dissection while preserving the breast" (49). This approach has been used for limited stage I and II carcinomas not exceeding 4 cm in diameter. In some centers, however, conservative treatment is limited to those with tumors 2 cm or less; in others, 3 cm is the maximum size allowed for conservative treatment.

While patient preferences, better cosmetic results, and psychosocial factors are important considerations in the selection of conservative therapy, certain clinical criteria and morphologic features of the tumor that may influence local-regional control of the tumor are invariably considered in the ultimate decision.

### *Conservative Therapy and its Implications*

Conservative therapy is defined as excision of the primary tumor and about 1 cm of adjacent breast tissue by procedures referred to as lumpectomy, segmental mastectomy, or partial mastectomy, followed by radiotherapy. Axillary node dissection is performed in order to obtain information of important prognostic significance; this would involve a routine dissection of levels I and II axillary nodes. To reduce the risk of local recurrence, the margins should be grossly and microscopically free of tumor. To obtain the optimal cosmetic results, excision of the overlying skin—except for superficial lesions—and suture reapproximation of mammary tissue preferably should be avoided.

Following surgery, 45 to 50 Gy megavoltage radiotherapy to the entire breast should be used routinely. Patients found to have focal microscopic involvement of the margins have been variably treated with either boost irradiation or mastectomy in reported trials.

Women who develop local recurrences following conservative therapy are treated by total mastectomy with good results in a substantial number of cases. While a majority of node-negative breast cancer patients treated by this conservative approach are cured, the risk of local and distant recurrences can be reduced from 30% to 20% by adjuvant tamoxifen (20 mg per day for at least two years) and combination chemotherapy. The benefits and side effects of adjuvant therapy should be discussed with the patient before any decision is made regarding its use.

### *Patient Selection*

It is important to be aware of the fact that some women are not candidates for conservative therapy. Women whose tumors have features often associated with increased likelihood of recurrence (multicentric malignancies, including grossly multifocal lesions or diffuse mammographically-detected microcalcifications) are not candidates for this approach. Women whose tumors are large relative to their breast size are not good candidates because of poor cosmetic results. Finally, women with a variety of collagen vascular diseases have been reported to develop massive fibrosis and disfiguration following radiotherapy and should be advised against this treatment option.

Women with small tumors (1 cm or less in diameter) and negative nodes in stages I and II are particularly good candidates for conservative therapy; their prognosis is excellent and they do not require adjuvant chemotherapy.

Preliminary results suggest that women whose carcinoma has an extensive in situ component are at higher risk for the development of recurrence and treatment failure. If confirmed by subsequent larger series, conservative therapy would not be appropriate for these patients. Controversies persist regarding the significance of extensive lymphatic involvement, and the patient's age (younger than 39 years).

### *Conservative Treatment of Breast Carcinomas Other than Infiltrating Duct Carcinoma*

The efficacy of conservative therapy for Stages I and II carcinomas other than infiltrating duct carcinoma was evaluated by Kurtz et al (36). Sixty-seven women so treated for infiltrating lobular carcinoma had an actuarial five-year survival of 100% if node negative and 77% if node positive. The probability of recurrence at five years was 13.5% for the infiltrating lobular carcinomas, compared to 8.8% for infiltrating ductal carcinomas. For 27 women with medullary carcinoma, a 90% five-year survival was obtained, with a 4% recurrence rate for the same period. None of the ten patients with colloid carcinoma developed recurrences, and the five-year survival was 100%. These findings suggest that conservative therapy may provide adequate local control for other histologic types as well.

## Infiltrating Carcinoma Presenting as an Axillary Mass

In 1907, Halsted (100) described three patients who presented with axillary node enlargement without a clinically palpable primary breast carcinoma; all three subsequently developed ipsilateral breast carcinoma. As a result he recommended radical mastectomy for these patients. Breast carcinoma presenting as an axillary mass in the absence of a clinically detectable breast tumor (occult primary), is now recognized as a rare manifestation of stage II disease (94,106,113,127).

About 10% of persistently enlarged axillary lymph nodes harbor a metastatic carcinoma (114). The most likely site of origin for a metastatic adenocarcinoma in the axillary lymph node is the ipsilateral breast. If the patient has had a carcinoma in one breast, rarely metastases to the contralateral axillary nodes do occur—4% in Haagensen's experience (98)—usually in women with advanced disease. If the morphology of the axillary mass is that of a classic mammary carcinoma, by convention, the lesion is interpreted as a primary breast carcinoma. In some cases, careful clinical examination along with mammography may disclose a carcinoma within the breast proper, but in at least 18% of cases, the primary lesion remains elusive (101). Melanoma, GI, kidney, lung, thyroid, and ovary are other sites that should be considered as possible sources of such a tumor.

The patients range in age from 33 to 83 years, with a median of 57 years; 45% have a positive family history of breast carcinoma (116). They present with an axillary mass of several months duration without any significant finding in the ipsilateral breast, and a negative mammography in 76% of the cases (117). About two to five years may elapse before a primary cancer becomes detectable in the ipsilateral breast (98a,99,108).

Morphologically, 65% of these tumors are infiltrating duct carcinomas; 20% are noninvasive (116, 117). A high proportion are characterized by a diffuse growth pattern and consist of relatively large cells with apocrine features (101,116). More typical breast carcinoma patterns are also observed with comedonecrosis, cribriform arrangements, along with trabeculae and gland-forming clusters. A positive reaction for cytokeratin would distinguish these tumors from melanoma and lymphoma, both of which are cytokeratin negative. Furthermore, melanoma would be S-100 protein and HMB-45 positive, while lymphoma would display a positive reaction for leukocyte common antigen (LCA) along with expression of other lymphoma-associated antigens. At the ultrastructural level, the presence of intracellular lumens and canaliculi, apical desmosomes, microvilli, and secretory vesicles favor an epithelial tumor (104). With the current availability of a variety of immunostains, however, ultrastructural evaluation is hardly ever indicated.

It is important to determine the hormone receptor status of the nodal tumor, as this may be the only tissue available for such studies (83,97). Bhatia et al (83) found both estrogen and progesterone receptors in three of 11 cases presenting with axillary nodal metastases.

Currently, most investigators believe that these women should be treated with the assumption that there is an invasive ipsilateral carcinoma. Therefore, mastectomy has been proposed for patients presenting with a breast carcinoma in the axillary nodes after other primary sites have been excluded (105). The mastectomy specimen reveals a small carcinoma in approximately 50% of the cases. In a very small number of patients, the only demonstrable carcinoma in the mastectomy specimen may be a non-invasive intraductal carcinoma or lobular neoplasia (116); but these may be totally unrelated to the axillary tumor.

A more conservative approach has been advocated by others, however. Feigenberg et al (93) proposed excision of upper outer quadrant initially. If there is no carcinoma in this quadrant, then block dissection of the axillary content and radiotherapy should follow. If the quadrant shows a carcinoma, however, modified radical mastectomy and radiotherapy were recommended. Vilcoq (124) also favors conservative treatment in the form of radiotherapy. Kemeny et al (106) found no significant difference in survival of patients treated by mastectomy and those treated by axillary dissection; they concluded that mastectomy is unnecessary.

The prognosis appears to be better than that of women with stage II, palpable breast carcinoma and axillary metastases (79). With a median follow-up of five years, 60% of the women who present with an axillary carcinoma are alive, without evidence of disease (117). Only about 9% to 29% of these women develop recurrences or die from the tumor (79,102, 124,127).

It is possible that some of these tumors actually arise from either the axillary tail of the breast, accessory breast tissue in the axilla, or heterotopic breast tissue in an axillary lymph node (125). The presence of normal breast tissue adjacent to the tumor would support one of the first two possibilities, while identification of heterotopic glands in other uninvolved lymph nodes would support the latter possibility.

## Axillary Node Morphology, With and Without Metastases

The smallest metastases are generally found in the subcapsular sinuses. With rare exceptions, the metastatic foci reflect the dominant morphology and degree of differentiation of the primary lesion (118). Extension of the carcinoma into extranodal stroma adversely affects the prognosis (109). The stromal alterations, such as elastosis observed in association with a primary breast carcinoma, do not accompany the tumor to the metastatic sites. Exceptions do occur, however, particularly in association with some of the special types of invasive carcinoma, ie carcinoma with osteoclastic giant cells.

The significance of axillary node morphology in the absence of metastatic carcinoma in patients with breast carcinoma has been evaluated in numerous studies (84,85,95,103,108,120,122). A variety of changes including sinus histiocytosis, germinal center and follicular hyperplasia, diffuse cortical hyperplasia (lymphocyte predominance), and lymphocyte depletion have been observed and interpreted as a reflection of tumor-host interactions. The prognostic significance of these changes remains controversial, however. Sinus histiocytosis and diffuse cortical hyperplasia have been reported to be associated with a lower frequency of axillary node metastases and better prognosis (84,103,119,120,122). Others have been unable to confirm a better prognosis or lower frequency of axillary node metastases in association with sinus histiocytosis (81,82,88). Germinal center and follicular hyperplasia, however, have been reported to have a possible adverse influence on the disease-free survival of women without lymph node metastases (95). The finding of lymphocyte-depleted axillary nodes has been interpreted as an ominous prognostic sign (122).

There are divergent viewpoints regarding the significance of a prominent lymphoplasmacytic response to the tumor. Some have associated this finding with a better prognosis (82,84,96), while others have reported a less favorable prognosis or no significant difference (59,60) associated with the presence of a lymphoplasmacytic infiltrate.

## Other Lesions in the Axillary Nodes

A variety of other lesions may present in the axillary lymph nodes. Biopsy of a persistently enlarged axillary lymph node shows nonspecific changes reflecting inflammation and hyperplasia in 69.5%, a lymphoma is identified in 13.9%, metastatic carcinoma in 9.7%, and 6.9% show granulomas (114). In addition to these findings, the axillary lymph nodes may contain benign breast tissue (123), epithelial inclusions of possible skin adnexal origin (89,98,102), nevus cells (92,105,111,112,115), angiomatosis, or display silicone lymphadenopathy associated with augmentation mammoplasty (121).

Nevus cells (Fig. 9.6) have been identified in 3% of serially-sectioned axillary lymph nodes (128). A majority of the melanocytic cells in this location are either nonpigmented or lightly pigmented and because of their cohesive and distinctive cell margins assume a mosaic appearance. Rarely, they may be deeply pigmented and sometimes the larger clusters dip into the nodal substance. These cells may give rise to blue nevi (80,91).

Benign epithelial inclusions resembling eccrine and apocrine sweat glands have been seen in the breast (Fig. 9.7). These are sometimes associated with the formation of large cysts lined partially or completely by keratinizing squamous epithelium and filled with keratinous debris. The presence of the various cell types (squamous in some cystic structures, apocrine and nonspecific-glandular-lining in others), and the bilayered (epithelial and myoepithelial) lining of the glandular structures (89) is an important clue to their benign nature. Differentiation from a metastatic adenocarcinoma becomes more difficult when epithelial proliferation is evident in the glandular structures as in Case 2 of Holdsworth et al (102). Identification of a myoepithelial cell layer around such hyperplastic glands is crucial to their interpretation as a benign inclusion; immunostains for actin will be helpful in unmasking the myoepithelial cells.

Apocrine gland cysts, adenomas, and adenocarcinomas do occur in the axilla and may extend to the adjacent nodes. Distinction from a mammary carcinoma (metastatic or originating in accessory breast tissue) can be difficult. Sweat gland carcinomas are noted for having a long duration (as many as 30 years) of existence prior to excision. Features that favor a primary axillary apocrine gland lesion include the presence of relatively mature tumor cells high in the dermis, transition from normal to neoplastic apocrine epithelium, and the demonstration of intracytoplasmic iron granules (126); iron granules are not present in mammary apocrine carcinomas.

Benign breast tissue is found occasionally within axillary lymph nodes (96,98,107,123). These mammary epithelial inclusions have the potential to develop the same range of pathology observed in the breast proper, and undoubtedly account for at least a fraction of the cases of mammary carcinoma presenting as a primary axillary mass with undetectable carcinoma in the ipsilateral breast.

The histogenesis of ectopic breast tissue in the axillary nodes is uncertain. Considering the fact that the milk line extends to the axillary region during developmental stages, this finding most probably reflects embryonic rests. An embolic phe-

A

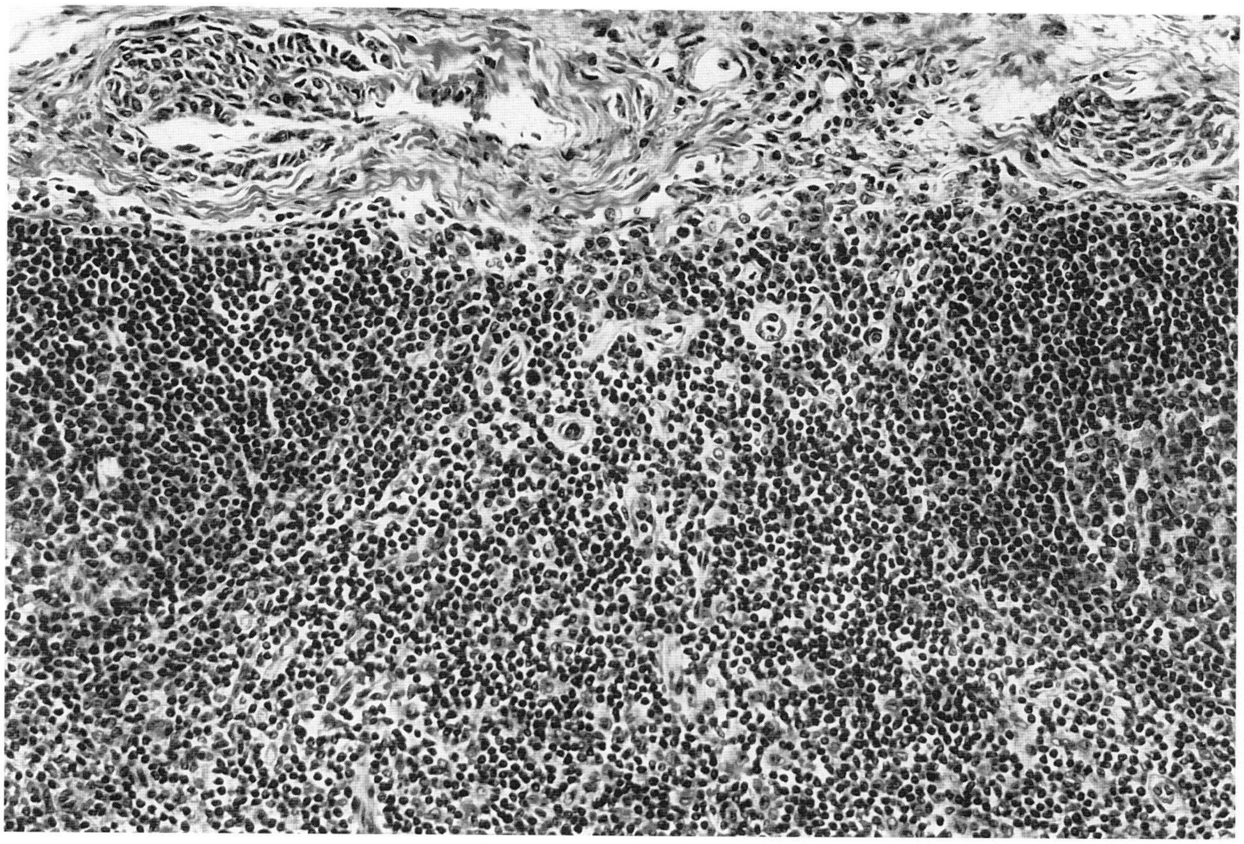

B

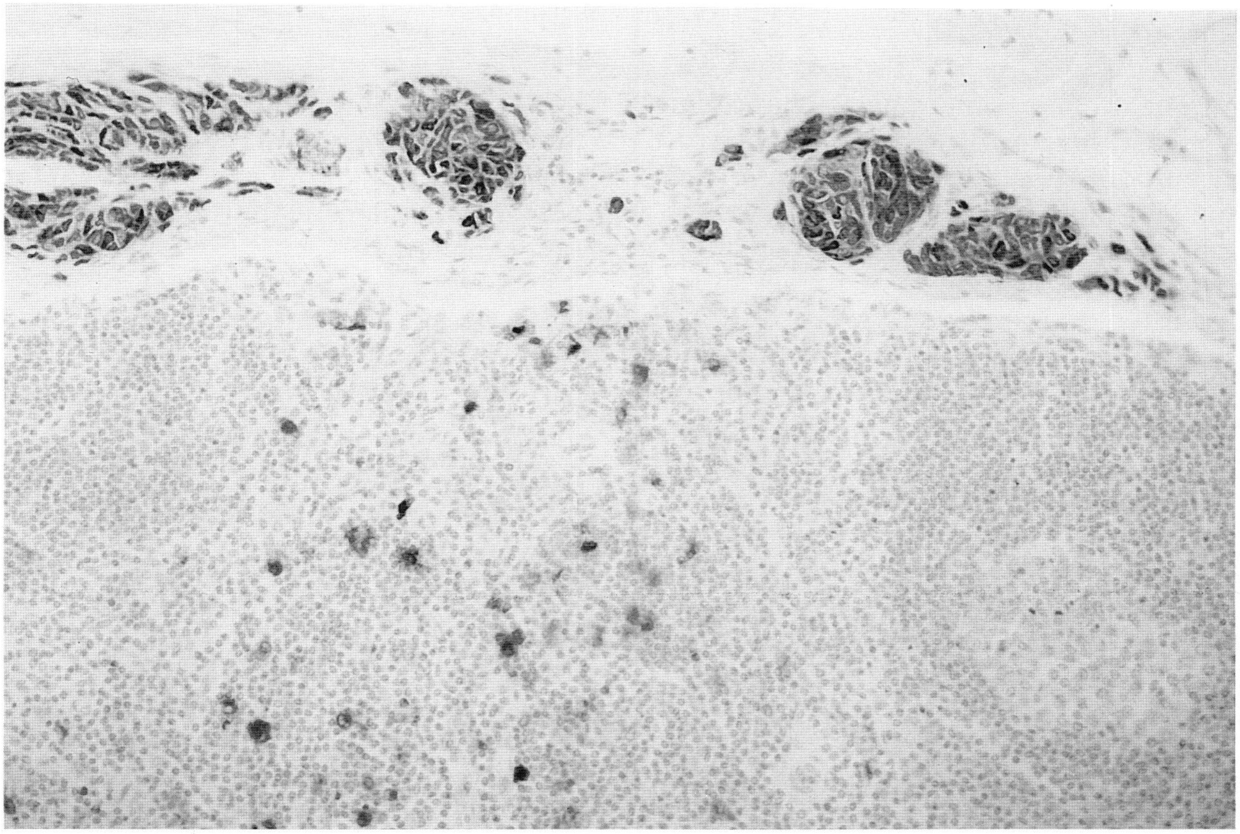

**Figure 9.6** Nevus cells forming small clusters beneath the capsule in an axillary node. A positive immunoreaction for S-100 protein is illustrated. (H&E, (a) X90; S-100 protein, (b) X90)

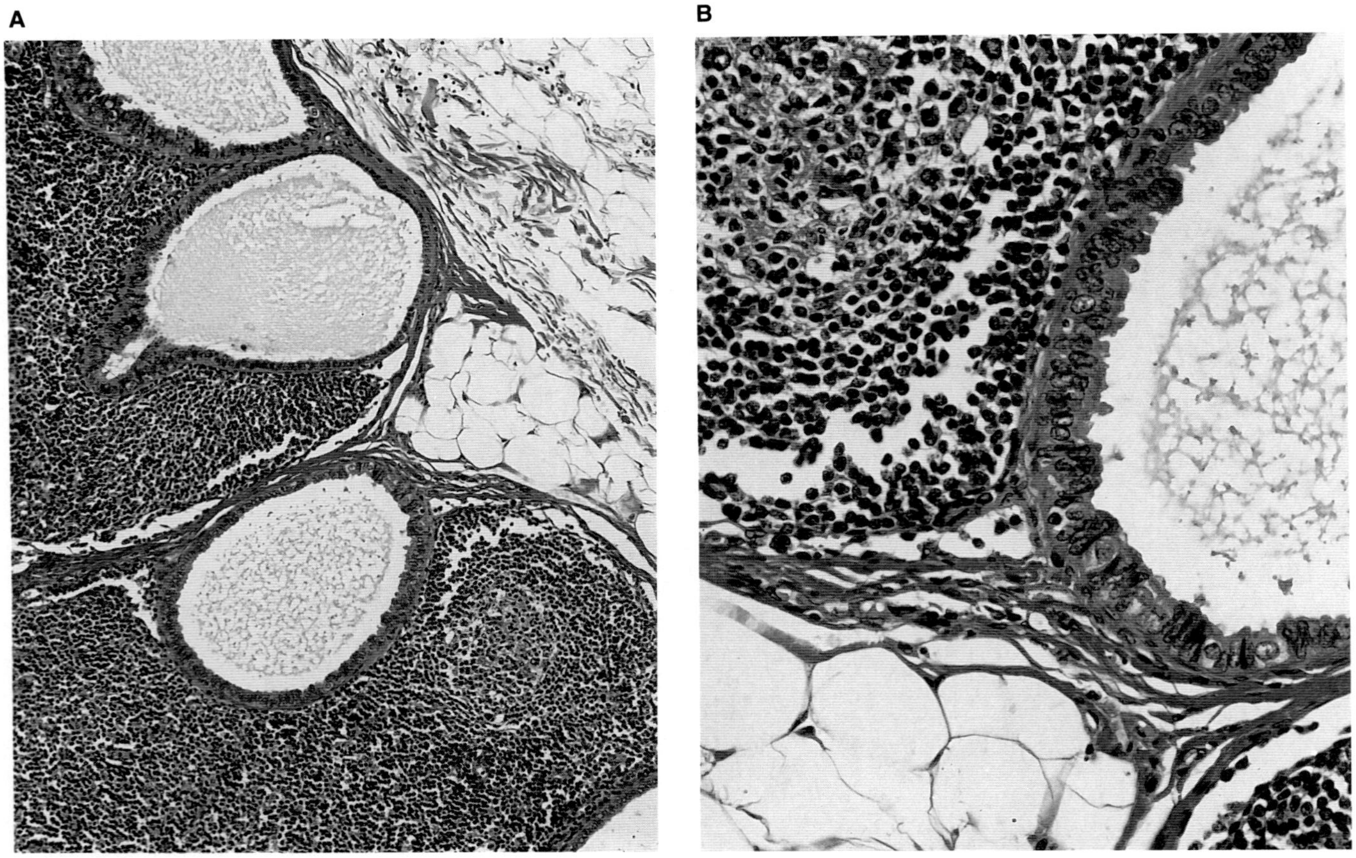

**Figure 9.7** Epithelial inclusions in the axillary nodes. (a & b) They are often multiple and lined by bland epithelium. (H&E, (a) X100; (b) X300)

nomenon—embolization of mammary glandular tissue during breast surgery—has also been proposed (123). If embolization were indeed involved in the histogenesis of this finding, I believe we should be seeing many more such cases considering the frequency and multiplicity of breast biopsies over the past ten years.

Regardless of the etiology, it is important to recognize these possibilities to prevent confusion with metastatic carcinoma.

## Morphologic Changes Induced by Radiation and Chemotherapy

Since radiation therapy is being used with increasing frequency as part of the conservative treatment option in the management of women with stage I and II breast carcinoma, it is important to become familiar with morphologic and functional alterations induced by this modality. Some of the women so treated may develop subsequent mammographic or clinically palpable lesions that will require excisional biopsy and microscopic evaluation. Familiarity with the range of morphologic alterations induced by radiotherapy will prevent misinterpretation of these changes as atypical or malignant.

The changes in the breast include alterations in the overlying skin which are identical to skin changes observed as a result of radiation to other parts of the body (131), as well as other general changes such as variable degrees of stromal fibrosis, hyalinization, vascular alterations (endothelial cell damage and fibrinoid necrosis of the vessel wall), fat and epithelial cell necrosis, as well as vacuolization of residual recognizable tumor cells (133). The fat necrosis may clinically simulate recurrent carcinoma (129,138).

Stromal fibrosis may be subtle or extensive. In some cases, atypical stromal cells with cytoplasmic vacuolization and enlarged hyperchromatic nuclei are also observed; sometimes these cells assume a florette-type appearance. Severe breast fibrosis has been noted as a serious complication of radiotherapy among breast cancer patients with collagen vascular disease—systemic lupus eythematosis, discoid lupus, progressive systemic sclerosis or scleroderma, rheumatoid arthritis (132,135,136). Simultaneous with the severe breast fibrosis, a worsening of the rheumatoid arthritis has occurred (136). Collagen vascular disease is now considered a contraindication to breast radiotherapy.

It has been proposed that radiotherapy causes vascular endothelial cell injury, resulting in exposure of the basement membrane and systemic antigen release. The released antigens provoke an autoimmune response which simultaneously causes progression of the systemic disease and attraction of inflammatory cells to the irradiated tissue. The inflammation is followed by fibroblastic proliferation, collagen synthesis, and eventual severe fibrosis (136).

Another significant change that could result in diagnostic problems deserves particular attention. A relatively common consequence of radiotherapy to the breast is the development of epithelial cells with enlarged hyperchromatic nuclei, inconspicuous nucleoli, and cystoplasmic vacuolization in the terminal duct-lobular unit (TDLU) (137) as well as in areas of adenosis (Fig. 9.8). These changes are not related to the presence or absence of recurrent cancer, patient age, interval between termination of radiotherapy and the subsequent biopsy, or the usual dosage of radiation. Similar changes may also affect the epithelial cells in larger ducts, but less frequently. Variable degrees of lobular sclerosis may also occur.

The radiation-induced atypia differs from carcinoma involving the lobules by the absence of epithelial hyperplasia, mitotic activity, and luminal necrosis. Furthermore, the cytoplasmic vacuolization and a history of prior radiotherapy should serve as additional clues. The absence of proliferative activity in the radiation-induced atypia helps distinguish it from spontaneous epithelial atypia which is frequently associated with hyperplasia. The radiation-induced atypia may appear rather subtle at low magnification, and could be entirely overlooked unless the pathologist has been forewarned about the history of radiation therapy.

At this time, it is not known whether or not radiotherapy may induce similar atypicalities in proliferating epithelial cells; if it does, it will prove to be a very difficult problem to resolve.

It is noteworthy that similar epithelial changes have also been observed secondary to chemotherapy. Close et al (130) described an increase in nuclear size, pleomorphism, vacuolization, and chromatin clumping in residual tumor cells after chemotherapy. Kennedy et al (134) described cytoplasmic vacuolization in the residual neoplastic cells imparting a histiocytoid appearance to the cells, and enlargement with nuclear atypia of non-neoplastic cells within the TDLU and larger ducts.

Illustrations of lobular atrophy and sclerosis described in association with both radiation and chemotherapy are identical to normal involutional changes in the lobules that are quite common in patients of breast carcinoma age. It is through comparison of the lobular appearance prior to and following therapy that a causal relationship can be established as accomplished by Kennedy et al (134). It is possible that these forms of therapy initiate or accelerate normal involutional changes.

Chemotherapy may induce nodular fibrosis and areas of fibrohistiocytic proliferation—most probably markers of the previous sites of carcinoma—in both the breast as well as in axillary lymph nodes. Chemotherapy does not induce the vascular and stromal changes associated with radiation therapy (134).

## INFILTRATING LOBULAR CARCINOMA

The origin of an invasive carcinoma characterized by a linear growth pattern of small cells and currently recognized as an infiltrating lobular carcinoma was traced to carcinoma within lobules by Cornil (143) and Waldeyer (178) in the 1860s and later confirmed by others (141,169). Haagensen (155) regarded these tumors as infiltrating small cell carcinomas and conceded that it is among the most frequent patterns of carcinoma that develop in women with lobular neoplasia.

Invasive lobular carcinoma accounts for 0.7% to 14% of all invasive breast carcinomas (146,148,157, 161,164,256); this range is in part due to differences in criteria. Inclusion of several subsequently-described variants has resulted in a higher percentage in more recent reports. The patients range in age from 26 to 86 years, with a median age ranging from 45 to 57 years (140,150,151,162,164,166,167,177). Among women less than 35 years of age, 2% of carcinomas are of this type, while it comprises 11% of carcinomas in women older than 75 years (55). Like other carcinomas, a majority of women present with a palpable mass. The larger tumors may become fixed to the overlying skin, or cause nipple retraction. Interestingly, Paget's

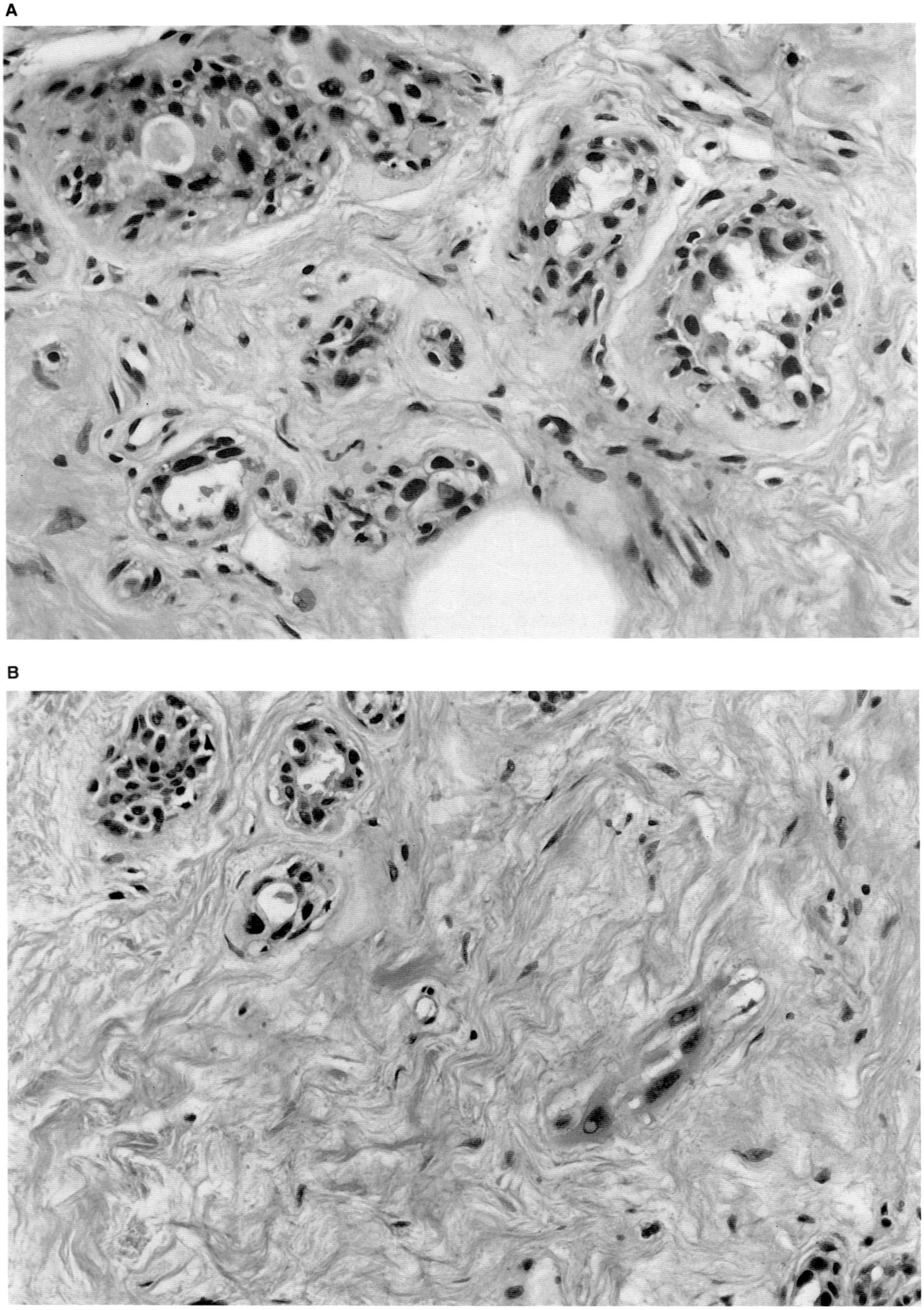


**Figure 9.8** Radiation effect. (a) The epithelial cells in the ductules show nuclear pleomorphism and cytoplasmic vacuolization. (H&E, X480) (b) The endothelial cells lining a small vascular space also show similar changes. (H&E, X480)

disease is not seen in association with infiltrating lobular carcinoma. Some tumors are hard to detect because of the diffuse growth pattern of the cellular infiltrate which may fail to produce a dominant or well-defined mass. Sometimes the lesion may be clinically palpable as an area of density, but mammography fails to delineate a mass. Further impediments to mammographic detection include frequent absence of calcification, lack of well-defined margins, and multifocality. Prior or concurrent bilateral carcinomas have been reported in 6% to 28% of cases (146,151,159,164). Subsequent contralateral carcinoma has been observed in 9% to 14% of the cases (146,147); 50% of these are invasive carcinomas (146,151,159).

## Macroscopic Features

Macroscopically, in addition to presenting either as an irregular, infiltrating or well-circumscribed, indurated mass, sometimes the lesion is not apparent to the naked eye. Infiltrating lobular carcinoma may form poorly-defined areas of density only a few millimeters in size, or it may become a massive tumor and occupy the entire breast. An unusual manifestation of the tumor is the formation of minuscule, dicrete, firm nodules, likened to "grains of sand" (167) within the breast tissue.

## Microscopic Features

Simultaneous with the description of lobular carcinoma in situ, Foote and Stewart (153) described the classic pattern of invasion associated with infiltrating lobular carcinoma. This classic pattern is characterized by cohesive and generally small cells diffusely invading the stroma (Fig. 9.9). The tumor cells display round to notched ovoid nuclei and a thin rim of cytoplasm with an occasional intracytoplasmic lumen. The tumor cells diffusely infiltrate the mammary stroma, entrapping normal structures and assuming a targetoid growth pattern around entrapped ducts. This classic pattern of infiltrating lobular carcinoma is associated with lobular neoplasia in around 90% or more of the cases (147,164). Subsequently, additional patterns of invasive lobular carcinoma were defined, including a solid pattern (150), alveolar pattern (161), and a mixed group composed of an admixture of one or more of these patterns (147); lobular neoplasia is identified in 40% to 60% of these variants (147). The solid variant consists of a closely-packed proliferation of cells forming large nests or wide trabeculae separated by very delicate vascular channels (Fig. 9.10). In the alveolar variant, a similar cell population forms rounded nests and islands of 20 or more cells separated by a minimal amount of stroma (Fig. 9.11). The mixed type shows admixtures of these patterns, sometimes with a cell population that is more atypical, displaying more numerous intracytoplasmic lumens and a tendency to form irregular aggregates. In a study by Dixon et al (147), the classic variant comprised 30% of the cases, the solid pattern 22%, the alveolar lesions 19%, and the mixed variety 29%. These variants are not commonly observed in Japan (165).

DiCostanzo et al (145) have suggested that the term infiltrating lobular carcinoma without further qualification should be used for tumors displaying the classic pattern in at least 85% of the tumor; the presence of the special variants should be noted following the diagnosis of infiltrating lobular carcinoma.

Another pattern designated as tubulolobular has been described (152,161). This variant displays tight or closed tubule formation along with cords of cells arranged in Indian files (Fig. 9.12). As mentioned in the introduction to this chapter, I would not accept a tumor forming tubules as a variant of lobular carcinoma. It could be considered as a tumor displaying both ductal and lobular patterns of invasion, however.

In cases of microinvasion from lobular neoplasia, a break in the continuity of the basement membrane is not apparent, and the invasive cells seem to have been sprayed into the surrounding stroma.

## Differential Diagnosis

All variants of infiltrating lobular carcinoma, particularly the solid variant, can closely simulate a lymphoma and are not infrequently misinterpreted as such when viewed under low magnification. The problem is compounded when the tissue fixation is suboptimal. Special stains for mucicarmine, Alcian

A

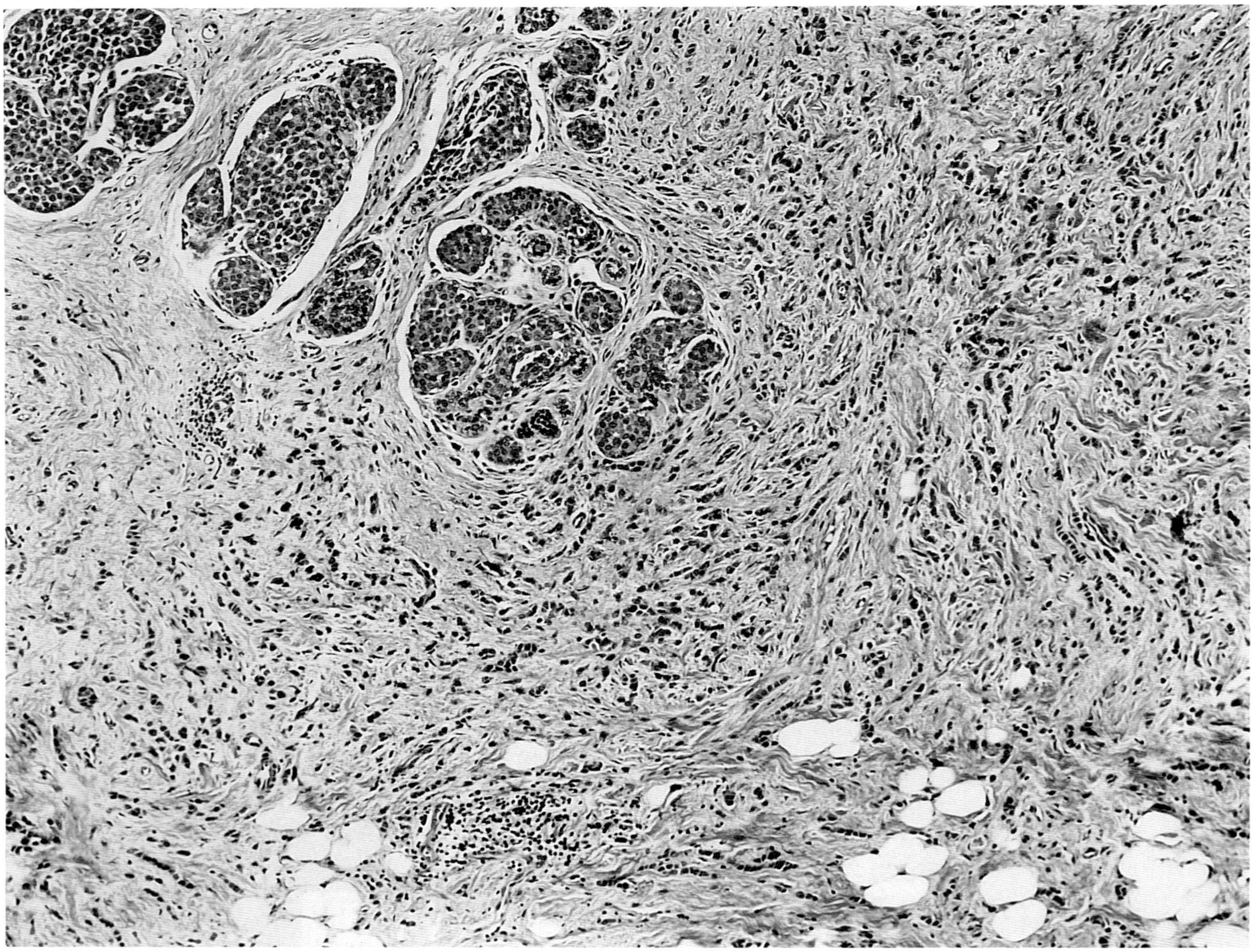

**Figure 9.9(a)** Infiltrating lobular carcinoma, classic pattern. There are isolated cells and small cords of cells invading the stroma around neoplastic lobules. (H&E, X150)

blue-PAS, or both are helpful in highlighting the intracytoplasmic lumen (ICL) containing cells. Lobular carcinomas contain predominantly neutral and sialomucins (154,163), but sulfated mucins have also been reported (232). Approximately 60% of primary and 50% of metastatic lobular carcinomas are mucin positive (177). Identification of ICL is also helpful in distinguishing a carcinoma from a lymphoma; ICL is not specific to lobular carcinomas (177), however, as occasionally even unequivocal ductal carcinomas may display abundant intracytoplasmic lumens. When cells with ICL are sparse or absent, immunostains for cytokeratin and leukocyte common antigen (LCA) unequivocally establish the nature of the neoplastic cells. Lymphomas are LCA positive, but negative for cytokeratin, while carcinomas show a positive reaction for cytokeratin and a negative reaction for LCA. Rarely, even inflammatory cells may simulate an infiltrating lobular carcinoma on frozen sections (176).

## Axillary Node Metastases

In Haagensen's series (155) of 76 Columbia Stage A small cell carcinomas (comparable to infiltrating lobular carcinoma), the frequency of axillary node metastases was 39.7%, compared to 30.8% for similar

B

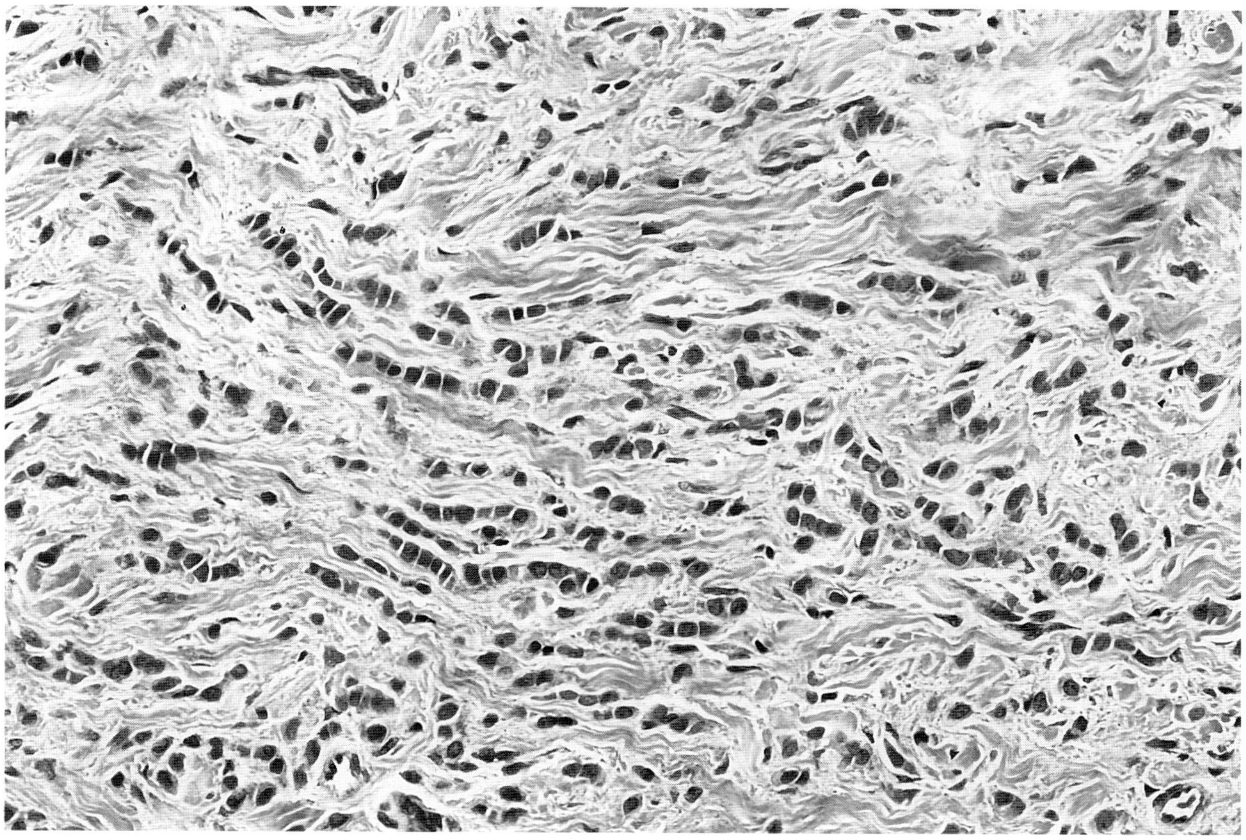

C

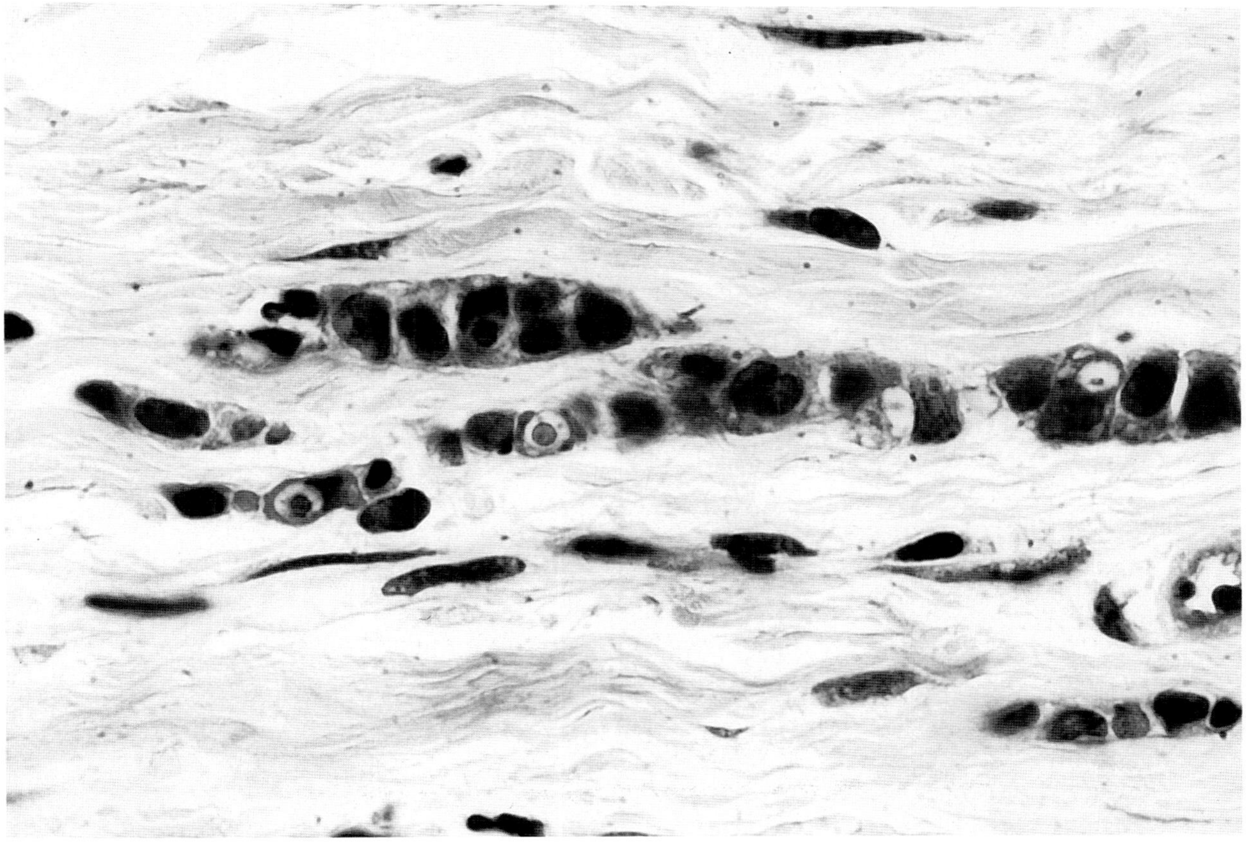

**Figure 9.9(b,c)** Infiltrating lobular carcinoma, classic pattern. (b) The cells form the characteristic "Indian files." (H&E, X400) (c) Intracytoplasmic lumens are apparent in the tumor cells forming an "Indian file." (H&E, X880)

A

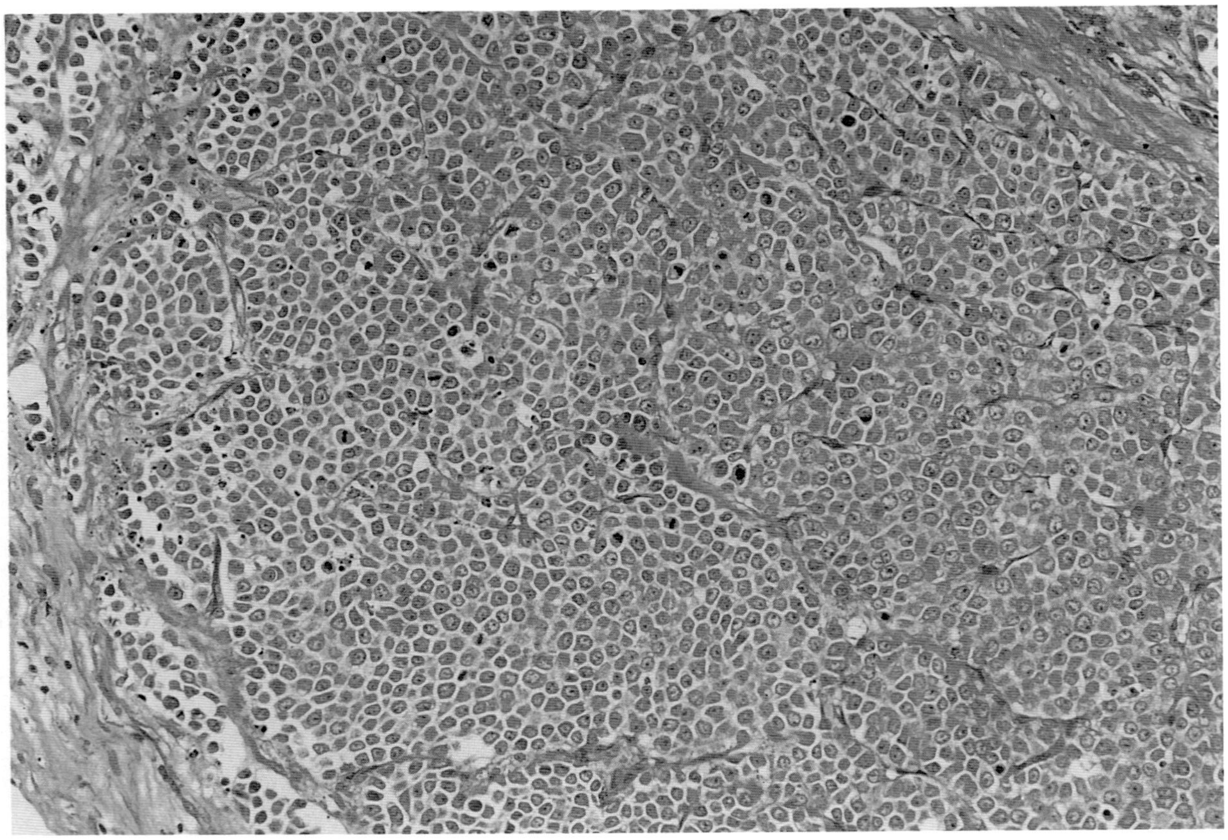

B

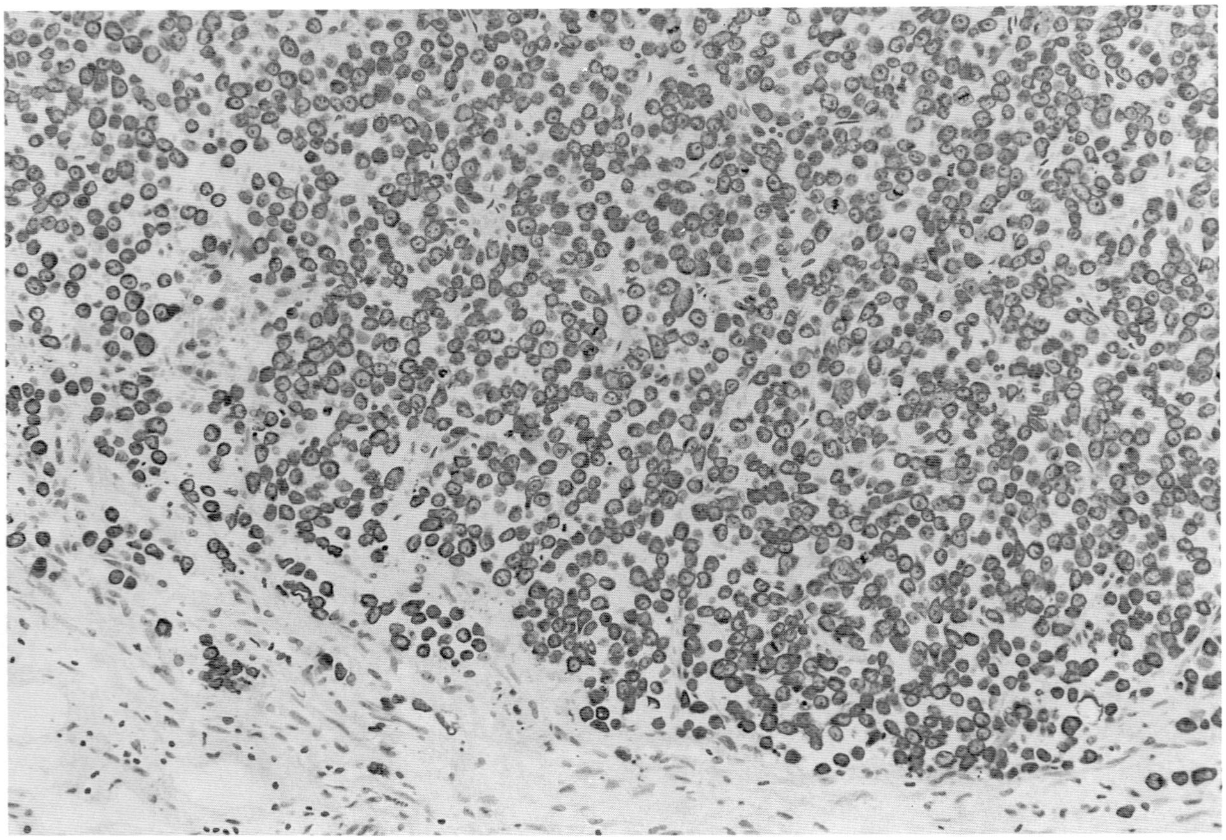

**Figure 9.10** (a) Solid variant of infiltrating lobular carcinoma shows loose cells proliferating and supported by a very delicate vascular stroma. This pattern is often mistaken for a lymphoma. (H&E, X240) (b) Immunostain for cytokeratin shows positivity confirming the epithelial nature of the tumor. (X240)

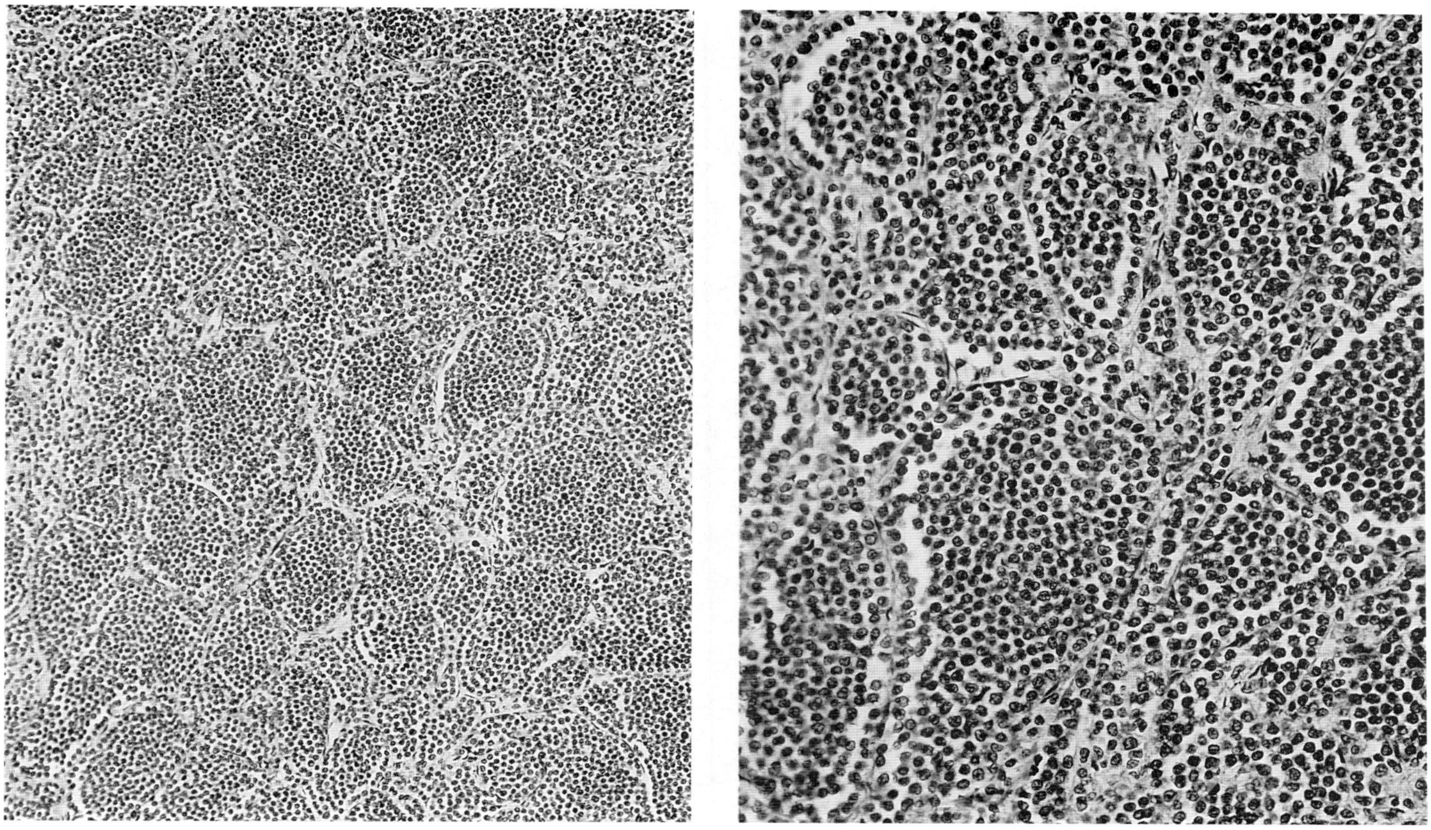


**Figure 9.11** Alveolar variant of infiltrating lobular carcinoma. (a&b) Closely-packed islands of uniform small cells. (H&E, (a) X120; (b) X240)

stage carcinomas of all types. Fechner (150) has suggested that the variant patterns may be associated with a lower frequency of axillary node metastases.

Infiltrating lobular carcinoma is notorious for simulating histiocytes in metastatic foci and when populating subcapsular and medullary sinuses in axillary lymph nodes (139,158). The sheet-like aggregation of the tumor cells and subtle distortion of the nodal architecture are helpful in arriving at the accurate diagnosis. When a distinction is difficult, special staining for mucin or immunostains for cytokeratin help resolve the issue; a positive reaction for mucin or cytokeratin would establish the diagnosis of carcinoma. In the eyelids, the histiocytic appearance of the metastatic tumor cells may cause misinterpretation of the lesion as a chalazion (158,180).

The metastatic pattern of lobular invasive carcinoma differs from that of invasive ductal carcinoma with a higher frequency of skeletal, visceral, diffuse serosal, and retroperitoneal metastases observed in lobular carcinomas (142,156). In the central nervous system, metastases from invasive lobular carcinoma form meningeal infiltrates, while ductal carcinomas show parenchymal deposits (172). Metastases to the ovary and uterus are common. In the endometrium, metastases cause bleeding, but because of the small cell size and diffuse pattern of infiltration in the endometrium, these metastases are easily overlooked. Furthermore, the pink metastatic tumor cells within the stroma are often misinterpreted as decidual reaction to progestins which many of the patients receive for their irregular bleeding prior to the curettage. Bone marrow metastases are particularly common (179), and constituted the most common site of metastases in DiCostanzo et al's series (145).

## Hormone Receptors and Ploidy

About 70 to 92% of lobular carcinomas are estrogen (ER) positive (2,46,52). ER positivity is observed in the classic and all other variants (163), with the alveolar variant appearing to have a greater likeli-

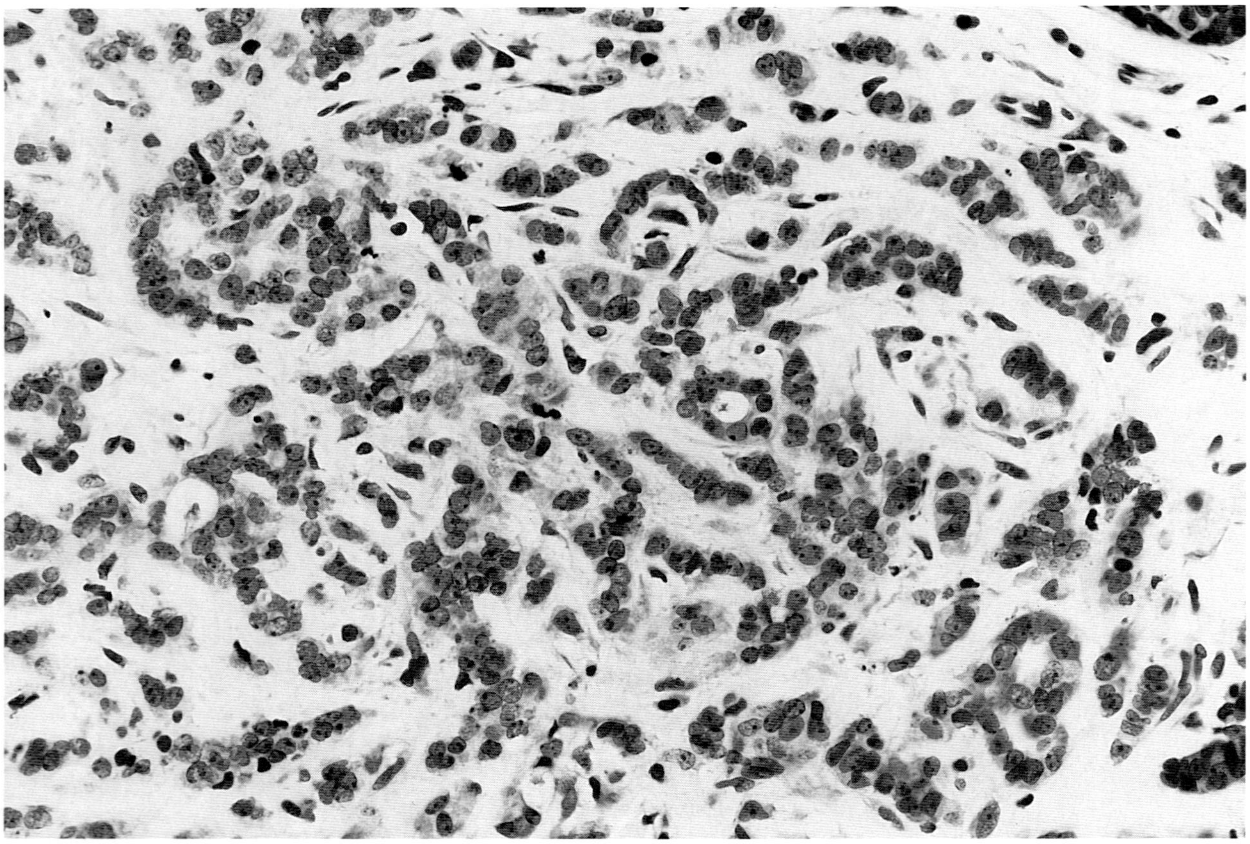

**Figure 9.12** The so-called tubulolobular infiltrating carcinoma which I would interpret as a ductal carcinoma based on the formation of small tubules. (H&E, X240)

hood of ER positivity (159). Progesterone (PR) receptors are found in 67% of the tumors (306). Carcinoembryonic antigen (CEA) has been reported in 33% to 63% of cases (34,163). Milk-related proteins such as lactalbumin and casein have been detected in some cases (149,174). Also, 60% of these tumors show a positive reaction for S-100 protein underscoring the lack of specificity of S-100 protein (13).

Approximately 22% of infiltrating lobular carcinomas are aneuploid. Among ER+ tumors, ploidy does not appear to influence the likelihood of PR positivity (306).

## Treatment and Prognosis

Treatment of infiltrating lobular carcinoma should parallel that of infiltrating mammary carcinomas in general and depends on the stage of the lesion.

The five- and ten-year survival rates for node-negative women are 86% and 74% respectively (140). Following radical mastectomy approximately 5.4% of the women develop local recurrences within ten years (155). About 50% of patients with positive nodes eventually die from their disease compared to 14% of the node-negative women (164).

While some pathologists have suggested a worse prognosis for infiltrating lobular carcinoma compared to ductal cancer (160), several studies have found no significant difference in survival of infiltrating duct and lobular carcinomas (140,144,173). When differences are observed, they are not substantial; about 6% of women with $T_1N_0M_0$ infiltrating lobular carcinomas treated by mastectomy died of their disease within ten years, compared to 14% of those with infiltrating ductal carcinoma (59). In Haagensen's experience (155), following radical mastectomy, women with Columbia Stage A infiltrating small cell carcinomas had a 75% probability of ten-year survival, compared to 72% for patients with all other types of breast carcinoma.

When the classic pattern is separated from the variants, a better disease-free interval has been noted for patients with stage I infiltrating lobular carcinoma, compared to women with the other patterns

(145,147). It has been reported that the variants may have a less favorable prognosis (147), but this needs to be confirmed in larger series. Variable extents of the lesions, and variations in the extent of the surgical treatment in the reported cases, weakens the conclusions. Unfortunately, the TNM stage is not provided in most studies, making comparison and analysis of the data difficult.

As mentioned before, the incidence of bilaterality is high for all types of infiltrating lobular carcinoma. The prognosis of the patient is unaffected, however, unless the tumors are synchronous (146,147).

## TUBULAR CARCINOMA

Tubular (well-differentiated) carcinoma, a distinctive variant of mammary carcinoma characterized by a deceptively bland appearance that continues to cause diagnostic problems, was recognized more than a 100 years ago (188). The term "tubular" refers to the distinctive microscopic feature of this tumor noted for a haphazard proliferation of angulated tubules separated from each other by a reactive, fibroblastic stroma. The tubules display open lumens and are lined by a single layer of epithelial cells. In order to qualify as tubular carcinoma, most authors require that a minimum of 75% of the lesion display this morphology (184,187,189,202,203,206), but I would insist on a 100% pure tubular arrangement for this diagnosis.

Considered a rare lesion in earlier reports, the increasing use of mammography and detection of smaller carcinomas have resulted in a dramatic increase in the frequency of tubular carcinomas (182). The reported incidence for the pure variant of tubular carcinoma ranges from 0.4% to 8% (181,184–186,199, 205,206,210), while a higher frequency of 2% to 21.2% has been noted for the mixed variety (181,184–186,199,205,206,209,210). The size of the tumor seems to be decreasing in more recent reports apparently due to mammographic detection of smaller tumors. Rosen et al (207) noted that tubular carcinoma accounts for 9% of carcinomas 1.0 cm or less in diameter. In another study, about 8% of mammographically-detected invasive carcinomas 1 cm or less in size were tubular carcinoma (183).

### Clinical Features

Tubular carcinoma occurs predominantly in women, though it has also been reported in the male breast (208). Patients with pure tubular carcinoma tend to be slightly younger than those with the mixed tubular carcinomas and regular infiltrating carcinomas (184, 185,189,206). They range in age from 23 to 87, with a median age of around 50 (184–186,189,195,202,203, 206). Most patients present with a palpable lesion; in one large series of 135 cases, 80% of the masses were discovered by the patient (202). In about 15% of the women, tumor fixation to the overlying skin and retraction occur (206). Multicentricity has been reported in up to 28% of the cases (199,203). Bilaterality has been observed in 12% to 38% of the pure and mixed varieties, compared to a 4.3% incidence of bilaterality in controls (185,187,199,203,206,208). A positive family history of carcinoma has been reported in 40% of patients with tubular carcinoma (199).

### Macroscopic Features

Tubular carcinomas range in size from 0.2 to 12 cm. In Haagensen's series (195), the mean size of pure (100%) tubular carcinomas was less than 2 cm, while the mean size of tumors with a 5% to 99% tubular component was over 2 cm. In some of the more recent series (202,203), a majority of the pure tumors (80% or more) have been 1 cm or less in diameter, while 52% of mixed tubular carcinomas were 1 cm or less in diameter. The cut surface (Fig. 9.13) of the tumor varies significantly from lesions displaying a stellate or scirrhous appearance to smaller ones that merely display areas of gray-white to chalky discoloration with induration and retraction.

### Microscopic Features

Microscopically, tubular carcinoma is characterized by a haphazard proliferation of angulated, oval, or elongated tubules within a reactive-appearing, fibroblastic stroma (Fig. 9.14). The tubules have open

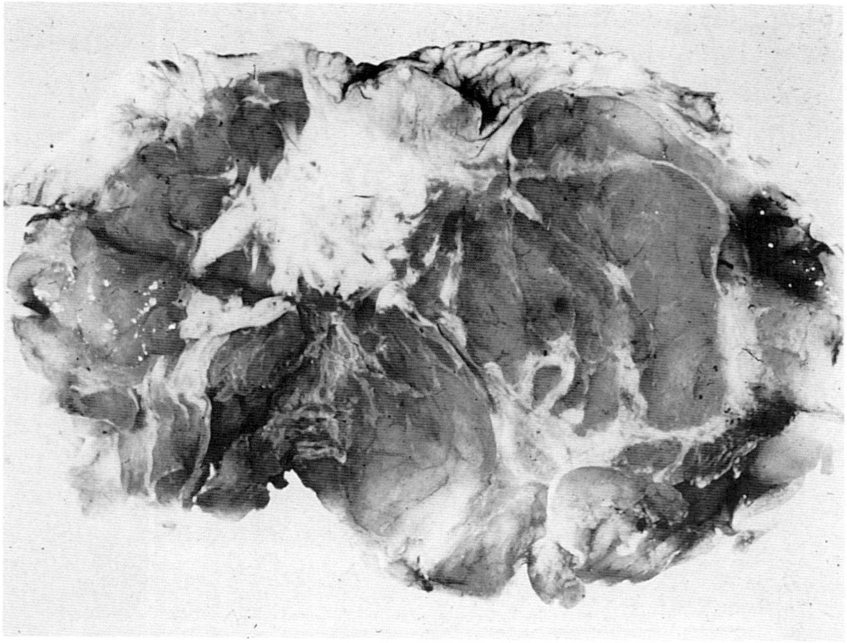

**Figure 9.13** Tubular carcinoma. When large enough to be grossly apparent, it does not look much different from a regular infiltrating duct carcinoma.

lumens and are lined by a single layer of epithelial cells (Fig. 9.15), and may extend into adipose tissue as well as around normal mammary structures. In general, the epithelial cells do not display significant atypia, and mitotic activity is rare. Apical snouts are observed in about a third of the cases. Calcification is present in half of the cases, either within the lumens of the neoplastic tubules or within the stroma. An intraductal carcinoma is evident in about 65% of the cases; a majority of the intraductal carcinomas are of the non-necrotic cribriform and micropapillary types (202). Lobular neoplasia is present in close proximity of the tumor in approximately 15% (range of 0.7% to 40%) (Fig. 9.16) of the cases (181,189,192,202,203). Perineural invasion does occur, but is not common. The stroma is most often reactive and fibroblastic in nature, but sometimes it is densely collagenous and even elastotic (211).

When the entire lesion is composed of tubules, the lesion qualifies as a pure tubular carcinoma. The lesion is referred to as a mixed tubular carcinoma when a minor component of the lesion consists of other types of infiltrating carcinoma; the second component is generally an infiltrating duct carcinoma. Opinions vary regarding the maximum proportion of the second type of carcinoma allowed to qualify the lesion as a mixed tubular carcinoma. While some have required less than 50% of regular infiltrating duct carcinoma for this designation, others allow less than 25% of a second type of carcinoma for a designation of mixed tubular carcinoma.

To determine the influence of the various proportions on patients' survival, Carsten et al (185), compared the long-term survival of patients with pure tubular carcinoma (carcinomas lacking any other pattern of invasive carcinoma) to that of patients having infiltrating duct carcinoma with a major tubular component (tubular component of 50% to 75%); patients with regular infiltrating duct carcinoma were used as controls for the two groups. The five, ten, and 20-year survival of women with tubular carcinoma far exceeded that of women from other groups. There was no significant difference in the survival of women with regular infiltrating duct carcinoma and those with a major tubular component. Therefore, Carsten et al (185) proposed to set 75% tubular carcinoma as a reasonable cut-off point for the mixed type of tubular carcinoma. Based on their approach, a pure tubular carcinoma is 100% tubular, a mixed tubular carcinoma is 75% or more tubular, an infiltrating duct carcinoma with a major tubular component is 50% to 74% tubular, and a regular infiltrating duct carcinoma may be up to 49% tubular in growth pattern. Since they found no significant difference in the survival of the latter two groups, there is no reason to distinguish them.

I also prefer Carstens cut-off point of 75% tubular for designating a lesion as a mixed tubular carcinoma.

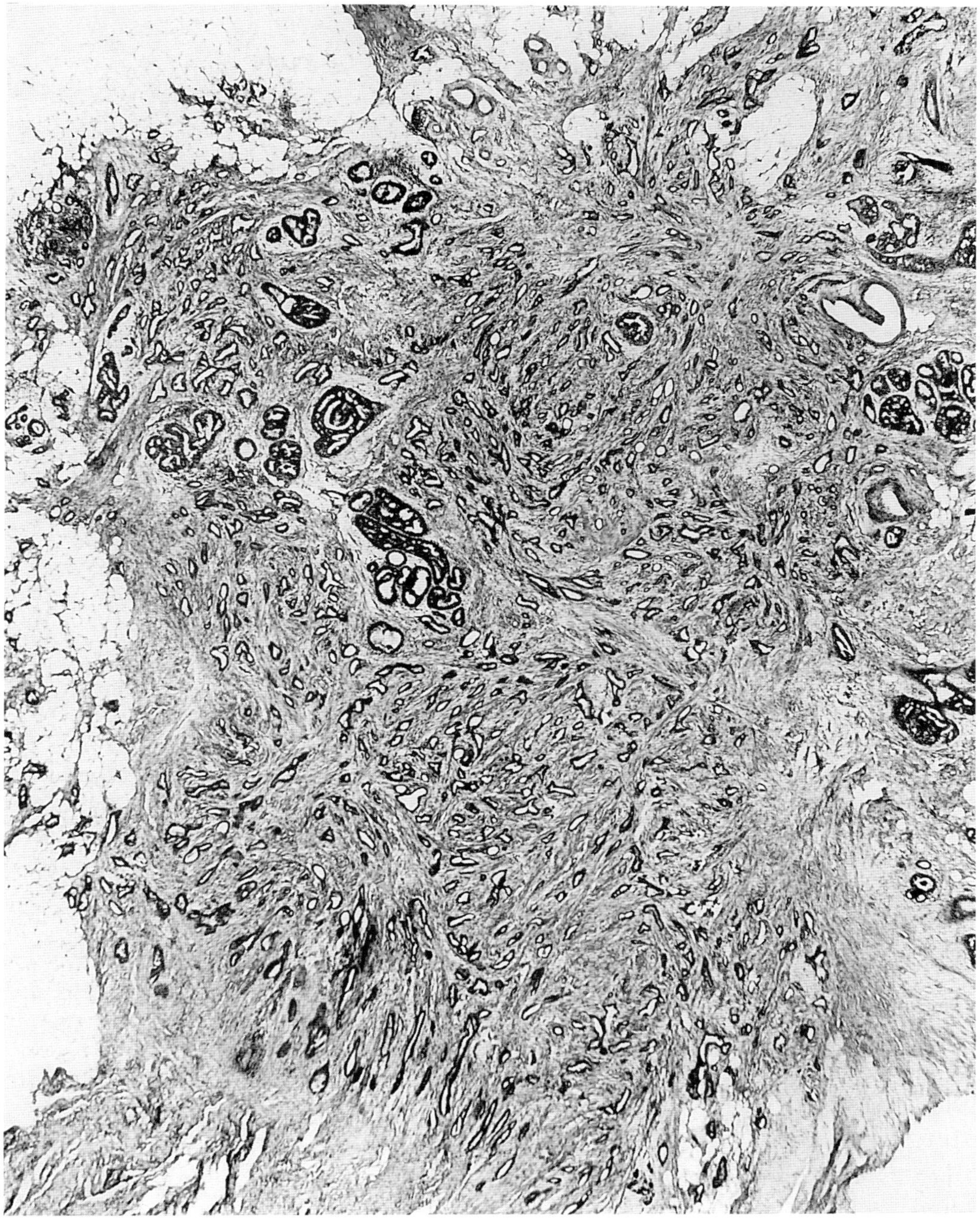

**Figure 9.14** Tubular carcinoma is characterized by a haphazard proliferation of tubules in a reactive-appearing fibroblastic stroma (H&E, X70)

## Differential Diagnosis

Lesions that can be mistaken for tubular carcinoma include sclerosing adenosis, microglandular adenosis and radial scar. The important features that can help distinguish tubular carcinoma from sclerosing adenosis and microglandular adenosis are tabulated in the section on microglandular adenosis in Chapter 4. Tubular carcinoma displays a haphazardous growth pattern in contrast to the lobulated outline of sclerosing adenosis. The tubules in tubular carcinoma are angulated or ovoid with open lumens and are lined by a single layer of epithelial cells, while the tubules in sclerosing adenosis are angulated with compressed lumens or round with practically obliterated lumens, and are lined by both epithelial and myoepithelial cells. A uniform layer of basement membrane can be demonstrated around the tubules of sclerosing adenosis using a PAS stain, while a basement membrane is either completely absent or present in a patchy fashion around the tubules of tubular carcinoma

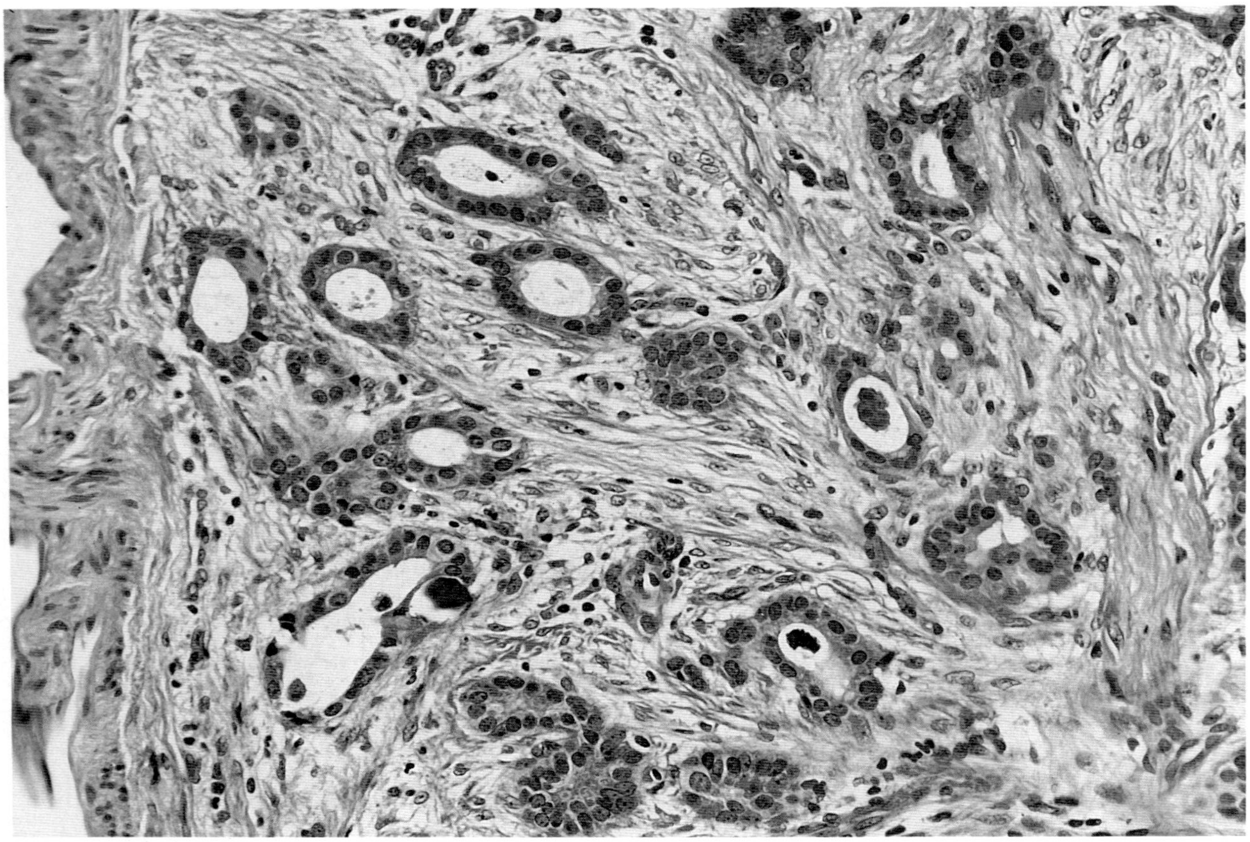

**Figure 9.15** Tubular carcinoma. The tubules have open lumen and are lined by a single line of epithelial cells. Calcification is rarely seen within the lumen and extending into the adjacent stroma. (H&E, X400)

(190,193). The minimal stroma in sclerosing adenosis is sclerotic in contrast to the fibroblastic, cellular stroma of tubular carcinoma.

In comparison with tubular carcinoma, the tubules in microglandular adenosis are rounded, with open lumens containing a colloid-like secretory material. The tubules are lined by a single layer of clear, or vacuolated epithelial cells. A myoepithelial cell layer is absent, but there is a multilayered basement membrane. The associated stroma is densely collagenous.

A radial scar has a stellate appearance, but the tubules entrapped in the collagenous or elastotic stroma are lined by both epithelial and myoepithelial cells. Linell et al proposed that radial scar reflects stage 0 of tubular carcinoma, and as tubular carcinoma progresses, it develops features of ordinary infiltrating duct carcinoma (200,201). Opinions regarding this proposal vary and at this time it has not been established that such a progression occurs in all, or even some, cases of tubular carcinoma (181,200, 212).

## Ultrastructural Features

Electron microscopy has confirmed the presence of only a single layer of epithelial cells lining the tubules in tubular carcinoma or the absence of the myoepithelial cell layer, as well as the complete absence or at most the presence of a patchy basement membrane around the tubules (191,196,198).

## Axillary Node Metastases and Recurrences

The reported incidence of axillary node metastases varies from 0% to 25%; the metastatic foci retain their tubular pattern. Tubular carcinoma rarely involves more than three low axillary nodes. None of the carcinomas with 76% to 100% tubular pattern in Haagensen's series metastasized (195). Only 1.4% of tubular carcinomas less than 1 cm in diameter display axillary nodal metastases, and none develop recur-

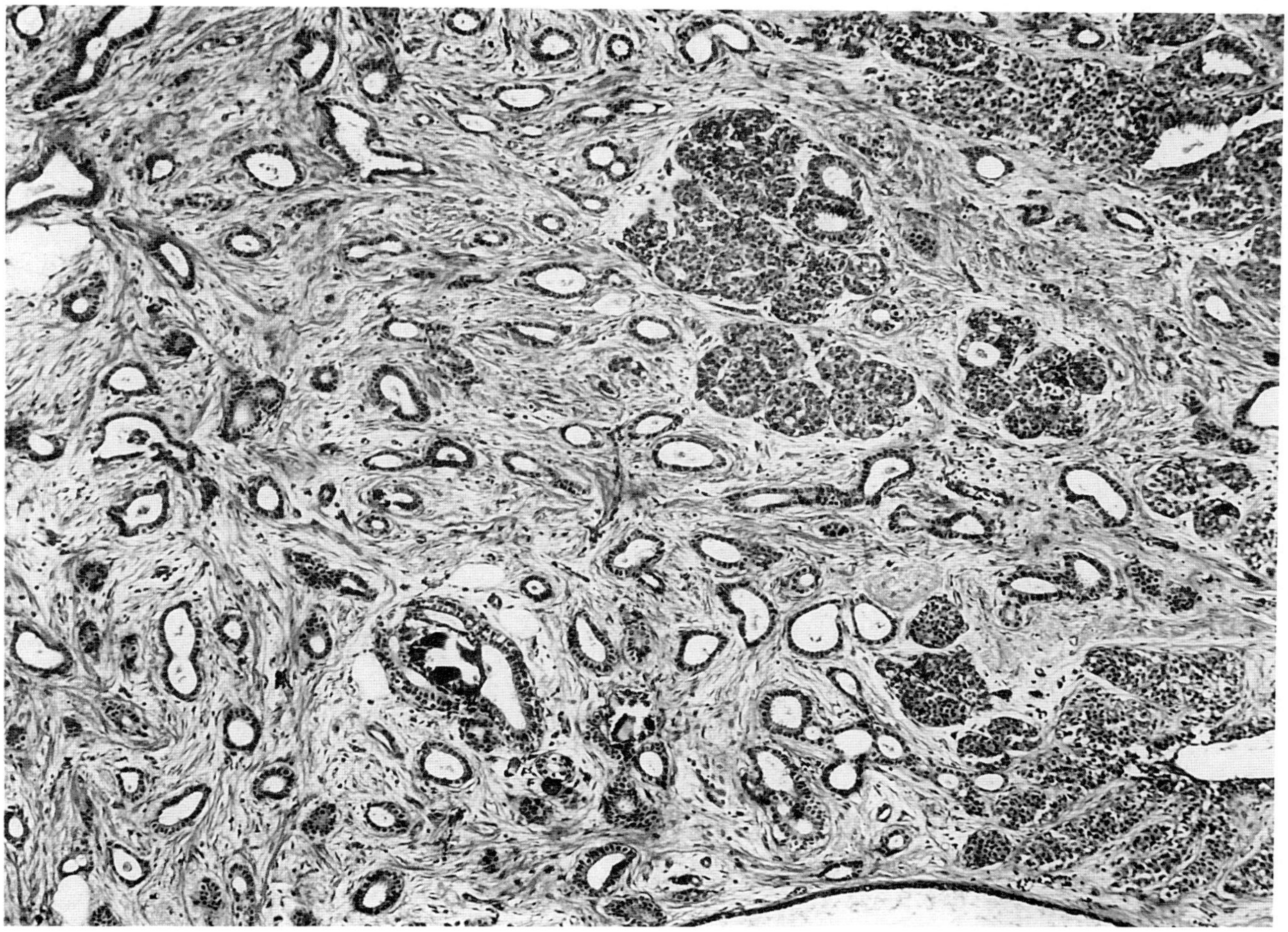

**Figure 9.16** Tubular carcinoma. Lobular carcinoma is present in association with this tumor in around 15% of cases. (H&E, X150)

rences or metastases within a five-year period after the diagnosis (202). In comparison, 21% to 29% of the mixed variety metastasizes (184,189). The latter is comparable to the 22% of a variety of carcinomas less than 1 cm that display axillary node metastases at the time of diagnosis; 8.4% of these women develop recurrences and metastases within five years (192). When size limits are removed, about 3.5% to 10.8% of patients with pure tubular carcinoma develop recurrences or metastases (167,202), compared to 52% of those without a tubular pattern (200). Recurrences and metastases are more likely to develop among women who have axillary node involvement; 25% of the women with axillary node metastases developed subsequent recurrence or died of the disease (202).

About 8% to 20% of women with tubular carcinoma develop metastases, compared to 50% to 60% of women with carcinoma in general (184,188,210).

When mixed tubular carcinomas of all sizes and various reported proportions are considered, about 21% to 29% of the patients have axillary node metastasis. Among women with the mixed variant, about 32% develop recurrences, and 6% to 28% die from the disease (167).

## Treatment and Survival

In view of the generally small size of the tumor and rarity of axillary node metastases, tubular carcinomas are ideally suited for conservative treatment. A majority of reported cases of tubular carcinoma (pure or mixed) have been treated with mastectomy, however. Even as recently as 1985 in a report from Denmark (185), simple mastectomy with optional postoperative radiation was the most common treatment, while modified radical mastectomy was the preferred option when there were clinically suspicious nodes. Since the option of lumpectomy with postoperative radiation is now offered as an equivalent of mastectomy in the treatment of stage I and II breast carcinomas, a large proportion of tubular carcinomas will be ideally suited for this option considering their small size and rarity of axillary node metastases.

The survival rate of tubular carcinoma far exceeds that of regular infiltrating duct carcinomas. Even the mixed tubular carcinomas have a better prognosis compared to regular infiltrating carcinomas, but their prognosis is not as favorable as that of the pure variety (187,204,206). Recurrences develop in less than 5% of pure tubular carcinomas, and may appear within months or up to 22 years after the treatment, but 32% of the patients with the mixed variety develop recurrences, and up to 28% die from their carcinoma (187,189,206). Death from pure tubular carcinoma is a rare event. In Denmark (185), the five-, ten-, and 20-year survival rates for pure tubular carcinoma were reported as 97.3%, 87.8%, and 77.3% respectively, compared to 44.8%, 32.6%, and 19.8% for regular infiltrating duct carcinomas. Cooper et al (187) reported a 100% 15-year survival rate for pure tubular carcinoma even with metastases, compared to 72% for the mixed type, and 33% for regular infiltrating duct carcinoma; the frequency of nodal metastases was 8%, 21%, and 67% in the three groups, respectively.

Recognition of tubular carcinoma is important because of the significantly better prognosis associated with this tumor when present in the pure form or the mixed variant.

## MUCINOUS (COLLOID) CARCINOMA

Mucinous (colloid) carcinoma, is defined here as a carcinoma that contains large amounts of extracellular mucus lakes in direct contact with the stroma, populated by clusters of tumor cell, and displaying a gelatinous gross appearance. The neoplastic cells seem to produce the mucus predominantly for the purpose of export to the extracellular spaces, as they are either completely devoid of, or contain only minimal amounts of, intracellular mucin. Rarely, however, a few signet-ring cell clusters are observed. Descriptions of colloid carcinoma were recorded in the 19th century by Robinson in 1852 (251), Larrey in 1853 (240), and Lange in 1896 (239). Subsequently, Gaabe (226) further elaborated regarding the better prognosis of mucinous carcinoma. These early descriptions questioned whether the mucus was epithelial or stromal in origin. Production of the mucin by the epithelial cells was eventually well-established at the ultrastructural level (257). Cheatle and Geschikter provided additional accounts of this tumor in the 1930s (219,228). In the numerous reports since then it has also been referred to by the alternate designations of gelatinous, mucoid, and mucin-producing carcinoma. None of these terms is quite satisfactory for this tumor as some refer to the macroscopic appearance of the lesion, while others would be equally appropriate for a variety of other mucin-producing carcinomas such as the signet-ring cell and secretory carcinomas; signet-ring cell carcinomas do not qualify as colloid carcinoma because of the lack of extracellular mucin.

The better prognosis of mucinous carcinoma was recognized as early as 1908 (226), and it has since been regarded as a low grade variant of mammary carcinoma.

### Clinical Features

Mucinous carcinoma constitutes about 1% to 6% of all breast carcinomas (215,225,241,243,244,255,260). The location of the tumor in the breast does not differ significantly from that of women with breast carcinoma in general. Rarely, nipple protrusion and a sensation of "swish" at the time of palpation have been recorded as distinctive signs of mucinous carcinoma (231). The tumor may adhere to the overlying skin. In some reports the median or mean age of patients with colloid carcinoma is over 60 years, and older than that of regular infiltrating carcinomas (220,248–250,255). In other reports a younger age or even no significant age difference (243,246) has been reported. Comparing breast carcinomas at extremes of age, Rosen et al (57) noted that colloid carcinomas account for 7% of the carcinomas in women older than 75 years of age, and only for 1% of cancers in those less than 35 years at the time of diagnosis.

### Macroscopic Features

Colloid carcinoma is noted for its gelatinous, glistening appearance and soft consistency. The consistency of the tumor varies with the degree of cellularity and the amount of extracellular mucin. The tumors vary in size from 0.5 cm to a massive 20 cm, but the average size is around 2.8 cm. The margins appear bosselated and pushing, rather than infiltrating.

## Microscopic Features

The typical colloid carcinoma displays small clusters of uniform, round cells with minimal amounts of eosinophilic cytoplasm floating in abundant lakes of mucus (Fig. 9.17). While some of these tumors appear very well-defined in their outline, others show smaller lakes of mucus-containing nests of tumor cells separated from the tumor mass by uninvolved breast tissue. These are probably irregular extensions of the tumor or, less likely, they may reflect multifocality. This finding is noted most often in cases where an in situ component is evident. It appears as if some of these foci reflect early disruption of the duct wall containing in situ carcinoma and spilling of the luminal mucinous material into the surrounding stroma. The cell clusters floating in the mucus lakes may be solid, form secondary lumen, or appear papillary. In general, they consist of a uniform population of small round cells (Fig. 9.18), but atypia, mitotic figures and signet-ring forms also occur. Calcification is rare, but does occur in association with the papillary pattern in particular. An in situ component is present in approximately 15% of the cases in the immediate vicinity of the tumor (Fig. 9.19). Intraductal carcinoma is observed more frequently in association with the cellular variant, and its argyrophilia may be similar to that of the invasive component. Delicate bands of fibrovascular connective tissue may be evident within the mucus lakes and may provide connections between the nests of tumor cells. Both neutral and acidic mucopolysaccharides have been detected in these tumors (257,259), while sulfated mucins are also present in infiltrating lobular and ductal carcinomas (232).

In 1963, carcinoid-like features were noted in two examples of colloid carcinoma by Feyrter (224). Subsequently, Capella et al (218) proposed subdivision of the pure mucinous carcinomas into two groups. Group A lesions are hypocellular with minimal intracellular mucin and no argyrophilic granules. Group B tumors are more cellular, with more intracytoplasmic mucin and are argyrophilic. Coady et al (221) have also suggested demonstration of argyrophilic granules in tumor cells as the basis for distinguishing two subtypes of pure mucinous carcinoma. The nonargyrophilic tumors were also devoid of S-100 protein, whereas, the argyrophilic lesions were S-100 positive. Ferguson et al (223) had difficulty utilizing this classification. In a review of 202 tumors, Rasmussen et al (250) found argyrophilic granules in 25% of the tumors; they found no significant morphologic or clinical difference between tumors containing neuroendocrine (NE) granules and those without them. Using immunostains for chromogranin, I have found that there is a great variation in the intracytoplasmic mucin and neuroendocrine granule content of the cells regardless of the degree of cellularity; either hypo or hypercellular variants may contain neuroendocrine granules, but not all hypercellular tumors display neuroendocrine granules.

Traditionally, a pure and mixed (Fig. 9.20) variant of mucinous carcinoma has been recognized. A regular infiltrating duct carcinoma is the most common tumor associated with the colloid pattern in the mixed tumors. It is of utmost importance to adhere to stringent criteria for separating the pure form from the mixed type because of the favorable prognosis of the pure variant. Silverberg et al (255) consider a carcinoma as mucinous only if it has at least 50% extracellular mucin. With the increasing number of cases reported, the pure form is further subdivided into hypocellular and hypercellular. Even the hypercellular variety should show separation of the clusters of cells from the surrounding stroma by extracellular mucus.

## Hormone Receptors and Ploidy

Estrogen receptor positivity has been reported in 43% to 75% of mucinous carcinomas (39,43,58). About 14% of the tumors are PR+ (43). Using paraffin-embedded archival tissues, the DNA stemline of colloid carcinoma has been found to be diploid in 25 of 26 pure colloid carcinomas, compared to over 50% (11 of 19 cases) aneuploid for the mixed variety (258); the latter is similar to infiltrating duct carcinoma which has been noted to be abnormal in 60% to 80% of cases.

A

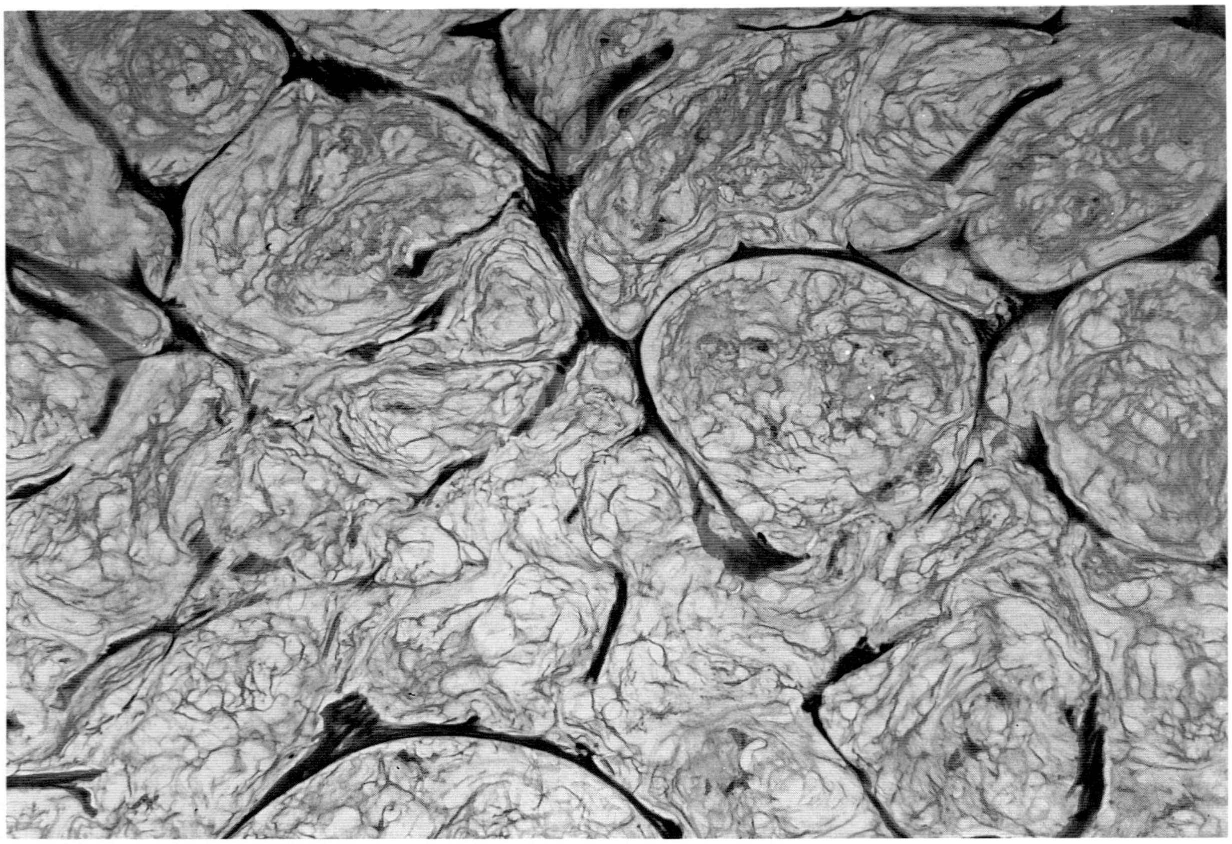

B

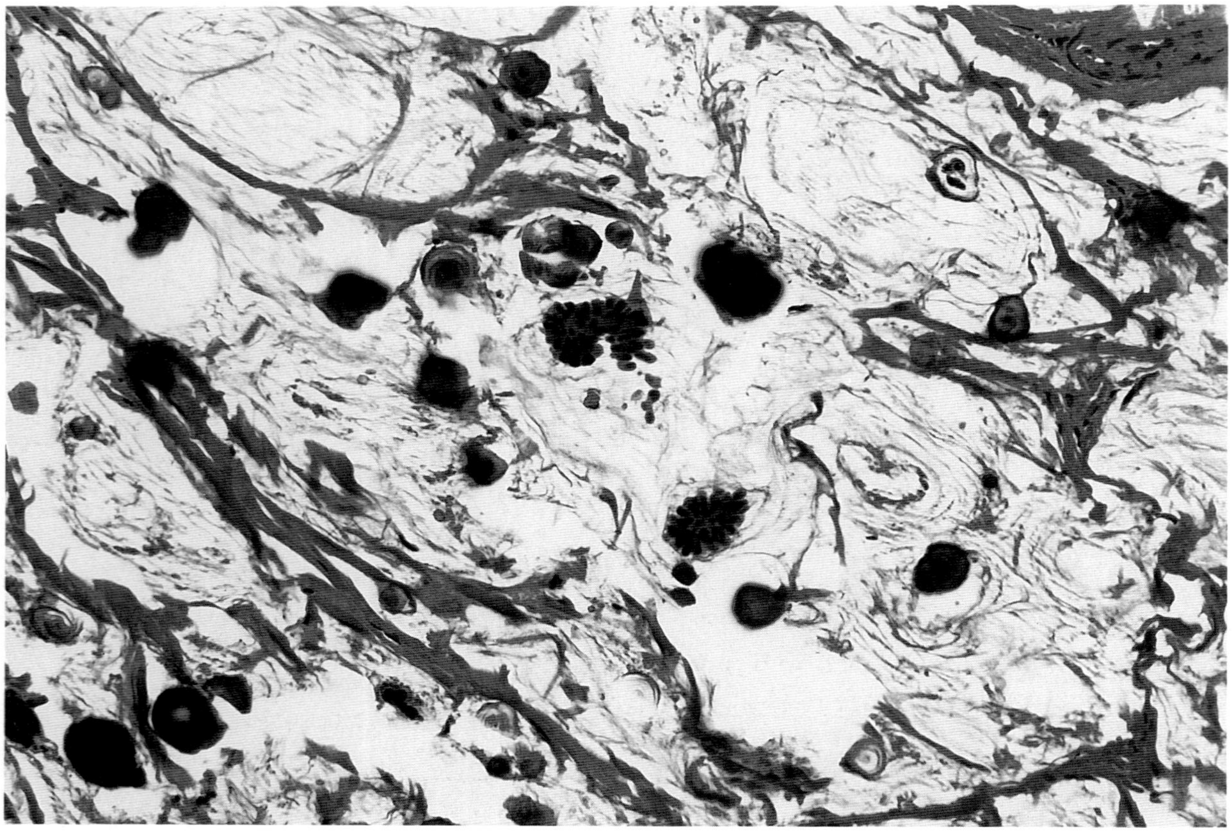

**Figure 9.17(a,b)** Colloid carcinoma. (a) Hypocellular variant. The almost complete absence of epithelial cells in the lakes of mucus and the septated organization had led to initial misinterpretation of this lesion as a myxoid fibroadenoma. (H&E, X150). (b) Hypocellular variant with only a few small cell clusters floating in the mucus lakes along with microcalcification. (H&E, X200)

C

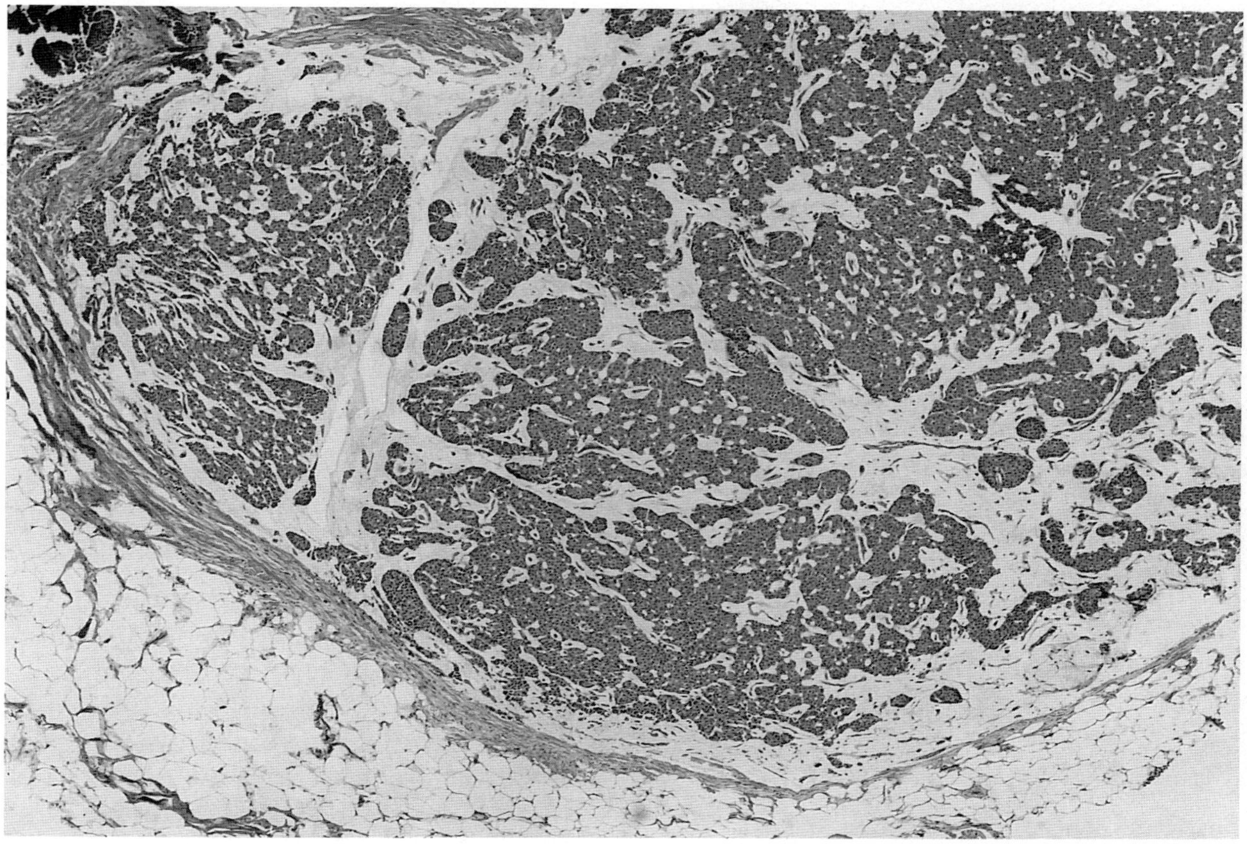

**Figure 9.17(c)** Colloid carcinoma. Cellular type with abundant neoplastic cell clusters surrounded by mucus. (H&E, X60)

## Ultrastructural Features

At the ultrastructural level, tightly-packed clusters of cells show microvillous cytoplasmic processes, mucin vacuoles, round to pleomorphic dense core granules, and aggregates of intracytoplasmic filaments (225,235, 236). Most of the mucin is extracellular, and intracytoplasmic lumens are quite rare.

## Differential Diagnosis

Colloid carcinoma should be distinguished from the rare mucocele (216,253) and myxoid fibroadenomas. I have seen examples of both of these lesions misinterpreted as colloid carcinoma.

Mucus lakes are occasionally seen in association with fibrocystic changes and reflect a ruptured cyst which, instead of the usual granular eosinophilic secretory material, contained mucus secretion (Fig. 9.21). These mucus lakes often contain no cells, and rarely exceed 2 to 3 mm in maximum diameter. There are, however, larger mucus lakes produced by the rupture of several adjacent ducts which may even contain strips of epithelium floating within them. These mucoceles can be distinguished from the hypocellular variants of mucinous carcinoma by the type of epithelial cells in the lakes. The strips of epithelium within these lakes reflects the epithelial lining of the disrupted duct. The epithelium may have been hyperplastic, and therefore may present as nests of cells. Invariably, however, in some of these nests, the myoepithelial cell layer is readily apparent even on H&E sections. If the myoepithelial cell layer is hard to discern on the H&E sections, immunostain for actin is extremely helpful. Often the presence of adjacent ducts in different stages of distension and disruption is a most helpful clue to the benign nature of the mucoceles. In general, if a lake of mucus material is less than 5 mm, is multifocal but each focus is less than 5 mm, or contains epithelial and myoepithelial cells in the cell floats, then it is regarded as a benign lesion.

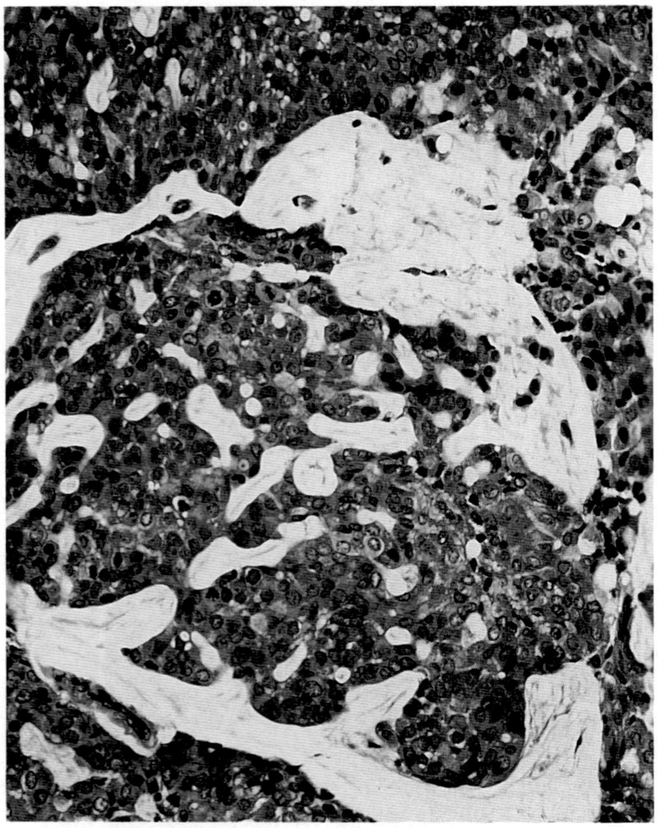

**Figure 9.18** Colloid carcinoma. The cells are uniform and lack significant atypia. (H&E, X240)

The myxoid fibroadenomas that have significant myxoid change can be mistaken for a colloid carcinoma both grossly and microscopically. The presence of attenuated layers of epithelial and myoepithelial cells lining compressed spaces, loose fibroblasts and myofibroblasts, and mast cells help distinguish the two.

## Axillary Node Involvement

The incidence of axillary node metastases varies significantly in various reports because of the lack of a delineation between pure and the mixed tumors in some of the older series. The incidence of nodal metastases dropped from a range of 28% to 36% in the older series (241,243,244,251,255,260) to a low of 4% in series applying stringent criteria for interpretation of the pure form (246). In studies comparing the incidence of nodal metastases in the pure and mixed variants, 3.1% to 15% of the pure variety showed axillary node metastases, compared to 33% to 46% of the mixed group (230,237,248).

Haagensen (230) noted axillary metastases in 11%, 33%, and 88% of patients with "mucoid carcinoma" in Columbia Stages A, B, and C&D (combined), respectively. In comparison, 31%, 72%, and 82% of women having all types of carcinoma had axillary node metastases in the same three groups, respectively. Unfortunately, Haagensen (230) included signet-ring cell carcinoma and secretory carcinoma in the category of mucoid carcinomas making it impossible to compare his findings with any other series.

## Clinical Behavior

Compared to the ordinary infiltrating breast carcinomas, mucinous carcinoma has been reported to have a far better short-term prognosis (213). In Norris and Taylor's series (246), 10% of the patients with pure mucinous carcinoma died from their tumors, whereas 29% of the patients with the mixed variant did so, but the follow-up did not exceed ten years in this study. With longer follow-up periods, nearly half of 41 women with pure mucinous carcinoma in one report (252) died from metastatic tumor 12 years or more after the diagnosis. Comparing the survival of the pure and mixed variants, Komaki et al (237) also reported a ten-year survival of 90.4% for pure colloid carcinoma, dropping to 83% at 20 years; the ten-year survival for the mixed group was 66%. At another institution, six of 15 women with mucinous carcinoma died of metastatic tumor 10 to 22 years after mastectomy (247). With an average follow-up of 15 years and up to 37 years, Clayton (220) reported a long-term survival of 68% excluding non-tumor related deaths. Haagensen (230) expressed the probability of survival of women with Columbia Stage A mucoid carcinoma (inclusive of colloid, secretory, and signet-ring cell carcinoma) as 83% compared to 80% for a series of women with all types of breast carcinoma. For stage B tumors, the probability of survival at ten years was 50% both for the women with mucoid carcinoma and those in the series with all types of breast carcinoma.

Factors that have been related to a more aggressive behavior include tumor cellularity, large size, and presence of axillary node metastases. All ten fatal cases in Clayton's series (220) were at least 2.5 cm, and had more than 10% cellularity. Four of the

A

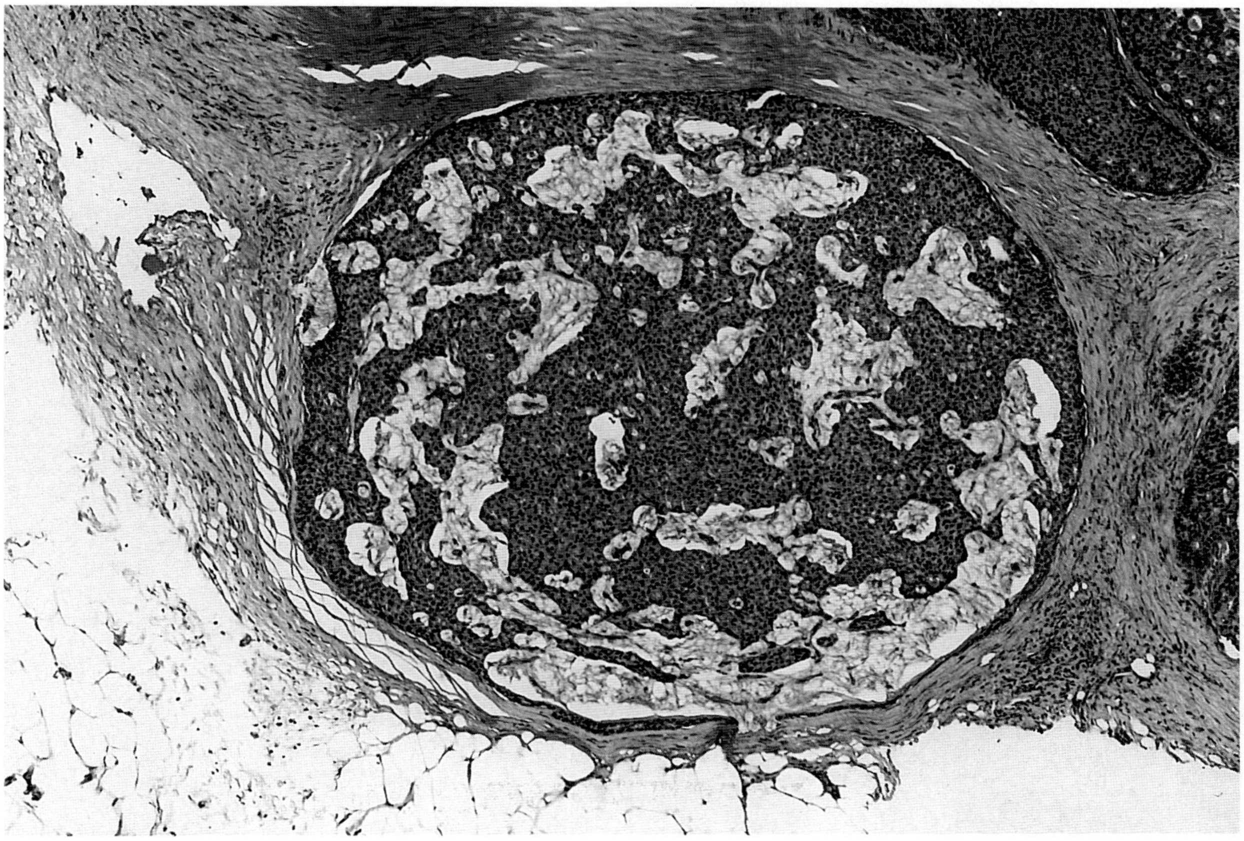

B

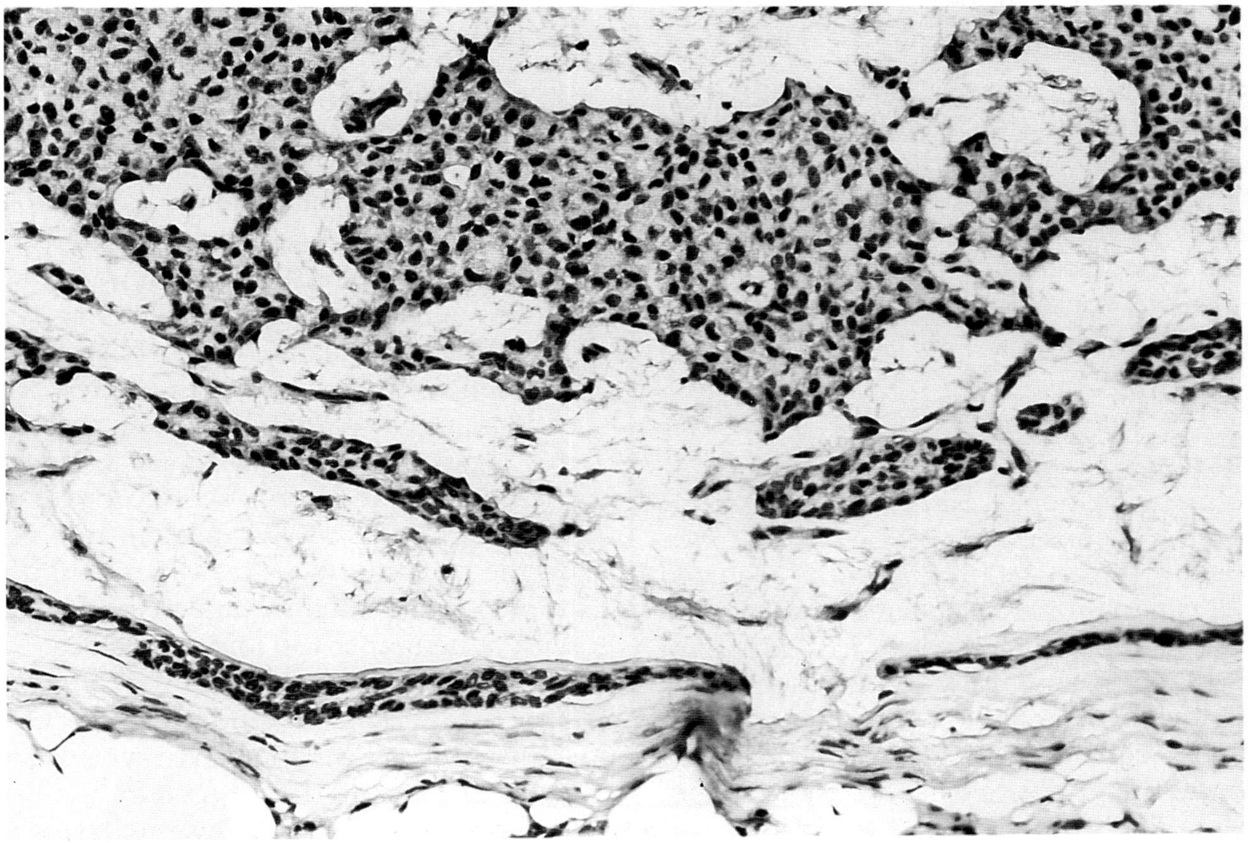

**Figure 9.19(a,b)** Intraductal colloid carcinoma. (a) There is a suggestion of early disruption of the duct wall. H&E, X120) (b) Higher magnification showing a break in the duct wall with mucous escaping through the opening. (H&E, X400)

C

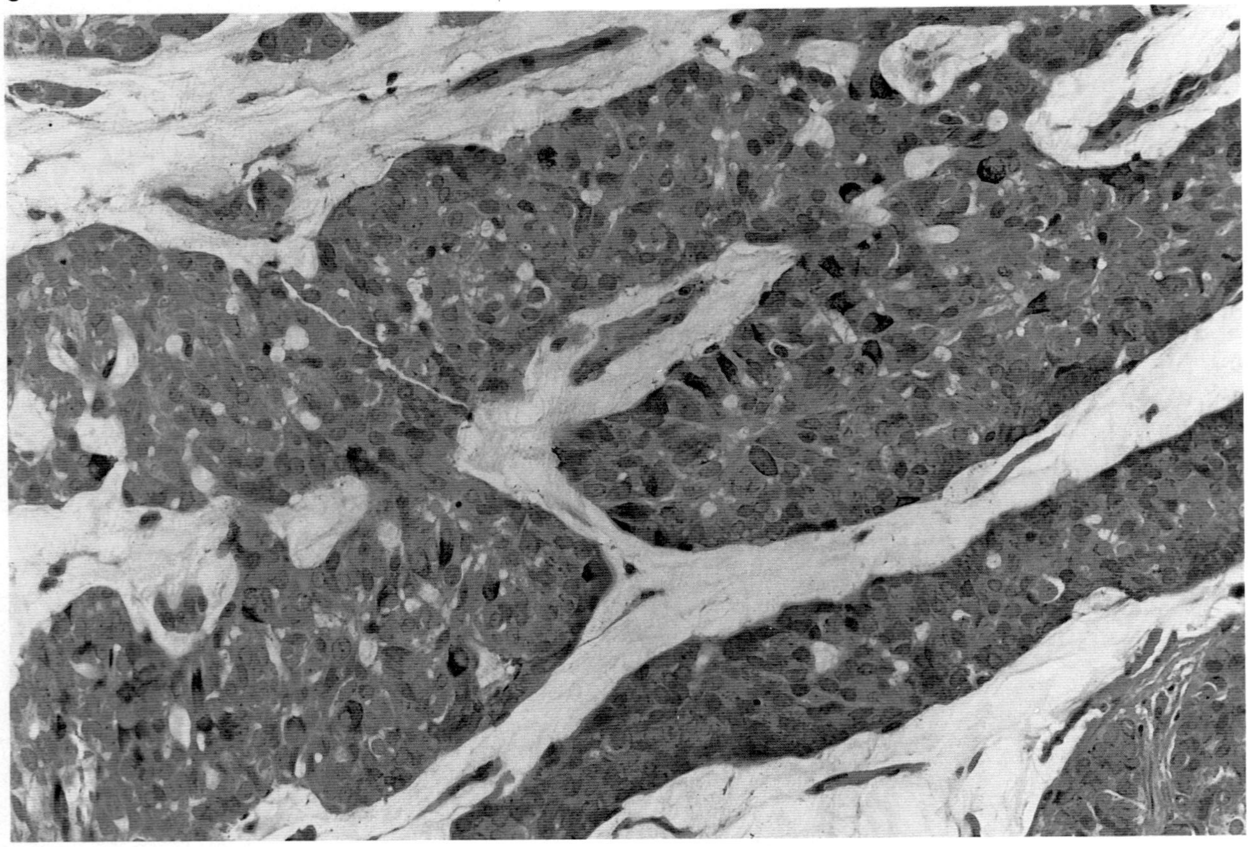

**Figure 9.19(c)** Intraductal colloid carcinoma. A Churukian-Schenk stain shows intracytoplasmic neuroendocrine granules. (X600)

women with disseminated disease had nodal metastases in contrast to one of the 27 long-term survivors (women free of cancer for more than ten years after the diagnosis).

An unusual pattern of metastases with mucin embolization to the cerebral arteries has been reported as a rare fatal complication of mucinous carcinoma (222,259).

## SIGNET-RING CELL CARCINOMA

The World Health Organization has not recognized signet-ring cell carcinoma as a specific entity. Signet-ring cell carcinoma has been described as a variant of infiltrating lobular carcinoma (217,227,256) as well as a subtype of mucinous carcinoma (243,254). While a high proportion of signet-ring cell carcinomas may be lobular in nature, the presence of intraductal carcinomas of the solid or cribriform types composed in part or in entirety of signet-ring type cells as well the presence of an admixture of signet-ring cells with typical infiltrating duct carcinomas indicate that signet-ring cell carcinomas may assume ductal patterns as well. As mentioned earlier, signet-ring carcinoma is not a variant of mucinous or colloid carcinoma. These two lesions are not only morphologically different, but there is also a significant difference in the clinical behavior of the two lesions.

The few available reports have noted that signet-ring cell carcinoma accounts for 2% (245) to 4% (235) of all mammary carcinomas. The precise frequency of this type of carcinoma is not known. The clinical presentation and macroscopic appearance of signet-ring cell carcinoma is similar to that of regular infiltrating carcinomas with the formation of firm, solid tumors. The patients range in age from 33 to 87 years with a median of the mid to late 50s. The criteria for the diagnosis varies. Tumors composed purely of signet-ring cells are indeed rare. Only two pure signet-ring cell carcinomas in which over 90% of the cells displayed this appearance were identified among 1,050 breast cancers reviewed at Edinburgh (51). The reported series included very few pure signet-ring cell carcinomas, but have applied this

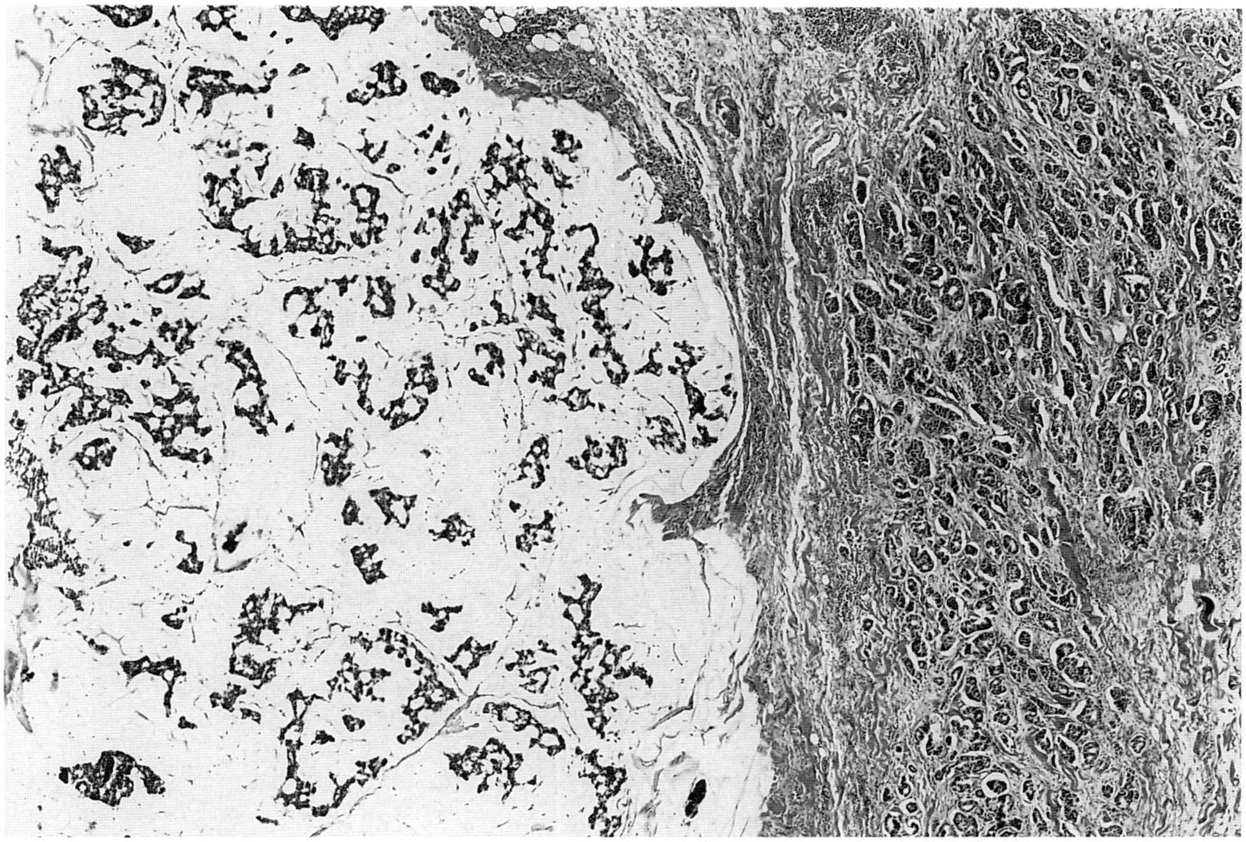

**Figure 9.20** Mixed colloid and infiltrating duct carcinoma. (H&E, X60)

designation to a variety of carcinomas ranging from lesions in which more than 20 signet-ring cells per high power field were identified in several foci, as well as lesions in which signet-ring cells composed 20% or more of the carcinoma.

Signet-ring cells should be distinguished from cells with intracytoplasmic lumens. Both can cause compression of the nucleus to a thin crescent, but the classic signet-ring cells are more likely to do so. While the secretory material may be washed out during processing, when present within intracytoplasmic lumens (ICL), it appears eosinophilic and does not completely fill the ICL. In contrast, the intracytoplasmic mucin in classic signet-ring cells resembles the secretory material in colloid carcinoma, with a clear to bluish tint on H&E stained sections. The distinction between the two cell types is not always easy. At the ultrastructural level, ICL are represented as an intracytoplasmic space with microvillous projections filled with granular secretory material. The mucin in signet-ring cells, however, is present either free within cisternae or as poorly-bound globules (214,233). Both cell types may be present within a tumor (Fig. 9.22), and breast carcinoma cells containing both types of secretory material have been reported (229). The in situ phase associated with signet-ring cell carcinoma may be lobular or ductal in type.

Analyzing the few available reports, it becomes obvious that regardless of their quantity, the presence of signet-ring cells within a carcinoma appears to impart a more aggressive behavior to the lesion.

Despite its secretory differentiation, signet-ring cell change reflects an aggressive transformation of the cells. This type of differentiation may develop in either ductal or lobular carcinomas, in situ or invasive. Because of its distinctive morphology and clinically more aggressive behavior, it should be designated as a specific variant of breast carcinoma when present in pure form. When signet-ring cells are present as a notable component of a typical infiltrating lobular (or ductal type of) carcinoma, the diagnosis should reflect the presence of signet-ring cells by stating infiltrating lobular carcinoma, with the percentage of signet-ring cell differentiation.

Recognition of the signet-ring cell component is important and it should be separated from mucinous (colloid) carcinoma (234), because it has been illustrated that carcinomas with a prominent signet-ring

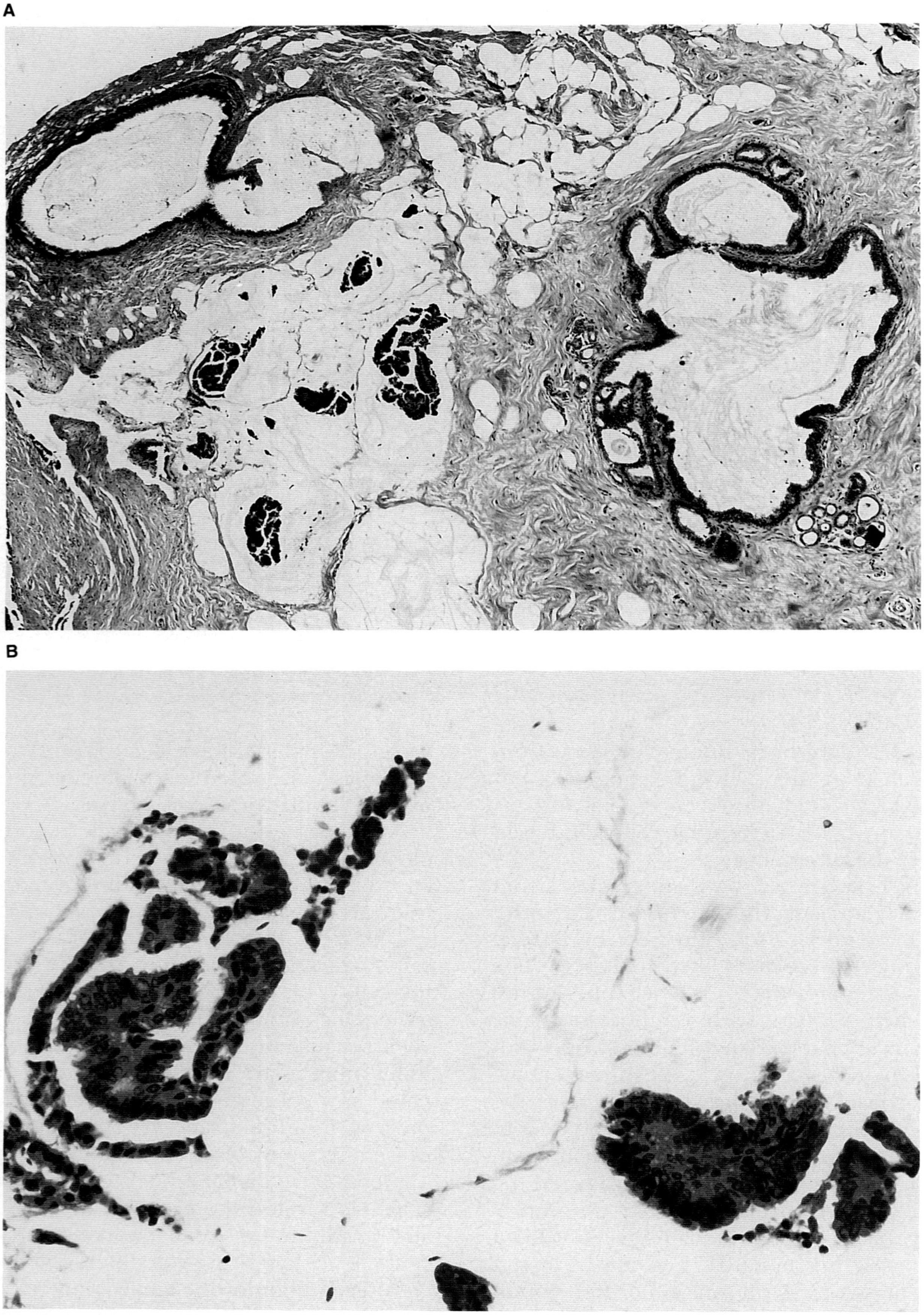


**Figure 9.21** Mucocele. (a) Several ruptured ducts with epithelial cells floating in them. (H&E, X300) (b) The presence of both epithelial and myoepithelial cells indicates a benign cell cluster. (H&E, X480)

A

B

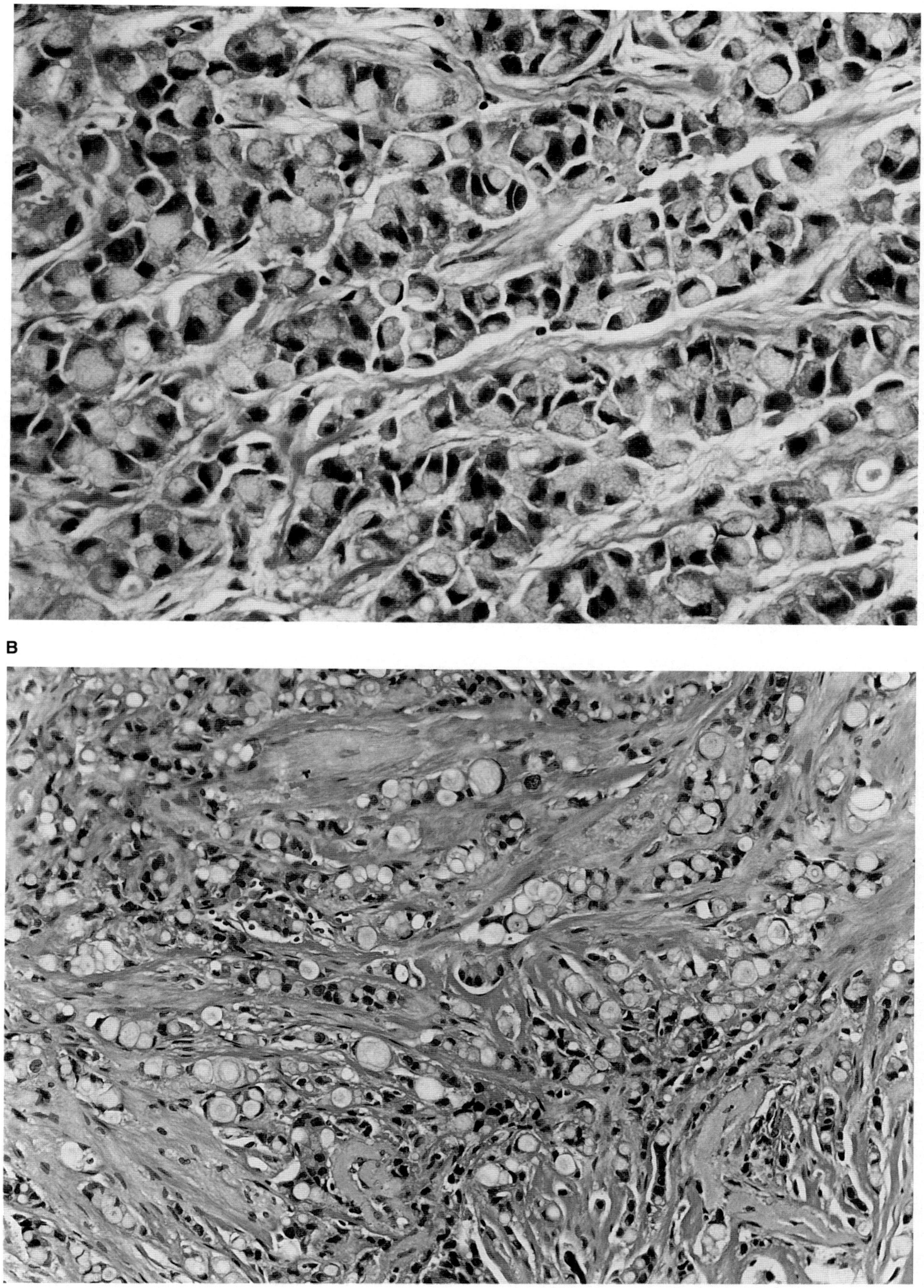

**Figure 9.22(a,b)** Signet-ring cell carcinoma. Two slightly different appearances of signet-ring cells with larger nuclei in (a), but more compressed nuclei in (b) along with a larger number of cells with targetoid secretion within intracytoplasmic lumens. (H&E, (a) X500; (b) X320)

C

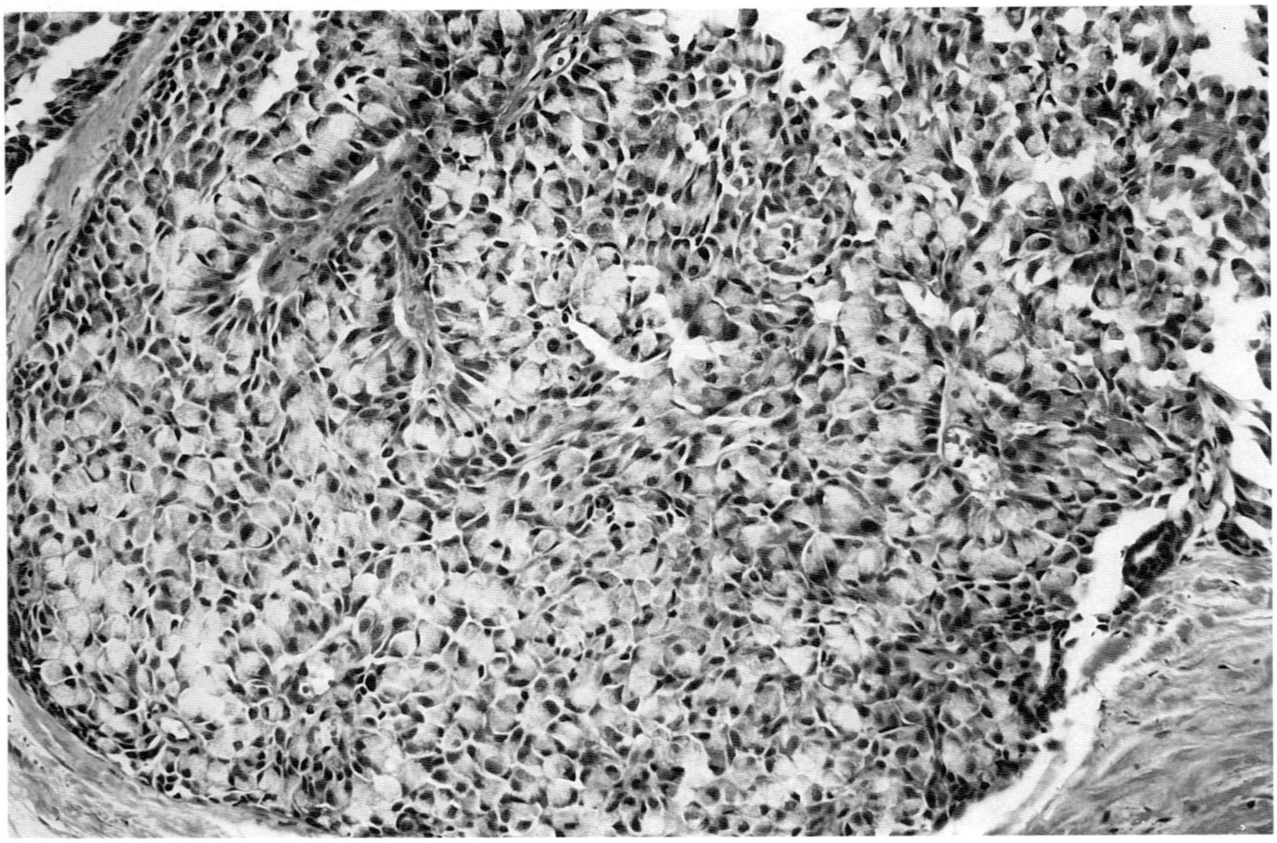

**Figure 9.22(c)** Intraductal signet-ring cell carcinoma. (H&E, X160)

cell component behave more aggressively. Furthermore, they are capable of metastasizing to unusual sites such as the bladder, stomach, and other gastrointestinal sites and serosal surfaces, where they may mimic a primary carcinoma of the organ involved (238,245).

## CARCINOMA WITH NEUROENDOCRINE DIFFERENTIATION

Feryter (224) is credited with the first description of a breast carcinoma with carcinoid features. He described two patients with colloid carcinoma. The tumor cells displayed argyrophilia and there were clinical manifestations of endocrine activity. Both tumors contained serotonin. He thought that these lesions were of myoepithelial origin since Vogler (292) had previously demonstrated argyrophilia in normal ductal cells that he interpreted as myoepithelial cells. It is now recognized that about 3% to 21% of mammary carcinomas display focal argyrophilic granules by light microscopy, and dense-core granules at the ultrastructural level (262,272,287,288,293). The tumors containing neuroendocrine (NE) granules encompass a wide range of patterns from infiltrating duct carcinoma to papillary and intraductal carcinomas. Neuroendocrine granules are not limited to female mammary carcinomas, as they have also been observed in male breast carcinomas (278,279). These granules show a positive reaction with Grimelius stain, immunostains for chromogranin, and sometimes more specific neuropeptides such as adrenocorticotropic hormone, ACTH, (268,277), prolactin (268), neurotensin (268), and norepinephrine (278). Some of these dense-core granules have been reported to contain lactalbumin, but this finding was subsequently attributed to a contaminant (267,282). Neuron specific enolase (NSE) and alpha chain of human chorionic gonadotropin (HCG) have also been observed in these tumors (291); in my experience, however, NSE does not appear to be a specific marker for anything.

At the ultrastructural level, the NE granules display dense cores and are often present in a closely aggregated cluster within the cytoplasm. In the breast, dense-core granules do not always represent neuroendocrine granules, however. Many of these are simply secretory granules. They are dispersed throughout the cytoplasm with concentration in the apical region. They are particularly abundant in cells stimulated to secrete during gestation and lactation. Ferguson and Anderson (271) considered the presence of abundant dense-core granules related to hormonal changes and a reflection of prelactational differentiation.

Occasionally, these tumors display patterns (Fig. 9.23) similar to those of carcinoid tumors that occur in other organs. This morphologic similarity has been the basis of designating some of these mammary carcinomas as carcinoid tumors (269,270). Currently, this term is avoided as there are many breast carcinomas lacking the morphologic features of a carcinoid tumor that also manifest such granules, and there are tumors morphologically similar to carcinoid tumors that lack any evidence of neuroendocrine granules. Furthermore, these tumors behave like a carcinoma.

Maluf et al (242) reported two examples of a predominantly intraductal, palisading spindle cell carcinoma of the breast with either intra or extracellular mucin production and argyrophilic signet-ring cells; both tumors occurred in women older than 70 years of age and both were associated with a bloody nipple discharge. I have seen several examples of cellular mucinous carcinomas with an abundance of spindle cells. The adjacent intraductal carcinoma was also composed predominantly or purely of spindle cells in some ducts; both the in situ and invasive spindle cells displayed a positive reaction for chromogranin indicating a neuroendocrine differentiation (Fig. 9.24). At the ultrastructural level, both mucin granules and dense-core NE granules may coexist within the cytoplasm of the tumor cells (242). An association between mucinous carcinomas containing NE granules and high levels of estrogen receptors has been reported (242,296).

When there is such a predominance of spindle cell proliferation within a cluster of ducts that also show unequivocal intraductal carcinoma, the lesion should be distinguished not only from a myoepithelial cell proliferation, but also from an ordinary intraductal hyperplasias. The negative reaction with actin and S-100 protein helps exclude a myoepithelial lesion. Distinction from ordinary patterns of intraductal hyperplasia can be quite difficult. In general, the intraductal spindle cell carcinomas are admixed with ducts showing more recognizable patterns of IDCA (Fig. 9.25a). Often there is transition from the nonnecrotic cribriform variant with rosette-like arrangement of the nuclei to the spindle cell population (Fig. 9.25b). In ordinary hyperplasia, the spindle cells are admixed with clearly benign-appearing epithelial cells. This pattern of intraductal carcinoma is a very difficult one to recognize and should not be diagnosed without special studies and consultation with a pathologist who has expertise in breast pathology. A positive chromogranin reaction in the absence of positivity for either actin or S-100 appears to favor an intraductal carcinoma, but this feature should be tested in a larger group of cases to include some ordinary hyperplasias with spindle cells.

Argyrophilic cells have been reported in the normal breast, albeit, rarely (263,294), as well as in fibrocystic changes (272). It is more likely, however, that the capacity to produce NE granules is attained during the neoplastic transformation (297). Not all carcinomas with NE granules produce hormonal substances.

Nesland et al (285,286) suggested that immunostain for neuron specific enolase (NSE) is the best screening marker of NE cells in breast carcinomas, but specific hormones are not present in all NSE positive tumors. They found that normal myoepithelial cells also show a positive reaction for NSE. This is important since ME cells can also show spindle cell intraductal proliferations that could be mistaken for a NE cell population on the basis of NSE positivity. Wilander (295), however, disputes the utility of NSE in screening for carcinomas, since many nonargyrophilic tumors also show NSE positivity. The presence of a positive immunoreaction for chromogranin, NSE, and/or E36 has been reported as evidence of neuroendocrine differentiation in breast carcinoma (263,284). The monoclonal antibody LICR-LON-E36 is normally distributed in cells exhibiting neural and neuroendocrine differentiation. An association between NE differentiation and ER positivity has been observed (265–267).

Carcinoid tumors can metastasize to the breast (275,276,280) and should be distinguished from primary breast carcinomas with neuroendocrine differentiation. The presence of an in situ carcinoma,

A

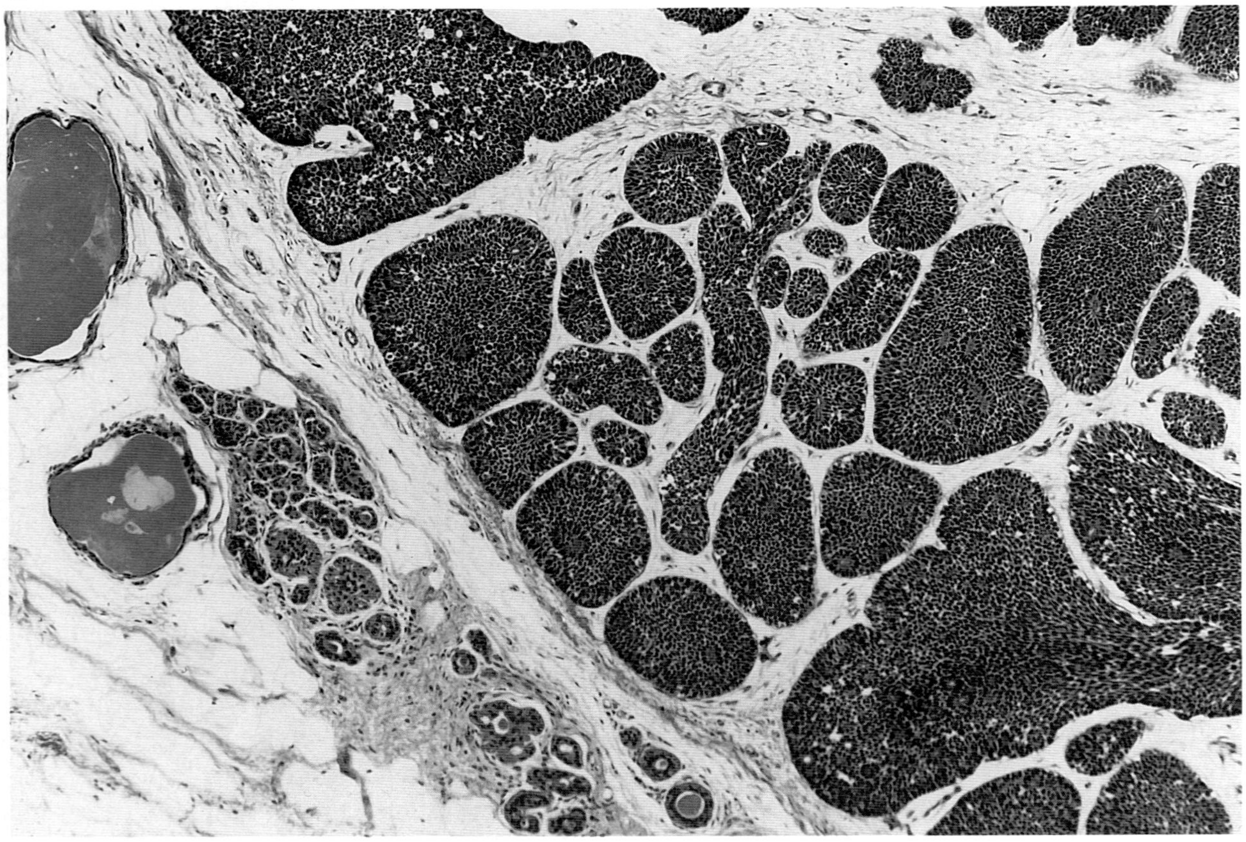

B

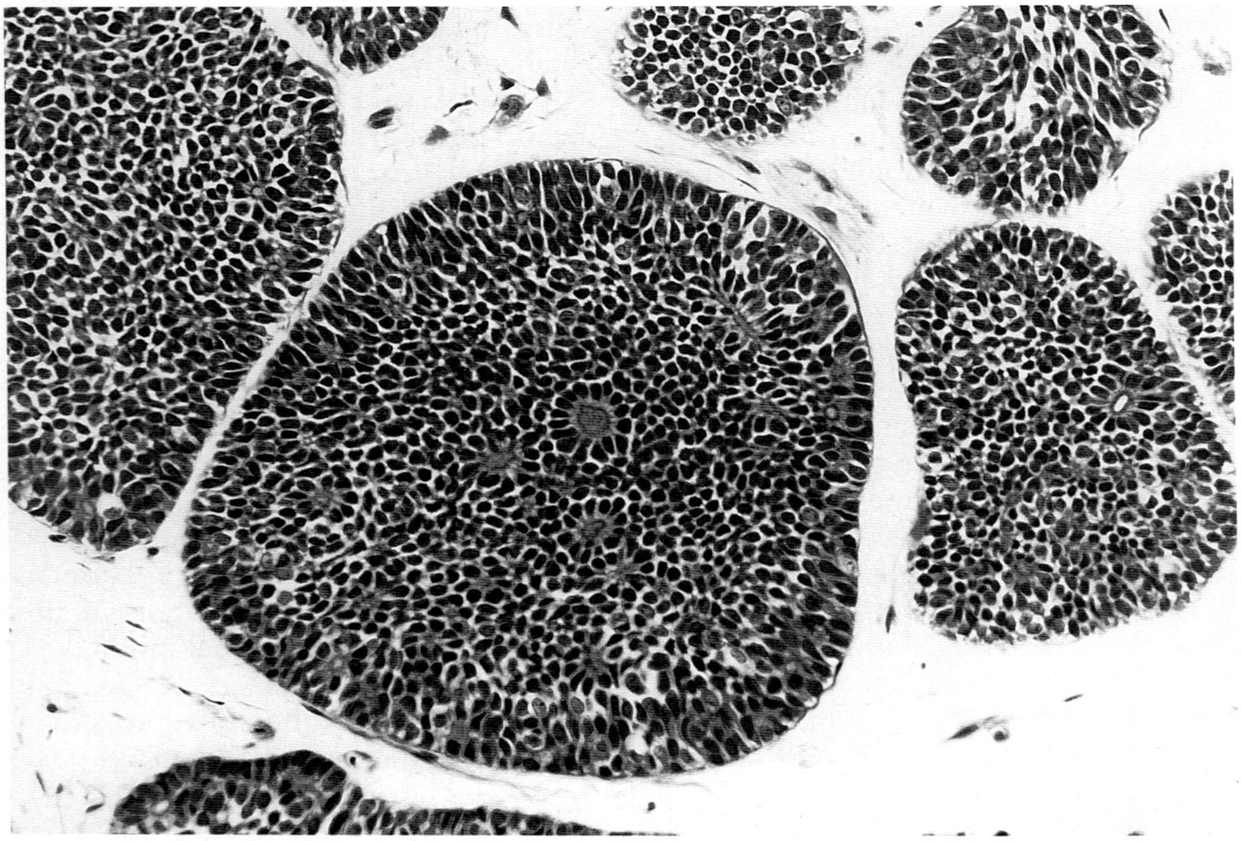

**Figure 9.23** Carcinoma (CA) with neuroendocrine (NE) differentiation. (a,b) The insular pattern of carcinoid tumor with rosette-like arrangement of nuclei is displayed here. (c) The delicate vascularity and trabecular arrangement between the longer nests reflect other distinctive features of carcinoid tumors. Both these tumors displayed a positive reaction for chromogranin. (H&E, (a) X75; (b) X240; (c) X150)

c

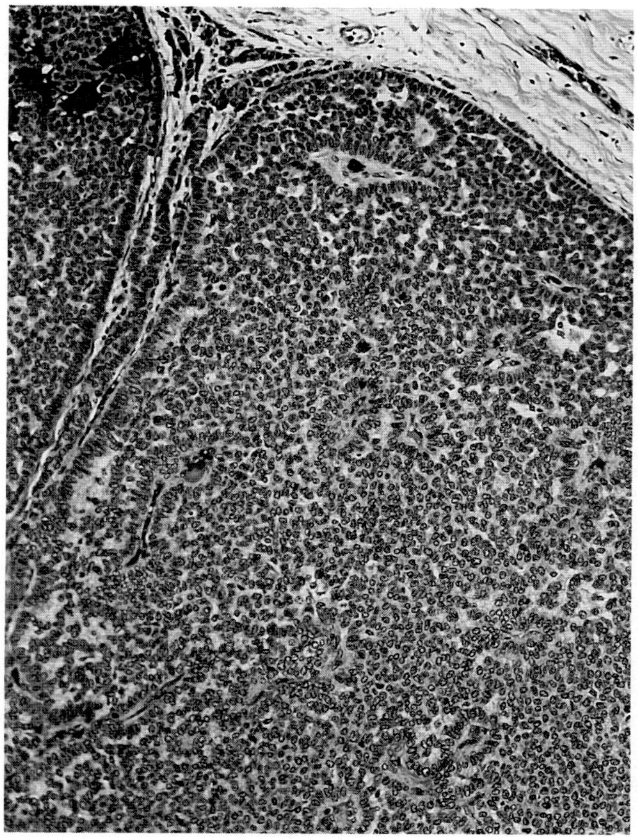

**Figure 9.23(c)** CA with NE differation. Legend on opposite page.

preferably with similar morphology, would support a primary mammary carcinoma. In the absence of an in situ component, careful attention to the patient's history and clinical findings is required to prevent misinterpretation of a metastatic carcinoid.

The term carcinoma with neuroendocrine granules should be reserved for mammary carcinomas displaying any of the growth patterns of a recognized carcinoid tumor (Fig. 9.23) (insular with or without rosettes, trabecular, spindle cell and oat cell), if it displays a strongly positive chromogranin positivity on immunostains. The presence of clusters of dense-core granules away from the apical portion of the cells would further support this designation. Care should be taken not to misinterpret normal secretory granules of the breast as NE granules. Some of these tumors may have variable amounts of extracellular mucin, and may also qualify as colloid carcinomas.

Whether or not these tumors behave differently from a morphologically comparable carcinoma lacking NE granules has not been established.

## MEDULLARY CARCINOMA

It was not until Geschikter's description (304) that medullary carcinoma was recognized as a specific entity even though Ewing (300) had used this designation for some mammary carcinomas. Ewing believed that the marked inflammatory reaction implied a defensive process, but did not necessarily mean that the effort would be successful. Geschikter described medullary carcinoma as a "neo-mammary" cancer, because he thought it originated from the primitive nipple pouch. He noted that large tumor cells grow in sheets or cords embedded in a lymphoid stroma as a characteristic feature of medullary carcinoma. While he did not particularly emphasize the lymphoplasmacytic infiltrate as a component of the tumor, he concluded that this group of carcinomas behave less aggressively than anticipated from their size and microscopic appearance.

In 1949, Moore and Foote (311) reported 52 medullary carcinomas among 1,000 consecutive mastectomy specimen. These patients had an excellent five-year survival rate of 82.7% compared to 50% for patients with ordinary infiltrating duct carcinomas. Axillary nodal metastases were identified in 43% of the women with medullary carcinoma compared to 60% of those with the ordinary infiltrating duct carcinoma. Moore and Foote suggested that the lymphoplasmacytic infiltrate may be responsible for the better prognosis of these patients.

Bloom et al (299) concluded that patients with medullary carcinoma did not have a prognostic advantage. But only 32% of tumors they designated as medullary carcinoma had a prominent lymphoid infiltrate. Therefore, the cases do not adhere to the definition of medullary carcinoma as originally defined by Moore and Foote (311).

Haagensen and Schwartz (305,317) used the term "solid, circumscribed" carcinoma for this tumor. The probability of survival at ten years for Columbia Stage A medullary carcinoma was 79%, compared to 80% for a series of breast carcinomas of all types. The stage B tumors, however, the probability was 86% for medullary carcinomas and 50% for the other group (305). Several subsequent studies have confirmed the better prognosis of medullary carcinoma (314,316, 318).

When patients with typical medullary carcinoma had contralateral carcinoma, it was more likely to

A

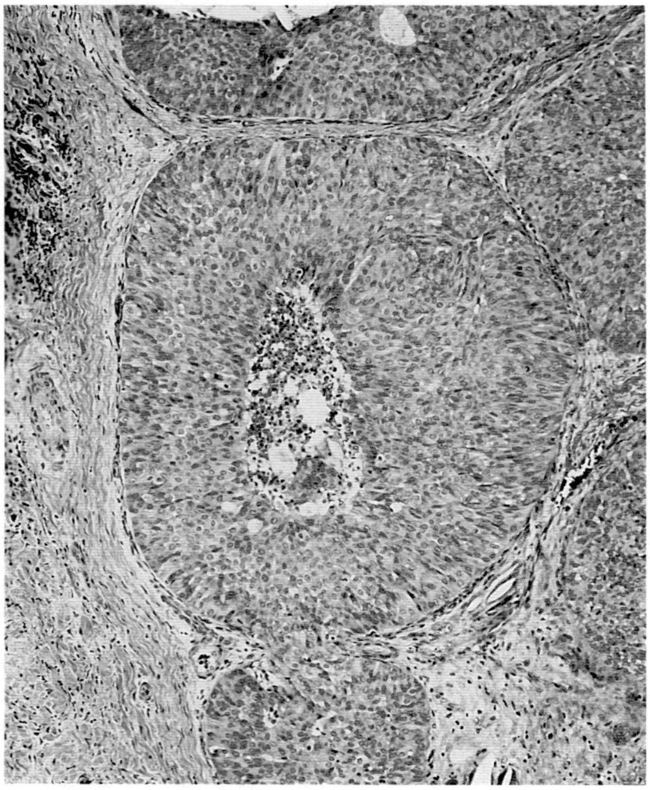

Figure 9.24 Carcinoma with NE differentiation and spindle cell dominance. (a) The in situ ductal carcinoma shows central necrosis and spindle cell predominance. (H&E, X240) (b) Chromagranin shows a positive reaction within a cluster of the intraductal cancer cells. (X480)

B

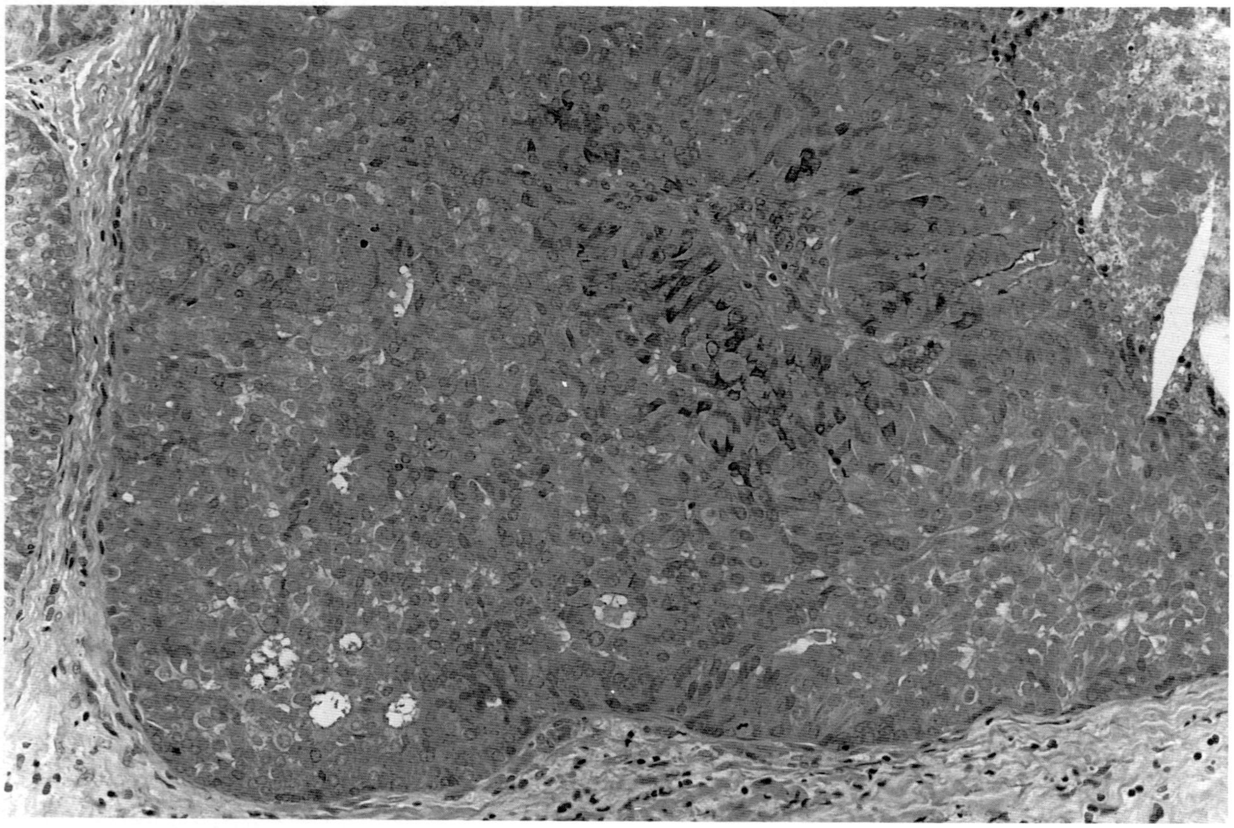

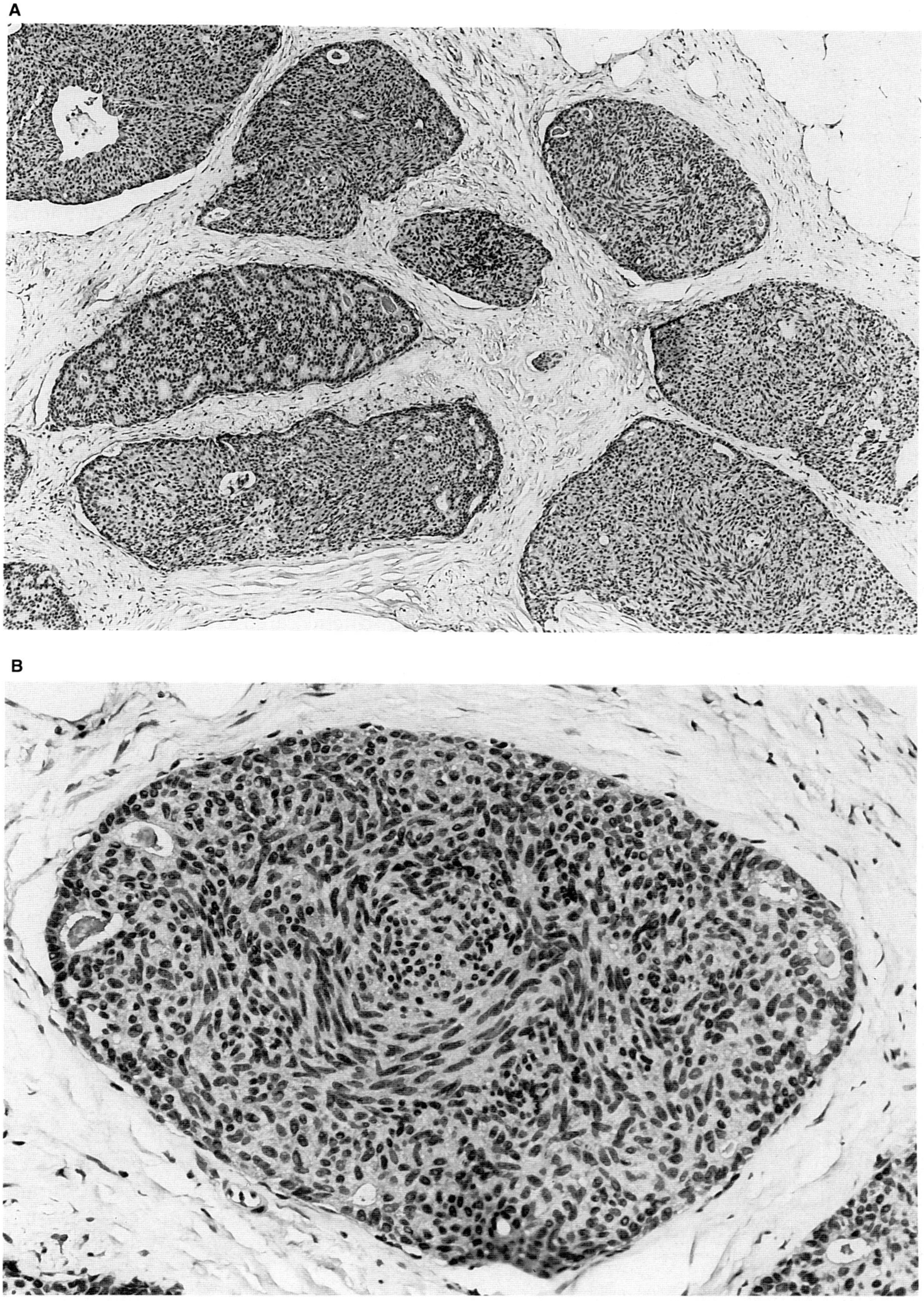


**Figure 9.25** Intraductal carcinoma with spindle cell transformation. Many ducts in this biopsy showed a cribriform pattern of intraductal carcinoma. (a) Focally, these ducts were admixed with others showing a pallisading spindle cell population. (b) The cells in the periphery of this duct show rosette-like arrangement as seen in the ducts with clear-cut cribriform carcinoma. The spindle cells were cytokeratin positive, S-100 and actin negative, confirming their epithelial nature. In isolation, this duct should not be interpreted as intraductal carcinoma without consultation. (H&E, (a) X120; (b) X400)

have been prior to the finding of medullary tumor. Bilateral medullary carcinoma is rare. The presence of intraductal carcinoma does not alter the prognosis.

## Clinical Features

Medullary carcinoma accounts for 5% to 7% of all breast carcinomas. The average age of women with medullary carcinoma ranges between 21 to 95 years (309,315,317), with a mean of around 50 years. This is comparable to that of atypical medullary and regular infiltrating duct carcinoma. The tumor is well-delineated on palpation and soft in consistency. The overlying skin may be reddened (305). Bilateral carcinomas were identified in 26 of 189 (13.4%) patients in Haagensen's series (305). Ten of these were bilateral medullary carcinomas.

## Macroscopic Features

Medullary carcinomas are distinctive spherical masses with well-circumscribed margins that may be confused with a fibroadenoma. Occasionally, they may appear encapsulated. The cut surface of the tumor is fleshy and bulges out in contrast to the shrinking cut surface of scirrhous carcinomas. It has a soft consistency. The tumor varies in color from tan to grayish-white with yellow zones of necrosis and red or brown hemorrhagic foci. Central necrosis may lead to cyst formation in some tumors. On the average, medullary carcinoma is larger than the ordinary infiltrating duct carcinoma. The mean diameter of stages A & B medullary carcinoma was 4.1 cm in Haagensen's series (305).

## Microscopic Features

Medullary carcinoma is well-defined with pushing, expansile margins (Fig. 9.26). A compressed fibrous zone partially, surrounding some of these tumors corresponds to the gross encapsulation observed in rare tumors.

The tumor cells grow as a syncytium, forming anastomosing cords and sheets separated by negligible amounts of loose fibroblastic connective tissue. The syncytial architecture comprises 75% of the tumor surface; the remaining area is occupied by the lymphoplasmacytic infiltrate and a loose stroma (Fig. 9.26b). Necrosis may be present in the center of the tumor.

The tumor cells are round with abundant cytoplasm, round, vesicular nuclei, containing one or more prominent nucleoli. Mitotic figures are common. Squamous metaplasia is observed in 10% to 16% of the tumors (305,316). Atypical tumor giant cells have been noted in 10% of the cases (316).

One of the most conspicuous features of this carcinoma is the presence of moderate to pronounced lymphoplasmacytic infiltrate in the supporting and surrounding stroma. The plasma cells in medullary carcinoma produce predominantly IgA and secretory component (SC), whereas, plasma cells associated with ductal carcinomas are of IgG type (308). An in situ carcinoma may be present in the adjacent breast tissue. Rarely, a granulomatous reaction may be evident in the stroma (300).

Histologic grading should not be applied to medullary carcinoma. If it were graded, the morphologic features would indicate a high grade tumor that would be expected to behave aggressively. It is well-known that the behavior of the tumor does not parallel its ominous morphology, however. The features of medullary carcinoma are listed in Table 9.2.

Formation of glandular, tubular, or cord-like structures by the tumor cells should not be present; the presence of these formations or any other pattern of ordinary infiltrating carcinoma disqualifies the lesion as a classic medullary carcinoma. Dense collagenous stroma is not a feature of medullary carcinoma either. A well-circumscribed lesion with syncytial proliferation of primitive carcinoma cells that shows either foci of ordinary infiltrating duct carcinoma, a paucity or absence of lymphoplasmacytic infiltrate, or dense fibrous bands has been designated as an atypical medullary carcinoma. The features used for a diagnosis of atypical medullary carcinoma are listed in Table 9.3. To avoid confusing clinicians in their therapeutic decisions, pathologists should refrain from using the designation of atypical medullary carcinoma since it has been shown that its behavior is not significantly different from that of ordinary infiltrating ductal carcinomas (314).

A

B

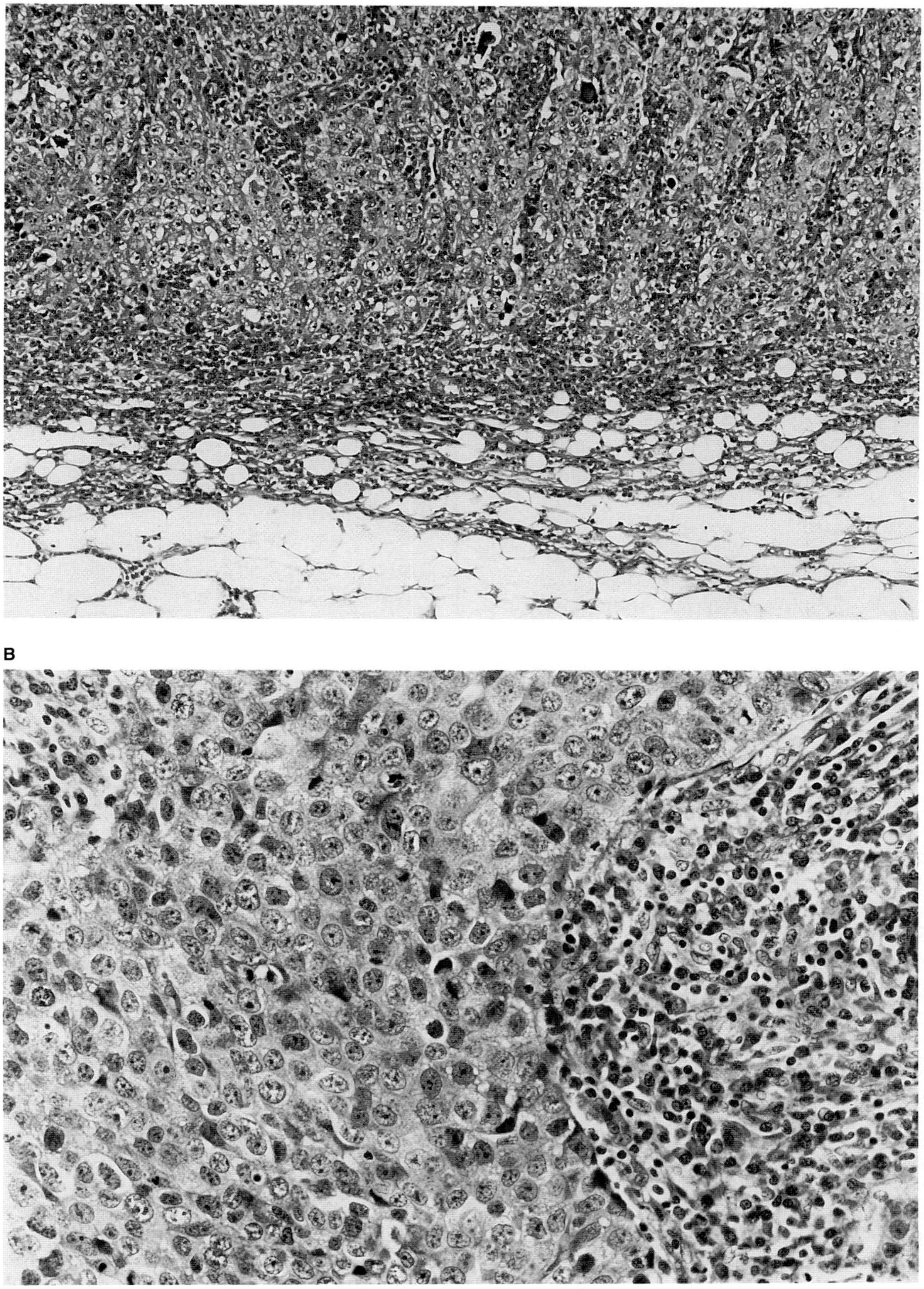

**Figure 9.26** Medullary carcinoma. (a) At low power, the pushing growth margin is readily appreciated. (b) At higher magnification, the primitive cells display a syncytial growth pattern, and there is a characteristic dense lymphoplasmacytic infiltrate. (H&E, (a) X20; (b) X240)

**Table 9.2** Microscopic Features of Typical Medullary Carcinoma

| |
|---|
| 1. Syncytial growth pattern (>75%) |
| 2. Circumscribed pushing margin |
| 3. Moderate to marked, diffuse lymphoplasmacytic infiltrate |
| 4. Absence of glandular arrangement |
| 5. Moderate to marked nuclear pleomorphism (nuclear grade 1 or 2) |
| 6. IDCA absent |

## Hormone Receptors and Ploidy

Medullary carcinomas have been reported to be ER+ in 2%, 28%, and 80% of cases—the latter figures reflect the proportion of tumor with less than 10 nm ER protein (46,58,73). Horsfall (307) reported a 29% ER and PR positivity for medullary carcinoma. Interestingly, four of five (80%) medullary carcinomas evaluated for S-100 protein have displayed a positive reaction for S-100 protein (13).

Medullary carcinomas have predominantly aneuploid DNA stemlines despite their favorable prognosis (301,307,313).

## Ultrastructural Features

Ultrastructural studies have yielded inconsistent results. Most viewers agree on the presence of light and dark cells, but then practically all tumors have light and dark cells at this level. Ahmad (298) suggested that medullary cancer cells have distinctive features. They exhibit well-developed Golgi complexes and contain abundant organelles, but no evidence of secretory granules. The stroma contains macrophages, lymphocytes, and plasma cells. The stromal vessels are lined by high endothelial cells which were thought to facilitate migration of lymphocytes. Harris (306), however, could not detect any significant differences between three medullary, eight atypical medullary, and four non-medullary carcinomas; he concluded that electron microscopy is neither useful in narrowing down the differential diagnosis, nor does it unmask a basis for its good prognosis.

**Table 9.3** Microscopic Features of Atypical Medullary Carcinoma

| |
|---|
| 1. Predominantly syncytial growth (>75%) |
| 2. Focal marginal irregularity or infiltrating margins |
| 3. Mild lymphoplasmacytic infiltrate |
| 4. Nuclear grade 3 |
| 5. Presence of glandular arrangement |
| 6. IDCA present |

## Features of Prognostic Significance and Survival

Tumor size appears to have prognostic significance as should be expected. In Ridolfi et al's series (316), medullary carcinomas less than 3 cm in diameter had a significantly better prognosis than larger medullary carcinomas or non-medullary carcinomas of equal size. No particular association with a family history of breast carcinoma antecedent to the diagnosis has been identified (316).

Of 95 lesions with abundant inflammatory infiltrate examined by Rapin et al (314) at the Institut Gustave-Roussy between 1960 and 1979, 26 had typical medullary carcinoma (TMC), 23 qualified as atypical medullary carcinoma (AMC), and 46 were non-medullary carcinomas (NMC). The TMC had a ten-year disease-free interval of 92% compared with 53% for AMC, and 51% for NMC. The five- and ten-year survival rate of 92% for medullary carcinoma in this report is the highest in the literature. The TMC was associated with a favorable prognosis despite large size and lymph node involvement, suggesting that the only therapy needed is the removal of all tumor. The AMC had a prognosis similar to other types of breast carcinoma without inflammatory stroma and adjuvant therapy may be justified for this group. These findings suggest that categorization of tumors as atypical medullary carcinoma is no longer justified.

In Ridolfi et al's (316) study, the ten-year survival for 57 women with medullary carcinoma was 84%, it was 74% for 79 women with atypical medullary carcinoma, and for the 56 patients with non-medullary, regular infiltrating carcinomas, it was 63%. Also, the medullary and non-medullary carcinomas had similar frequency of lymph node metastases, but medullary carcinoma had a more favorable prognosis even when nodal metastases were present.

It is noteworthy that in the 1990 National Surgical Adjuvant Breast and Bowel Project (NSABP) review (16) of eight-year survival for node-negative patients, atypical medullary carcinoma had the highest average mortality rate among all histologic types, and was classified among unfavorable tumor types, while medullary carcinoma was grouped with the favorable tumors.

Approximately 39% to 43.5% of women with medullary carcinoma manifest axillary node metastases at presentation, compared to 60% to 64% for other carcinomas (309,315). For "circumscribed" carcinomas, the frequency of axillary node metastases was 10.7% compared to 30.8% for a series of carcinomas of all other types in Haagensen's experience (305). The presence of axillary node metastases is an important prognostic feature within the group of medullary carcinomas. The five- and ten-year survival rates for patients with negative nodes are 77% and 61%; they drops to 55% and 38% respectively for women with positive nodes (309).

Most deaths from medullary carcinoma occur less than five years after the diagnosis.

## REFERENCES


1. Anastassiades OT, Bouropoulou V, Knotgeorges G, et al: Duct elastosis in infiltrating carcinoma of the breast. *Pathol Res Pract* 1979;165:411–421.

* 2. Antoniades K, Spector H: Correlation of estrogen receptor levels with histology and cytomorphology in human breast cancer. *Am J Clin Pathol* 1979;71:497–503.

3. Azzopardi JC: *Problems in Breast Pathology*. Philadelphia, WB Saunders, 1979, pp 244–274.

* 4. Azzopardi JG, Chepick OF, Hartmann WH, et al: Histologic typing of breast tumours. *Am J Clin Pathol* 1986;78: 806–816.

5. Bailey AJ, Sloan JP, Trichey BS, et al: An immunocytochemical study of alpha-lactalbumin in human breast tissue. *J Pathol* 1982;137:13–23.

6. Bedwani R, Vana J, Rosner D, et al: Management and survival of female patients with "minimal" breast cancer: As observed in the long-term and short-term surveys of the American College of Surgeons. *Cancer* 1981;47:2769–2778.

7. Black MM, Barclay THC, Hankey BF: Prognosis in breast cancer utilizing histologic characteristics of the primary tumor. *Cancer* 1975;36:2048–2055.

8. Brinton LA, Hoover R, Fraumeni JF: Epidemiology of minimal breast cancer. *JAMA* 1983;249:483–487.

* 9. Cedermark B, Askergren J, Alveryd A, et al: Breast-conserving treatment for breast cancer in Stockholm, Sweden, 1977–1981. *Cancer* 1984;53:1253–1255.

* 10. Contesso G, Delarue JC, Mouriesse H, et al: Anatomopathologie du cancer de sein et recepteurs hormonaux. *Pathol Biol* 1983;31:747–754.

11. Dixon JM, Page DL, Anderson TJ, et al: Long-term survivors after breast cancer. *Br J Surg* 1985;72:445–448.

* 12. Donegan WL, Spratt JS (eds): *Cancer of the Breast*. Philadelphia, WB Saunders, 1988.

13. Dwarakanath S, Lee AKC, Dellellis RA, et al: S-100 protein positivity in breast carcinomas: A potential pitfall in diagnostic immunohistochemistry. *Hum Pathol* 1987;18:1144–1148.

* 14. Fisher B, Bauer M, Margolese R, et al: Five-year results of a randomized clinical trial comparing total mastectomy and segmental mastectomy with or without radiation in the treatment of breast cancer. *N Engl J Med* 1985;312:665–673.

* 15. Fisher ER, Gregorio RM, Fisher B, et al: The pathology of invasive breast cancer. A syllabus derived from findings of the National Surgical Adjuvant Breast Project (Protocol no. 4). *Cancer* 1975;36:1–85.

* 16. Fisher ER, Redmond C, Fisher B, et al: Pathologic findings from the National Surgical Adjuvant Breast and Bowel Projects (NSABP). Prognostic discriminant for 8-year survival for node-negative invasive breast cancer patients. *Cancer* 1990;65:2121–2128.

* 17. Foote FW, Stewart FW: A histologic classification of carcinoma of the breast. *Surgery* 1946;19:74–99.

18. Fu YS, Maksem JA, Hubay CA et al: The relationship of breast cancer morphology and estrogen receptor protein status, in Fenoglio CM, Wolff M (eds): *Progress in Surgical Pathology*. New York, Masson, 1981, vol III, pp 65–76.

19. Gallager HS: Pathogenesis of early breast cancer, in Zander J, Blatzer J (eds): *Early Breast Cancer—Histopathology, Diagnosis and Treatment*. Berlin, Springer-Verlag, 1985, pp 14–19.

* 20. Gallager HS: Pathologic types of breast cancer and their prognosis. *Cancer* 1984;53:623–629.

21. Gallager HS, Martin JE: An orientation to the concept of minimal breast cancer. *Cancer* 1971;28:1505–1507.

22. Gilchrist KW, Kalish L, Gould VE, et al: Immunostaining for carcinoembryonic antigen does not discriminate for early recurrence in breast cancer. The ECOG experience. *Cancer* 1985;56:351–355.

23. Giorno R: Mononuclear cells in malignant and benign human breast tissue. *Arch Pathol Lab Med* 1983;107:415–417.

24. Glaubitz LC, Bowen JH, Cox ED, et al: Elastosis in human breast cancer. Correlation with sex steroid receptors and comparison with clinical outcome. *Arch Pathol Lab Med* 1984;108:27–30.

25. Gorton G, Linell F: Malignant tumours and sarcoid reactions in regional lymph nodes. *Acta Radiol* 1957;47:381–392.

* 26. Haagensen CD: *Diseases of the Breast*, ed 3. Philadelphia, WB Saunders, 1986.

* 27. Harris JR, Hellman S, Henderson IC, et al (eds): *Breast Diseases*. Philadelphia, JB Lippincott, 1987.

28. Hartmann WH: Minimal breast cancer. An update. *Cancer* 1984;53:681–684.

* 29. Helin EJ, Helle MJ, Kollioniemi O-P, et al: Immunohistochemical determination of estrogen and progesterone receptors in human breast carcinoma. Correlation with his-

topathology and DNA flow cytometry. *Cancer* 1989;63: 1761–1767.

* 30. Holland R, Solke H, Veling MSC, et al: Histologic multifocality of Tis, T1-2 breast carcinomas. Implications for clinical trials of breast-conserving surgery. *Cancer* 1985;56:979–990.

31. Horne CHW, Reid IN, Milne GD: Prognostic significance of inappropriate production of pregnancy proteins by breast cancers. *Lancet* 1976;2:279–282.

32. Hutter RVP: The pathologist's role in minimal breast cancer. *Cancer* 1969;24:1081–1085.

* 33. Jotti GS, Petit JY, Contesso G: Minimal breast cancer: A clinically meaningful term? *Sem Oncol* 1986;13:384–392.

34. Kuhajda FP, Offutt LE, Mendelsohn G: The distribution of carcinoembryonic antigen in breast carcinoma. *Cancer* 1983; 52:1257–1264.

35. Kouchoukos NT, Ackerman LV, Butcher HR: Prediction of axillary nodal metastases from the morphology of primary mammary carcinomas. *Cancer* 1967;20:948–960.

* 36. Kurtz JM, Jacquemier J, Thorhosrt J, et al: Conservation therapy for breast cancers other than infiltrating ductal carcinoma. *Cancer* 1989;63:1630–1635.

* 37. Lash RH, Bauer TW, Hermann RE, et al: Partial mastectomy: Pathologic findings and prognosis. *Hum Pathol* 1986; 17:813–822.

38. Lee AK, Rosen PP, Delellis RA, et al: Tumor marker expression in breast carcinomas and relationship to prognosis. An immunohistochemical study. *Am J Clin Pathol* 1985;84:687–696.

* 39. Lesser ML, Rosen PP, Senie RT, et al: Estrogen and progesterone receptors in breast carcinoma: Correlations with epidemiology and pathology. *Cancer* 1981;48:299–309.

* 40. Lippman ME, Lichter AS, Danforth DN (eds): *Diagnosis and Management of Breast Cancer*. Philadelphia, WB Saunders, 1988.

41. Masters JRW, Sangster K, Hawkins RA, et al: Elastosis and estrogen receptors in human breast cancer. *Br J Cancer* 1976;33:342–343.

* 42. Matsukuma A, Enjoji M, Toyoshima S: Ductal carcinoma of the breast. An analysis of proportions of intraductal and invasive components. *Pathol Res Pract* 1991;187:62–67.

* 43. McCarty KS Jr, Barton TK, Fetter BF, et al: Correlation of estrogen and progesterone receptors with histologic differentiation in mammary carcinoma. *Cancer* 1980;46:2851–2858.

44. McDivitt RW: Breast carcinoma. *Hum Pathol* 1978;9:3–21.

45. McDivitt RW, Stewart FW, Berg JW: *Tumors of the Breast*, Fasc 2. Atlas of Tumor Pathology, second series, Washington DC, Armed Forces Institute of Pathology, 1968.

* 46. Mohammed RJ, Lakatua DJ, Haus E, et al: Estrogen and progesterone receptors in human breast cancer. Correlation with histologic subtype and degree of differentiation. *Cancer* 1986;58:1076–1081.

47. Moskowitz M, Pemmaraju S, Fidler JA, et al: On the diagnosis of minimal breast cancer in screenee population. *Cancer* 1976;37:2543–2552.

48. Murad TM: A proposed histochemical and electron microscopic classification of human breast cancer according to the cell of origin. *Cancer* 1971;27:288–299.

* 49. NIH Consenses Conference. Treatment of early-stage breast cancer. *JAMA* 1991;265:391–395.

50. Oberman HA: Invasive carcinoma of the breast with granulomatous response. *Am J Clin Pathol* 1987;88:718–721.

* 51. Page DL, Anderson TJ: *Diagnostic Histopathology of the Breast*. New York, Churchill Livingstone, 1987, pp 198–205.

52. Pich A, Bussolati G, DiCarlo F: Production of casein and presence of oestrogen receptors in human breast cancers. *J Natl Cancer Inst* 1977;58:1483–1484.

53. Rasmussen BB, Pedersen BV, Thorpe SM, et al: Elastosis in relation to prognosis in primary breast carcinoma. *Cancer Res* 1985;45:1428–1430.

* 54. Rosen PP: The pathological classification of human mammary carcinoma: Past, present and future. *Ann Clin Lab Sci* 1979;9:144–156.

55. Rosen PP, Ashikari R, Thaler H, et al: A comparative study of some pathologic features of mammary carcinoma in Tokyo, Japan and New York, USA. *Cancer* 1977;39:429–434.

* 56. Rosen PP, Groshen S, Saigo PE, et al: Pathological prognostic factors in stage I (T1N0M0) and stage II (T1N1M0) breast carcinoma: A study of 644 patients with a median follow-up of 18 years. *J Clin Oncol* 1989;7:355–366.

* 57. Rosen PP, Lesser ML, Kinne DW: Breast carcinoma at the extremes of age: A comparison of patients younger than 35 years and older than 75 years. *J Surg Oncol* 1985;28:90–96.

58. Rosen PP, Mendez-Botet CJ, Nisselbaun JS, et al: Pathological review of breast lesions analyzed for estrogen receptor protein. *Cancer Res* 1975;35:3187–3194.

59. Rosen PP, Saigo PE, Braun DW Jr, et al: Predictors of recurrence in stage I (T1N0M0) breast carcinoma. *Ann Surg* 1981;193:15–25.

60. Roses DF, Bell DA, Flotte TJ, et al: Pathological predictors of recurrence in stage 1 (T1N0M0) breast cancer. *Am J Clin Pathol* 1982;788:817–820.

61. Sakamoto G: Histological classification of the breast cancer. *Jpn J Cancer Clin* 1985;31(Suppl):105–113.

62. Sakamoto G: Histologic classification of the breast cancer. *Jpn J Cancer Clin* 1986;32(Suppl 1):197–204.

63. Sakamoto G, Sugano H, Hartmann WH: Comparative pathological study of breast carcinoma among American and Japanese women, in McGuire WL (ed): *Breast Cancer. Advances in Research and Treatment*. New York, Plenum, 1981, vol 4, pp 211–231.

* 64. Sarrazin D, Le M, Rouesse J, et al: Conservative treatment versus mastectomy in breast cancer tumors with macroscopic diameter of 20 millimeters or less. The experience of the Institu Gustave-Roussy. *Cancer* 1984;53:1209–1213.

* 65. Schnitt SJ, Connolly JL, Harris JR, et al: Pathologic predictors of early local recurrences in stage I and II breast cancer treated by primary radiation therapy. *Cancer* 1984;53:1049–1057.

66. Shousha S, Lysiottis T, Godfrey VM, et al: Carcinoembryonic antigen in breast cancer tissue: A useful prognostic indicator. *Br Med J* 1979;1:777–779.

67. Schwartz GF, Feig SA, Patchefsky AS: Clinicopathologic correlations and significance of clinically occult mammary lesions. *Cancer* 1978;41:1147–1153.

* 68. Silverberg SG, Chitale AR: Assessment of significance of proportions of intraductal and infiltrating tumor growth in ductal carcinoma of the breast. *Cancer* 1973;32:830–837.

69. Symmers WSC: Localized tuberculoid granulomas associated with carcinoma. *Am J Pathol* 1951;27:493–521.

70. Van Bogaert LJ, Maldague P: Histologic classification of pure primary epithelial breast cancer. *Hum Pathol* 1978;9:175–180.

* 71. Veronesi U, Banfi A, Salvadori B, et al: Breast conservation is the treatment of choice in small breast cancer: Long-term results of a randomized trial. *Eur J Cancer* 1990;26:668–670.

72. Veronesi U, Saccozzi R, Del Vecchio M, et al: Comparing radical mastectomy with quadrantectomy, axillary dissection, and radiotherapy in patients with small cancers of the breast. *N Engl J Med* 1981;305:6–11.

* 73. Vollenweider-Zerargui L, Barrelet L, Wong Y, et al: The predictive value of estrogen and progesterone receptors' concentrations on the clinical behavior of breast cancer in women. Clinical correlation on 547 women. *Cancer* 1986;57:1171–1180.

74. Wallgren A, Silferersward C, Ecklung G: Prognostic factors in mammary carcinoma. *Acta Radiol* 1976;15:1–16.

75. Walker RA: Immunohistochemistry of biological markers of breast carcinoma, in Delellis RA (ed): *Advances in Immunohistochemistry*. New York, Masson Publishing, 1984, pp 223–241.

76. Wanebo HJ, Huvos AG, Urban JA: Treatment of minimal breast cancer. *Cancer* 1974;33:349–357.

* 77. Wise L, Mason AY, Ackerman LV: Local excision and irradiation: An alternative method for the treatment of early mammary cancer. *Ann Surg* 1971;174:392–401.

78. World Health Organization: *Histologic typing of breast tumors*, 2 ed. International Histologic Classification of Tumors, No. 2. Geneva, World Health Organization, 1981, p 19.

### Axillary Nodes

* 79. Ashikari R, Rosen PP, Urban JA, et al: Breast cancer presenting as an axillary mass. *Ann Surg* 1976;183:415–417.

80. Azzopardi JG, Ross CMD, Frizzera G: Blue nevi of lymph node capsule. *Histopathology* 1977;1:451–461.

81. Berg JW: Sinus histiocytosis: A fallacious measure of host resistance to cancer. *Cancer* 1956;9:935–939.

82. Berg JW: Morphological evidence of immune response to cancer—An historical review. *Cancer* 1971;28:1453–1456.

83. Bhatia SK, Saclarides JJ, Witt TR, et al: Hormone receptor studies in axillary metastases from occult breast cancers. *Cancer* 1987;59:1170–1172.

84. Black MM, Speer F: Lymph node reactivity in cancer patients. *Surg Gynecol Obstet* 1960;110:477–487.

85. Copeland EM, McBride CM: Axillary metastases from unknown primary sites. *Ann Surg* 1983;178:25–27.

86. Cutler SJ, Black MM, Mork T, et al: Further observations on prognostic factors in cancer of the female breast. *Cancer* 1969;24:653–667.

87. Devitt JE, Michalchuck AW: Significance of contralateral axillary metastases in carcinoma of the breast. *Can J Surg* 1969;12:178–180.

88. DiRe JJ, Lane N: The relationship of sinus histiocytosis in axillary lymph nodes to surgical curability of carcinoma of the breast. *Am J Clin Pathol* 1963;40:508–515.

* 89. Eldow DW, Carter D: Heterotopic epithelium in axillary lymph nodes: Report of a case and review of the literature. *Am J Clin Pathol* 1973;59:666–673.

90. Ellerbroeck N, Holmes F, Singletary E, et al: Treatment of patients with isolated nodal metastases from an occult carcinoma consistent with breast origin. *Cancer* 1990;66:1461–1467.

91. Epstein JI, Erlandson RA, Rosen PP: Nodal blue nevi. *Am J Surg Pathol* 1984;8:907–915.

92. Erlandson RA, Rosen PP: Electron microscopy of a nevus cell aggregate associated with an axillary lymph node. *Cancer* 1982;49:269–272.

93. Feigenberg Z, Zer M, Dintsman M: Axillary metastases from an unknown primary source. *Israel J Med Sci* 1976;12:1153–1158.

94. Feuerman L, Attie JN, Rosenberg B: Carcinoma in axillary lymph nodes as an indicator of breast cancer. *Surg Gynecol Obstet* 1962;114:5–8.

* 95. Fisher ER, Gregorio R, Redmond C, et al: Pathologic findings from the National Surgical Adjuvant Breast Project (Protocal No. 4). II. The significance of regional node histology other than sinus histiocytosis in invasive mammary cancer. *Cancer* 1976;22:21–30.

96. Garret R, Ada AEW: Epithelial inclusion cysts in an axillary lymph node. Report of a case simulating metastatic adenocarcinoma. *Cancer* 1957;10:173–178.

97. Grundfest S, Steiger E, Sebek B: Metastatic axillary adenopathy. Use of estrogen receptor protein as an aid in diagnosis. *Arch Surg* 1978;113:1108–1109.

98. Haagensen CD: *Diseases of the Breast*, ed 3. Philadelphia, WB Saunders, 1986, pp 653–663.

99. Haagensen CD, Bodian C, Haagensen DE Jr: *Breast Carcinoma, Risk & Detection*. Philadelphia, WB Saunders, 1981, pp 449–451.

100. Halsted WS: The results of radical operations for the cure of carcinoma of the breast. *Ann Surg* 1907;46:1–19.

*101. Haupt HM, Rosen PP, Kinne DW: Breast carcinoma presenting with axillary lymph node metastases. *Am J Surg Pathol* 1985;9:165–175.

*102. Holdsworth PJ, Hopkinson JM, Leveson SH: Benign axillary epithelial lymph node inclusions—a histological pitfall. *Histopathology* 1988;13:226–228.

103. Hunter RL, Ferguson DJ, Coppleson LW: Survival with mammary cancer related to the interaction of germinal center hyperplasia and sinus histiocytosis in axillary and internal mammary lymph nodes. *Cancer* 1975;36:528–539.

104. Iglehart JD, Ferguson BJ, Shingleton WW, et al: An ultrastructural analysis of breast carcinoma presenting as isolated axillary adenopathy. *Ann Surg* 1982;196:8–13.

* 105. Johnson WT, Helwig EB: Benign nevus cells in the capsule of lymph nodes. *Cancer* 1969;23:747–753.

* 106. Kemeny MM, Rivera DE, Terz JJ, et al: Occult primary adenocarcinoma with axillary metastases. *Am J Surg* 1986; 52:43–48.

107. Kempson RL: Consultation case. Benign glandular inclusions in iliac lymph nodes. *Am J Surg Pathol* 1978;2:321–325. A case of benign breast tissue in the axillary node seen by the author is mentioned in the discussion.

108. Klopp CT: Metastatic cancer of axillary lymph node without a demonstrable primary lesion. *Ann Surg* 1949;131:437–439.

109. Mambo NC, Gallagher HS: Carcinoma of the breast: The prognostic significance of extranodal extension of axillary disease. *Cancer* 1977;39:2280–2285.

* 110. Masse C, Chassaigne JP: Est-il possible de determiner le pronostic du cancer du sein d'apres l'examen histologique des ganglions axillaires? *J Med Bourdeaux* 1962;130:360–365.

111. McCarthy SW, Palmer AA, Bale PM, et al: Nevus cells in lymph nodes. *Pathology* 1974;6:351–358.

112. Micheau L, Contesso G: Formation d'aspect angioglomique dans les ganglion lymphatic axillaires. *Arch Anat Pathol* 1971;19:167–175.

* 113. Patel J, Nemoto T, Rosner D, et al: Axillary lymph node metastases from an occult breast cancer. *Cancer* 1981;47: 2923–2927.

114. Pierce EH, Gray HK, Dockerty MB: Surgical significance of axillary adenopathy. *Ann Surg* 1957;145:104.

* 115. Ridolfi RL, Rosen PP, Thaler H: Nevus cell aggregates associated with lymph nodes: Estimated frequency and clinical significance. *Cancer* 1977;39:164–171.

116. Rosen PP: Axillary lymph node metastases in patients with occult noninvasive breast carcinoma. *Cancer* 1980;46:1298–1306.

* 117. Rosen PP, Kimmel M: Occult breast carcinoma presenting with axillary lymph node metastases: A follow-up study of 48 patients. *Hum Pathol* 1990;21:518–523.

118. Sharkey FE, Greiner AS: Morphologic identity of primary tumor and axillary metastases in breast carcinoma. A quantitative study. *Arch Pathol Lab Med* 1985;109:256–259.

* 119. Silverberg, SG, Chitale AR, Hind AD, et al: Sinus histiocytosis and mammary carcinoma. Study of 366 radical mastectomies and an histological review. *Cancer* 1970;26: 1177–1185.

120. Syrjanen KL: Paracortical activity in the lymph nodes draining female breast carcinoma. *Neoplasma* 1979;26:95–102.

121. Truong LD, Cartwright J, Goodman MD, et al: Silicone lymphadenopathy associated with augmentiation mammoplasty. Morphologic features of nine cases. *Am J Surg Pathol* 1988;12:484–491.

122. Tsakrakildes V, Olson P, Kersey JH, et al: Prognostic significance of the regional lymph node histology in cancer of the breast. *Cancer* 1974;34:1259–1267.

* 123. Turner DR, Millis RR: Breast tissue inclusions in axillary lymph nodes. *Histopathology* 1980;4:631–636.

124. Vilcoq JR, Calle R, Ferme F, et al: Conservative treatment of axillary adenopathy due to probable subclinical breast cancer. *Arch Surg* 1982;117:1136–1138.

125. Walker AN, Fechner RE: Papillary carcinoma arising from extopic breast tissue in an axillary lymph node. *Diagn Gynecol Obstet* 1982;4:141–145.

126. Warkel RL, Helwig EB: Apocrine gland adenoma and adenocarcinoma of the axilla. *Arch Dermatol* 1978;114:198–203.

127. Westbrook KC, Gallager HS: Breast carcinoma presenting as an axillary mass. *Am J Surg* 1971;122:607–611.

128. Wilkinson EJ, Hause LL, Hoffman RG, et al: Occult axillary lymph node metastases in invasive breast carcinoma: Characteristics of the primary tumor and significance of metastases. *Pathol Annu* 1982;17:67–91.

### Radiation Induced Changes

129. Clarke D, Curtis JL, Martinez A, et al: Fat necrosis of the breast simulating recurrent carcinoma after primary radiotherapy in the management of early stage breast carcinoma. *Cancer* 1983;52:442–445.

130. Close PM, Tiltman AJ, Hacking EA: The effect of chemotherapy on the morphology of human breast carcinoma. *S Afr Med J* 1987;72:103–106.

131. Fajardo LF: *Pathology of Radiation Injury*. New York, Masson, 1982.

* 132. Fleck R, McNeese MD, Ellerbroek NA, et al: Consequences of breast irradiation in patients with pre-existing collagen vascular diseases. *Int J Radiat Oncol Biol Physic* 1989;17:829–833.

133. Haagensen CD: Diseases of the Breast, 3 ed. Philadelphia, WB Saunders, 1986, pp 954–971.

* 134. Kennedy S, Merino MJ, Swain SM, et al: The effects of hormonal and chemotherapy on tumoral and non-neoplastic breast tissue. *Hum Pathol* 1990;21:192–198.

* 135. Ransom DT, Cameron FG: Scleroderma: A possible contraindication to lumpectomy and radiotherapy in breast carcinoma. *Austral Radiol* 1987;31:317–318.

* 136. Robertson JM, Clarke DH, Pezner MM, et al: Breast conservation therapy. Severe breast fibrosis after radiation therapy in patients with collagen vascular disease. *Cancer* 1991;68:502–508.

* 137. Schnitt SJ, Connolly JL, Harris JR, et al: Radiation-induced changes in the breast. *Hum Pathol* 1984;15:545–550.

138. Stefanik DF, Brereton HD, Lee TC, et al: Fat necrosis following breast irradiation for carcinoma: clinical presentation and diagnosis. *Breast* 1982;8:4–6.

### Infiltrating Lobular Carcinoma

139. Allenby PA, Chowdhury LN: Histiocytic appearance of metastatic lobular breast carcinoma. *Arch Pathol Lab Med* 1986;110:759–760.

*140. Ashikari R, Huvos AG, Urban JA, et al: Infiltrating lobular carcinoma of the breast. *Cancer* 1973;31:110–116.

141. Cheatle GL, Cutler M: *Tumors of the Breast*. Philadelphia, JB Lippincott, 1931.

142. Cormier WJ, Gaffey TA, Welch JS, et al: Linitis plastica caused by metastatic lobular carcinoma of the breast. *Mayo Clin Proc* 1980;55:747–753.

143. Cornil A-V: Contributions a l'histoire du developpement histologique des tumeurs epitheliales (squirrhe, encephaloide, etc). *J Anat Physiol* 1865;2:266–273.

144. Davis RP, Nora PF, Kooy RG, et al: Experience with lobular carcinoma of the breast. Emphasis on recent aspects of management. *Arch Surg* 1979;114:485–488.

*145. DiCostanzo D, Rosen PP, Gareen I, et al: Prognosis of infiltrating lobular carcinoma. An analysis of "classical" and variant tumors. *Am J Surg Pathol* 1990;14:12–23.

*146. Dixon JM, Anderson TJ, Page DL, et al: Infiltrating lobular carcinoma of the breast: An evaluation of the incidence and consequence of bilateral disease. *Br J Surg* 1983;70:513–516.

*147. Dixon JM, Anderson TJ, Page DL, et al: Infiltrating lobular carcinoma of the breast. *Histopathology* 1982;6:149–161.

148. Donegan WL, Perez-Mesa CM: Lobular carcinoma: An indicator for elective biopsy of the second breast. *Am Surg* 1972;176:178.

149. Eusebi V, Pich A, Macchiorlatti E, et al: Morphofunctional differentiation of lobular carcinoma of the breast. *Histopathology* 1977;1:307–314.

*150. Fechner RE: Histologic variants of infiltrating lobular carcinoma of the breast. *Hum Pathol* 1975;6:373–378.

*151. Fechner RE: Infiltrating lobular carcinoma without lobular carcinoma in situ. *Cancer* 1972;29:1539–1545.

152. Fisher ER, Gregorio RM, Redmond C, et al: Tubulolobular invasive breast cancer: a variant of lobular invasive cancer. *Hum Pathol* 1977;8:679–683.

*153. Foote FW Jr, Stewart FW: Lobular carcinoma in situ: A rare form of mammary cancer. *Am J Pathol* 1941;17:491–498.

*154. Gad A, Azzopardi JG: Lobular carcinoma of the breast: A special variant of mucin-secreting carcinoma. *J Clin Pathol* 1975;28:711–716.

155. Haagensen CD: *Diseases of the Breast*, ed 3. Philadelphia, WB Saunders, 1986, pp 815–823.

156. Harris M, Howell A, Chrissohou M, et al: A comparison of the metastatic pattern of infiltrating lobular carcinoma and infiltrating duct carcinoma of the breast. *Br J Cancer* 1984; 50:23–30.

157. Henson D, Tarone R: A study of lobular carcinoma of the breast based on the Third National Cancer Survey in the United States of America. *Tumori* 1979;65:133–142.

158. Hood CL, Font RL, Zimmerman LE: Metastatic mammary carcinoma in the eyelid with histiocytoid appearance. *Cancer* 1973;31:793–800.

159. Lesser ML, Rosen PP, Kinne DW: Multicentricity and bilaterality in invasive breast carcinoma. *Surgery* 1982;91: 234–240.

160. McDivitt RW, Stewart FW, Berg JW: *Tumors of the Breast*, Fasc 2. Atlas of Tumor Pathology, second series, Washington DC, Armed Forces Institute of Pathology, 1968, p 82.

161. Martinez V, Azzopardi JG: Invasive lobular carcinoma of the breast: incidence and variants. *Histopathology* 1979;3: 467–488.

162. Miller HW Jr, Kay S: Infiltrating lobular carcinoma of the female mammary gland. *Gynecol Obstet* 1956;102:661–667.

163. Nesland JM, Holm R, Johannessen JV: Ultrastructural and immunohistochemical features of lobular carcinoma of the breast. *J Pathol* 1985;145:39–52.

*164. Newman W: Lobular carcinoma of the female breast. Report of 73 cases. *Ann Surg* 1966;164:305–314.

165. Noguchi S, Wada T, Nishizawa Y, et al: Clinicopathologic study of twenty-three infiltrating lobular carcinomas of the female breast with special reference to histologic variants and mucin-producing ability. *J Jpn Soc Cancer Ther* 1983;18: 1831–1839.

166. Richter GO, Dockerty MB, Clagett OT: Diffuse infiltrating scirrhous carcinoma of the breast. Special consideration of the single-filing phenomenon. *Cancer* 1967;20:363–370.

167. Rosen PP: in Harris JR, Hellman S, Henderson IC, et al: *Breast Diseases*. Philadelphia, JB Lippincott, 1987, pp 181–185.

*168. Rosen PP, Lesser ML, Senie RT, et al: Epidemiology of breast carcinoma. IV: Age and histologic tumor type. *J Surg Oncol* 1982;19:44–51.

169. Salomon A: Beitrage zur Pathologie und Klinik der mammacarcinome. *Arch Klin Chir* 1913;101:573–668.

170. Shousha S, Backhous CM, Alaghband-Zadeh J, et al: Alveolar variant of invasive lobular carcinoma of the breast. A tumor rich in estrogen receptors. *Am J Clin Pathol* 1986;85:1–5.

171. Shousha S, Bull B, Burn I: Alveolar variant of invasive lobular carcinoma of the breast: An electron microscopic study. *Ultrastruct Pathol* 1986;10:311–319.

172. Smith DB, Howell A, Harris M, et al: Carcinomatous meningitis associated with infiltrating lobular carcinoma of the breast. *Eur J Surg Oncol* 1985;11:33–36.

173. Smith DB, Howell A, Wagstaff J: Infiltrating lobular carcinoma of the breast: Response to endocrine therapy and survival. *Eur J Surg Oncol* 1987;23:979–982.

174. Toyoshima S, Inoshite S, Enjoji M: Invasive lobular carcinoma of the breast. An analysis of 29 cases. *Acta Pathol Jpn* 1986;36:161–171.

175. Tsuchiya S: Intracytoplasmic lumina of human breast cancer. A microscopic study and practical application in cytological diagnosis. *Acta Pathol Jpn* 1981;31:45–54.

176. Underwood JCE, Parsons MA, Harris SC, et al: Frozen section appearances simulating invasive lobular carcinoma in breast tissue adjacent to inflammatory lesions and biopsy sites. *Histopathology* 1988;13:232–234.

177. Van Bogaert L-J, Maldague P: Infiltrating lobular carcinoma of the female breast. Deviations from the usual histologic appearance. *Cancer* 1980;45:979–984.

178. Waldeyer W: Die Entwickelung der Carcinome. *Arch Pathol Anat Phys Klin Med* 1867;4:470–523.

179. Warren RB: Infiltrating lobular carcinoma metastatic to bone: An unusual morphologic pattern. *Breast* 1985;11:16–18.

180. Weinstein GW, Goldman JN: Metastatic adenocarcinoma of the breast masquerading as chalazion. *Am J Ophthalmol* 1970;69:259–264.

### Tubular Carcinoma

181. Andersen JA, Carter D, Linnell F: A symposium on sclerosing duct lesions of the breast. *Pathol Annu* 1986;21(2): 145–179.

182. Andersson I: Radiographic screening for breast carcinoma. II. Prognostic considerations on the basis of short-term follow-up. *Acta Radiol [Diagn]* 1981;22:227–233.

183. Beahrs O, Shapiro S, Smart C: Report of the working group to review the National Cancer Institute—American Cancer Society Breast Cancer Detection Demonstration Projects. *J Natl Cancer Inst* 1979;62:640–709.

184. Carstens PHB: Tubular carcinoma of the breast. A study of frequency. *Am J Clin Pathol* 1978;70:204–210.

185. Carstens PHB, Greenberg RA, Francis D, et al: Tubular carcinoma of the breast. A long-term follow-up. *Histopathology* 1985;9:271–280.

186. Carstens PHB, Huvos AG, Foote FW Jr, et al: Tubular carcinoma of the breast: A clinicopathologic study of 35 cases. *Am J Clin Pathol* 1972;58:231–238.

187. Cooper HS, Patchefsky AS, Krall RA: Tubular carcinoma of the breast. Association with multicentricity, bilaterality and family history of mammary carcinoma. *Am J Clin Pathol* 1981;73:25–30.

188. Cornil V, Ranvier L: *Manuel d'Histologie Pathologique*. Paris, Germer-Bailliere, 1869, pp 1167–1170.

*189. Deos PH, Norris HJ: Well-differentiated (tubular) carcinoma of the breast: A clinical pathologic study of 145 pure and mixed cases. *Am J Clin Pathol* 1982;78:1–7.

190. Ekblom P, Miettinen M, Forsman L, et al: Basement membrane and apocrine epithelial antigens in differential diagnosis between tubular carcinoma and sclerosing adenosis of the breast. *J Clin Pathol* 1984;37:357–363.

*191. Erlandson RA, Carstens PHB: Ultrastructure of tubular carcinoma of the breast. *Cancer* 1972;29:987–995.

192. Eusebi V, Betts CM, Bussolati G: Tubular carcinoma: A variant of secretory breast carcinoma. *Histopathology* 1979; 3:407–419.

193. Fisher B, Slack NH, Bross IDJ, et al: Cancer of the breast: Size of neoplasm and prognosis. *Cancer* 1969;24:1071–1097.

194. Flotte TJ, Bell DA, Greco MA: Tubular carcinoma and sclerosing adenosis. The use of basal lamina as a differential feature. *Am J Surg Pathol* 1980;4:75–77.

195. Haagensen CD: *Diseases of the Breast*, ed 3. Philadelphia, WB Saunders, 1986, pp 824–832.

*196. Harris M, Ahmed A: The ultrastructure of tubular carcinoma of the breast. *J Pathol* 1977;123:79–83.

197. Harris JR, Hellman S, Henderson IC, et al: *Breast Diseases*. Philadelphia, JB Lippincott, 1987, pp 164–166.

*198. Jao W, Recant W, Swerdlow MA: Comparative ultrastructure of tubular carcinoma and sclerosing adenosis of the breast. *Cancer* 1976;38:180.

199. Lagios MD, Rose MR, Margolin FR: Tubular carcinoma of the breast. Association with multicentricity, bilaterality and family history of mammary carcinoma. *Am J Clin Pathol* 1981;73:25–30.

200. Linell F, Ljungberg O: Breast carcinoma. Progression of tubular cancer and a new classification. *Acta Pathol Microbio Scand (A)* 1980;88:59–60.

201. Linell F, Ljungberg O, Andersson I: Breast carcinoma: Aspects of early stages, progression and related problems. *Acta Pathol Microbiol Scand (A)* (Suppl) 1980;272:4–233.

202. McDivitt RW, Boyce W, Gersell D: Tubular carcinoma of the breast. *Am J Surg Pathol* 1982;6:401–411.

203. Oberman HA, Fidler WJ Jr: Tubular carcinoma of the breast. *Am J Surg Pathol* 1979;3:387–395.

*204. Parl FF, Richardson LD: The histological and biological spectrum of tubular carcinoma of the breast. *Hum Pathol* 1983;14:694–698.

205. Patchefsky AS, Shaber GS, Schwartz GF, et al: The pathology of breast cancer detected by mass population screening. *Cancer* 1977;40:1659–1670.

*206. Peters GN, Wolff M, Haagensen CD: Tubular carcinoma of the breast—clinical pathological correlations based on 100 cases. *Ann Surg* 1981;193:138–149.

207. Rosen PP, Saigo PE, Braun DW Jr, et al: Prognosis in stage II (I1N1M0) breast cancer. *Ann Surg* 1981;194:576–584.

208. Taxy JB: Tubular carcinoma of the male breast. Report of a case. *Cancer* 1975;36:462–465.

*209. Taylor HB, Norris HJ: Well-differentiated carcinoma of the breast. *Cancer* 1970;25:687–692.

210. Tobon H, Salazar H: Tubular carcinoma of the breast. Clinical, histological and ultrastructural observations. *Archiv Pathol Lab Med* 1977;101:310–316.

211. Tremblay G: Elastosis in tubular carcinoma of the breast. *Arch Pathol* 1974;98:302–307.

212. Wellings SR, Alpers CE: Subgross pathologic features and incidence of radial scars in the breast. *Hum Pathol* 1984;15: 475–479.

### Mucinous (Colloid) Carcinoma and Signet-ring Cell Carcinoma

213. Adair F, Berg J, Toubert L, et al: Long-term follow-up of breast cancer patients: The 30 year report. *Cancer* 1974;22: 1145–1150.

214. Al-Hariri JA: Primary signet-ring cell carcinoma of the breast. *Virchows Arch (A) Path Anat and Histol* 1980;388:105–111.

215. Azzopardi JG: *Problems in Breast Pathology*. Philadelphia, WB Saunders, 1979, pp 294–296.

216. Bhargava V, Miller TR, Cohen MB: Mucocele-like tumors of the breast: Cytologic findings in two cases. *Am J Clin Pathol* 1091;95:875–877.

217. Breslow A, Brancaccio ME: Intracellular mucin production by lobular breast carcinoma cells. *Arch Pathol Lab Med* 1976;100:610–621.

*218. Capella C, Eusebi V, Mann B, et al: Endocrine differentiation in mucoid carcinoma of the breast. *Histopathology* 1980;4:613–630.

219. Cheatle GL, Cutler M: Gelatinous carcinoma of the breast. *Arch Surg* 1930;20:569–590.

*220. Clayton F: Pure mucinous carcinomas of breast. *Hum Pathol* 1986;17:34–38.

*221. Coady AT, Shousha S, Dawson PM, et al: Mucinous carcinoma of the breast: Further characterization of its three subtypes. *Histopathology* 1989;15:617–626.

222. Deck JH, Lee MA: Mucin embolism to cerebral arteries: A fatal complication of carcinoma of breast. *Can J Neurol Sci* 1978;5:327–330.

223. Ferguson DJP, Anderson TJ, Wells CA, et al: An ultrastructural study of mucoid carcinoma of the breast: Variability of cytoplasmic features. *Histopathology* 1986;10:1219–1230.

*224. Feyrter F, Hartmann G: Uber die carcinoide Wuchsform des Carcinoma mammae, insbesondere das carcinome dolidum (gelatinosum) mammae. *Frandf Z Pathol* 1963;73: 24–29.

225. Fisher ER, Palekar AS: Solid and mucinous varieties of so-called mammary carcinoid tumors. *Am J Clin Pathol* 1979;72:909–916.

226. Gaabe G: Der Gallertkrebs der Brustdruse. *Beitr z Klin Chir* 1908;60:760–807.

227. Gad A, Azzopardi JG: Lobular carcinoma of the breast: A special variant of mucin-secreting carcinoma. *J Clin Pathol* 1976;28:711–716.

228. Geschikter CF: Gelatinous mammary cancer. *Ann Surg* 1938;108:321–346.

229. Gilks B, Tavassoli FA: Coexistence of intracytoplasmic lumens and membrane-bound vesicles in an invasive carcinoma arising in a cystosarcoma phyllodes. *Ultrastruct Pathol* 1988;12:631–642.

230. Haagensen CD: *Diseases of the Breast*, ed 3. Philadelphia, WB Saunders, 1986, pp 798–807.

231. Halsted WS: A diagnostic sign of gelatinous carcinoma of the breast. *JAMA* 1915;64:1653.

232. Hanna WM, Corkill M: Mucins in breast carcinoma. *Hum Pathol* 1988;19:11–14.

233. Harris M, Vasudev KS, Anfield C, et al: Mucin-producing carcinomas of the breast: Ultrastructural observations. *Histopathology* 1978;2:177–188.

*234. Harris M, Wells S, Vasudev KS: Primary signet-ring cell carcinoma of the breast. *Histopathology* 1978;2:171–176.

*235. Hull MT, Seo IS, Battersby JS, et al: Signet-ring cell carcinoma of the breast. A clinicopathologic study of 24 cases. *Am J Clin Pathol* 1980;73:31–35.

236. Jao W, Lao IO, Chowdhury LN, et al: Ultrastructural aspects of mucinous (colloid) breast carcinoma. *Diagn Gynecol Obstet* 1980;2:83–92.

*237. Komaki K, Sakamoto G, Sugano H: Mucinous carcinoma of the breast in Japan. A prognostic analysis based on morphologic features. *Cancer* 1988;61:989–996.

238. Kondo Y, Akita T, Sugano I, et al: Signet-ring cell carcinoma of the breast. *Acta Pathol Jpn* 1984;34:875–880.

239. Lange F: Der Gallertkrebs der Brustdruse. *Beitr Klin Chir* 1896;16:1–60.

240. Larrey M: Tumeur gelatiniforme ou colloide de la mammelle. *Bull Soc Chir Paris* 1853;3:545–547.

241. Lee BJ, Hauser H, Pack GT: Gelatinous carcinoma of the breast. *Surg Gynecol Obstet* 1934;59:841–857.

*242. Maluf HM, Zukerberg LR, Dickersin GR, et al: Spindle-cell argyrophilic mucin-producing carcinoma of the breast. Histological, ultrastructural, and immunohistochemical studies of two cases. *Am J Surg Pathol* 1991;15:677–686.

243. McDivitt RW, Stewart JW, Berg FW: *Tumors of the Breast*, Fasc 2. Atlas of Tumor Pathology, second series, Washington DC, Armed Forces Institute of Pathology, 1968, p 55–57.

244. Melamed MR, Robbins GF, Foote FW Jr: Prognostic significance of gelatinous mammary carcinoma. *Cancer* 1961;14: 699–704.

*245. Merino MJ, Livolsi VA: Signet-ring carcinoma of the female breast: A clinicopathologic analysis of 24 cases. *Cancer* 1981;48:1830–1837.

*246. Norris HJ, Taylor HB: Prognosis of mucinous (gelatinous) carcinoma of the breast. *Cancer* 1965;18:879–885.

247. Peres-Mesa CM: Gross and Microscopic Pathology, in Donegan WL and Spratt JS (eds): *Cancer of the Breast*. Philadelphia, WB Saunders, 1988, pp 209–211.

*248. Rasmussen BB: Human mucinous breast carcinomas and their lymph node metastases. A histological review of 247 cases. *Pathol Res Pract* 1985;180:377–382.

*249. Rasmussen BB, Rose C, Christensen I: Prognostic factors in primary mucinous carcinoma of the breast. *Am J Clin Pathol* 1987;87:155–160.

*250. Rasmussen BB, Rose C, Thorpe SM, et al: Argyrophilic cells in 202 human mucinous breast carcinomas. Relation to histopathologic and clinical factors. *Am J Clin Pathol* 1985;84:737–740.

251. Robinson RR: Gelatinous cancer of the breast. *Trans Pathol Soc London* 1852;4:275–278.

*252. Rosen PP, Wang T-Y: Colloid carcinoma of the breast. Analysis of 64 patients with long-term follow-up. *Am J Clin Pathol* 1980;73(A):304.

253. Rosen PP, Mucocele-like tumors of the breast. *Am J Surg Pathol* 1986;10:464–469.

254. Saphir O: Mucinous carcinoma of the breast. *Surg Gynecol Obstet* 1941;72:908–914.

255. Silverberg SG, Kay S, Chitale AR, et al: Colloid carcinoma of the breast. *Am J Clin Pathol* 1971;55:355–363.

*256. Steinbrecher JS, Silverberg SG: Signet-ring cell carcinoma.

The mucinous variant of infiltrating lobular carcinoma? *Cancer* 1976;37:828–840.

257. Tellem M, Nedwick A, Amenta PS, et al: Mucin producing carcinoma of the breast: Tissue culture, histochemical and electron microscopic study. *Cancer* 1966;19:573–584.

*258. Toikkanen S, Eerola E, Ekfors T: Pure and mixed mucinous breast carcinomas: DNA stemline and prognosis. *J Clin Pathol* 1988;41:300–303.

259. Towfighi J, Simmonds MA, Davidson EA: Mucin and fat emboli in mucinous carcinomas causing hemorrhagic cerebral infarcts. *Arch Pathol Lab Med* 1983;107:646–649.

260. Veronesi U, Gennari L: II. Carcinoma gelatinoso della mammella. *Tumori* 1960;46:119–155.

261. Walker RA: Mucoid carcinomas of the breast: A study using mucin histochemistry and peanut lectin. *Histopathology* 1982;6:571–579.

### Carcinoma with Neuroendocrine Granules

*262. Azzopardi JG, Muretto P, Goddeeris P, et al: "Carcinoid" tumours of the breast: The morphological spectrum of argyrophil carcinomas. *Histopathology* 1982;6:549–569.

263. Bussolati G, Gugliotta P, Sapino A, et al: Chromogranin reactive endocrine cells in argyrophilic carcinomas ("carcinoids") and normal tissue of the breast. *Am J Pathol* 1985;120:186–192.

264. Bussolati G, Papotti M, Sapino A, et al: Endocrine markers in argyrophilic carcinoma of the breast. *Am J Surg Pathol* 1987;11:248–256.

265. Chabon AB, Costales F: Estrogen receptor activity in primary argyrophilic carcinoma of the breast. *Diagn Gynecol Obstet* 1980;2:93–97.

*266. Chen KTK: Breast carcinomas with carcinoid features. *Breast* 1981;7:2–5.

*267. Clayton F, Sibley RK, Ordonez NG, et al: Argyrophilic breast carcinomas: Evidence of lactational differentiation. *Am J Surg Pathol* 1982;6:323–333.

*268. Cross AS, Azzopardi JG, Krausz T, et al: A morphological and immunocytochemical study of a distinctive variant of ductal carcinoma in-situ of the breast. *Histopathology* 1985; 9:21–37.

*269. Cubilla AL, Woodruff JM: Primary carcinoid tumor of the breast. A report of eight cases. *Am J Surg Pathol* 1977;4:283–292.

270. Devitt PG: Carcinoid tumour of the breast. *Br Med J* 1978;ii,327.

*271. Ferguson DJP, Anderson TJ: Distribution of dense core granules in normal, benign and malignant breast tissue. *J Pathol* 1985;147:59–65.

*272. Fetissof F, Dubois MP, Arbeille-Brassart B, et al: Argyrophilic cells in mammary carcinoma. *Hum Pathol* 1983;14: 127–134.

*273. Fetissof F, Guilloteau D, Cornet M, et al: Association s'une forme solide et d'une forme colloide d'un carcinoide mammaire. *Ann Pathol* (Paris) 1981;1:213–220.

274. Fisher ER, Palekar AS, NSABP collaborators: Solid and mucinous varieties of so-called mammary carcinoid tumors. *Am J Clin Pathol* 1979;72:909–916.

275. Hawley PR: A case of secondary carcinoid tumors in both breasts following excision of primary carcinoid tumour of the duodenum. *Br J Surg* 1966;53:818–820.

276. Harrist TJ, Kalisher L: Breast metastasis: An unusual manifestation of a malignant carcinoid tumor. *Cancer* 1977;40: 3102–3106.

277. Juntti-Berggen L, Pitkanen P, Wilander E: Argyrophil endocrine cells with ACTH and HCG immunoreactivity in a carcinoma of the breast. *Virchows Arch (Cell Pathol)* 1983;43: 37–42.

278. Kaneko H, Hojo H, Ishikawa S, et al: Norepinephrine-producing tumors of bilateral breast. A case report. *Cancer* 1978;41:2002–2007.

279. Kaneko H, Sumida T, Sekiya M, et al: A breast carcinoid tumor with special reference to ultrastructural study. *Acta Pathol Jpn* 1982;32:327–332.

280. Kashlan RB, Powell RW, Nolting SF: Carcinoid and other tumors metastatic to the breast. *J Surg Oncol* 1982;20:25.

*281. McCutcheon J, Walker RA: The significance of argyrophilia in human breast carcinoma. *Virchows Arch (A)* 1987;410: 369–374.

282. Memoli VA, Nesland J, Warren WH, et al: Immunohistochemical and ultrastructural observations concerning the issue of neuroendocrine differentiation in breast carcinomas. *Lab Invest* 1984;50:39A.

283. Min K-W: Argyrophilia in breast carcinomas: Histochemical, ultrastructural and immunocytochemical study. *Lab Invest* 1983;48:58A.

*284. Monaghan P, Roberts JDB: Immunohistochemical evidence for neuroendocrine differentiation in human breast carcinomas. *J Pathol* 1985;147:281–289.

285. Nesland JM, Holm R, Johannessen JV: Neuroendocrine differentiation in breast lesions. *Pathol Res Pract* 1986;181: 524–530.

286. Nesland JM, Holm R, Johannessen JV, et al: Neuron specific enolase immunostaining in the diagnosis of breast carcinomas with neuroendocrine differentiation. Its usefulness and limitations. *J Pathol* 1986;148:35–43.

287. Papotti M, Macri L, Finzi G, et al: Neuroendocrine differentiation in carcinomas of the breast. A study of 51 cases. *Semin Diagn Pathol* 1989;6:174–188.

*288. Partanen S, Syrjanin K: Argyrophilic cells in carcinoma of the female breast. *Virchows Arch* (A) 1981;391:45–51.

289. Raju U, Fine G: The controversial mammary carcinoid tumor. *Lab Invest* 1983;48:69A.

*290. Santini D, Bazzocchi F, Pileri S, et al: Mammary carcinoma with argyrophilic cells: An immunohistochemical and ultrastructural study. *Tumori* 1985;71:331–338.

*291. Sariola H, Lehtonen E, Saxen E: Breast tumors with a solid and uniform carcinoid pattern. Ultrastructural and immunohistochemical study of two cases. *Pathol Res Pract* 1985; 178:405–411.

292. Taxy JB, Tischler AS, Insalaco SJ, et al: "Carcinoid" tumor of the breast. A variant of conventional breast cancer? *Hum Pathol* 1981;12:170–179.

293. Toyoshima S: Mammary carcinoma with argyrophil cells. *Cancer* 1983;52:2129–2138.

*294. Vogler E: Uber da basilare Helle-Zellen-organ der menschlichen Brustdruse. *Klin Med* 1947;129:37–42.

295. Wilander E, Pahlman S, Sallstrom J, et al: Neuron-specific enolase expression and neuroendocrine differentiation in carcinomas of the breast. *Arch Pathol Lab Med* 1987;111:830–832.

296. Wong SY, Kernohan NM, Walker F: Breast cancer with extremely high estrogen receptor protein status. *Histopathology* 1990;16:125–132.

297. Woodward BH, Eisenbarth G, Wallace NR, et al: Adrenocorticotrophic production by mammary carcinoma. *Cancer* 1981;47:1823–1827.


## Medullary Carcinoma


298. Ahmad A: The ultrastructure of medullary carcinoma of the breast. *Virchows Arch Path Anat and Histol (A)* 1980;388:175–186.

299. Bloom HJG, Richardson WW, Field JR: Host resistance and survival in carcinoma of breast. A study of 104 cases of medullary carcinoma in a series of 1,411 cases of breast cancer followed for 20 years. *Br Med J* 1970;3:181–187.

300. Daroca PJ: Medullary carcinoma of the breast with granulomatous stroma. *Hum Pathol* 1987;18:761–763.

301. Erhardt K, Auer G, Folin A, et al: Mammary carcinoma: Comparison between histologic type, estrogen receptor and nuclear DNA content. *Am J Clin Oncol* 1986;1:83–89.

302. Ewing J: *Neoplastic Diseases*, ed 4. Philadelphia, WB Saunders, 1940.

303. Flores L, Arlen M, Elguezabal A, et al: Host tumor relationships in medullary carcinoma of the breast. *Surg Gynecol Obstet* 1974;139:683–688.

304. Geschikter CF: *Diseases of the Breast: Diagnosis, Pathology, and Treatment*, ed 2. Philadelphia, JB Lippincott, 1945, p 565.

305. Haagensen CD: *Diseases of the Breast*, ed 3. Philadelphia, WB Saunders, 1986, pp 790–797.

306. Harris M, Lessells AM: The ultrastructure of medullary, atypical medullary and non-medullary carcinomas of the breast. *Histopathology* 1986;10:405–414.

307. Horsfall DJ, Telley WD, Orell SR, et al: Relationship between ploidy and steroid hormone receptors in primary breast cancer. *Br J Cancer* 1986;53:23–28.

*308. Hsu S, Raine L, Nayak RN: Medullary carcinoma of breast: An immunohistochemical study of its lymphoid stroma. *Cancer* 1981;48:1368–1376.

*309. Maier WP, Rosemon GP, Goldman LI, et al: A ten year study of medullary carcinoma of the breast. *Surg Obstet Gynecol* 1977;144:695–698.

310. Michaud J, Orin J: Ultrastructure d'un epitheliome medullaire de la glande mammaire. *Laval Medical* 1971;412:496–507.

311. Moore OS Jr, Foote FW Jr: The relatively favorable prognosis of medullary carcinoma of the breast. *Cancer* 1949;2:635–642.

312. Murad TM, Scarpelli DG: The ultrastructure of medullary and scirrhous mammary duct carcinoma. *Am J Pathol* 1967;50:335–360.

313. Olszewski W, Darzynkiewicz Z, Rosen PP, et al: Flow cytometry of breast carcinoma. I. Relation of DNA ploidy level to histology and estrogen receptors. *Cancer* 1981;48:980–984.

*314. Rapin V, Contesso G, Mouriesse H, et al: Medullary breast carcinoma. A reevaluation of 95 cases of breast cancer with inflammatory stroma. *Cancer* 1988;61:2503–2510.

315. Richardson RW: Medullary carcinoma of the breast: A distinctive tumour type with a relatively good prognosis following radical mastectomy. *Br J Cancer* 1956;10:415–423.

*316. Ridolfi RE, Rosen PP, Post A, et al: Medullary carcinoma of the breast. A clinical pathological study with 10 year follow-up. *Cancer* 1977;40:1365–1385.

317. Schwartz GF: Solid circumscribed carcinoma of the breast. *Ann Surg* 1969;169:165–174.

318. Wargotz ES, Silverberg SG: Medullary carcinoma of the breast: A clinicopathologic study with appraisal of current diagnostic criteria. *Hum Pathol* 1988;19:1340–1346.

# 10

# Infiltrating Carcinoma, Special Types



## METAPLASTIC CARCINOMA

Metaplastic carcinoma consists of a highly heterogeneous group of neoplasms characterized by an admixture of adenocarcinoma with areas of spindle, squamous, osseous or chondroid differentiation (27). The common denominator of these tumors is the presence of an epithelial or mesenchymal cell population other than and often in addition to an adenocarcinoma within the mammary neoplasm. The second and sometimes third cell population may be epithelial (squamous, etc) or mesenchymal (chondroid, osseous, etc) in nature; it may appear benign or malignant. The degree of differentiation as well as the proportion of the various elements within the tumors is highly variable.

An unusual ossified mammary tumor described by Bonet (6) in 1700 is often cited as the earliest recorded example of a metaplastic neoplasm. This lesion, hard as stone, was adherent to the skin and occurred in a young woman who eventually died from respiratory failure. During the autopsy, having put a knife between the ribs and the sternum, Bonet observed that a large quantity of water gushed out of the hole. He attributed the patient's misery and the respiratory difficulty to the accumulated fluid and concluded that had this disorder been clearly understood, the patient could have been easily and definitely cured of her disease and kept alive. More than two centuries later in 1938, a deep-seated epidermoid carcinoma of the breast with widespread metastases was described by Foot & Moore (17). In the interim occasional case reports alluding to metaplastic changes in unusual mammary carcinomas had appeared in the literature during the 18th, 19th and early 20th centuries (29). McDivitt et al (43) described metaplastic carcinoma as giving the illusion of being chondromyxoid, but with application of immunohistochemical (7) and ultrastructural analysis, it has become evident that there is no illusion but true chondroid (45,60), osseous and even rhabdomyosarcomatous differentiation in some of these tumors.

Furthermore, there are many cases in which the mesenchymal element is a chondrosarcoma, osteosarcoma (66) or a combination of a variety of indisputable sarcomas. Some of the metaplastic elements may even exhibit aneuploidy (16). The admixture of unequivocal sarcomatous areas with the carcinoma has complicated the selection of a proper designation for these neoplasms; the term carcinosarcoma, though appropriate, was not used for a long time because of the uncertainties and divergent viewpoints regarding the origin of the mesenchymal component in these tumors. The carcinosarcomas, along with fibroadenomas and cystosarcoma phyllodes, will be discussed in Chapter 11, Biphasic Tumors.

In contrast to the common occurrence of cartilage and bone in the mammary cancers of cats and dogs, cartilage and bone formation are relatively rare in human mammary carcinomas. This has led to considerable speculation regarding the origin of these tumors. While it is easy to accept the presence of squamous metaplasia within breast carcinomas, acceptance of metaplasia and transformation of epithelial cells to a mesenchymal cell population is more difficult. It should be underscored, however, that the capacity of cells of ectodermal origin to give rise to tissues of mesodermal appearance is well-recognized in certain sites and would not be unique or novel to the mammary epithelium. Schwann cells and glial cells are ectodermal in origin, yet histologically neurilemmomas and gliomas are mesodermal rather than epithelial in pattern. Bone and cartilage are seen in calcifying epithelioma of Malherbe, benign mixed tumors of the salivary glands and skin appendage tumors. Furthermore, the myoepithelial cell population in the breast is a hybrid cell population with partial epithelial and mesenchymal features. Because of the features it shares with both mesenchymal and epithelial cells, the myoepithelial cell seems to be a good candidate as a stem cell that could differentiate completely toward both epithelial and mesenchymal cell lines within a neoplasm. But since the neoplastic cell is no longer governed by the restrictions that mandate a given phenotypic expression in a normal cell, any neoplastic cell could theoretically transform or differentiate into a completely different cell line compared to its cell of origin.

Currently a metaplastic origin from epithelial or myoepithelial elements is favored for the mesenchymal component of these tumors; however, unequivocal evidence for this contention is lacking in the literature. In some earlier studies, the presence of transitional areas where the epithelial and mesenchymal elements merge at light microscopic level, or the presence of occasional tight junctions or "desmosomes" at the ultrastructural level in an otherwise typical or predominantly mesenchymal cell population (20) has been viewed as supporting an epithelial origin for the mesenchymal cells. Alternately, one might argue that in cases where the mesenchymal cells predominate, the presence of an occasional cell with epithelial features (expression of cytokeratin immunohistochemically, presence of desmosomes and tonofilaments at the ultrastructural level or both) indicates that it is the mesenchymal cell that is undergoing epithelial metaplasia and transformation rather than vice versa.

The inappropriate expression of epithelial antigens by mesenchymal tumors and the presence of occasional tight junctions and "desmosomes" in a variety of purely and unquestionably mesenchymal cells has been documented on numerous occasions (10,40,46). In general, however, this expression is limited to isolated cells and is sporadic in nature. Conventionally, in case of such mammary tumors, there has been a preference to interpret the lesion as epithelial even in the presence of features that are not that specific. For example, Harris (23) described a spindle cell mammary neoplasm which was composed of an admixture of fibroblasts and myofibroblasts at the ultrastructural level. The lesion was interpreted as epithelial in origin based on the presence of tonofilaments in some "myofibroblastic" cells. The relative proportion of the cells with tonofilaments in the tumor was not stated. An alternate explanation, however, could be that the cells with "tonofilaments" were mesenchymal cells undergoing epithelial metaplasia. The same argument could be extended to other cases and other types of metaplasia particularly when the predominant cell population in the tumor is mesenchymal in nature.

The evidence provided so far for a myoepithelial origin for metaplastic carcinomas with chondro/osseous differentiation (matrix producing) is not any more convincing, as it simply consists of the illustration of a large amount of classic bundles of tonofilaments around the nucleus of a neoplastic cell and interpretation of one of the smaller bundles as myofibrils (64). The partially illustrated cell shows no pinocytotic vesicles or patchy basal lamina to qualify it as a myoepithelial cell. Since intermediate filaments are present in many cells, their presence is not

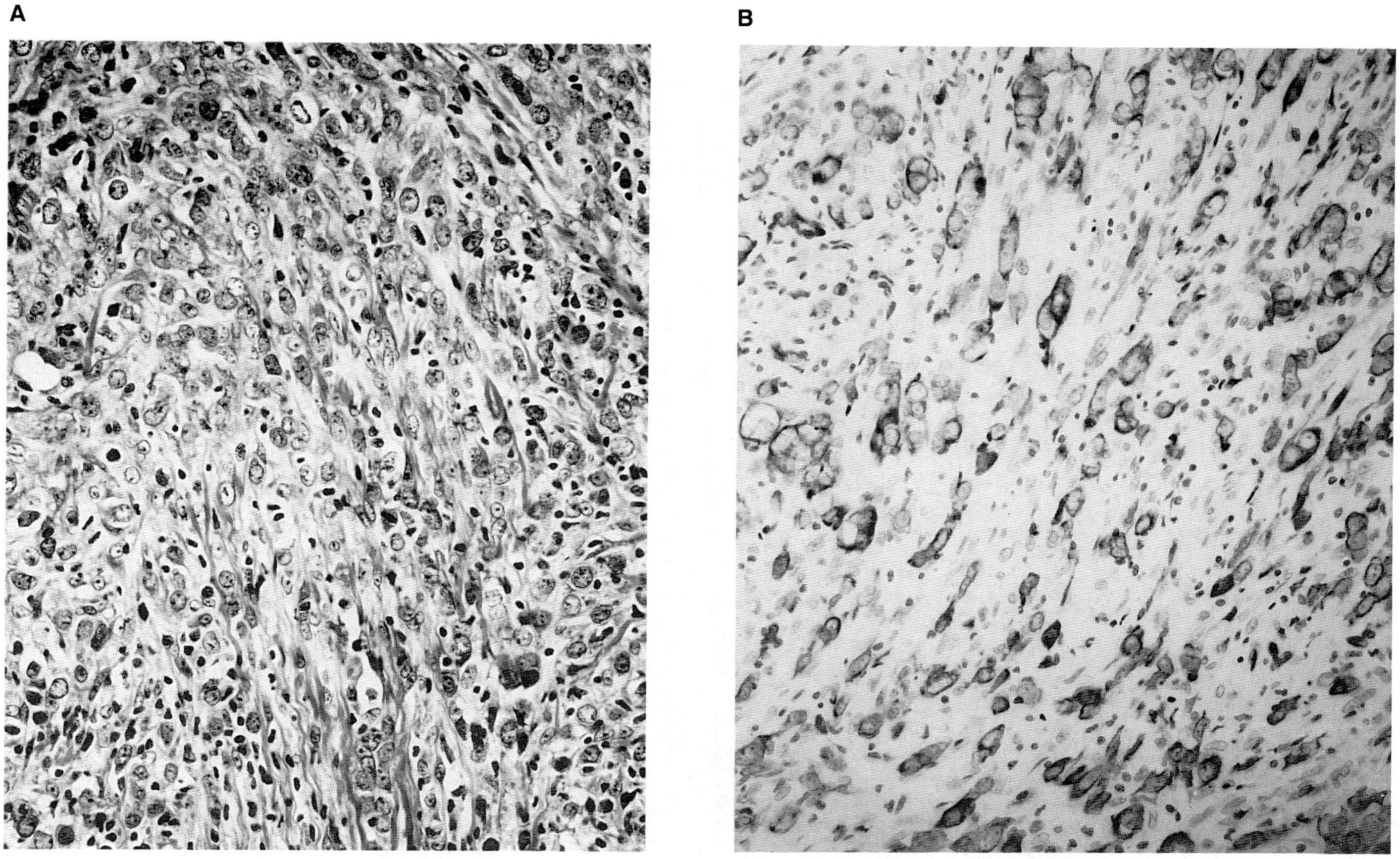


**Figure 10.1(a,b)** Pure spindle cell carcinoma. (a) The tumor is composed purely of mitotically-active spindle cells admixed with an inflammatory infiltrate. (H&E, X200) (b) The spindle cells react intensely with cytokeratin. (H&E, X250) (Figs 10.1a–e from Tavassoli FA: *Pathol Annu* 1992;27(pt 2): 89–119, with permission)

sufficient for designating a cell as myoepithelial in nature without other supportive features.

While resolution of the origin of these tumors may be difficult, it can be established with relative simplicity that the spindle cell or the mesenchymal-appearing component associated with the carcinoma in some of these neoplasms elaborates only epithelial antigens as confirmed by immunohistochemical analysis. Identification of epithelial features (numerous well-developed desmosomes and tonofilaments) at the ultrastructural level would further support their epithelial nature. Therefore, when the spindle cells reflect transformed epithelial cells (54), the lesion qualifies as metaplastic carcinoma.

In other carcinomas with a spindle cell component, the malignant spindle cells or other mesenchymal-appearing components fail to elaborate epithelial antigens immunohistochemically, and lack epithelial features ultrastructurally. The spindle cells in these tumors are indeed mesenchymal in nature and often show a positive reaction with desmin, actin or vimentin. These tumors qualify as carcinosarcoma regardless of the precise origin of the mesenchymal cell component.

A third group of carcinomas is composed purely of spindle cells (47), without recognizable squamous or adenocarcinoma within the lesion (Fig. 10.1). Some of these were recognized as myoepithelial lesions as early as 1931 (18), but others are epithelial in nature. These tumors can cause significant difficulty in classification particularly because they often have a prominent reactive stromal component admixed with the neoplastic cells. The neoplastic cells show a positive reaction to cytokeratin, while the reactive stromal cells display various degrees of positivity for actin, desmin and/or vimentin. The latter should not be mistaken for positivity in the neoplastic cells; this confusion could lead to the misinterpretation of these carcinomas as myoepithelial in nature or derivation. A true spindle cell myoepithelial carcinoma generally displays intense positivity for actin with or without a positive reaction for S-100 protein along with a generally less intense and often sporadic reaction for cytokeratin in the neoplastic cells. If immunoreac-

c

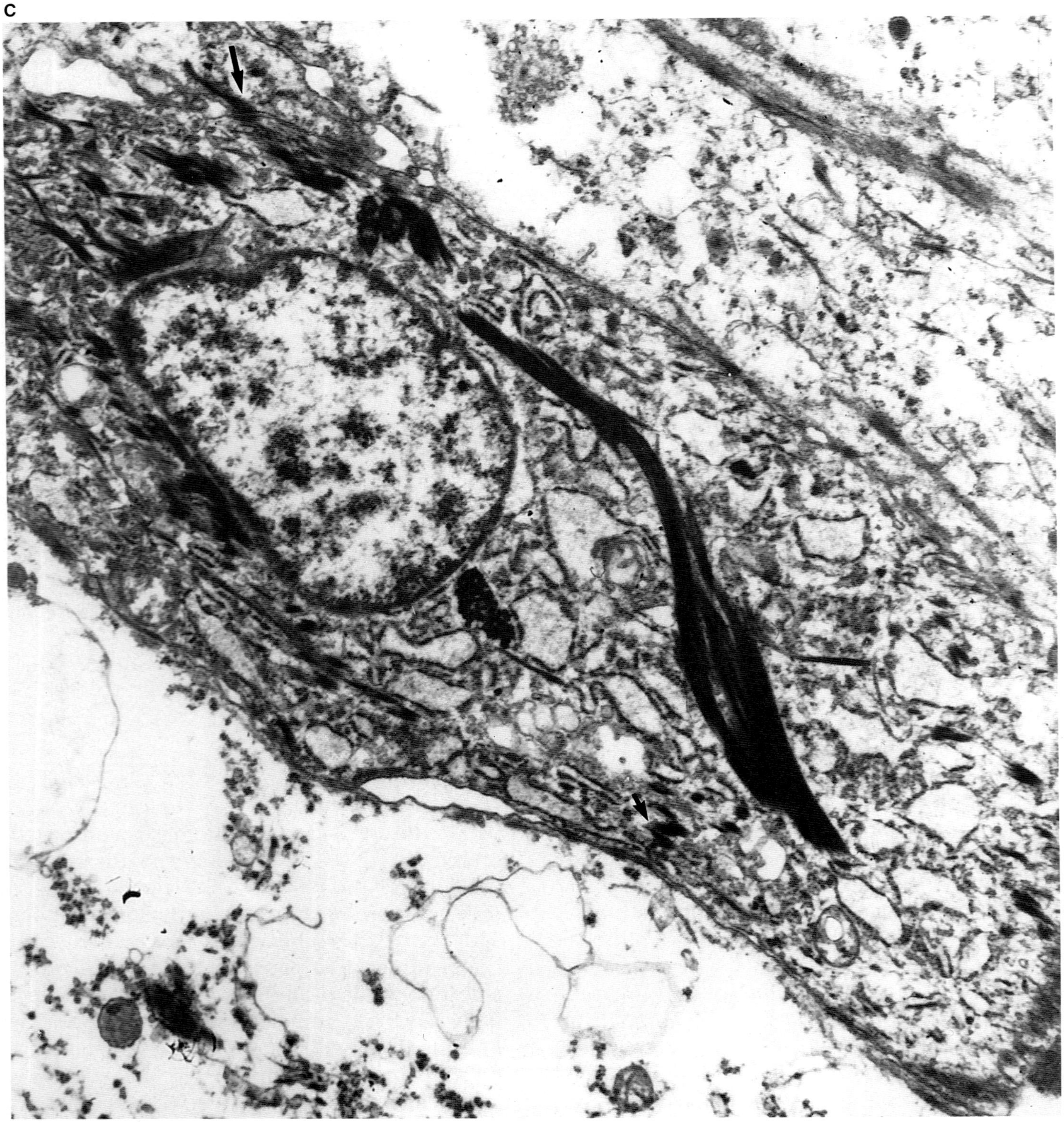

**Figure 10.1(c)** Spindle cell carcinoma. Tumor cells contain abundant tonofilaments, intracytoplasmic (short arrow) and intercellular (long arrow) desmosomes; the abundant tonofilaments indicate a squamous differentiation. (Uranyl acetate-lead citrate, X7,000)

tions are not valid for some reason, ultrastructural analysis can help resolve the problem.

Once it has been established that a pure spindle cell tumor is an epithelial neoplasm, it should be determined whether it is a squamous carcinoma or an adenocarcinoma. Electron microscopy can resolve this issue and also helps in the confirmation of a myoepithelial carcinoma. Desmosomes and tight

D

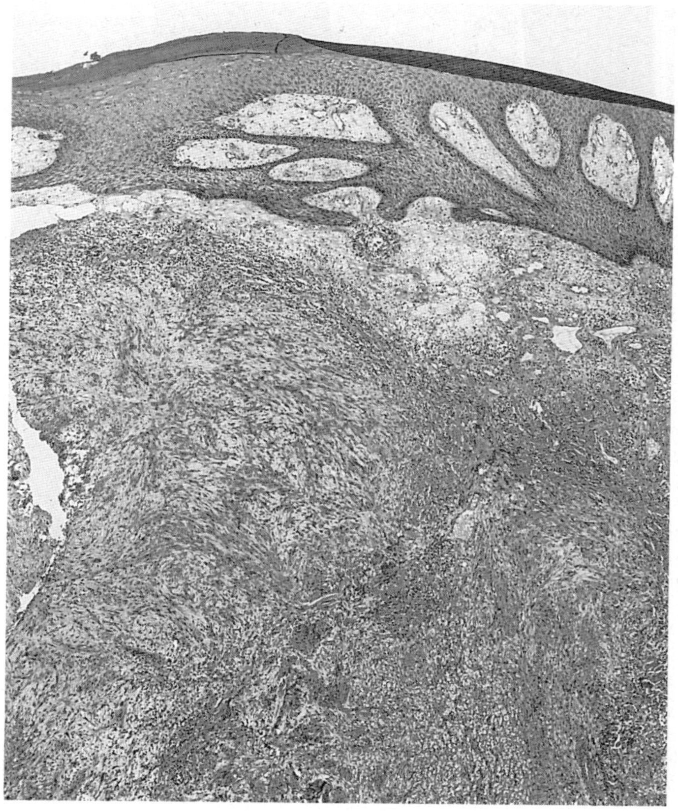

E

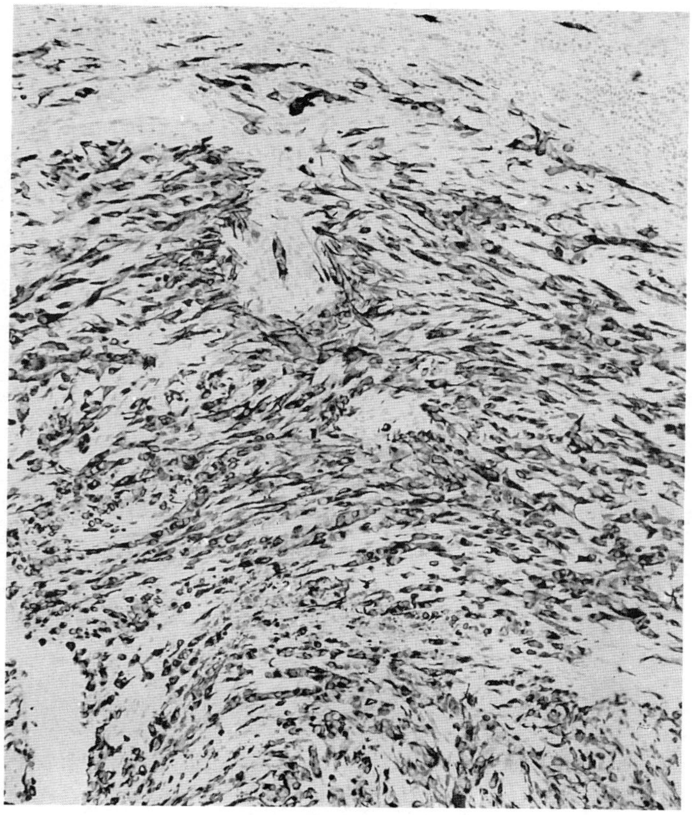

**Figure 10.1(d,e)** Spindle cell carcinoma. (d) Another pure spindle cell carcinoma extending to the subcutaneous region. (H&E, X75) (e) The cells show a positive reaction for cytokeratin. (Immunostain for cytokeratin, X100)

junctions are present in squamous carcinoma and adenocarcinoma, as well as in myoepithelial carcinomas. The presence of abundant tonofilaments in the tumor cells would favor a squamous differentiation, while the presence of microvilli and intracytoplasmic lumens would indicate an adenocarcinoma. A myoepithelial carcinoma is distinguished by the predominance of spindle cells that contain myofibrils with dense bodies, pinocytotic vesicles, and patchy basal lamina in addition to cells that also contain tonofilaments, generally in a perinuclear distribution. The ultrastructural findings would establish whether the spindle cell tumor is a squamous carcinoma with spindle cell metaplasia, an adenocarcinoma with spindle cell differentiation, or a myoepithelial carcinoma.

Among carcinomas with chondroid differentiation, there are some that resemble a pure chondroid tumor except for the fact that a majority of the neoplastic cells display a positive reaction for cytokeratin and S-100 protein simultaneously, but fail to react appreciably with actin. These tumors have been considered a variant of metaplastic carcinoma in the breast despite the dominance of chondroid features and the fact that skeletal chondrosarcomas with squamous differentiation and cytokeratin elaboration have been well documented (40).

To reduce the heterogeneity clearly evident in this category of metaplastic carcinomas and to obtain more reliable information concerning the prognosis and response to therapy, classification of these tumors based on the microscopic appearance of the lesion at the time of presentation is proposed (Table 10.1). This classification, which is supported by immunohistochemical and ultrastructural findings (60) encompasses all possible combinations that may occur within these tumors and is used here to discuss the various subtypes of metaplastic carcinoma.

## SQUAMOUS CARCINOMA

If a carcinoma is composed purely of squamous cells, then it should be designated as a squamous carci-

**Table 10.1** Classification of Metaplastic Carcinoma

**Squamous Carcinoma**

a. Large Cell, (keratinizing or non-keratinizing)
b. Squamous Carcinoma with Spindle Cell Metaplasia (with or without acantholytic features)

**Adenosquamous Carcinoma**

a. High Grade
b. Low Grade (including a syringomatous variant)

**Adenocarcinoma with Spindle Cell Metaplasia**

**Carcinoma with Chondroid Metaplasia**

a. Regular Infiltrating Duct or other types of Carcinoma with Focal Chondroid Differentiation
b. Chondroid Carcinoma (? Epithelioid Chondrosarcoma)

**Carcinoma with Osseous Differentiation**

noma regardless of its mode of development or the variation in the range of appearances of the neoplastic squamous cells (keratinizing, spindle cell, or acantholytic). Apocrine carcinomas and signet-ring cell carcinomas are also composed of a metaplastic cell population, but they are not referred to as metaplastic carcinoma. Furthermore, the origin of epidermoid carcinomas in the lungs is also through a metaplastic process, yet they are not designated as metaplastic carcinoma. To qualify as a primary mammary squamous carcinoma, the tumor should have no connection with the overlying cutaneous squamous epithelium. Squamous carcinomas arising within cystosarcomas (3) and metastatic squamous carcinoma from known primaries elsewhere in the body (38) are excluded from this group.

Primary squamous carcinomas are rare, accounting for less than 1% of all mammary carcinomas. While Fisher et al (15) noted squamous metaplasia in 3.7% of 1,665 invasive breast carcinomas, they did not observe a single case of pure squamous carcinoma. Haagensen (21) had not observed a single case of pure squamous carcinoma during a 54-year period between 1919 and 1973. At least 55 examples of pure squamous carcinoma can be found readily in the English literature (2,4,5,9,12–14,19,22,25,28,30,37,39, 48,56,61,63,65,67), however. There are around 40 pure squamous carcinomas in the AFIP files, 11 of which were included in a study of spindle cell carcinomas (63) and 22 of which were reported separately as squamous cell carcinoma (65). The average age of women with squamous carcinoma is around 54 years with patients ranging in age from the late 20s to the mid 80s.

## Macroscopic Features

The only distinctive gross feature of squamous carcinoma is the presence of cysts within many of the reported tumors. The lesions range in size from 2 to 12 cm with a median of 4 cm. They may appear well-circumscribed or highly irregular in outline. Areas of necrosis may be present in a small proportion of cases.

## Microscopic Features

Microscopically, squamous carcinomas may be large cell keratinizing, acantholytic, spindled or a combination of these cell types, often proliferating around a cyst (Figs. 10.2–10.3). Intercellular bridges, keratin

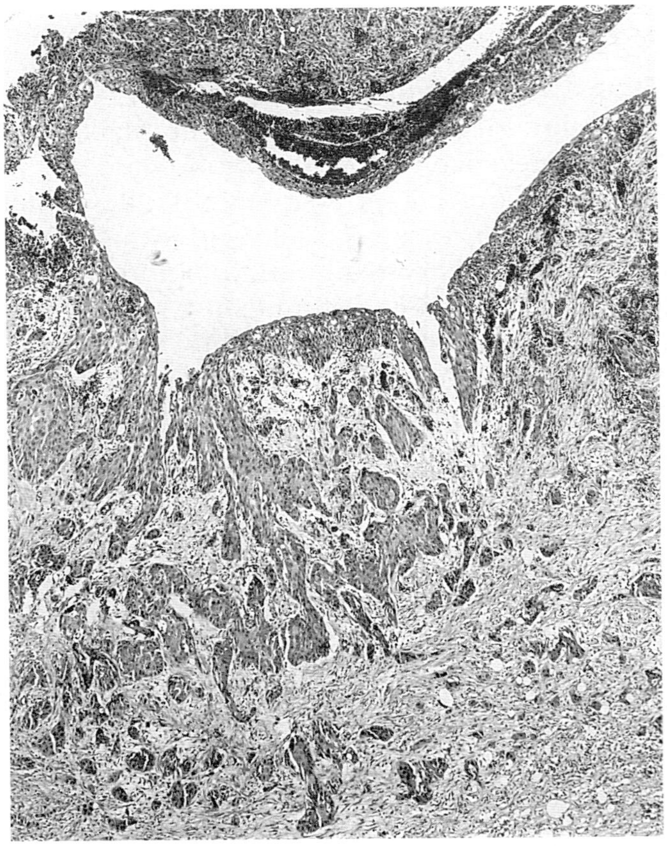

**Figure 10.2** Squamous carcinoma. A central cyst is lined by well-differentiated squamous epithelium. (H&E, X40) (From Tavassoli FA: *Pathol Annu* 1992;27(pt 2):89–119, with permission)

A

B

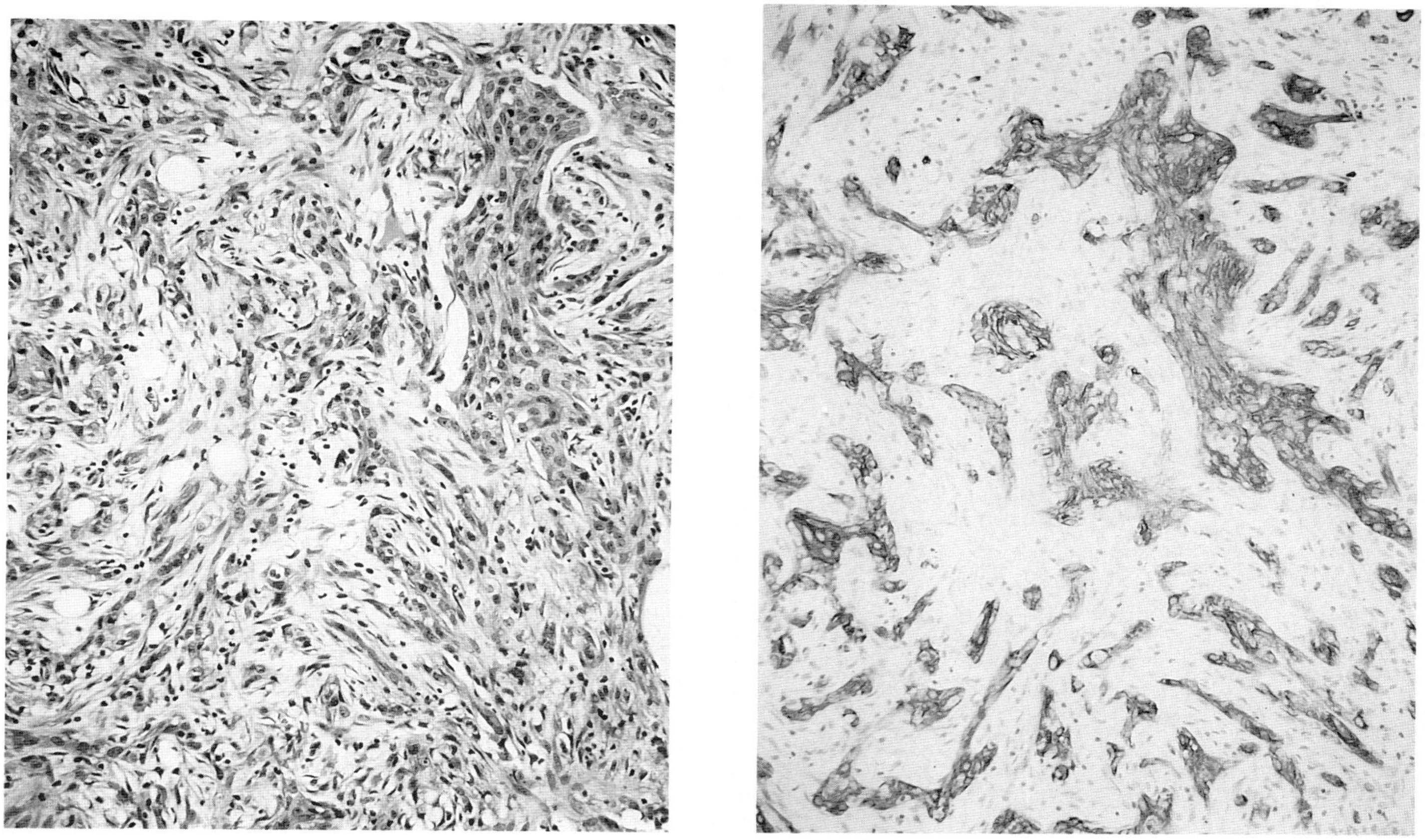

**Figure 10.3** Squamous carcinoma. (a) Farther away from the cyst, the cell clusters elongate and spindle out. (H&E, X160) (b) Immunoreaction with cytokeratin unmasks the actual epithelial component, separating it from the background of reactive stromal cells. (Immunostain for cytokeratin, X160) (From Tavassoli FA: *Pathol Annu* 1992;27(pt 2):89–119, with permission)

pearls, keratohyaline granules and areas of necrosis are common. The cystic portions of the tumor are often lined by banal-appearing squamous epithelium, but as branches of the tumor emanate from the cyst and infiltrate the surrounding stroma, the degree of atypia increases.

The proportion of spindle cell metaplasia within squamous carcinomas is highly variable when present; sometimes the tumor is composed predominantly of spindle cells with rare nests of squamous epithelium (Fig. 10.4). The acantholytic variant described by Eusebi et al (14) is characterized by an admixture of spindle cells and edematous-appearing "spongiotic" foci where channels of various sizes form an intricate network reminiscent of a vascular tumor (Fig. 10.5). The channels are either empty or filled with amorphous mucoid material. The cells lining the channels are attenuated or plump and cuboidal. They show a positive reaction to cytokeratin but are negative for factor VIII and epithelial membrane antigen (EMA). Nests of squamous epithelium may be present within the edematous and spongiotic areas.

When the spindle cells dominate, it is important to confirm the epithelial nature of the tumor by immunohistochemical stains for cytokeratin. A notable proportion of the spindle cells in many of these tumors reflect reactive stroma and these will not react with cytokeratin, but often display an intensely positive reaction with actin, vimentin, and/or desmin. The extracellular matrix of human breast tumor cells is mitogenic for the fibroblasts and also causes the spindle fibroblasts to become more elliptical and grow in whorls (31). A myofibroblastic cell population has also been identified in the pseudosarcomatous reaction in a polypoid carcinoma (34). Obviously, both fibroblasts and myofibroblasts can be identified in the supportive stroma of a carcinoma. As a rule it is not good practice to interpret a spindle cell tumor as spindle cell carcinoma when there is no immunohistochemical or ultrastructural confirmation that the spindle cells are indeed epithelial in nature. As alluded to in the introduction, in the absence of recognizable squamous epithelium, a positive reaction for cytokeratin or other epithelial antigens in the spindle cells does not necessarily imply a squamous

A

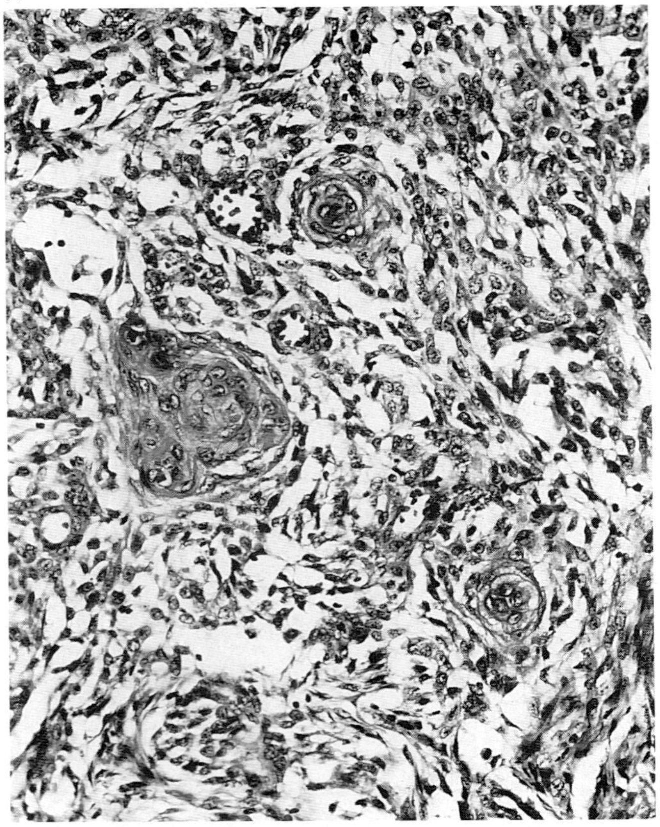

**Figure 10.4(a)** Squamous carcinoma, predominantly spindle cell type. Rare nests of squamous epithelium are surrounded by spindle cells. (H&E, X200) (Figs. 10.4a&b from Tavassoli FA: *Pathol Annu* 1992;27 (pt 2):89–119, with permission)

carcinoma since adenocarcinomas may also show a prominent spindle cell metaplasia. Electron microscopy in such cases would help establish the squamous nature of the tumor if abundant tonofilaments, intercellular bridges, or both are identified.

## Origin of Squamous Metaplasia

While squamous metaplasia is the most common metaplastic alteration in human breast carcinomas (43), the genesis of this change is not well understood. The possibility of origin from misplaced pluripotential embryonic cells has been raised by some (53). Currently however, a metaplastic origin from the glandular epithelium is favored. Squamous metaplasia with keratinization is prevalent in preneoplastic and neoplastic mammary glands of mice and rats following methylcholanthrene treatment (11,44). Mixtures of cyclic adenine nucleotide, prostaglandins and papaverine have induced extensive squamous metaplasia and excessive keratin production along with epithelial hyperplasia in nonmalignant breast tissue maintained in organ culture for ten days (55). These inducers are thought to elevate levels of 3′:5′-monophosphate in other systems. They appear to act synergistically, as, they have little or no activity individually, but their combination is highly active (55). The stage of the menstrual cycle at the time of breast biopsy strongly influences the responsiveness to the inducers. Mammary glands are most resistant during the first ten days of the cycle, very susceptible during the last ten days and intermediately sensitive after menopause. It has been proposed, therefore, that cyclic adenine nucleotides and prostaglandins may play a role in the spontaneous induction of squamous metaplasia in the human breast.

## Hormone Receptors

Estrogen receptor assays have shown only mild positivity in only two of the ten cases for which this information is available in the literature (4,48,56,63, 65). One of these was a spindle cell carcinoma, and it is not absolutely certain that it was indeed a spindled squamous carcinoma or a spindled adenocarcinoma (63).

## Prognosis

Opinions vary regarding the prognosis of squamous carcinoma. While some investigators believe the prognosis is comparable to that of typical invasive breast carcinoma (3,9,19), others (14,48,61) have suggested a worse prognosis for pure squamous carcinoma. The cases reported by Eusebi et al (14) were of the acantholytic type, and those reported by Toikannen (61) may have had similar areas. It is, therefore, possible that the acantholytic variant of squamous carcinoma reflects a poorly-differentiated tumor capable of a more aggressive behavior. Some squamous carcinomas, on the other hand, are very well-differentiated and low grade. One of the cases reviewed at AFIP consisted of a deep-seated tumor nodule in a 25-year-old woman. It was composed of solid nests of well-differenti-

B

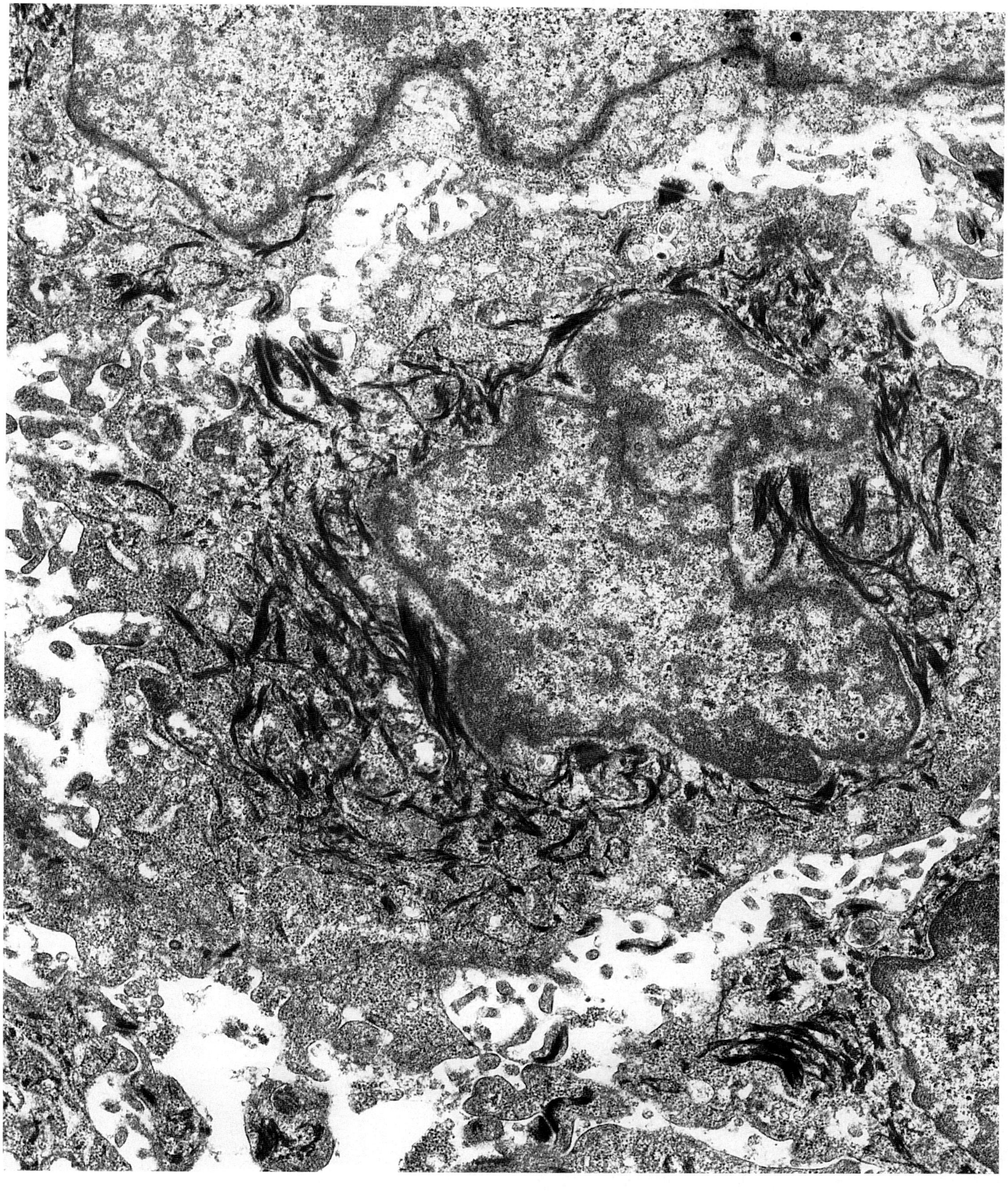

**Figure 10.4(b)** Squamous carcinoma. At the ultrastructural level, the spindle cells contain bundles of tonofilaments and display tight junctions and desmosomes; the presence of microvillous cytoplasmic projections is indicative of the metaplastic glandular origin of the cell. (Uranyl acetate-lead citrate, X5,500)

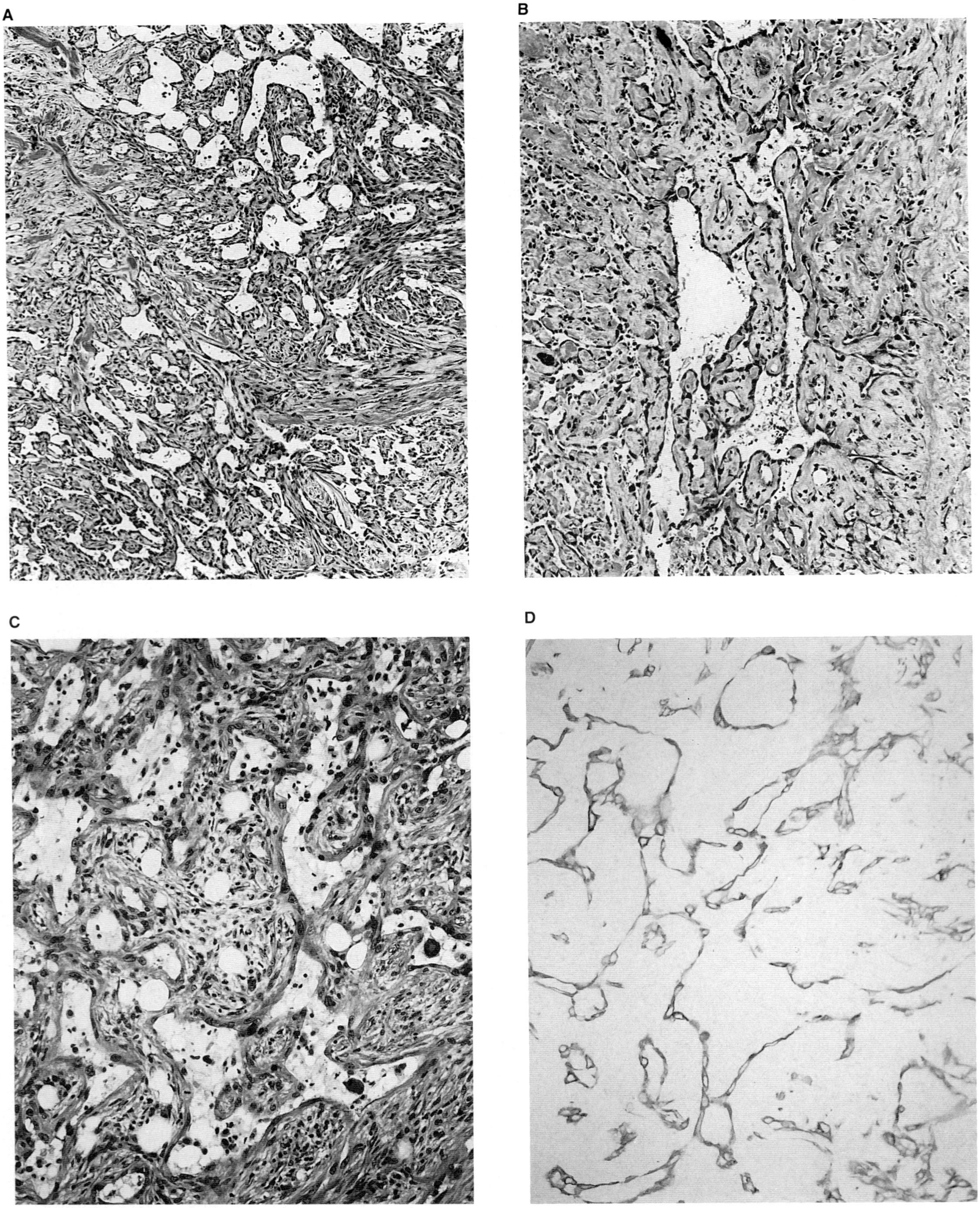


**Figure 10.5** Squamous carcinoma, acantholytic variant. (a) This densely cellular spindle cell neoplasm was initially interpreted as an angiosarcoma, based on the angulated, branching, anastomosing channels in the tumor. (H&E, X75) (b) Areas of interstitial sclerosis. (H&E, X100) (c) The actual diagnosis remained illusive even at higher magnification. (H&E, X160) (d) Immunoreaction for cytokeratin decorates the cells lining the channels, but these cells failed to react with factor VIII. (X160) (e) At the ultrastructural level, the cells contain abundant tonofilaments (small arrows) and are attached to one another by tight junctions (long arrows). A white cell is occupying the vascular-like space bound by the tapered squamous cells. (Uranyl acetate-lead citrate, X3,000) (From Tavassoli FA: *Pathol Annu* 1992;27(pt 2):89–119, with permission)

E

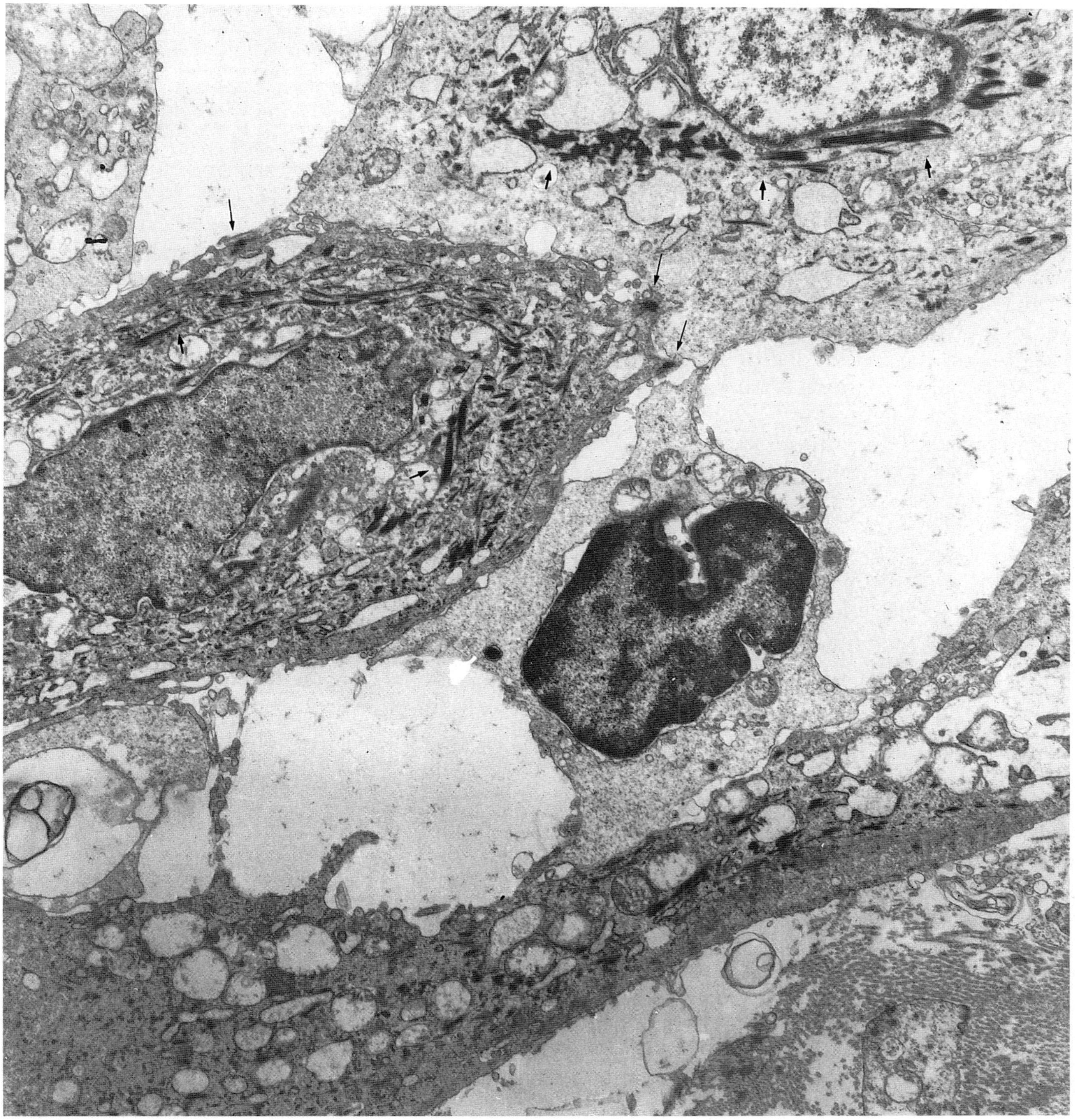

**Figure 10.5(e)** Squamous carcinoma, acantholytic variant. Legend on opposite page.

ated squamous cells. So bland was the appearance of this well-circumscribed tumor, that the patient had no further treatment following the excisional biopsy, despite a diagnosis of low grade squamous carcinoma. Six years later, an identical nodule appeared in the same location. At this time, mastectomy was performed and there was no evidence of lymph node metastasis. Lymph node metastases, morphologically similar to the primary tumor, do occur in some tumors, however.

## ADENOCARCINOMA WITH SQUAMOUS DIFFERENTIATION (ADENOSQUAMOUS CARCINOMA; MUCOEPIDERMOID CARCINOMA)

The terms adenosquamous carcinoma, mucoepidermoid carcinoma, adenoacanthoma sarcomatodes (49), and adenocarcinoma with squamous differentiation are all designations that have been used for this lesion. While Fisher et al (15) suggested an incidence of 0.3% for mucoepidermoid carcinoma, the precise incidence of this tumor is not known since the squamous component is often ignored when limited in amount, while those with extensive squamous differentiation could be easily misinterpreted as a pure squamous carcinoma as has been noted by Woodard et al (68). Several reports have referred to adenosquamous (mucoepidermoid) carcinoma of the breast as a specific entity (15,26,33,42,50), while others have simply included adenocarcinomas with squamous differentiation in the category of metaplastic carcinoma (27,48). The former have divided these neoplasms into high grade (26,33) and low grade (15,49) tumors and surprisingly have made no comment regarding similar lesions that have been reported under the category of metaplastic carcinoma. The term adenosquamous carcinoma is preferable to mucoepidermoid carcinoma since the adenocarcinoma in these tumors is generally an ordinary infiltrating duct carcinoma rather than the distinctive mucinous (colloid) carcinoma that occurs in the breast and might be implied by the use of the term "mucoepidermoid" carcinoma.

### Clinical Features

Women with adenosquamous carcinoma range in age from 31 to 87 with a median age of 57. Almost all patients present with a palpable breast mass. The tumor may have been present from a few weeks (26) to approximately 20 years (42) prior to excision. Overall, however, the clinical presentation does not differ appreciably from that of patients with regular infiltrating duct carcinoma.

### Macroscopic Features

The gross appearance of the tumor varies depending on the extent and degree of squamous differentiation in the tumor. When there is localization of keratinizing squamous carcinoma in the lesion, these appear as pearly white nodules (Fig. 10.6). The tumors range in size from 1.5 to 17 cm with a median of 2.5 cm. Most tumors have ill-defined margins, but a few have been described as well-circumscribed.

### Microscopic Features

Adenosquamous carcinoma is composed of an intimate admixture of various types of adenocarcinoma with squamous carcinoma. The proportion of the two components is highly variable within these neoplasms. The adenocarcinoma is generally an infiltrating duct carcinoma, but any other type of adenocarcinoma may be present theoretically. The squamous component may be spindled, but it is generally a well-differentiated, large-cell type with readily recognizable intercellular bridges and keratinization. Although stainable mucin may be present in the adenocarcinomatous component, none of the cases reported as mucoepidermoid carcinoma has had a classic mucinous or colloid carcinoma component. In many cases, the central portion of the tumor shows the most highly differentiated and banal keratinizing squamous element and becomes less differentiated and nonkeratinizing away from the center. The most peripheral areas have the most poorly-differentiated adenocarcinoma component. Areas of transition from adenocarcinoma to squamous carcinoma are readily evident within ducts and duct-like structures as one moves from the central squamous area to the peripheral aspects of the lesion (Figs. 10.7–10.9). The low grade variant shows tubules of well-differentiated adenocarcinoma and small nests of tumor cells containing both elements in a well-differentiated form, spread diffusely in a prominent reactive stroma with a pattern reminiscent of syringomas.

It is possible to accurately diagnose adenosquamous carcinomas by needle aspiration if both components of the lesion are represented in the aspiration sample (62).

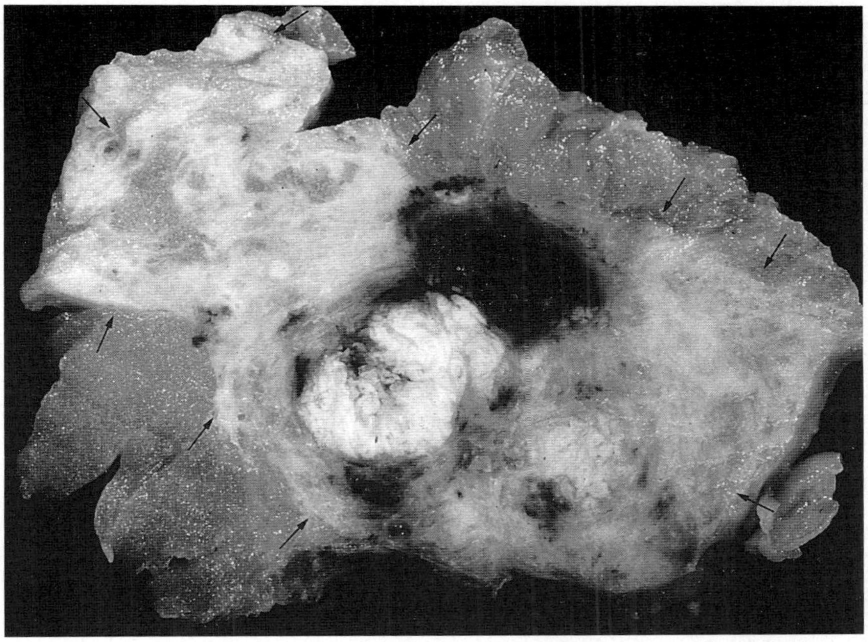

**Figure 10.6** Adenosquamous carcinoma. The entire gray area between the arrows reflects an invasive carcinoma. The central round nodule represents the keratinizing squamous carcinoma component. (From Tavassoli FA: *Pathol Annu* 1992;27(pt 2):89–119, with permission)

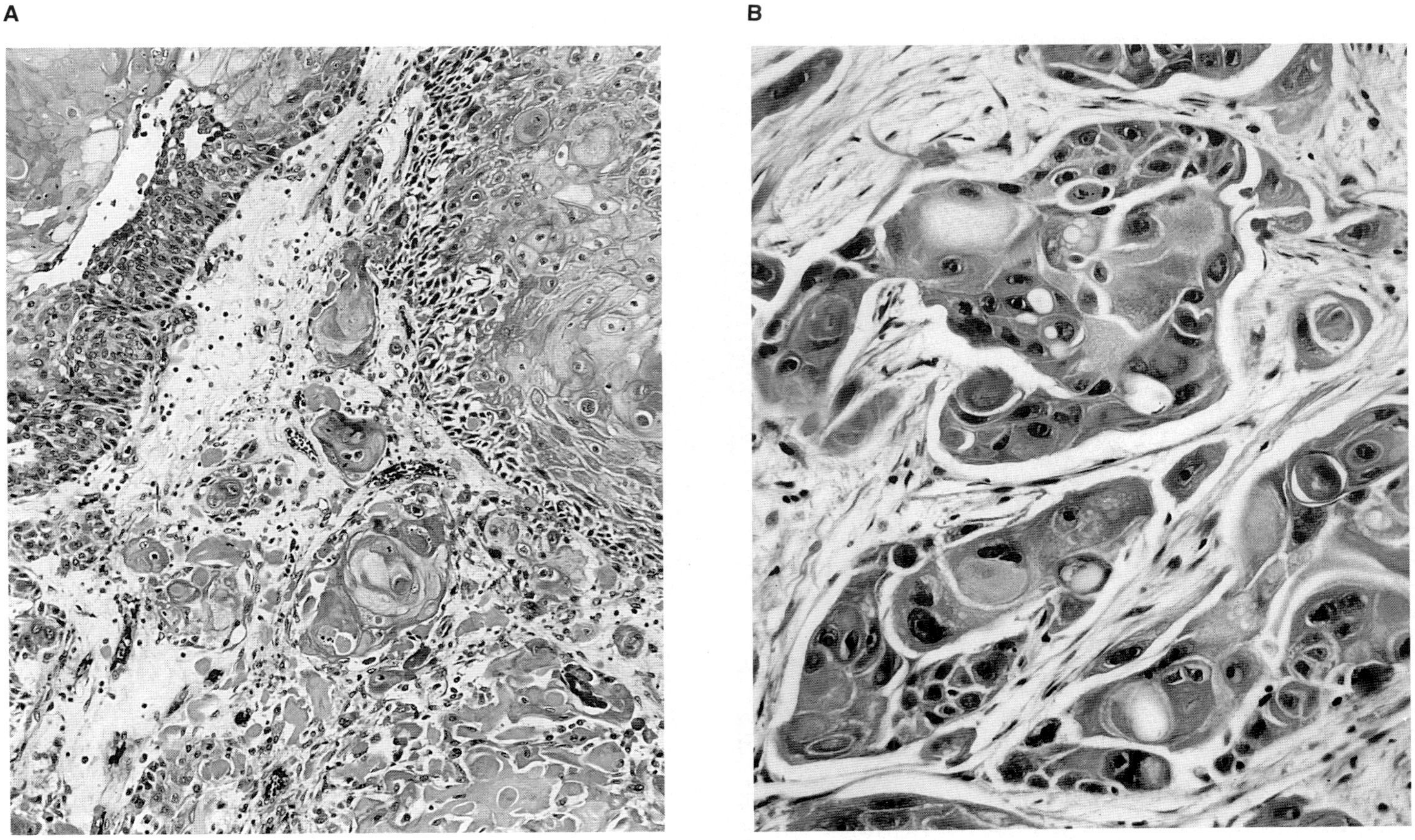

**Figure 10.7** Adenosquamous carcinoma, the same high grade lesion as pictured in Fig. 6. (a) An area with predominance of keratinizing squamous carcinoma. (H&E, 120) (b) The poorly-differentiated invasive areas are in the more peripheral aspects of the lesion. (H&E, X250) (From Tavassoli FA: *Pathol Annu* 1992;27(pt 2):89–119, with permission)

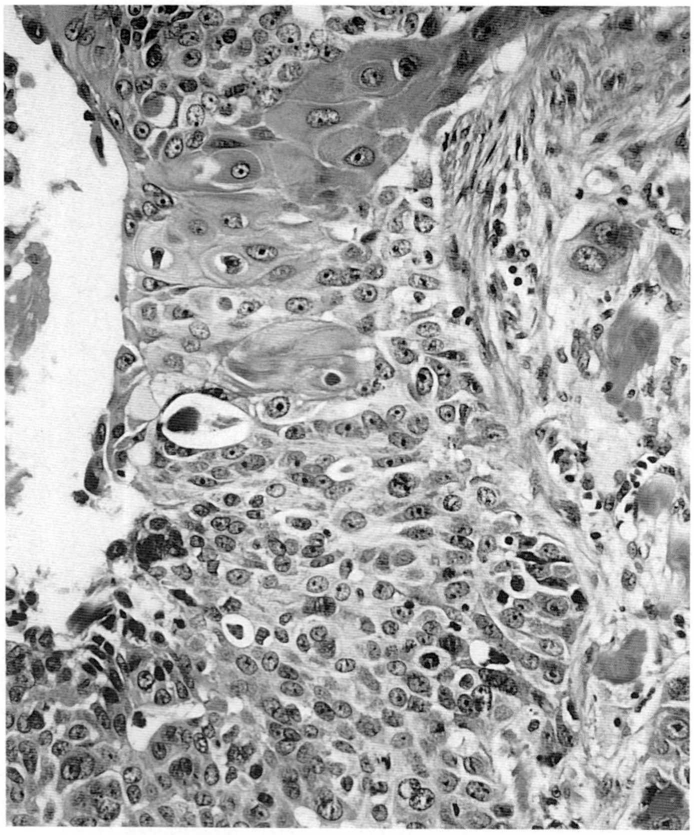

**Figure 10.8** Adenosquamous carcinoma, transitional areas of the same high grade lesion as Fig. 6. A duct with transition from the glandular epithelium to squamous epithelium. (H&E, X160) (From Tavassoli FA: *Pathol Annu* 1992;27(pt 2):89–119, with permission)

## Hormone Receptors

Two of the five cases reported by Woodard et al (68) had quantitatively low levels of saturable estrogen and/or progesterone binding proteins. In no case was there a qualitative or quantitative pattern of receptors indicative of hormonal response potential. The four carcinomas with predominance of squamous metaplasia in Oberman's study (48) were negative for hormone receptors.

## Prognosis

The prognosis of such combined tumors would depend on the degree of differentiation of their components. Both components of all of the low grade tumors reported by Fisher et al (15) and Rosen and Ernsberger (52) were well-differentiated; the eight patients with axillary node dissection in the two studies had no evidence of metastatic tumor. All patients with low grade adenosquamous carcinoma have survived without evidence of disease four to ten years after the diagnosis (15,52,68). Four of the eight patients with the low grade carcinoma who had local excision for their tumors did develop recurrences, (68), however, indicating that local excision is insufficient for the control of the low grade tumors.

The high grade mucoepidermoid carcinomas are aggressive tumors that often have lymph node metastases at the time of presentation. Even in the absence of nodal metastases and despite radiation therapy, chemotherapy and hormonal therapy, the patient described by Hastrup and Sehested (26) died with widespread systemic disease 25 months after mastectomy despite the small (1 cm) size of the primary tumor. In Oberman's 1987 review (48), one of the five patients with axillary node dissection had positive nodes; this patient and two others died from their carcinoma one year after the diagnosis.

# ADENOCARCINOMA WITH SPINDLE CELL METAPLASIA

This is one of the least recognized and discussed variants of metaplastic carcinoma. Although 72 of the 100 cases reported under the designation of spindle cell carcinoma in one study (63) had either an infiltrating duct or an intraductal component and no evidence of squamous carcinoma, these cases were not discussed in detail and the authors made no specific reference to the immunohistochemical or ultrastructural characteristics of the spindle cell element in this group as opposed to the spindle cells in the 11 cases with a squamous carcinoma. These neoplasms show an intimate admixture of adenocarcinoma with spindle cells, whereby tubules of adenocarcinoma appear to transform to a spindle cell population (Fig. 10.10).

Diagnosis of this tumor requires immunohistochemical and/or electron microscopic confirmation of the epithelial nature of the spindle cells. If the spindle cells show a positive reaction to cytokeratin, the epithelial nature of the entire lesion is confirmed. A positive reaction to a broad-based cytokeratin anti-

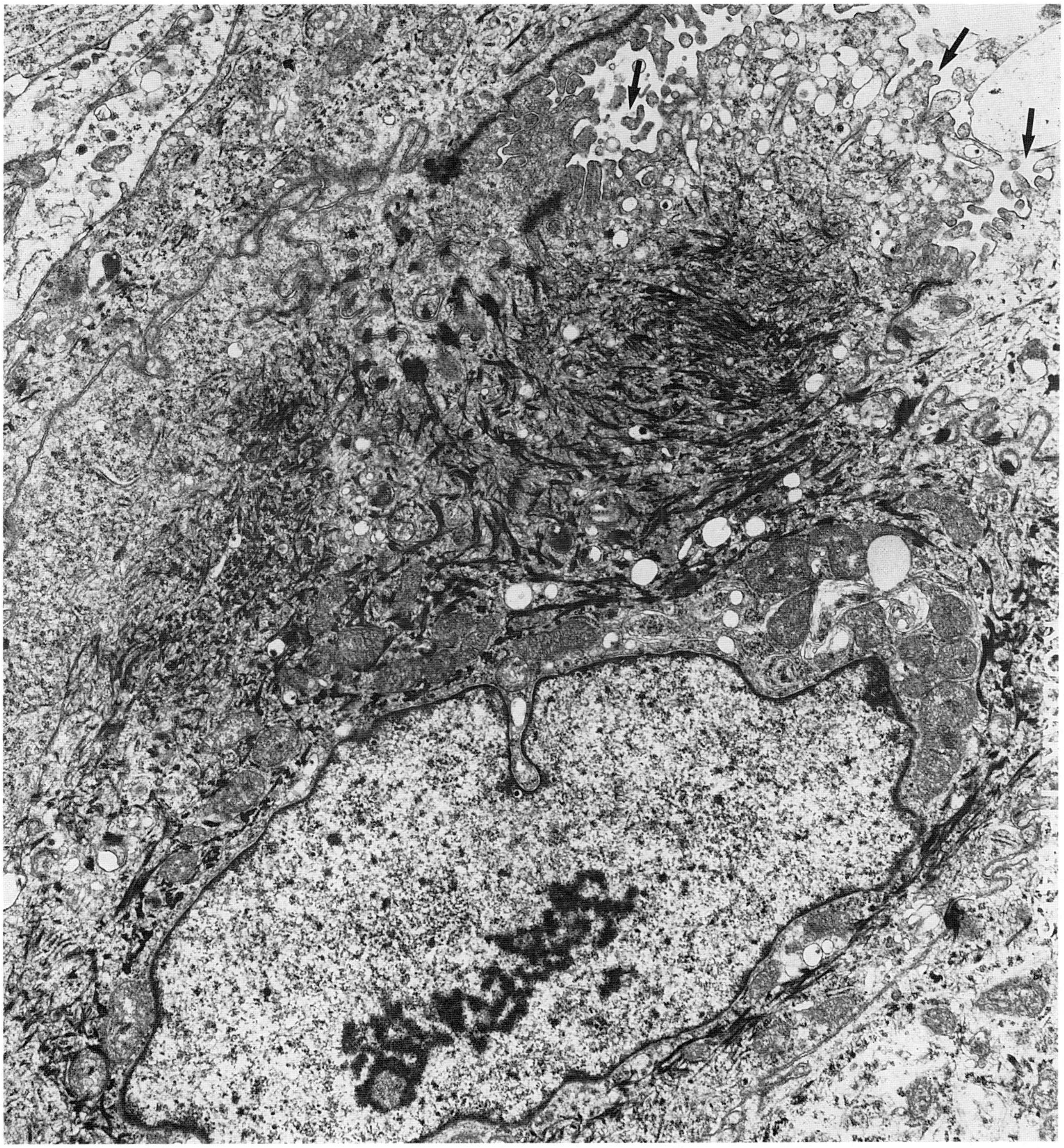

**Figure 10.9** Adenosquamous carcinoma, ultrastructural features, transitional area. The microvillous projections along the lumen reflect the glandular aspect of the cell (arrows), while the abundant tonofilaments within the cytoplasm of the cell depicted indicate early squamous differentiation. (Uranyl acetate-lead citrate, X4,400) (From Tavassoli FA: *Pathol Annu* 1992;27(pt 2):89–119, with permission)

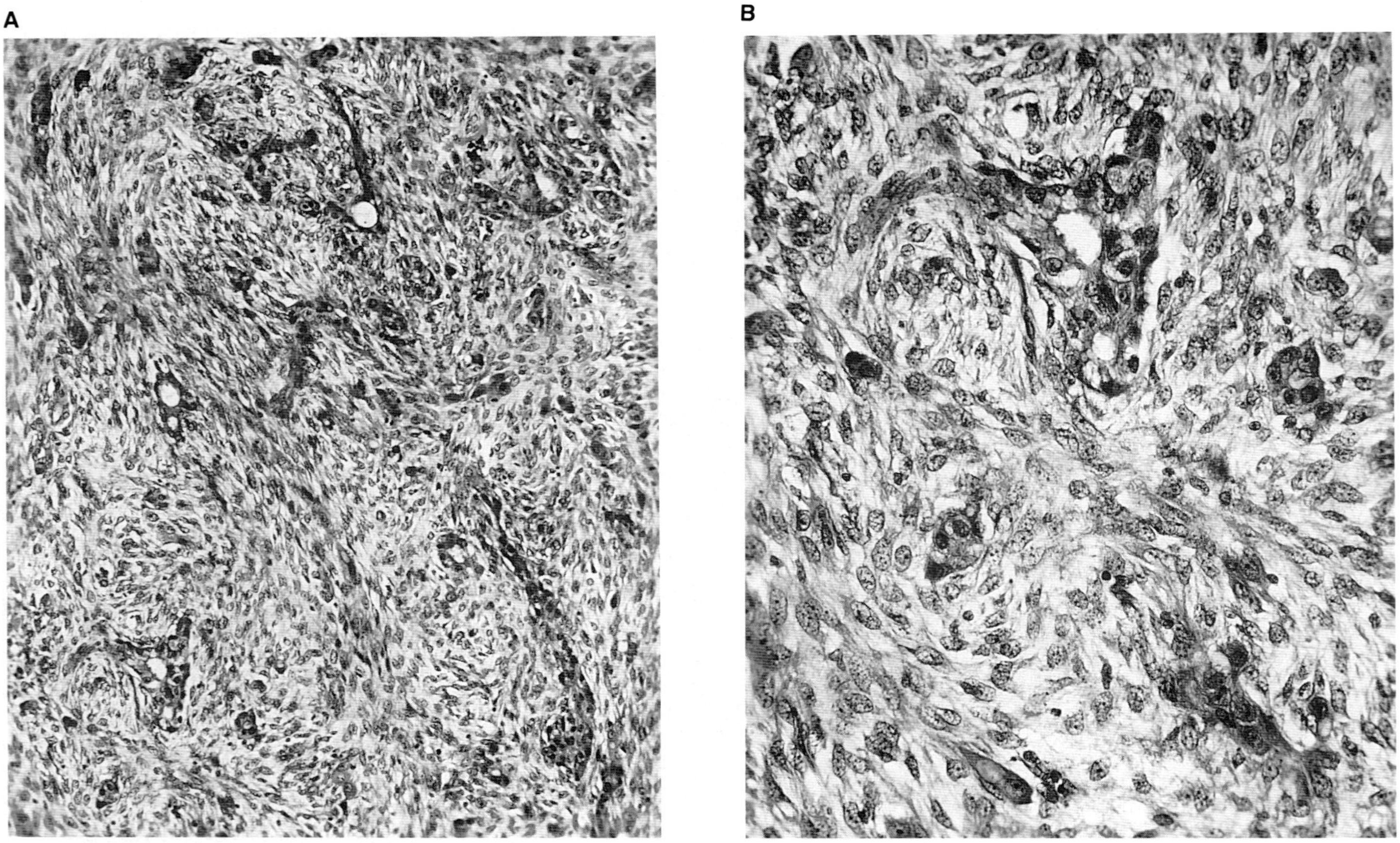

**Figure 10.10(a,b)** Adenocarcinoma with spindle cell metaplasia. (a) A predominantly spindle cell tumor may show well-formed ductal structures with open lumens, or compressed tubular structures. (H&E, X75) (b) Higher magnification of the latter shows an angulated tubule stretching out and merging with the surrounding spindle cells (H&E, X200) (Figs. 10.10a–b from Tavassoli FA: *Pathol Annu* 1992;27(pt 2):89–119, with permission)

body does not distinguish between squamous epithelium and glandular carcinomas, however. Therefore, until more specific antibodies become available for making this distinction reliably and reproducibly, ultrastructural analysis is required to determine whether the spindle cells reflect adenocarcinoma or squamous carcinoma. In addition to having well-developed desmosomes at the ultrastructural level, the spindled squamous cells will have abundant tonofilaments in their cytoplasm; spindled adenocarcinoma cells will also have desmosomes, but they lack abundant tonofilaments and some of them will actually contain intracytoplasmic lumens which will indisputably establish their glandular nature. In general, it would be highly unlikely for the spindle cell population in a tumor containing only adenocarcinoma, particularly those adenocarcinomas with a tubular arrangement, to reflect altered squamous epithelium. The behavior of this variant of metaplastic carcinoma has to be established in future studies. Rarely, even the adjacent intraductal carcinoma cells show a spindle cell transformation supporting the glandular nature of the invasive spindle cells (Fig. 10.11).

## CARCINOMA WITH CHONDROID METAPLASIA

These rare tumors are characterized by partial or complete chondroid differentiation (32,35,36,48,51, 59,64). Oberman (48) included these tumors under the category of invasive carcinomas with pseudosarcomatous metaplasia; he found chondroid metaplasia as the most common heterologous element in this group. Others have grouped this tumor together with carcinomas displaying osseous differentiation (58,64). These lesions occur in a wide age range (early 30s to late 80s) and can grow quite large leading to displacement of the nipple and ulceration of the overlying skin.

C

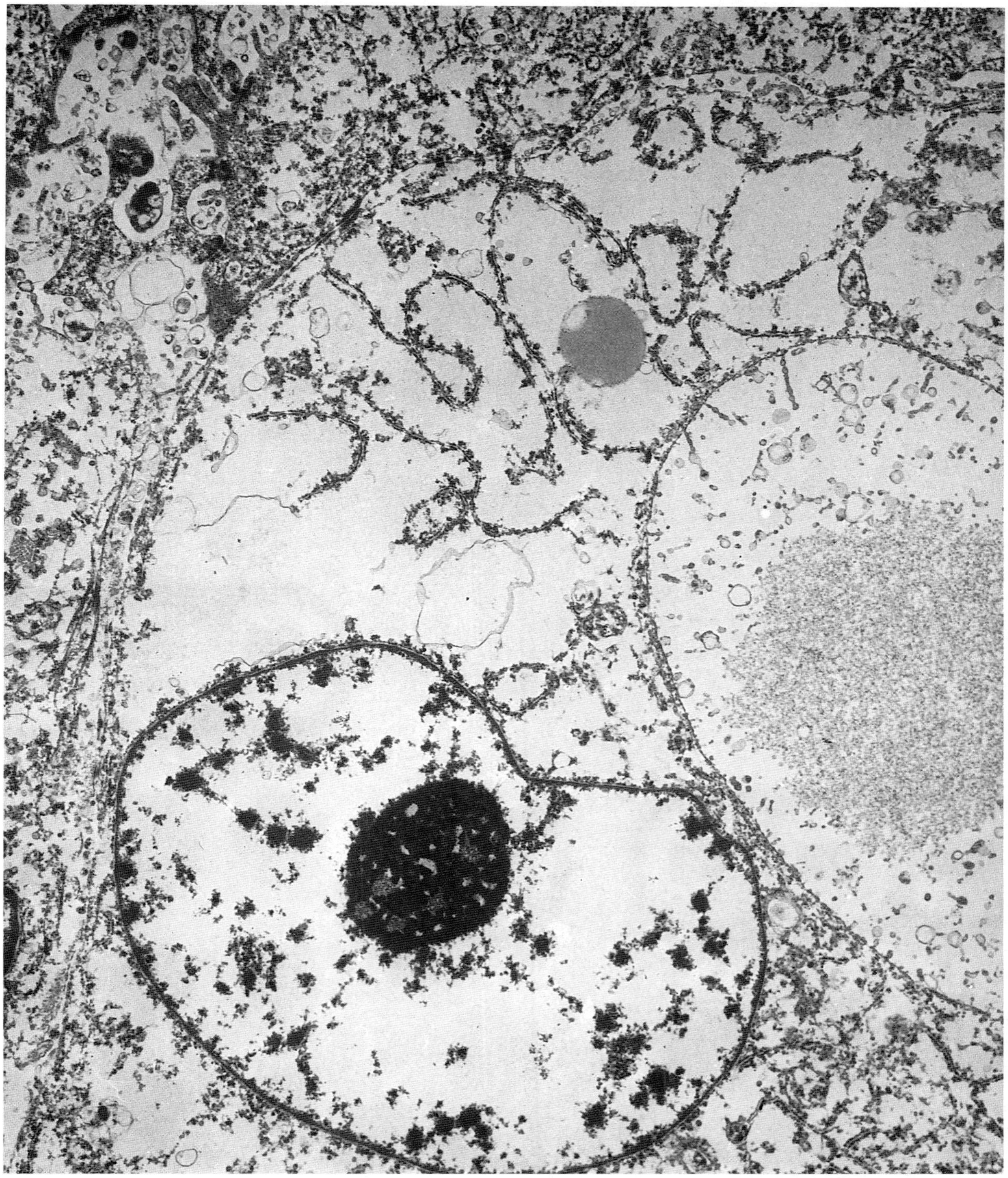

**Figure 10.10(c)** Adenocarcinoma with spindle cell metaplasia. At the ultrastructural level, some of the cells contain intracytoplasmic lumens (Uranyl acetate-lead citrate, X3,000)

## Macroscopic Features

Depending on the proportion of the chondroid differentiation, these tumors can appear similar to a regular infiltrating duct carcinoma with minor areas of firm, glistening tissue or appear as a well-circumscribed, firm, glistening chondroid mass. They can assume massive proportions of up to 20 cm in maximum diameter.

A

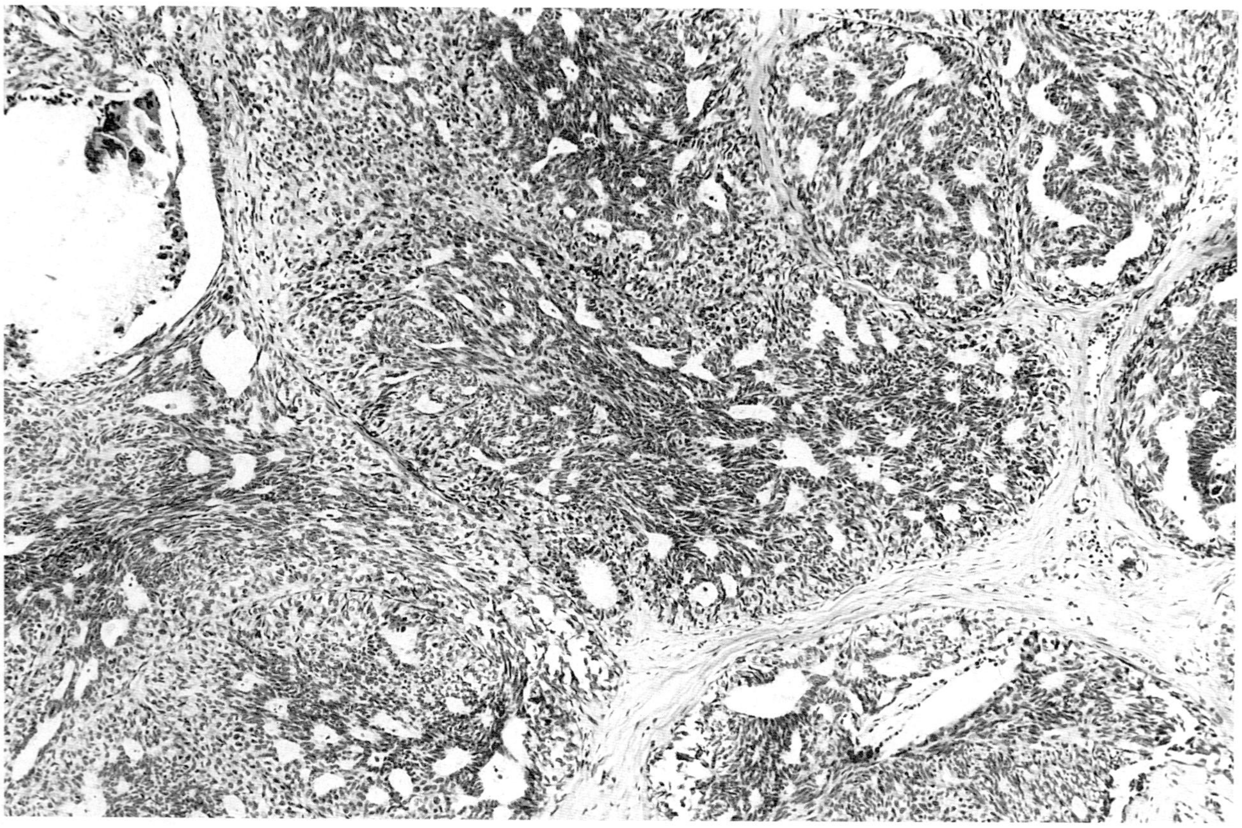

B

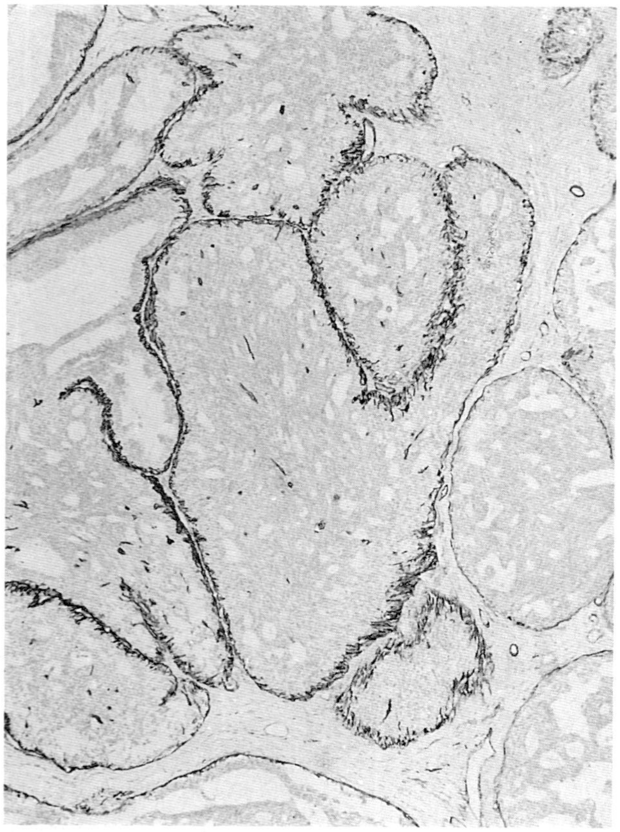

**Figure 10.11** Spindle cell intraductal carcinoma. (a) The proliferating cells are uniformly spindle shaped and form a cribriform arrangement. (H&E, X75) (b) The cancer cells fail to react with actin, while the surrounding myoepithelial cells show an intensely positive reaction. (X75)

A

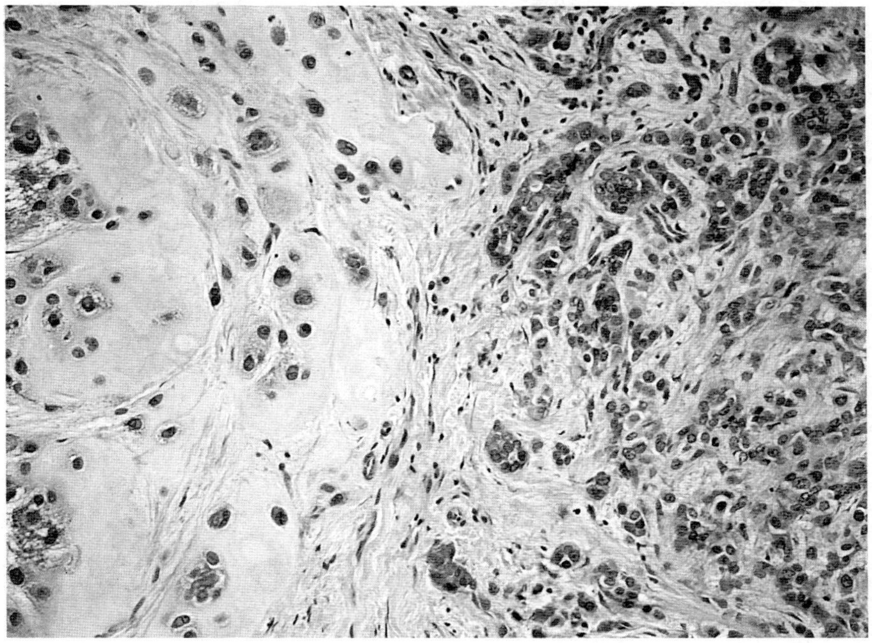

B

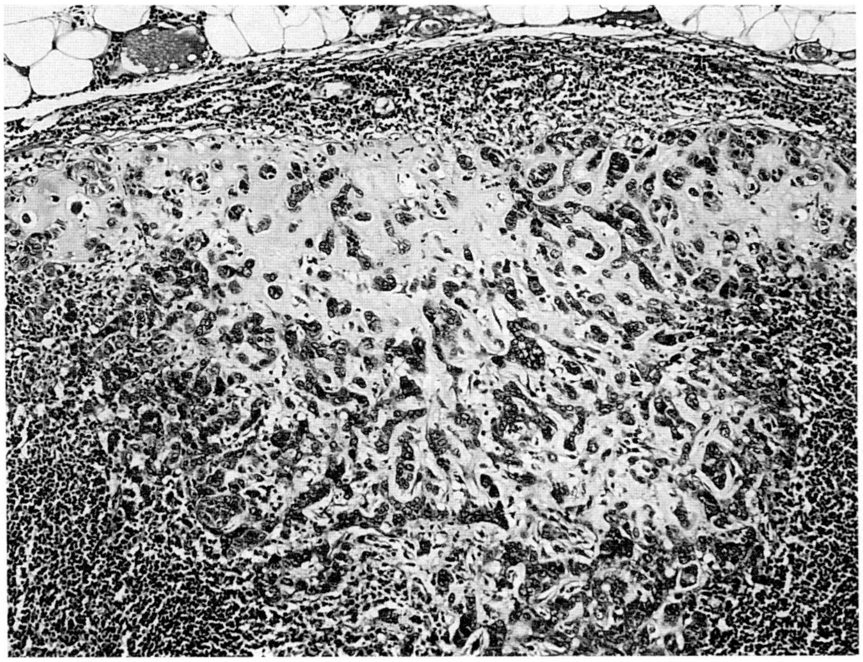

**Figure 10.12** Carcinoma with chondroid differentiation. (a) Nests of invasive duct carcinoma are present on the right side. (H&E, X160) (b) The metastatic carcinoma in the lymph node retained the chondroid differentiation. (H&E, X100) (Fig. 10.12a from Tavassoli FA: *Pathol Annu* 1992;27(pt 2):89–119, with permission)

## Microscopic Features

When readily recognizable, the carcinoma in this group is most frequently a regular infiltrating duct carcinoma (Fig. 10.12), but any type of carcinoma may be present. One variant has an overall chondroid appearance with the more cellular area distributed in the periphery of the neoplasm (Fig. 10.13). There is a paucity of thorough correlation of H&E, immunohistochemical, and ultrastructural findings in these tumors. In one recent study (64), carcinomas with chondroid and osseous differentiation were lumped together. Although immunohistochemical features of 13 cases were discussed in this study, it is not clear how many of these contained chondroid differentiation and how many had osseous or both types of change within them. The immunohistochemical and

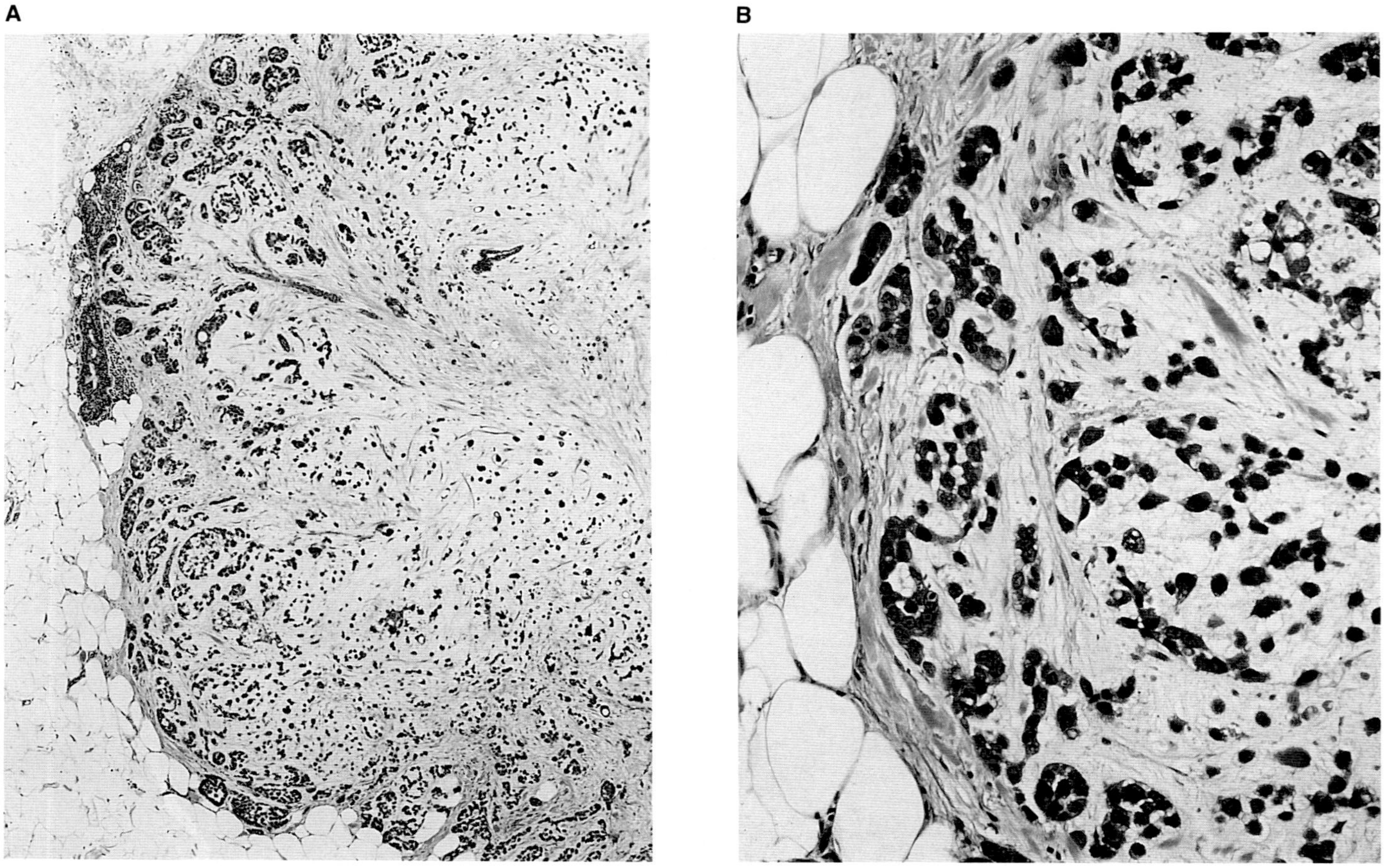

**Figure 10.13** Carcinoma with chondroid differentiation (chondroid carcinoma). (a) This variant has the appearance of a chondroid nodule with a lobulated margin. (H&E, X50) (b) Higher magnification displaying the cellular area in the periphery with occasional tubular arrangement. (H&E, X200) (Fro:n Tavassoli FA: *Pathol Annu* 1992;27(pt 2):89–119, with permission)

ultrastructural features of three cases of carcinoma with an overall chondroid appearance were reported recently (60). A majority of the tumor cells coexpressed S-100 protein and cytokeratin (Fig. 10.14), but none of the tumor cells displayed any positivity for actin. Since normal chondrocytes also react with S-100 protein, this positivity does not imply a myoepithelial origin for the tumor cells. A positive reaction for actin would have supported myoepithelial derivation, but the cells failed to react with actin.

## Ultrastructural Features

At the ultrastructural level, these tumors are composed of cells that have an overall chondrocytic appearance with short microvilli, abundant rough endoplasmic reticulum, prominent Golgi apparatus, and rare lipid droplets (60). Some of the tumor cells also contain abundant tonofilaments in their cytoplasm and are attached to each other by tight junctions or even well-formed desmosomes, indicating an epithelial differentiation (Fig. 10.15). Transitional cells with fewer bundles of tonofilaments distributed around the nucleus are abundant. None of the cells contain the myofilaments, pinocytotic vesicles, or patchy investiture by basement membrane necessary to even raise the possibility of myoepithelial cell origin. In the hypocellular regions of the tumor, individual neoplastic chondrocytes and transitional cells are surrounded by a territorial matrix, while in the more cellular areas, clusters of cells are surrounded by a common matrix.

While the abundance of tonofilaments and the numerous well-developed desmosomes support the designation of this tumor as an epithelial neoplasm, the possibility of a chondrosarcoma with epithelial differentiation cannot be totally dismissed. The predominance of chondrocytic-type cells at the light microscopic and ultrastructural levels does raise the possibility of a chondrosarcoma undergoing epithe-

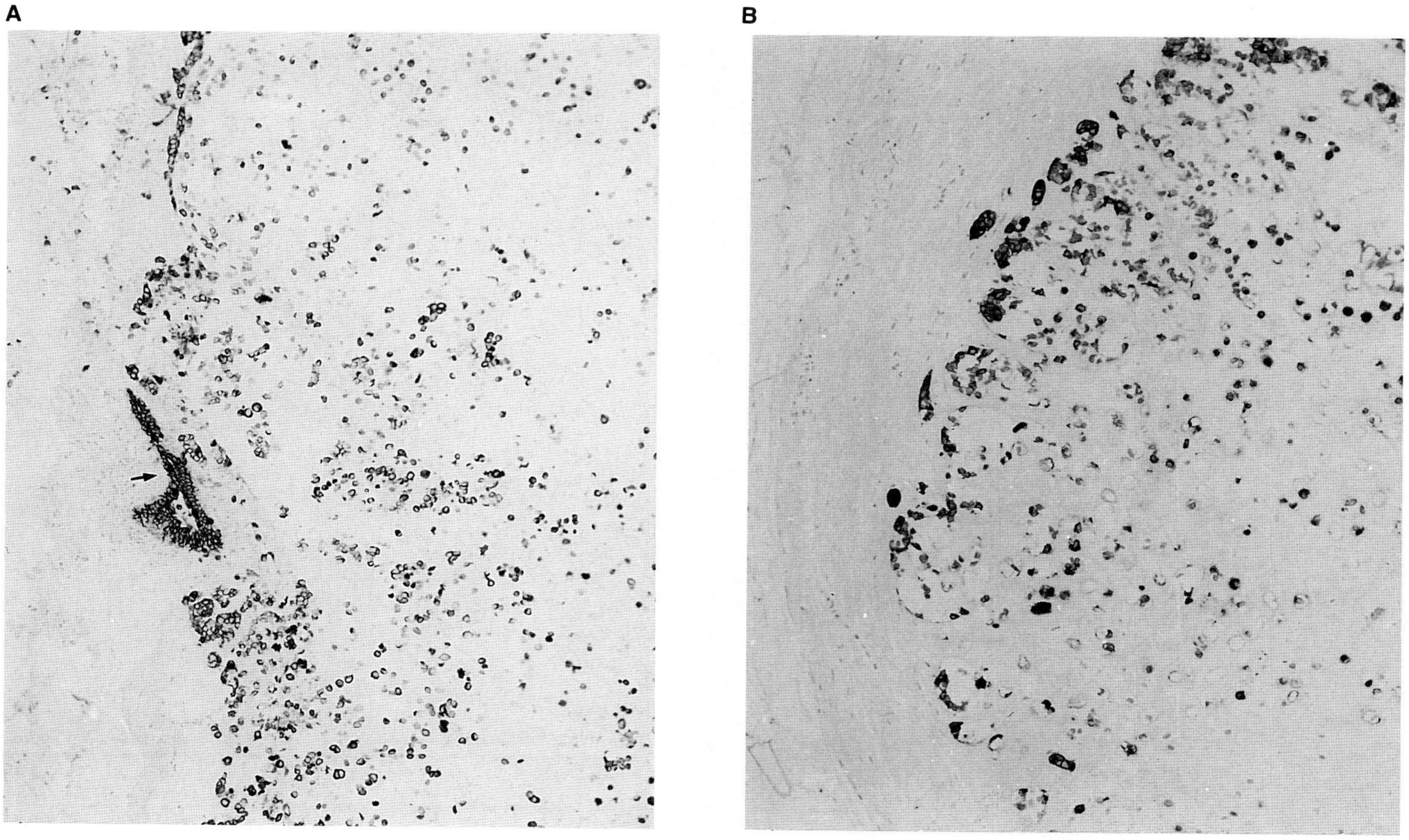


**Figure 10.14** Carcinoma with chondroid differentiation. (a) Immunoreaction shows positivity for cytokeratin in many tumor cells. A normal duct (arrow) adjacent to the tumor serves as a positive control. (X75) (b) Immunoreaction for S-100 protein displays positivity in many of the same tumor cells and additional cells indicating coexpression of cytokeratin and S-100 protein in many tumor cells. (X100) (From Tavassoli FA: *Pathol Annu* 1992;27(pt 2):89–119, with permission)

lial transformation. Interestingly, squamous differentiation in a primary chondrosarcoma of the proximal humerus, readily recognizable on H&E sections and confirmed by a positive immunoreaction for keratin and ultrastructural identification of tonofilaments and desmosomes, has been reported in a 68-year-old woman who had no evidence of a primary tumor elsewhere in the body (40).

Eventually, it may become necessary to separate these tumors from the typical infiltrating duct carcinomas displaying foci of benign chondroid differentiation and designate them as chondrosarcoma exhibiting epithelial features. The term "carcinoma with chondroid metaplasia" could be used when the chondroid element is intimately admixed with a readily recognizable carcinoma and the chondrocytes appear benign and/or display positivity for cytokeratin. Santeusanio et al (54), studied a carcinoma with areas of spindle, fibrosarcomatous, and cartilaginous differentiation. Monoclonal and polyclonal antibodies to keratin showed a positive reaction in the epithelial and chondroid areas. The cells failed to react with desmin, but S-100 protein was not utilized in the study. These findings were interpreted as reflecting mesenchymal differentiation (metaplasia) by the carcinoma.

In a background of an invasive carcinoma, if the chondrocytes appear clearly malignant and fail to react with cytokeratin or other epithelial antigens, then the lesion should be classified as a carcinosarcoma.

## Hormone Receptors

Only one of the eight tumors evaluated for estrogen receptors has been positive (64).

A

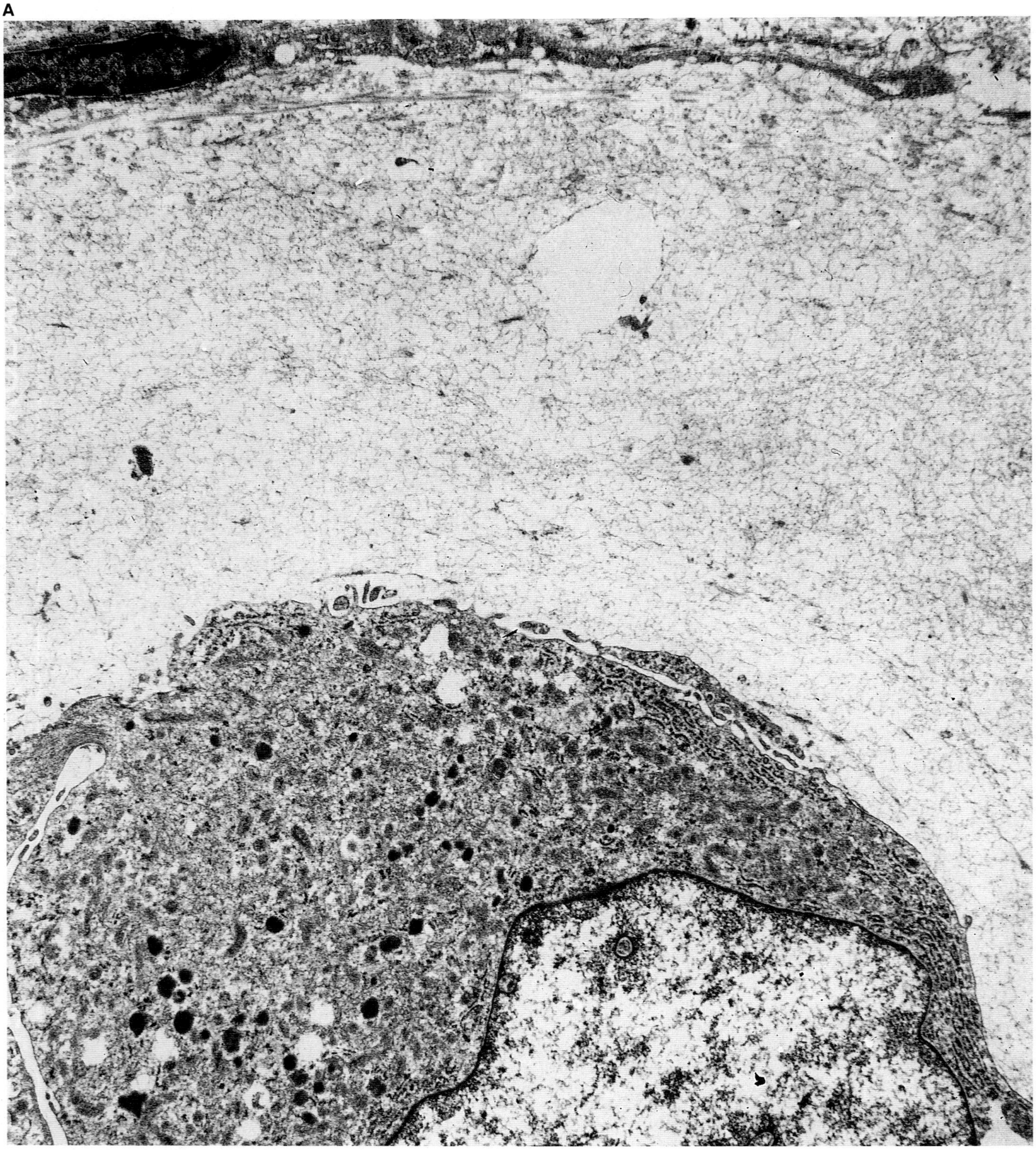

**Figure 10.15(a)** Carcinoma with chondroid differentiation. A cell with all of the features of a chondrocyte is surrounded by territorial matrix. (Uranyl acetate-lead citrate, X3,000)

B

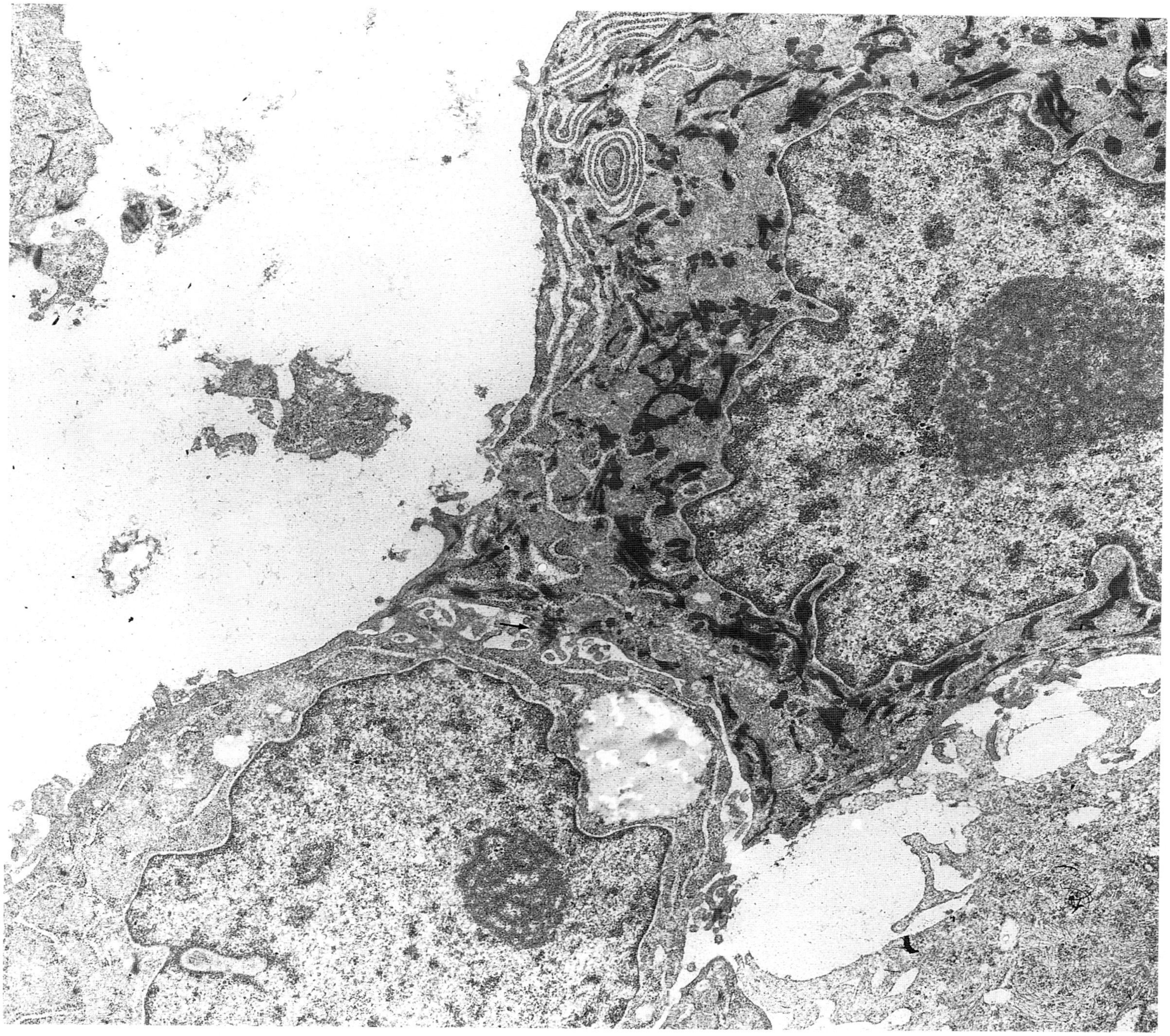

**Figure 10.15(b)** Two adjacent cells show the overall configuration of chondrocytes. One has abundant tonofilaments, the other is completely devoid of tonofilaments. The two cells are attached to one another by tight junctions (arrow). (Uranyl acetate-lead citrate, X4,400) (From Tavassoli FA: *Pathol Annu* 1992;27(pt 2):89–119, with permission)

## Prognosis

In one study, tumor size at the time of diagnosis correlated best with prognosis since the majority of patients whose carcinoma was less than 4 cm in diameter pursued a favorable course (48). The absence of nodal metastases and the circumscribed margins of the tumors were not associated with the favorable outcome anticipated, however. Six of the 15 patients in this series died from their tumors within 0.6 to 3.5 years after the initial diagnosis, and none of those who died had evidence of axillary node metastases (48). All but one of the 15 tumors had a

C

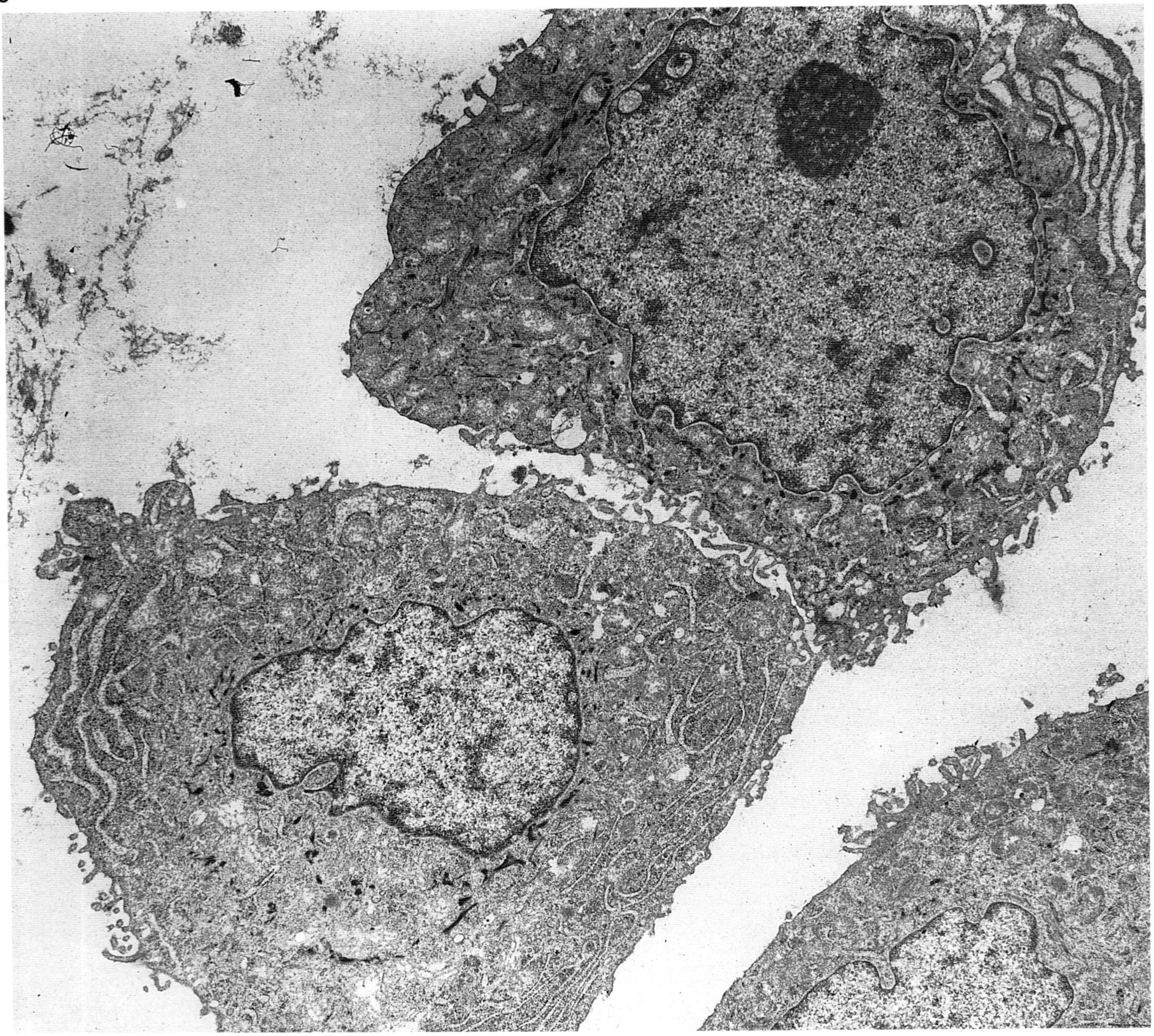

**Figure 10.15(c)** Two intermediate cells have prominent chondroid features and a small amount of tonofilaments in a perinuclear distribution (Uranyl acetate-lead citrate, X3,000)

circumscribed appearance grossly which corresponded to a pushing margin microscopically. Smith and Taylor (57) stated that adenocarcinomas with bone and cartilage are aggressive neoplasms since six of the ten patients in their study were dead of tumor at the time of follow-up inquiry, but they did not specify if the bone and cartilage appeared malignant or benign, and the length of follow-up was not provided.

The cumulative five-year survival in a group of 26 patients with carcinomas displaying chondroid or osseous differentiation was 68%, but again, it is not clear how many of these were carcinomas with chondroid differentiation, or how many had malignant versus benign-appearing chondroid differentiation (64).

The nodal metastases from these neoplasms may or may not contain the heterologous element. Five of

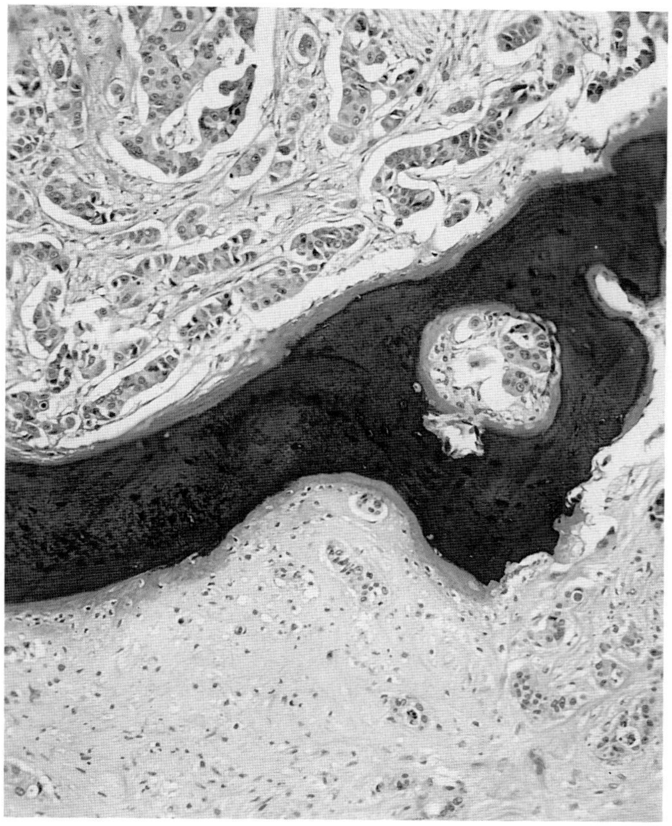

**Figure 10.16** Carcinoma with osseous differentiation. A fragment of mineralized bone is surrounded by clusters and cords of an invasive carcinoma (H&E, X160)

the 20 cases in Kaufman et al's study (32) had axillary node metastases; all lacked the metaplastic chondroid component. But chondroid differentiation does occur and has been observed in the axillary metastases in several cases reviewed at AFIP (Fig. 10.12).

## CARCINOMA WITH OSSEOUS DIFFERENTIATION

Carcinomas with osseous differentiation have generally been lumped together with those displaying chondroid differentiation (58,64), and it is not clear what proportion of these had malignant (osteosarcoma) or benign osseous differentiation. Occasionally, tumors with osseous differentiation are reported separately (1,8,41). While some of the osseous differentiation is through enchondral ossification, many of these tumors contain benign areas of bone formation within otherwise typical carcinoma, and transition from the carcinoma to the osseous elements with intermediate cells is not evident (Fig. 10.16). The carcinoma is most frequently an infiltrating duct carcinoma but other types of carcinoma including a colloid carcinoma have been seen (1,64). The carcinoma may be separated from the bone by reactive stromal cells, but in some cases, the osseous component appears to simply lodge itself in the middle of the tumor without a significant amount of intervening reactive stroma. Osteoblasts abound around the bone, but osteoclastic cells are less commonly observed in large numbers.

The rare example of this tumor that has been studied in detail with ultrastructural analysis supports origin of the osseous areas from stromal cells, without any evidence of epithelial transformation to the osseous component (1,4,58). The osteoblasts and osteoclasts in these tumors do not express cytokeratin. In my opinion, tumors showing a carcinoma admixed with osteogenic sarcoma qualify as carcinosarcoma and should be distinguished from carcinomas displaying mature bone.

The prognostic significance of mature bone formation within carcinomas is not well known, since these tumors have generally been grouped together with carcinomas displaying benign and malignant chondroid differentiation.

## APOCRINE CARCINOMA

*Definition:* Apocrine carcinoma is composed of cells with abundant, variably granular eosinophilic cytoplasm, round, centrally to eccentrically located nuclei, often containing prominent nucleoli and distinctive cell margins. Coarse eosinophilic granules or a yellow-brown pigment is often present within the copious cytoplasm. Apical snouts or cytoplasmic convexity may be present in some of the cells when luminal spaces are present within the tumor. The cells should be clearly recognizable as apocrine epithelium (73).

Cells with morphologic features of apocrine cells were noted in a malignant tumor in 1916 by Krompecher (95). In 1928, Ewing (84) provided a detailed description of apocrine carcinoma and later, he suggested that 25% of breast carcinomas arise in "sweat glands of the breast." More recently, Hamperl (93) stated that the term sweat-gland carcinoma of the breast should be abandoned. The various designations used for this tumor include apocrine carcinoma, carcinoma with apocrine metaplasia, sweat-gland carcinoma, and carcinoma with pink cells (69,73,78,79, 106,110,117,120).

While the World Health Organization (WHO) classification includes apocrine carcinoma as a special variant of breast carcinoma, the existence of apocrine carcinoma as a distinct clinicopathologic entity is still contested. The reluctance to recognize apocrine carcinoma as an entity stems from the apparent absence of distinctive features in the natural history of this variant of breast carcinoma. Discovery of a prognostic difference from the typical infiltrating duct carcinoma or other distinctive features affecting the management of the lesion would endorse establishment of apocrine carcinoma as a distinct clinicopathologic entity. So far, however, general agreement has not evolved regarding the behavior of apocrine carcinoma. Actually, several studies have concluded that the prognosis of apocrine carcinoma is not different from that of regular infiltrating duct carcinoma (69,87,98), while others have suggested a better prognosis for apocrine carcinomas (88,89). This dichotomy is in part due to variations in the definition and criteria for diagnosis of apocrine carcinoma which ranges from the presence of cells that simply exhibit cytoplasmic eosinophilia or display a positive reaction with gross cystic disease fluid protein (GCDFP) to the presence of cells clearly recognizable as apocrine-type epithelium.

The reported incidence ranges from the 0.3% to 0.4% of mammary cancers suggested by Azzopardi (73), Gadaleanu and Galatar (88), and Mossler et al (104); 1% of mammary carcinomas stated by Frable and Kay (87); 14.5% according to Bonser (74); to a rather high 60% suggested by Haagensen et al (91). This wide range reflects the lack of a uniform objective criteria for reliable and reproducible light microscopic identification of apocrine carcinoma. Mazoujian et al (101,102) have used specific antigenic markers of apocrine function to identify carcinomas with apocrine features. Gross cystic disease fluid protein, isolated from breast gross cyst fluid, is produced by the metaplastic apocrine cells lining the cysts and has three component proteins, 44, 24 and 15. The type 15 protein was the most extensively studied in their investigation and it was identified immunohistochemically in benign apocrine cells as well as carcinomas with apocrine features. Mazoujian et al (102) used immunostains for GCDFP-15 to evaluate a large number of breast carcinomas in a retrospective study of 562 patients with breast carcinoma. Of the 334 tumors with histologic features of apocrine differentiation, 75% displayed a positive reaction for GCDFP-15. In addition, 23% of tumors that were interpreted as nonapocrine also showed a positive reaction for GCDFP. This finding could be interpreted as implying that the functional differentiation of tumor cells precedes their morphologic differentiation.

Eusebi et al (82) evaluated 100 consecutive breast carcinomas to establish the incidence of apocrine carcinoma using morphologic as well as immunostaining for the detection of GCDFP-15 antiserum. Four cases met Azzopardi's (73) criteria for apocrine carcinoma. About 60% to 80% of the cells in these four tumors were positively stained with GCDFP-15. Focal staining of up to 10% was observed in an additional eight cases; the focal staining was confined to areas of intraductal carcinoma in four of these. They concluded that while the histologic and immunologic criteria for assessing apocrine differentiation in a tumor are broadly in agreement, the recognition of individual cells by either of the two methods is not always possible.

## Clinical Features

Considering the lack of a uniform definition and criteria for diagnosis of apocrine carcinoma and the failure of many pathologists to separate apocrine carcinoma from regular ductal carcinomas or carcinomas with early squamous metaplasia, the following statements regarding the clinical features of apocrine carcinoma are likely to be modified if and when a consensus is reached concerning the diagnostic criteria.

Pure apocrine carcinoma occurs in a wide age range (34 to 78 years). It is considered a tumor of advanced age, however, because its peak incidence occurs during the sixth and seventh decade of life. It occurs in both females (75,79,87,91,92,94,98,106,109, 116,118) and males (112). It presents as either a solid or a cystic (Taccagni et al, 1985) mass with varying duration of symptomatology.

## Gross and Microscopic Features

Apocrine carcinoma is generally about 2 cm in size but ranges from 0.5 to 5 cm (104). Grossly, it is often well-delineated and brown-tan in color; it may present as a cystic lesion.

Microscopically, apocrine carcinoma may arise in an apocrine cyst, but more frequently it appears as a solid, cellular tumor composed of cords and sheets of tumor cells. Apocrine carcinoma may have cystic areas within it. The neoplastic apocrine cells are large with abundant granular eosinophilic cytoplasm (Fig. 10.17). Where glandular arrangements are formed and lumens are present, the cells may exhibit apical cystoplasmic snouts along the luminal margin and there is sometimes a crescent-shaped concentration of eosinophilic granules within the apical cytoplasm. These coarse refractile granules are PAS-positive, diastase-resistant glycolipids that were demonstrated by Lendrum in apocrine cells back in 1945. The centrally to eccentrically located nuclei are round and vesicular with prominent eosinophilic nucleoli. Some tumors have a highly uniform cell population while others have bizzare multilobulated nuclei with very large and multiple nucleoli present in many cells. Actually, nucleoli frequently appear very prominent even in benign apocrine hyperplasias and when apocrine metaplasia extends to areas of sclerosing adenosis. Therefore, nucleolar prominence cannot be used as a feature of malignancy or even atypia in apocrine cells.

The in situ carcinoma associated with invasive apocrine carcinoma is generally an intraductal apocrine carcinoma, but apocrine differentiation has been described in lobular carcinoma as well (82).

## Histochemical and Immunohistochemical Characteristics

The granules in the apical cytoplasm are PAS-positive, diastase-resistant, Sudan black and toluidine-blue-positive glycolipids which have been well-illustrated and described by various investigators (70,99,107,112). Occasionally, the cytoplasm also contains hemosiderin, lipofuscin, crystalloid granules but rarely, if ever, iron.

As noted before, GCDFP-15 has been demonstrated in metaplastic apocrine cells as well as apocrine carcinomas of the breast (83,90,101,102). Additional studies are needed to determine the specificity of the commercially available antisera, however. Our initial trials with the commercially available antisera have not been very promising. Using commercial antisera for GCDFP-15, we have been unable to obtain a reliable staining of even normal metaplastic apocrine cells at AFIP. The tissue sections generally exhibited a diffuse staining which was only slightly more intense in some of the apocrine cells; some of the adjacent epithelial cells as well as some lactating cells also stained. Metaplastic apocrine cells have also shown a positive immunoreaction for prolactin (96).

Curiously, we have found the monoclonal antibody B72.3 to be consistently present in about 95% of metaplastic apocrine cells (114) whether they were benign or malignant (Fig. 10.18). Others have also made a similar observation (77).

In my personal experience, only about 50% of apocrine carcinomas and carcinomas with focal apocrine features stain positive for carcinoembryonic antigen (CEA). The case reported by Taccagni et al (112) exhibited a positive reaction for alpha-1-antichymotrypsin; these authors had observed the same marker in typical metaplastic apocrine cells also.

## Ultrastructural Features

There are only a limited number of studies on the ultrastructural features of apocrine carcinoma. The neoplastic apocrine cells have many features in common with metaplastic apocrine cells and the cells of the apocrine glands (104,108). They are basically characterized by the presence of numerous mitochondria that have simple or irregular cristae and collections of membrane-bound osmiophilic bodies within the cytoplasm. The osmiophilic bodies correspond to the coarse eosinophilic granules present at the light microscopic level (104). Some tumor cells contain empty vesicles of about the same dimension as the osmiophilic granules; these cells correspond to the cells with vacuolated cytoplasm on H&E sections. Eusebi et al (83) have suggested that the vesicles and dense granules correspond to GCDFP-15 content, while the mitochondrial content is responsible for the cytoplasmic eosinophilic granularity. The different studies on the ultrastructure of apocrine carcinoma are not always in agreement on the abundance of mitochondria, the presence of osmiophilic bodies, or the degree of the similarity of the neoplastic apocrine cells in the breast to the cells in the apocrine skin adnexal glands. This is expected since the criteria

A

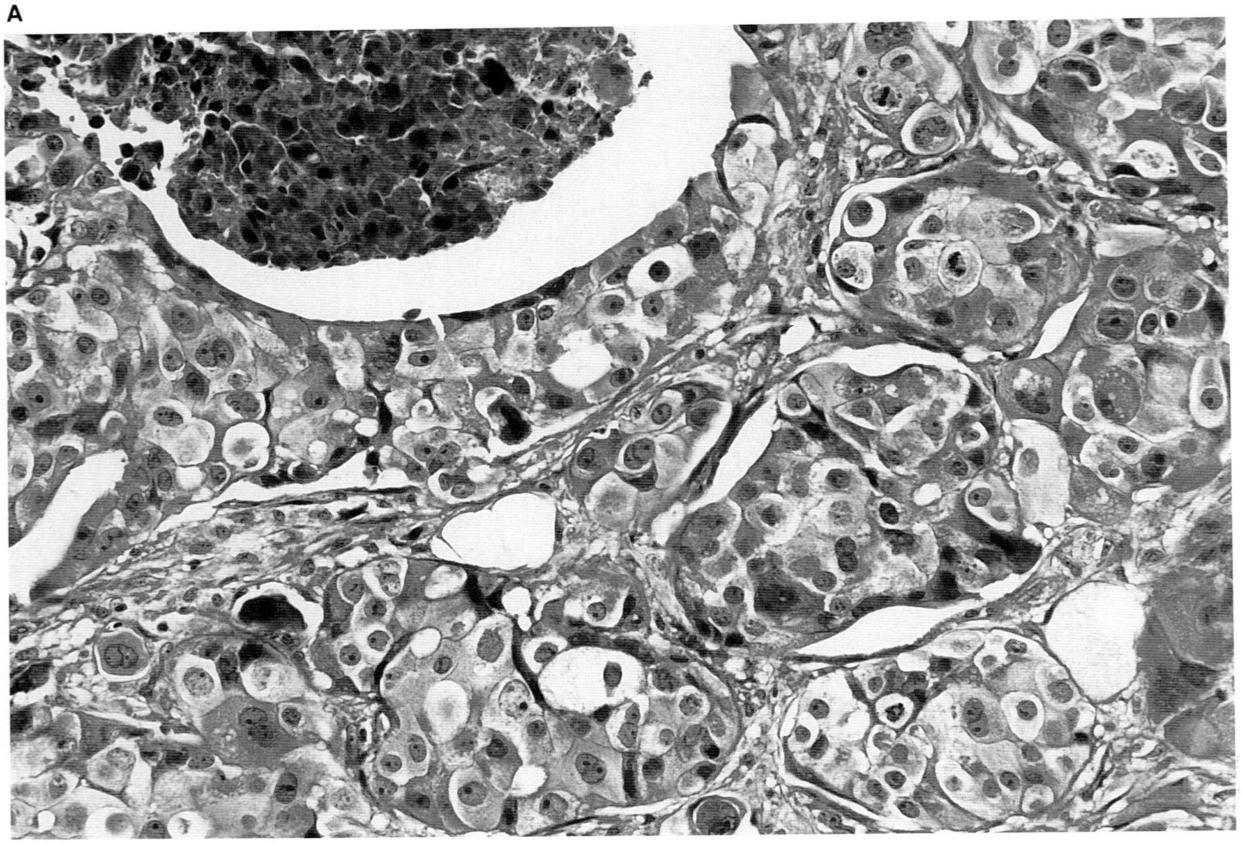

B

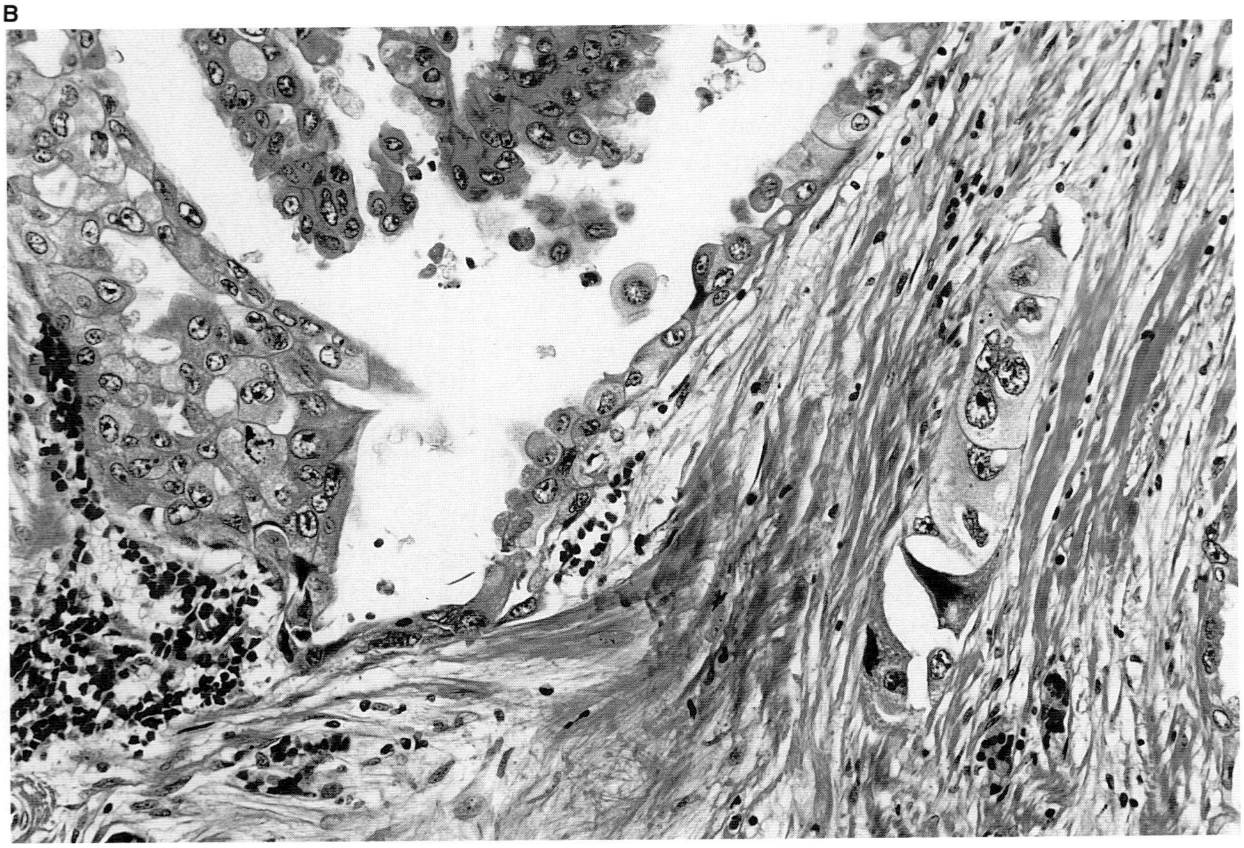

**Figure 10.17** Apocrine carcinoma, invasive. (a) Intraductal component with necrotic debris in its lumen along with invasive tumor in the form of rounded cell clusters. (b) The cells in the intraductal component show atypia and mitotic figures; the invasive cells form a cord-like pattern. (H&E, (a&b) X200)

A

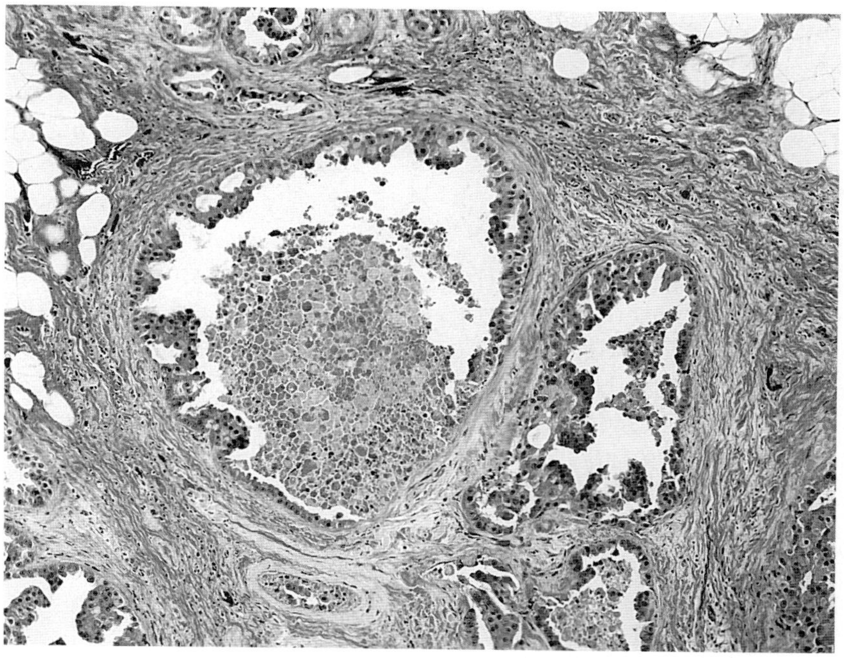

B

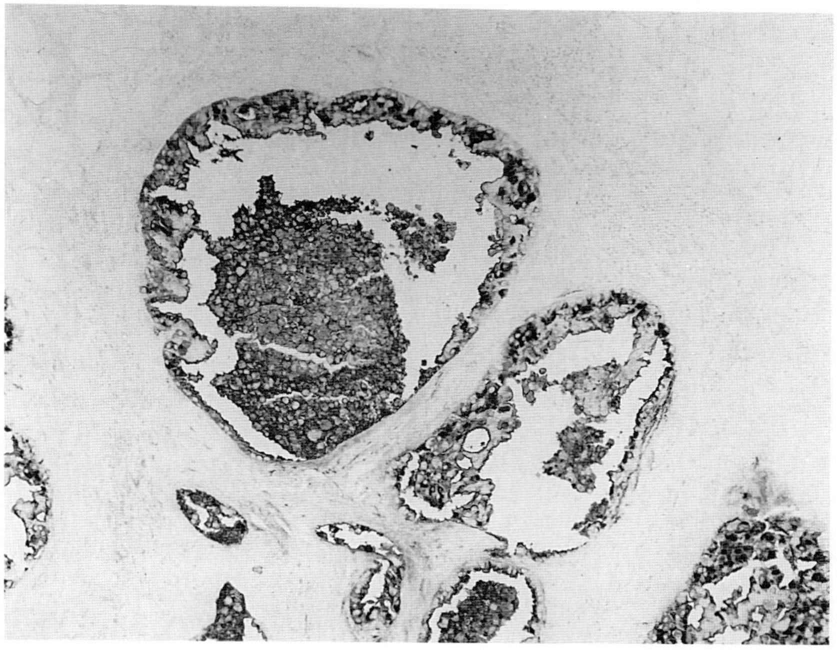

**Figure 10.18** (a) Intraductal apocrine carcinoma with central necrosis showing a positive reaction with B72.3 (b). (H&E, (a) X75; B72.3, (b) X75) (From Tavassoli FA, et al: *Am J Surg Pathol* 1990;14:128–133, with permission)

utilized by different pathologists for diagnosis of apocrine carcinoma are highly variable (71,72,85,104, 108). In general, the iron granules and decapitation secretion which are typically found in the skin apocrine glands have not been observed in the mammary apocrine cells.

## Differential Diagnosis

Lesions that enter the differential diagnosis include histiocytoid carcinoma, lipid-rich carcinoma, squamous carcinoma and granular cell tumor.

Histiocytoid carcinoma has a less granular to totally agranular and sometimes vacuolated cytoplasm and a paler staining eosinophilia as well as smaller and denser nuclei. Identification of intracytoplasmic lumens and demonstration of intracytoplasmic mucin in the histiocytoid tumor cells will distinguish histiocytoid carcinoma from apocrine carcinoma.

Lipid-rich carcinoma is also characterized by the presence of abundant foamy or vacuolated cytoplasm with very fine granularity. On H&E sections, it can be most difficult to distinguish this tumor from either apocrine or histiocytoid carcinomas. Absolute confirmation of this diagnosis would require fat stains on fresh or formalin-fixed tissue; fat stain on paraffin-embedded tissue is not very reliable. Lipid-rich carcinomas contain neutral lipids and lack intracytoplasmic mucin. Their rather vacuolated to foamy cytoplasm can be helpful in separating them from apocrine carcinomas. Furthermore, lipid-rich carcinomas have a more uniform nuclear appearance throughout the tumor and lack the multiple nucleoli often observed in apocrine carcinomas.

The distinction from carcinomas with squamous differentiation can be facilitated by demonstration of glycogen in the latter and its absence in apocrine carcinomas.

Another lesion that may be confused with apocrine carcinoma because of the prominent granularity of its abundant cytoplasm, is granular cell tumor. The nuclei of granular cells are smaller with dense chromatin and lack the nucleolar prominence typical of apocrine carcinoma cells. Furthermore, in contrast to apocrine carcinoma, granular cell tumors contain glycogen and show a positive reaction for S-100 protein.

## Hormone Receptors

Mossler et al (104) found only a low affinity, nonsaturable high capacity 4S progesterone-estrogen binding protein in their six cases. Several of the apocrine carcinomas studied by Eusebi et al (83) had ER reactivity and did not differ in this respect from the common breast carcinomas. The hormone receptor status was known for ten of the cases in Abati et al series (1990); six of these were estrogen receptor negative and four were positive. Two of the four with estrogen receptor positivity were progesterone receptor negative.

In vitro analysis of apocrine carcinomas have demonstrated an enhanced metabolism of testosterone precursors by this tumor compared to other types of carcinoma (103). The growth of cutaneous apocrine glands is stimulated by androgenic hormones (103) and analysis of human axillary apocrine gland secretions have shown the presence of dehydroepiandrosterone and androsterone sulfates (97). The enhanced metabolism of testosterone precursors by apocrine carcinoma could have significant clinical and therapeutic implications, and it should be correlated with the levels of androgen receptors as well as the clinical response to hormonal treatment. These findings may prove significant in establishing apocrine carcinoma as a distinct entity.

## Origin of Apocrine Cells

While the designation of sweat-gland carcinoma has been used for apocrine carcinoma (93,98), some have used this designation because they believed in the presence of true sweat glands or remnants thereof within the breast, while others did so because they regarded the breast as a modified sweat gland. Currently, it is generally believed that these tumors originate in cells with a potential to differentiate into apocrine cells. This potential is more frequently realized in the form of benign apocrine metaplasia, however. Interestingly, a number of studies have suggested that despite their resemblance to the cells of apocrine glands, the metaplastic apocrine cells actually have merocrine secretion (107). Some investigators have actually questioned the validity of the term apocrine for these mammary cells since, at the ultrastructural level, these cells lack iron granules and decapitation secretion, features typically observed in normal apocrine glands of the skin (76,108,115).

## Relationship to Apocrine Metaplasia

Yates and Ahmed (120) reported a case of apocrine carcinoma in a patient whose previous biopsy, 19 months earlier, had shown florid apocrine metaplasia intermingled with atypical apocrine cells. This sequence of events provides morphologic support to the suggestion that apocrine metaplasia is a "risk factor" for breast cancer, but the significance of apocrine metaplasia as a premalignant change is uncertain (96,120). Dixon et al (81) suggested that patients with cysts lined by metaplastic apocrine cells may be at greater risk for development of subsequent breast carcinoma compared to those patients who have cysts lined by nonapocrine cells. In its hyperplastic and papillary form, apocrine metaplasia is more common in breasts that harbour a carcinoma (119). Page and Dupont (105), however, have expressed reservations regarding the consideration of apocrine metaplasia as a premalignant change. In our own experience at AFIP, the presence of apocrine metaplasia, even when hyperplastic and papillary, in patients with either intraductal hyperplasia or atypical intraductal hyperplasia did not increase the chances for subsequent development of invasive breast carcinoma in either group when compared to those women with these hyperplastic changes who did not have apocrine metaplasia (113). The presence of cytologic atypia in metaplastic or hyperplastic apocrine cells, however, is a different issue and, in my opinion, probably constitutes an important risk factor of the same magnitude as atypical intraductal hyperplasia; this issue needs to be confirmed by appropriate studies.

### Prognosis

The prognosis of apocrine carcinoma has not been well established. Some contend it reflects a well-differentiated variant of breast carcinoma and has a better prognosis than ordinary infiltrating duct carcinoma. This contention is disputed by those who believe it shows no significantly different behavior from the regular infiltrating duct carcinoma (69,87).

If the presence of apocrine differentiation in mammary carcinomas is indeed of no clinical and prognostic significance, is it worthwhile to separate these tumors as a specific entity? Comparing these tumors to regular infiltrating duct carcinomas, the age distribution of patients and prognosis are not notably different. Some characteristics of apocrine carcinoma have emerged, however, which may prove to have therapeutic significance. In a study of 120 breast cancer explants, the presence of apocrine morphology correlated with the amount of GCDFP-15 released by the breast carcinoma and with androgen, rather than estrogen, receptor levels (103). In vitro observation of the effects of various hormones on the production of GCDFP-15 by carcinoma cells have shown that androgens apparently increase the rate of gene transcription of GCDFP-15 while inhibiting cell proliferation. Estrogens, in contrast, stimulate cellular proliferation and repress the rate of gene transcription of GCDFP-15 (111). Administration of androgens to patients with metastatic breast cancer has been shown to stimulate the production of GCDFP-15 in 52% of the patients (80,100). As Mazoujian has pointed out, one reason for segregating apocrine carcinomas would be the identification of a subgroup of tumors that appear to have a unique response to hormonal stimuli. As we continue to explore hormonal manipulations in the treatment of breast carcinoma, apocrine differentiation may emerge as an important feature that would influence therapeutic decisions and establish this lesion as a distinct entity.

## HISTIOCYTOID CARCINOMA

The term "histiocytoid carcinoma" was introduced by Hood et al in 1973 (127). In their analysis of 13 metastatic mammary carcinomas to the eyelid, they noted a pronounced histiocytoid appearance to the cells. This histiocytoid appearance had caused difficulty in arriving at the accurate diagnosis. The lesions in the eyelid had been confused for xanthoma, histiocytoma, xanthelesma, and even granular cell tumor. A subsequent report also concentrated on the morphology of the metastatic tumor in the eyelid (123). In 1989, Walford and ten Velden (128) described the morphologic features of two primary histiocytoid carcinomas along with a discussion of the histogenesis and associated diagnostic problems. Several additional cases of breast carcinoma with hystiocytoid features have also been reported in either the breast or in metastatic breast carcinoma (121,122,124,125).

Some authors believe that histiocytoid carcinoma is a variant of invasive lobular carcinoma characterized by a proliferation of cells that have abundant pale eosinophilic to finely vacuolated cytoplasm (Fig. 10.19) (126). The association with in situ lobular

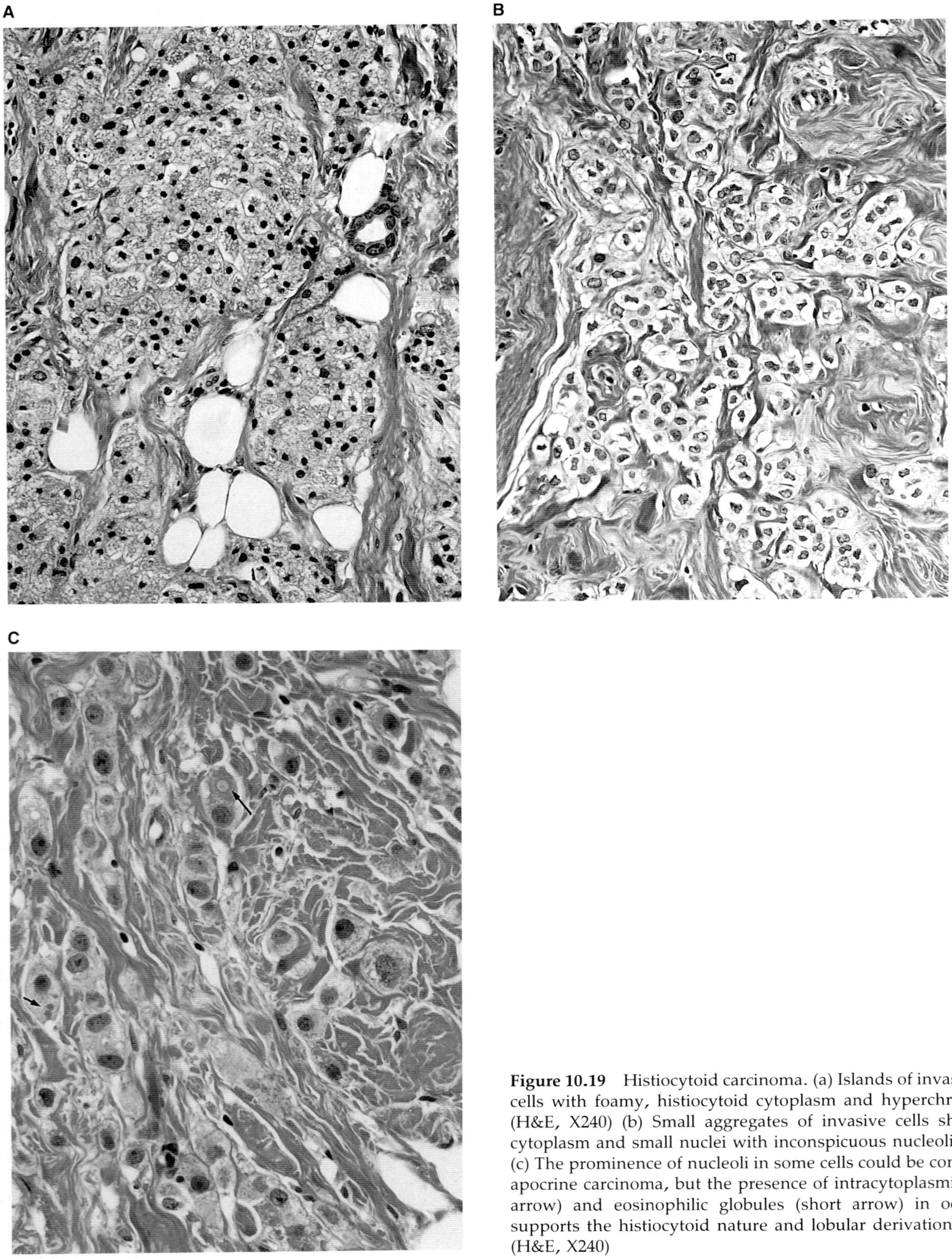


**Figure 10.19** Histiocytoid carcinoma. (a) Islands of invasive neoplastic cells with foamy, histiocytoid cytoplasm and hyperchromatic nuclei. (H&E, X240) (b) Small aggregates of invasive cells show abundant cytoplasm and small nuclei with inconspicuous nucleoli. (H&E, X200) (c) The prominence of nucleoli in some cells could be confused with an apocrine carcinoma, but the presence of intracytoplasmic lumen (long arrow) and eosinophilic globules (short arrow) in occasional cells supports the histiocytoid nature and lobular derivation of the lesion. (H&E, X240)

carcinoma and an invasive pattern characterized by "Indian filing" and "targetoid growth" supports lobular origin. Walford and ten Velden (128) observed transition from the typical in situ lobular carcinoma cell to apocrine-type cells and concluded that histiocytoid carcinoma is an apocrine variant of lobular carcinoma. The nuclei are small compared to those of apocrine carcinoma, however; they have dense chromatin and inconspicuous nucleoli. The presence of intracytoplasmic lumens and mucin along with the absence of intracytoplasmic lipid helps distinguish this tumor from lipid-rich carcinoma. Distinction of the invasive histiocytoid cells from granular cells, xanthomatous lesions, and an inflammatory lesion can be difficult; granular cells display positive immunoreaction for S-100 protein and xanthoma cells lack mucin droplets, however. For a more detailed description of the differential diagnosis, see the differential diagnosis of apocrine carcinoma.

## LIPID-RICH CARCINOMA

One of the least-frequently diagnosed variants of breast carcinoma, lipid-rich or lipid-secreting carcinoma was first described by Aboumrad, Horn and Fine in 1963. Subsequently, 13 examples of this lesion were studied by Ramos and Taylor (133) and ten additional cases were reported by Van Bogaert and Maldague (134) who used the designation of lipid-secreting carcinoma in a broad sense. They subdivided lipid-secreting carcinomas into histiocytoid, sebaceous, and apocrine types. The general trend, however, is to separate apocrine carcinomas into a different category. While there are a few examples of adenoid cystic carcinoma with sebaceous differentiation, a pure sebaceous cell carcinoma of the breast proper has not been defined or described. A few additional cases have appeared in the literature sporadically since then.

The incidence of this tumor ranges from 1.4% in Ramos and Taylor's (133) study to 1.6% in Van Bogaert and Maldague's (134) report. Only 15 well-documented cases have been reported. Over the past 12 years at AFIP (1976–1988), only one additional example of lipid-rich carcinoma has been diagnosed.

### Clinical Features

Patients with lipid-rich carcinoma range in age from 33 to 81 years. They present with a mass or an ill-defined induration in the breast. The tumor may become ulcerated when large and induce peau d'orange appearance in the overlying skin of the breast.

### Gross and Microscopic Features

The tumors range in size from 1.2 to 15 cm and have ill-defined margins. Cut surface of the tumors generally lacks chalky streaks or umbilication.

Lipid-rich carcinoma is composed of large cells with abundant foamy cytoplasm containing neutral lipid (Figs. 10.20–10.21). Neutral lipids should be demonstrable in at least 80% and preferably 100% of the cells for the lesion to qualify as lipid-rich carcinoma. Rigid adherence to this 80% to 100% lipid-rich cell population is mandatory to define a distinct group of tumors since a high proportion of breast carcinomas have some cells that will have stainable neutral fat within them. The tumor cells do not contain mucin. Either ductal or lobular in situ carcinoma may be associated with this invasive pattern. It is noteworthy that Ramos and Taylor (133) demonstrated lipid in only four cases for which unfixed tissue was available. The other nine cases were identified retrospectively on the basis of histologic pattern alone in a review of 900 breast carcinomas.

Van Bogaert and Maldague (134) described three variants of lipid-secreting carcinoma. They designated these as histiocytoid, sebaceous, and apocrine types. The sebaceous variant had greater nuclear pleomorphism and more bubbly cytoplasm than the histiocytoid type. The apocrine type had "apocrine extrusion of nuclei." Since this terminology could cause additional confusion rather than clarification of the nature of the lesion and because subtle differences can be explained on the basis of nuclear grade, this subclassification is unnecessary. The apocrine variant of Van Bogaert and Maldague resembles the tumors described by Hamperl (93) characterized by hobnail appearance of neoplastic cells lining glandular lumens brought about by protrusion towards the lumen of the apically-oriented, pleomorphic nuclei;

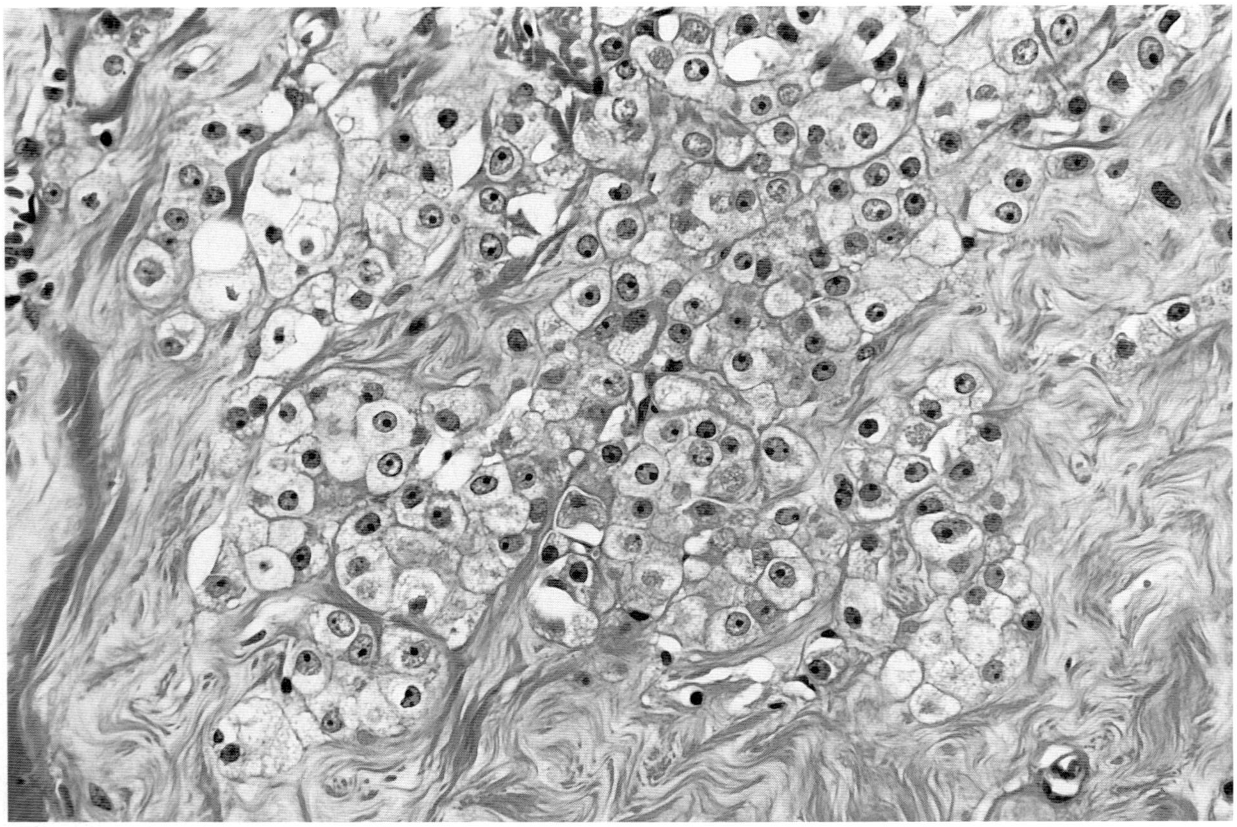

**Figure 10.20** Lipid-rich carcinoma. The large cells with round nuclei form cord-like arrangement or sheets and nests. The nuclei have prominent nucleoli. (H&E, X240)

the patients had received estrogen-progesterone preparations.

The distinctive feature of lipid-rich carcinoma is the presence of abundant intracytoplasmic neutral fat demonstrated by oil red O stain in tumors that may, but do not invariably, display an unusually foamy or vacuolated cytoplasm.

Intracytoplasmic lipid accumulation is not uncommon and may be quite marked in some of the regular breast carcinomas (130). Up to 75% of 87 consecutive breast carcinomas stained with oil red O show slight to marked staining (130). It is not simply the presence of stainable lipid within some tumor cells that would qualify the tumor as lipid-rich, however. The tumors must have some cytoplasmic vacuolization in addition to abundant intracytoplasmic lipid within 80% to 100% of the neoplastic cells to warrant a designation of lipid-rich carcinoma. Since Ramos and Taylor (133) demonstrated that the lipid within these cells is a secretory product and does not reflect a degenerative change, Van Bogaert and Maldague have recommended the term "lipid-secreting" carcinoma as originally suggested by Aboumrad et al (129). Considering Fisher et al's finding of lipid within such a high proportion of breast carcinomas, however, the term lipid-rich carcinoma would seem more appropriate. The advantages of a designation of lipid-rich versus lipid-secreting carcinoma have been discussed by Vera-Sempere and Llombart-Bosch (135).

Ultrastructurally, lipid-rich carcinoma is distinguished by the presence of abundant intracytoplasmic lipid droplets that may coalesce into irregular globules with no degenerative changes (131). The lipid droplets appear first around the nucleus and gradually indent and compress the nucleus to the periphery. Glycogen is present in some tumor cells. Intramitochondrial crystals may be observed in some degenerating cells (132). In my personal experience, the sporadic finding of a few lipid droplets within breast carcinoma cells is very common at the ultrastructural level, but rarely do the droplets constitute a prominent intracytoplasmic element. Therefore, it is not surprising that routine staining of breast carcinomas with oil red O would pick up a high proportion that show some neutral lipids in their cytoplasm. The difference between the carcinomas that assume the typical foamy cytoplasm of lipid-rich carcinomas and

A

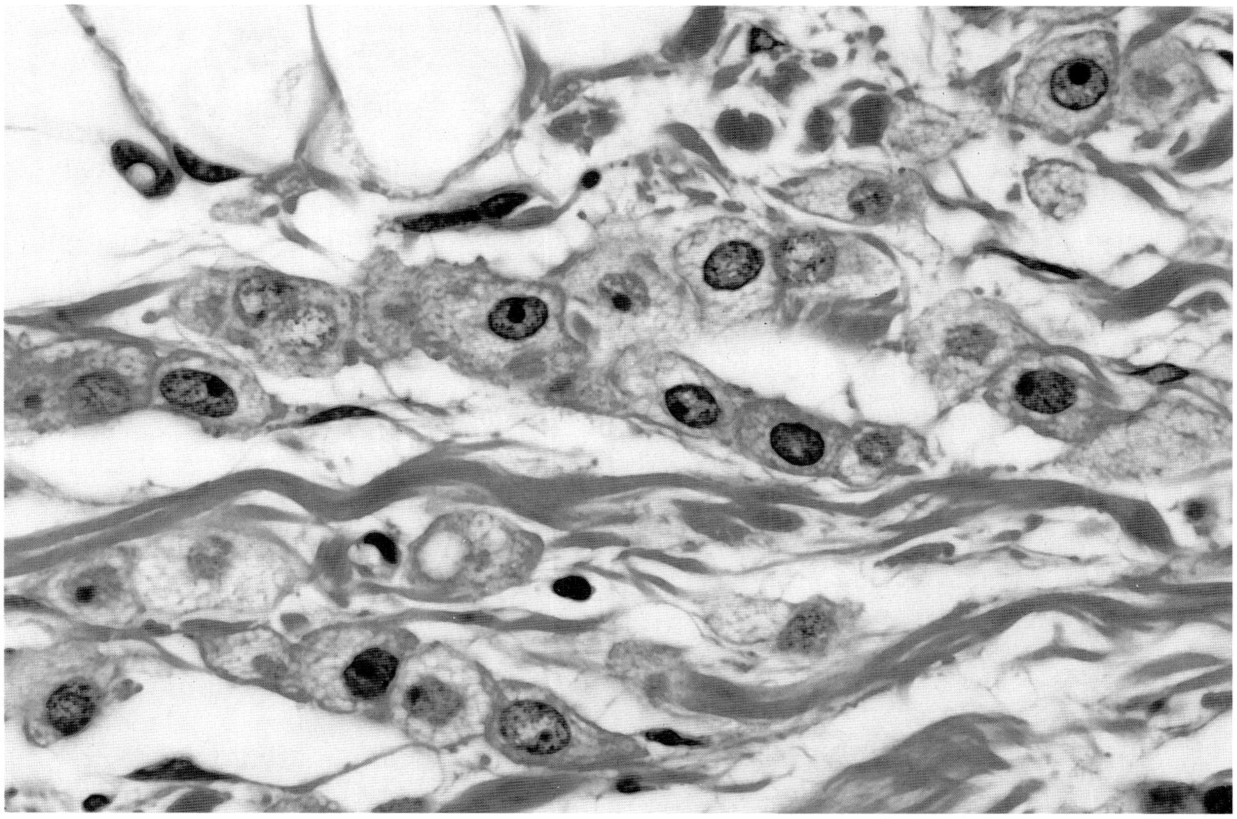

B

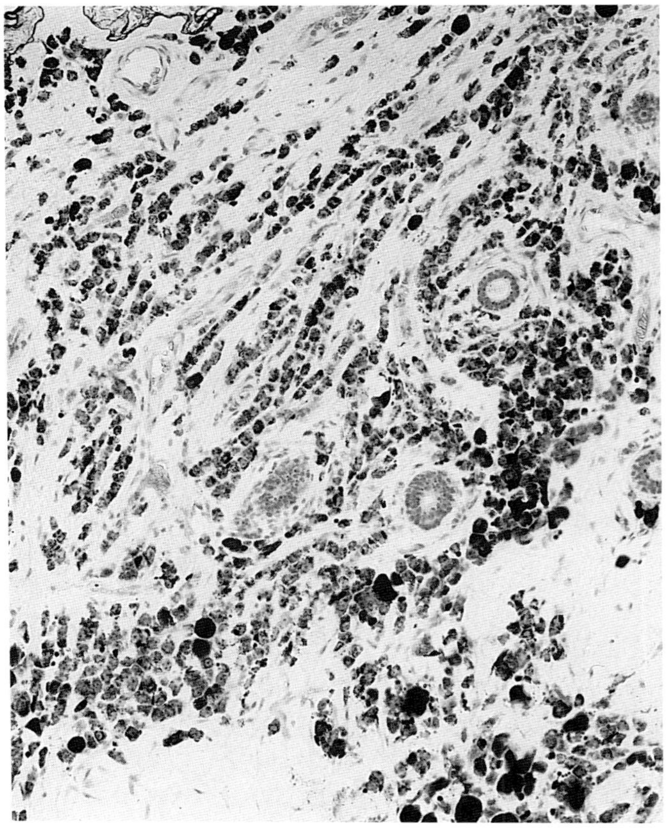

**Figure 10.21** Lipid-rich carcinoma. (a) At higher magnification, many cells display numerous small round vacuoles in the cytoplasm. The nuclei retain their round to oval shape and are not compressed by the cytoplasmic vacuoles. (H&E, X630) (b) The tumor cells show diffuse and intensely positive reaction on Oil-red-O for neutral lipids. (H&E, X120)

those that lack the foamy cytoplasm may be due to the size of the lipid droplets and the clustering pattern of the lipid droplets within the tumor cells. Wrba et al (136), found most of the intracytoplasmic lipid in autophagic vacuoles. While a well-developed Golgi complex suggestive of secretory activity by tumor cells was described by Ramos & Taylor (133), the Golgi complex and profiles of rough endoplasmic reticulum were inconspicuous in the five cases evaluated by Wrba et al (136).

Immunohistochemically, the tumor cells display diffuse, intense reaction with alpha-lactalbumin (ALA) and lactoferrin (LFr), whereas, only isolated cells react with human milk fat globule membrane antigen (HMFG-2) (136). All of the seven lipid-rich carcinomas evaluated for receptors were negative for steroid receptors (131,136).

## Prognosis

In Ramos and Taylor's study (133), 11 of the 12 patients treated by radical mastectomy had axillary lymph node metastases. During the first two years following the diagnosis of their tumors, 50% of the patients in Ramos and Taylor's study (133) died prompting Van Bogaert and Maldague (134) to suggest that this tumor may be associated with a worse prognosis compared to other types of breast carcinoma. In Wrba et al's (136) group of five cases, three of the four patients who had axillary node excision had positive nodes. Two of the five patients developed metastases, one of whom died within three weeks from generalized metastases. Another patient died of cardiac insufficiency. The follow-up on one case was too short, and the fifth patient was alive without evidence of disease 2.5 years following surgery. Neither vascular invasion nor lymph node metastases were present in either of the two tumors reported by Kurebayashi et al (131). The possibility that lipid-rich carcinoma may be more aggressive than regular infiltrating duct carcinomas has not been established with certainty.

It is also important to compare the behavior of the lipid-rich carcinoma with foamy cytoplasm with the type of tumor described by Fisher et al (130) characterized by marked intracytoplasmic lipid content but without the foamy cytoplasm to determine if indeed the presence of intracytoplasmic lipid, associated or unassociated with cytoplasmic vacuolization on H&E sections has any prognostic significance.

Disagreements persist on the issue of whether these are lipid-secreting or lipid-rich carcinomas. Those who have identified prominent Golgi complexes in their ultrastructural analysis favor a secretory cell type, but others argue against active secretion by the tumor cells. The latter opinion is advanced by those who have encountered inconspicuous Golgi complexes at the ultrastructural level. The absence of extracellular secretory material (lipid) is presented as further supportive evidence of the lack of secretory activity. Therefore, for the time being, the term lipid-rich carcinoma would seem more appropriate.

# SECRETORY CARCINOMA

The first detailed description of secretory carcinoma was published in 1966 by McDivitt and Stewart (147). The seven tumors that constituted the basis of their report occurred in children ranging from 3 to 15 years in age. Impressed by the young age of the patients, McDivitt and Stewart suggested the designation of "juvenile" carcinoma. Subsequently, several clusters of cases and isolated case reports noted the occurrence of this lesion in a much wider age range than anticipated from the initial report as well as development of axillary node and rare distal metastases (140,143,151). Nonetheless, an outstanding clinical feature of this tumor is its tendency to occur relatively more frequently during the first three decades of life. It is by no means exclusive to children, however. Therefore, the designation of juvenile carcinoma has been replaced by the descriptive term of secretory carcinoma.

## Clinical Features

Patients with secretory carcinoma range in age from 3 to 73 years with a median age of 25 (138,139,145–149,151,154–156). About one third of the reported cases have occurred in women 30 years of age or older. Although a majority of the reported cases have occurred in females, several cases have been reported in both prepubertal and adult males (140,143–145,149,150,153,156). Also a majority of the tumors have occurred in caucasians. Most patients present with a breast mass. The distribution of the mass throughout the breast is not unusual; the tumor may be located in the subareolar region or the axillary tail of the breast as well. We have also seen a case of secretory carcinoma arising in accessory breast tissue in the inner thigh/vulvar region. Nipple discharge has been observed in association with some of the subareolar lesions.

## Gross Pathologic Features

The tumors range in size from 1 to 12 cm with a median of 3 cm. They are firm, discrete, or circumscribed lesions appearing as densely fibrous masses simulating fibroadenomas. Infiltrating margins also occur, however. The cut surface of the tumors is grayish-white to tan in color. Rarely, a central papillary component may be present.

## Microscopic Features

Secretory carcinoma is characterized by the presence of abundant extracellular and intracellular secretory material (Fig. 10.22) which stain pink to intensely eosinophilic on H&E sections. The neoplastic cells lack significant atypism or mitotic activity and can appear deceptively bland. Depending on the amount of the intracellular secretory content, the cells may appear bulging with secretions, vacuolated with secretory droplets, vacuolated without apparent secretory droplets, or granular. Although based on the cytoplasmic features, Tavassoli and Norris (152) distinguished two major cell types (A and B); both cell types are present in almost every tumor and predominance of one or the other has no prognostic significance. The nuclei are round to oval with small and generally inconspicuous nucleoli. The tumor cells may proliferate as a densely cellular, solid mass composed of nests of cells separated by fibrous septae and with a pushing growth margin; this pattern corresponds to the grossly fibroadenomatous appearance. The central portion of these well-circumscribed tumors sometimes assumes a papillary pattern. In one of Tokunaga et al's (155) cases, the secretory carcinoma appeared to arise from juvenile papillomatosis. The tumor may also show an infiltrating growth pattern associated with areas of intraductal carcinoma. The secretory character of the cells is apparent even when the tumor invades with a cord-like pattern. These distinctive cytologic features can be helpful in arriving at an accurate diagnosis even on samples removed for aspiration cytology (141).

A single case of noninvasive secretory carcinoma has been reported in a 33-year-old Japanese woman (152) who complained of nipple discharge. This patient did not have a palpable lesion or a mammographic abnormality. Suspicious tumor cells were detected in the smears of the nipple discharge. She had no evidence of axillary node metastases. In the AFIP files, there is an intraductal proliferation identical to secretory carcinoma that was observed in a background of gynecomastia in a 47-year-old man (Fig. 10.23); because it was confined to a small duct less than 2 mm in size, it was designated as atypical secretory intraductal hyperplasia. The patient had no further treatment since most of his breast tissue had already been removed for gynecomastia.

When secretory carcinoma metastasizes to axillary lymph nodes or recurs, the secretory pattern is retained (151,153,155).

## Histochemical and Immunohistochemical Characteristics

The secretory material exhibits tremendous variation and does not always stain uniformly in different cases or even within a given tumor. Majority of cases evaluated by Tavassoli and Norris (153) stained as sulfated acid mucopolysaccharides, while others persistently stained as a sialomucin. Generally, the secretory material was PAS-positive, diastase-resistant, alcian-blue-positive and exhibited a highly sporadic positivity with mucicarmine.

Six cases of secretory carcinoma from adult females subsequent to those previously reported from AFIP, were evaluated for the presence of alphalactalbumin; a strongly positive reaction was observed in both the intracellular and the extracellular secretory material. Botta et al (139) also evaluated one case for a variety of milk proteins such as alphalactalbumin, beta-casein, and milk-fat globule membrane antigen, as well as CEA and actin. The secretory material, regardless of its location, was strongly

A

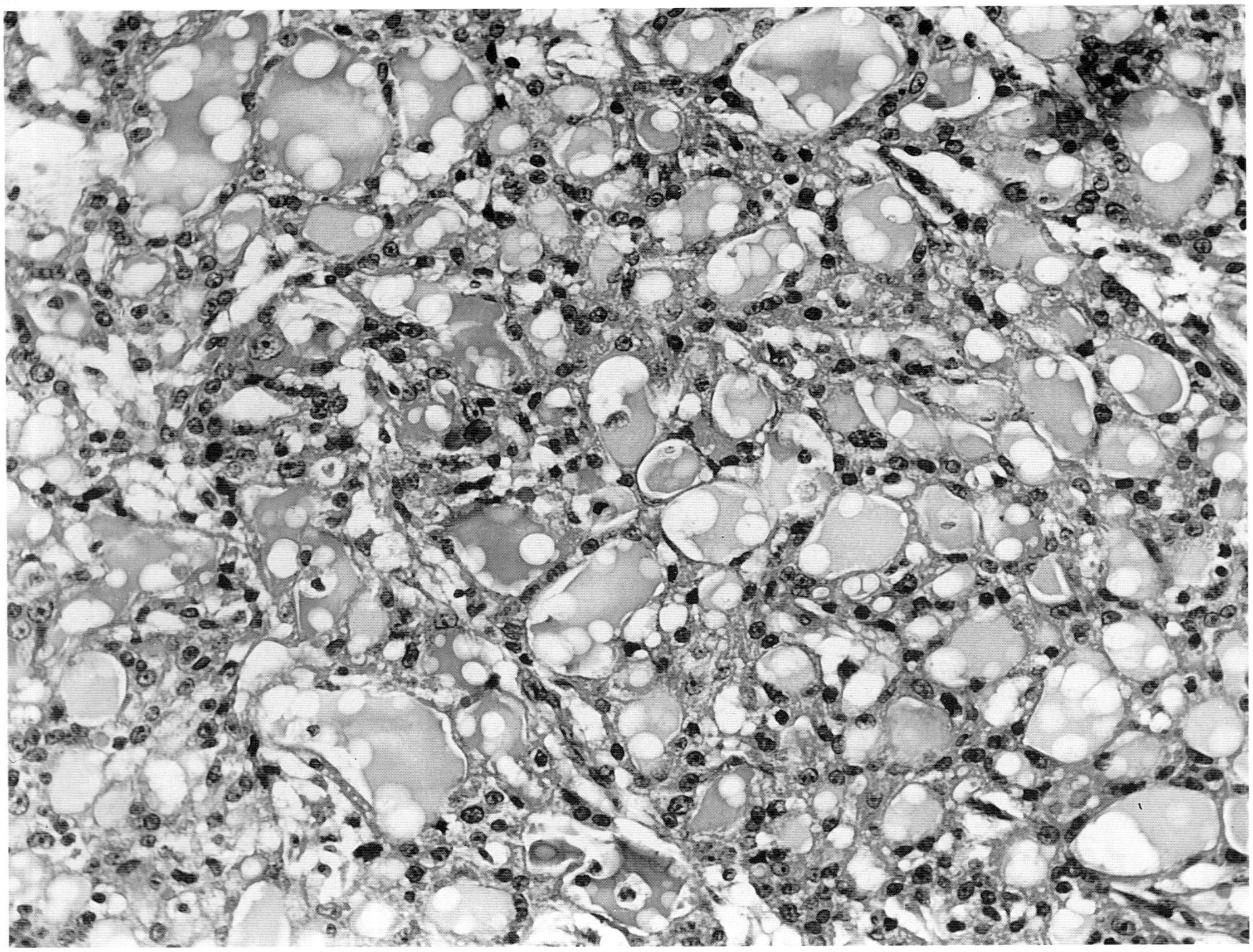

B

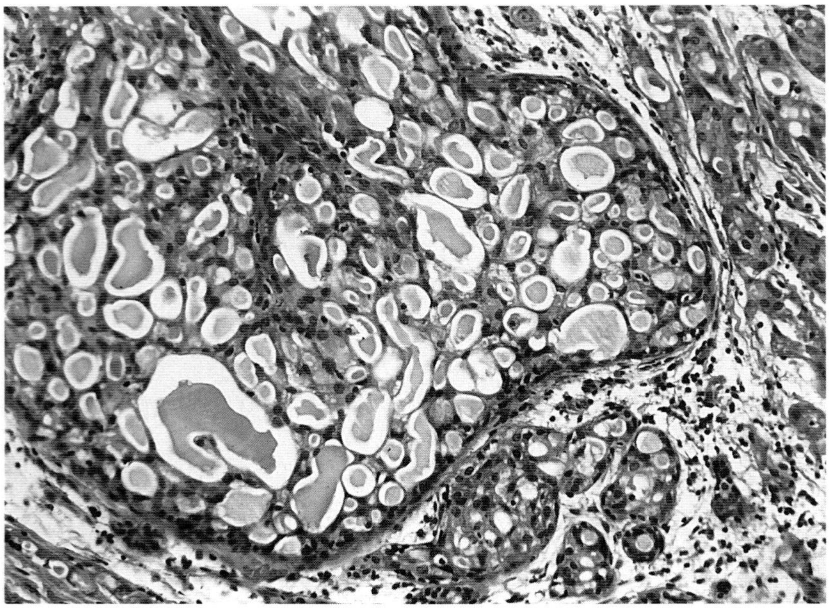

**Figure 10.22** Secretory carcinoma. (a) There is extensive extra and intracellular secretory material in the tumor. The nuclei are relatively monotonous and round; mitotic figures are rare. (H&E, X150) (b) The intraductal component is also characterized by the presence of abundant secretory material. (H&E, X60) (Figs. 10.22 a&b from Tavassoli FA, Norris HJ: *Cancer* 1980;45:2404–2413, with permission)

c

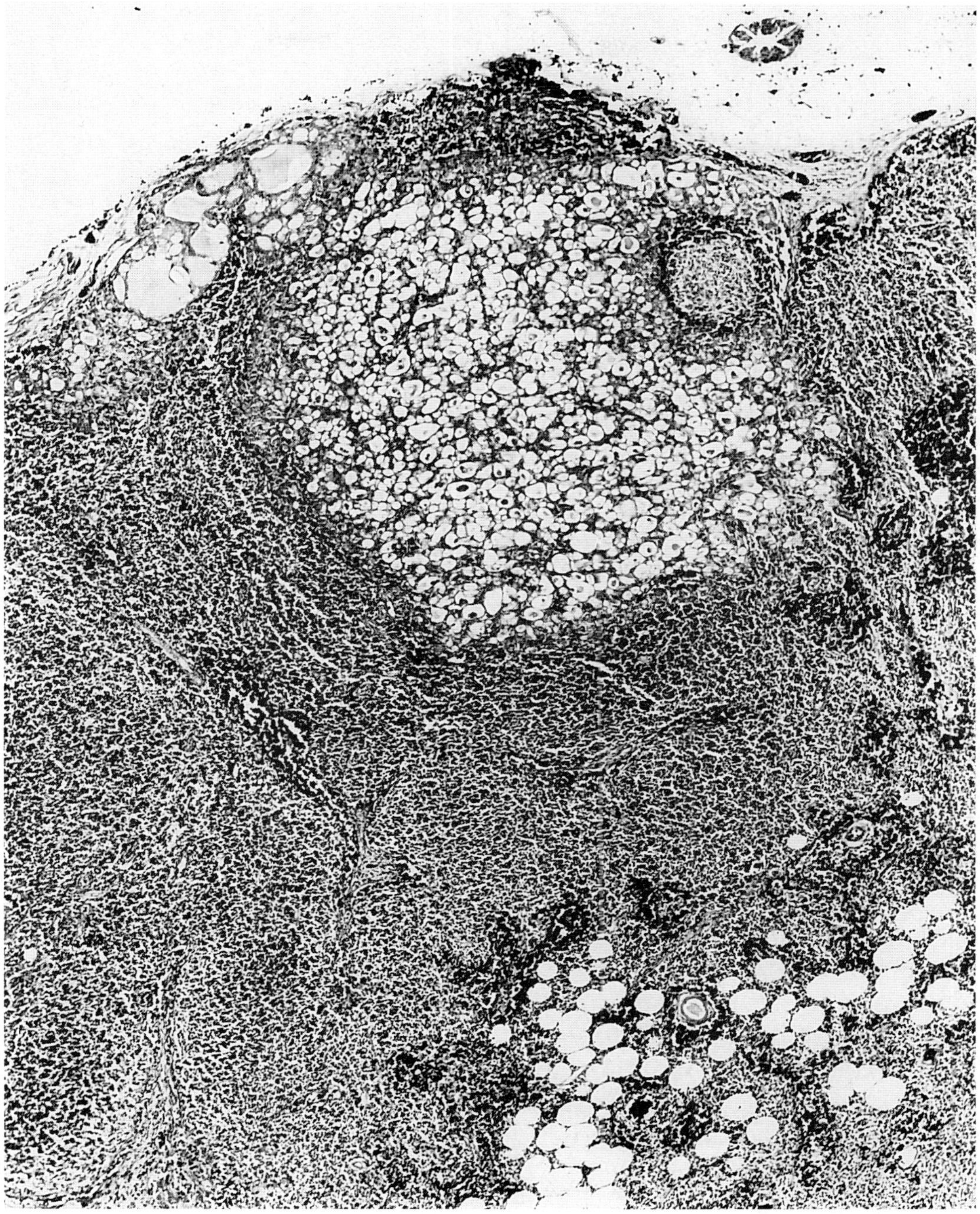

**Figure 10.22(c)** Secretory carcinoma metastatic to an axillary lymph node. The same pattern is retained. (H&E, X75)

positive for all the milk proteins. The neoplastic cells were intensely stained by the immunoperoxidase method for CEA. The case occurring in a 23-year-old male (149) also had some cells that stained strongly positive for alpha-lactalbumin, but there was no staining in the secretory material and there was no CEA reactivity. The negative reaction for actin confirmed absence of myoepithelial cells in the infiltrating carcinoma, but focal positivity in the areas of intraductal carcinoma indicated persistence of residual myoepithelial cells.

## Ultrastructural Features

The abundant secretory material is also apparent at the ultrastructural level both in extracellular spaces as well as within intracytoplasmic lumens (ICL) (Fig. 10.24). Almost every cell has one or more intracytoplasmic lumens. The extracellular secretory material has a targetoid appearance with a more electron-dense central area. The neoplastic cells have microvil-

A

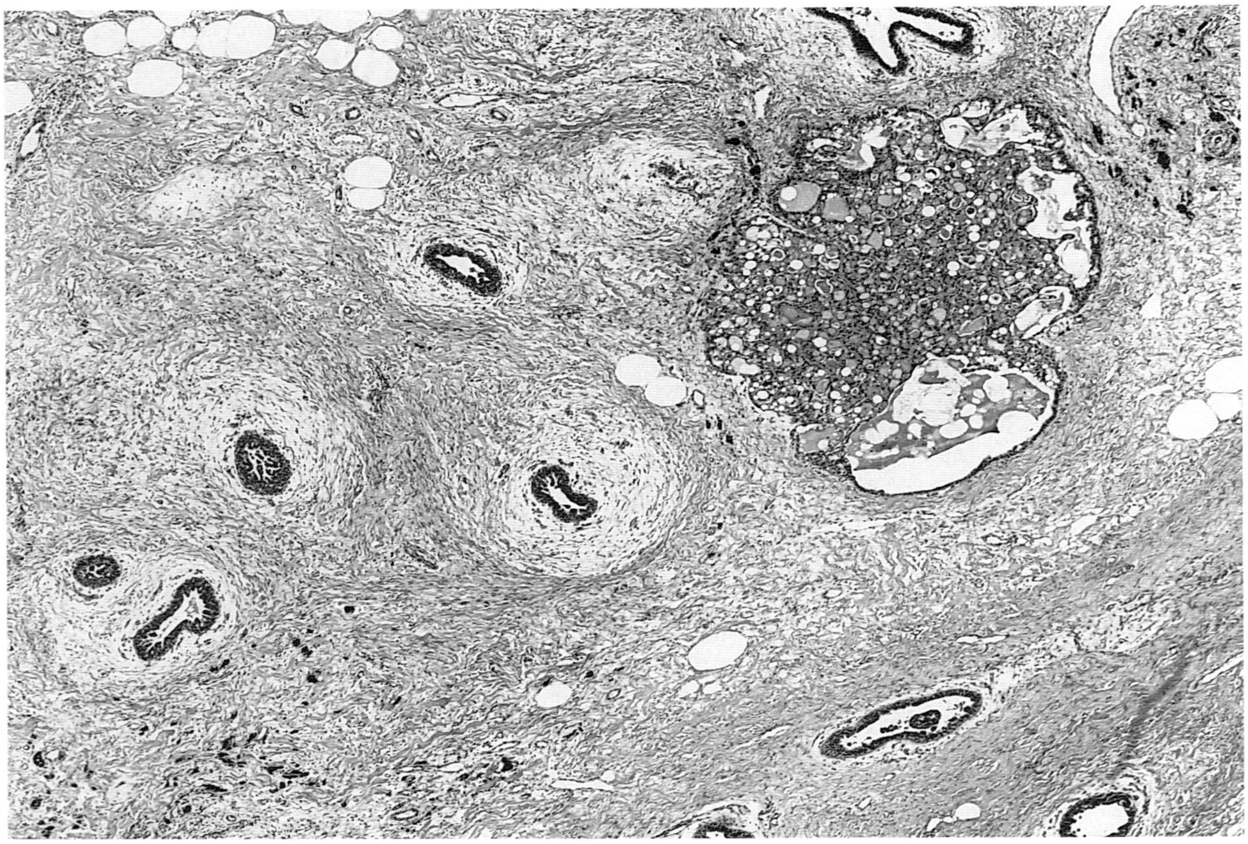

**Figure 10.23** (a&b) Atypical intraductal secretory hyperplasia in a male breast with gynecomastia. (H&E, (a) X60; (b) X200)

lous cytoplasmic processes protruding into the extracellular spaces and into the intracytoplasmic lumens. The cells are attached to one another by desmosomal junctions. Other carcinomas also have intracytoplasmic lumens (ICL) but they are not as abundant as those found in secretory carcinoma; an origin from the Golgi apparatus has been proposed for the ICL (142).

## Hormone Receptors

Information is available on five cases from AFIP; three of these were ER-positive, the other two were negative; all of these patients were over 20 years of age. The assays for both ER and PR were negative in a 33-year-old woman reported by Abe and Masuda (137). Both cases reported by Tokunaga et al (155) were ER- and PR-negative; one patient was a 13-year-old prepubertal girl, the other was an 18-year-old pubertal girl. The tumor from the 16-year-old pubertal girl reported by Masse et al had an estrogen receptor assay value of 12.4 fentomoles per mg (146).

## Treatment and Prognosis

Judging from the small number of reported cases, the behavior of this tumor appears to be age dependent. The tumor seems to have limited aggressiveness when it occurs in patients less than 20 years of age; in older patients, its behavior more closely parallels that of regular infiltrating duct carcinoma. The seven children in McDivitt and Stewart's (146) report were all alive and well from 3 to 15 years after the initial diagnosis; their surgical excision ranged from local resection, and simple mastectomy to radical mastectomy. Three of the five patients who were less than 20 years of age in Tavassoli and Norris's report (153) had local excision (two) or partial mastectomy (one); these patients were alive 0.5, 1.75 and 10 years after the diagnosis without evidence of recurrent or meta-

B

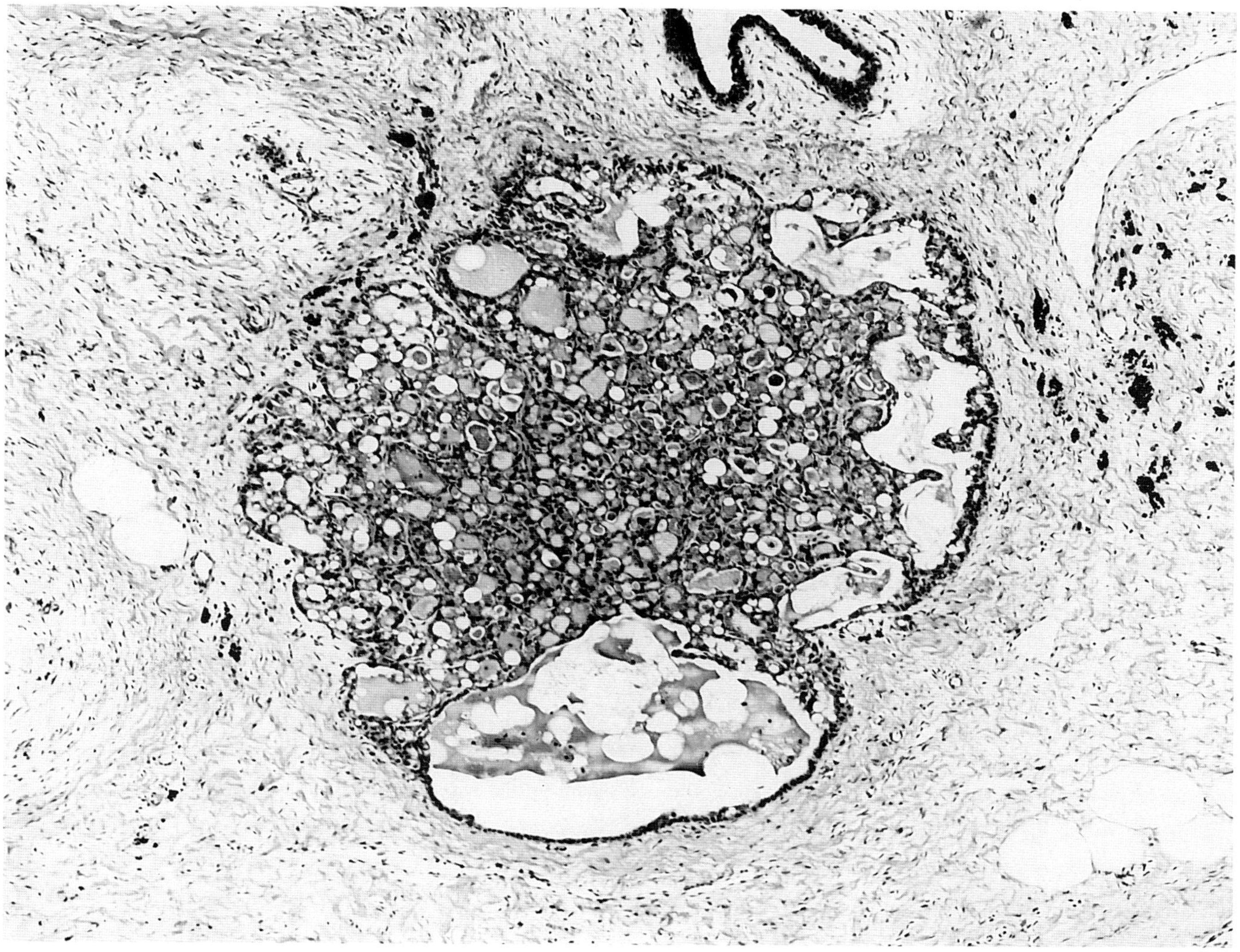

**Figure 10.23(b)** Legend on opposite page.

static disease. One of these patients, a 9-year-old boy who had been free of disease 1.75 years after the diagnosis at the time of the report, subsequently developed a recurrent tumor and had a simple mastectomy 6.5 years after the initial diagnosis.

Two more recent reports also suggest that longer follow-up on patients with secretory carcinoma is needed to more accurately assess the biologic behavior of the neoplasm. The 19-year-old patient reported by Botta et al (139) developed a recurrent tumor seven years after incomplete excision of the initial tumor which had been misinterpreted as an atypical proliferation. She had mastectomy and axillary node dissection for the recurrence; one of 14 axillary nodes had metastatic tumor. She has had no recurrences one year after mastectomy. Another patient who had a simple mastectomy for a 6 cm secretory carcinoma when she was 13 years of age developed recurrences three years later. A radical operation with resection of axillary nodes and pectoral muscle was performed. The recurrent carcinoma had metastasized to axillary lymph nodes; the secretory pattern was retained in the recurrent and metastatic tumors. She died 12 years after the initial diagnosis with extensive metastatic tumor (155). Four of the five patients reported by Krausz et al (145) developed recurrences following simple mastectomy (two cases) or local excision (two cases); two patients had axillary node metastases.

When secretory carcinoma occurs in patients less than 20 years of age, wide local excision is advocated as the initial treatment. Because of the infrequency of axillary node metastases in this age group, axillary node dissection is indicated only if nodal involvement is clinically suspected. Due to the indolent nature of the lesion and possibility of recurrences, long-term follow-up of these patients is required. In

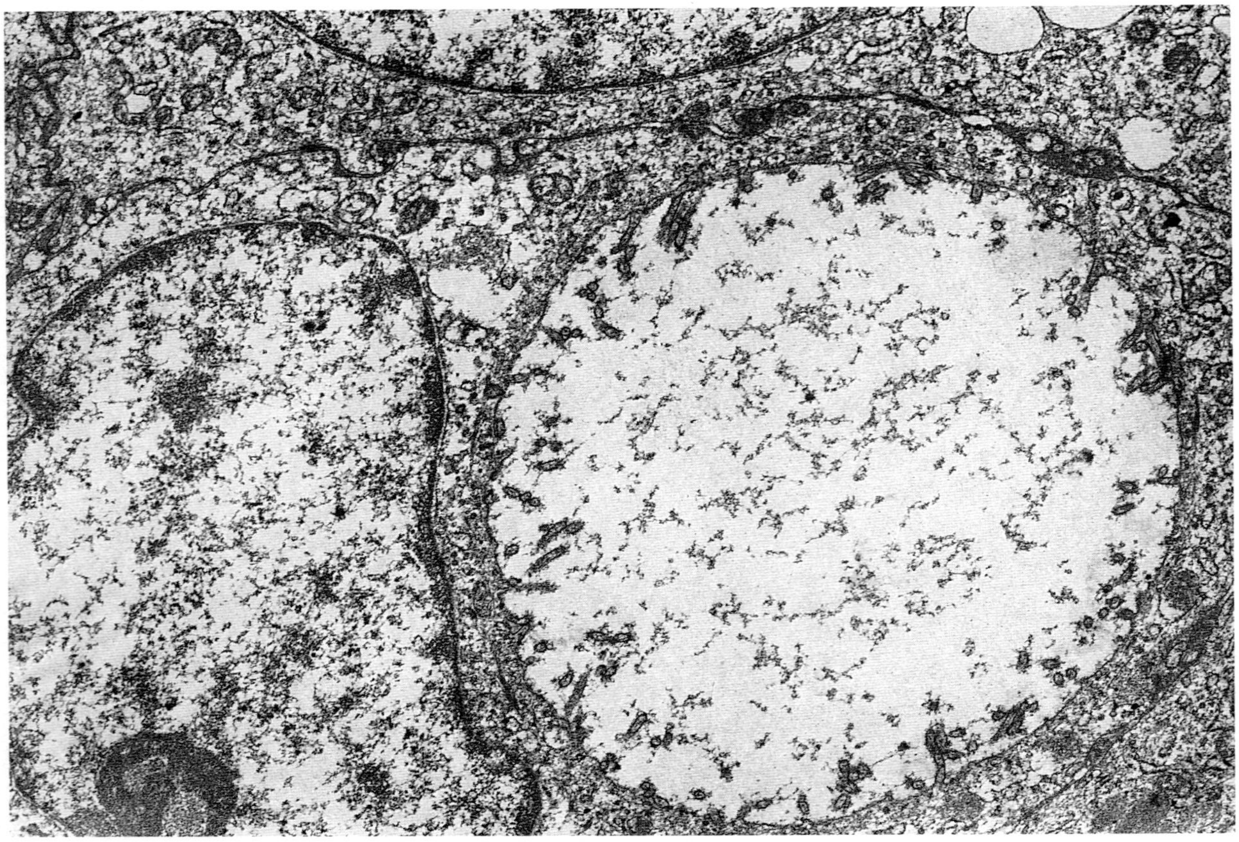

**Figure 10.24** Secretory carcinoma. At the ultrastructural level, the cytoplasm is distended by an intracytoplasmic lumen; microvillous processes project into the cytoplasmic lumens. (Uranyl acetate-lead citrate, X23,500)

view of the changing concepts in treatment of mammary carcinoma and the increasing use of lumpectomy, radiotherapy, or both, particularly for smaller tumors, there is no reason why a similar approach could not be used for secretory carcinoma when it occurs in patients 20 years of age or older. Considering the higher frequency of nodal involvement in the older women, axillary node dissection should be performed regardless of the extent of the initial surgical procedure. For larger tumors, mastectomy should be considered.

## GLYCOGEN-RICH (CLEAR-CELL) CARCINOMA

Clear-cell carcinomas occur in many organs. These tumors are characterized by either a solid, tubular, or papillary growth pattern and cells that are columnar and polygonal with abundant clear cytoplasm (Fig. 10.25). This variant of carcinoma has been recognized only recently in the breast, with about 20 examples reported in the literature (157,158,161). In their review of 1,555 invasive breast carcinomas, Fisher et al (158) identified 45 cases in which the dominant (more than 50%) neoplastic cells contained optically clear cytoplasm and centrally located nuclei. All of these tumors contained glycogen compared to 58% of the remaining 1,510 tumors that were composed of nonclear cells. The glycogen-rich, clear-cell carcinomas constituted 3% of the 1,555 invasive carcinomas in their review. The incidence of glycogen-rich, clear-cell carcinomas was 1.4% in a study from Finland (162). A more strict criteria in this study required the presence of cells with predominantly clear and occasional finely granular cytoplasm containing periodic acid-Schiff (PAS) positive, diastase labile material in 90% of the tumor area seen microscopically. I also require the presence of these changes in 90% of the tumor cells for a diagnosis of glycogen-rich, clear-cell carcinoma.

Patients with glycogen-rich carcinoma present with a palpable mass which may be associated with skin dimpling or nipple retraction (160). The original case reported by Hull et al (159) is unusual in its

A

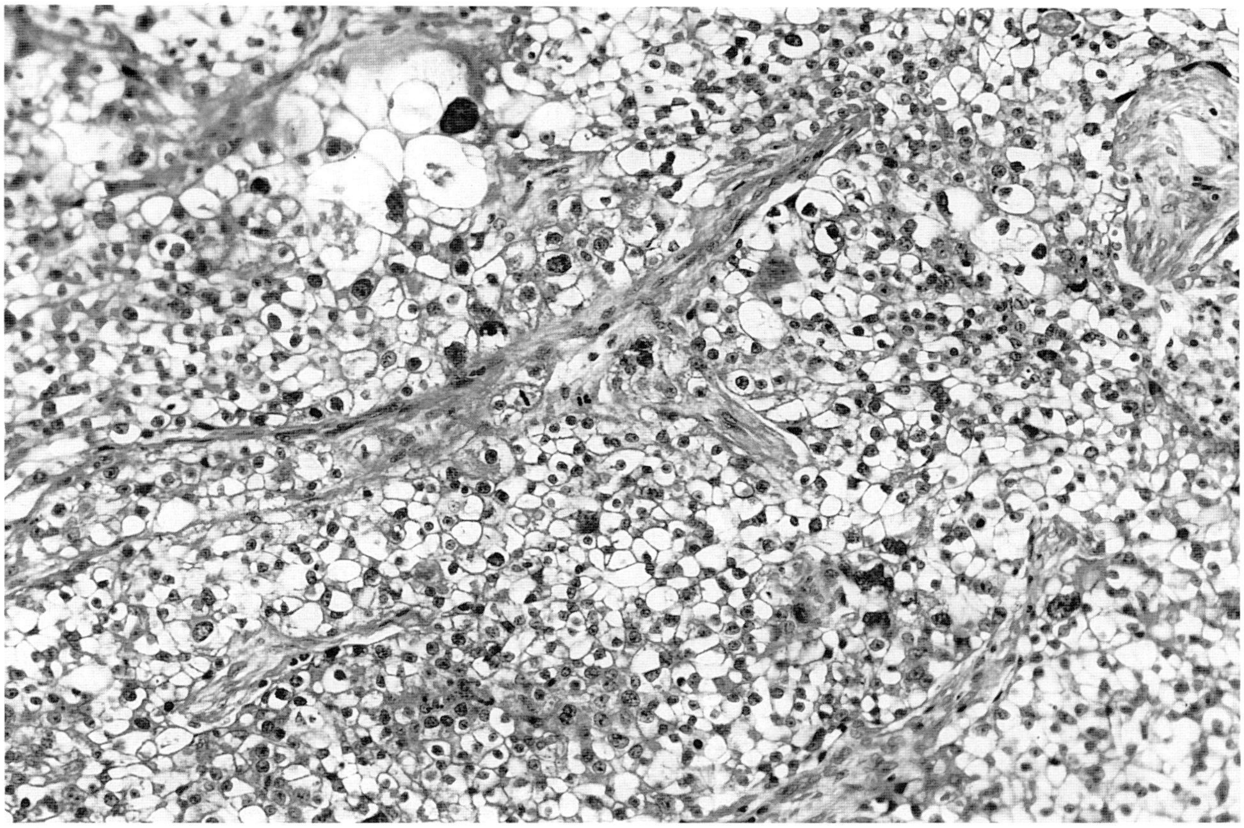

B

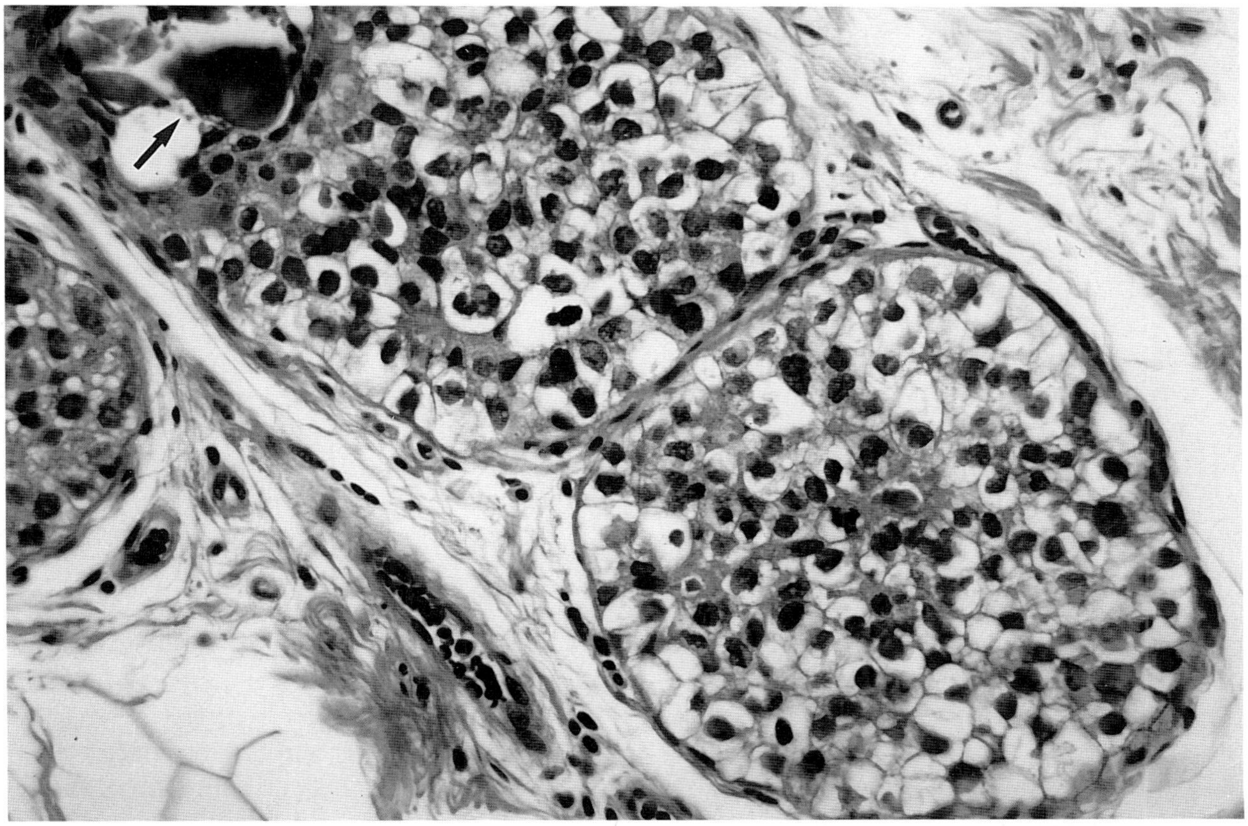

**Figure 10.25** Clear-cell (glycogen-rich) carcinoma. (a) Large solid nests of clear cells with distinct cell membranes characterize this tumor. (H&E, X150) (b) The in situ component is also characterized by a solid proliferation of clear cells within terminal ductules; microcalcification (arrow) may be present. (H&E, X250)

presentation; the mass had been present for 20 years with gradual enlargement. Because of this history and the absence of any axillary node metastases, Fisher et al dispute their diagnosis and have suggested that it may reflect a benign eccrine acrospiroma or some other benign lesion. The tumor occurs in women 41 to 78 years of age with median age of 57 years. The neoplasms range from 1.8 to 8 cm in size.

Microscopically, they are characterized by proliferation of cells in a generally solid, but occasionally papillary, and rarely, a tubular growth pattern. The tumor cells form clusters of various sizes and may be either circumscribed and well-delineated, or have a typical infiltrating pattern. The neoplastic cells are characterized by an optically clear cytoplasm which contains glycogen but no lipids or mucin. The labile nature of glycogen in aqueous solutions accounts for some of the variability of PAS staining within identical clear cells of a given neoplasm. The nuclei are hyperchromatic and centrally or eccentrically located; they may be round, ovoid, or irregular in shape. In 60% of the cases studied by Fisher et al (158), the glycogen-rich carcinomas were grade 2, a frequency that was comparable to the cancers lacking clear cells in their study. Pure glycogen-rich carcinomas lack mucosubstances, but the tumor may be admixed with other types of carcinoma. Mucosubstances may be found in the second cell population admixed with the glycogen-rich cells. The small amounts of extracellular secretory material rarely present in these tumors may stain positively for mucin. Among the glycogen-rich clear-cell carcinomas studied by Fisher et al (158), 78% were regular infiltrating duct carcinomas, 11% appeared as invasive lobular carcinoma, and the rest were a combination of tubular and regular infiltrating duct carcinoma, pure tubular or medullary in type. While an intraductal component was present in all 45 tumors studied by Fisher et al (158), none of the previously reported cases consisted of a purely intraductal neoplasm. At AFIP, several examples of pure intraductal clear-cell carcinomas have been observed (see Chapter 7, Intraductal Carcinomas); about 70% of these had other types of intraductal carcinoma present in the same biopsy. The clear-cell features are retained in axillary node metastases.

The differential diagnosis includes all tumors that may be characterized by the presence of a clear-cell cytoplasm including lipid-rich carcinoma, histiocytoid carcinoma, adenomyoepithelioma and clear-cell hidradenoma. The presence of abundant lipid along with the absence of glycogen in lipid-rich carcinoma, the presence of intracytoplasmic mucin in histiocytoid carcinoma, and the presence of a positive reaction for actin, S-100 protein, or both in adenomyoepitheliomas would distinguish these lesions from glycogen-rich clear-cell carcinoma. The presence of two cell types in parts of a clear-cell hidradenoma could help distinguish the two lesions. A more thorough analysis of all breast tumors with clear-cell features including immunohistochemical evaluation is required to more clearly define and delineate this group and its mixed variants; future studies may obviate any need for separating some of these from regular infiltrating duct carcinomas.

At the ultrastructural level, the distinctive characteristic of glycogen-rich, clear-cell carcinoma is the presence of lakes of membrane-bound glycogen in the cytoplasm; some cells have abundant small aggregates of glycogen admixed with other cytoplasmic organelles.

Only two of the reported patients have had hormone receptor studies, and in both, the neoplasms were estrogen-receptor-positive and progesterone-receptor-negative (157,159).

Despite initial impressions to the contrary (157), data from subsequent reports suggest that glycogen-rich carcinoma is as aggressive as—and probably more aggressive than—typical ductal carcinoma with frequent lymph node metastases and high mortality. Seven of the nine patients who had axillary node dissection had lymph node metastases in Hull and Warfel's report (160); five of the nine patients with follow-up in the same series died from their carcinomas and one was alive with residual disease three years after the initial diagnosis. Using contingency table analyses, Fisher et al (158) found significantly ($p < 0.05$) greater frequencies of positive nodal metastases, high histologic grade (III), moderate to marked tumor necrosis, and dense (non-myxoid) tumor stroma in the glycogen-rich, clear-cell carcinomas compared to those lacking these cytoplasmic features. Life table analysis showed disease-free survival for 12 years for all patients to be significantly less ($p = 0.0038$) in patients with glycogen-rich cancers than those whose cancers lacked clear-cell features; survival appeared to be dependent on nodal status and histologic grade of the tumor (158). Five of the six patients reported by Toikkanen and Joensu (162) had axillary node metastases, and all of these five

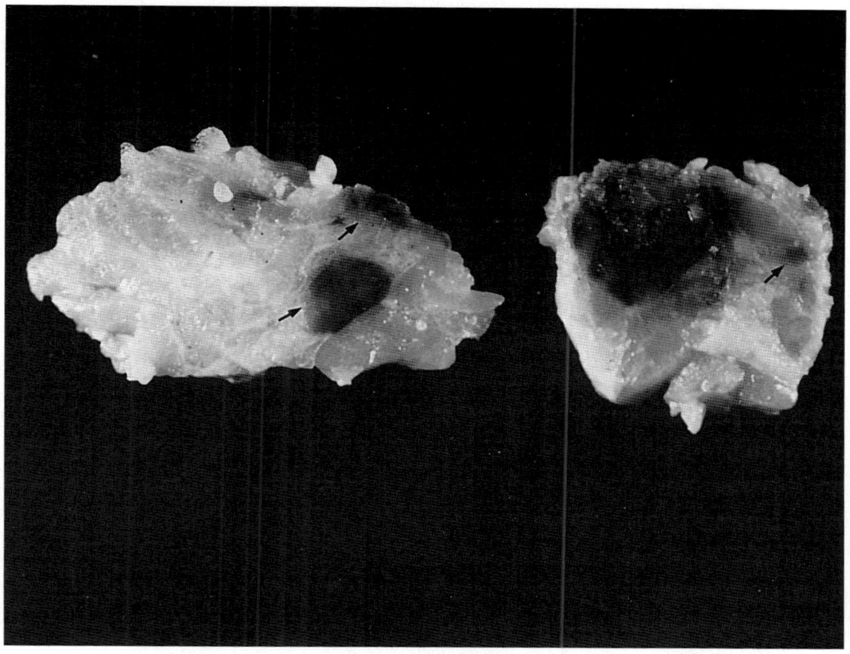

**Figure 10.26** Carcinoma with osteoclastic giant cells characterized by formation of satellite nodules (arrows) around the main tumor mass and a hemorrhagic appearance. (From Tavassoli FA, Norris HJ: *Arch Pathol Lab Med* 1986;110:636–639, with permission)

patients succumbed to the disease within seven years of the diagnosis. All tumors in this study were nondiploid, whereas 68% of other infiltrating carcinomas were nondiploid. The mean S-phase fraction of clear-cell, glycogen-rich carcinomas was 19.2%, compared to 11.2% for the other infiltrating carcinomas. The five-year corrected survival for patients with glycogen-rich carcinoma was 33% compared to 56% for patients with other types of invasive breast carcinoma.

## CARCINOMA WITH OSTEOCLASTIC GIANT CELLS

Osteoclastic giant cells have been observed in breast carcinomas and some mesenchymal tumors of the breast (osteoclastomas). When present in carcinomas, they are often located in a reactive-appearing, hypervascular, and often hemorrhagic stroma that surrounds a variety of invasive breast carcinomas, within the lumen of the intraductal and invasive ductal carcinomas, or both. A number of ultrastructural and immunohistochemical studies have confirmed the histiocytic nature of the giant cells (167,176,180,181).

Carcinoma with osteoclastic giant cells occurs most frequently in the upper outer quadrant, but they may be found in any of the four quadrants, as well as the axillary tail of the breast and in a subareolar location where they can cause inversion of the nipple. Two of the seven lesions in Tavassoli and Norris's (181) study fluctuated in size during the menstrual cycle.

Grossly, the tumors are striking because of the soft consistency and hemorrhagic appearance of a majority of the lesions. They may be ill-defined or sharply-circumscribed ovoid nodules (Fig. 10.26). The tumors range from 0.5 to 10 cm in diameter and all but one of the reported cases have been solitary. One of the tumors in Tavassoli and Norris's series was a multinodular lesion composed of nodules which ranged from 0.2 to 2.2 cm in diameter spread over a 3-cm radius.

Microscopically, a majority of the neoplasms are invasive ductal carcinomas. The carcinoma may be any of the known patterns of breast carcinoma including tubular, metaplastic, invasive cribriform (181), squamous (169), infiltrating lobular (178), papillary (163), and mucinous (177). The common denominator to all these various patterns of carcinoma in this interesting variant is the presence of osteoclastic giant cells in the surrounding stroma which often appears fibroblastic, reactive, and hypervascular with extravasated red blood cells, lymphocytes, monocytes and hemosiderin-laden macrophages (165,166, 168–175,178).

The giant cells are highly variable in size and shape and are usually found abutting nests of epithe-

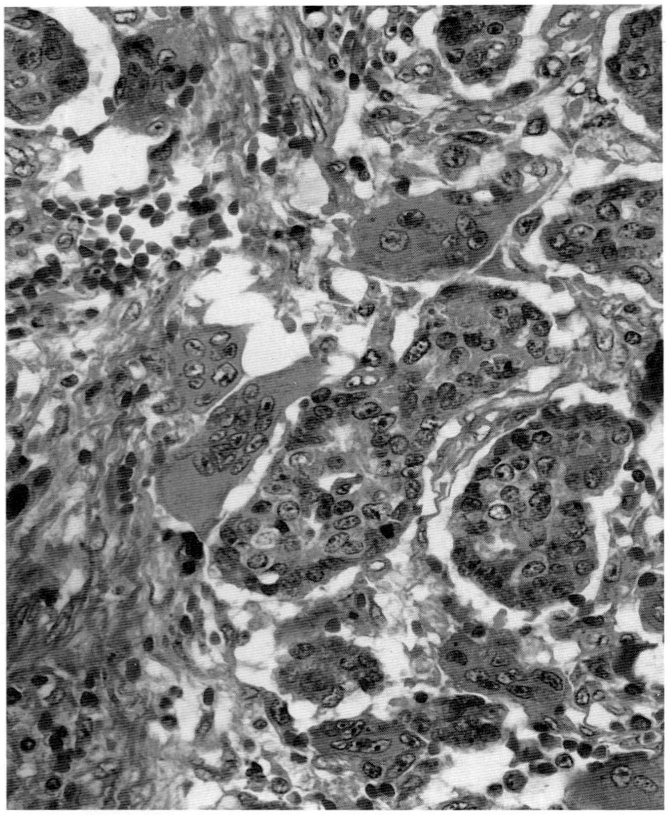

**Figure 10.27** Carcinoma with osteoclastic giant cells. The giant cells often abut against the clusters of cancer cells. (H&E, X250) (From Tavassoli FA, Norris HJ: *Arch Pathol Lab Med* 1986;110:636–639, with permission)

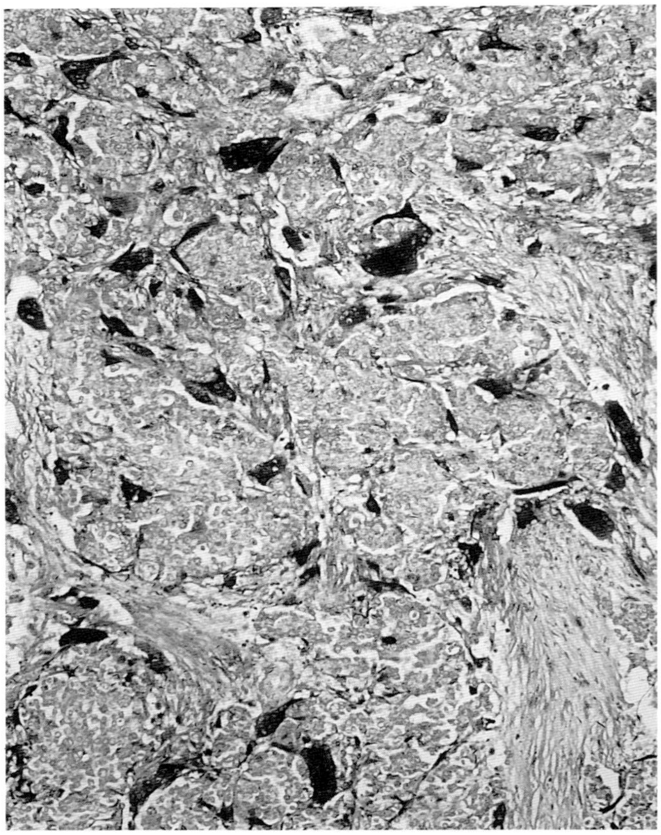

**Figure 10.28** Carcinoma with osteoclastic giant cells. The giant cells show a positive reaction with acid phosphatase. (X160) (From Tavassoli FA, Norris HJ: *Arch Pathol Lab Med* 1986;110:636–639, with permission)

lial tumor cells (Fig. 10.27). Although predominantly in the stroma, giant cells are also identified within lumens formed by the cancer cells. The giant cells show a positive reaction for acid phosphatase (Fig. 10.28) and fail to react with epithelial markers (181); the mono and multinucleated (giant) cells exhibit a variable positivity for muramidase and alpha-1-antitrypsin, and are negative for Factor VIII (177). The carcinoma cells show an intensely positive reaction for cytokeratin (Fig. 10.29) and CEA but fail to react with other antisera (177,181). Since the giant cells are often numerous, they can be easily picked up along with the carcinoma by aspiration cytology (164,178, 181,183). The multinucleated giant cells, as well as the hypervascular reactive stroma, occur in lymph node and distant metastases as well as in recurrences (181). Not all metastatic foci contain the giant cells or the hemorrhagic stroma, however. Factors responsible for the induction of angiogenesis and giant cell formation in these tumors have not been specified yet. It is known, however, that breast carcinomas produce factors such as prostaglandins. Some of the subtypes of prostaglandins or other angiogenesis and chemotactic factors may be responsible for the induction of vascularity and migration of histiocytes and their subsequent transformation into giant cells in these tumors.

Ultrastructural evaluation of several of these tumors has confirmed the histiocytic nature of the giant cells and their resemblance to osteoclastic giant cells (167,181). Some of the giant cells contain aggregates of vesicles and vacuoles corresponding to secondary lysosomes in their cytoplasm, while others have numerous mitochondria and no lysosomes (Fig. 10.30). The number of lysosomes is far less than anticipated from the strong acid phosphatse reaction; a similar disparity has also been observed in normal osteoclasts and in osteoclasts of giant-cell tumors of the bone (182).

Hormone receptors were evaluated in three of the cases reported by Tavassoli and Norris in 1986 (181). Both estrogen and progesterone receptor levels were negative in one case. The second case had an estrogen receptor level of 41.7 fmol/mg of protein.

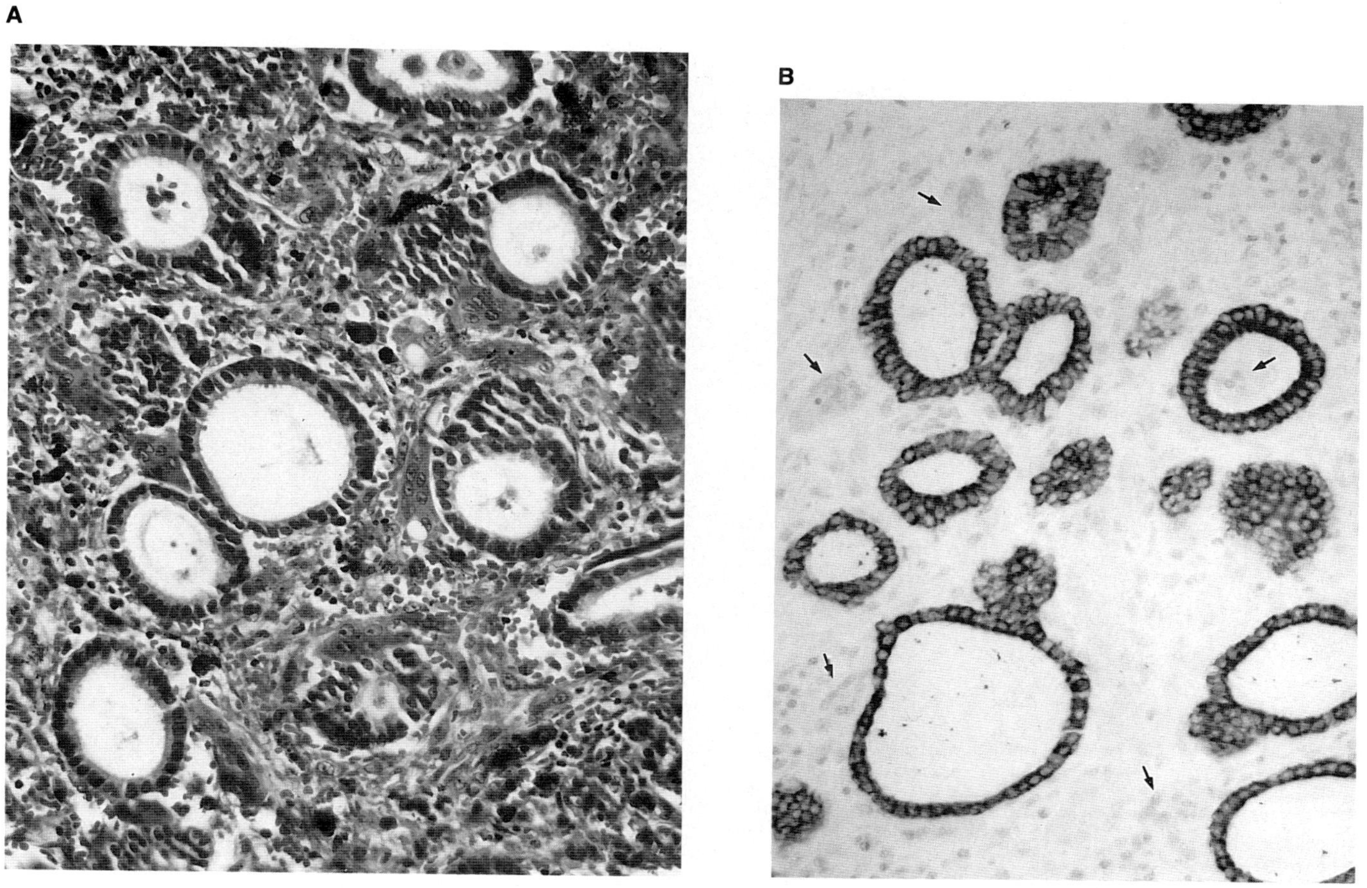


**Figure 10.29** Carcinoma with osteoclastic giant cells. (a) The carcinoma is a tubular carcinoma in this cases. (H&E, X250) (b) Immunostain for cytokeratin shows a positive reaction in the cancer cells, but the giant cells (arrows) fail to react. (X250) (Fig. 10.29b from Tavassoli FA, Norris HJ: *Arch Pathol Lab Med* 1986;110:636–639, with permission)

The third case had an estrogen receptor level of less than 5 fmol/mg protein, and a negative level of progesterone receptor in the primary tumor; when the tumor recurred in the chest wall, however, the estrogen receptor level was 19 fmol/mg protein while the progesterone receptor level was 149 fmol/mg protein. Holland and Van Haelst's (171) cases also had relatively low levels of estrogen receptors but several had remarkably high levels of progesterone receptors.

About a third of the reported cases have had axillary node metastases. Local recurrences and distant metastases have been reported in several cases. The follow-up in a majority of reported cases rarely exceeds five years, and about two-thirds of the patients have been reported to be alive. It would be of interest to determine if the varieties of invasive carcinomas that share the capacity to elicit an unusual stromal response with giant cell reaction will ultimately differ in their prognosis and behavior from the same pattern of carcinoma without these stromal features.

## INVASIVE CRIBRIFORM CARCINOMA

Recently described by Page et al (185) as a specific subtype of breast carcinoma with an excellent prognosis, invasive cribriform carcinoma (ICC) is uncommon, accounting for 1.7 to 3.5% of breast carcinomas (185–187). The classic ICC consists entirely of an invasive pattern that has the same cribriform arrangement as is characteristic of intraductal cribriform carcinoma (Fig. 10.31). Also included among classic ICC in Page et al's series were tumors in which the same cribriform pattern predominates, but less than 50% of the lesion is composed of tubular carcinoma. When less than half of the tumor consisted of areas of less well-differentiated invasive carcinoma, as judged by a solid pattern and cytologic features, however, it was designated as a mixed invasive cribriform carcinoma. Since the main difference between the classic and mixed variant is the degree of cytologic differentiation, it is possible that the mixed variant in Page et

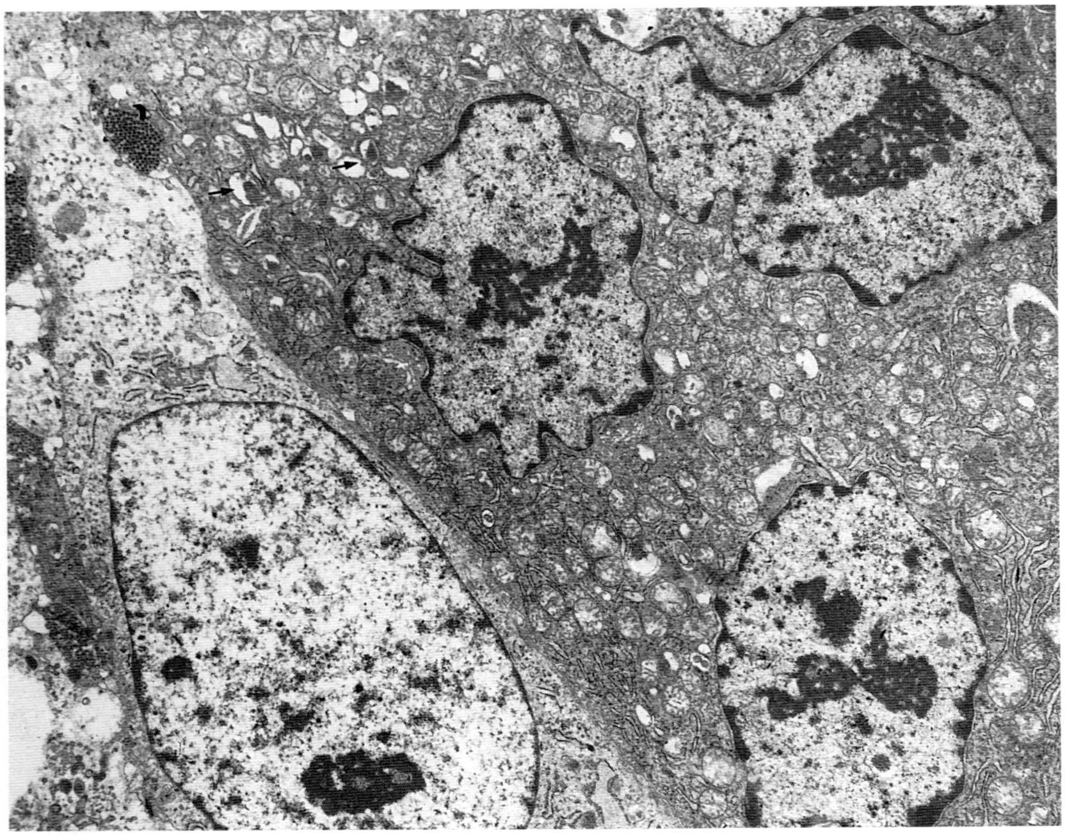

**Figure 10.30** At the ultrastructural level, some of the giant cells have abundant mitochondria and a small number of vesicles corresponding to secondary lysosomes (arrows). (Uranyl acetate-lead citrate, X3,300)

al's series simply reflects a higher grade of the same lesion. In Venable et al's series, tumors were either pure ICC or "mixed"; the latter group included an admixture of ICC with a variety of other carcinomas, including tubular carcinoma.

Patients with classic invasive cribriform carcinoma range in age from 33 to 86 years with an average age of 53; those patients with a mixed invasive cribriform carcinoma range in age from 39 to 85 years, with an average age of 62 (185). Venable et al's (186) series included a 19-year-old patient and a 73-year-old man.

The average size of the classic type, as defined by Page et al (185), is 2.6 cm, while the average size of the pure ICC as defined by Venable et al is 3.1 cm compared to 4.2 cm for the mixed type in Page et al's series and 3.2 cm for the mixed type in Silverberg et al's series. Seven of the 35 classic invasive cribriform carcinomas were multifocal in contrast to one of the mixed group in Page et al's study. Lymph node metastases occurs in pure and classic ICC, but rarely involves more than three axillary nodes. None of the patients with classic ICC had distant metastases at presentation, while four of the mixed group had positive nodes and two had distant metastases at presentation (185).

Follow-up for the classic group in Page et al's study averaged 14.5 years; only one patient died from breast carcinoma. This patient developed a contralateral squamous carcinoma seven years after treatment for the cribriform carcinoma and died four years later from disseminated squamous carcinoma. Three patients died from other causes and 30 were alive at follow-up; only one of these developed recurrent tumor in the axillary and supraclavicular lymph nodes one and five years after the initial diagnosis. The cribriform pattern was retained in the metastases. The average follow-up for the mixed group in the same study was 12.5 years. Six patients died from breast cancer, although three of these survived ten years. Four patients died of other causes and six were alive. The adjusted ten-year survival rate for the mixed group was 75% which compared quite favorably with a 40% ten-year survival rate previously observed for invasive carcinoma by the same group (184).

A

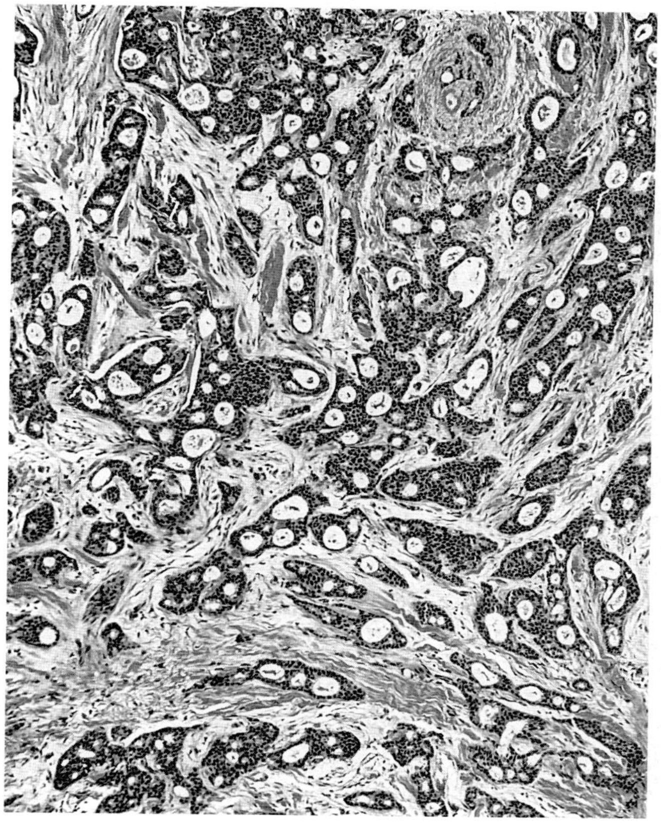

Figure 10.31 (a) Invasive cribriform carcinoma characterized by angulated clusters of tumor cells forming a cribriform arrangement; (b) the tumor cells lack significant pleomorphism or mitotic activity. (H&E, (a) X75; (b) X240) (Courtesy of Dr. Mark A. Ashton)

B

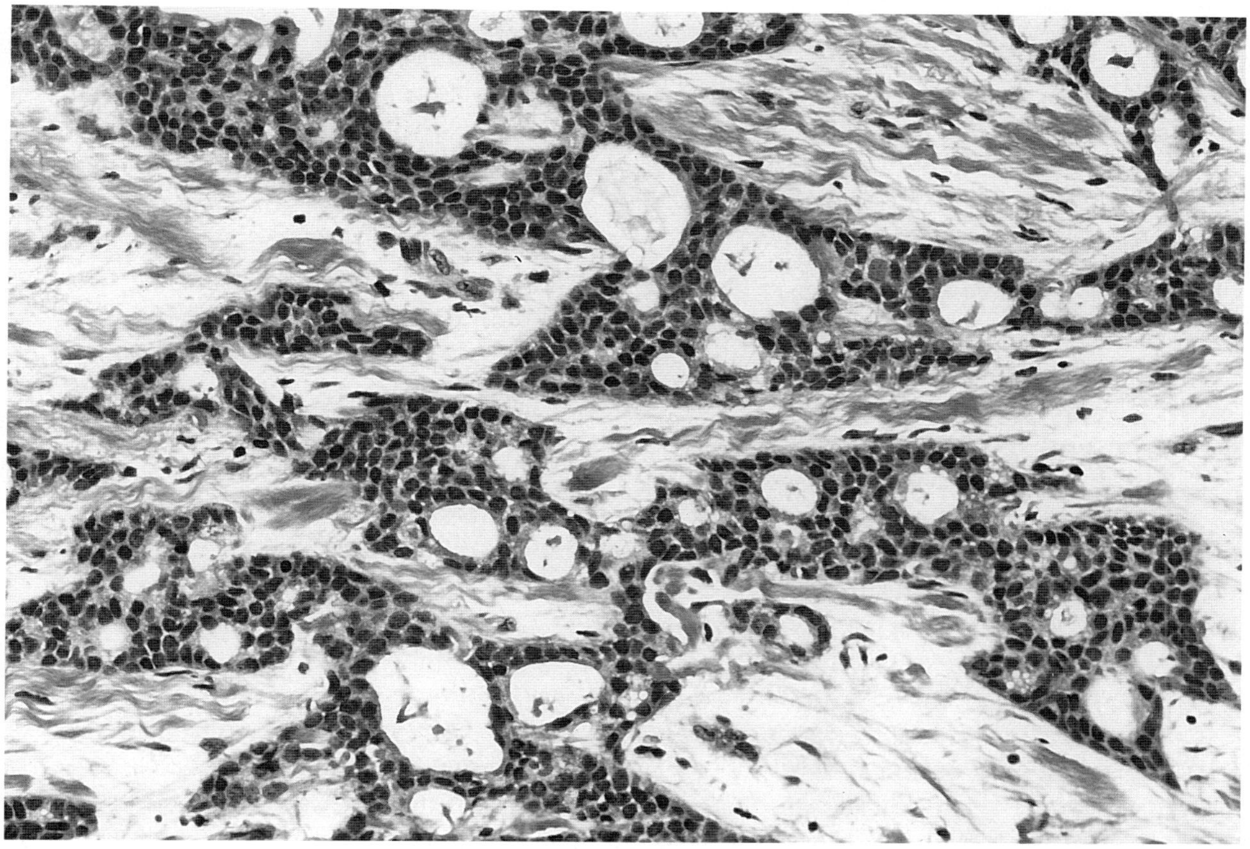

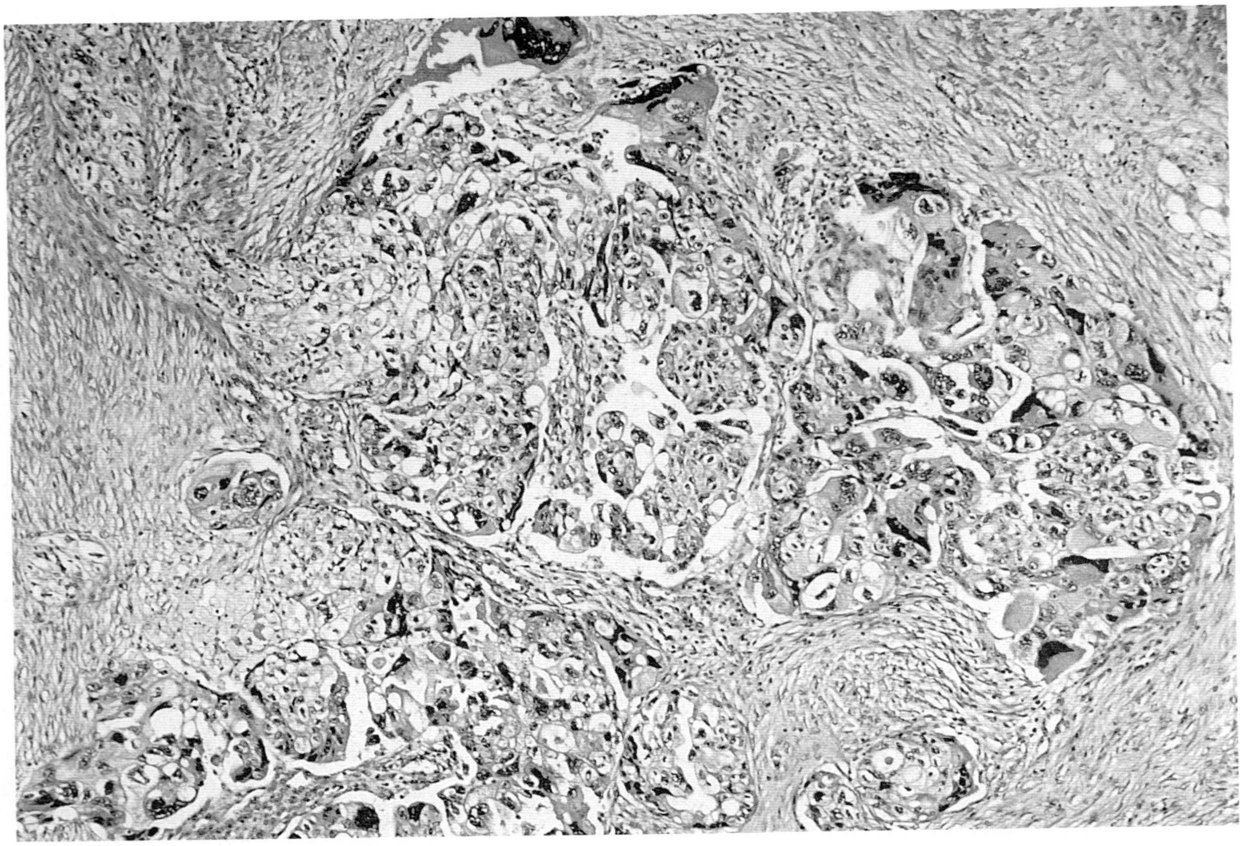

**Figure 10.32** Carcinoma with choriocarcinomatous features. Irregular aggregates of an anaplastic cell type characterize this tumor. (H&E, X60)

Five-year survival rates were 100% for the pure group, 88% for <50% ICC, and 78% for the infiltrating duct carcinoma controls in Venable et al's study.

Of 16 cases evaluated for estrogen receptors (ER) and progesterone receptors (PR), all were ER-positive, and 11 (69%) were PR-positive (186).

## CARCINOMAS WITH "CHORIOCARCINOMATOUS" FEATURES

Breast carcinomas are capable of producing a variety of hormones such as human chorionic gonadotropin (HCG) (188,189,193–197,199,201), adrenocorticotropic hormone (ACTH) (190,202), placental lactogen (194), and norepinephrine (192), not ordinarily considered native to the mammary gland. Horne et al (191) evaluated 50 examples of breast carcinoma for the presence of a variety of pregnancy-associated proteins using immunohistochemical methods. Pregnancy-specific beta-1-glycoprotein was present in 76% of the tumors, placental lactogen was identified in 82%, and 60% exhibited chorionic gonadotropin. Patients whose tumors were negative for placental lactogen and beta-1-glycoprotein had significantly longer survival rates compared to those whose cancers stained positive for these proteins. None of these tumors were described as having the morphologic features of a choriocarcinoma, however.

Saigo and Rosen (198) reported an unusual breast carcinoma occurring in a 55-year-old woman. The 2.5 cm tumor was grossly hemorrhagic in part. Microscopically, it was composed of areas of moderately-differentiated infiltrating duct carcinoma admixed with areas strongly resembling choriocarcinoma; the latter areas corresponded to the grossly hemorrhagic areas. The presence of beta-HCG in the regions resembling choriocarcinoma was confirmed immunohistochemically. The patient died seven months later from disseminated carcinoma. Recently, a rather pleomorphic carcinoma with diffuse choriocarcinomatous features was reviewed at AFIP (Fig. 10.32); syncytiotrophoblastic-type giant cells were abundant in the tumor and they stained positively for HCG and cytokeratin (Fig. 10.33).

A choriocarcinomatous pattern has been ob-

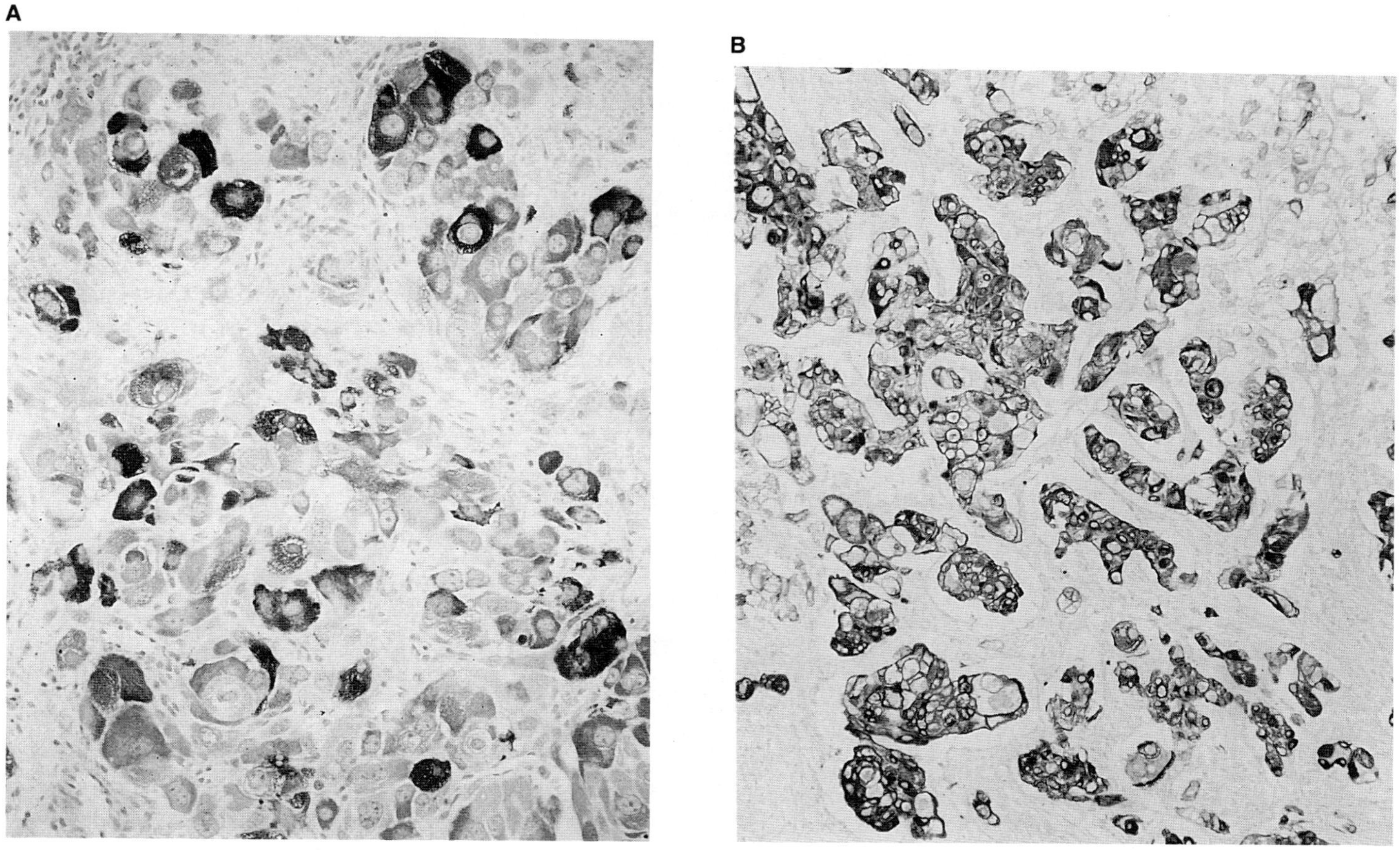

**Figure 10.33** Carcinoma with choriocarcinomatous features. (a) Positive immunostain for HCG is evident in many of the giant cells as well as some of the mononucleated cells. (X160) (b) Immunostain for cytokeratin shows a positive reaction in all tumor cells. (X100)

served solely or in association with adenocarcinoma in a variety of gastrointestinal tumors in the stomach, jejunum, colon, and esophagus. The most plausible explanation for this finding is that a metaplastic process occurs in these tumors resulting in partial or complete transformation to a choriocarcinomatous pattern. Clearly, breast carcinomas have a potential for a wide variety of biochemical and morphologic expressions.

Since many trophoblast-specific products are thought to have immunosuppressive properties, it is likely that the production of such proteins by malignant tumors could be one method by which these tumors escape immunologic surveillance mechanisms and continue to proliferate incognito. If this were true, then the production of such proteins by malignant tumors could ultimately influence the length of survival. Viewpoints regarding the prognostic significance of elaboration of HCG by mammary carcinomas are conflicting, however. Tormey et al (200) reported that 95% of those without elevated serum HCG levels responded to chemotherapy as compared to 71% of those with elevated serum levels. Horne et al (191), however, did not find a difference in survival between tumors expressing HCG and those that did not; they found production of pregnancy-specific beta-1-glycoprotein as the best indicator of prognosis, however.

## INFLAMMATORY CARCINOMA

The clinical features of inflammatory carcinoma as we recognize it today were defined by Lee and Tannenbaum (223) and Taylor and Meltzer (241). One of the earliest descriptions of inflammatory carcinoma has been ascribed to Charles Bell who in 1807 observed that a purple discoloration of the skin overlying a tumor reflects an unfavorable sign. A variety of terms such as mastitis carcinomatosa (220) and carcinoma mastitoides were proposed to describe this lesion. The term inflammatory carcinoma was proposed by

Lee and Tannenbaum. In 1909, Leitch (224) attributed peau d'orange to lymph stasis and noted subdermal lymphatic spread in acute mammary carcinoma.

Considered by Haagensen (217) as the most malignant type of breast carcinoma, inflammatory carcinoma represents 1% to 2% of breast carcinomas (223,225,238,240). In a review of 94 breast carcinomas in Tunisia, however, 28% of the cases in which the skin was examined showed dermal lymphatic involvement (211). In Lee and Tannenbaum's series (223), the patients ranged in age from 24 to 62 years, with an average age of 44 years. In Robbins et al's (235) series, the median age of patients was 55 years with 69% of patients being postmenopausal, while the average age of patients in Stocks and Patternson's series (240) was 48 years with 53% of them postmenopausal. Three examples of inflammatory carcinoma have been described in male breasts (242) and a case in a 12-year-old girl was reported by Nichini et al (230). The typical patient presents with pain, tenderness, firmness, and enlargement of the breast. Characteristically, the skin of the breast is reddened, warm, edematous and thickened (Fig. 10.34a); a ridge is often palpable at the margin of the discoloured skin. The edema is frequently accompanied by peau d'orange (Fig. 10.34b) in the dependent region of the breast (205,214,235). During the early stages, an underlying mass may not be palpable and this could lead to misinterpretation of the lesion as an inflammatory process (232). In a group of 83 patients with inflammatory carcinoma, two thirds of the patients had a palpable mass and the remainder showed diffuse breast involvement (235).

Rarely, cutaneous metastases from breast carcinoma assume an inflammatory, erysipelatoides appearance due to plugging of the dermal lymphatics by tumor cells (206,239,243).

## Clinical versus Pathologic Definition

Clinicians have generally used the clinical appearance to define this entity, while pathologists often insist on the presence of dermal lymphatic involvement to confirm the clinical diagnosis. In a majority of cases, the clinical picture and the pathologic picture of dermal lymphatic involvement coincide. Not all patients with the clinical disease have dermal lymphatic involvement, however, and there are also cases with the dermal lymphatic involvement but without the clinical inflammatory features. The criteria for clinical diagnosis of inflammatory carcinoma include diffuse erythema, edema extending to greater than two thirds of the breast, peau d'orange, tenderness, induration, warmth, enlargement, and diffuseness of tumor by palpation. Not all of these features are required to be prominent in each case (226). The pathologic diagnosis of inflammatory carcinoma requires the presence of tumor in the dermal lymphatics (Fig. 10.35). The significance of dermal lymphatic involvement as a prognostic factor has been evaluated by different investigators using various approaches. Without describing the clinical features, Ellis and Teitelbaum (215) reviewed the pathologic material and/or reports on eight patients reported to be free of disease at least five years following radical mastectomy for inflammatory carcinoma; none of these patients had dermal lymphatic invasion either present in the slides available for evaluation or noted in the surgical pathology reports.

Salzstein (237) echoed Ellis and Teitelbaum's conclusion after studying four patients with clinically occult inflammatory carcinoma (patients without clinical signs of inflammatory carcinoma but with tumor involvement of dermal lymphatics); these patients followed rapid downhill courses similar to inflammatory carcinoma.

Lucas and Perez-Mesa (226) evaluated three groups of patients: those with clinical inflammatory carcinoma only (19 patients), those with both the clinical and pathologic features of the disease (39 patients) and finally those who had only dermal lymphatic invasion but none of the clinical features (15 patients). They concluded that occult inflammatory carcinomas have a slightly better prognosis but nonetheless had almost as fulminant a clinical course as clinically apparent inflammatory carcinoma in agreement with Saltzstein. Furthermore, inflammatory carcinomas behave aggressively even in the absence of dermal lymphatic invasion. A poor short-term prognosis is implicated by either the clinical or the pathologic features; therefore, use of the term inflammatory carcinoma is justified in either case. Using a similar stratification scheme, Levine et al (225) reviewed data abstracted from medical records of a larger population of patients diagnosed with breast cancer between 1975 and 1981 in nine geographic areas covered by the National Cancer Institute's Surveillance, Epidemiology, and End Result (SEER) program. The patients

A

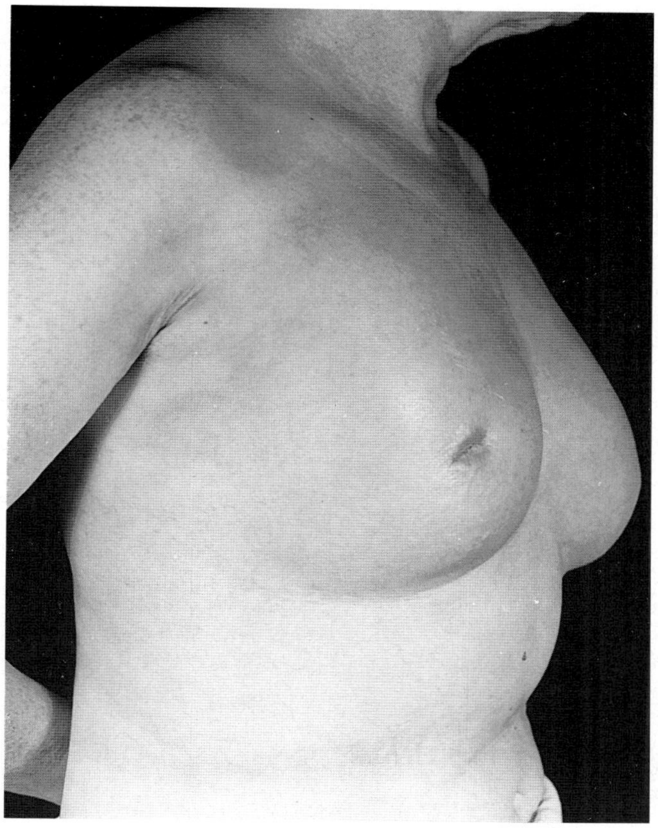

B

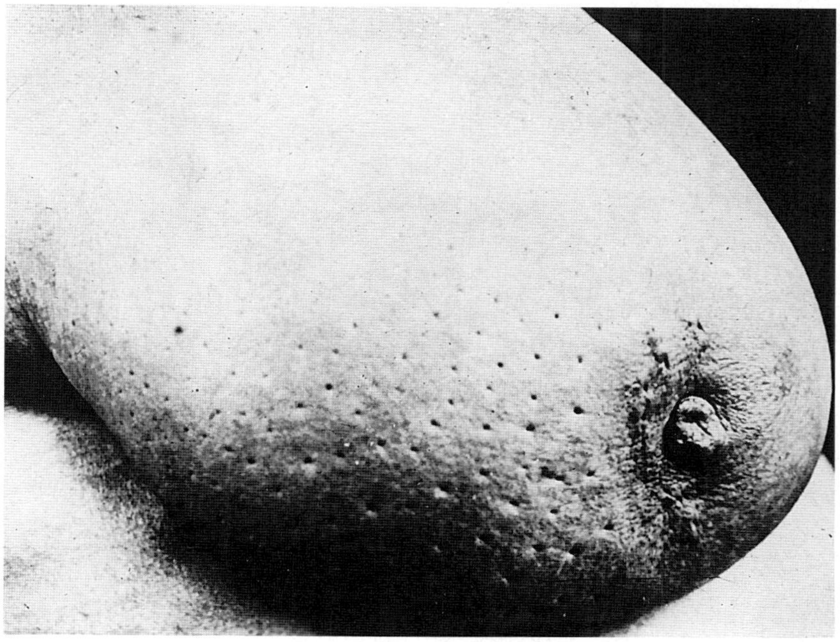

**Figure 10.34** Inflammatory carcinoma. (a) The skin over the surface of the breast is reddened and edematous; note the inverted nipple. (b) The lesion may also display pea d'orange.

with occult inflammatory carcinoma were generally younger. Three years after diagnosis, the survival rates for patients with clinical features only, pathologic features only, and those with combined clinical and pathologic features were 60%, 52%, and 34% respectively. This compared with a 90% survival at three years for other types of breast cancer. This study has the advantage of a large number of patients but suffers to an unknown extent from the lack of uniformity inherent in a study of this

A

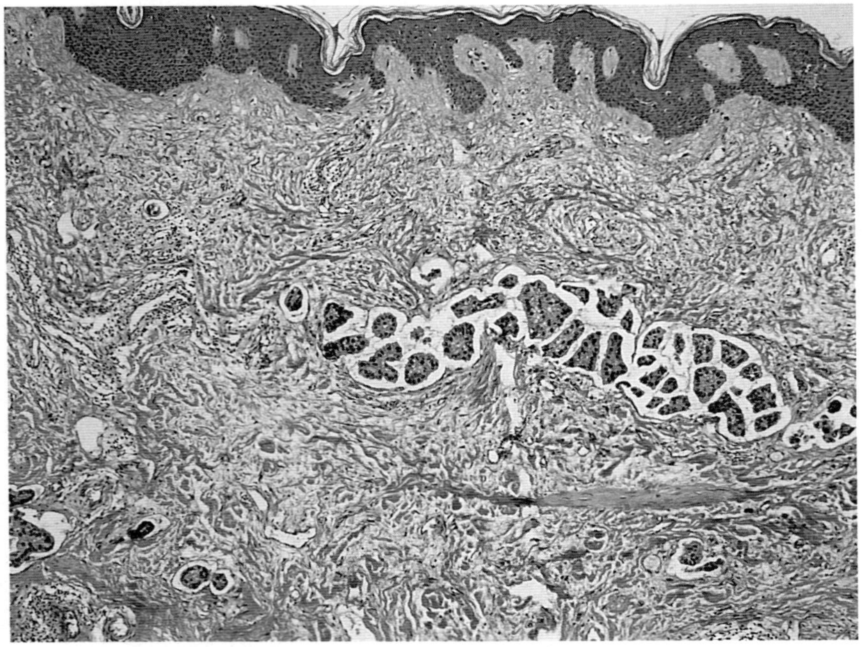

Figure 10.35 Inflammatory carcinoma. Tumor cells are present as multiple clusters (a), or in the form of solitary cell clusters in dermal lymphatics (b). (H&E, (a) X15; (b) X40)

B

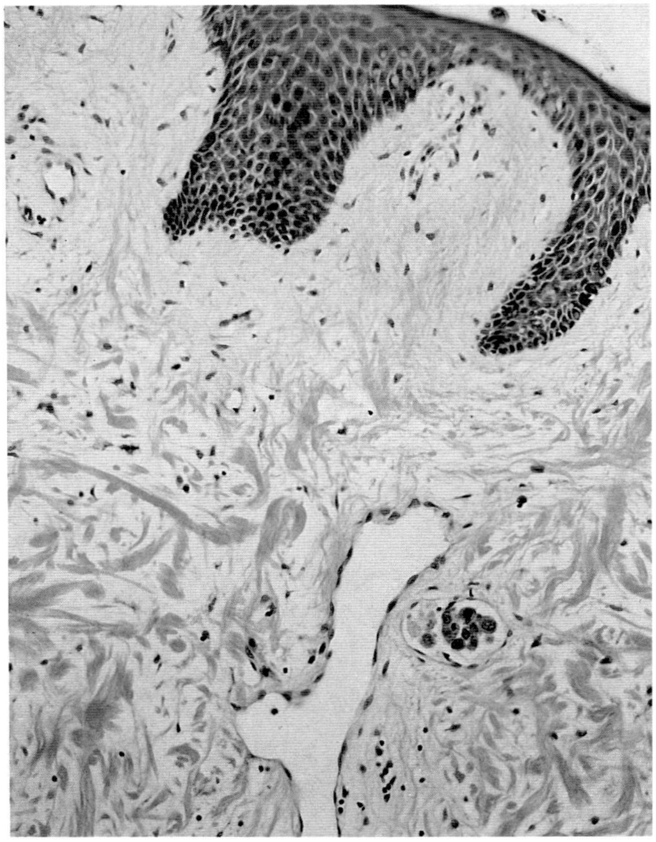

proportion which utilizes multiple institutions with multiple pathologists over a long period of time.

## Behavior and Treatment

Inflammatory carcinoma is a lesion with ominous prognostic implications. Most patients die of metastatic tumor within two years following the diagnosis (204,208,212,234). Kokal et al (221) reviewed 64 patients comparing the behavior of inflammatory carcinoma and locally advanced breast carcinoma; their results suggested that inflammatory carcinoma behaves as an ER− subtype of locally advanced breast carcinoma. Inflammatory carcinoma was usually fatal within two years regardless of the mode of therapy. The actuarial three-year survival for a group of 64 patients treated for primary inflammatory breast carcinoma was 38% and the median disease-free time was 19 months in a study utilizing a combination of chemotherapy and radiation therapy (209). The age at diagnosis, menopausal status, and type of chemotherapy did not influence prognosis but erythema involving the entire breast at presentation or erythema present after initial chemotherapy and lymph node involvement were isolated as bad prognostic factors by these investigators. The mean survival of 40 patients in Haagensen's practice was 16.3 months. The five-year survival has ranged from 3% to 10% (203,235,240).

Various approaches to the treatment of inflammatory carcinoma have been used (208,210,212,216, 231,236).

While some have considered inflammatory carcinoma an inoperable disease, mastectomy may be beneficial in improving five-year survival when combined with multiagent chemotherapy (218). Droulias et al (214) have suggested that while in most patients surgery other than biopsy is contraindicated, those patients whose breast mass does not involve the entire breast and whose breast mass had been present prior to the sudden onset of inflammatory signs, as well as those who lack dermal lymphatic invasion (biopsy proven) in erythematous areas not overlying the mass and show no evidence of dissemination at presentation or for several weeks after completion of radiotherapy should be considered for surgery following supervoltage radiotherapy.

Mastectomy may also assist local control of the disease and improve the quality of life in patients who have responded well to preoperative radiotherapy or chemotherapy (229). A surgical approach to therapy has been utilized in the past (203,228,236). More recent literature emphasizes other means including a combined modality approach to treatment using chemotherapy and radiation therapy with or without surgery (204,207,209,222,231,235,240,244). With a combined modality approach, approximately 30% of patients can be expected to be relapse-free five years after treatment (216,227,238). In comparison, only 3.2% of 63 patients treated at Memorial Hospital prior to 1967 were clinically free of disease longer than five years (235). This approach has opened new vistas in management of a tumor that for a long time had been considered rapidly fatal. The pessimism formerly associated with this disease may no longer be warranted.

## Hormone Receptors and Cell Kinetics

Considering the heterogenous nature of inflammatory carcinoma, hormone receptors and cell kinetics could be helpful in identifying patients for an individualized therapeutic approach. Forty-seven percent of the 59 women reported by Delarue et al (213) were ER+; 34% of the 59 women were PR+. In a study by Paradiso et al (233), 44% of 28 inflammatory carcinomas were estrogen receptor positive (ER+) and 30% had progesterone receptors (PR). Of 16 patients reported by Harvey et al (219), 31% were ER+. In contrast, of 50 locally advanced ordinary carcinomas, 64% were ER+ and 51% were PR+. Inflammatory carcinoma also had a higher median labelling index value for proliferative activity.

# ADENOID CYSTIC CARCINOMA

Accounting for less than 0.1% to 0.2% of breast carcinomas (281), adenoid cystic carcinoma (ACC) is of special interest because of its favorable prognosis and distinctive histologic appearance (245,248). It is possible that these percentages have been inflated by inclusion of some of the now well-recognized cribriform ductal carcinomas in the older series. Mammary ACC is morphologically identical to similar tumors

A

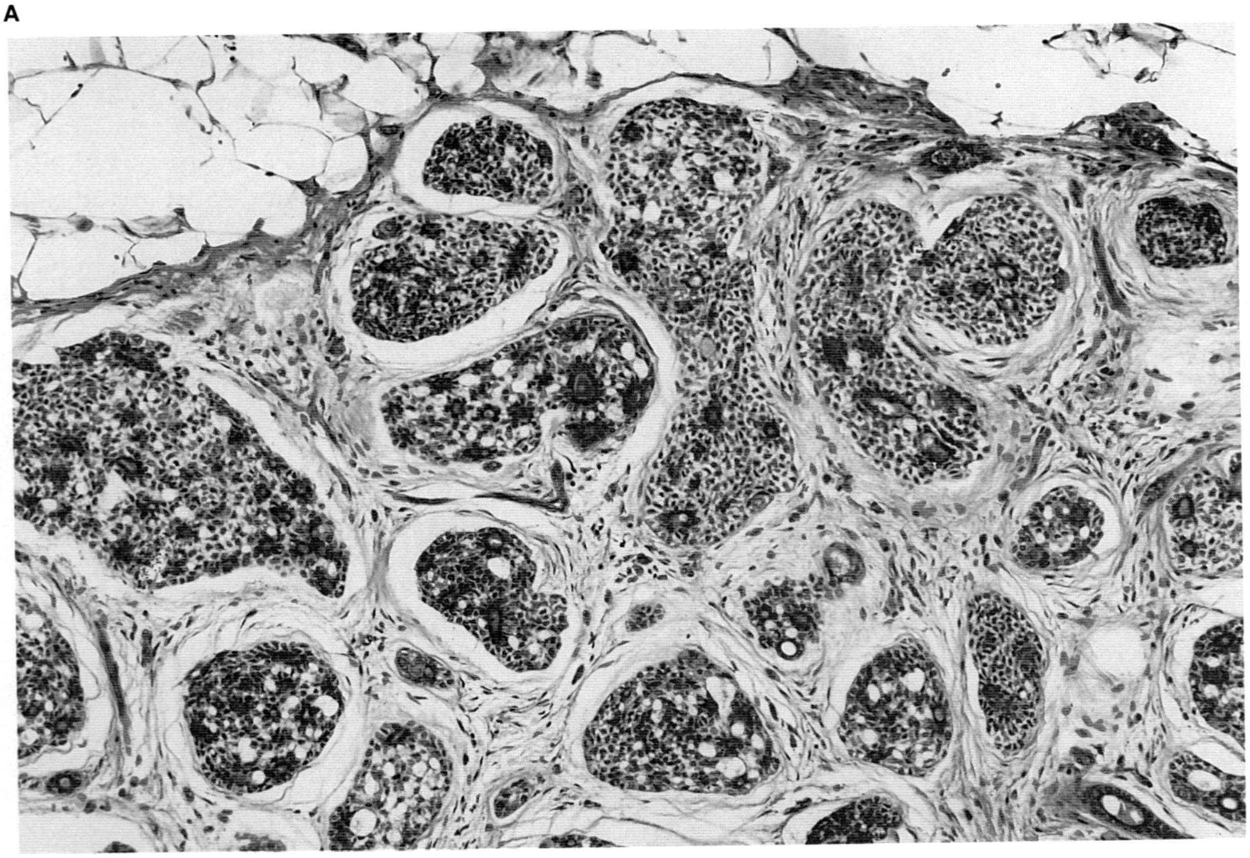

B

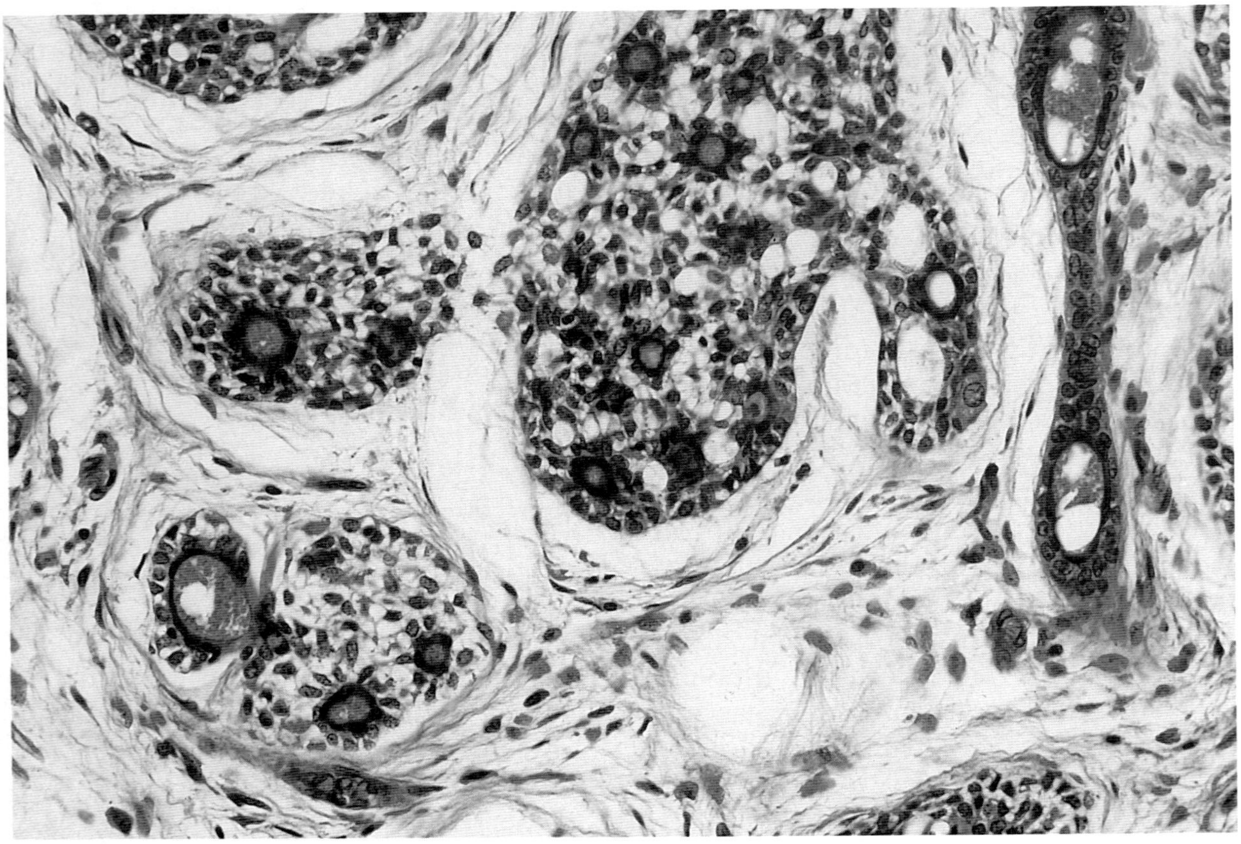

**Figure 10.36** Adenoid cystic carcinoma. Two cell types are identified in adenoid cystic carcinoma. (a) Most islands show dominance of basaloid cells with rare spaces surrounded by an intensely eosinophilic cell population. (b) The basaloid cells may be loosely cohesive. (H&E, (a) X100; (b) X240)

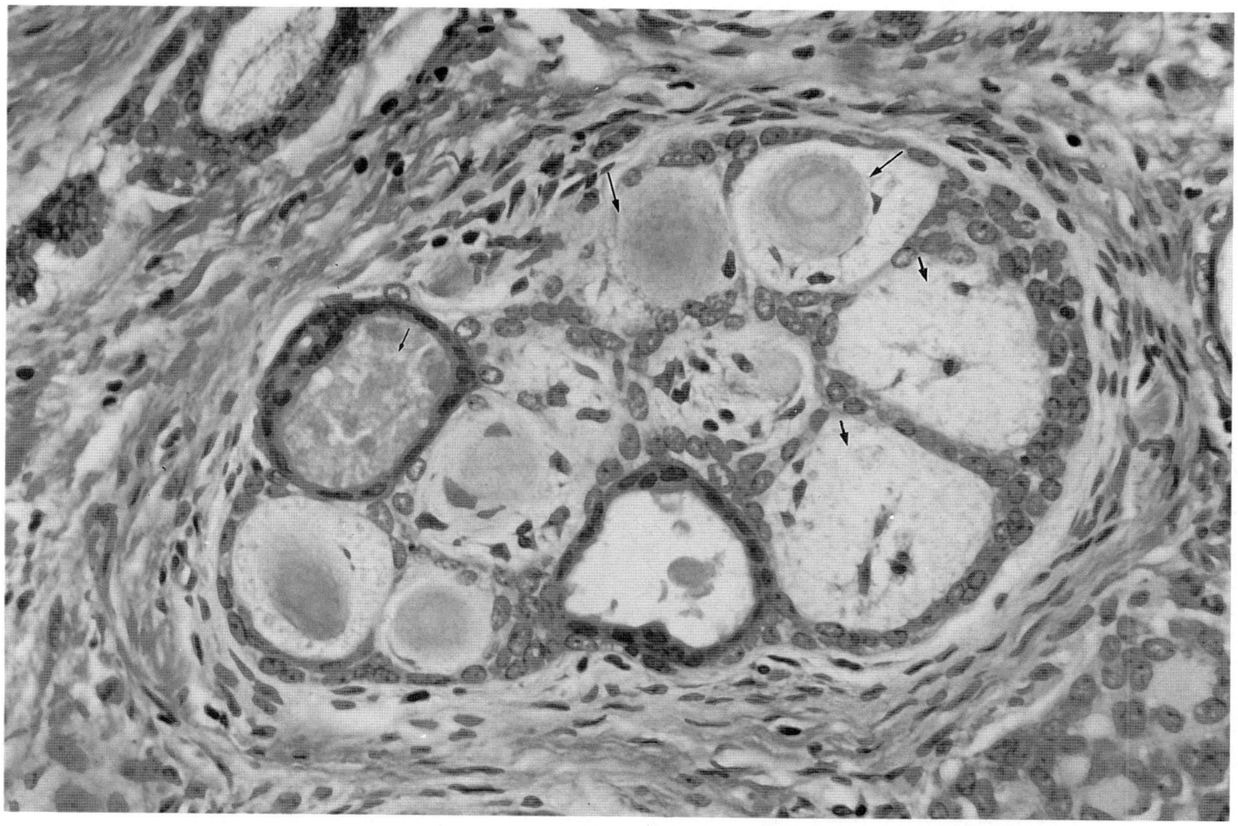

**Figure 10.37** Adenoid cystic carcinoma characterized by three types of intraluminal content: hyaline bodies (long arrow), mucoid secretion (short arrow) and granular eosinophilic material (small, thin arrow). (H&E, X300)

that occur most frequently in the salivary glands and has also been referred to by the alternate designation of cylindroma (274).

The term adenoid cystic carcinoma was first used in reference to breast carcinoma by Geschickter (259) who used the term "adenocystic basal cell cancer" when describing four breast lesions in 1945. Subsequently, three additional examples of adenoid cystic carcinoma were described by Foote and Stewart in 1946 (256). Two decades later, the first series of nine cases was reported by Galloway et al (258) from the Mayo Clinic with a summary of the 12 previously reported examples.

In contrast to the aggressive behavior manifested by their salivary gland counterparts, mammary adenoid cystic carcinomas have an excellent prognosis. The reason for this dichotomous behavior has remained an enigma.

## Clinical Features

Patients with adenoid cystic carcinoma range in age from 25 to 80 years with a median that varies from 50 to 63 years in different reports (245,278,281). While the lesion occurs predominantly in women, several cases have been described in the male breast (263,279). The lesion occurs with greater frequency in the subareolar region, but shows no predilection for either breast. Despite its central and subareolar location, it is not generally associated with nipple discharge. Patients often present with a tender tumor mass of a few days to a few weeks duration. Occasionally, patients have been aware of the presence of a mass for many months and even up to 15 years (245,258). When the tumor is large or superficial, the overlying skin may be ulcerated and exhibit peau d'orange or dimpling.

## Gross Pathologic Features

Adenoid cystic carcinoma ranges from 1 to 5 cm in size (median, 2.2 cm), but may be only a few mm or up to 12 cm in diameter (250,281). The lesion has well-demarcated margins and is grey to yellow on cut surface. Cystic areas do occur in some tumors but are not common.

A

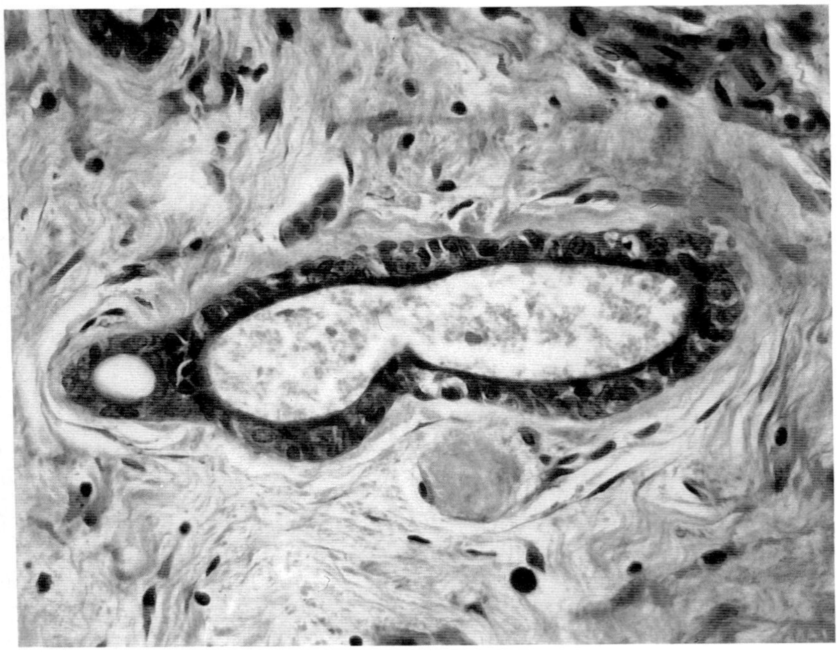

B

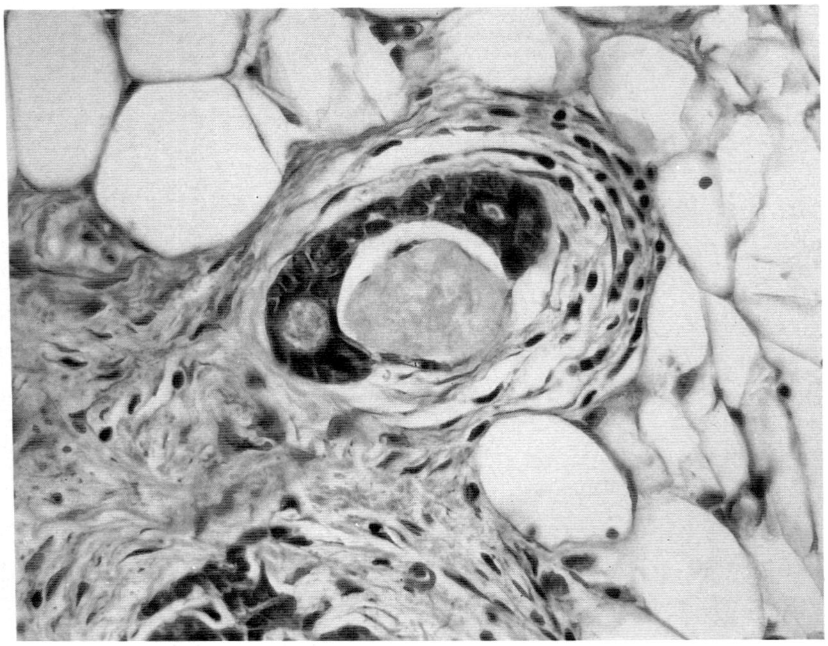

**Figure 10.38** Adenoid cystic carcinoma. (a–d) The various illustrations display different stages in the incorporation of hyaline bodies from the stroma into the cell clusters by growth of tumor cells around the hyaline globules and their gradual engulfment. (H&E, (a) X400; (b) X400; (c) X250; (d) X400) (Figs. 10.38a,b,&d from Tavassoli FA, Norris HJ: *Arch Pathol Lab Med* 1986;110:1045–1053, with permission)

## Microscopic Features

Despite its grossly circumscribed appearance, adenoid cystic carcinoma is characterized by an invasive proliferation of circumscribed nests, islands, and cord-like clusters of tumor cells forming solid, cribriform, tubular, and trabecular arrangements. While one of these patterns may dominate in a tumor, often all patterns coexist. Within these islands, there are two cell types, a basaloid cell population which predominates and a smaller population of cells with

C

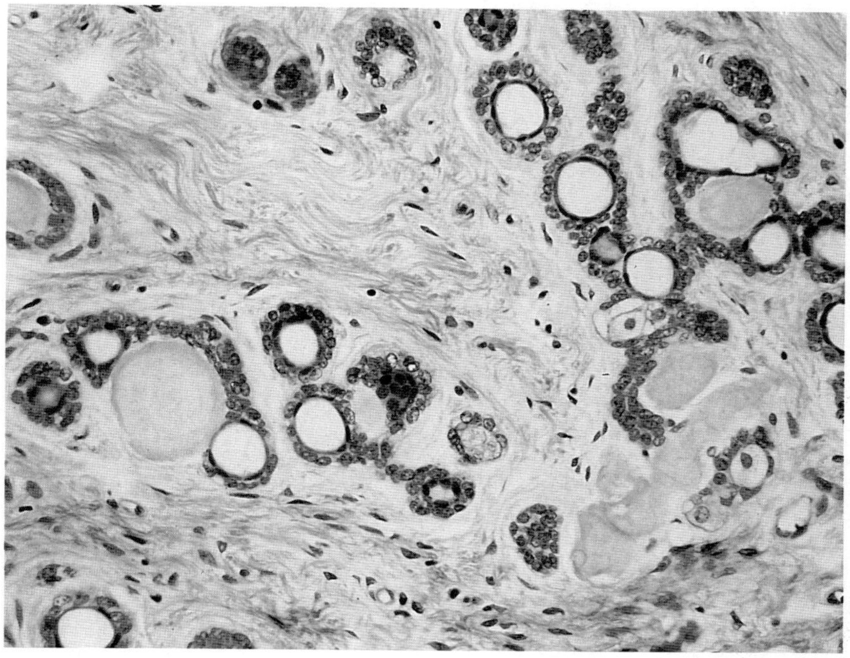

D

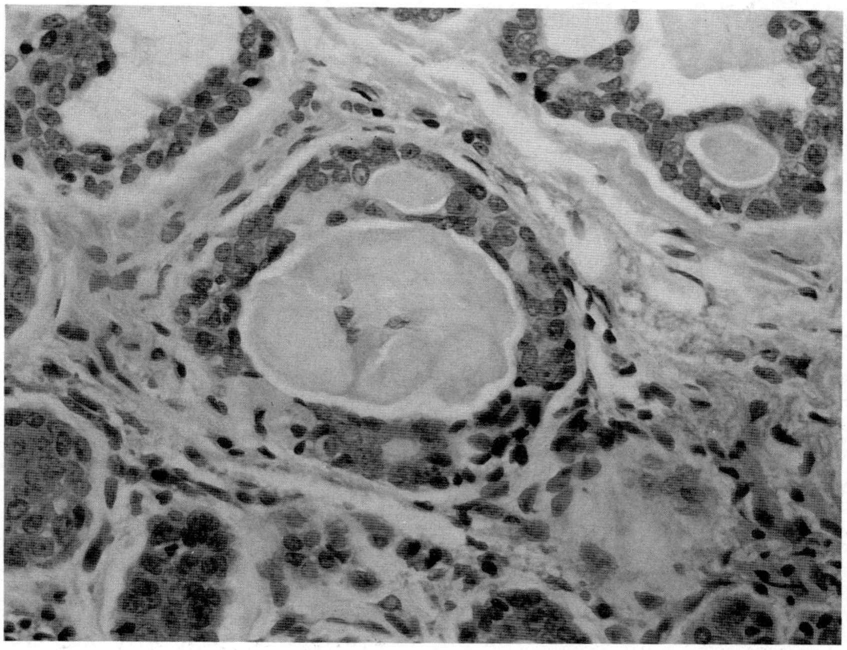

**Figure 10.38(c,d)** Adenoid cystic carcinoma. Legend on opposite page.

bright eosinophilic cytoplasm (Fig. 10.36). At AFIP, the presence of these two cell types is required for a diagnosis of ACC. Among various reports on mammary ACC, the presence of these two cell types is specifically noted in only some (245,257,269,280,282, 284,286,289). The appearance of ACC is highly variable depending of the proportion of the basaloid cell population and the patterns formed by the islands of tumor cells. The cribriform islands are punctated by spaces filled with eosinophilic basement-membrane-like material (hyaline bodies), mucoid secretory material, or a bright eosinophilic band deposited on the lining cells with or without granular eosinophilic material in the lumen (Fig. 10.37). The lumens of tubules may also have similar contents. Most tumors have one or more of these luminal contents, but the proportion and distribution of each type is highly variable within different islands in a given tumor and

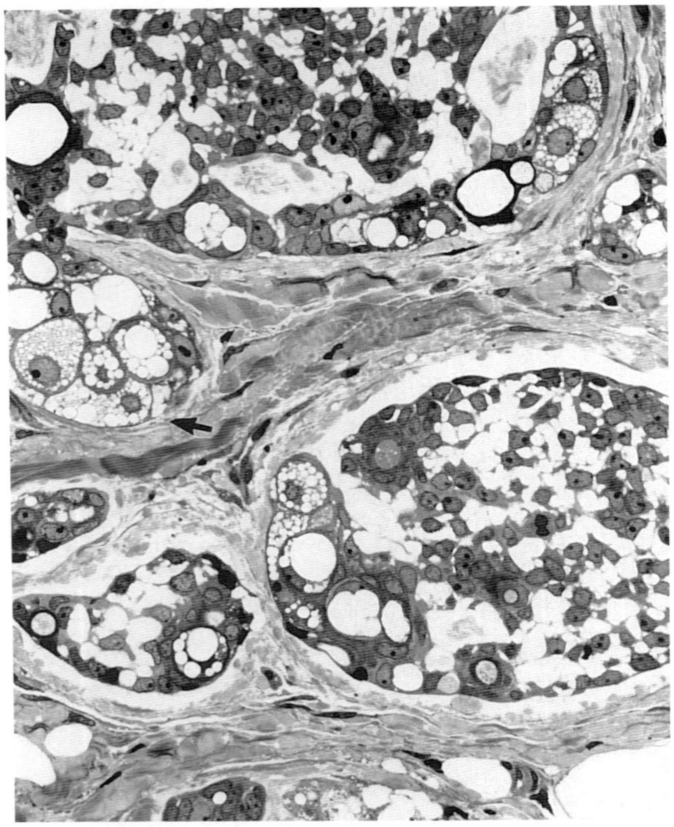

**Figure 10.39** Adenoid cystic carcinoma with sebaceous cells with thick cell membranes (arrow) evident in small clusters. (Toluidine blue, X400) (From Tavassoli FA, Norris HJ: *Arch Pathol Lab Med* 1986;110:1045–1053, with permission)

in different tumors. The predominantly solid tumors contain rare and often very small lumens within the nests of tumor cells; these lumens may be completely devoid of any noticeable content. Hyaline bodies may be present in the surrounding stroma as well and it appears that the tumor cells proliferate around and eventually engulf these hyaline bodies, gradually incorporating them into the nests of tumor cells (Fig. 10.38). The cords of tumor cells also spiral helically around portions of stroma as well as nerve fibers; the cylindrical nerve fibers serve to channel the spiraling cords.

The stroma in ACC may be composed of fibroblasts or may be edematous, hyalinized, or vaguely chondroid in appearance.

About 15% of adenoid cystic carcinomas have a third cell type, sebaceous cells (284), within the nests and tubules of the tumor (Fig. 10.39). The presence of these sebaceous cells does not alter the prognosis. Sebaceous cells have also been reported in adenoid cystic carcinomas of the salivary glands (252).

## Immunohistochemical Features

Adenoid cystic carcinomas show a variably positive reaction for actin and S-100 protein in the basaloid cells and a positive reaction for cytokeratin in the second, densely eosinophilic, cell population (269,284). Adenoid cystic carcinomas of the salivary gland have shown coexpression of keratin and vimentin (249). Caselitz et al (249) observed a stronger reaction for keratin in the "inner layer" of tumor cells. This stronger reaction probably corresponds to the staining of the bright eosinophilic cells which has been shown to have adenosquamous characteristics with a tremendous amount of tonofilaments at the ultrastructural level (284) compared to the paucity of any cytoplasmic organelles including tonofilaments in the basaloid cells. Keratin has also been demonstrated in an adenoid cystic carcinoma of the uterine cervix (270,273). Staining with laminin shows a thin line of positivity within some of the lumens and a strongly positive reaction in areas where hyaline bodies are present (252,286). Some of the luminal spaces are lined by type IV collagen (254), confirming the previous ultrastructural description of basement membrane-like material within some of the lumens (284).

## Ultrastructural Features

The presence of two cell types in mammary adenoid cystic carcinoma has been confirmed in several studies (270,276,279,284). The nature of these two cell types has been interpreted differently by various investigators, however. The basaloid cells are highly uniform in their appearance. They are mainly cuboid with a centrally-located oval nucleus containing finely-dispersed chromatin, with one or two nucleoli. Their cytoplasm contains a paucity of organelles (Fig. 10.40). These cells have short cytoplasmic projections which extend in various directions where well-developed desmosomes connect them to similar processes of adjacent cells. While an occasional cell contains fine cytoplasmic fibrils, fibrillar and cell membrane densities or pinocytotic vesicles which are characteristically present in myoepithelial cells were not identified in any of the six cases evaluated by Tavassoli and Norris (284). The basaloid cells are dominant in the nests of tumor cells and surround some of the lumens. The bright eosinophilic cells surrounding a smaller number of the lumens within the cell clusters are spindle-shaped or cuboid with abundant tonofilaments in their cytoplasm, sometimes concentrated in a linear fashion along the luminal cytoplasmic margin. Numerous blunt microvilli are present along the luminal margin; microvilli are more widely spaced along the remaining margin of the cells. A band-like concentration of granular secretory material is often present overlying the microvilli projecting into the lumen. Numerous well-developed desmosomes attach these eosinophilic cells to each other and to adjacent basaloid cells. Intracytoplasmic lumens are occasionally observed in these cells. Because of the simultaneous presence of prominent tonofilaments and desmosomes, along with well-developed luminal microvillous projections and occasional intracytoplasmic lumens (Fig. 10.41), Tavassoli and Norris (284) have designated these cells as adenosquamous cells. The abundant tonofilaments observed in these cells are not characteristic of ductal epithelial cells unless they are undergoing squamous metaplasia which is rather uncommon.

Some reports have interpreted one of these two cell types (generally the basaloid cells) as myoepithelial (ME) in nature (245,257,260,264,268,280). While derivation from the ME cells is quite likely, claims of myoepithelial differentiation at the ultrastructural level are not convincing. Intracytoplasmic fibrils with dense bodies and pinocytotic vesicles, features characteristic of mammary myoepithelial cells, are scant if present at all in most reports, and in one case, the light microscopic appearance of the tumor was not illustrated (260).

The presence of myoepithelial differentiation has been documented in extramammary ACC (265,266). Not a single neoplastic cell with typical features of a myoepithelial cell (desmosomes, intracytoplasmic fibrils with dense bodies, densities along the cytoplasmic margin and pinocytotic vesicles) was observed in any of the six cases studied at the ultrastructural level by Tavassoli and Norris (284), however. Wells et al (286) were also unable to identify a typical myoepithelial cell population in the neoplasm they studied ultrastructurally.

The spaces seen within the clusters of tumor cells in ACC reflect both true lumens and "pseudocysts," (246). The latter reflect extracellular spaces enclosed by tumor cells and lined by intact basal lamina. The true lumens are formed by the tumor cells attached to each other by tight junctions and desmosomes; the cells display prominent microvilli along the luminal margin. Some of the adenosquamous cells with abundant tonofilaments, microvilli and occasional intracytoplasmic lumens also line the true lumens.

The positive immunoreaction for S-100 and/or actin in some of the basaloid cells in the absence of convincing ultrastructural features of myoepithelial differentiation can be explained in two ways. Either the functional differentiation and expression of certain antigens for intermediate filaments precede morphologic differentiation in neoplastic cells or functional capabilities persist even when all morphologic characteristics are lost in an undifferentiated cell population.

## Hormone Receptors

There is very limited data on hormone receptors in adenoid cystic carcinoma. With rare exceptions, ACC has been negative for estrogen and progesterone receptors (254,267,280,281,289). Both estrogen and progesterone receptor positivity was documented in one of the six cases reported by Rosen, and another was positive for progesterone and negative for estrogen receptors (267,281); both of these were low grade tumors.

## Differential Diagnosis

Adenoid cystic carcinoma should be distinguished from intraductal and invasive cribriform carcinoma on the malignant side, and from collagenous microspherulosis (251) on the benign side. The term "pseudoadenoid cystic carcinoma" has been used for carcinomas mimicking the sieve-like pattern of ACC (262). The easiest way to make a distinction between adenoid cystic carcinoma and the other lesions is by strict adherence to the requirement of the presence of two cell types for a diagnosis of ACC. None of the other lesions has these two cell types. Occasionally, lymphocytes or histiocytes migrate into the proliferating neoplastic cells of the invasive cribriform carcinoma. These lymphocytes may appear as clear cells

A

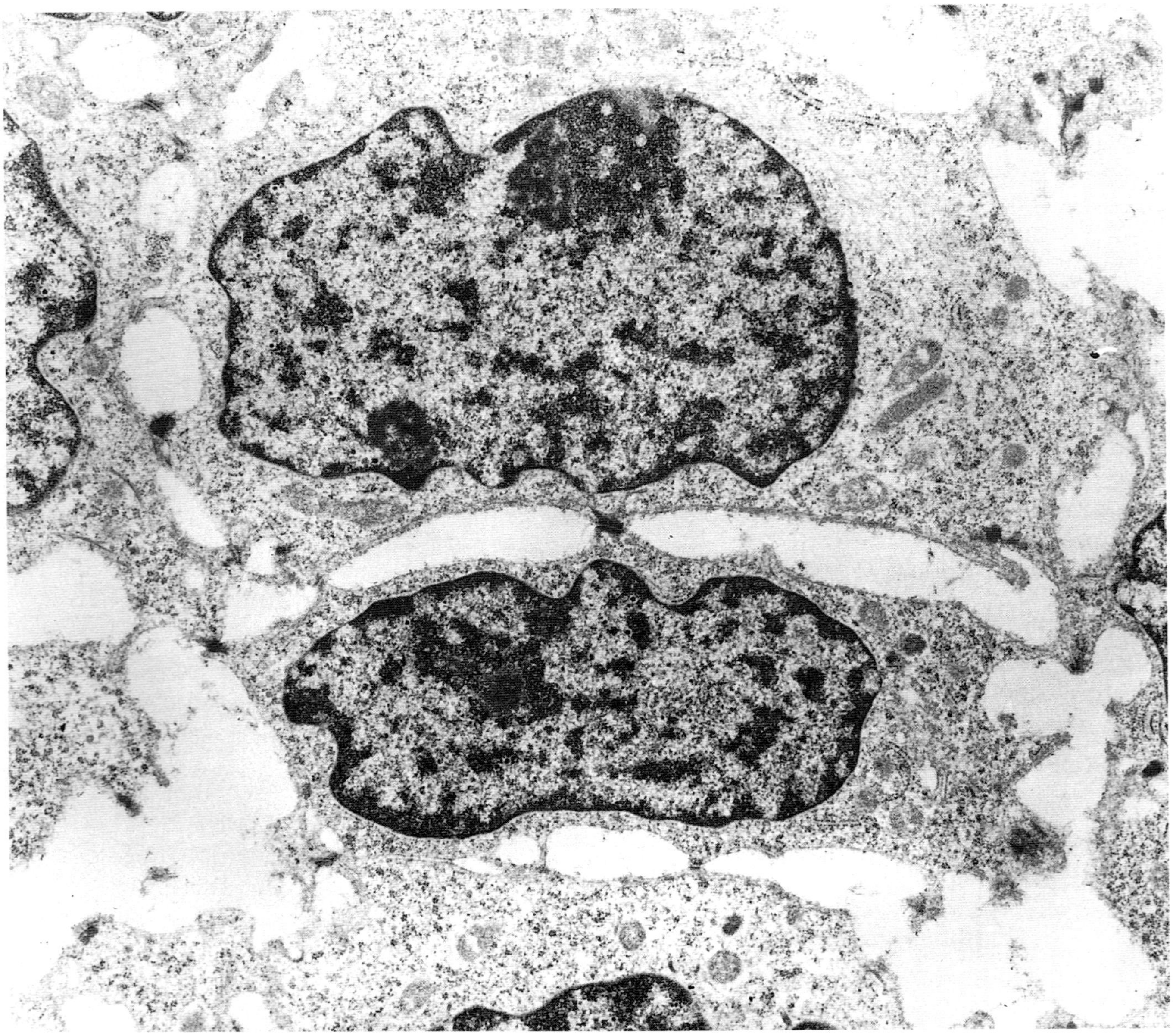

**Figure 10.40** Adenoid cystic carcinoma. (a) The dominant basaloid cells show a paucity of intracytoplasmic organelles and are attached to one another by desmosomes. (b) Secondary lumens are lined and filled by a fibrillar, basal laminar type of material corresponding to the hyaline globules seen on H&E sections. (Uranyl acetate-lead citrate, (a) X3,000; (b) X4,500) (From Tavassoli FA, Norris HJ: *Arch Pathol Lab Med* 1986;110:1045–1053, with permission)

which could be confused with the presence of a myoepithelial cell population within the tumor; immunoreaction for leukocyte common antigen (LCA) and any of the antisera for histiocytic cells would help establish the nonepithelial nature of these cells.

Contrary to claims that mucin histochemistry may be of diagnostic value in distinguishing ACC from pseudo-ACC (279), we have found it of little, if any, use. One reason is that not all ACC have the three or even two different types of luminal content within the various luminal spaces. For example, the predominantly solid basaloid variant has few if any lumens, and of those that are present only a few contain any secretory material. Furthermore, even regular infiltrating duct carcinomas may have variably staining secretory material within their glandular spaces which could lead to their misinterpretation as ACC if one were to rely on mucin histochemistry.

Aside from lacking the two cell types of ACC, collagenous microspherulosis (Fig. 10.42) is generally confined to two or three ducts in contrast to the invasive and extensive nature of ACC.

B

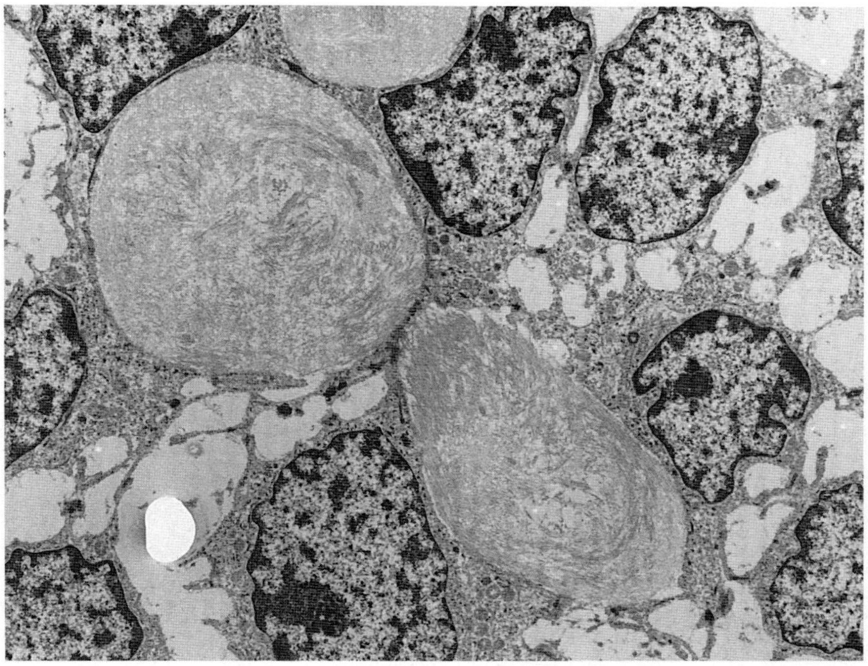

**Figure 10.40(b)** Adenoid cystic carcinoma. Legend on opposite page.

## Behavior and Prognosis

Adenoid cystic carcinoma is one of the least aggressive mammary carcinomas. It rarely ever metastasizes to the axillary nodes, but it does recur and may develop distant metastases years after the diagnosis. Recurrences often develop following local excision (248,250,272,288), but recurrent tumor has also been documented following simple mastectomy (287). The first report of an ACC with lymph node metastasis appeared in 1973 (285), but Azzopardi (247) and Peters and Wolff (278) have questioned the authenticity of this case. A well-documented example of ACC with axillary node metastases has been reported recently by Wells et al (286), however.

Data is available on several patients who developed distant mestastases even after radical mastectomy, four of whom died with pulmonary metastases (274,275,289). Metastatic lung lesions may appear up to nine years after the initial diagnosis and may be multiple and bilateral (255,271,274,287).

Since both recurrences and metastases have been reported many years following the initial diagnosis, long-term follow-up of the patients is necessary (263).

Grading mammary ACC using the same system utilized for the salivary gland tumors (277,283) may be of assistance in predicting the behavior of these lesions (280). The tumors are stratified into three grades. Grade I tumors are characterized by the presence of glandular and cystic areas lacking a solid component. Grade II tumors contain solid areas which constitute less than 30% of the tumor, and grade III tumors have a solid growth pattern in more than 30% of the lesion. Ro et al (280) graded 12 mammary ACC in this manner resulting in five grade I tumors, six grade II lesions and only one grade III neoplasm. All patients with grade I tumor were either alive without tumor or had died of other causes within an average of five years. One of the six patients with grade II tumor developed a recurrence five years after the diagnosis and subsequent pulmonary metastases and one died of metastatic ACC 13 years after the diagnosis. The only patient with grade III tumor had axillary lymph node metastases and she died of her disease two years later.

Alternatively, the tumors may be subdivided into low grade showing prominence of the cribriform pattern, or high grade with predominance of solid, basaloid areas (281). Of 23 adenoid cystic carcinomas reported by Rosen (281), 18 were low grade and five were high grade. None of the 23 had axillary node metastases. All women were well with no evidence of recurrence or metastases 14 to 155 months following the diagnosis. The only difference between the two groups was the larger size of the high grade lesions.

A

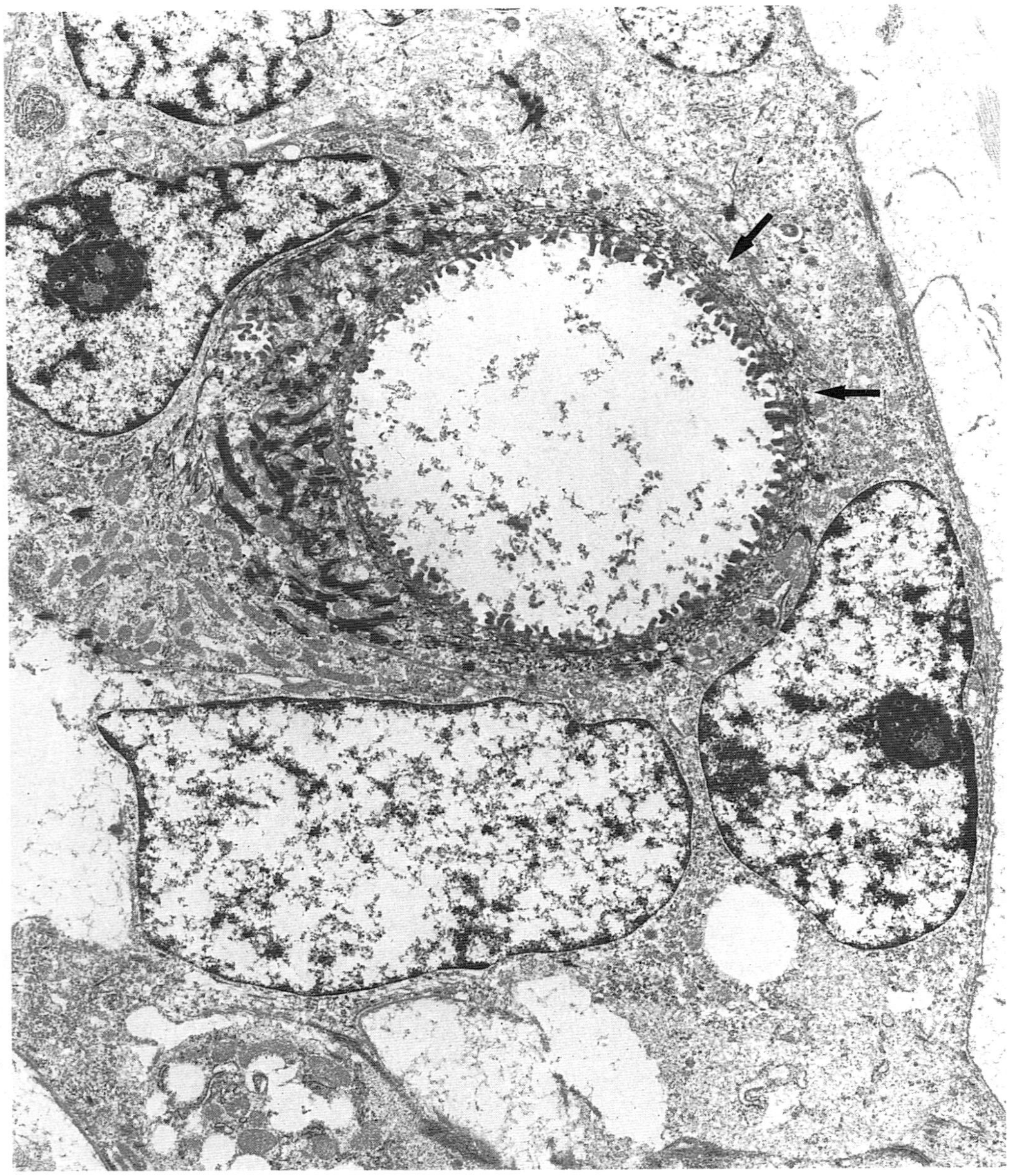

**Figure 10.41(a)** Adenoid cystic carcinoma. Elongated processes of adenosquamous cells with well-developed microvilli surround a space filled with granular material (arrow). These cells correspond to the intensely eosinophilic second cell population seen in adenoid cystic carcinomas. (Uranyl acetate-lead citrate, X4,500) (Fig. 10.41a from Tavassoli FA, Norris HJ: *Arch Pathol Lab Med* 1986;110:1045–1053, with permission)

The two groups did not differ in their clinical presentation or prognosis.

Rosen (281) divided adenoid cystic carcinomas into low grade and high grade tumors. The low grade neoplasms (18 cases) were characterized by gland or tubule formation (adenoid component) and varying amounts of stromal or basement membrane material (cylindromatous component). Syringomatous, adenomyoepitheliomatous, squamous, and sebaceous differentiation occurred in this variant, but solid growth was absent or minimal. The high grade variant (five cases) was characterized by a predominantly solid growth pattern, with areas of poorly-formed adenoid cystic configuration. The high grade tumors were larger, but they did not differ otherwise. Eighteen patients had mastectomy. Sixteen of the 23 patients had excision of the axillary nodes and none had any evidence of metastatic tumor. None of the 23 patients developed metastases or recurrences; follow-up ranged from 14 to 155 months with a median of 53 months. This study did not reveal a prognostic significance between the low and high grade tumors.

B

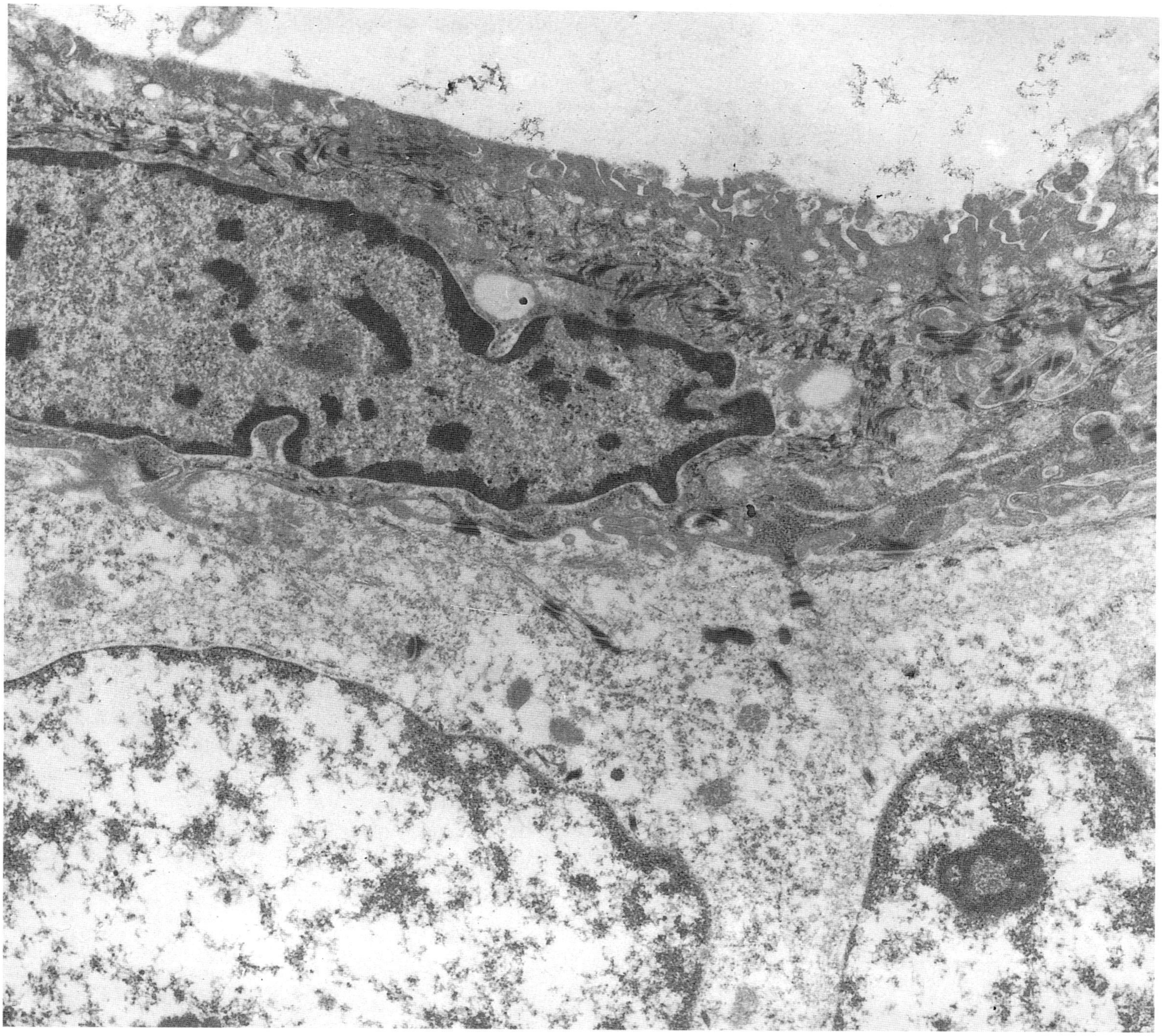

**Figure 10.41(b)** Adenoid cystic carcinoma. At higher magnification, the cells contain abundant tonofilaments and well-developed microvillous processes. The adenosquamoid cell is attached to two adjacent basaloid cells by desmosomal junctions. (Uranyl acetate-lead citrate, X7,000)

Longer follow-up may be necessary to reveal differences between various grades of this tumor since we are dealing with a basically low grade carcinoma.

The literature has predominantly described patients who have had either modified or radical mastectomy for ACC. Recurrences do develop after local excision and may occur up to seven or eight years postoperatively (250,278). Chest wall recurrence has been reported after simple mastectomy (287). Haagensen (261) considered simple mastectomy as a reasonable method of treatment for ACC and noted that it would cure 90% of the patients if performed promptly and would prevent local recurrence. Grading the tumors may eventually aid in selecting a group of patients who could be treated conservatively with lumpectomy rather than mastectomy. Because

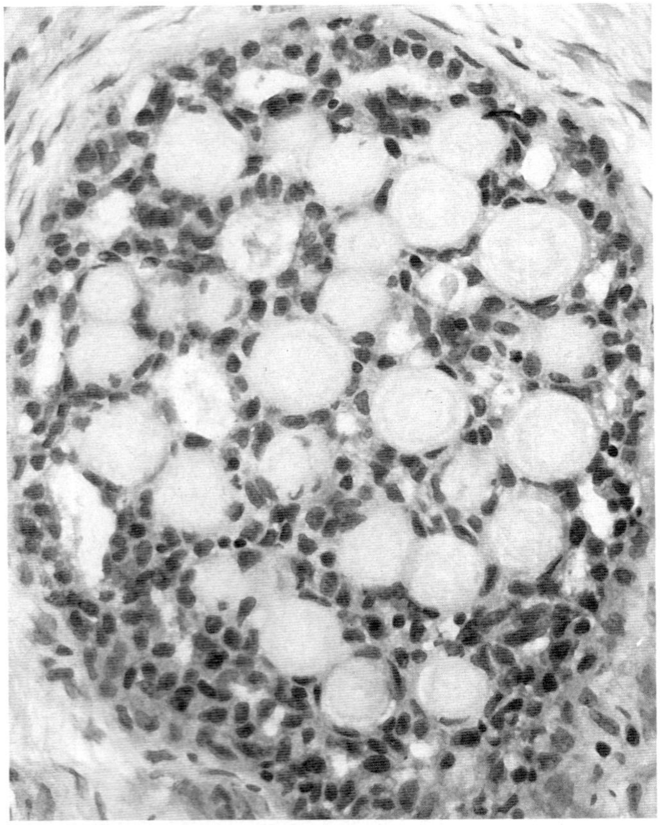

**Figure 10.42** Collagenous spherulosis. Multiple collagenous spherules are surrounded by a monotonous population of cells proliferating in a duct; the peripheral myoepithelial cell layer persists. Note early lamination in the spherules. A second proliferating cell type, characteristically observed in adenoid cystic carcinoma, is not present. (H&E, X115)

of the frequent extension of this tumor beyond the gross margins, a margin of uninvolved tissue should be allowed when considering conservative treatment.

## METASTATIC CARCINOMA

Recognition of metastatic carcinoma in the breast is important as it would prevent unnecessary mutilation of the breast and result in directing attention to treatment against the primary tumor. The most common metastatic carcinoma of the female breast is metastatic cancer from the contralateral breast (320), while the most common one to the male breast is carcinoma of the prostate (307,317,318). Metastases to the breast from extramammary carcinomas are uncommon (293–305,311,320,326); they represented only 1.2% of cancers identified in the breast during a ten-year period at the Memorial Hospital (302). Metastases to the breast often present as part of or following a disseminated disease; the patient often dies within a year or two. Occasionally, however, the mammary lesion reflects the first manifestation of a clinically occult malignancy (292,293,302,307,310,314, 320,322,325). While metastases from the contralateral breast are thought to involve the lymphatic channels of the anterior chest ("cross lymphatic metastases") (315), metastases from extramammary cancers are through the hematogenous route.

Aside from hematopoietic and lymphoreticular malignancies, the three most common tumors metastasizing to the breast are malignant melanoma (302, 316), lung cancer, and prostatic carcinoma. Ovarian (319), stomach, and cervical carcinoma (323) are next in that sequence. Several metastatic carcinoids to the breast have also been reported (297,303,321), as well as a rare metastatic bladder carcinoma (320). While melanoma is most frequently a metastatic tumor in the breast, it is noteworthy that rarely primary melanocytic lesions do occur in the breast. Several cases of primary melanoma have been reported in the breast (301,316,324). Even a case of malignant blue nevus has been described (290); this lesion occurred in a 58-year-old woman and consisted of a diffuse infiltration of the breast by spindle cells containing coarse melanin pigment. Making matters even more difficult for pathologists, melanocyte colonization and pigmentation of breast carcinoma does occur (291), and actually breast carcinoma metastatic to the skin can rarely simulate melanoma (306). A distinction, though difficult in these cases, can be made using a simple mucin stain in some cases and a panel of immunostains for epithelial (EMA and cytokeratin) and melanocytic (S-100 protein and HMB-45) antigens can help resolve the issue. A positive mucin stain in the tumor cells supports interpretation of the lesion as a carcinoma, so does a positive immunoreaction for cytokeratin or EMA. A positive reaction for S-100 and/or HMB-45, in the absence of any reaction with cytokeratin or EMA, would support the diagnosis of a melanocytic lesion.

The symptomatology of metastatic carcinoma is similar to those of primary mammary carcinoma. Patients present with a palpable tumor mass of varying duration. The tumors are generally superficially located and multinodular. Nipple retraction and discharge are not usually observed. Rarely, bilateral metastases simulate primary inflammatory carcinoma (313). Some metastatic ovarian carcinomas rich in psammoma bodies may mimic a primary breast cancer on mammography (294,308).

Microscopically, metastatic carcinomas are sharply demarcated and lack an intraductal carcinoma or lobular neoplasia component; necrosis and calcification are also absent. The presence of an in situ carcinoma is the only absolute proof of the primary nature of breast cancer, but it is not identified in all cases of primary breast carcinoma either. Some metastatic carcinomas may display distinctive features that help in their recognition; serous carcinoma of the ovary sometimes metastasizes in the form of micropapillary structures often within vascular spaces. Ovarian carcinomas may also grow within ducts and lobules, however, making distinction from a primary tumor difficult (312,315,319). Linitis plastica of the stomach can mimic a primary signet-ring cell carcinoma of the breast (298), and is one of the more difficult lesions for which a primary site needs to be established.

As a rule, whenever a well-circumscribed carcinoma is identified in the breast without an in situ component and the morphology appears even slightly unusual for a breast primary, the possibility of a metastatic carcinoma should be considered and excluded.

## REFERENCES

### Metaplastic Carcinoma

* 1. An T, Grathwohl M, Frable WJ: Breast carcinoma with osseous metaplasia: An electron microscopic study. *Am J Clin Pathol* 1984;81:127–132.
2. Arffman E, Hojgaard K: Squamous carcinoma of the breast: Report of a case. *J Pathol Bacteriol* 1965;90:319–320.
3. Azzopardi JG: *Problems in Breast Pathology*. Philadelphia, WB Saunders, 1979, pp 297–301.
* 4. Bauer TW, Rostock RA, Eggleston JC, et al: Spindle cell carcinoma of the breast: Four cases and review of the literature. *Hum Pathol* 1984;15:147–152.
* 5. Bogomoletz WV: Pure squamous cell carcinoma of the breast. *Arch Pathol Lab Med* 1982;106:57–59.
* 6. Bonet T: *Sepulchretum: Sive anatomia practica, ex cadaveribus. Morbo Denatis*, Vol 2, bk 3, chap 61. Geneva, Cramer and Perachon, 1700, p 522.
* 7. Christensen L, Nielsen M, Holund B, et al: Differentiation between metaplastic carcinomas and sarcomas of the human female breast by fibronectin. *Virchows Arch (Pathol Anat)* 1985;407:465–476.
8. Cook SS, DeMay R: Adenocarcinoma of the breast with osseous metaplasia. Report of a case with needle aspiration cytology. *Acta Cytol* 1984;28:318–324.
* 9. Cornog JL, Mobini J, Steiger E, et al: Squamous carcinoma of the breast. *Am J Clin Pathol* 1971;55:410–417.
* 10. Dervan PA, O'Loughlin J, Hurson BJ: Dedifferentiated chondrosarcoma with muscle and cytokeratin differentiation in the anaplastic component. *Histopathology* 1988;12: 517–526.
11. Dunning WF, Curtis MR, Eisen MJ: The carcinogenic activity of methylcholanthrene in rats. *Am J Cancer* 1940;40: 85–127.
* 12. Eggers JW, Chesney TM: Squamous cell carcinoma of the breast: A clinicopathologic analysis of eight cases and review of the literature. *Hum Pathol* 1984;15:526–531.
13. Essex WB, Rigg BM: Squamous cell carcinoma of the breast: Report of a case. *Aust NZ J Surg* 1965;34:207–210.
* 14. Eusebi V, Lamovec J, Cattani MG, et al: Acantholytic variant of squamous-cell carcinoma of the breast. *Am J Surg Pathol* 1986;10:855–861.
* 15. Fisher ER, Palekar AS, Gregorio RM, et al: Mucoepidermoid and squamous cell carcinoma of breast with reference to squamous metaplasia and giant cells. *Am J Surg Pathol* 1983;7:15–27.
16. Flint A, Oberman HA, Davenport RD: Cytophotometric measurements of metaplastic carcinoma of the breast: Correlation with pathologic features and clinical behavior. *Mod Pathol* 1988;1:193–197.
* 17. Foot NC, Moore SW: A fatal case of deep-seated epidermoid carcinoma of the breast with widespread metastasis. *Am J Cancer* 1938;34:226–233.
* 18. Gaudier, Grandclaude, Lambert M: Tumeur Maligne du sein a type myoepithelial. *Ann d'Anat Path* 1931;VIII:68–70.
* 19. Gersell DJ, Katzenstein A-LA: Spindle cell carcinoma of the breast. A clinicopathologic and ultrastructural study. *Hum Pathol* 1981;12:550–561.
20. Gonzales-Licea A, Yardley JH, Hartmann WH: Malignant tumor of the breast with bone formation. *Cancer* 1967;20: 1234–1247.
21. Haagensen CD: *Diseases of the Breast*, ed 3. Philadelphia, WB Saunders Co, 1986, pp 843–844.
* 22. Harrington SW, Miller JM: Intramammary squamous-cell carcinoma. *Proc Mayo Clin* 1939;14:484–487.
23. Harris M: Spindle cell squamous carcinoma: Ultrastructural observations. *Histopathology* 1982;6:197–210.
* 24. Harris M, Persaud V: Carcinosarcoma of the breast. *J Pathol* 1974;112:99–105.
25. Hasleton PS, Misch KA, Vasudev KS, et al: Squamous carcinoma of the breast. *J Clin Pathol* 1978;31:116–124.
* 26. Hastrup N, Sehested M: High grade mucoepidermoid carcinoma of the breast. *Histopathology* 1985;9:887–892.
* 27. Huvos AG, Lucas JC, Foote FW: Metaplastic breast carcinoma. Rare form of mammary cancer. *NY State J Med* 1973;73:1078–1082.
28. James TGI, Treip C: Squamous-celled carcinoma of the breast. *Br J Surg* 1955;42:650–654.
29. Johnson R, Lawrence TWP: Two cases of squamous epithelial tumour of the breast. *Br J Surg* 1917;5:417–421.

* 30. Jones EL: Primary squamous-cell carcinoma of breast with pseudosarcomatous stroma. *J Pathol* 1969;97:383–385.
31. Kao RT, Hall J, Engel L, et al: The matrix of human breast tumor cells is mitogenic for fibroblasts. *Am J Pathol* 1984; 115:109–116.
* 32. Kaufman MW, Marti JR, Gallager HS, et al: Carcinoma of the breast with pseudosarcomatous metaplasia. *Cancer* 1984;53:1908–1917.
33. Kovi J, Duong HD, Leffall LD Jr: High grade mucoepidermoid carcinoma of the breast. *Arch Pathol Lab Med* 1981;105: 612–614.
* 34. Lagace R, Schurch W, Seemayer TA: Carcinome polypoide pseudosarcomateux. Histogenese. Evidence d'une reponse myofibroblastique. *Ann Pathol* (Paris) 1981;1:27–37.
35. Lanzafame S, Basile G: Metaplasia condrosarcomatosa nel carcinoma della mammella umana: Sulla natura mioepiteliale. Studio morfologico ed immunoistochimico di un caso con revisione della litteratura. *Pathologica* 1985;77:525–538.
36. Lawler RG: Cartilaginous metaplasia in a breast tumour. *J Pathol* 1969;97:385–387.
37. Lazarevic B, Katatikarn V, Marks RA: Primary squamous cell carcinoma of the breast. Diagnosis by fine needle aspiration cytology. *Acta Cytol* 1984;28:321–324.
38. Leiman G: Squamous carcinoma of the breast: Diagnosis by aspiration cytology. *Acta Cytol* 1982;26:201–209.
39. Li Z, Yu-tian L: Squamous cell carcinoma of the breast. *Am J Surg* 1984;147:701–702.
* 40. Ling LL, Steiner GC: Primary multipotential malignant neoplasm of bone: Chondrosarcoma associated with squamous cell carcinoma. *Hum Pathol* 1986;17:317–320.
* 41. Llombart-Bosch A, Peydro A: Malignant mixed osteogenic tumors of the breast: An ultrastructural study of two cases. *Virchows Arch A* 1975;31:116–124.
* 42. Luchtrath H: Mucoepidermoid cancer of the breast. *Pathologe* 1984;5:282–284.
43. McDivitt RW, Stewart FW, Berg JW: *Tumors of the Breast*, Fasc 2. *Atlas of Tumor Pathology*, second series, Washington, DC, Armed Forces Institute of Pathology, 1968, p 82.
44. Medina D: Mammary tumorigenesis in chemical carcinogen-treated mice. VI. Tumor producing capabilities of mammary dysplasia in BALB/c Grgl mice. *J Natl Cancer Inst* 1976;57:1185–1189.
45. Meis JM, Ordonez NG, Gallager HS: Sarcomatoid carcinoma of the breast: An immunohistochemical study of six cases. *Virchows Arch A* 1987;410:415–421.
46. Miettinen M, Soini Y: Malignant fibrous histiocytoma—heterogenous patterns of intermediate filament proteins by immunocytochemistry. *Hum Pathol* 1986;17:317–320.
* 47. Nesland JM, Holm R, Johannesen JV: Spindle cell tumor in the breast. *Ultrastruc Pathol* 1986;10:415–419.
48. Oberman HA: Metaplastic carcinoma of the breast. A clinicopathologic study of 29 patients. *Am J Surg Pathol* 1987;11:918–929.
* 49. Pasternack JG, Wirth JE: Adenoacanthoma sarcomatoides of the mammary gland. *Am J Pathol* 1936;12:423–435.
50. Patchefsky AS, Frauenhoffer CM, Krall RA, et al: Low grade mucoepidermoic carcinoma of the breast. *Arch Pathol Lab Med* 1979;103:196–198.
51. Reddy DJ, Sivasankaran P: Chondromatous metaplasia in mammary adenocarcinoma. *Indian J Med Sci* 1969;23:245–248.
* 52. Rosen PP, Ernsberger D: Low-grade adenosquamous carcinoma. A variant of metaplastic mammary carcinoma. *Am J Surg Pathol* 1987;11:351–358.
* 53. Rottino A, Wilson K: Osseous, cartilaginous and mixed tumors of the human breast. A review of the literature. *Arch Surg* 1945;50:184–193.
* 54. Santeusanio G, Pascal RR, Bisceglia M, et al: Metaplastic breast carcinoma with epithelial phenotype of pseudosarcomatous components. *Arch Pathol Lab Med* 1988;112:82–85.
55. Schaefer FV, Custer RP, Sorof S: Squamous metaplasia in human breast culture: Induction by cyclic adenine nucleotide and prostaglandin, and influence of menstrual cycle. *Cancer Res* 1983;43:279–286.
56. Shousha S, James AH, Fernandez D, et al: Squamous cell carcinoma of the breast. *Arch Pathol Lab Med* 1984;108:893–896.
* 57. Smith BH, Taylor HB: The occurrence of bone and cartilage in mammary tumors. *Am J Clin Pathol* 1969;51:610–618.
* 58. Spagnolo DV, Shilkin KB: Breast neoplasms containing bone and cartilage. *Virchows Arch (Pathol Anat)* 1983;400: 287–295.
59. Surakiatchanukul S, Brown HW, Sielger E: Carcinoma of the breast with cartilagenous metaplasia. *Int Surg* 1973;58: 138–140.
* 60. Tavassoli FA: Classification of metaplastic carcinomas of the breast, in Rosen PP, Fechner RD (eds): *Pathology Annual 1992*, 1992;27(pt 2):89–119. Norwalk, CT, Appleton & Lange.
* 61. Toikkanen S: Primary squamous cell carcinoma of the breast. *Cancer* 1981;48:1629–1632.
62. Trapasso RL, McCarty KS, Proia AD, et al: Adenosquamous differentiation: Mammary needle aspiration cytology. *Acta Cytol* 1981;25:196–198.
63. Wargotz ES, Deos PH, Norris HJ: Metaplastic carcinomas of the breast. II. Spindle cell carcinoma. *Hum Pathol* 1989; 20:732–740.
64. Wargotz ES, Norris HJ: Metaplastic carcinomas of the breast. I. Matrix-producing carcinoma. *Hum Pathol* 1989;20: 628–635.
* 65. Wargotz ES, Norris HJ: Metaplastic carcinoma of the breast. IV. Squamous cell carcinoma of ductal origin. *Cancer* 1990;65:272–276.
66. Wayte DM, Stewart JB, Mckenzie CE: A composite malignant tumor of the elderly female breast. *J Clin Pathol* 1970;23:414–422.
* 67. Willis RA: Squamous-cell mammary carcinoma of predominantly fibrosarcoma-like structure. *J Pathol Bacteriol* 1958; 76:511–515.
* 68. Woodard BH, Brinkhous HT, McCarty KS Sr, et al: Adenosquamous differentiation in mammary carcinoma. An

ultrastructural and steroid receptor study. *Arch Pathol Lab Med* 1980;104:130–133.

## Apocrine Carcinoma

* 69. Abati AD, Kimmel M, Rosen PP: Apocrine mammary carcinoma: A clinicopathologic study of 72 cases. *Am J Clin Pathol* 1990;94:371–377.

70. Ahmed A: Apocrine metaplasia in cystic hyperplastic mastopathy. Histochemical and ultrastructural observations. *J Pathol* 1975;115:211–214.

71. Ahmed A: *Atlas of the Ultrastructure of Human Breast Diseases*. Edinburgh, Churchill Livingstone, 1978, pp 130–133.

72. Archer F, Omar M: Pink cell (oncocytic) metaplasia in a fibroadenoma of the human breast: Electron microscopic observation. *J Pathol* 1969;99:99–124.

* 73. Azzopardi JD: *Problems in Breast Pathology*. London, WB Saunders, 1979, pp 341–344.

* 74. Bonser GM, Dossett JA, Jull JW: *Human & Experimental Breast Cancer*. London, Pitman Medical, 1961, pp 288–298.

75. Bryant J: Male breast cancer: A case of apocrine carcinoma with psammona bodies. *Hum Pathol* 1981;12:751–753.

* 76. Bussolati G, Cattani MG, Gugliotta P, et al: Morphologic and functional aspects of apocrine metaplasia in dysplastic and neoplastic breast tissue. *Ann NY Acad Sci* 1986;464:262–274.

77. Castagna M, Nuti M, Squartini F: Mammary cancer antigen recognized by monoclonal Ab B72.3 in apocrine metaplasia of human breast. *Cancer Res* 1987;47:902–906.

* 78. D'Amore ESG, Terrier-Lacombe MJ, Travagli JP, et al: Invasive apocrine carcinoma of the breast: A long-term follow-up study of 34 cases. *Breast Cancer Res Treat* 1988;12: 37–44.

* 79. Dawson EK: Sweat gland carcinoma of the breast. A morpho-histological study. *Edinburgh Med J* 1932;39:409–438.

80. Dilley WG, Haagensen DE Jr, Leight GS, et al: Fluoxymesterone stimulation of tumor marker secretion in patients with breast carcinoma. *Breast Cancer Res Treat* 1986;8:205–215.

81. Dixon JM, Lumsden AB, Miller WR: The relationship of cyst type to risk factor for breast cancer and the subsequent development of breast cancer in patients with breast cystic disease. *Eur J Cancer Clin Oncol* 1985;21:1047–1050.

82. Eusebi V, Betts C, Haagensen DE Jr, et al: Apocrine differentiation in lobular carcinoma of the breast. A morphologic, immunologic and ultrastructural study. *Hum Pathol* 1984;15:134–140.

* 83. Eusebi V, Millis RR, Cattani MG, et al: Apocrine carcinoma of the breast. A morphologic and immunocytochemical study. *Am J Pathol* 1986;123:532–541.

* 84. Ewing J: *Neoplastic Diseases*, ed 3. Philadelphia, WB Saunders, 1928.

85. Fisher ER: Ultrastructure of the human breast and its disorders. *Am J Clin Pathol* 1976;66:291–375.

* 86. Fisher ER, Gregorio RM, Fisher B, et al: The pathology of invasive breast cancer. *Cancer* 1975;36:1–78.

* 87. Frable WJ, Kay S: Carcinoma of the breast—histologic and clinical features of apocrine tumors. *Cancer* 1968;21:756–763.

88. Gadaleanu V, Galatar N: Apocrine carcinoma of the breast. *Morphol Embryol* (Bucur) 1986;32:33–38.

* 89. Geschickter CF: *Diseases of the Breast*. Philadelphia, WB Saunders, 1943, p 422.

* 90. Haagensen CD: *Diseases of the Breast*, ed 3. Philadelphia, WB Saunders, 1986, pp 82–102.

* 91. Haagensen DE Jr, Dilley WG, Mazcujian G, et al: Review of GCDFP-15. An apocrine marker protein. *NY Acad Sci* 1990;586:161–173.

* 92. Hamperl H: Onkociten und Geschwulste der Speicheldrusen. *Virchow Arch F (Anat Path)* 1931;282:724.

* 93. Hamperl H: The so-called sweat-gland carcinoma of the human breast. A review. *Z Krebsforsch* 1977;88:105–119.

* 94. Higginson JF, McDonald JR: Apocrine tissue, chronic cystic mastitis and sweat gland carcinoma of the breast. *Surg Gynecol Obstet* 1949;88:1–11.

* 95. Krompecher E: Zur Histogenese und Morphologie der Cystenmamma (maladie Kystique reclus, cystadenoma Schimmelbuscin, mastitis chronica cystic Konig) des intrakanaliken Kystadenomas und der Kystadenokarzinome der Brustdruse (Hidro-Kystoma, Kystadenoma, Hidrokystadenocarzinoma mammae). *Beitr Pathol Anat* 1916;62:403.

96. Kumar S, Mansel RE, Jasani B: Presence and possible significance of immunohistochemically demonstrable prolactin in breast apocrine metaplasia. *Br J Cancer* 1987;55: 307–309.

97. Labows JN, Hoelzle E, Leyden J, et al: Steroid analysis of human apocrine secretion. *Steroids* 1979;34:249–258.

* 98. Lee BJ, Pack GT, Scharnagel I: Sweat gland cancer of the breast. *Surg Gynecol Obstet* 1933;56:975–996.

* 99. Lendrum AC: On the "pink" epithelium of the cystic breast and the staining of its granules. *J Pathol* 1945;57:267–273.

100. Manni A, Santen RJ, Boucher AE, et al: Evaluation of CEA and GCDFP-15 plasma levels during hormonally induced cancer stimulation. *Anticancer Res* 1984;4:141–144.

*101. Mazoujian G, Pinkus GS, Davis S, et al: Immunohistochemistry of breast gross cystic disease fluid protein (GCDFP-15): A marker of apocrine epithelium and breast carcinomas with apocrine features. *Am J Pathol* 1983;110: 105–111.

*102. Mazoujian G, Bodian C, Haagensen DE Jr, et al: Expression of GCDFP-15 in breast carcinomas. Relationship to pathologic and clinical factors. *Cancer* 1989;63:2156–2161.

103. Miller WR, Shivas AA, Franchimont P, et al: Breast gross cystic disease fluid protein-15 in human breast cancer in culture. *Eur J Cancer Clin Oncol* 1988;24:223–228.

*104. Mossler JA, Barton TK, Brinkhous AD, et al: Apocrine differentiation in human mammary carcinoma. *Cancer* 1980;46:2463–2471.

105. Page DL, Dupont WD: Are breast cysts a premalignant marker? *Eur J Cancer Clin Oncol* 1986;22:635–636.

106. Paikova LV: Cancer of the mammary glands with apocrine metaplasia. *Archiv Patol* 1973;I:49–52.

107. Pier WJ, Garancis JC, Kuzma JF: The ultrastructure of apocrine cells in intracystic papilloma and fibrocystic disease of the breast. *Arch Pathol* 1970;89:446–452.

108. Roddy HJ, Silverberg SG: Ultrastructural analysis of apocrine carcinoma of the human breast. *Ultrastruc Pathol* 1983;63:385–393.

109. Roncalli M, Servida E: Carcinoma apocrino della mammella. *Istocitopatologia* 1981;3:247–250.

110. Shousha S, Bull TB, Southall PJ, et al: Apocrine carcinoma of the breast containing foam cells. An electron microscopic and immunohistological study. *Histopathology* 1987; 11:611–620.

111. Simard J, Hatton AC, Labrie C, et al: Inhibitory effect of estrogens on GCDFP-15 on RNA levels and secretion in ZR-75-1 human breast cancer cells. *Mol Endocrinol* 1989;3: 694–702.

112. Taccagni GL, Sironi M, Dell'Antonio G, et al: Pure apocrine carcinoma of the female breast presenting as a cyst: A case report. *Pathologica* 1985;77:91–99.

113. Tavassoli FA, Norris HJ: A comparison of the results of long-term follow-up for atypical intraductal hyperplasia and intraductal hyperplasia of the breast. *Cancer* 1990;65: 518–529.

*114. Tavassoli FA, Jones MW, Majeste RM, et al: Immunohistochemical staining with monoclonal Ab B72.3 in benign and malignant breast disease. *Am J Surg Pathol* 1990;14: 128–133.

115. van Bogaert LJ: Recent progress in the histological typing of human breast tumors. *Diagn Histopathol* 1981;4:349–353.

116. Wahren B, Lidbrink E, Wallgren A, et al: Carcinoembryonic antigen and other tumor markers in tissue and serum or plasma of patients with primary mammary carcinoma. *Cancer* 1978;42:1870–1878.

117. Wald M, Kakulas BA: Apocrine gland carcinoma (sweat gland carcinoma) of the breast. *Aust NZ J Surg* 1964;33:200–204.

118. Walker RA: Demonstration of CEA in human breast carcinomas by the immunoperoxidase technique. *J Clin Pathol* 1980;33:356–360.

119. Wellings SR, Alpers CE: Apocrine cystic metaplasia: Subgross pathology and prevalence in cancer associated versus random autopsy breasts. *Hum Pathol* 1987;18:381–386.

*120. Yates AJ, Ahmed A: Apocrine carcinoma and apocrine metaplasia. *Histopathology* 1988;13:228–231.

### Histiocytoid Carcinoma

121. Allenby PA, Chowdery LN: Histiocytic appearance of metastatic breast carcinoma. *Arch Pathol Lab Med* 1986;110: 759–760.

*122. Azzopardi JG: *Problems in Breast Pathology*. Philadelphia, WB Saunders, 1979, pp 301–302.

123. Dabski K, Milgrom H, Stoll HL: Breast carcinoma metastatic to the eyelids: Case report and review of the literature. *J Surg Oncol* 1985;29:233–236.

*124. Eisenberg BL, Bagnall JW, Harding CT: Histiocytoid carcinoma: A variant of breast cancer. *J Surg Oncol* 1986;31:271–274.

125. Filototico M, Trabucco M, Gallone D, et al: Histiocytoid carcinoma of the breast. A problem of differential diagnosis for the pathologist. Report of a case. *Pathologica* 1983;75: 429–433.

126. Gad A, Azzopardi JG: Lobular carcinoma of the breast: A special variant of mucin-secreting carcinoma. *J Clin Pathol* 1975;28:711–716.

*127. Hood CI, Font RL, Zimmerman LE: Metastatic mammary carcinoma in the eyelid with histiocytoid appearance. *Cancer* 1973;31:793–800.

128. Walford N, ten Velden J: Histiocytoid breast carcinoma: An apocrine variant of lobular carcinoma. *Histopathology* 1989; 14:515–522.

### Lipid-rich Carcinoma

*129. Aboumrad MH, Horn RC, Fine G: Lipid-secreting mammary carcinoma: Report of a case associated with Paget's disease of the nipple. *Cancer* 1963;16:521–525.

130. Fisher ER, Gregorio R, Kim WS, et al: Lipid in invasive cancer of the breast. *Am J Clin Pathol* 1977;68:558–561.

*131. Kurebayashi J, Izuo M, Ishida T, et al: Two cases of lipid-secreting carcinoma of the breast: Case reports with an electron microscopic study. *Jpn J Clin Oncol* 1988;18:249–254.

132. Lim-co RY, Gisser SD: Unusual variant of lipid-rich mammary carcinoma. *Arch Pathol Lab Med* 1978;102:192–195.

*133. Ramos CV, Taylor HB: Lipid-rich carcinoma of the breast: A clinicopathological analysis of thirteen examples. *Cancer* 1974;33:812–819.

*134. Van Bogaert LJ, Maldague P: Histologic variants of lipid-secreting carcinoma of the breast. *Virchows Arch A (Path Anat Histol)* 1977;375:345–353.

*135. Vera-Sempere F, Llombart-Bosch A: Lipid-rich versus lipid-secreting carcinoma of the mammary gland. *Pathol Res Pract* 1985;190:553–556.

*136. Wrba F, Ellinger A, Reiner G, et al: Ultrastructural and immunohistochemical characteristics of lipid-rich carcinoma of the breast. *Virchows Arch A Pathol Anat* 1988;413: 381–385.

### Secretory (Juvenile) Carcinoma

137. Abe R, Masuda T: Secretory carcinoma of the breast in a Japanese woman. *Jpn J Surg* 1986;16:52–55.

138. Akhtar M, Robinson C, Ali MA, et al: Secretory carcinoma of the breast in adults: Light and electron microscopic study of three cases with review of the literature. *Cancer* 1983;51:2245–2254.

139. Botta G, Fessia L, Ghiringhello B: Juvenile milk protein secreting carcinoma. *Virchows Arch (Pathol Anat)* 1982;395: 145–152.

140. Byrne MP, Fabey MM, Gooselaw JG: Breast cancer with axillary metastasis in an 8 1/2 year old girl. *Cancer* 1973;31: 726–728.

141. Craig JP: Secretory carcinoma of the breast in an adult. Correlation of aspiration cytology and histology on the biopsy specimen. *Acta Cytol* 1985;29:589–592.

142. Harris M, Vasudev KS, Anfield C, et al: Mucin-producing carcinomas of the breast: Ultrastructural observations. *Histopathology* 1978;2:177–188.

143. Heydenrych JJ, Villet WT, Von der Heyden U: Carcinoma of the breast in children. *S Afr Med J* 1980;57:1005–1008.

144. Karl SR, Ballantine TVN, Zaino R: Juvenile secretory carcinoma of the breast. *Hum Pathol* 1981;12:1044–1046.

*145. Krausz T, Jenkins D, Grontoft O, et al: Secretory carcinoma of the breast in adults: Emphasis on late recurrence and metastasis. *Histopathology* 1989;14:25–36.

146. Masse SR, Rioux A, Beauchesne C: Juvenile carcinoma of the breast. *Hum Pathol* 1981;12:1044–1045.

*147. McDivitt RW, Stewart FW: Breast carcinoma in children. *JAMA* 1966;195:388–390.

*148. Oberman HA: Secretory carcinoma of the breast in adults. *Am J Surg Pathol* 1980;4:465–470.

*149. Roth JA, Discafani C, O'Malley M: Secretory breast carcinoma in a man. *Am J Surg Pathol* 1988;12:150–154.

150. Simpson JS, Barson AJ: Breast tumors in infants and children. *Can Med Assoc J* 1969;101:100–102.

*151. Sullivan JJ, Magee HR, Donald KJ: Secretory (juvenile) carcinoma of the breast. *Pathology* 1977;9:341–346.

152. Tamura G, Kaizuka H, Iwasaki T, et al: Non-invasive secretory carcinoma of the breast. *Gan No Rinsho* 1987;33:723–728.

*153. Tavassoli FA, Norris HJ: Secretory carcinoma of the breast: A clinicopathologic study with ultrastructural findings. *Cancer* 1980;45:2404–2413.

154. Teasdale C, Baum M: Breast cancer in a school girl. *Lancet* 1976;2:627.

155. Tokunaga M, Wakimoto J, Muramoto Y, et al: Juvenile secretory carcinoma and juvenile papillomatosis. *Jpn J Clin Oncol* 1985;15:457–465.

*156. Tournemaine N, Audouin AF, Anguill C, et al: Le carcinoma secretoire juvenile. Cinq nouveaux cas chez des femme d'age adulte. *Arch Anat Cytol Pathol* 1986;34:146–151.

### Glycogen-rich Carcinoma

*157. Benisch B, Peison B, Newman R, et al: Solid glycogen-rich clear cell carcinoma of the breast (a light and ultrastructural study). *Am J Clin Pathol* 1983;79:243–245.

*158. Fisher ER, Tavares J, Bulatao IS, et al: Glycogen-rich clear cell breast cancer: With comments concerning other clear cell variants. *Hum Pathol* 1985;16:1085–1090.

*159. Hull MT, Priest JB, Broadie TA, et al: Glycogen-rich clear cell carcinoma of the breast: A light and electron microscopic study. *Cancer* 1981;48:2003–2009.

*160. Hull MT, Warfel KA: Glycogen-rich clear cell carcinomas of the breast. A clinicopathologic and ultrastructural study. *Am J Surg Pathol* 1986;10:553–559.

*161. Sorensen FB, Paulsen SM: Glycogen-rich clear cell carcinoma of the breast: A solid variant with mucus. A light microscopic, immunohistochemical and ultrastructural study of a case. *Histopathology* 1987;11:857–869.

*162. Toikkanen S, Joensuu H: Glycogen-rich clear-cell carcinoma of the breast: A clinicopathologic and flow cytometric study. *Hum Pathol* 1991;22:81–83.

### Carcinoma with Osteoclastic Giant Cells

*163. Agnantis NT, Rosen PP: Mammary carcinoma with osteoclast-like giant cells. *Am J Clin Pathol* 1979;72:383–389.

164. Bondeson L: Aspiration cytology of breast carcinoma with multinucleated reactive stromal giant cells. *Acta Cytol* 1984;28:313–316.

165. Chilosi M, Bonetti F, Menestrina F, et al: Breast carcinoma with stromal multinucleated giant cells. *J Pathol* 1987;70:787–791.

*166. Duboucher H, Montpellier J, Laffarque F: Epitheliome mammaire avec reaction de type myeloplazique. *Ann Pathol* 1933;70:787–791.

*167. Factor SM, Biempical L, Ratner I, et al: Carcinoma of the breast with multinucleated reactive stromal giant cells. *Virchows Arch* 1977;374:1–12.

168. Ferlito A: L'epitheliome a cellules geantes du sein. *Arch Anat Pathol* 1974;22:99–104.

169. Fisher ER, Gregorio RM, Paleka AS, et al: Mucoepidermoid and squamous cell carcinomas of breast with reference to squamous metaplasia and giant cell tumors. *Am J Surg Pathol* 1983;7:15–27.

170. Frappart L, Berger G, Raudrant D, et al: Les adenocarcinomes mammaires a cellules geantes. Etude anatomo-clinique d'un cas et revue de la literature. *Senologia* 1980;5:131–136.

170a. Hinoura Y, Marutsuka K, Hayashi T, et al: Breast cancer with stromal osteoclast-like multinucleated giant cells. A case report. *J Jpn Soc Clin Cytol* 1991;30:1109–1114.

*171. Holland R, van Haelst UJGM: Mammary carcinoma with osteoclast-like giant cells: Additional observations on six cases. *Cancer* 1984;53:1963–1973.

172. Ichijima K, Kobashi N, Samoto T, et al: Breast cancer with osteoclast-like multinucleated giant cells. *Acta Pathol Jpn* 1984;34:1475–1484.

173. Lecene P: Les tumeurs mixtes du sein. *Rev Chir* 1906;33:434–449.

174. Leroux R: Reaction giganto cellulaire du stroma dans un epitheliome mammaire. *Bull Cancer* 1931;20:692–697.

175. Leven A, Rywlin AM, Tachmes P: Carcinoma of the breast with stromal epulis-like giant cells. *South Med J* 1981;74:889–891.

176. McMahon RFT, Ahmed A, Connolly CE: Breast carcinoma with stromal multinucleated giant cells. A light microscopic, histochemical and ultrastructural study. *J Pathol* 1986;150:175–179.

*177. Nielsen BB, Kiaer HW: Carcinoma of the breast with stromal multinucleated giant cells. *Histopathology* 1985;9:183–193.

178. Pettinato G, Manivel JC, Picone A, et al: Alveolar variant of infiltrating lobular carcinoma of the breast with stromal osteoclast-like cells. *Path Res Pract* 1989;185:388–394.

179. Pettinato G, Petrella G, Manco A, et al: Carcinoma of the breast with osteoclast-like giant cells. Fine needle aspiration cytology, histology and electron microscopy of 5 cases. *Appl Pathol* 1984;2:168–178.

180. Sugano I, Nagao K, Kondo Y, et al: Cytologic and ultrastructural studies of a rare breast carcinoma with osteoclast-like giant cells. *Cancer* 1983;52:74–78.

* 181. Tavassoli FA, Norris HJ: Breast carcinoma with osteoclastic giant cells. *Arch Pathol Lab Med* 1986;110:636–639.

* 182. Steiner GC, Ghosh L, Dorfman HD: Ultrastructure of giant cell tumors of bone. *Hum Pathol* 1972;3:569–586.

183. Volpe R, Carbone A, Nicolo G, et al: Cytology of a breast carcinoma with osteoclast-like giant cells. *Acta Cytol* 1983; 27:184–187.

### Invasive Cribriform Carcinoma

184. Dixon JM, Anderson TJ, Page DL, et al: Infiltrating lobular carcinoma of the breast. *Histopathology* 1982;6:149–161.

* 185. Page DL, Dixon JM, Anderson TJ, et al: Invasive cribriform carcinoma of the breast. *Histopathology* 1983;7:525–536.

* 186. Venable JG, Scwartz AM, Silverberg SG: Infiltrating cribriform carcinoma of the breast: A distinctive clinicopathologic entity. *Hum Pathol* 1990;21:333–338.

187. Wells CA, Ferguson DJ: Ultrastructural and immunocytochemical study of a case of invasive cribriform breast carcinoma. *J Clin Pathol* 1988;41:17–20.

### Carcinoma with Choriocarcinomatous Features

188. Bellet D, Arrang JM, Contesso G, et al: Localization of the beta-subunit of human chorionic gonadotropin on various tumors. *Eur J Cancer* 1980;16:433–439.

189. Castro A, Bauschbaum P, Nadji M, et al: Ectopic human chorionic gonadotropin in breast carcinoma. *Experimentia* 1979;35:1392–1393.

190. Cohle SD, Tschen JA, Smith FE, et al: ACTH-secreting carcinoma of the breast. *Cancer* 1979;43:2370–2376.

191. Horne CHW, Reid IM, Milne GD: Prognostic significance of inappropriate production of pregnancy proteins by breast cancers. *Lancet* 1976;2:279–282.

192. Kaneko H, Hojo H, Ishikawa S, et al: Norepinephrine producing tumors of bilateral breasts. *Cancer* 1978;41:2002–2007.

193. Kuida CA, Braunstein GD, Shintaku P, et al: Human chorionic gonadotropin expression in lung, breast, and renal carcinomas. *Arch Pathol Lab Med* 1988;112:282–285.

194. Lee AK, Rosen PP, DeLellis RA, et al: Tumor marker expression in breast carcinomas and relationship to prognosis. *Am J Clin Pathol* 1985;84:687–696.

195. McManus LM, Naughton MA, Martinez-Hernandez A: Human chorionic gonadotropin in human neoplastic cells. *Cancer Res* 1976;36:3476–3481.

196. Monteiro JCMP, Ferguson KM, McKinna JA, et al: Ectopic production of human chorionic gonadotrophin-like material by breast cancer. *Cancer* 1984;53:957–962.

197. Nishiyama T, Stolbach LL, Rule AH, et al: Expression of oncodevelopmental markers (regan isozyme, Beta-HCG, CEA) in tumor tissues and uninvolved bronchial mucosa: An immunohistochemical study. *Acta Histochem Cytochem* 1980;13:245–253.

* 198. Saigo PE, Rosen PP: Mammary carcinoma with "choriocarcinomatous" features. *Am J Surg Pathol* 1981;5:773–778.

199. Sheth NA, Sarmiga JN, Ranadive KT, et al: Ectopic production of human chorionic gonadotropin by breast tumors. *Br J Cancer* 1974;30:566–570.

200. Tormey DC, Waalkes TP, Simon RM: Biologic markers in breast carcinoma. II. Clinical correlations with human chorionic gonadotropin. *Cancer* 1977;39:2391–2396.

201. Wachner R, Wittekind C, von Kleist S: Immunohistochemical localization of beta-HCG in breast carcinoma. *Eur J Cancer Clin Oncol* 1984;20:679–684.

202. Woodard BH, Eisenbarth G, Wallace NR, et al: Adrenocorticotropin production by a mammary carcinoma. *Cancer* 1981;47:1823–1827.

### Inflammatory Carcinoma

203. Barber KWJ, Dockerty MB, Clagett OT: Inflammatory carcinoma of the breast. *Gynec Obstet* 1961;112:406.

204. Barker JL, Montague ED, Peterson LJ: Clinical experience with irradiation of inflammatory carcinoma of the breast with and without elective chemotherapy. *Cancer* 1980;45: 625–629.

205. Barker JL, Nelson AJ, Montague ED: Inflammatory carcinoma of the breast. *Radiology* 1976;121:173–176.

206. Brownstein MH, Helwig EB: Spread of tumors to the skin. *Arch Dermatol* 1973;107:80–86.

* 207. Buzdar AU, Montague ED, Barker JL, et al: Management of inflammatory carcinoma of breast with combined modality approach—An update. *Cancer* 1981;47:2537–2542.

208. Camp E: Inflammatory carcinoma of the breast—the case for conservatism. *Am J Surg* 1976;131:583–586.

* 209. Chevalier B, Asselain B, Kunlin A, et al: Inflammatory breast cancer. Determination of prognostic factors by univariate and multivariate analysis. *Cancer* 1987;60:897–902.

210. Chu Am, Wood WC, Doucette JA: Inflammatory breast carcinoma treated by radical radiotherapy. *Cancer* 1980;45: 2730–2737.

211. Costa J, Weber BL, Levine PH, et al: Histopathological features of rapidly progressing breast carcinoma in Tunisia: A study of 94 cases. *Int J Cancer* 1982;30:35–37.

212. Dao TL, McCarthy JD: Treatment of inflammatory carcinoma of the breast. *Surg Gynecol Obstet* 1957;105:289–294.

* 213. Delarue JC, May-Levin F, Mouriesse H, et al: Estrogen and progesterone receptors in clinically inflammatory tumors of the human breast. *Br J Cancer* 1981;44:911–916.

* 214. Droulias CA, Sewell CW, McSweeney MB, et al: Inflammatory carcinoma of the breast: A correlation of clinical

radiologic and pathologic findings. *Ann Surg* 1976;184:217–222.

*215. Ellis DL, Teitelbaum SL: Inflammatory carcinoma of the breast. A pathologic definition. *Cancer* 1974;33:1045–1047.

*216. Fastenberg NA, Martin RG, Buzdar AU, et al: Management of inflammatory carcinoma of the breast. A combined modality approach. *Am J Clin Oncol* 1985;8:134–141.

*217. Haagensen CD: *Diseases of the Breast*, ed 3. Philadelphia, WB Saunders, 1986, pp 808–814.

218. Hagelberg RS, Jolly PC, Anderson RP: Role of surgery in the treatment of inflammatory breast carcinoma. *Am J Surg* 1984;148:125–131.

*219. Harvey HA, Lipton A, Lawrence BV, et al: Estrogen receptor status in inflammatory carcinoma. *J Surg Oncol* 1982;21:42–44.

220. Klotz HH: Uber Mastitis Carcinomatosa Gravidarum et Lactantum. *Halle*. Apr 1869.

*221. Kokal WA, Hill LR, Porudominsky D, et al: Inflammatory breast carcinoma: A distinct entity. *J Surg Oncol* 1985;30:152–155.

222. Krutchik AN, Buzdar Au, Blumenschein GR, et al: Combined chemoimmunotherapy and radiation therapy of inflammatory breast cancer. *J Surg Oncol* 1979;11:325–332.

*223. Lee BJ, Tannenbaum NE: Inflammatory carcinoma of the breast. *Surg Gynecol* 1924;39:580–595.

*224. Leitch A: Peau d'orange in acute mammary carcinoma: Its cause and diagnostic value. *Lancet* 1909;1:861–863.

*225. Levine PH, Steinhorn SC, Ries IG: Inflammatory breast cancer: The experience of the Surveillance, Epidemiology and End Results (SEER) Program. *J Natl Cancer Inst* 1985; 74:291–297.

*226. Lucas FV, Perez-Mesa C: Inflammatory carcinoma of the breast. *Cancer* 1978;41:1595–1605.

*227. McBride CM, Hortobagyi GN: Primary inflammatory carcinoma of the female breast: Staging and treatment possibilities. *Surgery* 1985;98:792–798.

*228. Meyer AC, Dockerty MD, Harrington SW: Inflammatory carcinoma of the breast. *Surg Gynecol Obstet* 1948;87:417–424.

229. Morris DM: Mastectomy in the management of patients with inflammatory breast cancer. *J Surg Oncol* 1983;23:255–258.

230. Nichini FM, Goldman L, Lapayowker MS, et al: Inflammatory carcinoma of the breast in a 12-year-old girl. *Arch Surg* 1972;105:505–508.

231. Noguchi S, Keisuki M, Nishizawa Y, et al: Management of inflammatory carcinoma of the breast with combined modality therapy including intraarterial infusion chemotherapy as an induction therapy. Long-term follow-up results of 28 patients. *Cancer* 1988;61:1483–1491.

232. Nussbaum H, Kagan AR, Gilbert H, et al: Management of inflammatory carcinoma. *Dis Breast* 1977;3:25–28.

*233. Paradiso G, Tommasi S, Brandi M, et al: Cell kinetics and hormonal receptor status in inflammatory breast carcinoma. Comparison with locally advanced disease. *Cancer* 1989;64:1922–1927.

234. Richards FJ, Lewison EF: Inflammatory carcinoma of the breast. *Surg Gynecol Obstet* 1961;113:729.

235. Robbins GF, Shah J, Rosen P, et al: Inflammatory carcinoma of the breast. *Surg Clin North Am* 1974;54:801–810.

236. Rogers CS, Fitts WT: Inflammatory carcinoma of the breast: A critique of therapy. *Surgery* 1956;39:367–370.

237. Salzstein SL: Clinically occult inflammatory carcinoma of the breast. *Cancer* 1974;34:382–388.

238. Sherry MM, Johnson DH, Page DL, et al: Inflammatory carcinoma of the breast. *Am J Med* 1984;79:355–364.

239. Siegel JM: Inflammatory carcinoma of the breast. *Arch Dermatol Syphilol* 1952;66:710–716.

240. Stocks LH, Patternson FM: Inflammatory carcinoma of the breast. *Surg Gynecol Obstet* 1976;143:885–889.

*241. Taylor GW, Metzler A: Inflammatory carcinoma of the breast. *Am J Cancer* 1938;33:33–49.

*242. Treves N: The inoperability of inflammatory carcinoma of the breast. *Surg Gynecol Obstet* 1959;109:240–242.

243. Tschen EH, Apisarnthanarax P: Inflammatory metastatic carcinoma of the breast. *Arch Dermatol* 1981;117:120–121.

244. Zylberberg B, Salat-Baroux J, Ravina JH, et al: Initial chemoimmunotherapy in inflammatory carcinoma of the breast. *Cancer* 1982;49:1537–1543.

### Adenoid Cystic Carcinoma

*245. Anthony PP, James PD: Adenoid cystic carcinoma of the breast: Prevalence, diagnostic criteria, and histogenesis. *J Clin Pathol* 1975;28:647–655.

246. Ahmed A: *Atlas of Ultrastructure of Human Breast Disease*. London, Churchill-Livingstone, 1978, pp 134–138.

*247. Azzopardi JG: *Problems in Breast Pathology*. Philadelphia, WB Saunders, 1979, pp 335–339.

248. Cammoun H, Contessou G, Rouesse J: Les adenocarcinomes cylindromateux du dein. *Ann Pathol* 1972;17:143–154.

249. Caselitz J, Becker J, Seifert G, et al: Coexpression of keratin and vimentin filaments in adenoid cystic carcinoma of salivary glands. *Virchows Archiv A* 1984;403:337–344.

*250. Cavanzo FJ, Taylor HB: Adenoid cystic carcinoma of the breast: An analysis of 21 cases. *Cancer* 1969;24:740–745.

251. Clement PB, Young RH, Azzopardi JG: Collagenous spherulosis of the breast. *Am J Surg Pathol* 1987;11:411–417.

252. Cramer SF, Gnepp DR, Kiehn CL, et al: Sebaceous differentiation in adenoid cystic carcinoma of the parotid gland. *Cancer* 1980;46:1405–1410.

253. D'Ardenne AJ, Kirkpatrick P, Wells CA, et al: Laminin and fibronectin in adenoid cystic carcinomas. *J Clin Pathol* 1986;39:138–144.

*254. Due W, Herbst H, Loy V, et al: Characterization of adenoid cystic carcinoma of the breast by immunohistology. *J Clin Pathol* 1989;42:470–476.

255. Elsner RA: Adenoid cystic carcinoma of the breast: Review of the literature and clinicopathologic study of seven patients. *Pathol Eur* 1970;5:357–364.

256. Foote FW, Stewart FW: A histologic classification of carcinoma of the breast. *Surgery* 1946;19:74–99.

* 257. Friedman BA, Oberman HA: Adenoid cystic carcinoma of the breast. *Am J Clin Pathol* 1970;54:1–14.

258. Galloway JR, Woolner LB, Clagget OT: Adenoid cystic carcinoma of the breast. *Surg Gynecol Obstet* 1966;122:1289–1294.

259. Geschikter CF: *Diseases of the Breast*, ed 2. Philadelphia, JB Lippincott, 1945, pp 421–422.

260. Gould VE, Miller J, Jao W: Ultrastructure of medullary, intraductal, tubular, and adenoid cystic breast carcinomas: Comparative differentiation and basal lamina deposition. *Am J Pathol* 1975;78:401–416.

* 261. Haagensen CD: *Diseases of the Breast*. ed 3. Philadelphia, WB Saunders, 1986, pp 833–842.

* 262. Harris M: Pseudoadenoid cystic carcinoma of the breast. *Arch Pathol Lab Med* 1977;101:307–309.

263. Hjorth S, Magnusson PH, Blomquist P: Adenoid cystic carcinoma of the breast. Report of a case in a male and review of the literature. *Acta Clin Scand* 1977;143:155–158.

264. Hopkins GB, Tullis RH: Adenoid cystic carcinoma of the breast. *Calif Med* 1972;117:9–11.

265. Hoshino M, Yamamoto I: Ultrastructure of adenoid cystic carcinoma. *Cancer* 1970;25:186–198.

266. Iwamoto T, Jakobiec FA: A comparative ultrastructural study of normal lacrimal gland and its epithelial tumors. *Hum Pathol* 1982;13:916–924.

267. Kern WH: Morphologic and clinical aspects of estrogen receptors in carcinoma of the breast. *J Clin Pathol* 1986;39:138–144.

* 268. Koss LG, Brannan CD, Ashikari R: Histologic and ultrastructural features of adenoid cystic carcinoma of the breast. *Cancer* 1970;26:1271–1279.

* 269. Lamovec J, Us-Krasovec M, Zidar A, et al: Adenoid cystic carcinoma of the breast: A histologic, cytologic, and immunohistochemical study. *Sem Diagn Pathol* 1989;6:153–164.

270. Lawrence JB, Mazur MT: Adenoid cystic carcinoma: A comparative study of tumors in salivary gland, breast, lung, and cervix. *Hum Pathol* 1982;13:916–924.

271. Lim SK, Kovi J, Warner OG: Adenoid cystic carcinoma of breast with metastasis: A case report and review of the literature. *J Natl Med Assoc* 1971;71:329–330.

272. Lusted D: Structural and growth patterns of adenoid cystic carcinoma of the breast. *Am J Clin Pathol* 1970;54:419–425.

273. Mazur MT, Battifora HA: Adenoid cystic carcinoma of the uterine cervix: Ultrastructure, immunofluorescence, and criteria for diagnosis. *Am J Clin Pathol* 1982;77:494–500.

274. Nayer HR: Cylindroma of the breast with pulmonary metastases. *Chest* 1957;31:324–327.

275. O'Kell RT: Adenoid cystic carcinoma of the breast. *Missouri Med* 1964;61:855–858.

276. Orenstein JM, Dardick I, van Nostrand AWP: Ultrastructural similarities of adenoid cystic carcinoma and pleomorphic adenoma. *Histopathology* 1985;9:623–638.

277. Perzin KH, Gullane P, Clairmont AC: Adenoid cystic carcinoma arising in salivary glands: A correlation of histologic features and clinical course. *Cancer* 1978;42:265–282.

* 278. Peters GN, Wolff M: Adenoid cystic carcinoma of the breast: Report of 11 new cases: Review of the literature and discussion of biological behavior. *Cancer* 1979;52:1752–1760.

* 279. Qizilbash A, Patterson MC, Oliviera KF: Adenoid cystic carcinoma of the breast: Light and electron microscopy and a brief review of the literature. *Arch Pathol Lab Med* 1977;101:302–306.

* 280. Ro JY, Silva EG, Gallagher HS: Adenoid cystic carcinoma of the breast. *Hum Pathol* 1987;18:1276–1281.

* 281. Rosen PP: Adenoid cystic carcinoma of the breast. A morphologically heterogenoeus neoplasm. *Pathol Annu* 1989;24(2):237–254.

282. Sumpio BE, Jennings TA, Sullivan PD, et al: Adenoid cystic carcinoma of the breast. Data from the Connecticut Tumor Registry and a review of the literature. *Ann Surg* 1987;205:295–301.

* 283. Szanto PA, Luna MA, Tortoledo ME, et al: Histologic grading of adenoid cystic carcinoma of the salivary glands. *Cancer* 1984;54:1062–1069.

* 284. Tavassoli FA, Norris HJ: Mammary adenoid cystic carcinoma with sebaceous differentiation. A morphologic study of the cell types. *Arch Pathol Lab Med* 1986;110:1045–1053.

285. Verani RR, van der Bel-Kahn J: Mammary adenoid cystic carcinoma with unusual features. *Am J Clin Pathol* 1973;59:653–658.

* 286. Wells CA, Nicoll S, Ferguson DJP: Adenoid cystic carcinoma of the breast: A case with axillary lymph node metastasis. *Histopathology* 1986;10:415–424.

287. Wilson WB, Spell JP: Adenoid cystic carcinoma of breast: A case with recurrence and regional metastasis. *Ann Surg* 1967;166:861–864.

288. Woyke S, Domogala W, Olszewski W: Fine structure of mammary adenoid cystic carcinoma. *Pol Med J* 1970;9:1140–1148.

* 289. Zaloudek C, Oertel YC, Orenstein JM: Adenoid cystic carcinoma of the breast. *Am J Clin Pathol* 1984;81:297–307.


### Metastatic Carcinoma


290. Ackerman LV, Taylor HB: Seminars on lesions of the breast, in *Proceedings of the American Society of Pathologists*. Chicago, 1956, pp 10–11.

* 291. Azzopardi JG, Eusebi V: Melanocytic colonization or pigmentation of breast carcinoma. *Histopathology* 1977;1:21–30.

292. Bardram L, Jensen NB, Pedersen NT: An unusual manifestation of carcinoma of the stomach. *Acta Chir Scand* 1982;148:389–392.

293. Barker JNWN, Girling AC: A case of metastatic malignant melanoma masquerading as disseminating mammary carcinoma. *Histopathology* 1989;14:219–221.

* 294. Bohman LG, Bassett LW, Gold RH, et al: Breast metastases from extramammary malignancies. *Radiology* 1982;144:309–312.

* 295. Charache H: Metastatic tumors in the breast. *Ann Surg* 1942;115:47–50.

* 296. Charache H: Metastatic tumors in the breast. *Surgery* 1953;33:385–390.
297. Chodoff RJ: Solitary breast metastasis from carcinoid of the ileum. *Am J Surg* 1965;109:814–815.
298. Cormier WJ, Gaffey TA, Welch JM, et al: Linitis plastica caused by metastatic lobular carcinoma of the breast. *Mayo Clin Proc* 1980;55:747–753.
299. Dawson EK: Metastatic tumour of the breast, with report of a case. *J Pathol Bacteriol* 1936;43:53–60.
* 300. Di Bonito L, Luchi M, Giarelli L, et al: Metastatic tumors to the female breast. An autopsy study of 12 cases. *Pathol Res Pract* 1991;187:432–436.
301. Gatch WD: A melanoma, apparently primary in the breast. *Arch Surg* 1956;73:266–268.
* 302. Hajdu S, Urban JA: Cancers metastatic to the breast. *Cancer* 1972;20:1691–1696.
303. Harrist T, Kalisher L: Breast metastasis: An unusual manifestation of a malignant carcinoid tumor. *Cancer* 1977;40:3102–3106.
* 304. Harwood TR: Metasatic carcinoma to the breast. *JAMA* 1971;218:97.
305. Ibach JR Jr: Carcinoma of the ovary metastatic to the breast. *Arch Surg* 1964;88:410–414.
306. Jacoby R, Roses DF, Valensi Q: Carcinoma of the breast metastatic to the skin and simulating malignant melanoma, in Ackerman AB (ed): *Pathology of Malignant Melanoma*. Chicago, Yearbook Medical Publishers Inc, 1981, pp 263–267.
307. Kelly C, Henderson D, Corris P: Breast lumps. Rare presentation of oat-cell carcinoma of lung. *J Clin Pathol* 1986;24:97–102.
308. Laifer S, Buscema J, Parmley TH, et al: Ovarian cancer metastatic to the breast. *Gynecol Oncol* 1986;24:97–102.
309. Lo MC, Chomat B, Rubenstone AI: Metastatic prostatic adenocarcinoma of the male breast. *Urol* 1978;11:641–646.
* 310. McCrea ES, Johnston C, Haney PJ: Metastases to the breast. *AJR* 1983;141:685–690.
* 311. McIntosh IH, Hooper AA, Millis RR, et al: Metastatic carcinoma within the breast. *Clin Oncol* 1976;2:393–401.
* 312. Moncada R, Cooper RA, Garces M, et al: Calcified metastases from malignant ovarian neoplasm. *Radiology* 1974;113:31–35.
313. Nance FC, MacVaugh H III, Fitts WT Jr: Metastatic tumor to the breast simulating bilateral primary inflammatory carcinoma. *Am J Surg* 1966;112:932–935.
* 314. Nielsen M, Andersen JA, Henriksen FW, et al: Metastases to the breast from extramammary carcinoma. *Acta Pathol Microbiol Scand* 1981;89:251–256.
* 315. Paulus DD, Libshitz HI: Metastasis to the breast. *Radiol Clin North Am* 1982;20:561–568.
316. Pressman PI: Malignant melanoma and the breast. *Cancer* 1973;31:784–788.
317. Pribe WA: Prostatic metastasis to the breast and the role of estrogens. *J Urol* 1963;11:891–899.
* 318. Pribe WA, Ockuly EA: Prostatic metastasis to the breast and the role of estrogens: Case report and review. *J Am Geriatr Soc* 1963;11:891–898.
319. Royen PM, Ziter FMH: Ovarian carcinoma metastatic to the breast. *Br J Radiol* 1974;47:354–357.
* 320. Sandison AT: Metastatic tumors in the breast. *Br J Surg* 1959;47:54–58.
321. Schurch W, Lamoureux E, Lefebvre R, et al: Solitary breast metastasis: First manifestation of an occult carcinoid in the ileum. *Virchows Arch A Anat and Histol* 1980;386:117–124.
* 322. Silverman EM, Oberman HA: Metastatic neoplasms in the breast. *Surg Gynecol Obstet* 1974;138:26–28.
323. Speert H, Greeley AV: Cervical cancer with metastasis to the breast. *Am J Obstet Gynecol* 1948;55:894–896.
324. Stephenson SE, Boyd BF: Malignant melanoma of the breast. *Am J Surg* 1959;97:232–235.
* 325. Toombs BD, Kalisher L: Metastatic disease to the breast. Clinical pathologic and radiographic features. *AJR* 1977;129:673–676.
326. Truesdale BH, Johnson RD, Evins SO: Carcinoma of bladder metastatic to breast. *Urol* 1979;13:430–431.

# 11

# Biphasic Tumors



Biphasic tumors of the breast are composed of various combinations of proliferating epithelial and stromal elements. Depending on the benign or malignant nature of each element, various possible combinations may occur. Three major categories of biphasic tumors occur, two of which—fibroadenoma and cystosarcoma phyllodes—are well recognized. In fibroadenoma, both the epithelial and the mesenchymal elements are benign. In cystosarcoma phyllodes, the epithelial component is benign, but the stroma is hypercellular or sarcomatous, and sometimes overtly malignant. Carcinosarcoma, a tumor in which both components are malignant, has not been well defined as an entity and disagreements persist on the type of breast lesion that deserves this designation.

## FIBROADENOMA

Fibroadenoma (FA) is the third most common lesion of the breast following fibrocystic changes and carcinoma. In his study of entire breasts, Cheattle (14) reported fibroadenomas, some barely visible to the naked eye, in 25% of all normal breasts examined microscopically at post mortem. In 225 autopsies, Frantz et al (26) found 21 fibroadenomas (9% of the cases), seven of which were microscopic lesions. Fibroadenomas in general (27), and the juvenile variant in particular (4), appear to be more prevalent in black patients.

Fibroadenomas constitute a mild risk factor for subsequent development of carcinoma. In Oliver and Major's (69) review of 175 patients with fibroadenoma followed from 4 to 25 years, only one developed carcinoma. Semb (83) did not find even a single case of subsequent cancer among the 142 patients with fibroadenoma followed for 4 to 27 years.

More recently, however, Kodlin et al (44) followed 849 women with fibroadenomas. Sixteen of these women developed carcinoma during the follow-up period when only 2.3 were expected to do so in the general population. This study contradicts current belief that fibroadenomas have only a low significance as a risk factor (See Chapter 2).

### Clinical Features

Fibroadenoma occurs most often in women of childbearing age; it is the most frequently observed neoplasm in women under age 25 (14). In Oliver and Major's (69) review of 400 fibroadenomas, the highest incidence in white women was observed between ages 20 and 24; the incidence in blacks reached a peak between 15 and 19 years of age. Geschickter (28) found an average age of 20 to 25 years in his review of 500 examples of fibroadenoma. Giacomelli and Re (30) reported a mean age of 31 years for those with the intracanalicular pattern, and a mean age of 21 for

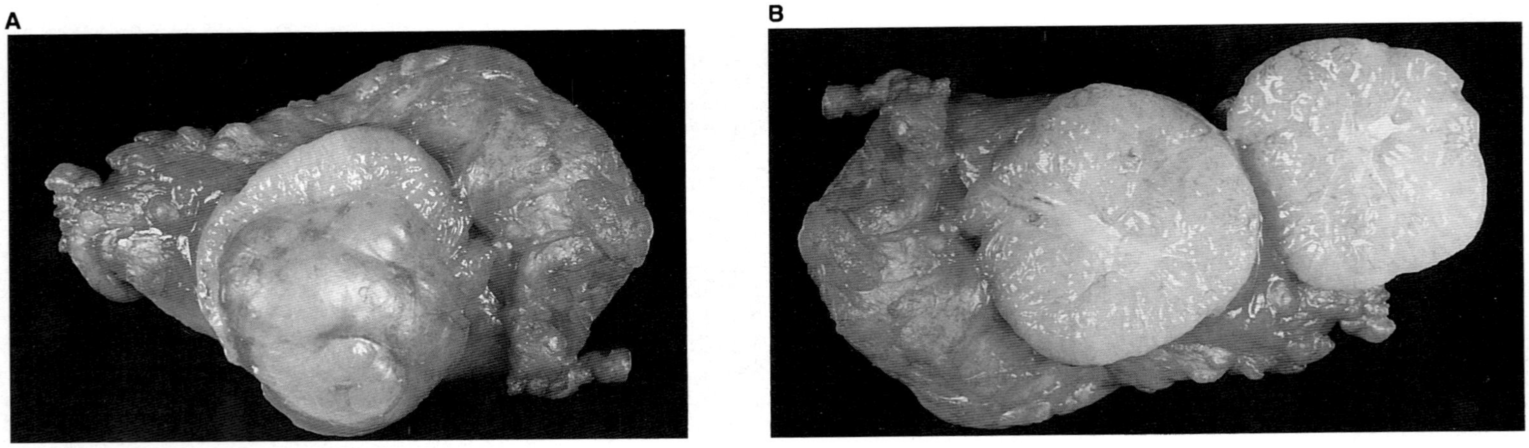

**Figure 11.1** (a) The bosselated appearance of the nodule is typical of fibroadenomas. (b) The bulging cut surface of the lesion shows a uniformly solid tumor.

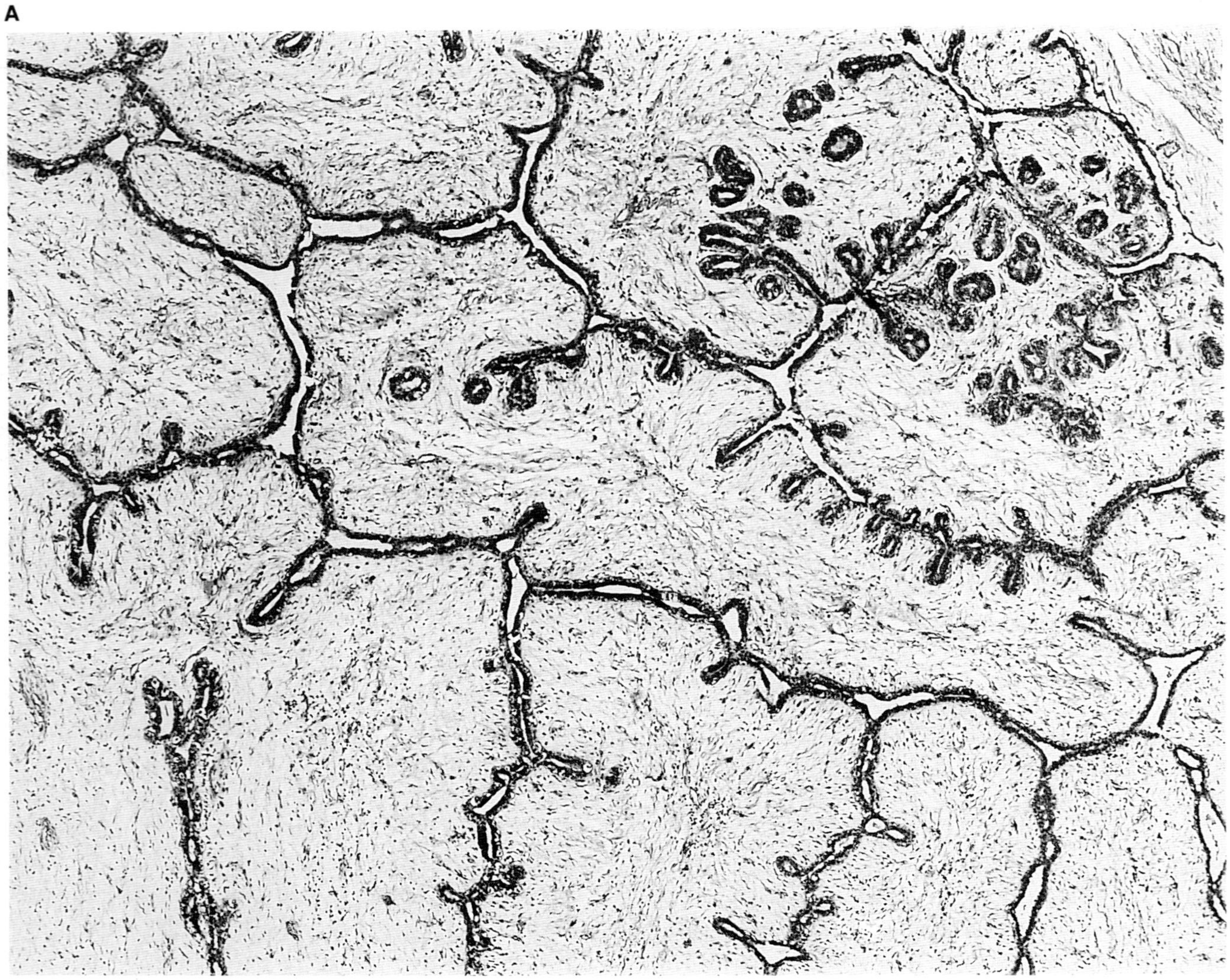

**Figure 11.2(a)** Fibroadenoma, intracanalicular type. Note the compressed ductal structures. (H&E, X600)

33 patients with the pericanalicular variant of fibroadenoma in a series of 496 patients from Milan. Only 2.5% of patients with fibroadenomas in Haagensen's experience (35) were postmenopausal; their average age was 33.9 years.

The development of fibroadenoma is believed to be a result of the unopposed estrogenic influence on susceptible tissue (8,28,47,69). The occurrence in young women, the high levels of urinary estrogen in the absence of progesterone, and the high estrogen content in occasional cases (8,54) support this contention. Some fibroadenomas show a slight increase in size during pregnancy; this minimal alteration is followed by regression following parturition.

Generally presenting as a solitary neoplasm, multiple fibroadenomas may develop simultaneously or successively in one or both breasts. In Haagensen's (35) series of 402 patients, 16% had more than one lesion. The incidence of multiplicity in three other series was 7% (28,83) and 15.7% (69). Fibroadenoma presents as a painless small nodule which grows slowly up to 2 to 3 cm after which there is an arrest in further growth in most cases. Sometimes however, they assume massive proportions (over 10 cm) (8,16, 53,71,90). These massive tumors generally occur in adolescent females, may become as large as 19 cm (35) and are seen more frequently in blacks. Five of the seven patients in Haagensen's experience were black. The term giant fibroadenoma would be appropriate for these tumors based on their size only. In some adolescent girls, there is a tendency for the development of numerous successive fibroadenomas in both breasts. Each excision may be followed by the development of one or more new ones.

B

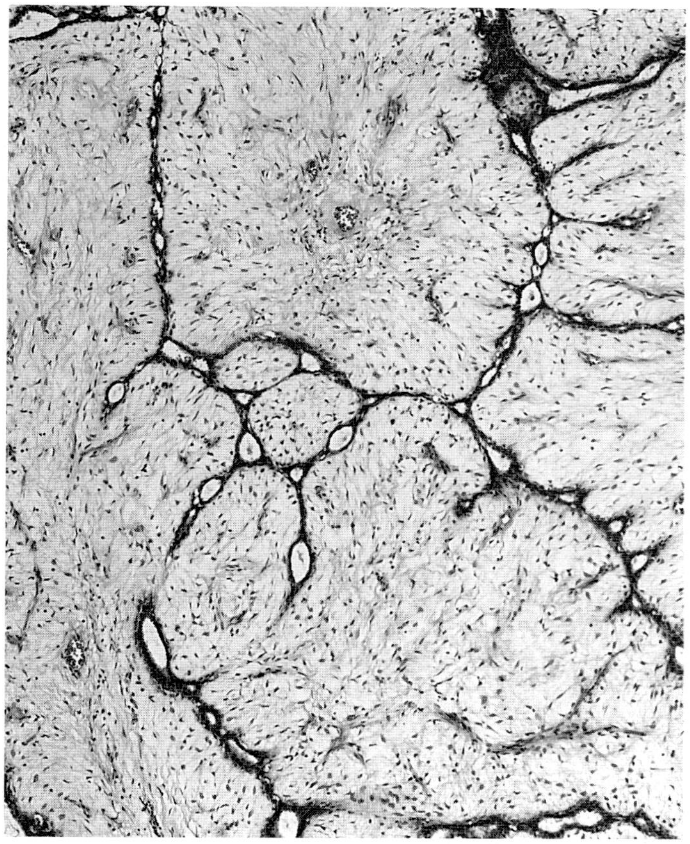

**Figure 11.2(b)** Fibroadenoma, intracanalicular type. The stromal cells exhibit a radial growth with their long axis perpendicular to the epithelial elements. (H&E, X75)

## Gross Pathology

Characteristically, fibroadenoma is sharply demarcated from surrounding tissue (Fig. 11.1) and often appears encapsulated. It is generally 2 to 3 cm in size but may become massive. Cut surface of the tumor is bulging, firm, and white; this appearance varies, however, depending of the amount of hyalinization and myxoid change. Cysts, apparent to the naked eye, are not a characteristic feature of fibroadenomas, but they are present rarely.

## Microscopic Features

Fibroadenoma consists of a combined proliferation of epithelial and mesenchymal elements. The stroma proliferates around tubular (pericanalicular) or compressed cleft-like (intracanalicular) ducts. In the pericanalicular pattern, there is a random or concentric proliferation of the stromal elements around the epithelial structures; silver stains demonstrate the random or concentric deposition of reticulin around the ducts. In the intracanalicular pattern (Fig. 11.2), the stroma exhibits a radial growth with deposition of reticulin fibers perpendicular to the epithelial elements on silver stain. The two patterns do coexist within some lesions but one often dominates. The ducts are generally lined by two cell layers, a luminal epithelial cell layer and an underlying layer of myoepithelial cells (Fig. 11.3). A pushing growth margin is observed in a majority of fibroadenomas, but focal irregularities are seen in some cases. A well-formed capsule is seen around some tumors (Fig. 11.4). Fibroadenomas are generally within breast paren-

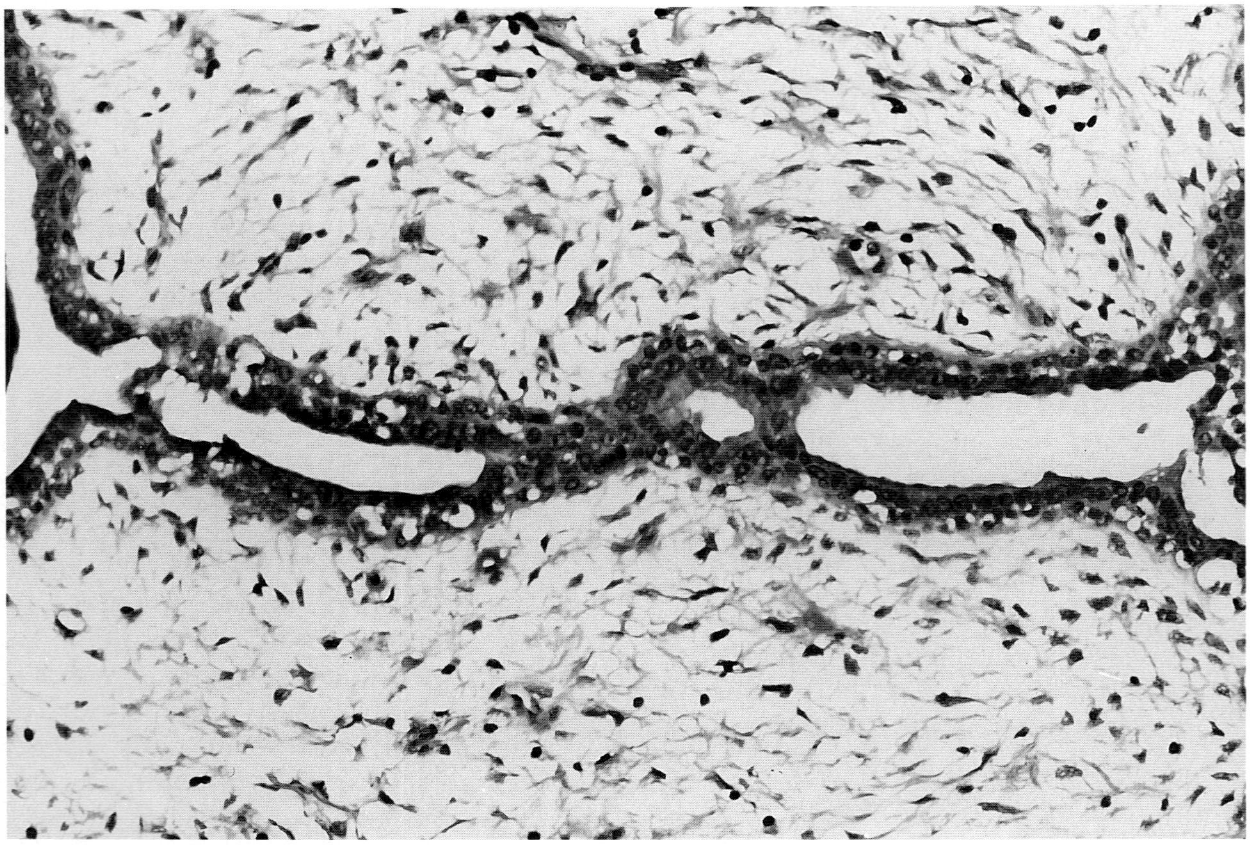

**Figure 11.3** Fibroadenoma, intracanalicular type. Note the presence of epithelial and myoepithelial cell layers lining the slit-like ductal spaces. (H&E, X300)

chyma, but there is a single case in the AFIP files of a fibroadenoma that presented as a subareolar mass; the fibroadenoma was located within one of the lactiferous ducts (Fig. 11.5).

A variety of metaplastic changes and differentiations occur in the epithelium and the stroma. The epithelial cells may rarely show squamous metaplasia (80). In a review of 100 consecutive fibroadenomas at AFIP, I found apocrine metaplasia in 11% of the intracanalicular and 18% of the pericanalicular types. Oberman and French (67) noted apocrine change in 35% of their fibroadenomas. Pink cell (oncocytic metaplasia) was also noted by Archer and Omar (3). Azzopardi (5) found apocrine metaplasia in 14% of fibroadenomas. The epithelium becomes attenuated and atrophic in elderly women. Neuroendocrine cells have been identified in several fibroadenomas (5,82, 98).

The stromal component may show focal or diffuse hypercellularity, extensive myxoid or mucinous (46) change (Fig. 11.6) transforming the tumor to a gelatinous nodule, or hyalinization (Fig. 11.7); calcification is observed in the hyalinized lesions. Among our recent consultation cases at AFIP, several examples of fibroadenoma with myxoid stroma occurring in women less than 40 years of age were associated with the development of multiple recurrences. The myxoid change was often patchy in nature and the original tumor had a lobulated margin with mildly increased focal cellularity, but not of a degree to even raise the possibility of a cystosarcoma phyllodes. The recurrent lesions often had similar morphology with focal cellularity of a mild degree. Myxoid mammary fibroadenomas have been observed in some patients suffering from a complex of cardiac and cutaneous myxomas, spotty pigmentation and endocrine overactivity (11,12). Therefore, it would be prudent to inquire about other components of this complex when a patient presents with myxoid fibroadenomas. In elderly women, fibroadenomas show lesser degrees of stromal cellularity and increased hyalinization. Atypical and bizarre multinucleated giant cells are occasionally identified in the stroma (7,64,78). These may be present focally or diffusely, but they are benign and have no prognostic significance. Adipose tissue or fatty change is rarely found in the stroma (50). Chondroid and osseous metaplasia also occur (89). Bone was identified in 1.1% of fibroade-

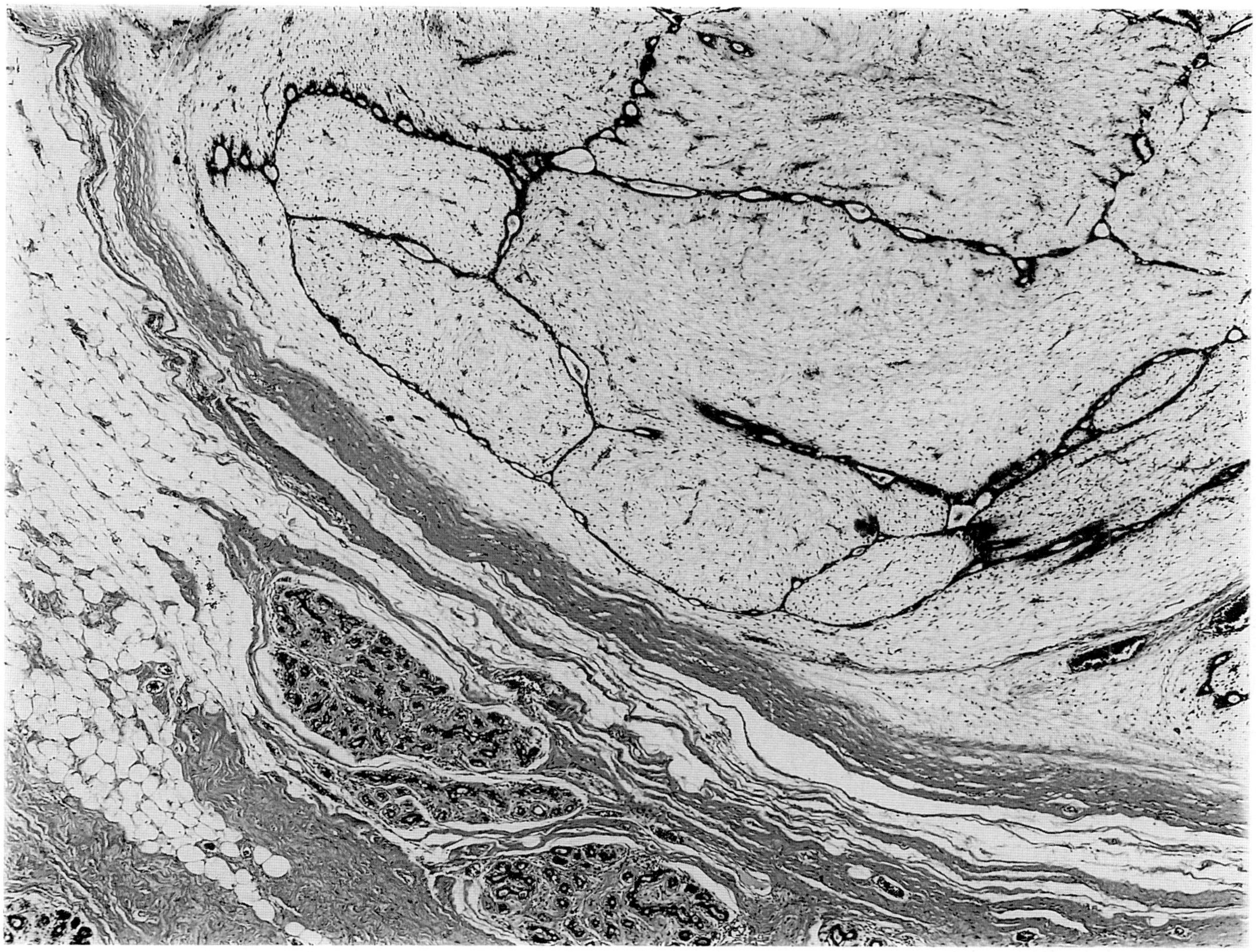

**Figure 11.4** Fibroadenoma, intracanalicular type. A dense capsule surrounds the tumcr. (H&E, X140)

nomas reviewed by Spagnola and Shilkin (85). One of the less common stromal alterations is smooth muscle metaplasia (5,34,51,77). Only eight fibroadenomas with smooth muscle metaplasia were identified in the AFIP files over the past ten years, but one of these was particularly extensive with replacement of almost two-thirds of the stroma by the metaplastic cells (Fig. 11.8). As a rule, elastic tissue is not found in the stroma except when it remains as residue from the interlobular connective tissue and is incorporated into a developing fibroadenoma during the coalescence of fibroadenomatous nodules (see origin of fibroadenoma). Sarcoma developing in fibroadenoma is extremely rare and of a highly aggressive nature when it occurs (79). Such a tumor is distinguished from a cystosarcoma phyllodes by the absence of leaf-like processes in the biphasic component of the lesion.

Epithelial prominence, proliferative changes, atypia, and infarction are observed in fibroadenomas. Some lesions show predominance of the epithelial component in the form of adenosis which may be confused with an invasive carcinoma. The presence of myoepithelial cells around some of the tubules and a concentrically oriented collagen or basement membrane around other tubules identifies them as benign (Fig. 11.9). The epithelium lining the ducts may show various degrees of hyperplasia with or without atypia. As a rule, epithelial hyperplasias when confined to fibroadenomas are believed to be of no significant consequence but do require follow-up when atypia is present (58).

Sometimes the myoepithelial (ME) cells become prominent or hyperplastic. They may assume an unusually myoid appearance and give the impression of blending with the surrounding stromal cells. Of-

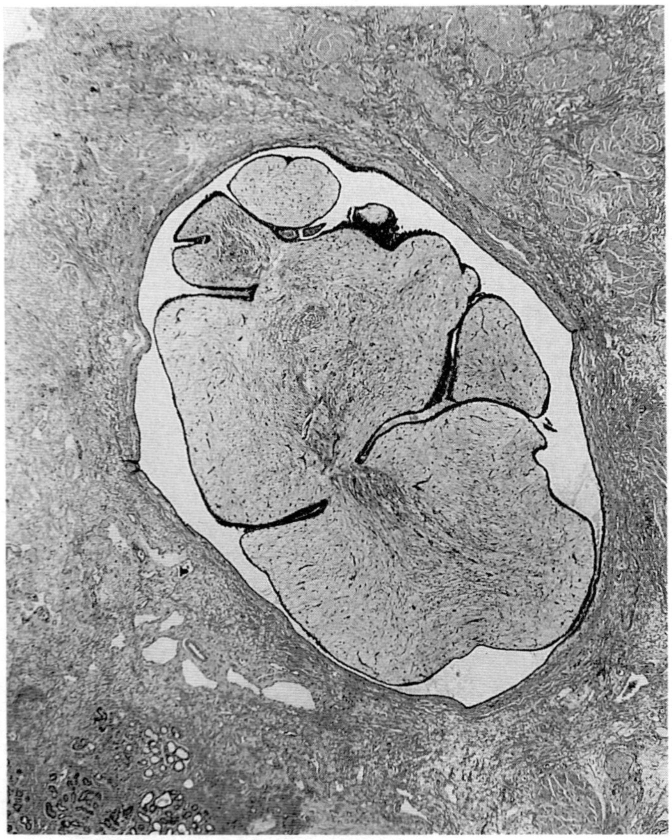

**Figure 11.5** Subareolar fibroadenoma. This tumor presented as a subareolar nodule and was located within a distended lactiferous duct. (H&E, X25)

ten, a basement membrane can be seen separating the ME cells from the surrounding stromal cells, however. The myoid transformation and proliferation of the ME cells should not be confused with smooth muscle metaplasia which takes place within the stromal component.

Rarely, metaplastic neuroendocrine cells may also develop and proliferate, assuming a pattern similar to lobular neoplasia (5,82,98,101). The neuroendocrine cells are round or polygonal with round, centrally located nuclei and sharp cytoplasmic margins. The cytoplasm appears clear, pale or finely granular. They proliferate in solid or a pagetoid fashion. The proliferating cells bud toward the stroma rather than into the lumens. The proliferating cells may also form tubular arrangements; these tubules are lined by a single layer of neuroendocrine-type cells in contrast to the two cell types observed in the ductal structures of the breast. Argyrophilia requiring more than one type of silver impregnation method for its demonstration, dense core granules or both have been demonstrated in these cells (98). Whether these proliferating cells reflect hyperplasia or neoplasia is not established at this time.

Fibrocystic changes, adenosis, and sclerosing adenosis (Fig. 11.10) do occur in fibroadenomas as well. Less than 10% of 100 consecutive tumors reviewed by Azzopardi had sclerosing adenosis (5); this feature was conspicuous in 8% of 100 consecutive fibroadenomas I reviewed at AFIP.

Occasionally, spontaneous infarction occurs during pregnancy and lactation (18,35,38,88). Thrombosed vessels may be seen in the areas of infarction. The possibility that the thrombosis may be secondary to the infarction rather than its cause cannot be excluded, however. In Haagensen's (35) review of 1,000 fibroadenomas, the incidence of spontaneous infarction was 0.5% (5 of 1,000 cases), three of the patients were pregnant or lactating. Infarction in this setting has been attributed to relative vascular insufficiency during phases of increased metabolic activity and nutritional requirement (52). Two cases of infarction associated with thrombo-occlusive vascular changes in the feeding vessels have been documented by Newman and Kahn (62).

## Hormonal and Drug Influences

Minor alterations in the epithelial and stromal cells of fibroadenoma have been reported during the menstrual cycle. Although not as well developed, the changes parallel but lag behind changes that occur in the surrounding breast. Geschikter et al (28) found variation in size with menstrual cycle to be rare, but enlargement with pregnancy was not uncommon in their experience. The most distinctive changes are observed in the myoepithelial cells during the menstrual phase. They become highly vacuolated while the epithelial cells show some swelling and the stroma becomes edematous. Secretory changes of pregnancy are also reflected in fibroadenomas, but again the changes are generally not as fully developed as in the adjacent breast tissue.

Reports on the effect of oral contraceptives on fibroadenomas are few. Neither Taylor (86) nor Fechner (23) found any difference in the incidence of fibroadenoma, the patient's age, or the tumor pathology between patients taking oral contraceptive hormones and those not taking contraceptive hormones. The epithelial proliferation and predominance re-

A B

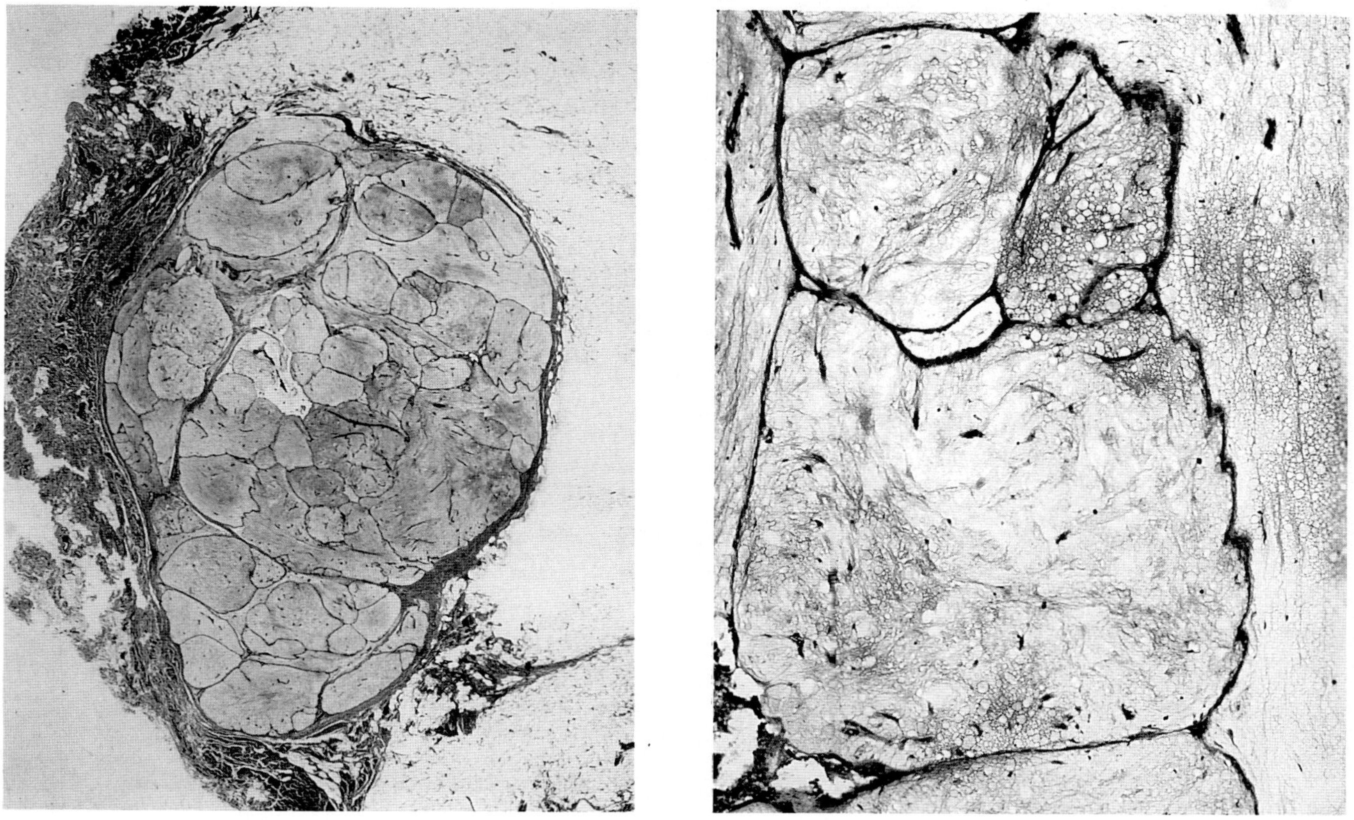

**Figure 11.6** Fibroadenoma with myxoid stromal change. (a&b) The stroma appears particularly hypocellular. (H&E, (a) X10; (b) X75)

ported earlier by Brown (10) and Goldenberg et al (33) in fibroadenomas removed from patients on oral contraceptive steroids may have been fortuitous. Neither increased atypical epithelial proliferation (49), nor differences in the rate of cellular proliferation (57) have been observed in association with the use of oral contraceptive hormones. Azzopardi (5) has observed secretory changes in the epithelial component of fibroadenomas associated with the use of large doses of contraceptive hormones, particularly in patients on Depo-Provera® (medroxy progesterone).

The hormonal milieu in which fibroadenoma develops is of interest. Martin et al (54) found higher than normal levels of plasma estradiol in 84 patients with fibroadenoma but observed that plasma progesterone levels were significantly lower. They also demonstrated high concentration of estrogen-binding sites in 35 of 84 patients.

A single case of bilateral massive fibroadenomatoid hyperplasia in a 69-year-old man, after using spironolactone for four years, has been reported (63).

## Differential Diagnosis

Fibroadenoma should be distinguished from cystosarcoma phyllodes (CP). The typical cystosarcoma phyllodes has leaf-like processes projecting into cystic spaces and a densely cellular stroma. There are many borderline lesions with only minimal and localized areas of cellularity. If the lesion lacks or has rare and poorly-formed leaf-like processes, and the stroma shows minimally increased cellularity, the designation of cellular fibroadenoma would be appropriate. If the stroma is hypocellular or of the degree of cellularity expected in a typical fibroadenoma but the lesion contains well-formed leaf-like processes, the term fibroadenoma phyllodes (Fig. 11.11), to convey the leafy growth pattern, would be suitable. Squamous, chondroid, and osseous metaplasia occur more frequently in cystosarcomas, and their presence would favor this diagnosis (Table 11.1). As a rule, in borderline lesions, the more conservative diagnosis

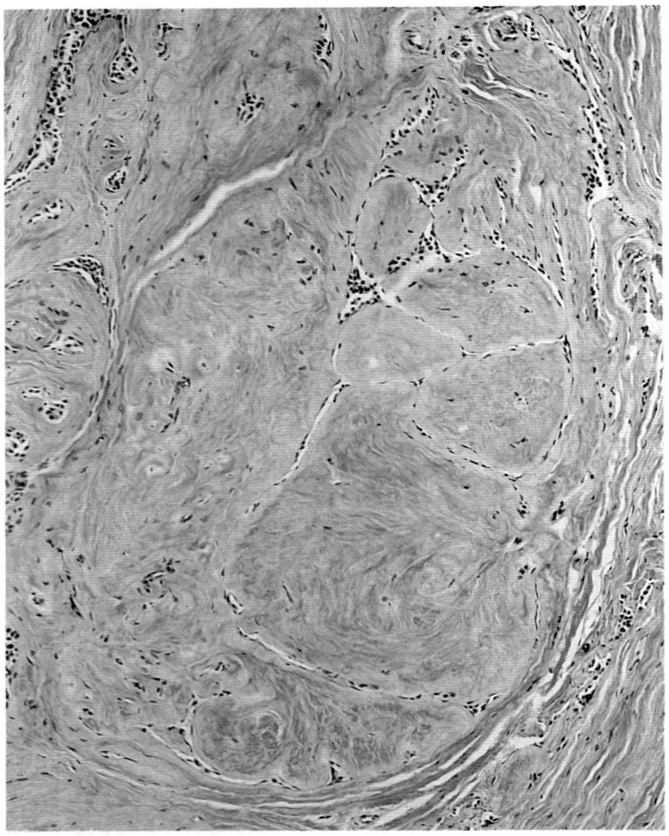

**Figure 11.7** Hyalinized fibroadenoma. Extensive hyalinization is generally observed in fibroadenomas from older women and is associated with atrophy of the epithelial elements. (H&E, X100)

of fibroadenoma is favored particularly when the patient is less than 15 years of age.

Distinction from tubular adenoma is easy because of the abundant stromal component of fibroadenomas. Frequently, however, we see fibroadenomas that have a minor component of a tubular adenoma, or tubular adenomas with focal fibroadenomatous features; in such cases, the diagnosis is based on the dominant component with a comment regarding the other element. If both components are equally represented or prominent, then the designation of a combined tubular-fibroadenoma (Fig. 11.12) would be appropriate.

## Juvenile Fibroadenoma

Fibroadenoma is the most common mammary lesion in the adolescent female (17,22,66,81). In about 7% of adolescent females (ages 10 to 20) with fibroadenoma, the tumor is characterized by rapid growth, massive size, stretching of the overlying skin and dilatation of superficial veins. Juvenile fibroadenomas may grow so rapidly that the involved breast may double in size within a month (42) and may assume giant proportions (20,39,61,84). All 21 patients in Fekete et al's series (24) were black females. They ranged in age from 10 to 39 years with a median of 15 years. Thirteen of these patients presented with solitary lesions while eight had successive and multiple lesions. Microscopically, these tumors often, but not exclusively, display a pericanalicular growth pattern (Fig. 11.13), with numerous irregularly proliferating duct-like and tubular structures. The stroma is generally dense and more cellular than the adult type (21,24,75). Intracanalicular stromal proliferation, myxoid degeneration and metaplastic changes may occur but are generally rare and focal when present.

Juvenile fibroadenomas often display an epithelial hyperplasia with irregular tufts overlying a stratified epithelium similar to that seen in gynecomastia (Fig. 11.14b). Other patterns of hyperplasia may also occur less frequently (Fig. 11.14). Epithelial hyperplasia in juvenile fibroadenoma, when of a borderline nature, should be interpreted conservatively. Follow-up of these patients, in the form of annual examination of the breasts by palpation, should be advised when the proliferation is atypical in nature.

There is no histologic difference between those occurring as solitary or multiple lesions, or between lesions occurring in patients younger and older than age 20 (24). Designated as juvenile fibroadenoma, these tumors should be distinguished from juvenile hypertrophy and cystosarcoma phyllodes. In juvenile hypertrophy, there is a diffuse enlargement of the entire breast; discrete palpable masses are absent. Cystosarcoma phyllodes has a more cellular stroma and leaf-like processes, rarely displays a prominent pericanalicular growth pattern, and occurs in an older age group. It should be emphasized that a majority of fibroadenomas in adolescent females are of the adult type.

## Fibroadenoma Variant

Fibroadenoma variant has a highly collagenous and cellular stroma which also grows in a pericanalicular pattern; the epithelial cells show an increased nuclear/cytoplasmic (N/C) ratio and increased vesicularity

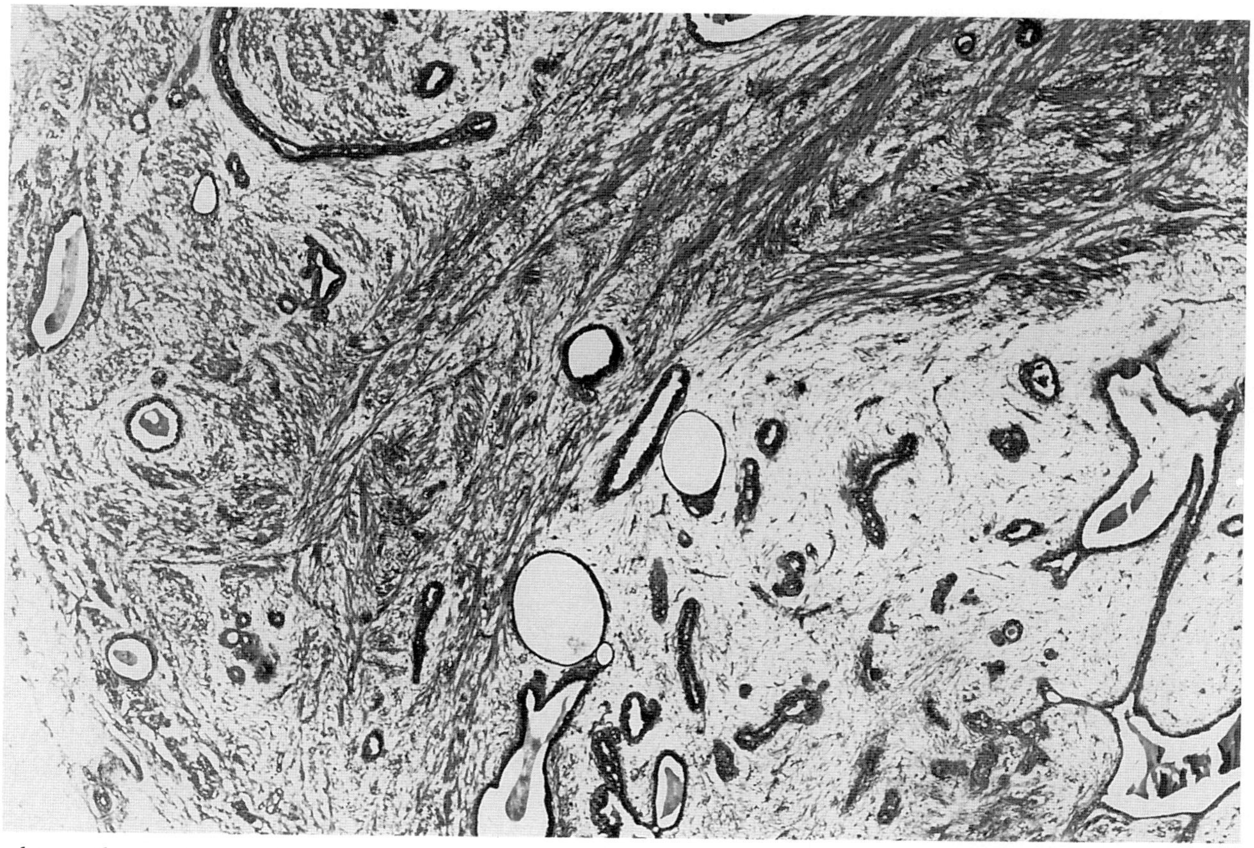

**Figure 11.8** Stromal smooth muscle metaplasia. Abundant bundles of smooth muscle replaced a prominent portion of this fibroadenoma. (H&E, X120)

of the nuclei (5). The tumor size and the average age of the patient with fibroadenoma variant are similar to that of regular fibroadenoma.

## Treatment

Fibroadenomas are easily shelled out and do not recur except for the occasional patients who have a predisposition for development of multiple fibroadenomas. As noted before, several fibroadenomas with myxoid stroma occurring in young women developed multiple recurrences and the recurrent tumor occasionally had a more cellular stroma. Therefore, follow-up of patients whose neoplasms demonstrate a myxoid stroma, whether patchy or diffuse, is advised.

## Carcinoma Arising in a Fibroadenoma

Carcinoma arising in a fibroadenoma is rare and should be distinguished from secondary involvement of a fibroadenoma by an invasive carcinoma from the adjacent breast. At least 225 carcinomas involving a fibroadenoma have been reported (72,91–113). Over half of the carcinomas were confined to the fibroadenoma. The presence of carcinoma in situ (CIS) within fibroadenomas is associated with in situ carcinoma in the adjacent breast tissue in 21% of the cases (96). The age range of the patients varies from 15 to 86 years. The average age of women with carcinoma arising in a fibroadenoma is 43 years, or 20 years older than the peak incidence of fibroadenoma in the general female population (97).

Detailed histologic descriptions were provided on 209 of the 225 reported cases. Lobular neoplasia (LN)/lobular carcinoma in situ (LCIS) was the most common lesion (Fig. 11.15) found in more than 50% of the tumors (126 cases), followed by 59 examples of in situ ductal carcinoma (Figs. 11.16 and 11.17). In situ ductal and lobular carcinoma coexist in about 5% of the cases. Atypical intraductal hyperplasia also occurs in fibroadenomas (Fig. 11.18). A variety of pure or combined invasive carcinomas, including a squamous carcinoma, were present in the remaining cases. We have even seen a small colloid carcinoma

A

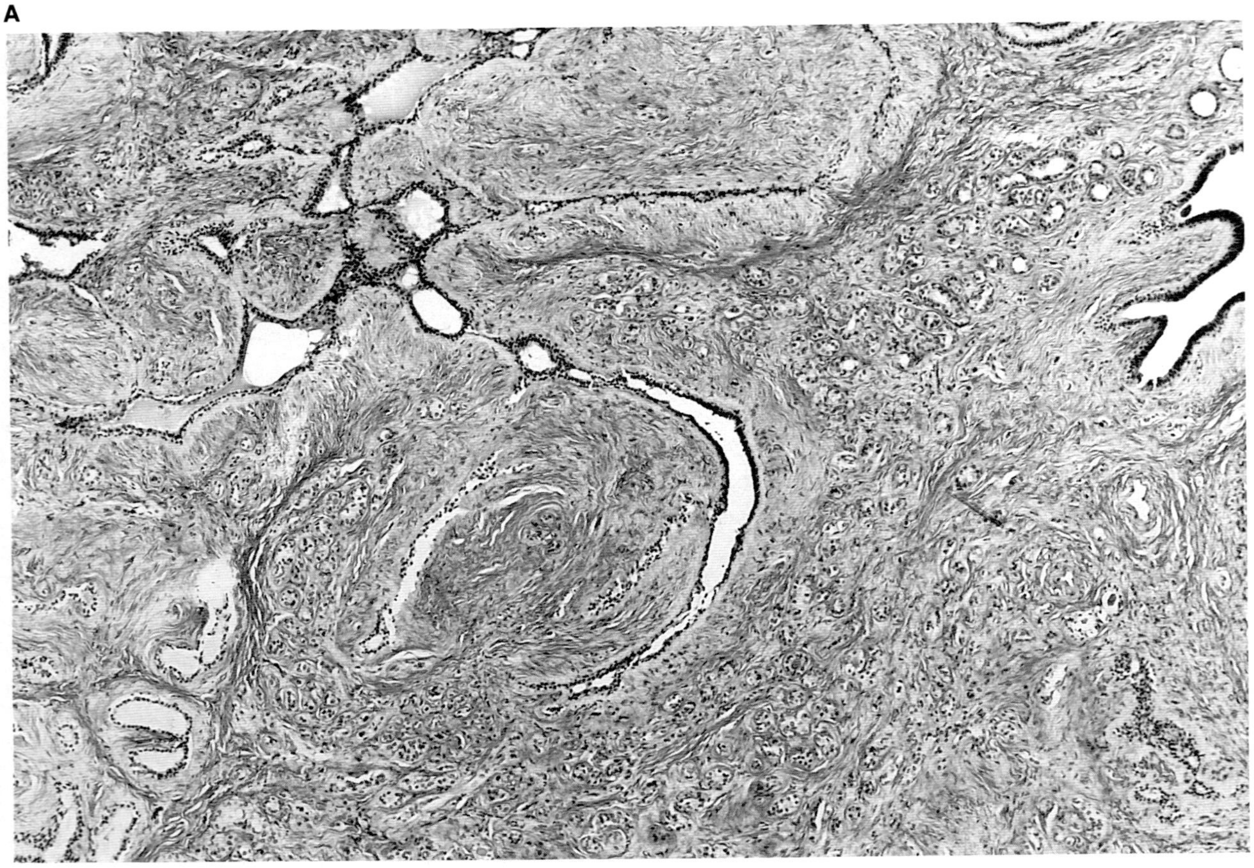

B

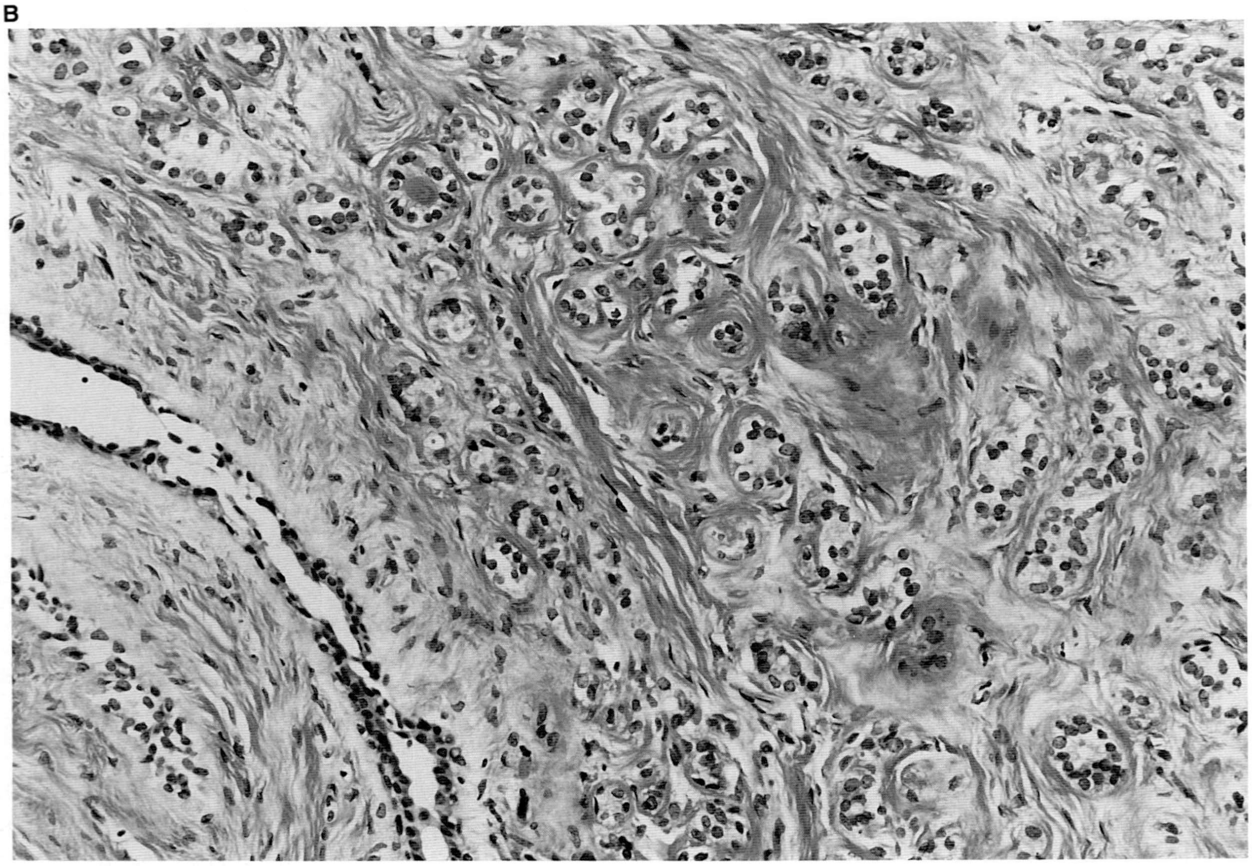

**Figure 11.9** Fibroadenoma with adenosis. (a&b) Part of the stroma is replaced by small tubules, superficially reminiscent of carcinoma. The concentric distribution of collagen and basement membrane around the tubules identifies them as benign. (H&E, (a) X200; (b) X600)

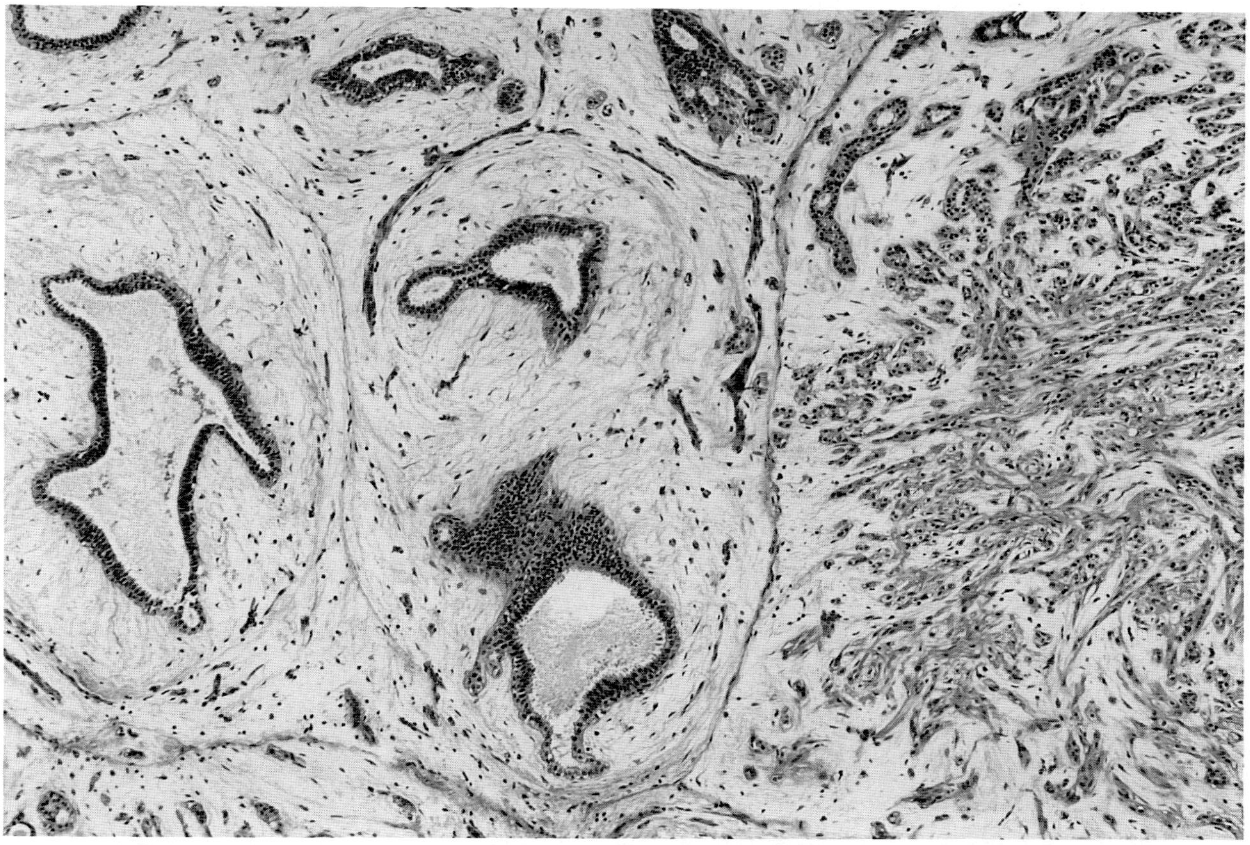

**Figure 11.10** Fibroadenoma with sclerosing adenosis. Sclerosing adenosis with streaming of the myoepithelial cells. (H&E, X240)

confined to a fibroadenoma (Fig. 11.19), as well as various other invasive carcinomas (Figs. 11.20, 11.21). Atypical intraductal hyperplasia, sometimes bordering a non-necrotic intraductal carcinoma, is not uncommon in fibroadenomas (Figs. 11.20, 11.21).

The predominance of lobular neoplasia is in sharp contrast to the rarity of lobules within fibroadenomas, and the fact that lobular lesions account for only 5% to 15% of all breast carcinomas. This finding has been related to the lobular origin of fibroadenomas. Moreover, the higher frequency of in situ as opposed to invasive lesions in fibroadenomas suggests that the progression of carcinomas in this setting is interrupted at an earlier stage due to their presentation within a readily detectable nodule. Also, most fibroadenomas develop in women less than 30 years of age, while approximately 1% of invasive carcinomas occur in this age group.

Among patients with lobular neoplasia (LN) within a fibroadenoma, some have shown excellent survival despite limited therapy, while others have subsequently developed invasive carcinomas in either breast (72,96), a behavior which parallels that of lobular neoplasia when identified within the breast proper. Of 152 patients whose operative procedures were recorded, surgical therapy consisted of radical, modified, or simple mastectomy in 96 cases and local excision in 56 cases. In McDivitt et al's series (105), two patients developed infiltrating carcinoma following local excision of fibroadenomas containing LN. In two other patients who had mastectomy for fibroadenomas containing LN, additional areas of LN were found in other quadrants. Haagensen treated four patients—two with lobular neoplasia and two with intraductal carcinoma confined to fibroadenomas—conservatively; none developed recurrences 4.5 to 21 years after the local excision. Only one of 26 women with carcinoma in situ (lobular or ductal) within a fibroadenoma who was treated conservatively developed an ipsilateral carcinoma in Diaz et al's series (96). None of the 26 patients treated conservatively developed contralateral carcinoma, but 3 of 23 women with carcinoma in situ within fibroadenoma who had mastectomy developed subsequent carcinoma in the contralateral breast.

The management of carcinomas arising in a fibroadenoma should follow accepted current principles for that type of carcinoma were it to occur in its usual setting within the breast proper. A majority of the reports concerning carcinomas within fibroade-

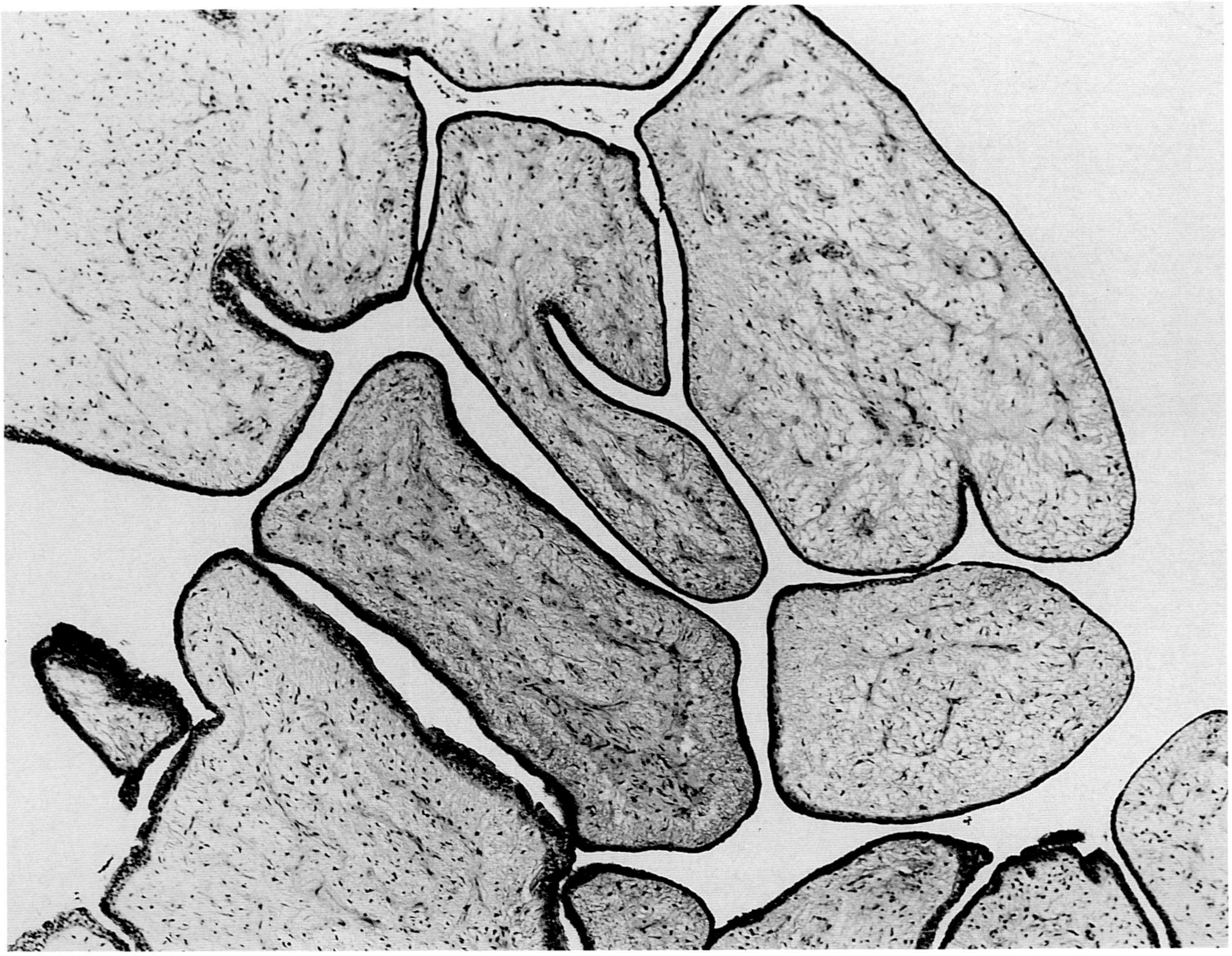

**Figure 11.11** Fibroadenoma phyllodes (benign phyllodes tumors). In this lesion, the stroma is hypocellular as that of a fibroadenoma but leaf-like processes are readily identifiable. (H&E, X600)

nomas have appeared prior to the publication of Haagensen's viewpoints regarding conservative treatment of lobular neoplasia (102). This fairly widespread conservative attitude toward management of lobular neoplasia will undoubtedly influence future management of lobular neoplasia or carcinoma in situ arising in fibroadenomas. Conservative therapy has been recommended for carcinoma in situ arising in fibroadenoma in a more recent study (96). Regardless of the extent of the surgical treatment, only rarely have patients with carcinoma arising in a fibroadenoma died of the tumor; the deaths have generally been due to invasive ductal carcinomas (72,109).

**Table 11.1** Cellular Fibroadenoma vs Cystosarcoma Phyllodes

| | FA | CP |
|---|---|---|
| Leaf-like processes | − | + |
| Age less than 15 yrs | + | − |
| Squamous metaplasia | − | + |
| Chondroid metaplasia | − | + |
| Osseous metaplasia | − | + |
| Adipose tissue | − | + |
| Infiltrating margins | − | + |

*Note:* (−) = rare to absent; (+) = present; yrs = years.

## Origin of Fibroadenomas

Fibroadenomas originate in lobules (87). Orcel and Douvin (70) have defined four evolutionary stages in the development of a fibroadenoma (Fig. 11.22). The initial process is a proliferation of both the epithelial and stromal components of multiple lobules either spontaneously or precipitated by hormonal alterations (hyperestrogenic states). Next, there is a gradual confluence of the hyperplastic nodules. This is

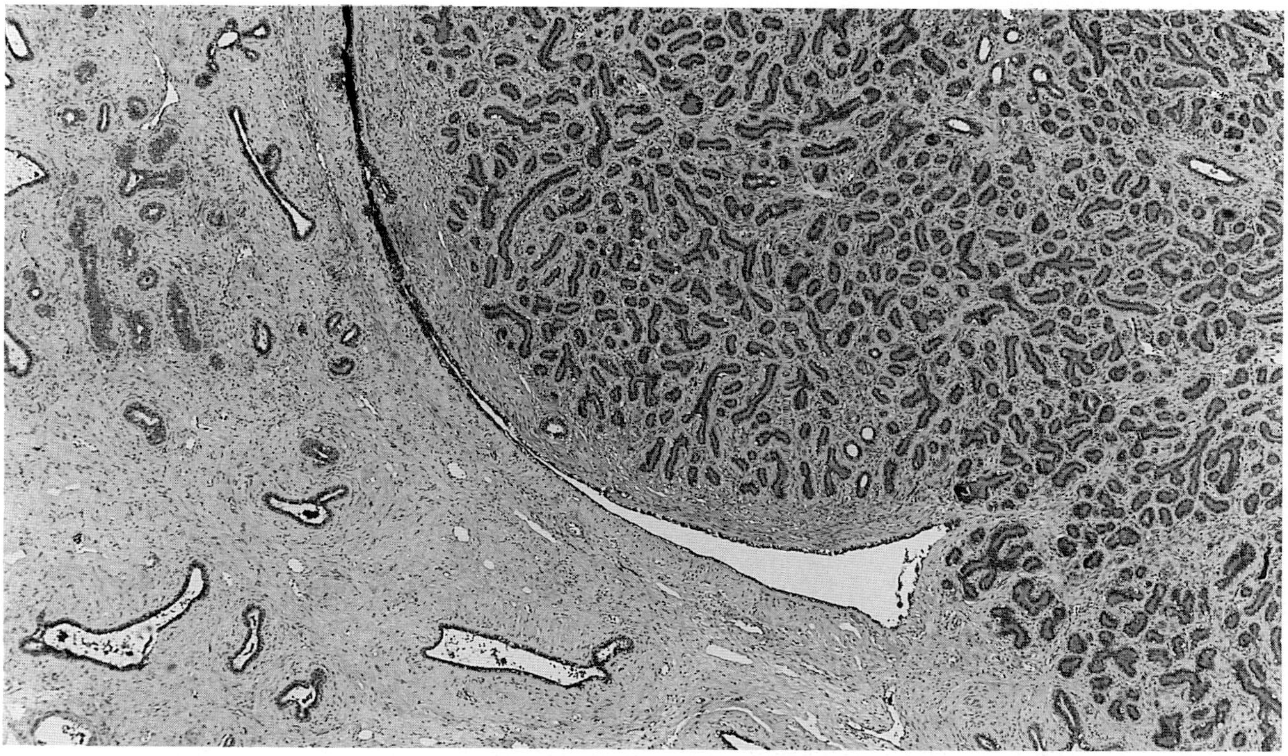

**Figure 11.12** Combined tubular-fibroadenoma. A combination of tubular adenoma pattern and fibroadenoma is present in this tumor. (H&E, X60)

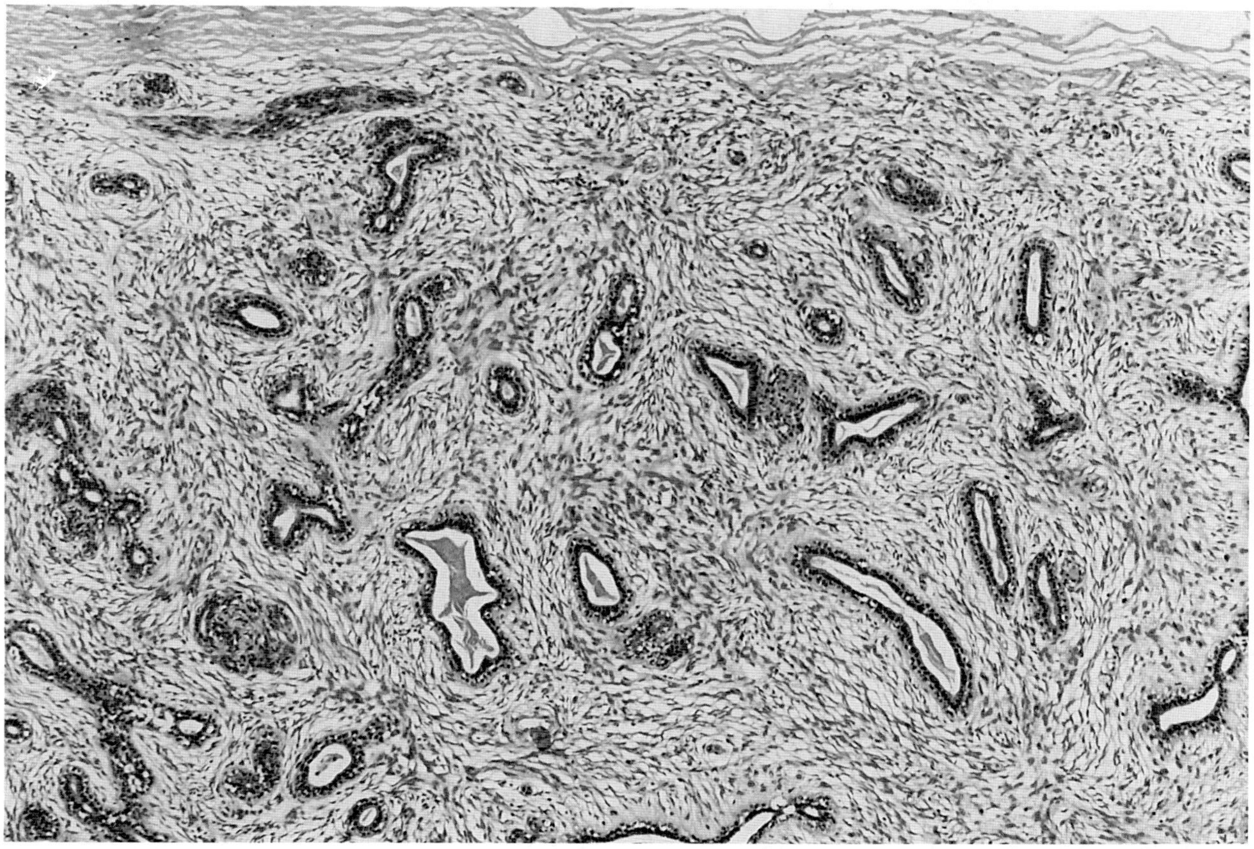

**Figure 11.13** Juvenile fibroadenoma. The stroma is more cellular than that of a classic fibroadenoma and the growth pattern is pericanalicular. (H&E, X300)

A

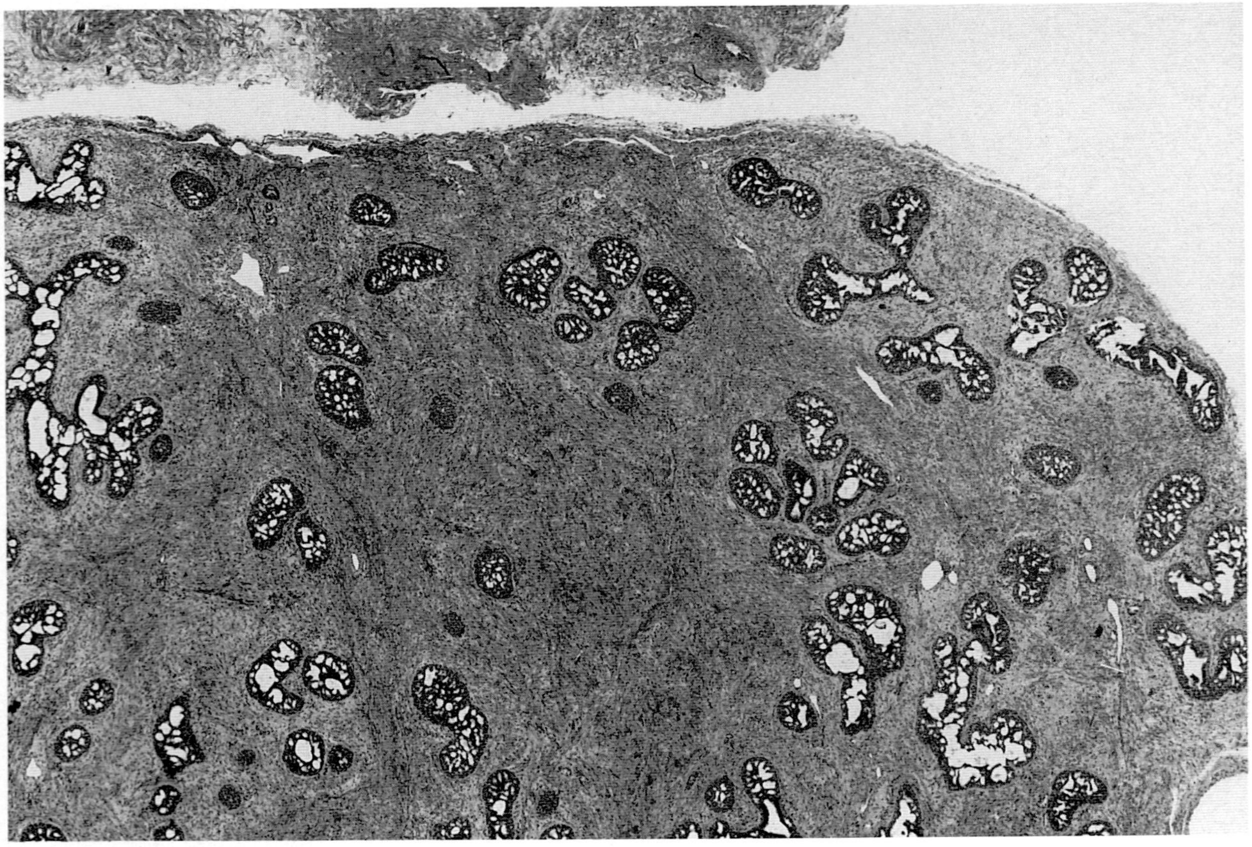

B

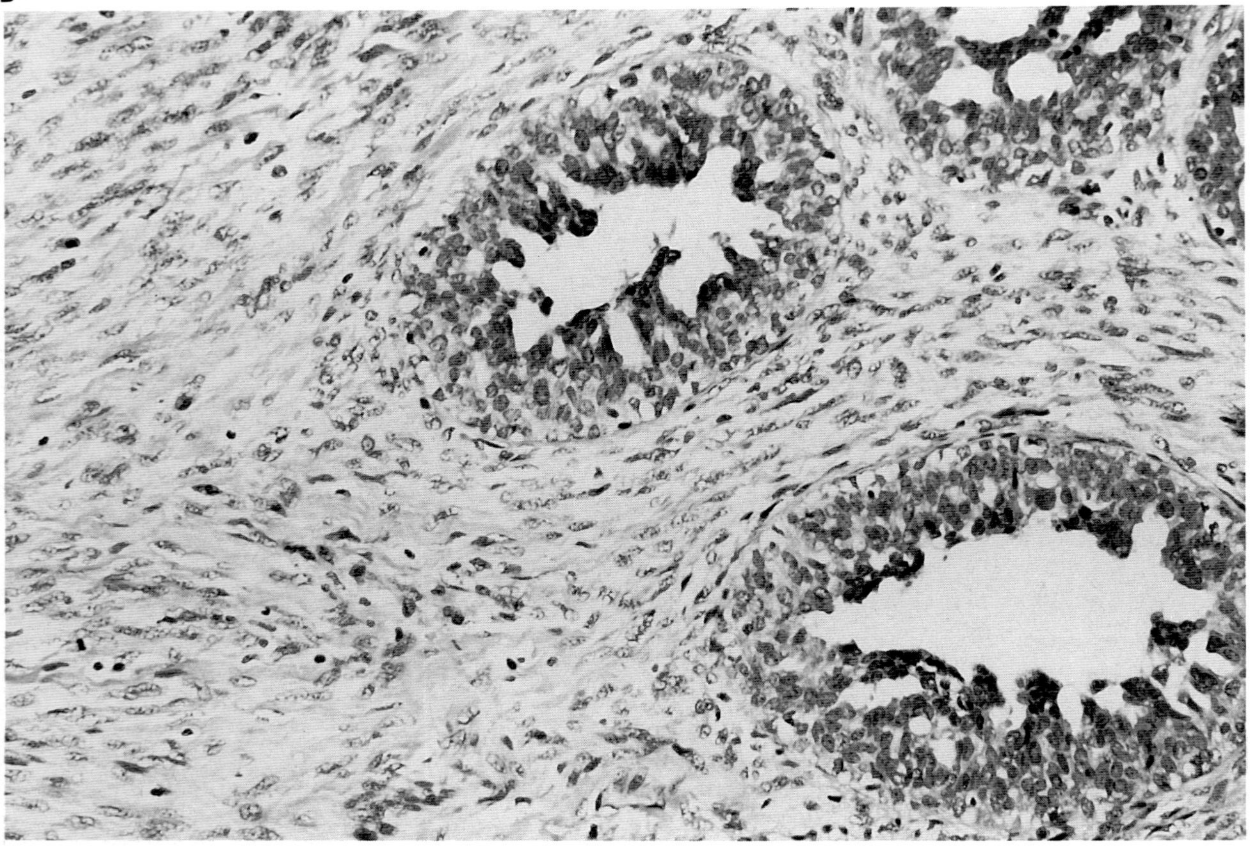

**Figure 11.14** (a) Juvenile fibroadenoma with epithelial hyperplasia. (b) The irregular tufts overlying the stratified epithelium in the ducts is similar to the pattern of hyperplasia in gynecomastia. (c) Ordinary intraductal hyperplasia in a juvenile fibroadenoma. (H&E, (a) X320; (b) X30; (c) X240)

c

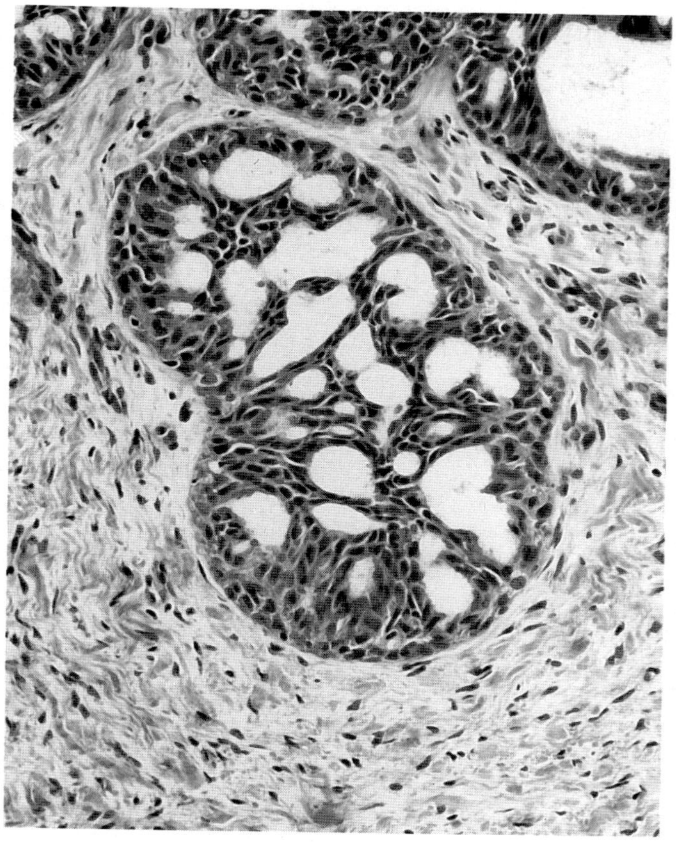

**Figure 11.14(c)** Legend on opposite page.

followed by formation of fibroadenomatous nodules of various age, size, and histologic appearances. Hanson et al, (36) have referred to these changes as fibroadenomatosis; the term fibroadenomatous hyperplasia (Fig. 11.23) is preferred at AFIP. Finally, there is coalescence of the fibroadenomatous nodules and formation of a fully developed fibroadenoma (Fig. 11.24). Fibroadenomas, therefore, enlarge by central expansion, as well as accretion (Fig. 11.25); the initial process of proliferation of epithelial and stroma components continues while additional altered lobules are added to the periphery of the lesion. The process may be arrested or undergo hyalinization at any stage. The histologic variations observed in fibroadenoma result from either an exaggeration of one of the evolutionary stages or from the quantitative dominance of one of the proliferating constituents of the biphasic tumor.

Meanwhile, the interlobular adipose tissue generally atrophies and disappears completely about the time of confluence. Rarely, some of the adipose tissue may persist and may even proliferate assuming a lipomatous appearance resulting in a defect in the confluence of the fibroadenomatous nodules and creating irregularities in the margin.

Three-dimensional reconstruction of FA by serial sectioning of a small lesion has shown continuity of its compressed ductal structures with the adjacent normal duct system. The junction of the FA with the adjacent normal breast is associated with the gradual merger of the proliferating stroma with the normal periductal connective tissue (19). While the connective tissue is the dominant proliferating component of FA, morphometric analysis supports participation of the epithelial element in the proliferative process (74).

## Immunohistochemical and Ultrastructural Findings

The ultrastructural features of fibroadenoma have been studied by a number of investigators (1,3,6,41, 60).

Based on immunohistochemical and ultrastructural studies, the stromal cells have been variably interpreted as fibroblasts (1) and myofibroblasts (41). Ohtani and Sasano (68) designated the stromal cells as fibroblasts, but emphasized that they use this term in a broader sense to include myofibroblasts. In one of the earlier ultrastructural studies of fibroadenomas, Murad et al (60) speculated that the stromal cells are derived from pericytes based on the finding of cytoplasmic microfilaments and basal lamina around the cells. This speculation has been refuted, however, in subsequent studies (1,13,25,72).

Recent immunohistochemical evaluations of fibroadenomas have shown that the stromal cells express a positive reaction for actin in most tumors (32). In fibroadenomas with a fibroblastic or cellular stroma, the stromal cells display strongly-positive reaction for actin, while in tumors with either a myxoid or sclerotic stroma, the stromal cells display a weakly-positive reaction for actin (68). The multinucleated giant cells rarely observed in fibroadenomas fail to react with a variety of epithelial and mesenchymal markers. The reaction of the epithelial cells in fibroadenoma to a variety of epithelial antigens parallels that of the epithelial cells elsewhere in the breast.

At the ultrastructural level, the stroma contains fibroblasts, myofibroblasts, blood vessels, and collagen. Groups of lysosome-like bodies were described in a minority of the stromal cells by Harris & Kahn (37). A Z-line-like band is present in some cells; these

A

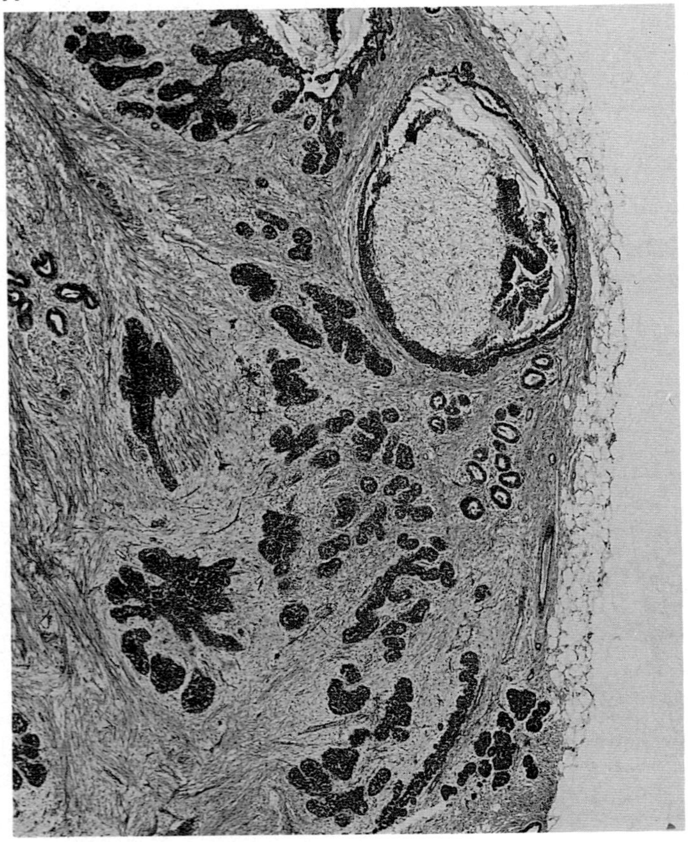

B

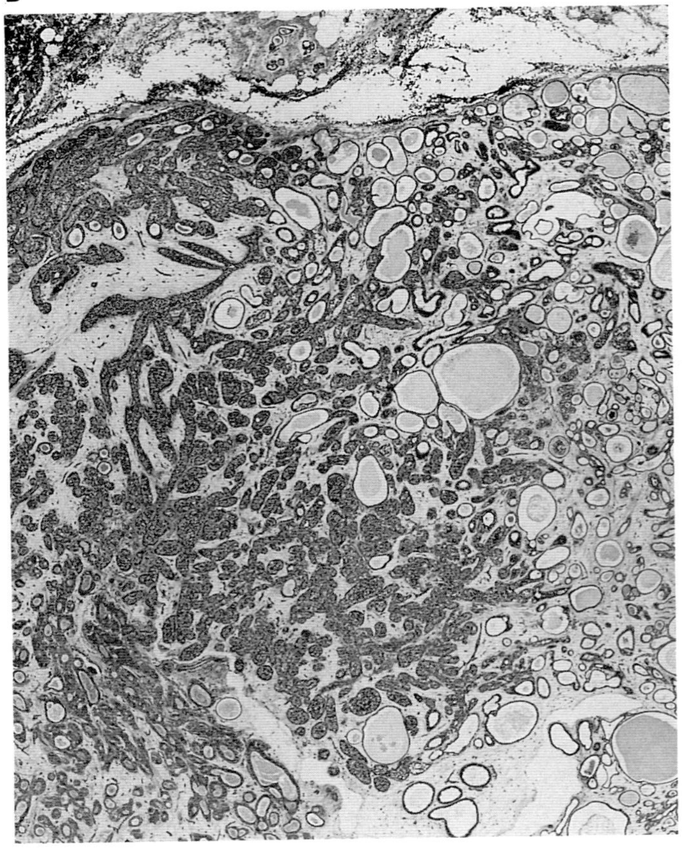

C

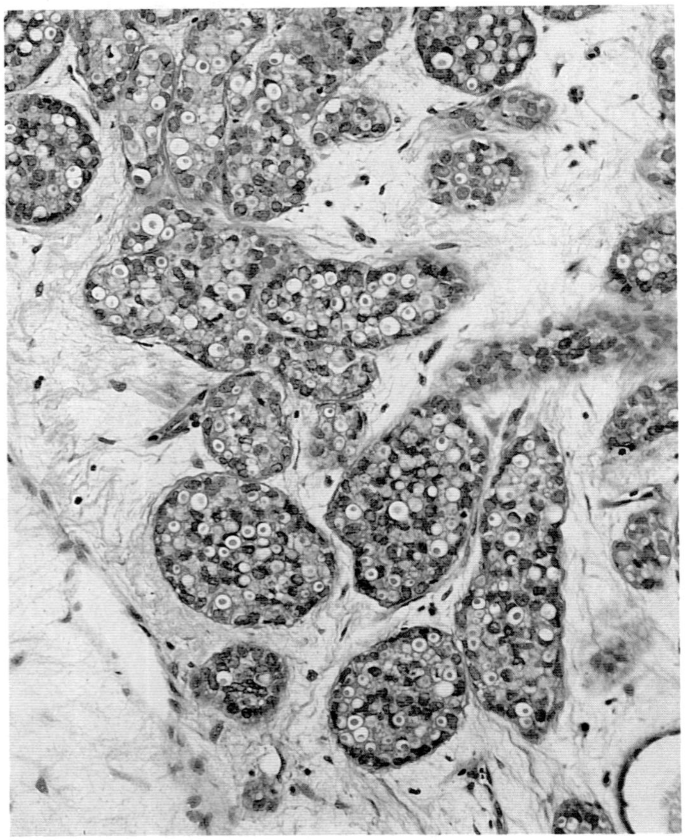

**Figure 11.15** Lobular neoplasia in fibroadenoma. (a) There is proliferation of small, uniform, round cells occluding epithelial-lined spaces in the fibroadenoma. There was no lobular disease in the surrounding breast tissue. (b&c) Another fibroadenoma with a secretory variant of lobular neoplasia. (H&E, (a) X15; (b) X25; (c) X200)

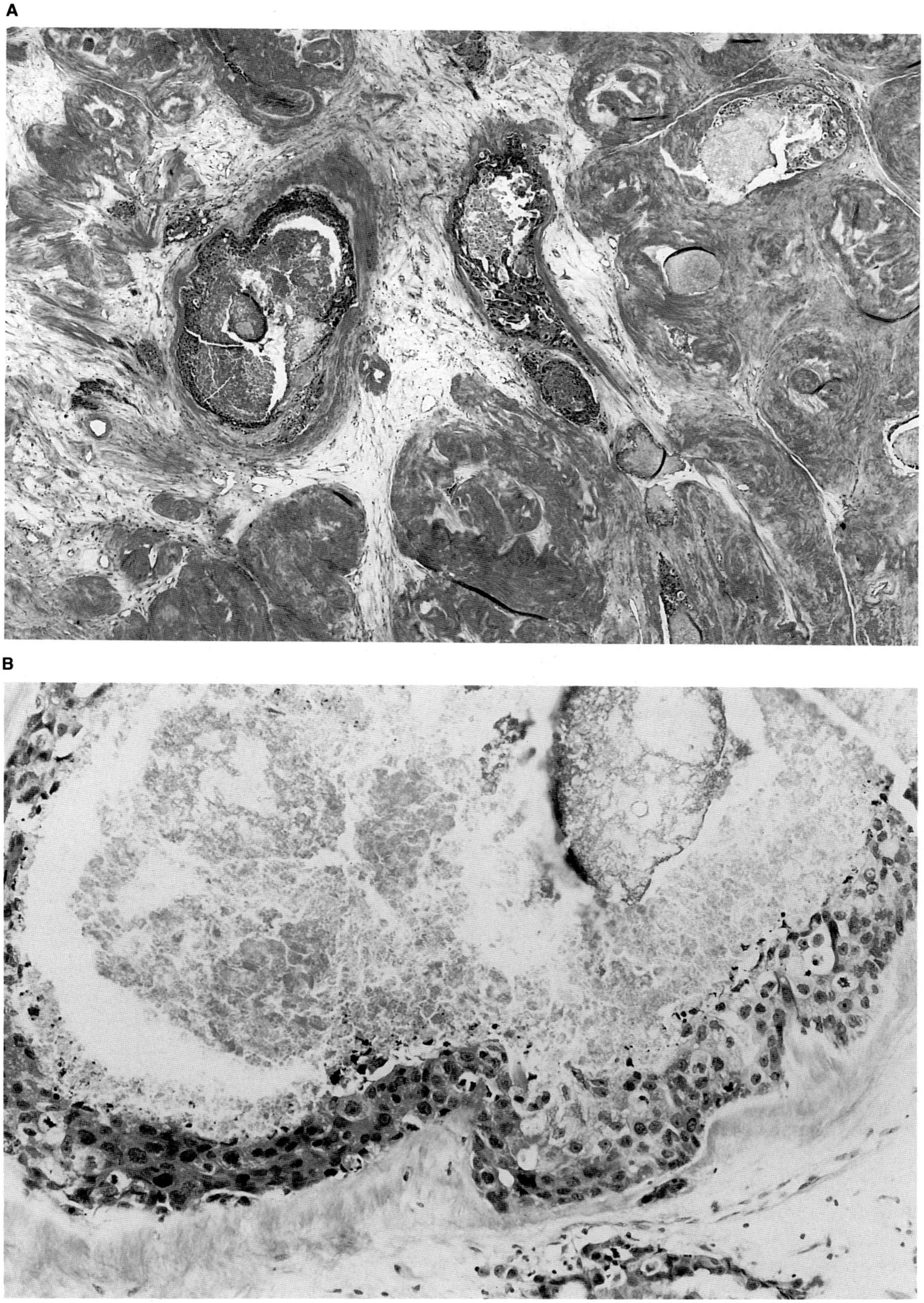

Figure 11.16 Intraductal carcinoma in a hyalinized fibroadenoma. (a&b) Much of the tumor is hyalinized with epithelial atrophy, except for areas where the epithelial component displays a comedocarcinoma. (H&E, (a) X60; (b) X150)

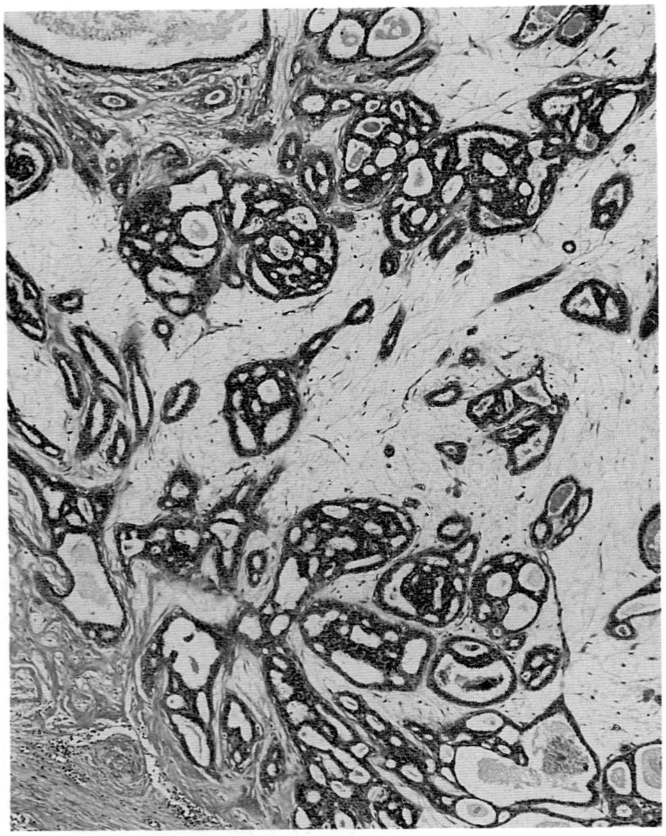

**Figure 11.17** Fibroadenoma with IDCA. A cribriform intraductal proliferation of uniform cells and minimal necrotic debris is evident in this fibroadenoma. Patient also had extensive comedo intraductal carcinoma in the surrounding breast. (H&E, X75)

bands are intermediate between the Z-lines of striated muscle and the dense bodies of smooth muscle. Desmosome-like junctions have been observed between the stromal cells and their cytoplasmic processes. The ductal structures have a luminal epithelial cell layer, an interrupted myoepithelial cell layer and a distinct basal lamina which may be multilayered (1).

Ultrastructurally, the multinucleated stromal giant cells resemble multinucleated fibroblasts. Even though a myoepithelial origin has been proposed by Nielsen and Ladefoged (64), their evidence is not convincing. Their electron micrographs show no evidence of cystoplasmic fibrils with dense bodies or basal laminae, features characteristic of myoepithelial cells. They do illustrate a desmosome, but isolated desmosomes and desmosome-like junctions do occur occasionally in stromal cells of fibroadenomas (68). These giant cells appear identical to similar stromal giant cells occasionally observed in the mammary stroma in association with fibrocystic changes (see Chapter 13, Mesenchymal Lesions of the Breast).

## Hormone Receptors in Fibroadenomas

Eleven of 13 fibroadenomas evaluated by Rao et al (76), had progesterone receptor (PR) but only two of the 13 cases had estrogen receptor (ER). Mechtersheimer et al (56) found PR+ ER− ductal epithelium in 9 of 13 fibroadenomas. Using a biochemical approach, Mohammed et al (59) found a PR content higher than that of ER in fibroadenomas, while Rao et al (54) found PR in 11 of 13 fibroadenomas and ER in only two of the 13 cases.

## CYSTOSARCOMA PHYLLODES

Cystosarcoma phyllodes (CP) is a biphasic tumor that is composed of benign epithelial elements and a cellular, spindle-cell stroma. Early descriptions of this lesion have been attributed to Cumin (129) and Chelius (125), but it was Johannes Mueller (166) who introduced the term cystosarcoma phyllodes. In 1838, Mueller described a breast tumor characterized by proliferation of fleshy leaf-like processes into cystic spaces; this he designated cystosarcoma phyllodes, sarcoma for the fleshy nature of the lesion and phyllodes for the leaf-like processes. Either phyllodes (leaf-like) or phylloides (leafy) is utilized in the designation.

In the original description of cystosarcoma phyllodes, Mueller actually emphasized the benign nature of this often massive tumor. Subsequently, cystosarcomas with clearly malignant behavior were documented and the term sarcoma attained a malignant connotation. Since a majority of cystosarcomas are not clinically malignant, however, it is generally acknowledged that CP is not an ideal designation. Consequently, over 60 different names have been proposed for this lesion (134) adding confusion to the literature and making a thorough review of the subject practically impossible. The term CP has remained the standard designation for this lesion despite its inherent flaws as it is already firmly established in the literature and is the most widely used designation. The term phyllodes tumor, proposed by WHO, is preferable as it avoids the designation of sarcoma with its deceptive implication of malignancy for a majority of these tumors. This term, with further qualification as low grade or malignant, is an accept-

A

B

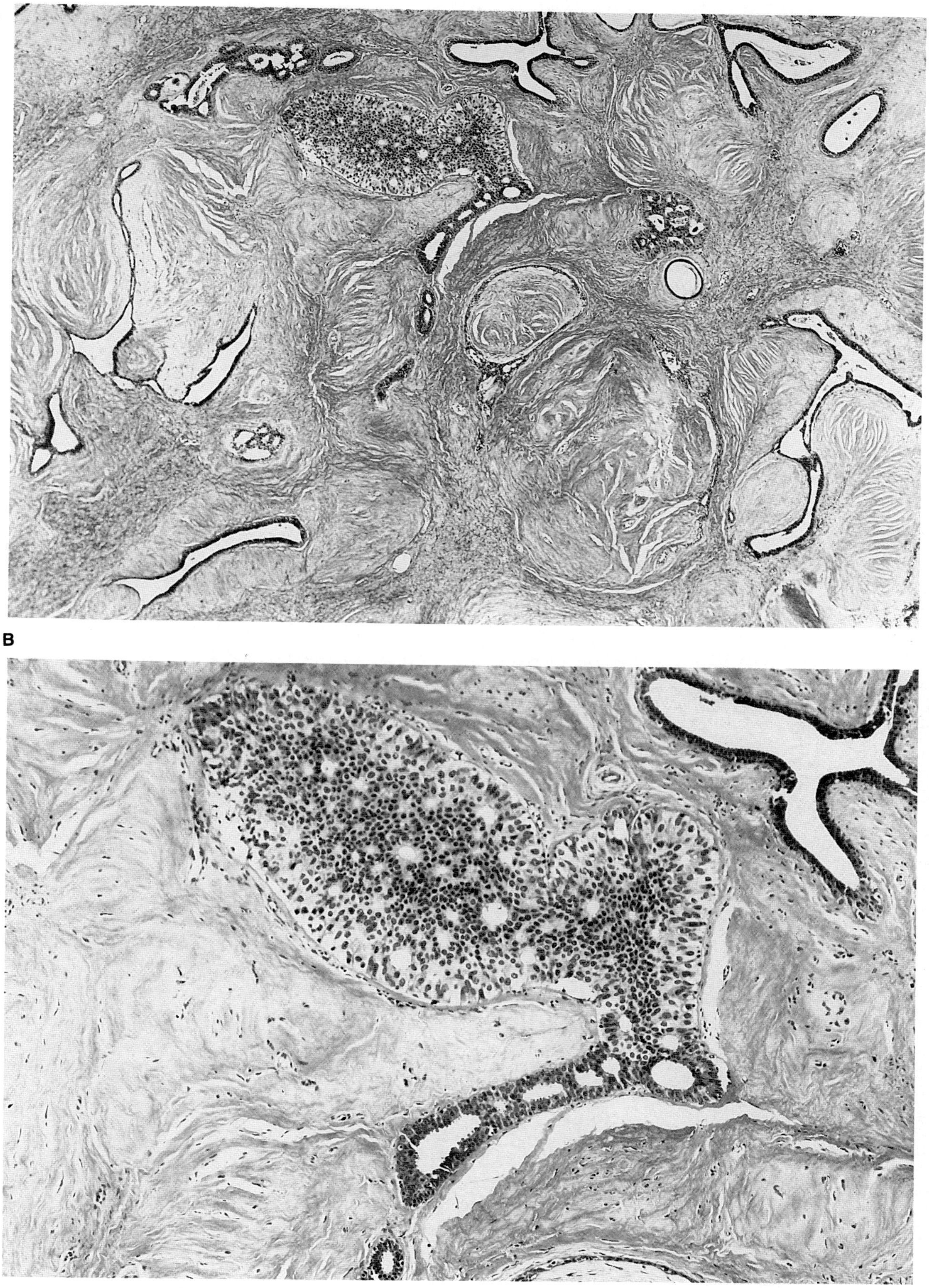

**Figure 11.18** Fibroadenoma with atypical intraductal hyperplasia (AIDH). (a&b) A cribriform proliferation composed of two cell types partially distends a ductal space in this hyalinized fibroadenoma. (H&E, (a) X60; (b) X150)

A

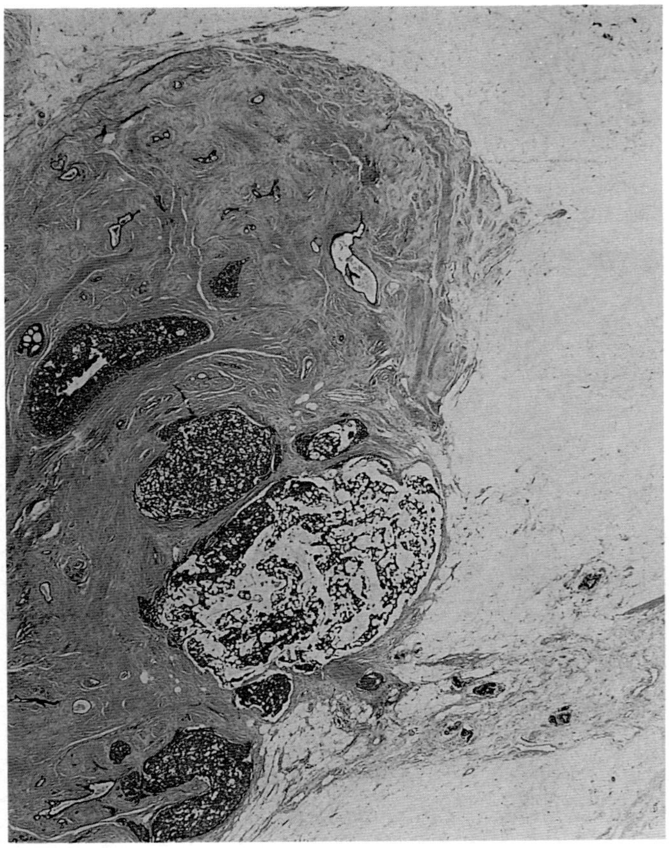

B

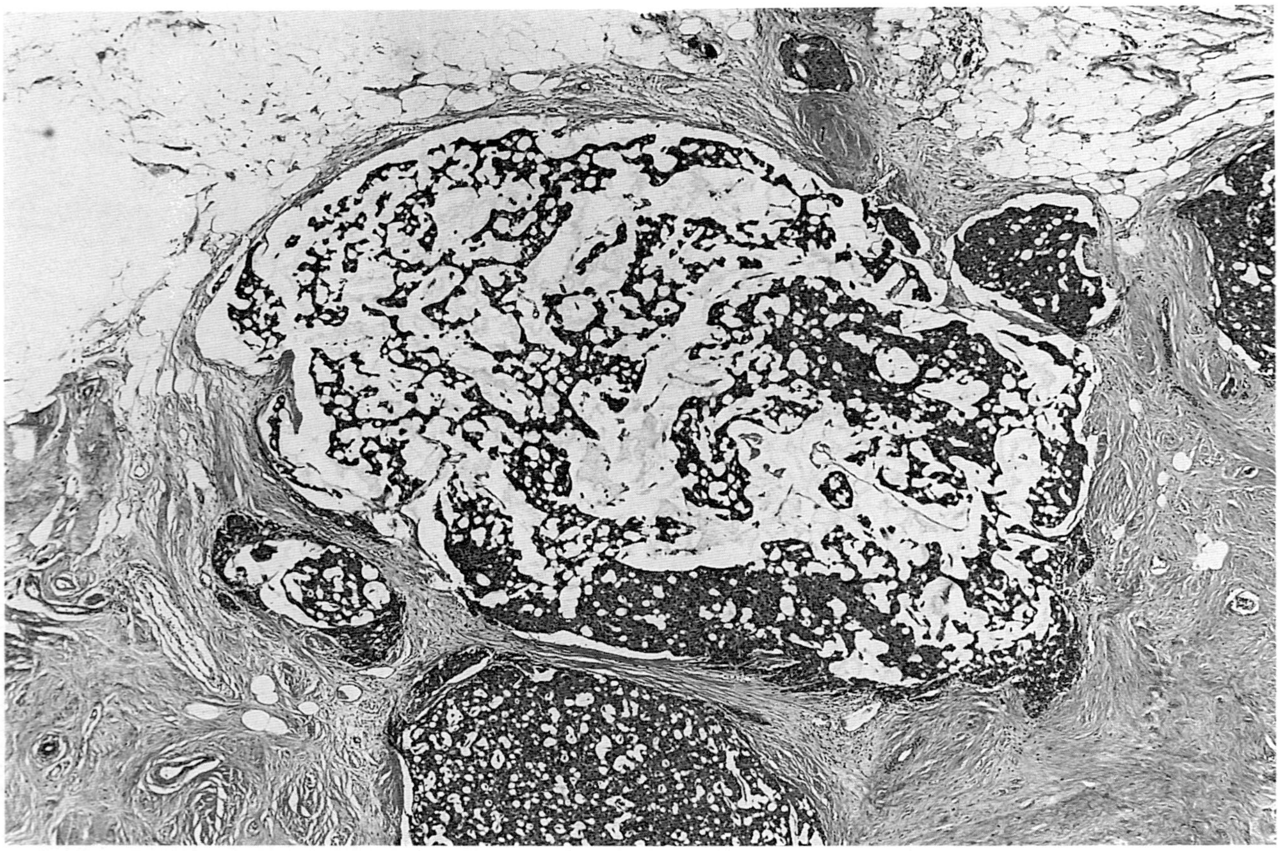

**Figure 11.19** Fibroadenoma with colloid carcinoma. (a,b) A hyalinized fibroadenoma is evident with several areas of epithelial proliferation, one of which appears disrupted. (c) Higher magnification shows irregular clusters of epithelial cells floating in abundant mucous. (H&E, (a) X15; (b) X30; (c) X150)

c

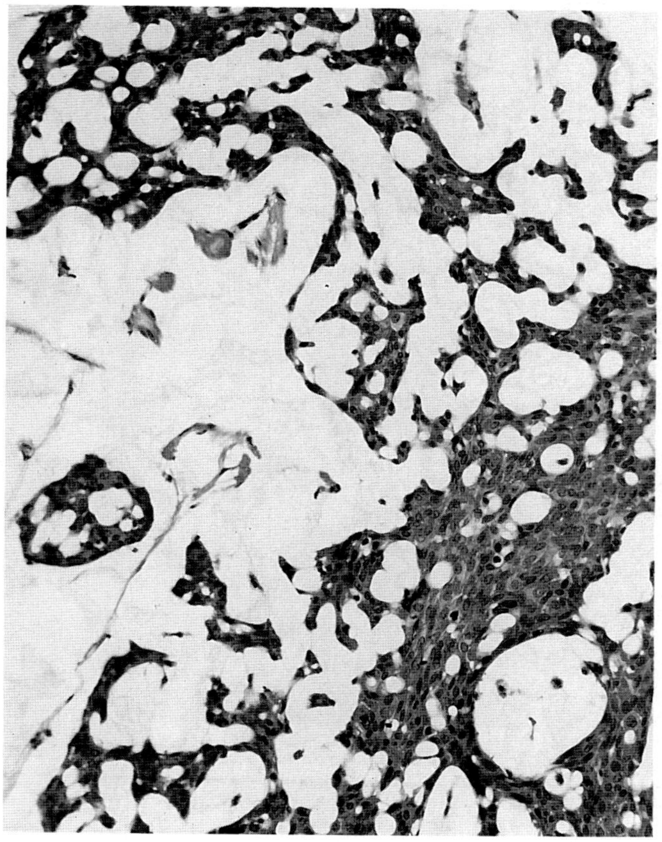

**Figure 11.19(c)** Legend on opposite page.

able alternative to the designation of CP. It is anticipated that within 5 to 10 years application of the term "phyllodes tumor" will gain significant popularity.

The incidence of cystosarcoma phyllodes is quite low. It constitutes 0.3% of all breast tumors (118), and approximately 2.5% of all fibroepithelial tumors of the breast (156,185). The dominance of the stroma relative to the epithelial component in CP is similar to that of fibroadenoma, but the stroma is often more cellular and hyperplastic. The distinction between the two is based on a subjective estimation of the degree of stromal cellularity and the presence of leaf-like processes. Exactly what degree of stromal cellularity is required to qualify a lesion as a CP is difficult to define at its lower limit, and the capability to make this distinction improves with experience. Leaf-like processes apparent to the naked eye or microscopic leaf-like processes are more common in cystosarcomas and their presence would favor a CP when the degree of stromal cellularity is borderline. The presence of leaf-like processes alone is not sufficient to warrant a diagnosis of CP, in my opinion. Tumors that display a hypocellular, edematous stroma with formation of leaf-like processes better qualify as fibroadenoma phyllodes or low grade phyllodes tumor rather than a CP.

Until 1931 when Lee and Pack (155) reviewed a large series of 111 cases and noted histologically malignant features in one, CP was considered innocuous. Actually, Friend (135) had reported a case which was probably a malignant CP but it had been designated an intracanalicular fibroma undergoing sarcomatous change. In 1940, White (190) reported an example of metastatic CP and since then about 100 cases of metastatic CP have appeared in the English literature. The aggressive potential of CP is now well recognized, but it is extremely difficult to reliably predict the behavior of CP on the basis of its histologic features.

Interestingly, there are records of histologically benign tumors that have metastasized (114), as well as many histologically malignant tumors that have not recurred.

## Clinical Features

The average age of women with CP is 45 with a wide range, occurring in the adolescent, albeit rarely, as well as the octagenerian. Patients with CP are on the average 15 to 20 years older than patients with fibroadenoma. Those with histologically malignant tumors are about three years older than patients with the benign variety (162). Women dying of metastatic disease have a median age seven years older than the median for all patients with CP (168).

The racial origin of patients with CP has been recorded in many studies. In Norris and Taylor's series (168), 87% were caucasian, 8% black and 5% of other racial extractions. About 8% of the patients in Treves and Sunderland's series (186) were black, the remaining patients were caucasian. In a review of metastatic CP by Kessinger et al (152), there were 51 caucasians (85%), eight blacks (13%), and one Alaskan indian (1.6%). Treves and Sunderland (186) found that 22% of their histologically malignant cases occurred in blacks.

Patients generally present with a breast mass. Some relate the presence of a small hard mass for many years followed by the onset of rapid growth of the tumor; this was observed by more than a third of the patients with histologically malignant lesions in

A

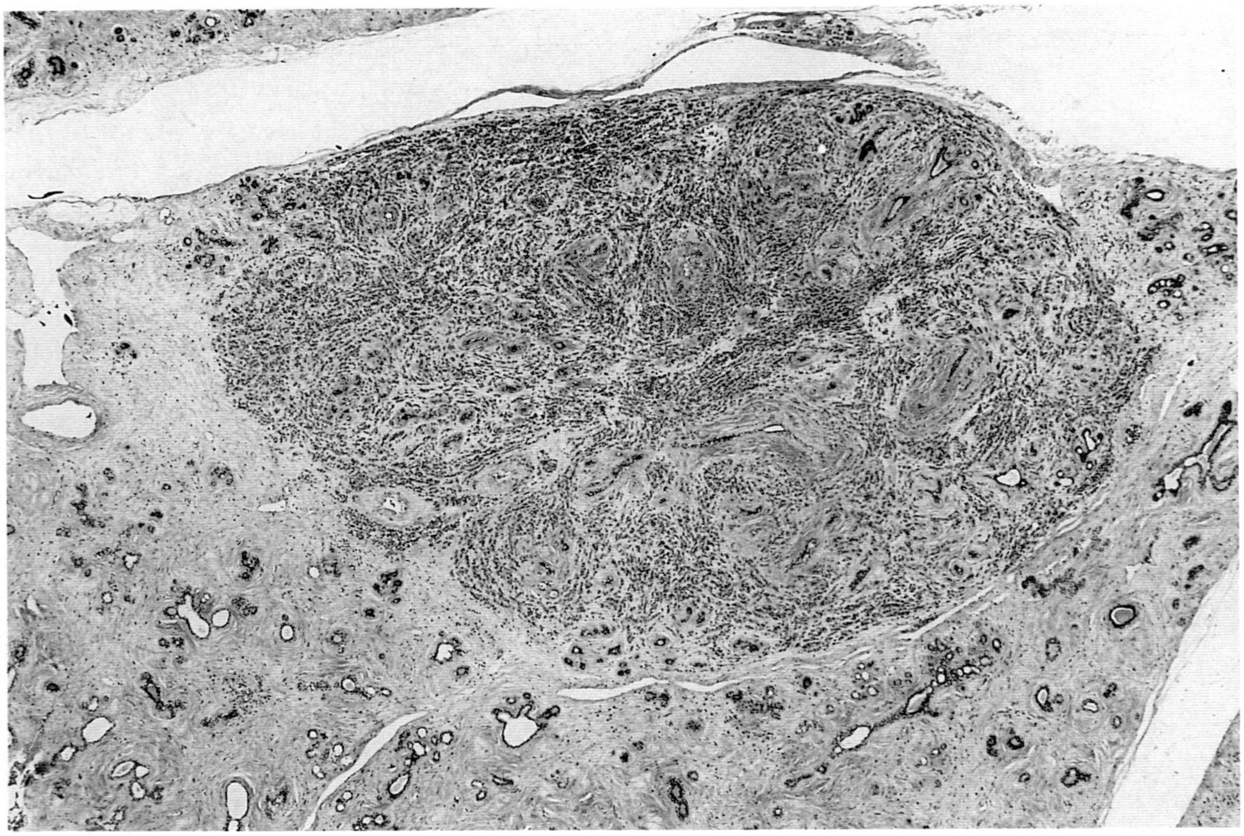

B

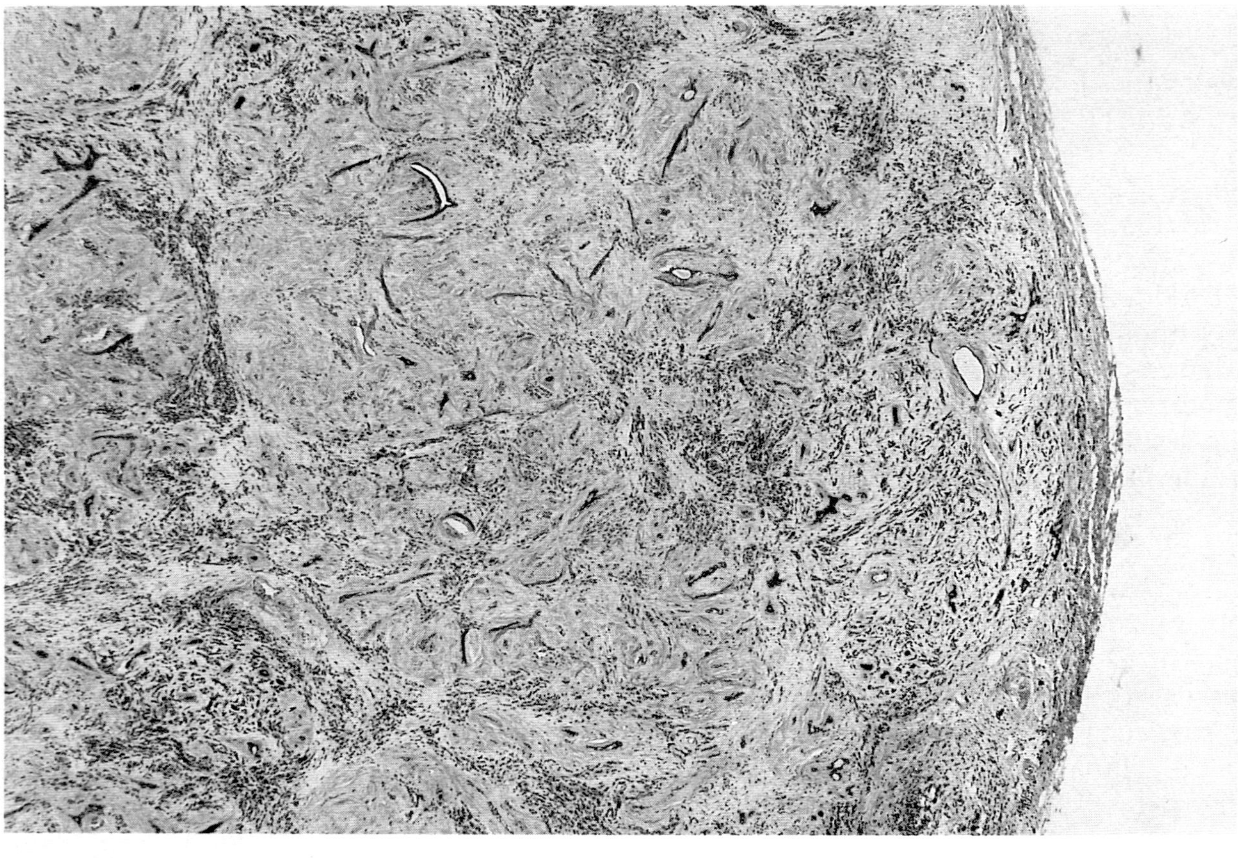

**Figure 11.20** Fibroadenoma with infiltrating lobular carcinoma. (a,b) There are diffuse and concentrated areas of small cell infiltration in this large fibroadenoma. (c) At higher magnification, there is Indian-file arrangement of the small invasive cells, typical of infiltrating lobular carcinoma. (H&E, (a) X20; (b) X24; (c) X300)

c

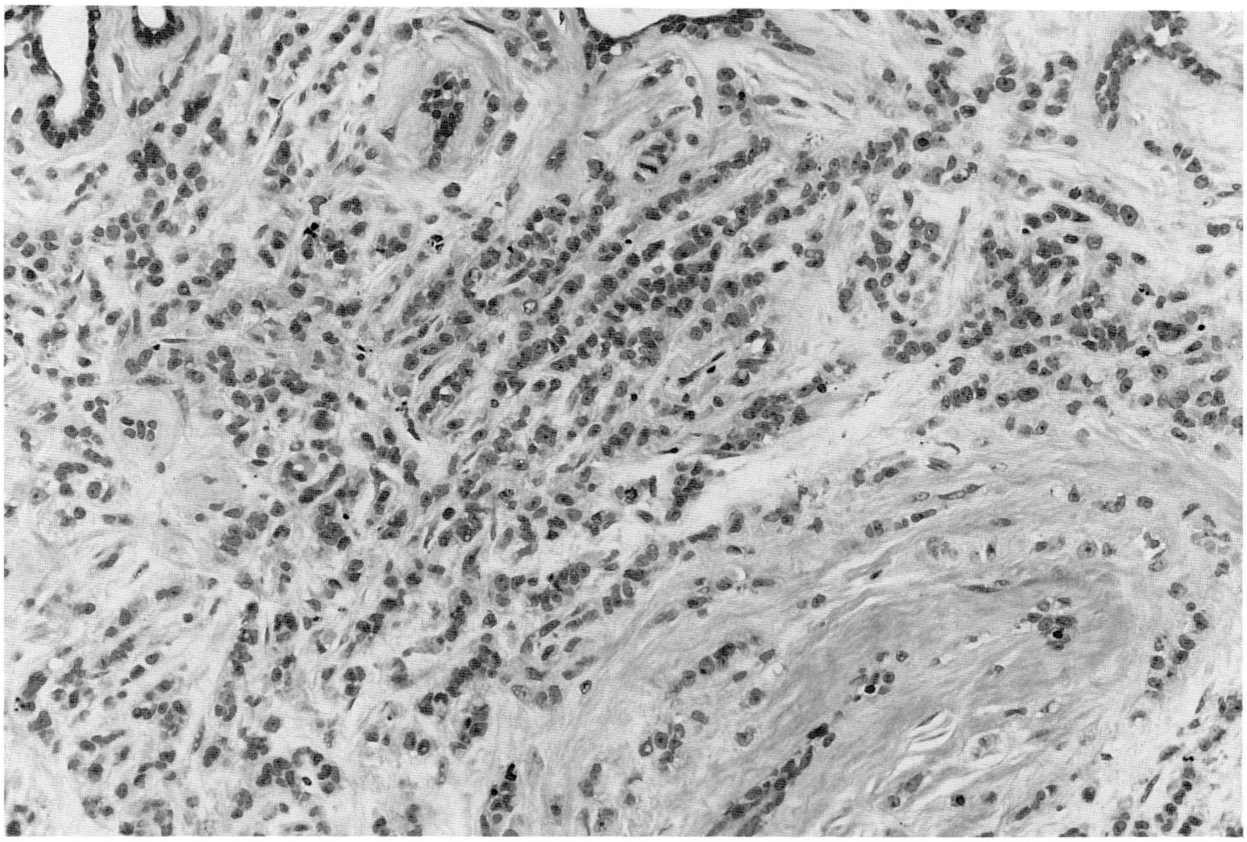

**Figure 11.20(c)** Legend on opposite page.

McDivitt et al's series (162). These tumors can progress rapidly to assume massive proportions displacing the nipple (Fig. 11.26); Treves and Sunderland (186) reported a benign neoplasm that grew to a 20-cm size in three months. Large tumors may cause stretching of the overlying skin with distension of the superficial vein. Ulceration occurs in some patients but this is not an indication of malignancy. Most patients have no complaint of pain. Usually the tumor is multilobular, not attached to the skin and freely movable.

Regional lymph node enlargement is not uncommon having been noted in 17% of patients in Norris and Taylor's report (168), but it is generally due to reactive changes rather than metastatic tumor. Bilaterality is rare (139,156,168,186), but even bilateral malignant CP occurs (176). Bilateral tumors are not generally simultaneous, with intervals of months to years between manifestation of the two lesions. Some bilateral "cystosarcomas" reported in children (144) probably reflect giant fibroadenomas. Multiplicity is even more uncommon (165).

## Macroscopic Features

Cystosarcoma phyllodes is highly variable in its gross appearance but a majority display a solid, fleshy mass with cystic areas (Fig. 11.27). In a series of unselected cases, most neoplasms were between 3 to 5 cm in one study (185) and the median was 6.4 cm in another (168). The tumors range in size from 1 to 45 cm, however. The average size of tumors that metastasized was 11.8 cm in Kessinger's review (152), but very small lesions have also metastasized, the smallest being 1.5 cm (162). While some cystosarcomas have the classic fleshy leaf-like processes, others appear rather solid with barely visible cysts. A

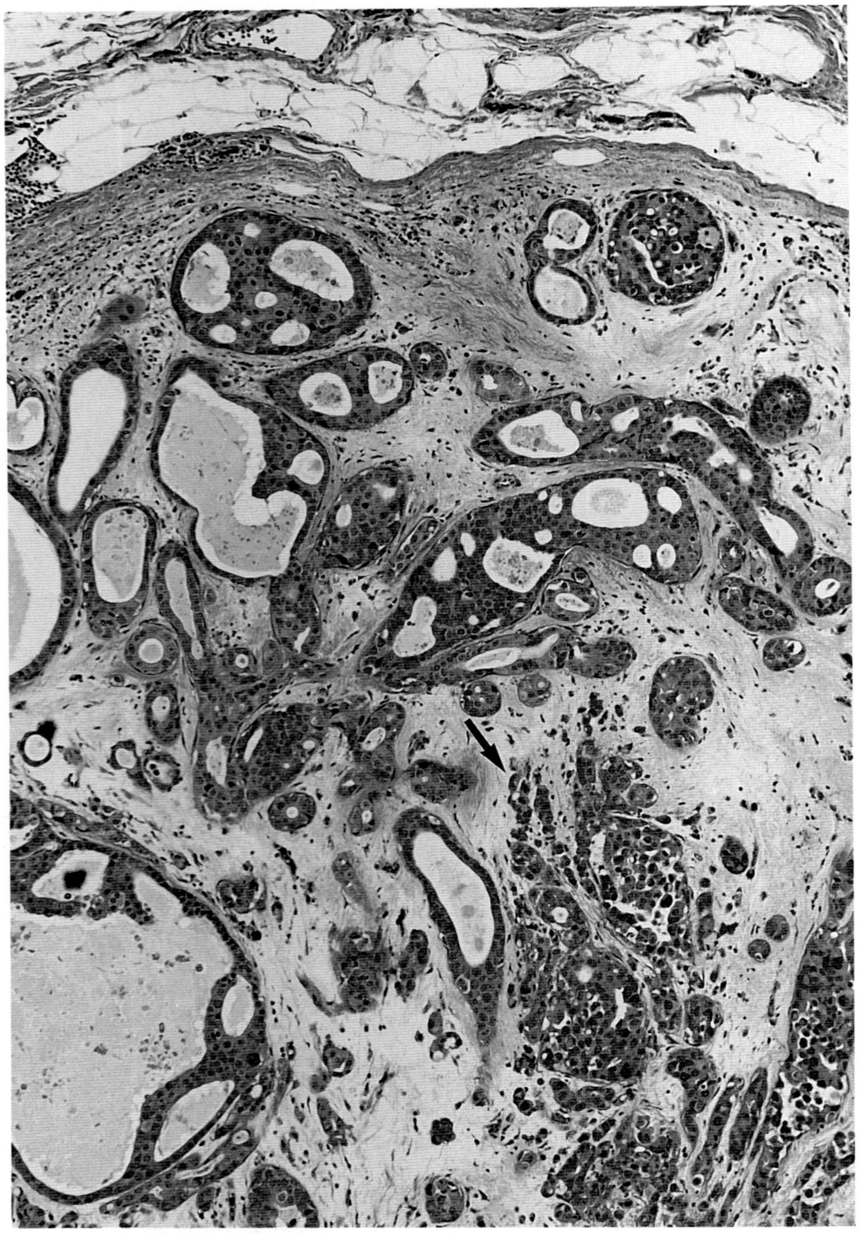

**Figure 11.21** Fibroadenoma with early infiltrating duct carcinoma. In addition to multiple ducts with AIDH in this field, there is focal invasion (arrow) in this fibroadenoma. (H&E, X75)

majority of these tumors are well circumscribed and are grey-white or yellow with foci of hemorrhage and necrosis in the larger lesions. The consistency varies from fleshy to mucoid and the cut surface generally bulges out.

## Microscopic Features

Histologically, cystosarcoma phyllodes is composed of a benign epithelial component and a cellular, spindle-cell stroma; the tumor is characterized by formation of leaf-like processes protruding into cystic spaces (Fig. 11.28). The epithelial elements lining the ducts and slit-like spaces and covering the leaf-like processes consist of the two cell types characteristic of the mammary duct system, the luminal epithelial cells and the myoepithelial cells. As a rule the stroma is more cellular than that of fibroadenomas and it is generally fibrosarcomatous in appearance. The formation of leaf-like processes is a crucial feature that helps separate cellular fibroadenoma from low grade cystosarcoma phyllodes.

Spindle-shaped fibroblastic cells (Fig. 11.29) generally constitute the stroma but highly atypical and multinucleated cells also occur (Fig. 11.30). In

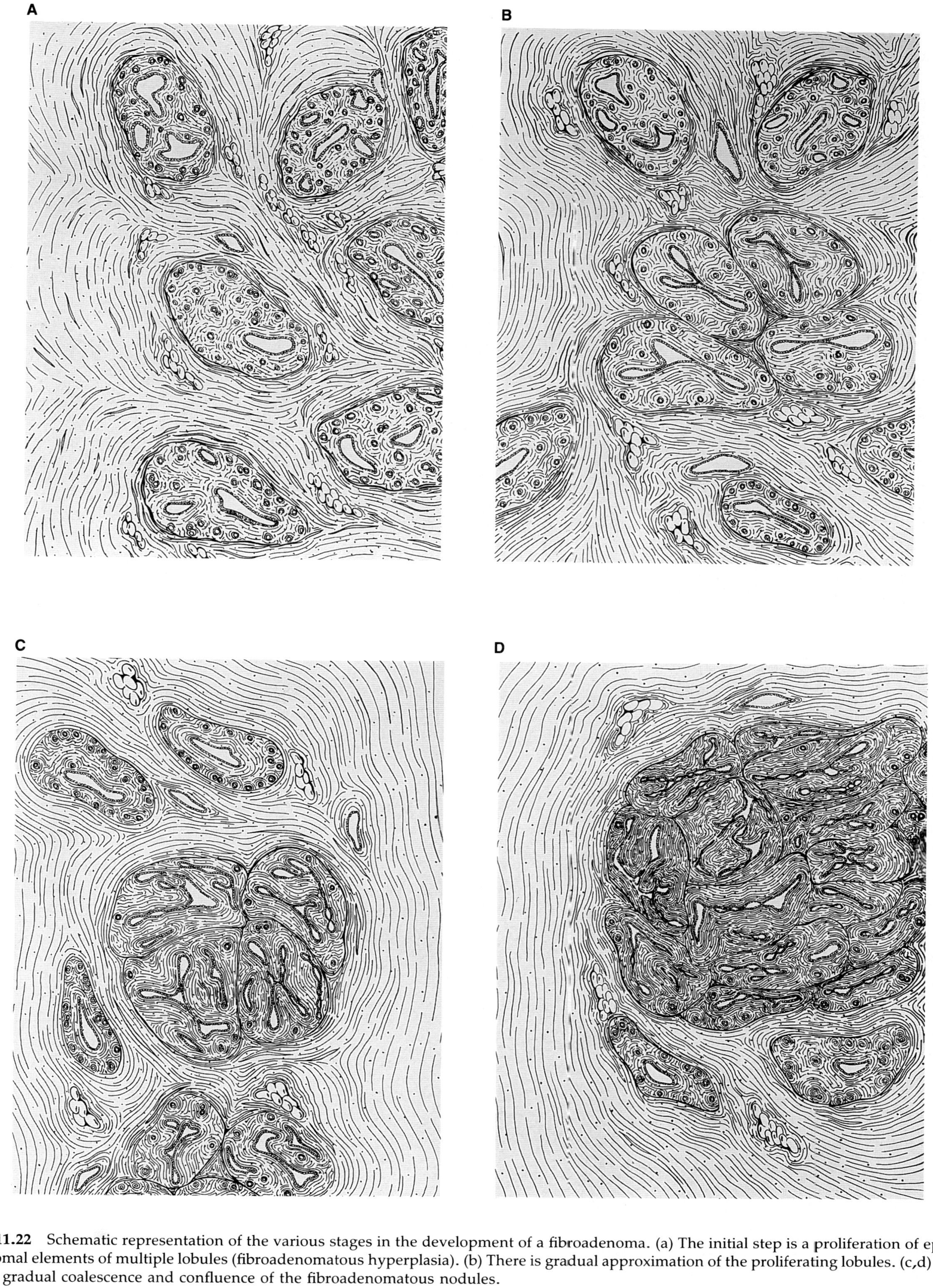


**Figure 11.22** Schematic representation of the various stages in the development of a fibroadenoma. (a) The initial step is a proliferation of epithelial and stromal elements of multiple lobules (fibroadenomatous hyperplasia). (b) There is gradual approximation of the proliferating lobules. (c,d) Finally, there is gradual coalescence and confluence of the fibroadenomatous nodules.

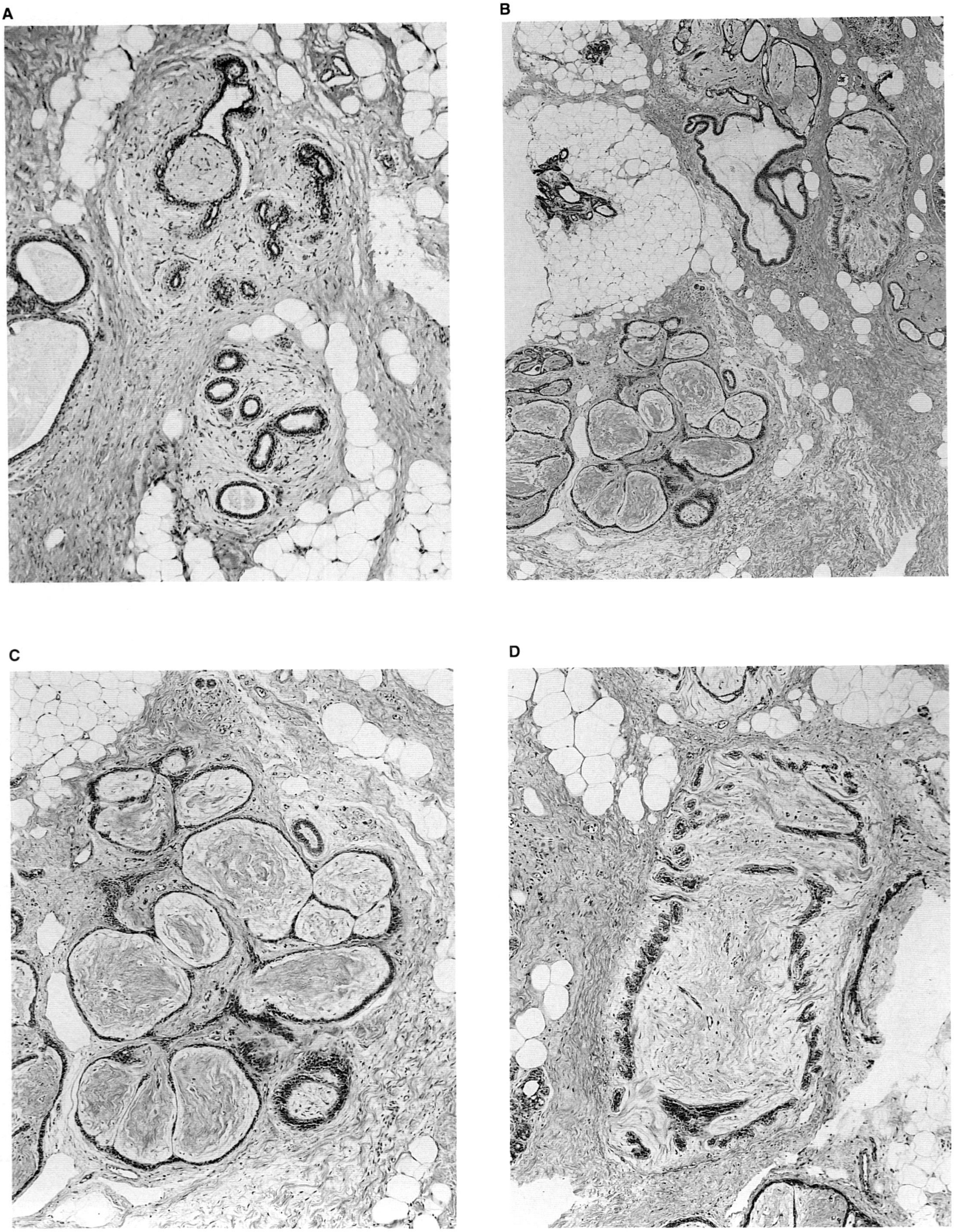


**Figure 11.23** Fibroadenomatous hyperplasia. (a,b) Several lobules show fibroadenomatous hyperplasia. (H&E, (a) X60; (b) X40) (c,d) Higher magnification shows hyalinization of the stromal component in some of these lobules. (H&E, (c,d) X75)

A

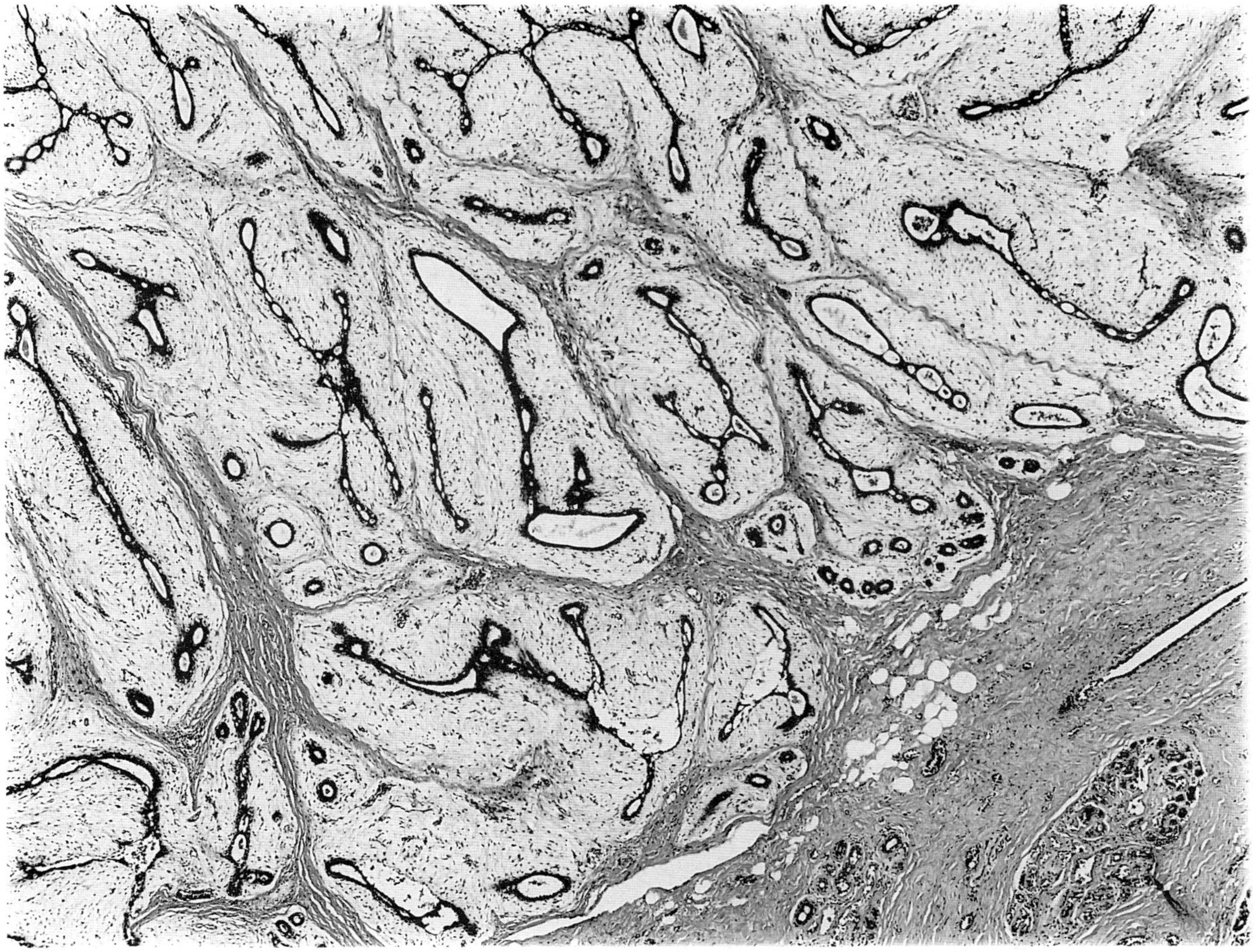

**Figure 11.24(a)** Fibroadenoma, development. A relatively uniform appearance is apparent in the coalescent nodules in this case. (H&E, X60)

their review of 94 cases at AFIP, Norris and Taylor (168) noted focal areas of lipoid (seven cases), chondroid (six cases), chondroid and osseous (five cases) (Fig. 11.31), rhabdomyoblastic (two cases) and smooth muscle (one case) differentiation in a relatively small number of cases. While the aggressive stromal component is often fibrosarcomatous in appearance, other types of sarcoma such as liposarcoma (Fig. 11.32), (119,168,173,174), chondrosarcoma, osteosarcoma, rhabdomyosarcoma (Fig. 11.33) (173), hemangiopericytoma as well as malignant fibrous histiocytoma also develop in CP (164,173). Furthermore, it is not uncommon to find more than one type of differentiation within the sarcomatous component. Pietruszka and Barnes (173) advocate classification of the sarcomatous component on the basis of its differentiation. While I would endorse their recommendation, in a relatively high proportion of cases reviewed at AFIP, we have found that the sarcomatous component defies classification as a distinct soft tissue sarcoma, even though we routinely utilized the expertise of the Soft Tissue Pathology Department in attempts to classify the sarcomas.

Overgrowth of the sarcomatous component occurs in some cases but this feature has been quantitated only recently (146,188). Generally, it is the sarcomatous component that is present at the margin of the neoplasm and it shows either a pushing (Fig. 11.34) or an infiltrating (Fig. 11.35) growth pattern.

B

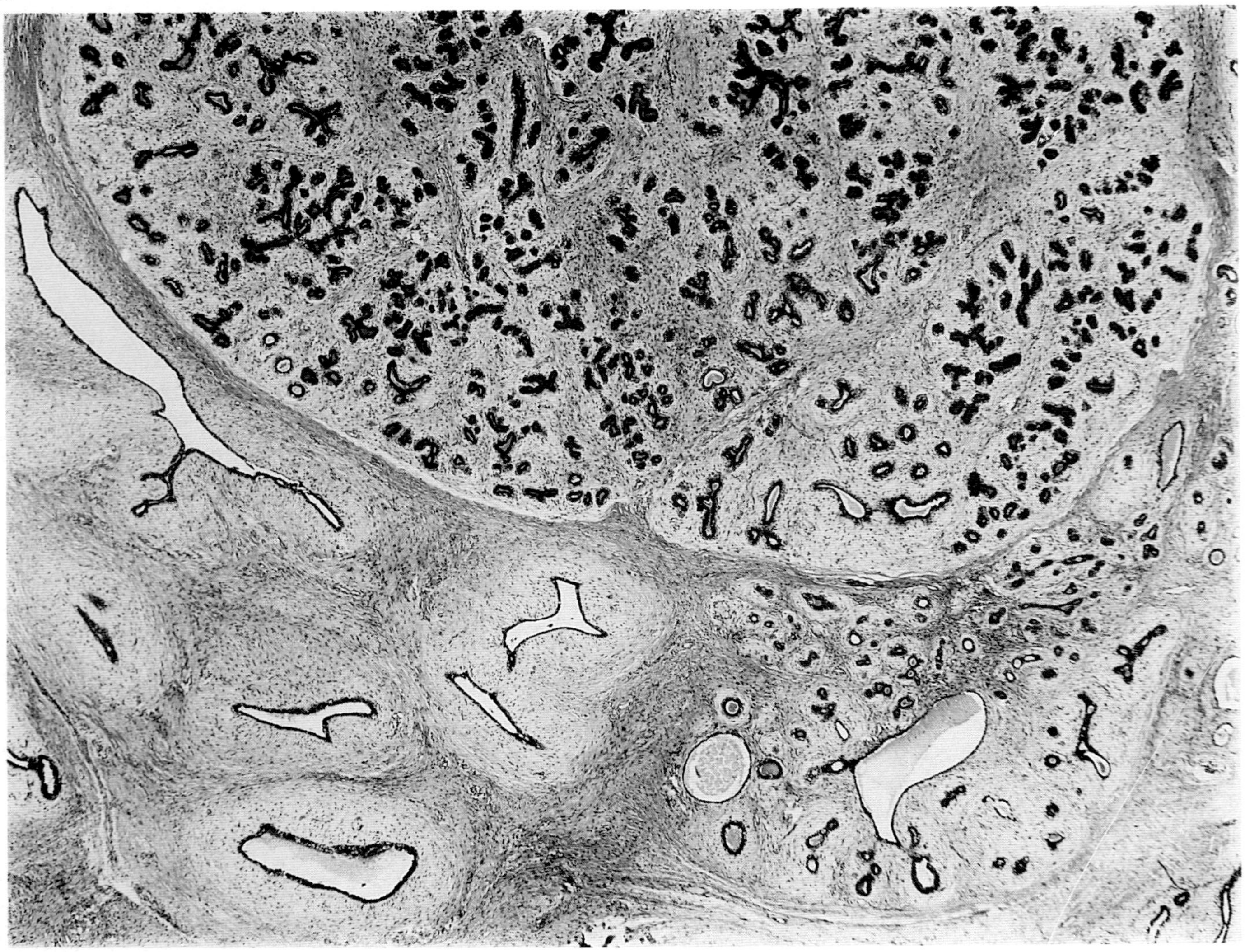

**Figure 11.24(b)** Fibroadenoma, development. Gradual coalescence and confluence of fibroadenomatous nodules at various stages of development. (H&E, X120)

Since sarcomatous overgrowth may severely diminish the epithelial elements to a few minuscule foci, thorough evaluation and sampling of all apparently pure sarcomas is required to exclude their origin in a CP.

The epithelial element of a CP may also show a variety of alterations. Areas of adenosis and cystic change develop occasionally. Metaplastic changes including apocrine (162) and squamous metaplasia (Fig. 11.36) (120,139,168) have been observed also. Hyperplasia, including areas of atypia, is not uncommon (162,168). The development of in situ and invasive carcinomas within cystosarcomas will be discussed later in this chapter.

## Correlation of Histologic Features with Clinical Behavior

Opinions vary regarding the prognostic significance of various gross and histologic parameters. Many pathologists divide cystosarcomas into benign and malignant. McDivitt et al (162) stated that the main difference between the two was that the degree of pleomorphism in the fibrous, myxoid, and fatty stromal growth was significantly less in the benign lesions. Of 59 benign tumors in their series, local recurrences developed in ten patients all of whom

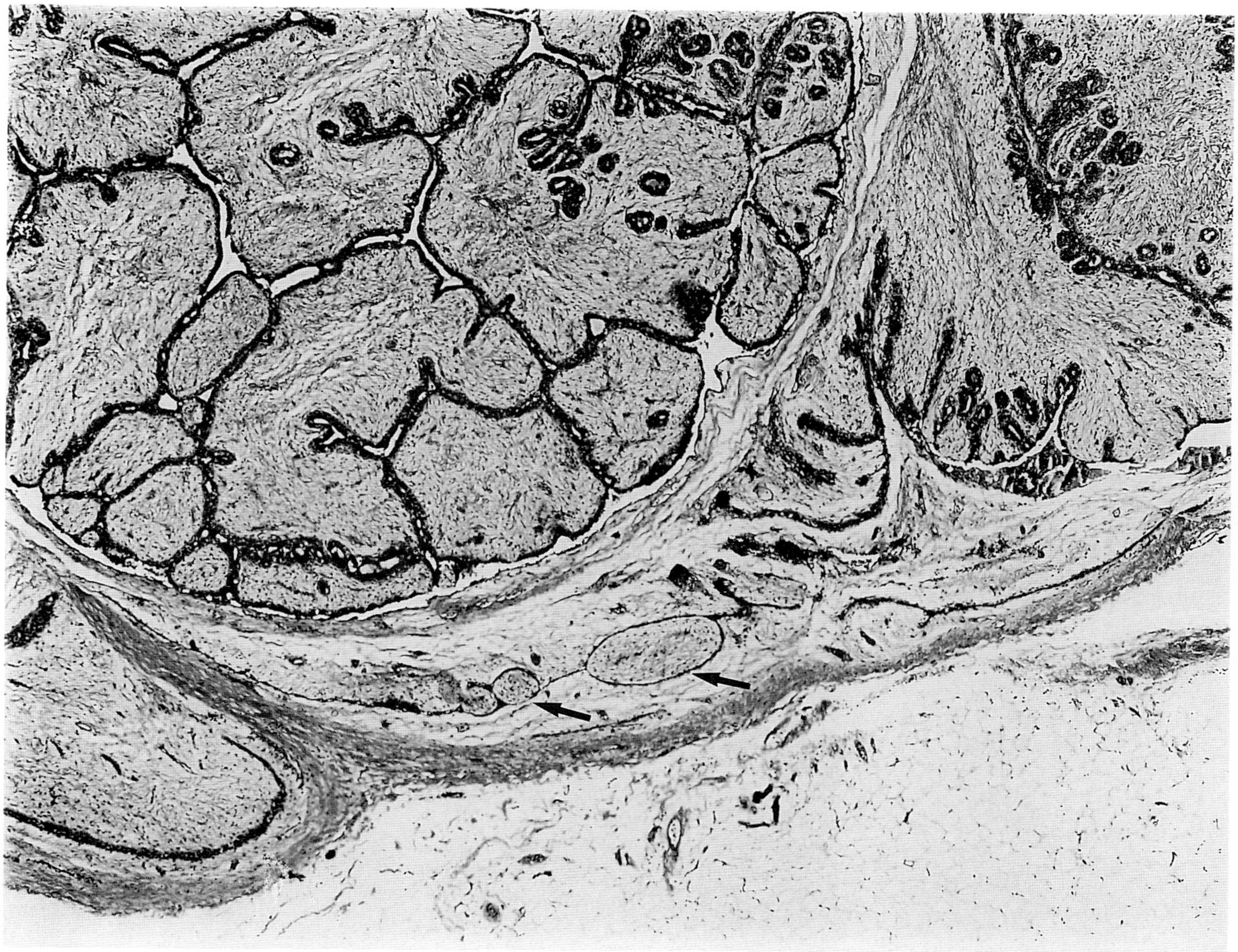

**Figure 11.25** The expansile nodule on the right is surrounded by smaller fibroadenomatous nodules (arrows) which add on to the periphery of the lesion, increasing the size of the tumor within the fibrous capsule. (H&E, X120)

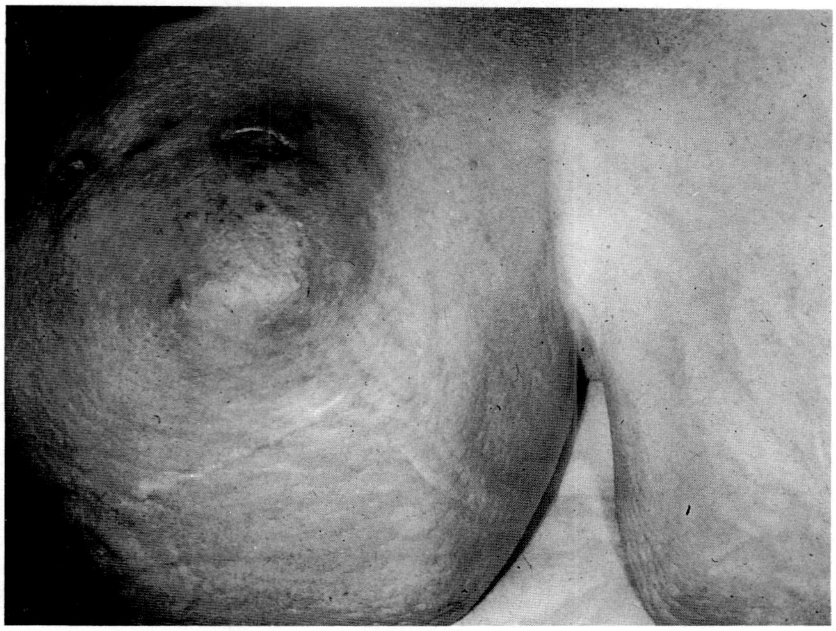

**Figure 11.26** This massive CP totally distorted the breast, with ulceration through the skin and displacement of the nipple.

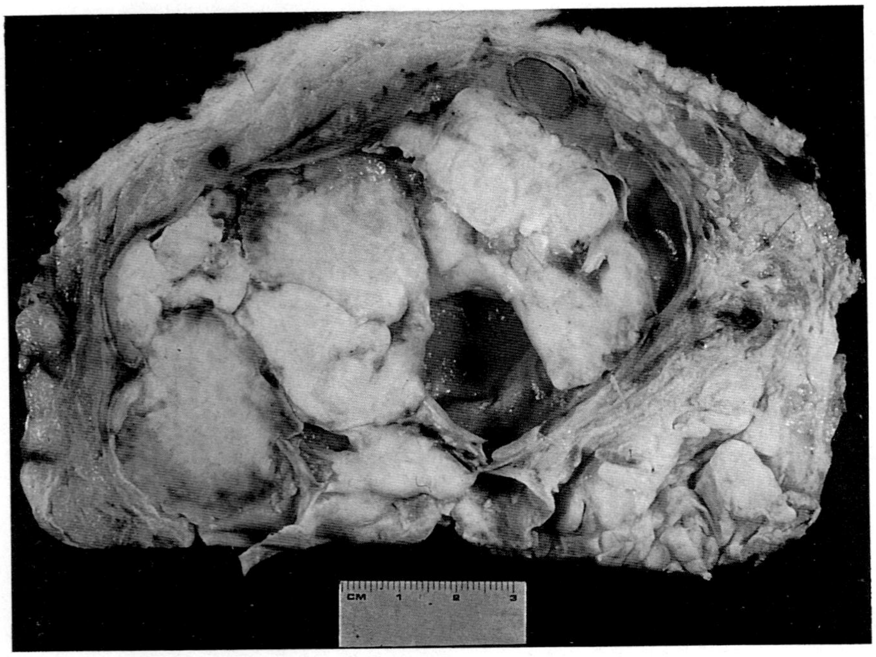

**Figure 11.27** Cystosarcoma phyllodes. A large cystic and solid mass occupies much of the breast.

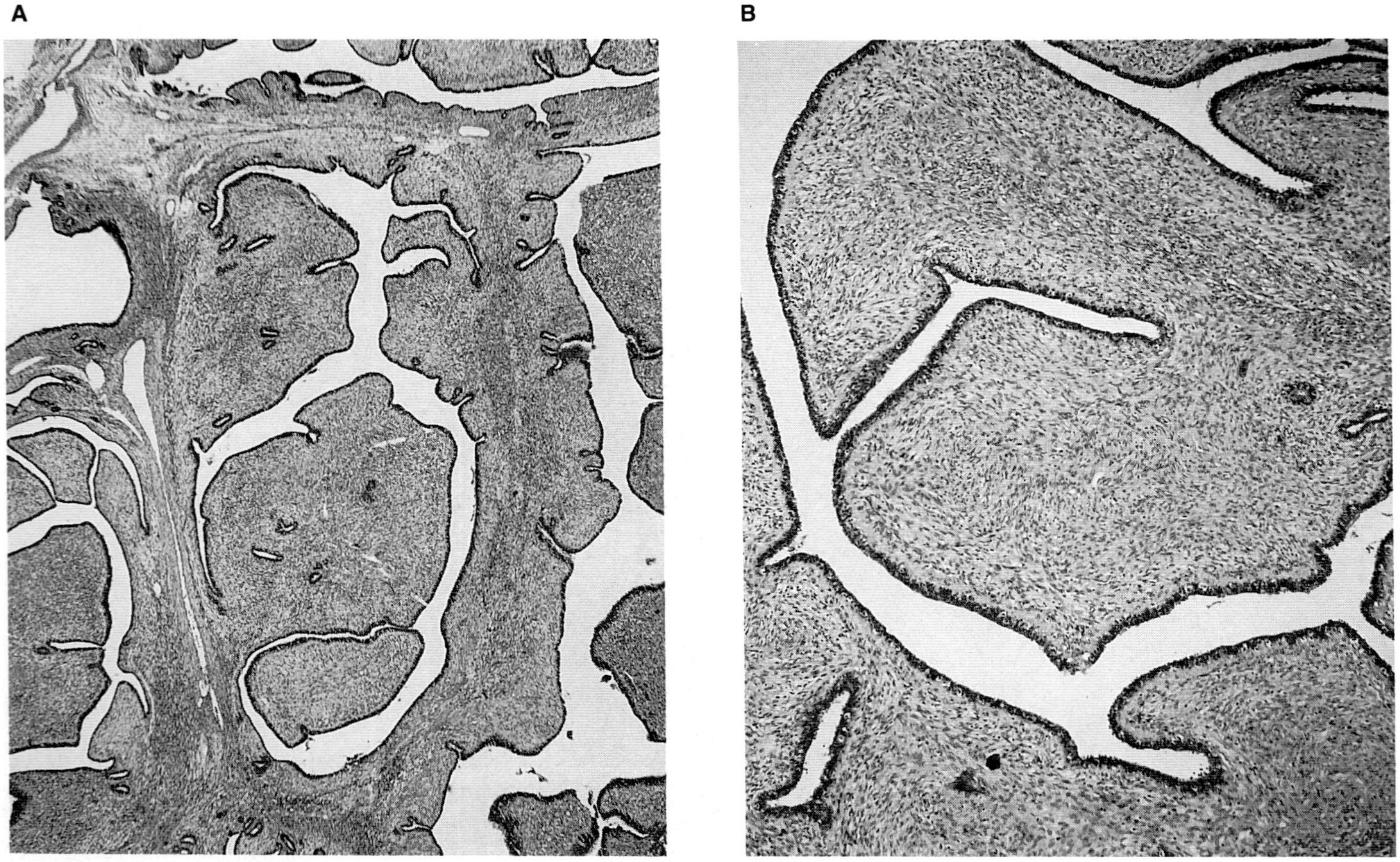


**Figure 11.28** Cystosarcoma phyllodes. (a&b) The tumor consists of leaf-like processes with a moderately cellular stroma. The epithelial cells do not display hyperplastic changes. (H&E, (a) X25, (b) X60)

A

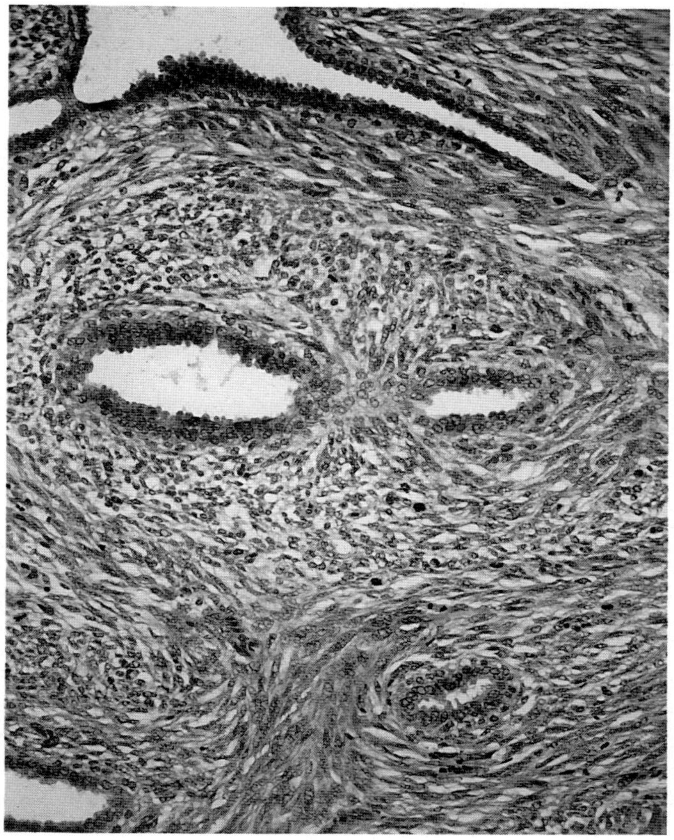

**Figure 11.29(a)** Cystosarcoma phyllodes. A cellular spindle cell stroma with several mitotic figures is the most common mesenchymal component of this tumor. (H&E, X200)

were initially treated by local excision. A clinically malignant course was not observed in any of the histologically benign tumors. Only one of the 14 patients with a histologically malignant tumor developed recurrences and multiple pulmonary metastases and died from disseminated tumor; another patient developed a local recurrence. All of the other 12 patients had remained free of disease since their initial treatments which varied from local excision (four cases) to mastectomy of various extents (four simple, four radical and one modified radical). In their evaluation of 26 cystosarcomas, Hart et al (145) regarded tumors with stromal cells that had microscopic features resembling those of soft-tissue sarcomas as malignant; neoplasms with less ominous-appearing stromal cells were designated as histologically benign. None of their 12 histologically benign tumors metastasized, but two did recur. Of the 14 malignant tumors, four developed recurrences and one of these caused death by direct extension to the lung. Three other patients developed pulmonary metastases, two of whom died, while the third survived 16 years after pulmonary lobectomy.

Norris and Taylor (168) reported that a fairly good estimate of the behavior of cystosarcoma phyllodes can be made by evaluating several pathologic features including tumor size, contour, stromal atypia, and mitotic activity. None of the 15 tumors that proved fatal was less than 4 cm. Lesions less than 4 cm in diameter had a lower rate of recurrence (11%) than larger ones (37%). Tumors with "pushing" margins recurred in 15% of patients and were lethal in only 3%, whereas tumors with infiltrating margins had a recurrence rate of 38% and killed 35% of the patients. Increasing degrees of cytologic atypism were associated with increasing incidence of recurrence and fatal outcome. Of the 15 tumors that proved fatal, only five had 3+ atypia (scale of 1 to 3), while of the 30 lesions with 1+ atypia, 27% recurred and 7% proved fatal. Tumors with five or more mitotic figures per 10 high power fields (HPF) accounted for 11 of the 15 deaths. Of tumors with 0 to 2 mitotic figures per 10 HPF, 17% developed recurrence and 18% of those with only 3 to 4 mitotic figures per 10 HPF died from their tumors despite radical mastectomy in one case. Consequently, it was concluded that no single histologic feature could reliably predict the behavior of this neoplasm and that a combination of tumor size, margin, atypia, and mitotic activity would be helpful as a guide in predicting the behavior of these lesions but clearly not in an absolute way.

Because of the difficulty in predicting the behavior of CP and since even histologically benign tumors are capable of at least recurrence, at AFIP the qualification of benign is not used for CP. Lesions are designated as low grade if they have a pushing growth margin, mild (1+) atypia, and less than three mitotic figures per 10 HPF; these tumors have a potential for local recurrence but are very unlikely to metastasize. The term high grade cystosarcoma phyllodes is used to designate a tumor with potential for distant metastasis and characterized by invasive or pushing margin, moderate to severe atypia (2+ to 3+), and three or more mitotic figures per 10 HPF.

Based on a composite evaluation of the number of mitotic figures, atypia, and tumor contour, several investigators have proposed subdivision of CP into benign, intermediate (borderline), and malignant groups (126,143,173,186). The criteria proposed by various investigators are different, however. The dif-

B

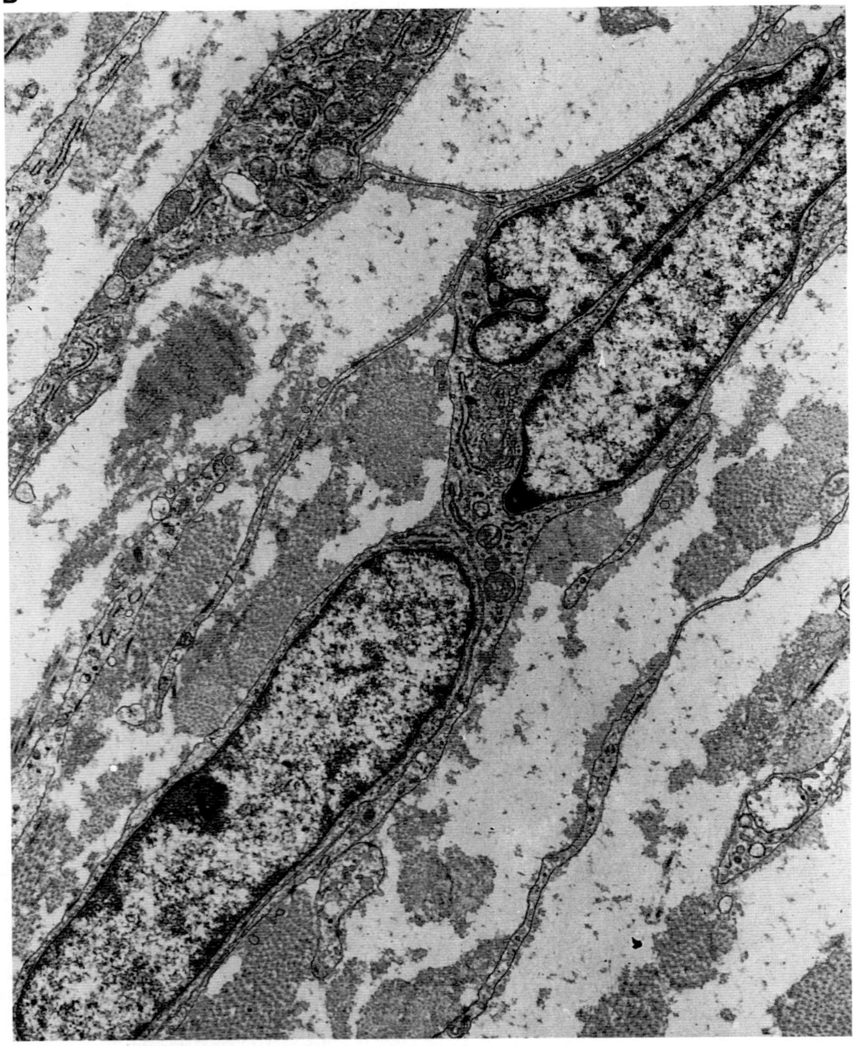

**Figure 11.29(b)** Spindled stromal cells in cystosarcoma phyllodes. At the ultrastructural level the stromal cells in this tumor were predominantly fibroblasts. (Uranyl acetate-lead citrate, X3,000)

ference is primarily in the number of mitotic figures allowed for each subgroup; but there are also differences in the type of cases studied, the extent of surgical excision, and the length of follow-up contributing to variable outcomes for the patients in different studies. For example, in one study (126) there were no recurrences in either the benign or the borderline group. Furthermore, there were no metastases but only recurrences in five of the seven patients with follow-up in the malignant group. In another study (173), four of the 18 benign tumors developed recurrences and one of the three patients followed with a borderline tumor died with direct extension of the tumor to the lungs 23.5 years later and after 14 recurrences. Interestingly, only four of the 17 patients with malignant tumors and follow-up developed metastasis, three of whom died of their tumors. The remaining patients were alive and well without evidence of disease from one month to 23.5 years after the diagnosis with the exception of one patient who died from an unrelated cause ten years later without evidence of disease.

In conclusion, while addition of a borderline category may appear useful, the criteria advanced so far seem more helpful in creating an arbitrary histologic separation than in having clinical predictive values. Salvadori et al (181) found no difference between borderline and malignant tumors in terms of local recurrence or distant metastases.

Stromal overgrowth is another factor which has prognostic significance. While Hart et al (145) had noted this feature only in malignant cystosarcomas, it has been quantitated only recently (146,189). Ward and Evans (188), defined stromal overgrowth as overgrowth of the sarcomatous component to the point that epithelial elements are absent in at least one

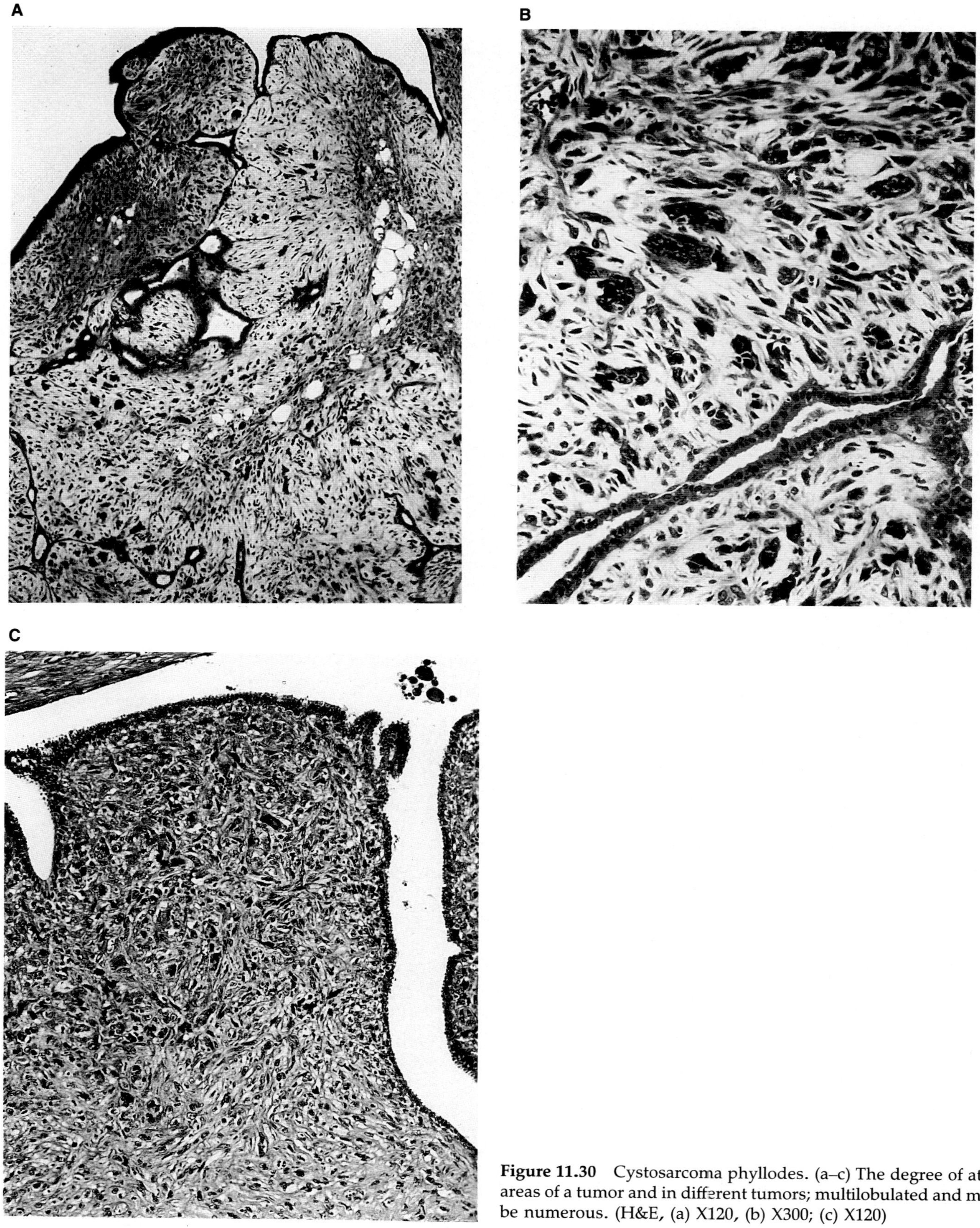


**Figure 11.30** Cystosarcoma phyllodes. (a–c) The degree of atypia varies in different areas of a tumor and in different tumors; multilobulated and multinucleated cells may be numerous. (H&E, (a) X120, (b) X300; (c) X120)

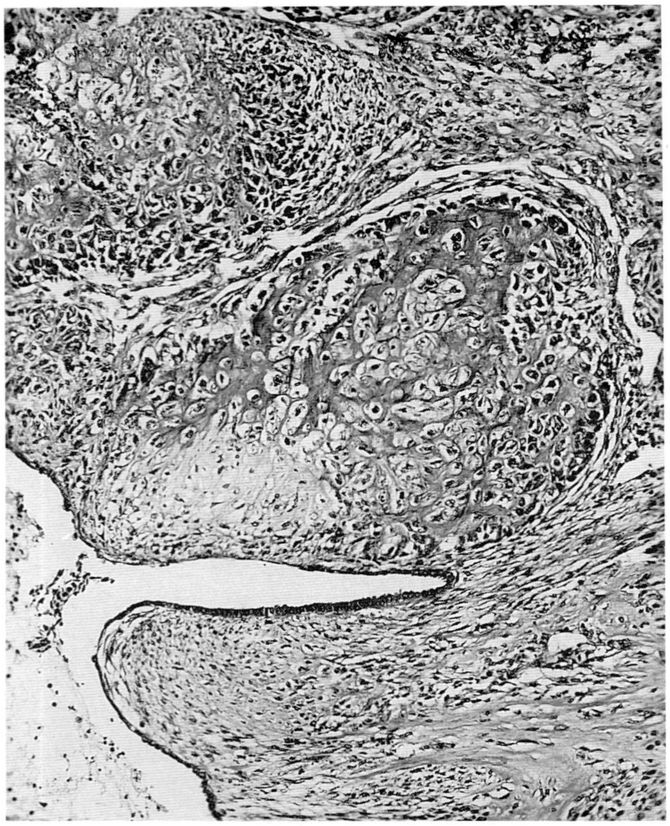

**Figure 11.31** Osseous metaplasia in cystosarcoma phyllodes. (H&E, X100)

low-power field (X40 magnification). In a review of 26 cystosarcomas, Ward and Evans (188) found stromal overgrowth in six of the seven patients who died of tumor, including all five with metastasis; they concluded that stromal overgrowth is a significant morphologic indicator of malignant behavior. While I agree that sarcomatous overgrowth is a significant prognostic variable, I believe that the threshold should be raised significantly to refer only to neoplasms that display predominance of a pure sarcoma on multiple sections with residual CP elements barely identifiable (Fig. 11.37). In my experience at AFIP, overgrowth of even bland-appearing stroma to the exclusion of the epithelial component in two or more low power fields is not uncommon in tumors larger than 5 cm.

## Differential Diagnosis

In cases where there is extensive stromal overgrowth, distinction from a pure sarcoma becomes important.

A

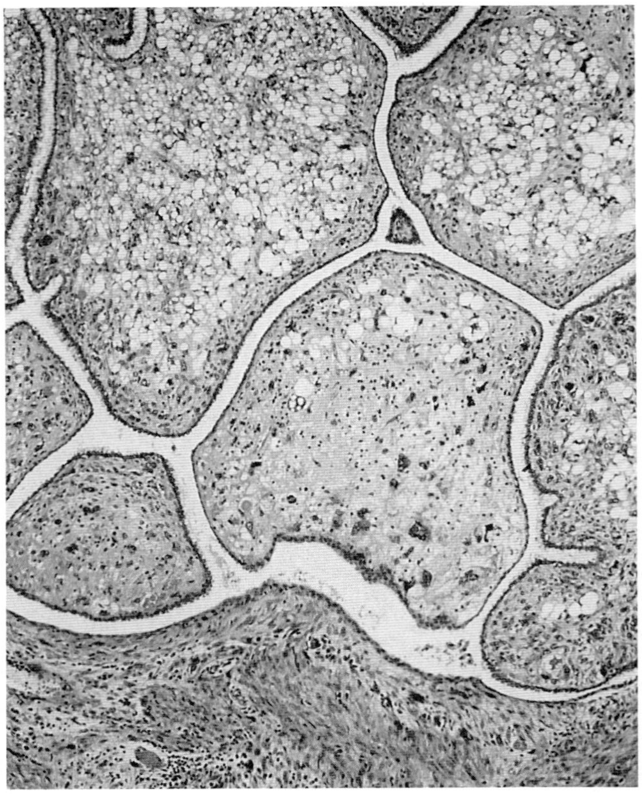

B

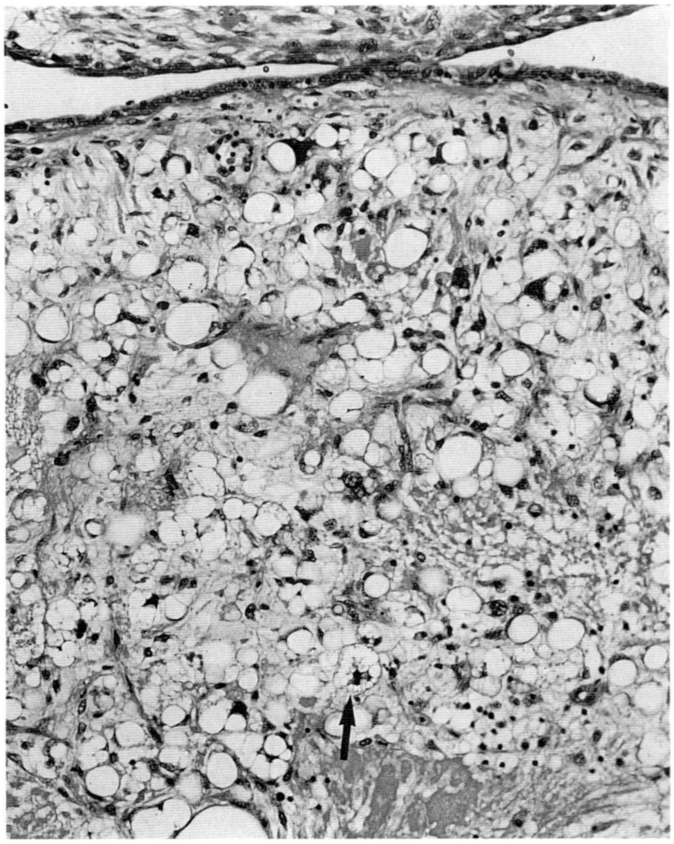

**Figure 11.32** Cystosarcoma phyllodes with liposarcomatous stroma. (a) Much of the stroma consists of liposarcoma. (b) A classic lipoblast is evident. (H&E, (a) X75; (b) X150)

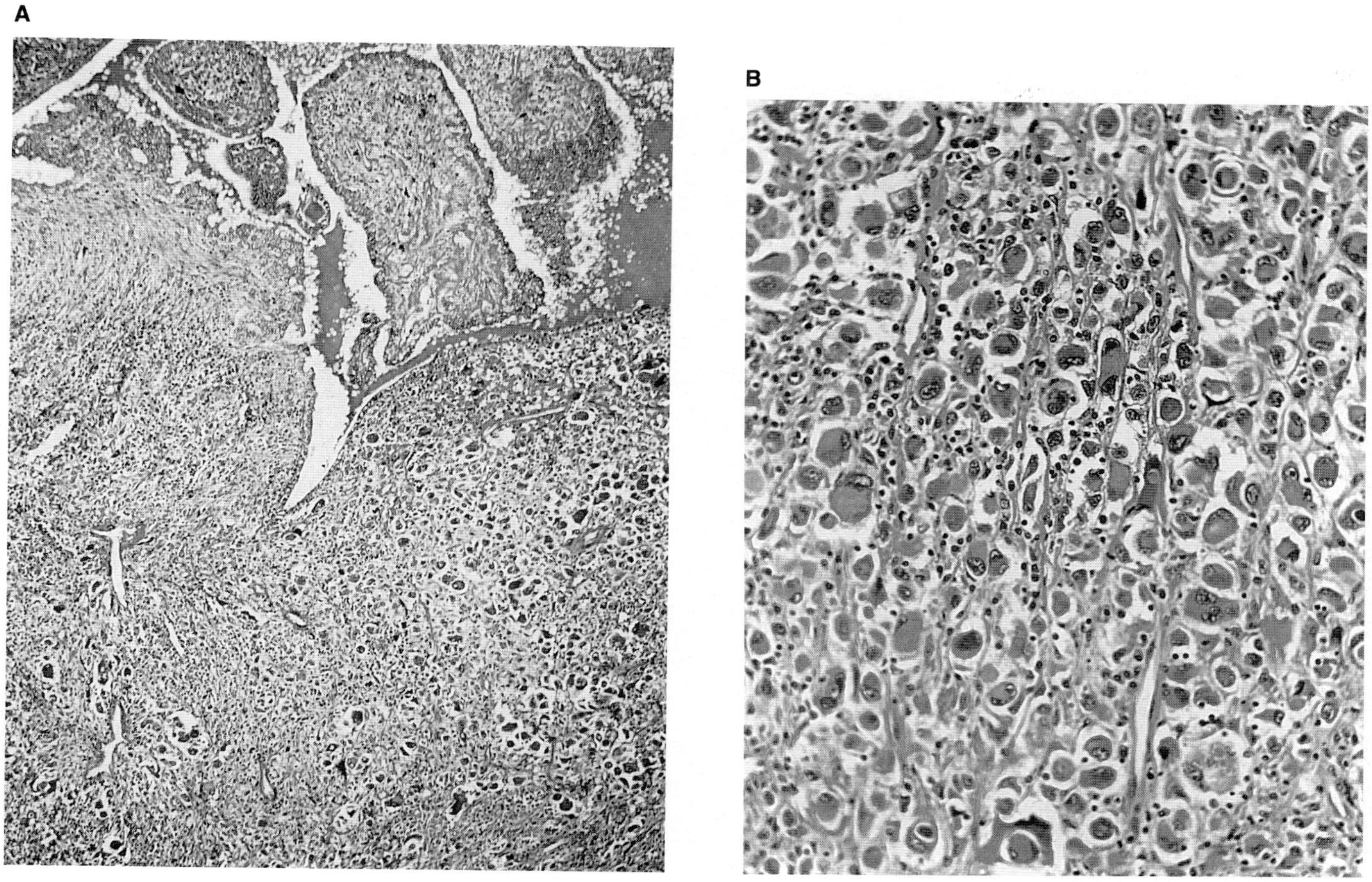

**Figure 11.33** Cystosarcoma phyllodes with rhabdomyosarcoma. (a) At low magnification, parts of the stroma show a concentration of large isolated cells. (b) At higher magnification, the rhabdomyosarcomatous nature of the cells is evident. (H&E, (a) X60; (b) X160)

In such cases, adequate sampling of the tumor (one tissue section per each cm of maximum tumor diameter) is necessary to identify the epithelial elements which may be reduced to an occasional focus within a large neoplasm. Furthermore, since some cystosarcomas recur as a pure sarcoma, it is important to obtain a thorough history when dealing with what appears to be a pure sarcoma, and review any previous biopsies to exclude the possibility of cystosarcoma.

The distinction from cellular fibroadenomas has been discussed earlier in this chapter under the differential diagnosis of fibroadenomas.

## Recurrence and Metastases

Recurrences develop in approximately 30% of cystosarcomas and the majority of them develop within two years after the diagnosis. Multiple recurrences —up to 14 recurrences over a 23-year period—have been reported (173). Subsequent recurrences often retain the histologic features of the original neoplasm, but they may become more cellular, atypical, and mitotically active. Local recurrences develop in about 50% of patients with metastasizing cystosarcomas. Fatality due to extension of the recurrent tumor to vital organs in the absence of distant metastasis occurs rarely (173).

Metastases occur in less than 10% of unselected cases, although there is a wide range reported in the literature. Metastases occur through the blood stream. Lymph node metastases are not common, having been described in about 15% of metastatic cystosarcomas (114,165,168). A majority of the tumors (66%) metastasize to the lungs, while the skeleton is involved in 28%, the heart in 9.4%, and liver in 5.6% of cases with metastases. Metastases have been reported to almost all organ sites (Fig. 11.38) including intraneural and central nervous system (138), the adrenal, pancreas, spleen, omentum, stomach, larynx, cervical and paraaortic lymph nodes, pleura, subpleura, gum, scalp, vulva, and even the

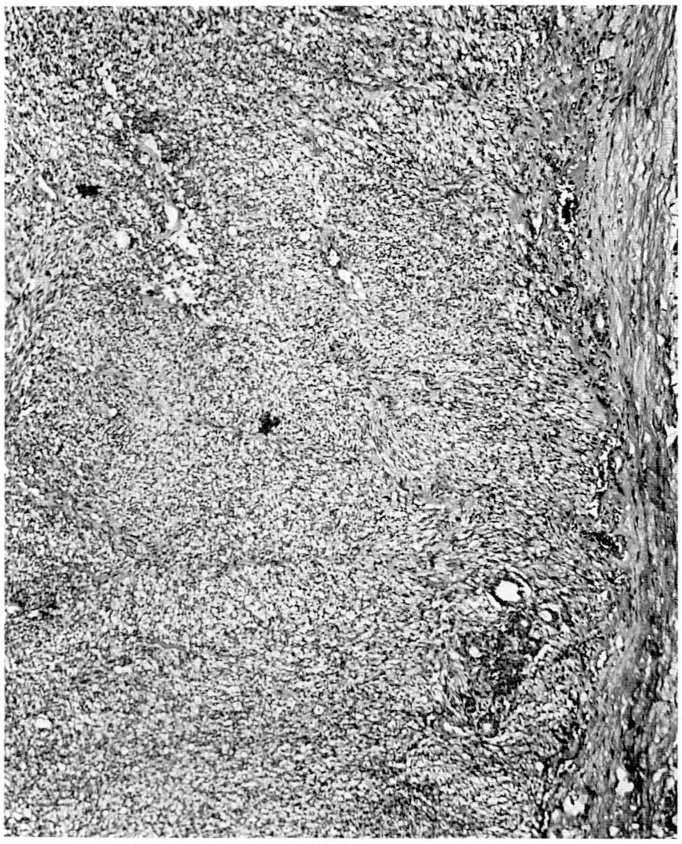

**Figure 11.34** Cystosarcoma phyllodes with an expansible, pushing margin. (H&E, X60)

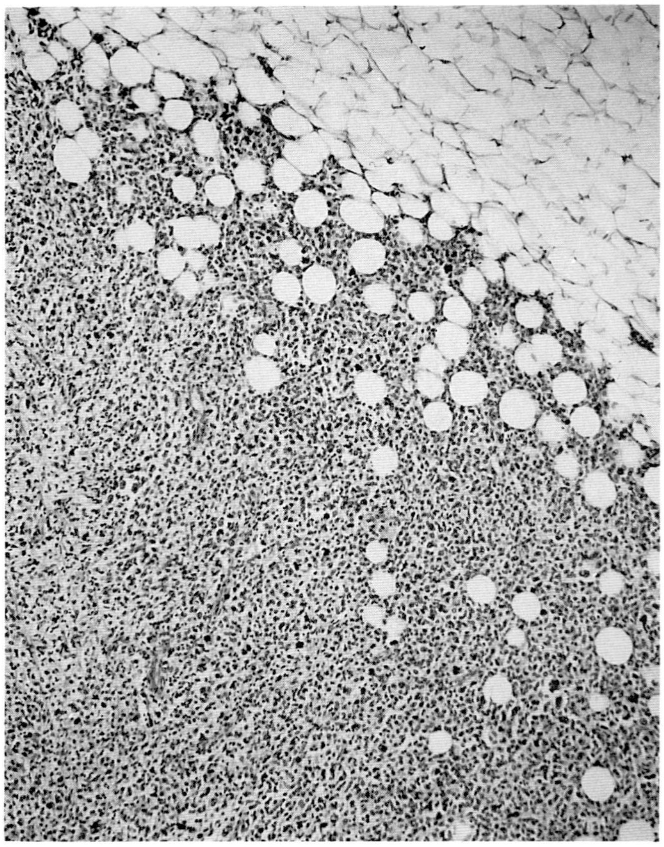

**Figure 11.35** Cystosarcoma phyllodes with an infiltrating margin. (H&E, X60)

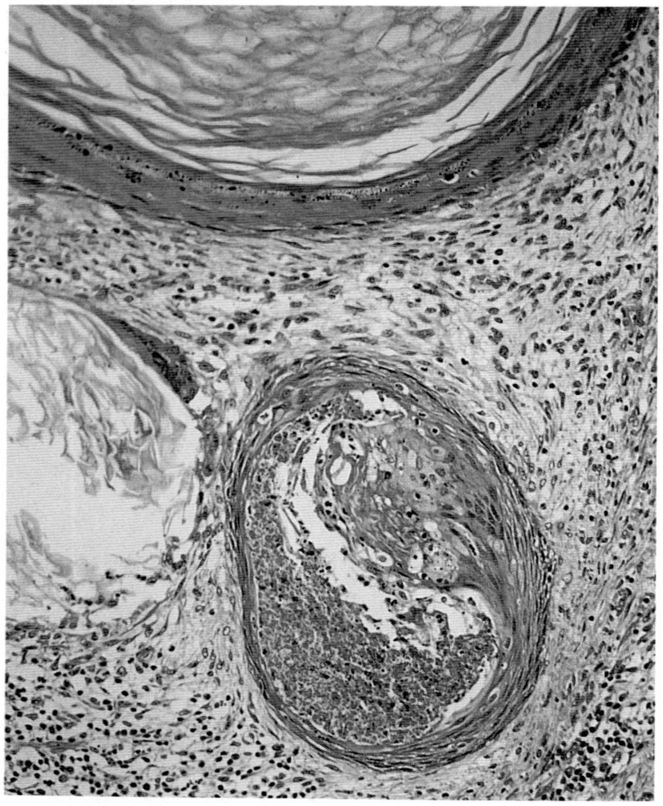

**Figure 11.36** Squamous metaplasia in cystosarcoma phyllodes. (H&E, X160)

sole of the foot (152). With one rare exception (189), the metastatic tumors have been devoid of epithelial elements. In general, metastases become evident within two years of the initial treatment but variations exist in this time interval. Cure and survival over ten years are rare after metastases have occurred (158,176).

## Treatment

There has been divergence in the recommendations for treatment of cystosarcomas. While simple, modified, and radical mastectomy have been used in many cases and mastectomy remains the initial treatment in some cases, a more conservative approach (wide local excision) is now advocated as primary treatment (181). In Haagensen's experience (139), local excision has been remarkably successful in treatment of CP. He objects to radical mastectomy since the axillary dissection included in the operation is superfluous—CP almost never metastasizes to axillary lymph

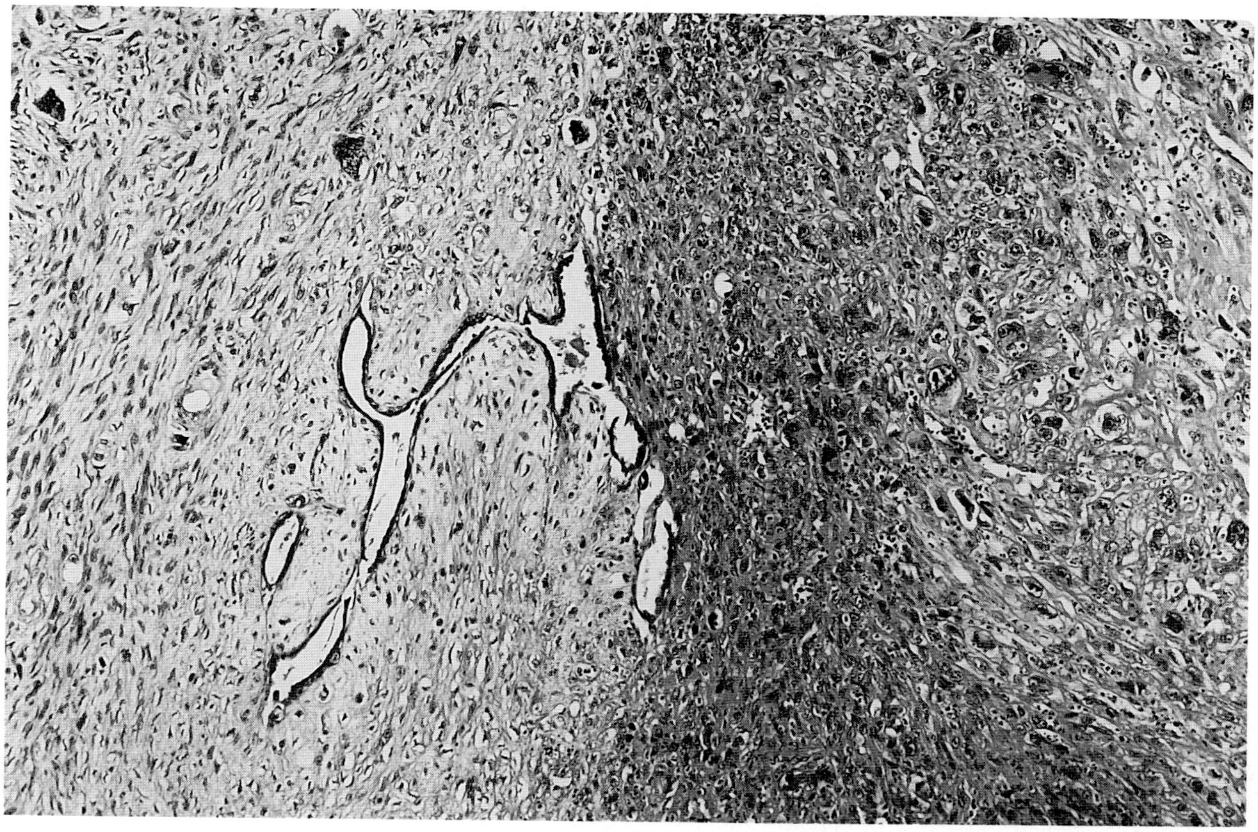

**Figure 11.37** Sarcomatous overgrowth in a CP. The epithelial component was identified only after extensive search. (H&E, X150)

nodes and the highly malignant tumors prove fatal despite the extent of excision. Norris & Taylor (168) also advocated total excision of the tumor, unless a large tumor size or invasive margins required mastectomy for total excision of the tumor.

The extent of the surgical excision is determined in part by the size and margin of the neoplasm. Because of the lobulations in the margin of many neoplasms, excision of the tumor with a margin of uninvolved breast tissue is preferable. If the tumor has unusual marginal irregularities detectable mammographically, it is worthwhile to do specimen mammography to ascertain complete removal of the lesion prior to cutting the specimen (Fig. 11.39). Recurrences should be resected in a similar way. Simple mastectomy should be reserved for massive tumors or lesions with infiltrating margins and aggressive histologic features that would defy total excision with a clear margin by a lesser procedure. Total mastectomy is also indicated for local recurrences of borderline and malignant lesions (181). The effectiveness of other treatment modalities has not been established, but a combination of cisplatin and etoposide chemotherapy and radiation therapy has been reported to be effective in the management of three patients with symptomatic metastases (124). While pulmonary metastases may be resectable (133,145), therapy for metastatic disease has been rather discouraging. A variety of therapeutic approaches including radiation, hormonal manipulation, and chemotherapy have failed to sustain remission.

## Conclusion

Considering the relatively small number of patients who actually develop metastases, a comparatively higher number that develop recurrences, and our inability to accurately predict either event, it is best to separate cystosarcomas into two groups: the low grade cystosarcoma phyllodes having a potential for local recurrence, and the high grade tumors, with a potential for metastases. The terms benign and malignant should be avoided in the diagnosis. If there are recognizable patterns of specific sarcomas, however, they should be included in the diagnosis. Uti-

A

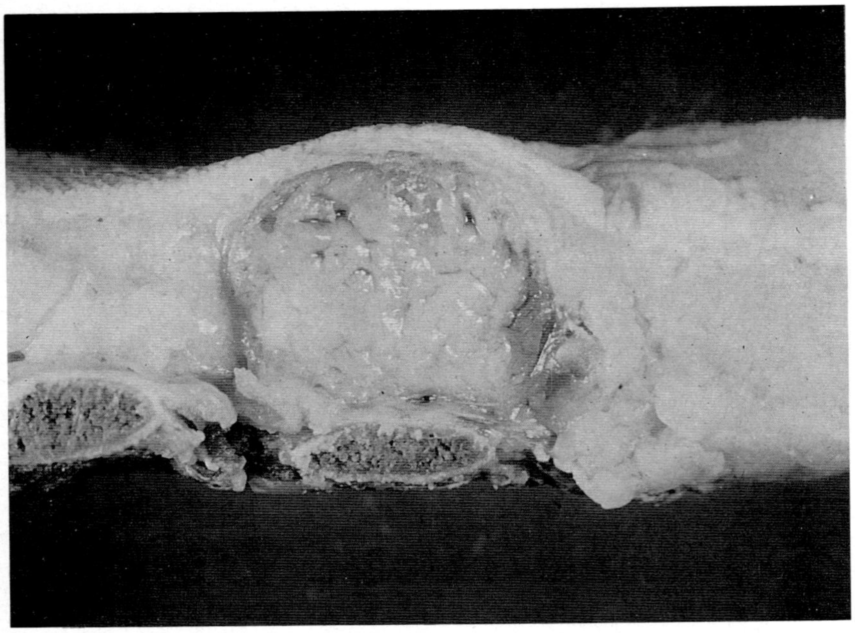

B

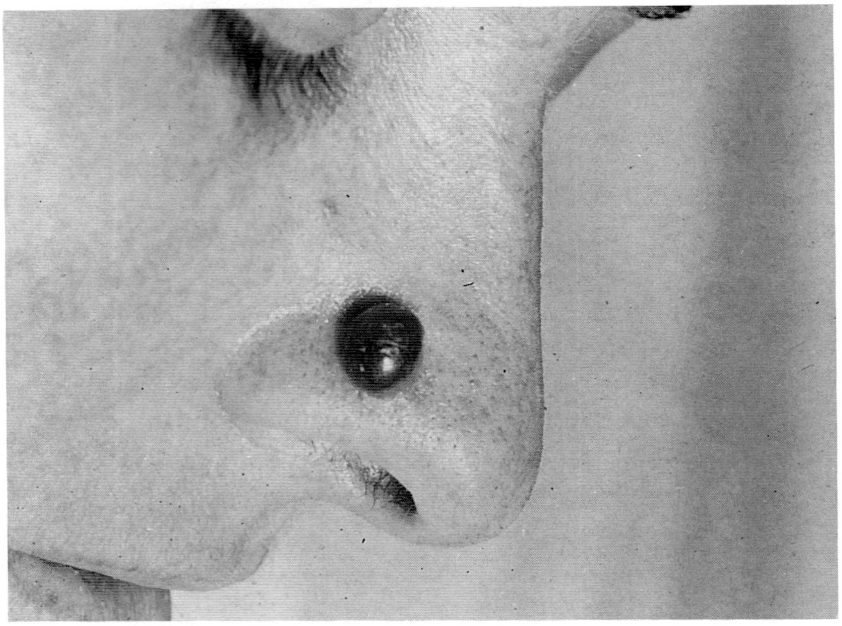

**Figure 11.38** (a) Recurrence of cystosarcoma in the soft tissue of the anterior chest wall. (b) Cutaneous metastasis from cystosarcoma phyllodes. (c) Metastasis of the sarcomatous component to the axillary region adjacent to a lymph node. (H&E, (c) X160)

lizing Norris and Taylor's criteria (168), tumors with less than three mitotic figures per 10 HPF, mild to moderate atypia, cellular stroma, and predominantly pushing margins would be designated as low grade CP. Neoplasms with three or more mitotic figures per 10 HPF, moderate to severe stromal atypia, cellular stroma, and infiltrating margins would be designated as CP without further qualification, implying a high grade group. Also tumors with sarcomatous overgrowth—whether a nonspecific or a specific soft tissue sarcoma—and a minor residual recognizable CP component would be placed in the latter group.

## Carcinoma Arising in Cystosarcoma Phyllodes

Both in situ (including LCIS or lobular neoplasia) and invasive carcinomas occur in CP but they are rather

c

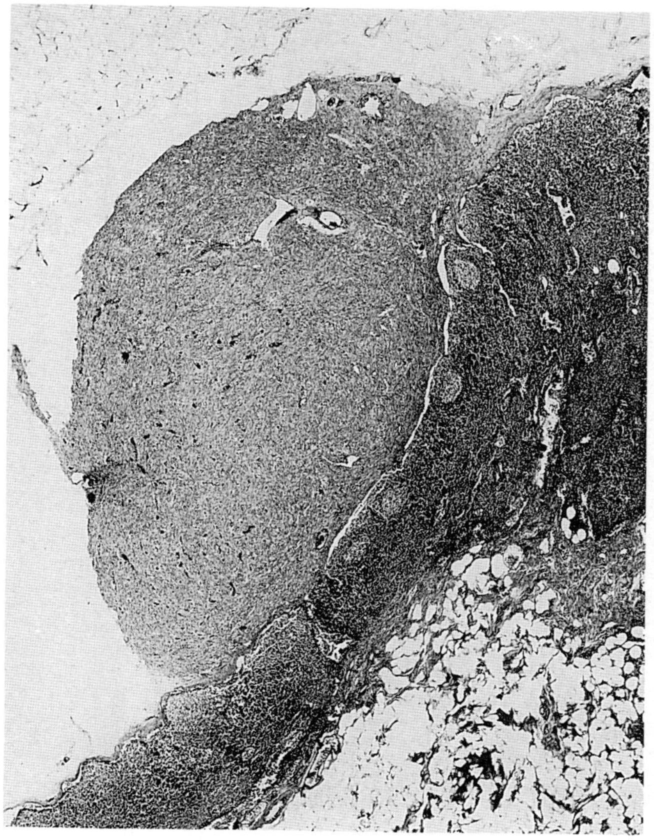

**Figure 11.38(c)** Legend on opposite page.

uncommon (139,168,185,195–202). Intraductal carcinoma was identified in one tumor in Norris and Taylor's series (168) from AFIP. In the same study, two examples of invasive ductal carcinoma involving CP were identified. Squamous carcinoma (194,195) has also been reported in cystosarcomas. There are many more reported examples of carcinoma (both in situ and invasive) arising in fibroadenoma (FA), than there are of carcinomas arising in CP; this is probably due to the rarity of CP and abundance of FA.

Recently, I had the opportunity to review several cases of invasive carcinomas confined to cystosarcomas. In one, a highly pleomorphic carcinoma replaced a significant portion of the almost bland-appearing stroma in a CP (Fig. 11.40 a–c). There were abundant areas of atypical ductal epithelial hyperplasia, but only focally did the changes qualify as cribriform variant of intraductal carcinoma; the patient had a regular infiltrating duct carcinoma in the contralateral breast. The second CP had an infiltrating duct carcinoma (Fig. 11.40d) as well as sarcomatous overgrowth. The third lesion displayed an adenocarcinoma with squamous metaplasia within a high grade CP that also had hemangiopericytoma areas within the stroma. Consideration of some of these complex tumors as carcinosarcoma will be discussed later in this chapter. Both in situ and invasive carcinoma are more common in the breast tissue adjacent to a CP than within it. Furthermore, lobular neoplasia is the tumor most commonly observed in association with CP both within the CP and in the adjacent breast tissue.

## Cystosarcoma in Children and Men

Rarely does CP affect children. There were only three patients less than 20 years of age among the 94 cases reported by Norris and Taylor (168). McDivitt et al (162), had three such cases, while Haagensen had four (139). There has not been a single case of CP in girls less than ten years of age diagnosed at AFIP. In general, CP does not behave aggressively in children, but a few cases of metastasizing CP in children have been reported (137,173,194) including a 14-year-old girl who died from metastasizing CP (149).

Cystosarcoma phyllodes has rarely been reported in men (see also Chapter 16, Male Breast Lesions). Three such cases were in the series of Lee and Pack (155). There were none in McDivitt et al's report (162), nor were there any in Norris and Taylor's series of 94 cases (168). A single case was reported by Reingold and Ascher in a man with gynecomastia (177). A massive (30 cm) tumor which had been present for 50 years in a 70-year-old man was reported by Pantoja et al (172); the contralateral breast had moderately advanced gynecomastia.

In a review of the AFIP files on cystosarcoma phyllodes, only two definite cases of CP were identified in men. Both of these tumors were low grade, considering the mild degree of stromal cellularity (Fig. 11.41). Both of these patients had gynecomastia in the adjacent breast tissue. A third case which may also reflect a highly aggressive cystosarcoma phyllodes was characterized by a massive leiomyosarcomatous growth with a few areas displaying a questionable cystosarcomatous growth pattern in a 40-year-old black man. Following mastectomy for the initial lesion, this patient developed five recurrences within a five year period, three of which contained only the sarcomatous component. Two of the recurrences included sarcomatous nodules excised from

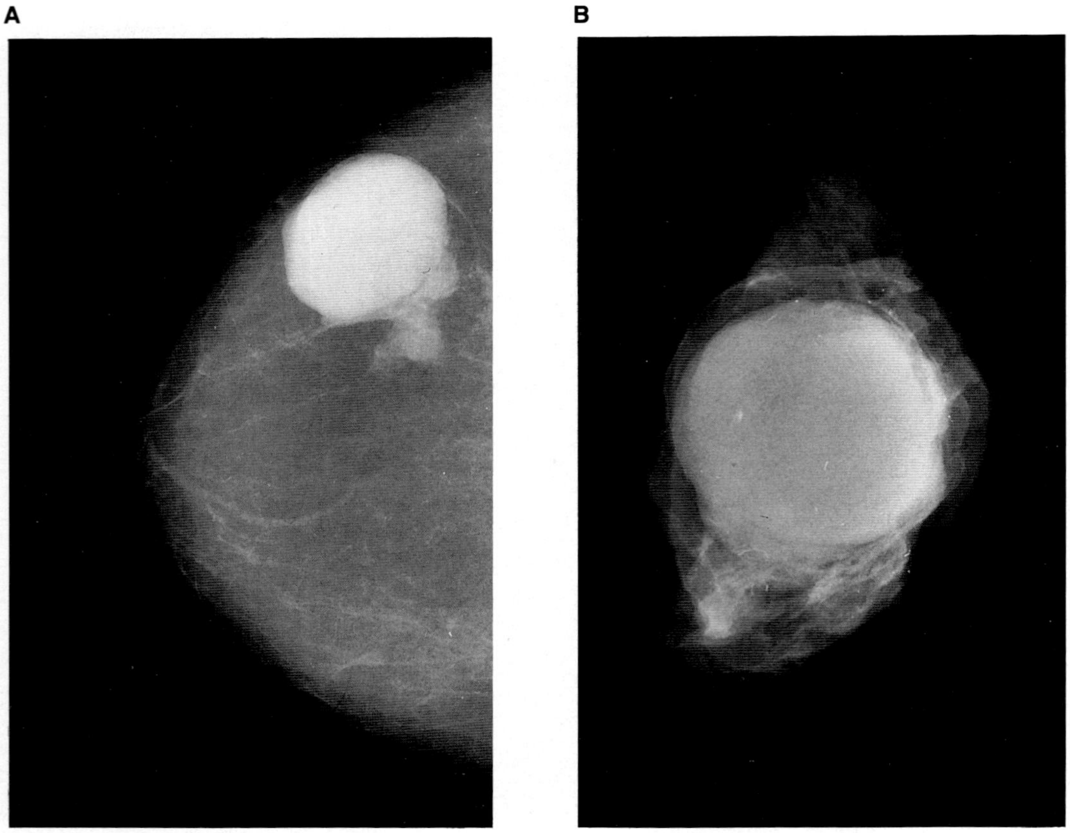


**Figure 11.39** (a) Mammographically, an irregular extension of this otherwise round mass of cystosarcoma is readily apparent. (b) Specimen mammography confirms that the entire tumor, including the irregular extension has been removed.

the axilla. While these could reflect total replacement of lymph nodes, several nodes adjacent to these nodules showed no evidence of metastatic tumor.

Treatment of CP in children and male patients should be directed at total excision of the lesion. Special care should be taken to avoid damaging uninvolved developing breast tissue in children and adolescent females. Follow-up of the patients is necessary particularly if morphologic features of an aggressive neoplasm are identified.

## Origin of Cystosarcoma Phyllodes

The pathogenesis of cystosarcoma phyllodes has remained an enigma. Some authors believe CP arises de novo from breast parenchyma (131,140,185); the developmental process may be similar to that described earlier for fibroadenomas with simultaneous proliferation of the epithelial and stromal components within the lobules.

It is also possible that some CPs arise from pre-existing fibroadenomas (128,131,147,155). Occasional reports of patients who have noted a sudden onset of growth in small breast nodules that had been present for up to 45 years (159), and the rare finding of small but typical CP areas within an otherwise classic fibroadenoma lend support to this mode of development.

The possible role of radiation in malignant transformation of fibroadenoma has been suggested in a report describing a cystosarcoma with fibroadenomatous areas which appeared in a 48-year-old woman 15 years after radiation for a breast nodule (154).

A variety of factors have been implicated in stimulating growth of CP. Trauma, lactation, pregnancy, and increased estrogenic activity (120,137,176, 193) have all been noted as factors affecting the growth of CP.

A B

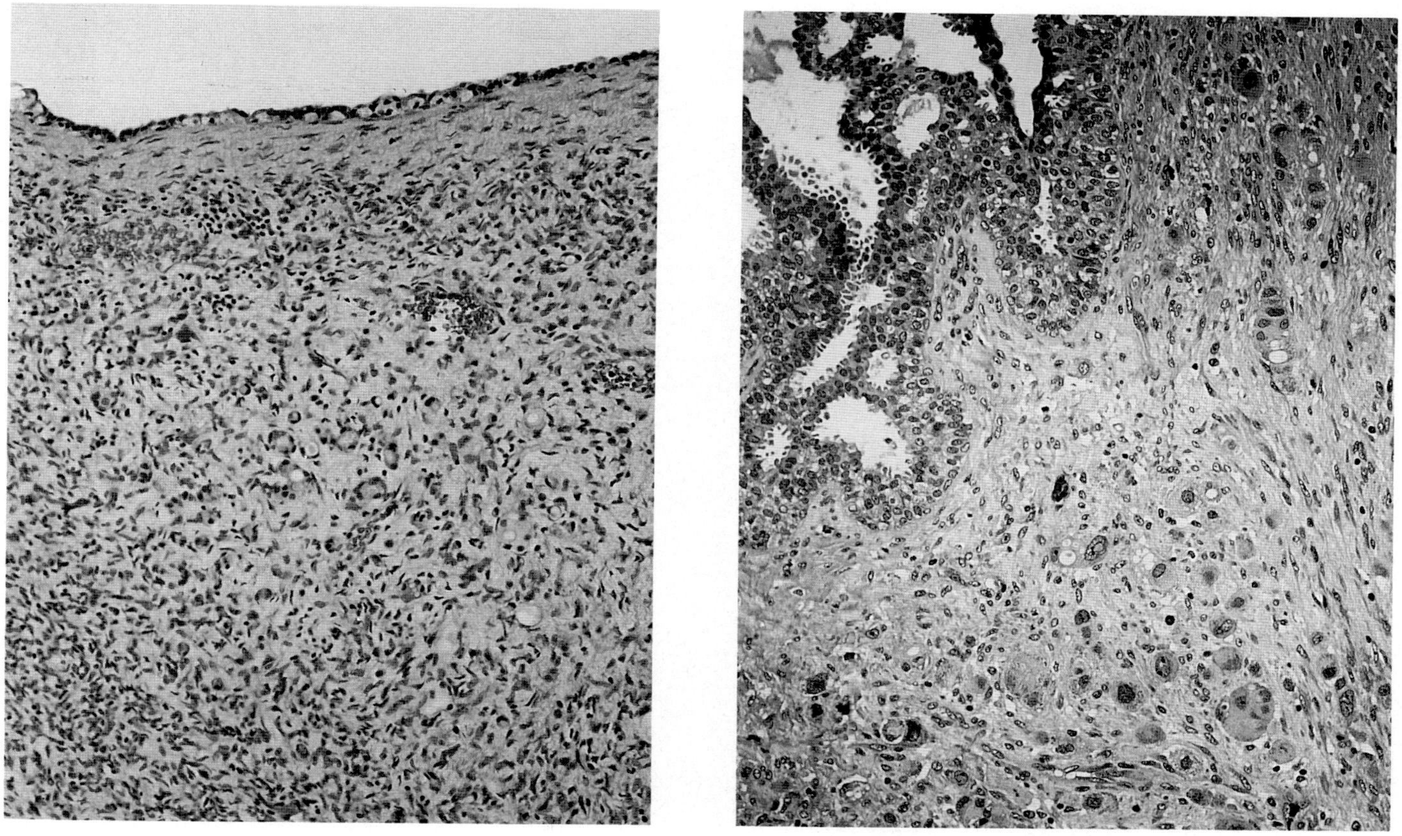

**Figure 11.40(a,b)** Invasive carcinoma in cystosarcoma phyllodes. The stroma is invaded by isolated carcinoma cells, but these cells are not readily apparent on H&E sections. (H&E, (a) X150; (b) X250)

## Ultrastructural Features, Hormone Receptors and DNA Ploidy

The spindle stromal cells of CP are generally of the fibroblastic/myofibroblastic type (Fig. 11.29), unless a more specific type of soft tissue sarcoma develops in the stroma.

The small number of cystosarcoma evaluated for ER and PR have displayed positivity for PR more frequently (175). Forty percent of cystosarcomas studied by Giani et al (31) were ER− PR+. The three cases of CP evaluated by Mechtersheimer et al (56) had a very heterogeneous degree of PR and ER expression leading them to conclude that neither estrogen, nor progesterone plays a major role in the histogenesis of CP.

El-Naggar et al (132) performed flow cytometric DNA and cell cycle analysis on 30 cystosarcomas to determine the potential prognostic utility of these procedures. Multivariate regression analysis of their results showed that DNA content is a significant predictor of the patient's clinical outcome.

## PERIDUCTAL STROMAL SARCOMA

Some pathologists have used "cellular periductal stromal tumor" as an alternate designation for cystosarcoma phyllodes (170,171). I prefer to use the term periductal stromal sarcoma for a specific and rare biphasic neoplasm characterized by a cellular, sarcomatous spindle cell proliferation around tubules that retain open lumens and absence of leaf-like processes (Fig. 11.42). The spindle cell nodules are separated by irregular aggregates of adipose tissue. While the tumor is generally at least partially well-delineated, occasionally it dissects irregularly into breast tissue.

C

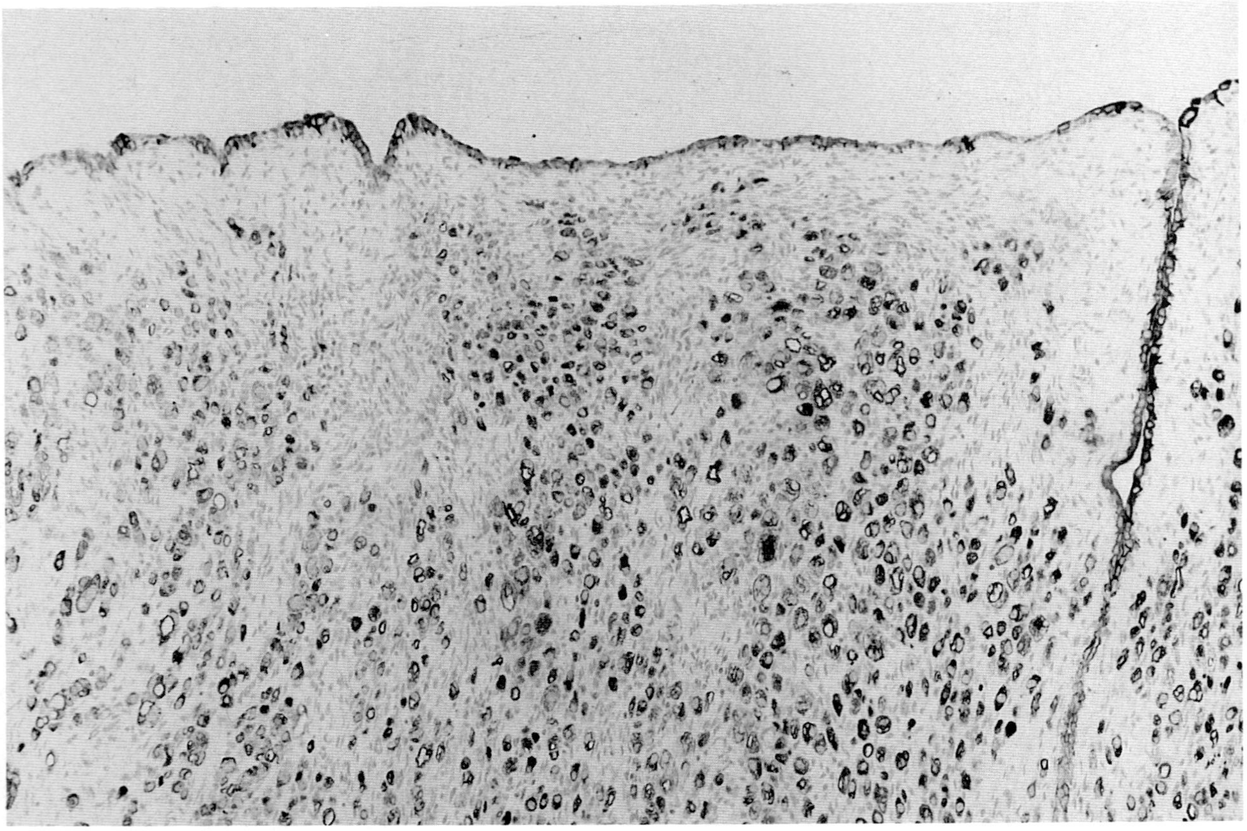

D

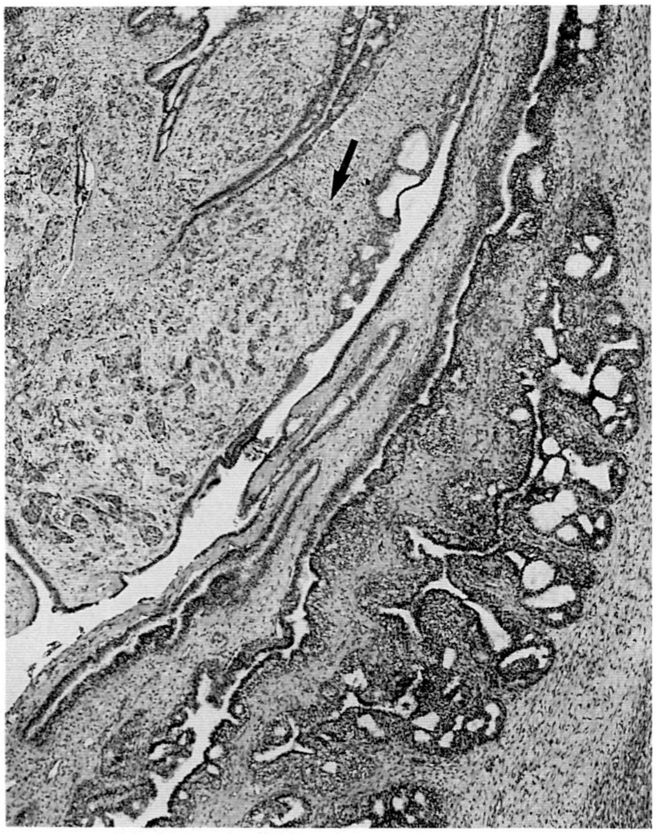

**Figure 11.40(c,d)** (c) Immunoreaction for cytokeratin unmasks the abundant invasive carcinoma cells in the stroma. (d) A regular infiltrating duct carcinoma (arrow) is present in this CP. (H&E, (c) X160; (d) X40)

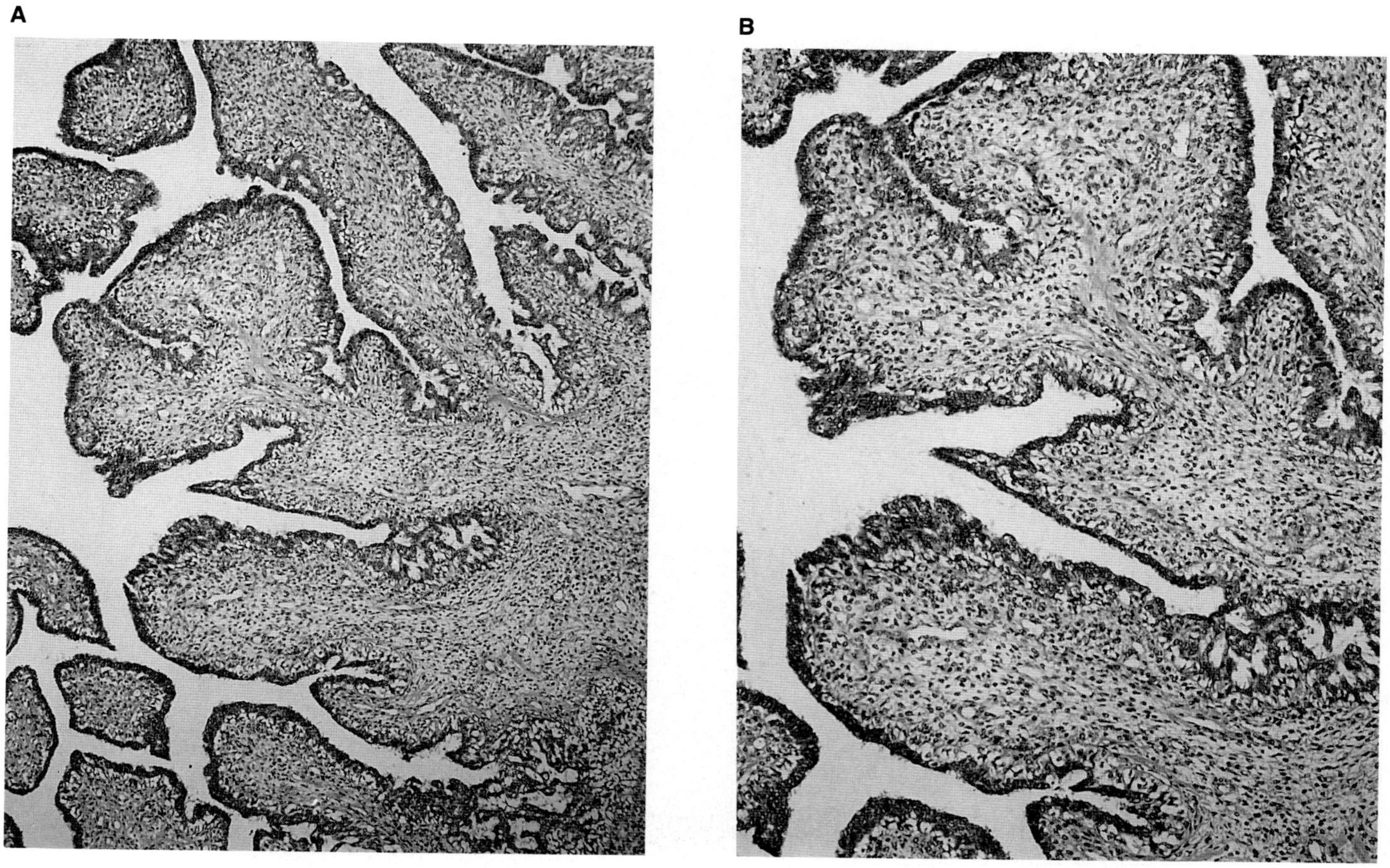

**Figure 11.41** (a&b) Cystosarcoma phyllodes in male breast. The typical leaf-like processes are evident. (H&E, (a) X60; (b) X100)

The behavior of this tumor is probably dependent on the grade of the spindle cell sarcoma, but that has not been established.

## CARCINOSARCOMA

Carcinosarcoma consists of an admixture of malignant epithelial and mesenchymal elements. Excluding carcinomas arising in cystosarcoma phyllodes, mammary carcinosarcoma is rare. Only a few reported cases were accepted by Azzopardi (204). One major problem in accepting a diagnosis of carcinosarcoma in the breast has been the widely and strongly held viewpoint regarding the potential of malignant epithelial cells to undergo metaplastic change transforming into spindle cells and possibly even cartilagenous and osseous elements (127,208,210–212,214,219, 222). The origin of the sarcomatous component in these tumors has also been attributed to the metaplastic potential of the myoepithelial cells (205,213, 221). Designation of carcinomas with a wide variety of metaplastic changes as metaplastic carcinoma in the past has led to the creation of a highly heterogeneous group of tumors both in regard to histomorphology as well as the clinical behavior of the neoplasms. Only the presence of a malignant striated muscle component as reported in Bird's case in 1970 has been regarded as definitive proof of a true sarcomatous component by some pathologists (204). On the other hand, if malignant epithelium or myoepithelium is capable of undergoing metaplasia and forming so many other mesenchymal cell types, there is no reason why one or the other could not also give rise to a malignant striated muscle as well.

Since the occurrence of biphasic tumors in the forms of fibroadenoma and cystosarcoma phyllodes has been well recognized, it seems only logical to assume that a biphasic tumor in which both the epithelial and the mesenchymal components are malignant also occurs. Therefore, cystosarcomas containing a carcinomatous component appear to be the most logical and acceptable manifestation of a carci-

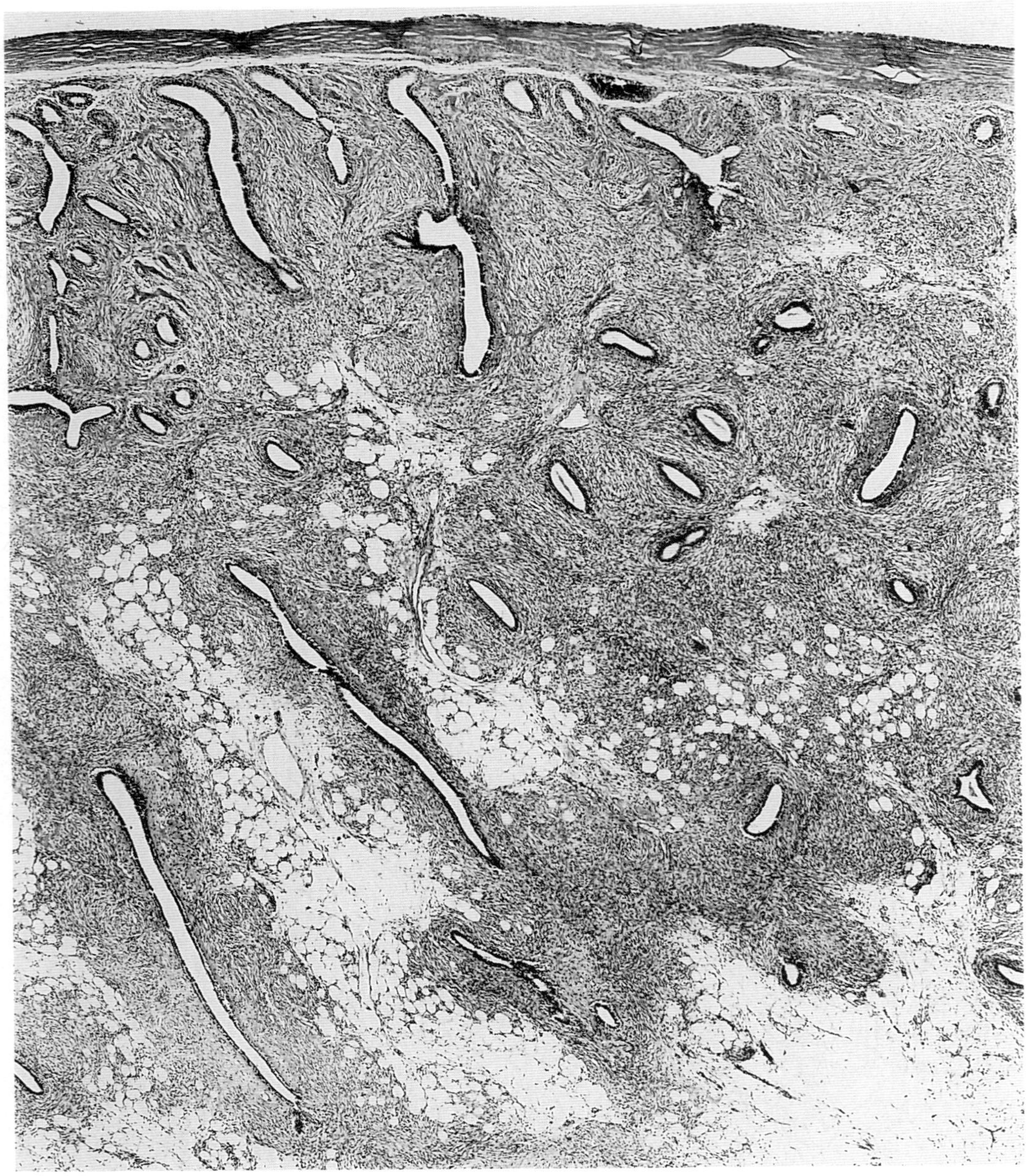

**Figure 11.42** Periductal stromal sarcoma. Tubules with open lumens are surrounded by a cellular, spindle cell proliferation. Aggregates of adipose tissue separate the nodules of spindle cells proliferating around the tubules. (H&E, X120)

nosarcoma. In 1974, Harris and Persaud (197) tabulated 16 well-documented carcinosarcomas reported since 1937 including two of their own cases; six of these were regarded as originating in either a fibroadenoma or a cystosarcoma phyllodes. One of these cases, however, is not well documented and is probably better classified as a cystosarcoma as noted previously by Azzopardi (204). Even though some reports (168) state that carcinomas arising in CP are not aggressive, the behavior of this type of lesion would undoubtedly depend on the grade of the cystosarcoma phyllodes as well as the relative amount of the carcinoma within the CP. These tumors are best designated as carcinomas arising in cystosarcoma phyllodes (see cystosarcoma phyllodes) to differentiate them from those carcinosarcomas that have no cystosarcoma phyllodes in the background.

The following discussion refers to a second group of carcinosarcomas that have no evidence of origin in either a cystosarcoma or a fibroadenoma.

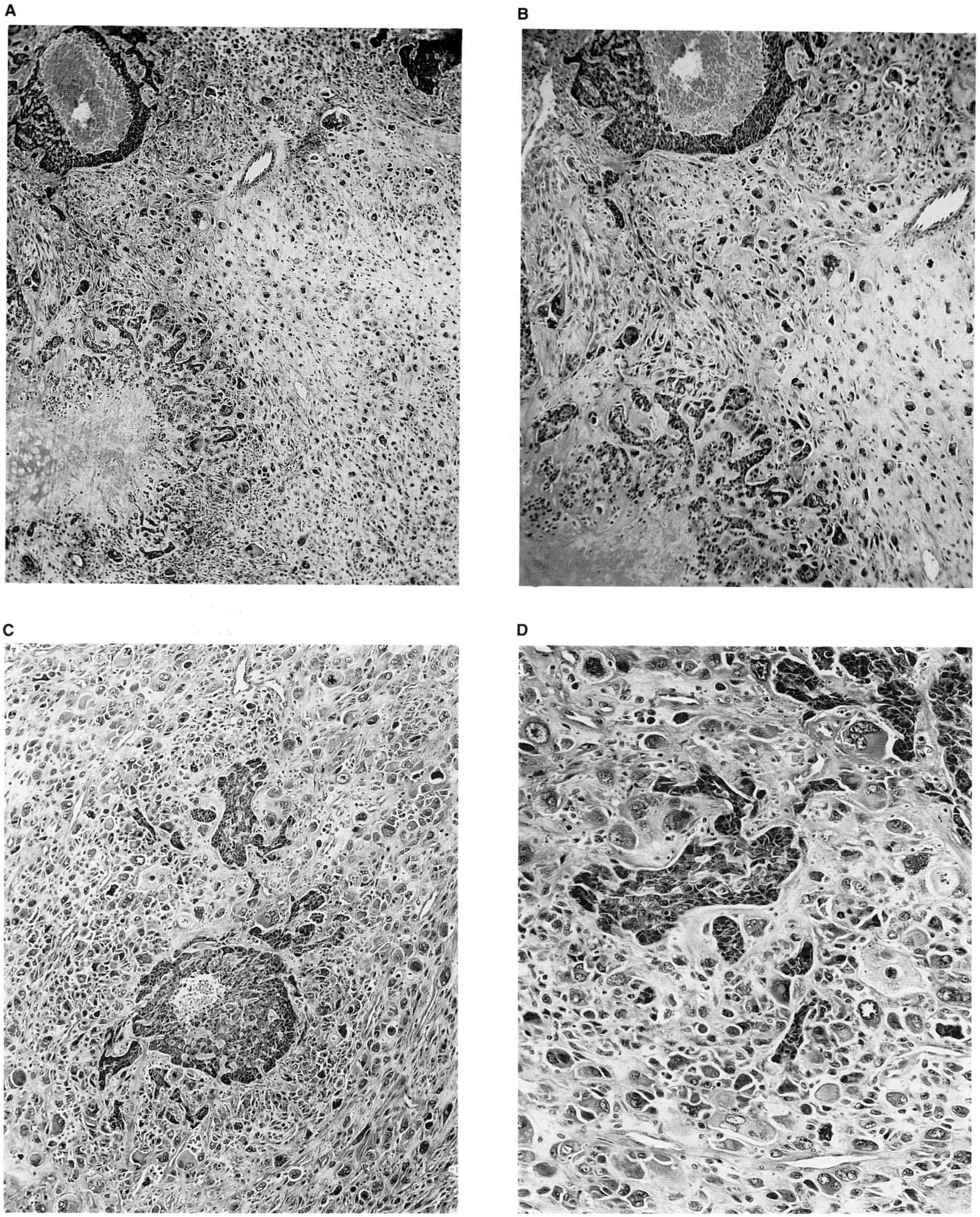


**Figure 11.43** Carcinosarcoma. (a–d) An infiltrating duct carcinoma is admixed with a highly pleomorphic sarcoma. (H&E, (a) X40; (b,c) X75; (d), X150)

## Clinical Features

Patients with carcinosarcoma range in age from 27 to 95 years with a median age of 57 years. They present with a solitary palpable mass which may become fixed to the skin or the underlying chest wall in case of large tumors in particular. Nipple discharge, retraction and ulceration may occur. Application of a more precise diagnostic criteria could lead to the establishment of a more restricted patient population in the future.

## Macroscopic Features

The gross appearance of carcinosarcoma is highly variable as anticipated from the variety of possible components and combinations thereof. The tumor size varies from less than 1 cm to 20 cm, with a median of 6.5 cm. It may be well circumscribed or highly irregular in its margin. The cut surface of the tumor often appears fleshy with patchy areas of gritty, hard tissue. Necrosis and hemorrhage are present in many of the tumors larger than 5 cm.

## Microscopic Features

Carcinosarcomas are composed of an admixture of unequivocal carcinoma with areas of unquestionable sarcoma (Fig. 11.43). With our better understanding of breast lesions today, lesions composed of squamous carcinoma and spindle cell elements which may have been mistaken for a carcinosarcoma in the past are now recognized as reflecting squamous carcinoma with spindle cell metaplasia. The acceptance of a lesion as carcinosarcoma or metaplastic carcinoma based on the evaluation of hematoxylin-eosin (H&E) stained sections alone is no longer acceptable and does not constitute adequate documentation of the nature of these tumors.

Clearly, certain ground rules should be established for distinguishing a carcinosarcoma from a metaplastic carcinoma. All tumors that show a clearcut carcinoma or even areas vaguely suggestive of carcinoma admixed with a mesenchymal-appearing spindle or pleomorphic cells should be evaluated immunohistochemically for the presence of epithelial and mesenchymal antigens. If the sarcomatous-appearing areas show a positive reaction for epithelial antigens (ie, cytokeratin), then the lesion should be classified as a metaplastic carcinoma. If the sarcomatous-appearing component fails to display positivity for cytokeratin, then it qualifies as a carcinosarcoma (Fig. 11.44).

Any type of carcinoma may be present as a component of a carcinosarcoma, but most are an infiltrating duct, squamous, or adenosquamous carcinoma. The sarcoma may be a fibrosarcoma, malignant fibrous histiocytoma (MFH, including its giant cell variant), pleomorphic sarcoma, osteogenic sarcoma (spindle cell, osteoblastic or osteoclastic variants), rhabdomyosarcoma, or a combination of two or more of these sarcomas (220). The epithelial component displays a positive reaction for cytokeratin, while the mesenchymal component may react with actin, vimentin, or S-100 protein, but fails to react with cytokeratin. In some tumors, the mesenchymal-appearing sarcomatous cells may show rare cells that display a positive reaction for cytokeratin; these tumors would still qualify as a carcinosarcoma since even pure sarcomas may have a rare cell which expresses epithelial antigens.

At the ultrastructural level, the epithelial component shows desmosomes or tight junctions with tonofilaments, but the sarcomatous element generally fails to display any epithelial features, except for rare tight junctions. Again it is important to emphasize that at the ultrastructural level, poorly-formed intercellular bridges and desmosomes are occasionally observed in a rare cell even in pure and indisputible sarcomas. Therefore, these neoplasms are best included in the biphasic category of breast neoplasms rather than metaplastic carcinomas.

Anytime a clearly recognizable soft-tissue-type sarcoma such as a liposarcoma, chondrosarcoma, osteosarcoma, rhabdomyosarcoma, or a malignant fibrous histiocytoma is admixed with a carcinoma, then the neoplasm should be classified as a carcinosarcoma. If there is obviously benign bone and cartilage within the carcinoma, the lesion should be designated as a carcinoma with osseous or chondroid metaplasia. This is the only way to determine with accuracy if tumors with benign mesenchymal elements behave differently from those that have a malignant mesenchymal component.

## Behavior and Prognosis

Carcinosarcomas are invariably highly aggressive neoplasms. Metastases from these tumors may contain any combination of the various elements or only the carcinomatous component. A patient with mammary carcinosarcoma recently referred to AFIP presented with liver metastasis six months after mastectomy; the morphology of the primary and metastatic tumor were identical with prominent rhabdomyosarcomatous differentiation confirmed by electron microscopy present in both. The aggressive behavior manifested by all carcinosarcomas is in sharp contrast to the rarity of aggressive behavior by cystosarcoma phyllodes.

## Hormone Receptors

Only about 10% of cases evaluated for estrogen receptor are positive and about 10% of the tumors positive for estrogen receptor are also positive for progesterone receptors (221).

## Synovial Sarcoma—A Connective-Tissue-Derived Carcinosarcoma

So far, I have described two types of carcinosarcoma: those that are of biphasic origin arising in a background of a cystosarcoma phyllodes, and those in which the mesenchymal component is believed to be either epithelial or myoepithelial derived through a metaplastic process. Another biphasic tumor that rarely occurs in the breast is a synovial sarcoma. Only one example of this tumor has been observed in the breast over the past 15 years at the AFIP. This lesion occurred in the right breast of a 25-year-old woman. It was located close to the axilla, and the woman remained disease-free five years after an excisional biopsy.

Microscopically, the neoplasm was a typical biphasic "synovial sarcoma," (Fig. 11.45). The cleft-lining cells showed positive reaction for cytokeratin. A rare cell in the spindle cell areas showed a positive reaction for cytokeratin as well, probably reflecting cells undergoing epithelial metaplasia.

At the ultrastructural level, the cleft-lining cells were at least partially, and often completely, surrounded by basal lamina (Fig. 11.46). Light and dark cells were present lining the clefts of various sizes and shapes; the dark cells were often more elongated than the light cells. The cleft-lining cells had microvilli and occasionally cilia on the luminal margin and were attached to one another by desmosomes and tight junctions (Fig. 11.47); these cells were identical to epithelial cells. Abundant whorled aggregates of intracytoplasmic microfibrils were present in some of these epithelial cells (Fig. 11.48). The epithelial cells were surrounded by fibroblastic spindle cells that lacked any epithelial features. Small amounts of collagen separated some of these cells from each other.

While some pathologists favor a synovioblastic origin for the monophasic variant of synovial sarcoma (215), more recent studies have raised doubts as to whether "synovial sarcoma" deserves to be called as such. These doubts are based on the constant occurrence of terminal bars, basal lamina, and true microvilli in this neoplasm when such structures do not occur in the normal or pathologic human synovium (209), and on the elaboration of epithelial antigens by the cleft-lining cells of the tumor (217). Furthermore, immunohistochemical studies of this tumor have demonstrated cytokeratin in the epithelial component of the neoplasm and vimentin in the sarcomatous component; human synovial cells contain vimentin but no cytokeratin. As a result of these studies, a number of investigators (209,216,218) have emphasized the biphasic nature of synovial sarcoma, and some have suggested the designation of carcinosarcoma for this neoplasm.

Synovial sarcoma would then constitute a third variant of carcinosarcoma derived from connective tissue and totally different from those originating in CP or those of metaplastic epithelial or myoepithelial derivation. The behavior of carcinosarcomas arising in a CP would depend on the grade of the CP and the relative quantity of the carcinoma compared to the CP. While the metaplastic carcinosarcomas of epithelial or myoepithelial derivation are highly aggressive neoplasms, those of connective tissue origin (synovial sarcomas) are so rare that enough data is not yet available on their behavior. Nonetheless, synovial sarcoma would be expected to behave like similar tumors occurring elsewhere in the body. Among these three variants, only the epithelial/myoepithelial-derived carcinosarcomas exhibit the aggressive behavior anticipated from a comparable carcinosar-

A

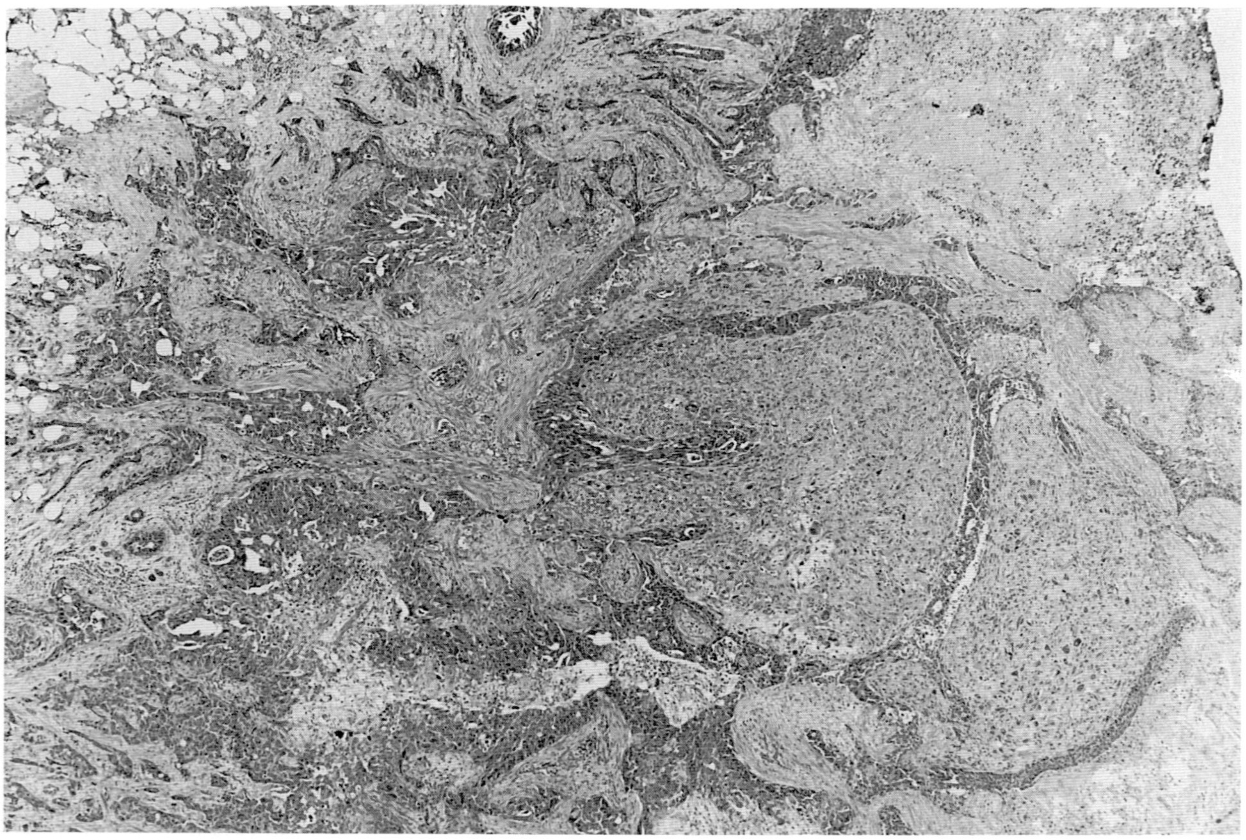

B

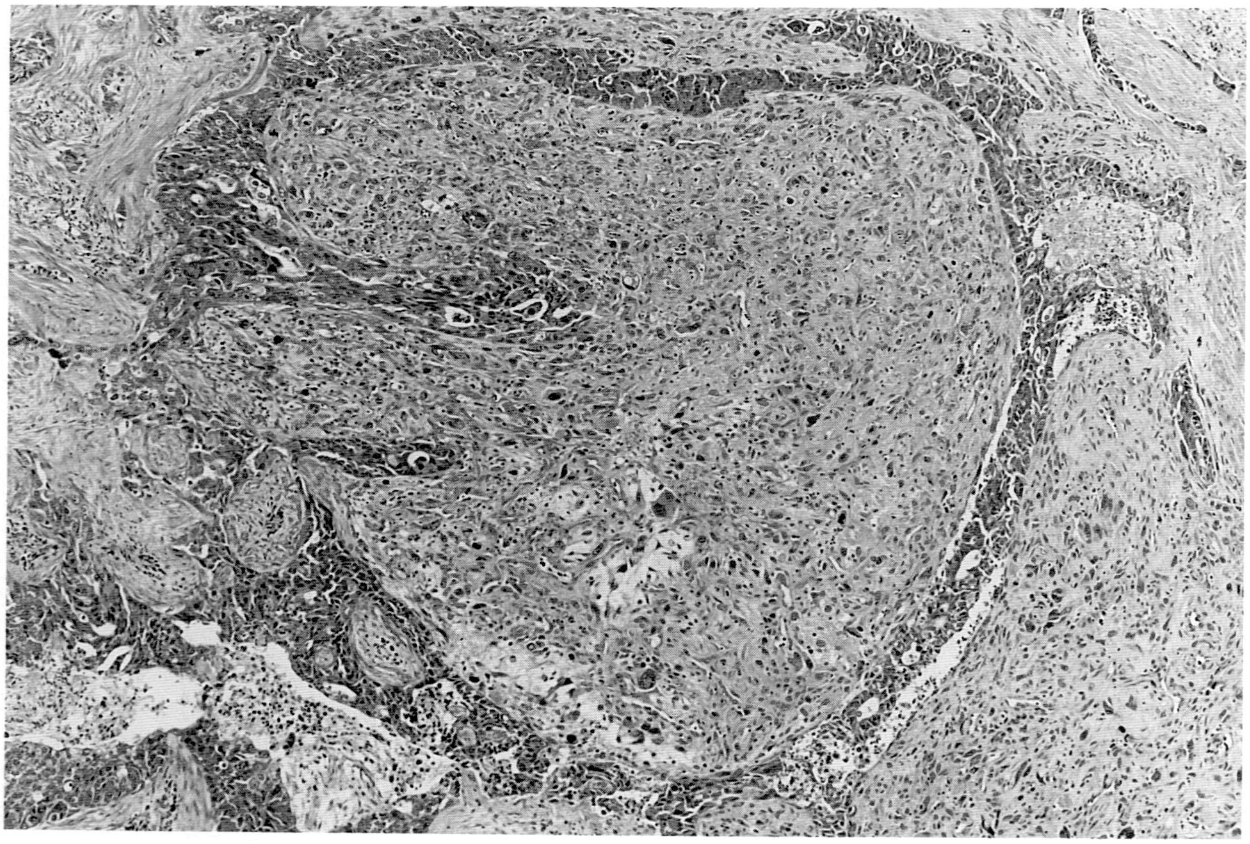

**Figure 11.44** Carcinosarcoma. (a–c) Another classic carcinosarcoma shows an admixture of the two malignant components (H&E, (a) X24; (b) X100). (c) Immunoreaction for cytokeratin decorates the epithelial elements and confirms the biphasic nature of the tumor (Immunoperoxidase reaction for cytokeratin, X100) (Figs. 11.44b&c from Tavassoli FA: *Pathol Annu* 1992;27(pt 2):89–119, with permission)

C

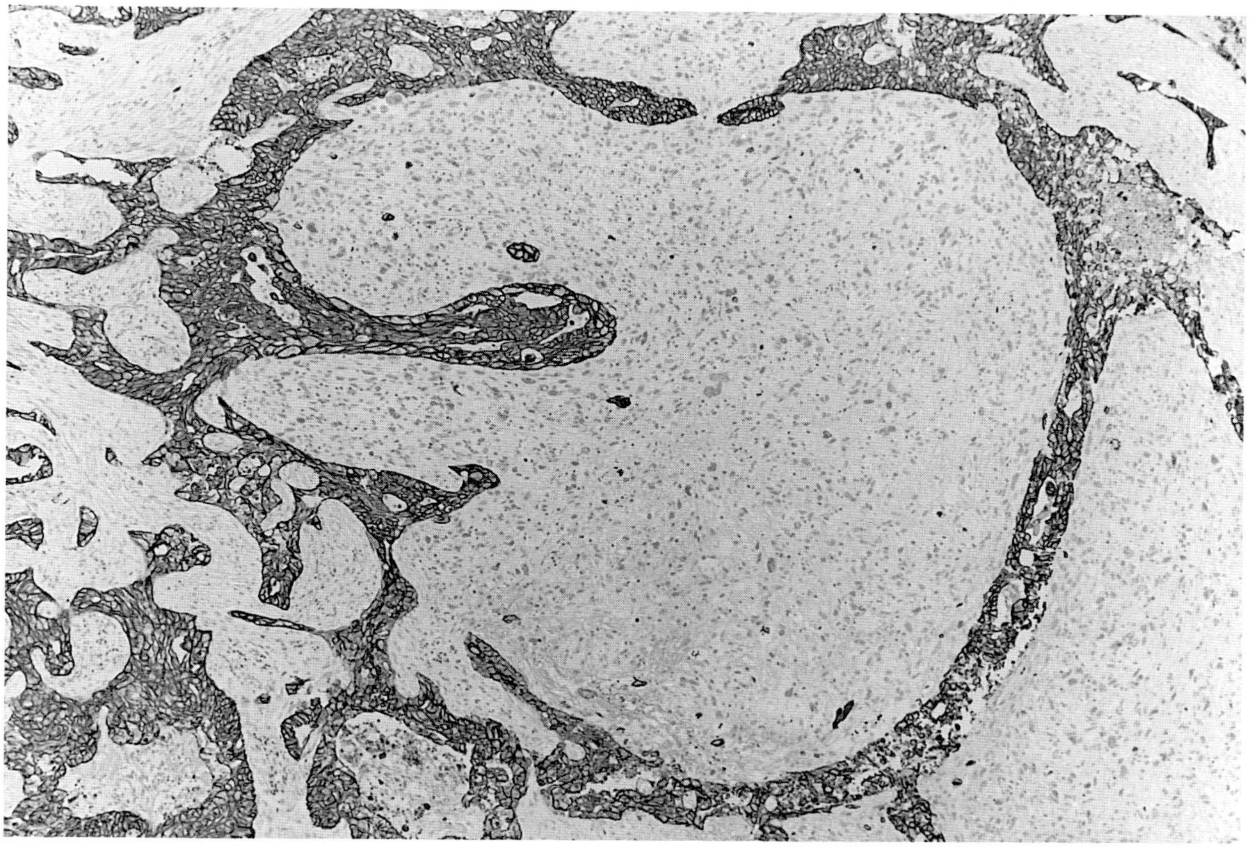

**Figure 11.44(c)** Legend on opposite page.

A B

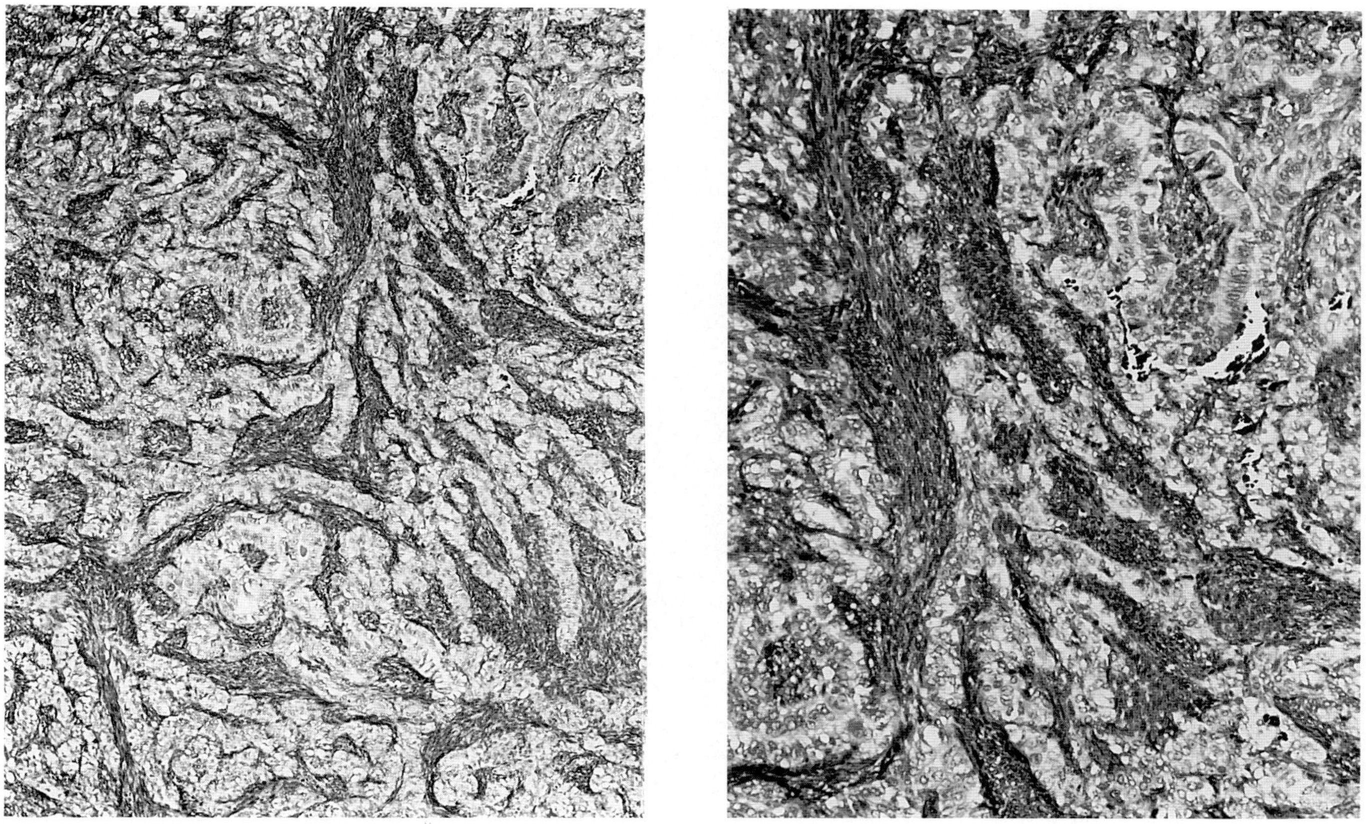

**Figure 11.45** Synovial sarcoma, biphasic variant. (a) A network of epithelioid cords proliferates in a spindle cell background. (H&E, (a) X160) (b) Immunostain for cytokeratin decorates the epithelial elements and not the stromal component. (Immunoreaction for cytokeratin, (b) X160)

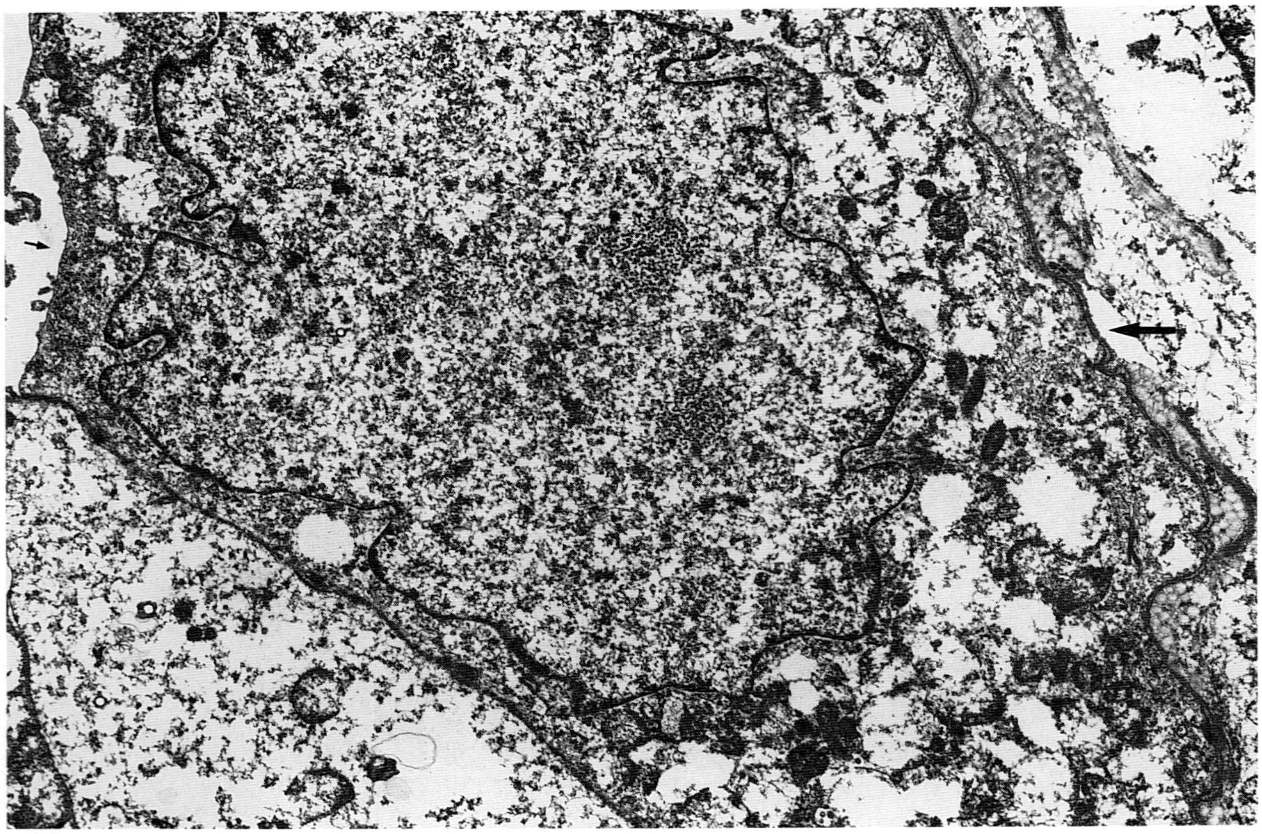

**Figure 11.46** Synovial sarcoma. At the ultrastructural level, a well-developed basal lamina (long arrow) surrounds an epithelial-lined space. The truncated luminal margin of this cell is apparent at the left (short arrow). (Uranyl acetate-lead citrate, X3,000)

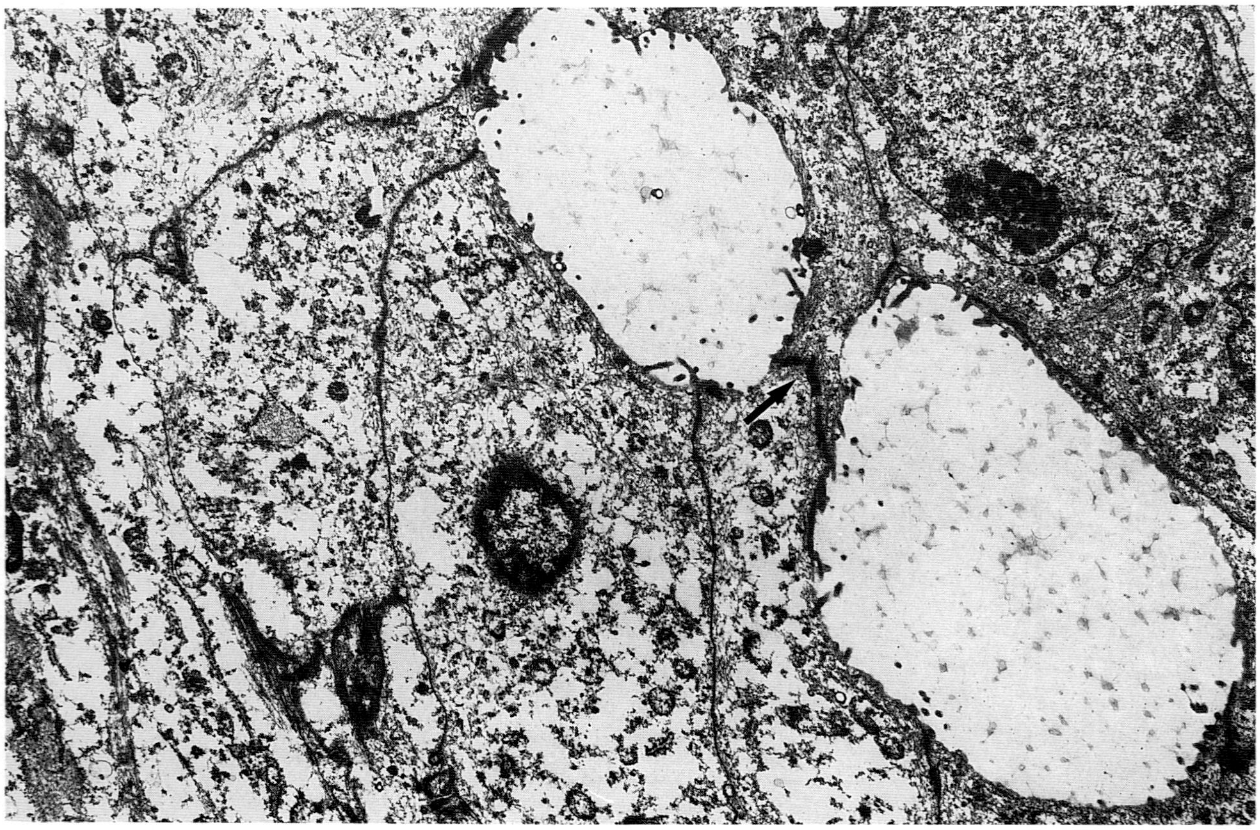

**Figure 11.47** Synovial sarcoma. Microvilli and desmosomal attachments (arrow) are evident in the epithelial tubules formed by the cells. (Uranyl acetate-lead citrate, X4,400)

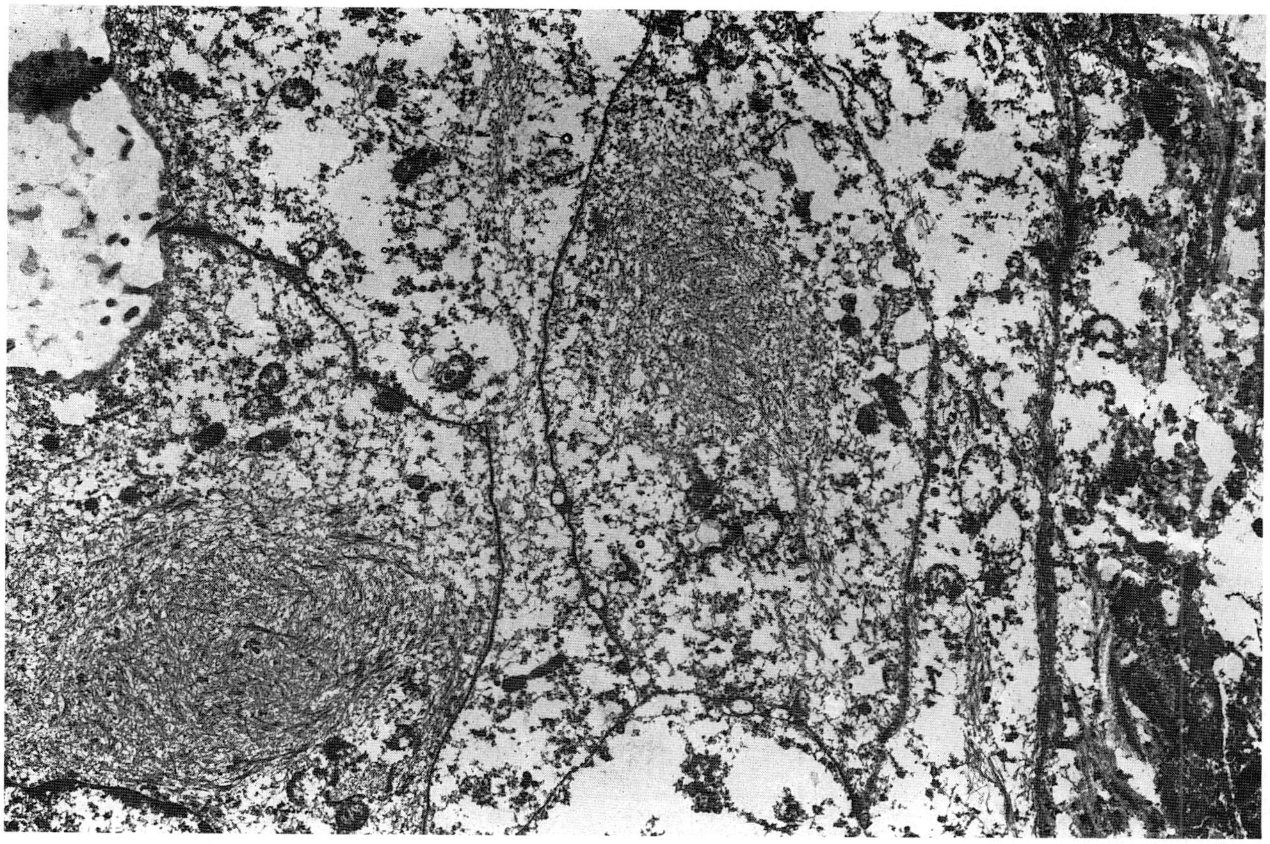

**Figure 11.48** Synovial sarcoma. Some of the epithelial cells contain abundant whorls of intracytoplasmic fibrils. (Uranyl acetate-lead citrate, X4,400)

coma occurring elsewhere in the body. Therefore, it is important to separate the mammary carcinosarcomas into three types: Type 1, carcinoma arising in a CP; Type 2, carcinosarcoma, metaplastic (epithelial or myoepithelial derived); Type 3, synovial sarcoma (carcinosarcoma, metaplastic of connective tissue origin). The various subtypes of carcinosarcoma are listed in Table 11.2.

**Table 11.2** Three Variants of Carcinosarcoma

| |
|---|
| 1. Carcinomas arising in cystosarcoma phyllodes |
| 2. Carcinosarcoma, metaplastic, of epithelial or myoepithelial origin |
| Infiltrating carcinoma with fibrosarcoma |
| Infiltrating carcinoma with malignant fibrous histiocytoma |
| Infiltrating carcinoma with pleomorphic sarcoma |
| Infiltrating carcinoma with osteogenic sarcoma |
| Infiltrating carcinoma with chondrosarcoma |
| Infiltrating carcinoma with rhabdomyosarcoma |
| Infiltrating carcinoma with two or more sarcoma variants |
| 3. Synovial sarcoma, (carcinosarcoma, metaplastic, of connective tissue origin) |

From Tavassoli (220)

## REFERENCES

### Fibroadenoma Classic Type and Variants


1. Ahmed A: *Atlas of the Ultrastructure of Human Breast Diseases*. Edinburgh, Churchill Livingstone, 1978, pp 58–64.
2. Ansah-Boateng Y, Tavassoli FA: Fibroadenoma and cystosarcoma phyllodes of the male breast. *Mod Pathol* 1992; 5:in press.
3. Archer F, Omar M: Pink cell (oncocytic) metaplasia in a fibroadenoma of the breast: Electron microscopic observations. *J Pathol* 1969;99:99–124.
4. * Ashikari R, Farrow JH, O'Hara J: Fibroadenomas in the breast of juveniles. *Surg Gynecol Obstet* 1971;132:259–262.
5. * Azzopardi JG: *Problems in Breast Pathology*. Philadelphia, WB Saunders, 1979, pp 39–56.
6. Barton AA: An electron microscope study of human breast cells in fibroadenosis and carcinoma. *Br J Cancer* 1964;18: 682–685.
7. Berean K, Tron VA, Churg A, et al: Mammary fibroadenoma with multinucleated stromal giant cells. *Am J Surg Pathol* 1986;10:823–827.
8. Block GE, Zlatnik PA: Giant fibroadenomata of the breast in a prepubertal girl. *Arch Surg* 1960;80:155–159.

9. Bonser GM, Dossett JA, Jull JW: *Human and Experimental Breast Cancer*. London, Pitman Medical Publishing Company, 1961, pp 212–236.
10. Brown JM: Histological modification of fibroadenoma of the breast associated with oral hormonal contraceptives. *Med J Aust* 1970;1:276–277.
11. Carney JA, Gordon H, Carpenter PC, et al: The complex of myxomas, spotty pigmentation, and endocrine overactivity. *Medicine* 1985;64:270–283.
12. Carney JA, Toorkey BC: Myxoid fibroadenoma and allied conditions (myxomatosis) of the breast. A heritable disorder with special associations including cardiac and cutaneous myxomas. *Am J Surg Pathol* 1991;15:713–721.
13. Carstens PHB: Ultrastructure of fibroadenoma. *Arch Pathol* 1974;98:23–32.
* 14. Cheatle GL: Hyperplasia of epithelial and connective tissues in the breast: Its relation to fibroadenoma and other pathologic conditions. *Br J Surg* 1923;10:436–455.
* 15. Cheatle GL, Cutler M: *Tumours of the Breast. Their Pathology, Symptoms, Diagnosis and Treatment*. London, Arnold & Co, 1931, pp 455–475.
16. Clarke JC: Giant intracanalicular fibroadenoma of the breast. *Ann Surg* 1948;127:372–376.
17. Daniel WA, Mathews MD: Tumors of the breast in adolescent females. *Pediatrics* 1968;1:743–749.
18. Delarue J, Redon H: Les Infarctus des fibroadenomes mammaires. Problem clinique et pathogenique. *Semaine d' Hop Paris* 1949;25:2991–2996.
19. Demetrakopoulos NJ: Three-dimensional reconstruction of a human mammary fibroadenoma. *Bull North Western U Med School* 1958;32:221–228.
20. Devitt JE: Juvenile giant fibroadenoma of the breast. *Can J Surg* 1974;17:205–207.
21. Duray PH, Holahan K, Merino M, et al: Adolescent cellular fibroadenomas: A clinical and pathologic study, abstracted, *Lab Invest* 1985;50:17A.
22. Farrow JH, Ashikari H: Breast lesions in young girls. *Surg Clin No Am* 1969;49:261–269.
* 23. Fechner RE: Fibroadenomas in patients receiving oral contraceptives: A clinical and pathologic study. *Am J Clin Pathol* 1970;53:857–864.
24. Fekete P, Petrek J, Majmudar B, et al: Fibroadenomas with stromal cellularity. *Arch Pathol Lab Med* 1987;111:427–432.
25. Fisher ER: Ultrastructure of human breast and its disorders. *Am J Clin Pathol* 1976;66:291–375.
* 26. Frantz VK, Pickren JW, Melcher GW, et al: Incidence of chronic cystic disease in so-called "normal breast." A study based on 225 postmortem examinations. *Cancer* 1951;4:762–783.
27. Funderburk WW, Rosero E, Leffall LD: Breast lesions in blacks. *Surg Gynecol Obstet* 1972;135:58–60.
* 28. Geschickter CF: *Diseases of the Breast. Diagnosis, Pathology, Treatment*, ed 2. Philadelphia, J.B. Lippincott, 1945, pp 291–324.
* 29. Geschickter CF, Lewis D, Hartman CG: Tumors of the breast related to the oestrin hormone. *Am J Cancer* 1934;21:828–859.
30. Giacomelli V, Re A: Studio statisico sulle affezioni displastiche della mammella in rapporto all'eta. *Tumori* 1951;25:213–222.
31. Giani C, D'Amore E, Delarue JC, et al: Estrogen and progesterone receptors in benign breast tumors and lesions: Relationship with histological and cytological features. *Int J Cancer* 1986;37:7–10.
32. Gibert MA, Noel P, Faucon M, et al: Comparative immunohistochemical localization of fibronectin and actin in human breast tumor cells in vivo and in vitro. I. Fibroadenoma. *Virchows Arch (Cell Pathol)* 1982;40:99–112.
33. Goldenberg VE, Wiegenstein L, Mottet NK: Florid breast fibroadenoma in patients taking hormonal oral contraceptives. *Am J Clin Pathol* 1968;49:52–59.
34. Goodman ZD, Taxy JB: Fibroadenomas of the breast with prominent smooth muscle. *Am J Surg Pathol* 1981;5:99–101.
* 35. Haagensen CD: *Diseases of the Breast*, ed 3. Philadelphia, WB Saunders Co, 1986, pp 267–283.
36. Hanson CA, Snover DC, Dehner LP: Fibroadenomatosis (fibroadenomatoid mastopathy): A benign breast lesion with composite pathologic features. *Pathology* 1987;19:393–396.
37. Harris M, Kahn MK: Phyllodes tumour and stromal sarcoma of the breast: An ultrastructural comparison. *Histopathology* 1984;8:315–330.
38. Hasson J, Pope CH: Mammary infarcts associated with pregnancy presenting as breast tumors. *Surgery* 1961;49:313–316.
39. Hines JR, and Geurkink RE: Giant breast tumor in the adolescent. *Am J Surg* 1965;109:810–813.
40. Ingleby H: Relation of fibro-adenoma and chronic mastitis to sexual cycle changes in the breast. *Arch Pathol* 1932;14:21–41.
41. Jao W, Vazquez LT, Keh PC, et al: Myoepithelial differentiation and basal lamina deposition in fibroadenoma and adenosis of the breast. *J Pathol* 1978;126:107–112.
42. Jordal K, Sorenson B: Giant fibroadenoma of the breast. Report of two cases, one treated with mammoplasty. *Acta Chir Scand* 1961;122:147–151.
43. Kern WH, Clark RW: Retrogression of fibroadenomas of the breast. *Am J Surg* 1973;126:59–62.
44. Kodlin D, Winger EE, Morgestern NL, et al: Chronic mastopathy and breast cancer. A follow-up study. *Cancer* 1977;39:2603–2607.
* 45. Lacombe MJ, Llombart-Bosch A, Lecluse Y, et al: Fibroadnome du sein avec hyperplasie epitheliale atypique a cellule claire. A propos de 7 cas. Etude immunohistochimique. *Ann Pathol* 1986;1:37–44.
46. Lefer LG: Fibroadenoma of the breast with prominent mucinous stromal component. *Arch Pathol Lab Med* 1982;106:649–650.
47. Lewis D, Hartman CG: Tumors of the breast related to the oestrin hormone. *Am J Cancer* 1934;21:828–859.

48. Linsk J, Kreuzer G, Zajicek J: Cytologic diagnosis of mammary tumors from aspiration biopsy smears. II. Studies on 219 fibroadenomas and 219 cases of benign dysplasia. *Acta Cytol* 1972;16:130–138.

* 49. LiVolsi VA, Stadel BV, Kelsey JL, et al: Fibroadenoma in oral contraceptive users. A histopathologic evaluation of epithelial atypia. *Cancer* 1979;44:1778–1781.

* 50. Lubarsch O, Henke F: *Handbuck der Speziellen Pathologischen Anatomie*. Berlin, Springer, 1933, vol 7, p 241.

51. MacKenzie DH: A fibro-adenoma of the breast with smooth muscle. *J Pathol Bacteriol* 1968;96:231–232.

52. Majmudar B, Rosales-Quintana S: Infarction of breast fibroadenomas during pregnancy. *JAMA* 1975;231:963–964.

53. Markowitz B, Howell HL: Rapid growth of a large breast fibroma in a young girl. *JAMA* 1936;107:1043–1044.

54. Martin PM, Kuttenn F, Serment H, et al: Studies on clinical, hormonal, and pathological correlations in breast fibroadenomas. *J Steroid Biochem* 1978;9:1251–1255.

55. McFarland J: Adenofibroma and fibro-adenoma of the female breast. *Surg Gynecol Obstet* 1927;45:729–746.

* 56. Mechtersheimer G, Kruger KH, Born IA, et al: Antigenic profile of mammary fibroadenoma and cystosarcoma phyllodes. A study using antibodies to estrogen and progesterone receptors and to a panel of cell surface molecules. *Pathol Res Pract* 1990;186:427–438.

57. Meyer JS: Cell proliferation in normal human breast ducts, fibroadenomas, and other ductal hyperplasias measured by nuclear labeling with tritiated thymidine. Effects of menstrual phase, age, and oral contraceptive hormones. *Hum Pathol* 1977;8:67–81.

58. Mies C, Rosen PP: Juvenile fibroadenoma with atypical epithelial hyperplasia. *Am J Surg Pathol* 1987;11:184–190.

59. Mohammed RH, Lakatua DJ, Haus E, et al: Estrogen and progesterone receptors in human breast cancer. *Cancer* 1986;58:1076–1081.

60. Murad TM, Greider MH, Scarpelli DG: The ultrastructure of human mammary fibroadenoma. *Am J Pathol* 1967;51:663–669.

61. Nambiar R and Kutty MK: Giant fibro-adenoma (cystosarcoma phyllodes) in adolescent female—a clinicopathological study. *Br J Surg* 1974;61:113–117.

62. Newman J, Kahn LB: Infarction of fibro-adenoma of the breast. *Br J Surg* 1973;60:738–740.

* 63. Nielsen BB: Fibroadenomatoid hyperplasia of the male breast. *Am J Surg Pathol* 1990;14:774–777.

64. Nielsen BB, Ladefoged C: Fibroadenoma of the female breast with multinucleated giant cells. *Pathol Res Pract* 1985;180:721–724.

* 65. Oberman HA: Benign breast lesions confused with carcinoma, in McDivitt RW, Oberman HA, Ozzello L, (eds): *The Breast*. Baltimore, Williams and Wilkins, 1984.

* 66. Oberman HA: Breast tumors in the adolescent female. *Pathol Annu* 1979;14:175–201.

67. Oberman HA, French AJ: Chronic fibrocystic disease of the breast. *Surg Gynecol Obstet* 1961;112:647–652.

* 68. Ohtani H, Sasano N: Stromal cells of the fibroadenoma of the breast. *Virchows Arch (Pathol Anat)* 1984;404:7–16.

69. Oliver RL, Major RC: Cyclomastopathy: A physio-pathological conception of some benign breast tumors, with an analysis of four hundred cases. *Am J Cancer* 1934;21:1–85.

* 70. Orcel L, Douvin D: Contribution a l'etude histogenetique des fibroadenomes mammaries. *Ann Anat Path* 1973;18:255–276.

71. Owens FM, Adams WE: Giant intracanalicular fibroadenoma of the breast. *Arch Surg* 1941;43:588–598.

72. Ozzello L, Gump FE: The management of patients with carcinomas in fibroadenomatous tumors of the breast. *Surg Gynecol Obstet* 1985;160:99–104.

73. Pambakian H, Tighe JR: Mammary infarction. *Br J Surg* 1971;58:601–602.

74. Pesce C, Colacino R: Morphometry of the breast fibroadenoma. *Pathol Res Pract* 1986;181:718–720.

* 75. Pike AM, Oberman HA: Juvenile (cellular) adenofibromas: A clinicopathologic study. *Am J Surg Pathol* 1985;9:730–736.

76. Rao BR, Meyer JS, Fry CG: Most cystosarcoma phyllodes and fibroadenomas have progesterone receptors but lack estrogen receptor: Stromal localization of progesterone receptor. *Cancer* 1981;47:2016–2921.

77. Riddell RH, Davis JD: Muscular hamartomas of the breast. *J Pathol* 1973;111:209–211.

78. Rosen PP: Multinucleated mammary stromal giant cells. A benign lesion that stimulates invasive carcinoma. *Cancer* 1979;44:1304–1308.

79. Rottino A, Howley CP: Osteoid sarcoma of the breast: A complication of fibroadenoma. *Arch Pathol* 1945;40:44–50.

* 80. Salm R: Epidermoid metaplasia in mammary fibroadenoma with formation of keratin cysts. *J Pathol Bacteriol* 1957;74:221–222.

* 81. Sandison AT, Walker JC: Diseases of the adolescent female breast. A clinicopathological study. *Br J Surg* 1968;55:443–448.

82. Scarani P, Bondi A, Calderoni A, et al: Neoplasia lobulare endocrina in fibroadenoma mammario. *Pathologica* 1981;73:657–667.

* 83. Semb C: Pathologico-anatomical and clinical investigation of fibroadenomatosis cystica mammae and its relation to other pathological conditions in the mamma, especially cancer. *Acta Chir Scandinavia* 1928;64(suppl 10):1–482.

84. Simpson TE, Van Dervoort RL Jr, Lynn HB: Giant fibroadenoma (benign cystosarcoma phyllodes): Report of a case in 13-year-old girl. *Surgery* 1969;65:341–342.

85. Spagnola DV, Shilkin KB: Breast neoplasms containing bone and cartilage. *Virchows Arch (Pathol Anat)* 1983;400:287–295.

* 86. Taylor HB: Oral contraceptive and pathologic changes in the breast. *Cancer* 1971;28:1388–1390.

* 87. Wellings SR, Jensen HM, Marcum RG: An atlas of subgross pathology of the human breast with special reference to possible precancerous lesions. *J Natl Cancer Inst* 1975;55:231–273.

* 88. Wilkinson L, Green WO Jr: Infarction of breast lesion during pregnancy and lactation. *Cancer* 1964;17:1567.

89. Willis RA: *Pathology of Tumors*, ed 4. London, Butterworths, 1967, pp 215–216.

90. Wulsin JH: Large breast tumors in adolescent females. *Ann Surg* 1960;152:151–159.


### Lobular Neoplasia and Carcinoma Arising in FA


* 91. Austin WE, Fidler HK: Carcinoma developing in fibroadenoma of the breast. *Amer J Clin Path* 1953;23:688–690.

* 92. Azzopardi JG: *Problems in Breast Pathology*. Philadelphia, W.B. Saunders, 1979, pp 253–254.

93. Botta P-G, Cosimi MF: Breast lobular carcinoma in a fibroadenoma. *Eur J Surg Pathol* 1985;11:283–285.

94. Bosincu L, Eusebi V: Carcinoma della mammella insorto in fibroadenoma. *Tumori* 1972;58:195–202.

95. Buzonowski-Konakry K, Harrison EG, Payne WS: Lobular carcinoma arising in fibroadenoma of the breast. *Cancer* 1975;35:450–456.

96. Diaz NM, Palmer JO, McDivitt RW: Carcinoma arising within fibroadenomas of the breast. A clinicopathologic study of 105 patients. *Am J Clin Pathol* 1991;95:614–622.

97. Durso EA: Carcinoma arising in fibroadenoma: A case report. *Radiology* 1972;102:565.

98. Eusebi V, Azzopardi JG: Lobular endocrine neoplasia in fibroadenoma of the breast. *Histopathology* 1980;4:413–428.

* 99. Fondo EY, Rosen PP, Fracchia AA, et al: The problem of carcinoma developing in a fibroadenoma. Recent experience at Memorial Hospital. *Cancer* 1979;43:563–567.

100. Goldman RL, Friedman NB: Carcinoma of the breast arising in fibroadenoma with emphasis on lobular carcinoma. A clinicopathologic study. *Cancer* 1969;23:544–550.

101. Govoni E, Bazzocchi F, Pileri S, et al: Lobular endocrine neoplasia in a fibroadenoma of the breast. *Virchows Arch (Pathol Anat)* 393:299–306.

102. Haagensen CD, Lane N, Lattes R, et al: Lobular neoplasia (so-called lobular carcinoma in situ) of the breast. *Cancer* 1978;42:737–769.

*103. Harrington SW, Miller JM: Malignant changes in fibroadenoma of the mammary gland. *Surg Gynecol Obstet* 1940;70: 615–619.

*104. Kellett HS, Stewart FW, Farrow JH: Breast carcinoma arising in solitary fibroadenoma. *Br J Surg* 1958;45:620–622.

*105. McDivitt RW, Stewart FW, Farrow JH: Breast carcinoma arising in solitary fibroadenomas. *Surg Gynecol Obstet* 1967; 125:572–576.

106. More IAR, Sandison AT: Triple carcinoma of the breast, one arising within a fibroadenoma. *J Pathol* 1973;109:263–265.

107. Netto D, Satchidanand SK, Gaeta JF: Carcinomas arising in fibroadenomas: A report of two cases and a review of the literature. *J Surg Oncol* 1980;13:367–372.

108. Parache RM, Poisson P, Barlier C: Lobular carcinoma in situ in a breast fibroadenoma. *Arch Anat Cytol Pathol* 1978; 26:47–49.

*109. Pick PW, Iossifides IA: Occurrence of breast carcinoma within a fibroadenoma. A review. *Arch Pathol Lab Med* 1984;108:590–594.

*110. Rose K: Uber die Mastopathia chronica cystica und das Fibroadenoma mammae und ihre Umwandlung in Carzinom und Sarkom. *Frankfurt Z Path* 1942–1943;57:62–83.

111. Shinde SR, Jusscavalla DJ: Lobular carcinoma arising in a fibroadenoma. *J Surg Oncol* 1982;20:59–61.

112. Walter P, Kuentz Cl: Epitheliomas (lobulaires) developes dans un fibroadenome. Etude d'une observation et revue de la litterature. *Ann Anat Pathol* 1978;23:153–160.

113. Yoshida Y, Takaoka M, Fukumoto M: Carcinoma arising in fibroadenoma: Case report and review of the world literature. *J Surg Oncol* 1985;29:132–140.


### Cystosarcoma Phyllodes


114. Ackerman LV, Taylor HB: Seminar on lesions of the breast, in *Proceedings of the American Society of Clinical Pathologists*. Chicago, 1956.

115. Adami HG, Hakelius L, Rimsten A, et al: Malignant locally recurrent cystosarcoma phyllodes in an adolescent female. *Acta Chir Scand* 1984;150:93–100.

116. Al-Jurf A, Hawk WA, Crile G: Cytosarcoma phyllodes. *Surg Gynecol Obstet* 1978;146:358–364.

117. Amerson JR: Cystosarcoma phyllodes in adolescent females: A report of seven patients. *Ann Surg* 1970;171:849–858.

118. Ariel L: Skeletal metastases in cystosarcoma phyllodes. *Arch Surg* 1961;82:275–280.

119. Aronson W: Malignant cystosarcoma phyllodes with liposarcoma. *Wisconsin Med J* 1966;65:184–187.

120. Baader E, Isaacson C: Bilateral malignant cystosarcoma phyllodes. *Br J Surg* 1960;48:519–521.

*121. Blichert-Toft M, Hansen JPH, Hansen OH, Schiodt T: Clinical course of cystosarcoma phyllodes related to histologic appearance. *Surg Gynecol Obstet* 1975;140:929–932.

122. Blumenkranz PW, Gray GF: Cystosarcoma phyllodes: Clinical and pathologic study. *NY State J Med* 1978;78:623–627.

123. Brodie BC: *Lectures on Various Subjects in Pathology and Surgery*. London, Longmans Green & Co, 1846, p 148.

124. Burton GV, Hart LL, Leight GS, et al: Cystosarcoma phyllodes. Effective therapy with cisplatin and etoposide chemotherapy. *Cancer* 1989;63:2088–2092.

*125. Chelius MJ: *Neue Jahrbuecher der Teutschen. Medicin und Chirurgie*. Heidelberg, Naegele und Puchelt, 1827, pp 517–521.

126. Chowdhury C, Chattopadhyay TK, Pramanik M, et al: Cystosarcoma phyllodes—A clinicopathologic analysis of 32 cases. *Ind J of Cancer* 1984;21:23–30.

127. Cohn-Cedermark G, Rutquist LE, Rosendahl T, et al: Prognostic factors in cystosarcoma phyllodes. A clinicopathologic study of 77 patients. *Cancer* 1991;68:2017–2022.

128. Cooper WG, Ackerman LV: Cystosarcoma phyllodes, with a consideration of its more malignant variant. *Surg Gynecol Obstet* 1943;77:279–283.

*129. Cumin W: The general view of the diseases of the mamma;

with cases of some of the more important affections of the gland. *Edinb Med J* 1827;27:225–240.

130. Curran RC, Dodge OG: Sarcoma of breast, with particular reference to its origin from fibroadenoma. *Am J Clin Pathol* 1972;57:431–437.
131. Dyer NH, Bridger JE, Taylor RS: Cystosarcoma phylloides. *Br J Surg* 966;53:450–455.
132. El-Naggar AK, Ro JY, McLemore D, et al: DNA content and proliferative activity of cystosarcoma phyllodes of the breast. Potential prognostic significance. *Am J Clin Pathol* 1990;93:980–985.
133. Fernandez BB, Hernandez FJ, Spindler W: Metastatic cystosarcoma phyllodes. *Cancer* 1976;37:1737–1746.
134. Fiks A: Cystosarcoma phyllodes of the mammary gland—Mueller's tumor. *Virchows Archiv (Pathol Anat)* 1981;392: 1–6.
135. Friend E: Intracanalicular fibroma of the female breast undergoing sarcomatous change. *JAMA* 1909;53:1485–1487.
136. Fruhling L, Le Gal Y: La transformation sarcomateuse de la tumeur phyllode. *J Chir* 1954;70:16–29.
137. Gibbs BF, Roe RD, Thomas DF: Malignant cystosarcoma phyllodes in a pre-pubertal female. *Ann Surg* 1968;167:229–231.
138. Grimes MM, Lattes R, Laretzki A III: Cystosarcoma phyllodes. Report of an unusual case, with death due to intraneural extension to the central nervous system. *Cancer* 1985;56:1691–1695.
*139. Haagensen CD: *Diseases of the Breast*, ed 3. Philadelphia, WB Saunders Co, 1986, pp 284–312.
140. Hafner CD, Mezger E, Wylie JH Jr: Cystosarcoma phyllodes of the breast. *Surg Gynecol Obstet* 1962;115:29–34.
141. Hajdu SI, Espinosa MH, Robbins GF: Recurrent cystosarcoma phyllodes: A clinicopathologic study of 32 cases. *Cancer* 1976;38:1402–1406.
142. Halverson JD, Hori-Rubaina JM: Cardiac metastasis from cystosarcoma phyllodes. *Missouri Med* 1972;69:923.
143. Halverson JD, Hori-Rubaina JM: Cystosarcoma phyllodes of the breast. *Am Surgeon* 1974;40:295–301.
144. Harrington SW, Miller JM: Malignant changes in fibroadenoma of the mammary gland. *Surg Gynecol Obstet* 1940;70: 615–619.
*145. Hart WR, Bauer RC, Oberman HA: Cystosarcoma phyllodes: A clinicopathologic study of 26 hypercellular periductal stromal tumors of the breast. *Am J Clin Pathol* 1978;70:211–216.
146. Hawkins RE, Schofield JB, Fisher C, et al: The clinical and histologic criteria that predict metastases from cystosarcoma phyllodes. *Cancer* 1992;69:141–147.
*147. Hill RP, Stout AP: Sarcoma of the breast. *Arch Surg* 1942;44:723–759.
148. Hines JR, Gordon RT, Widget C, et al: Cystosarcoma phyllodes metastatic to a Brenner tumor of the ovary. *Arch Surg* 1976;111:299–300.
149. Hoover HC, Trestioreanu A, Ketcham AS: Metastatic cystosarcoma phyllodes in an adolescent girl: An unusually malignant tumor. *Ann Surg* 1975;88:243–247.
150. Horie A: Fine structure of cystosarcoma phyllodes with reference to smooth muscle tumors. *Acta Pathol Jpn* 1981; 31:1015–1028.
151. Kay S: Light and electron microscopic study of a malignant cystosarcoma phyllodes featuring stromal cartilage and bone. *Am J Clin Pathol* 1971;55:770–776.
152. Kessinger A, Foley JF, Lemon HM, et al: Metastatic cystosarcoma phyllodes: A case report and review of the literature. *J Surg Oncol* 1972;4:131–147.
*153. Lamonoco F: Il tumore della mammella (Cistosarcoma filloide di Muller). *Tumori* 1960;46:156–184.
154. Lamovec J, Us-Krasovec M: Malignant phyllodes tumor following irradiation of the breast. *Pathol Res Pract* 1985;180: 727–732.
*155. Lee BJ, Pack GT: Giant intracanalicular fibro-adenomyxoma of the breast. The so-called cystosarcoma phyllodes mammae of Johannes Muller. *Am J Cancer* 1931;15:2583–2595.
*156. Lester J, Stout AP: Cystosarcoma phyllodes. *Cancer* 1954;7: 335–353.
*157. Lindquist KD, Van Heerden JA, Weiland LH, et al: Recurrent and metastatic cystasarcoma phyllodes. *Am J Surg* 1982;144:341–343.
158. Long RTL, Hesker AE, Johnson RE: Surgical management of cystosarcoma phyllodes with a report of eight cases. *Missouri Med* 1962;59:1179–1181.
159. Maier WP, Rosemond GP, Wittenbert P, et al: Cystosarcoma phyllodes mammae. *Oncology* 1968;22:145–158.
160. Manivel C, Shenoy BV, Wick MR, et al: Cystosarcoma phyllodes of the prostate. A pathologic and immunohistochemical study. *Arch Pathol Lab Med* 1986;110:534–538.
161. McCullough K, Lynch JM: Metastatic sarcoma of the heart from cystosarcoma phyllodes of the breast. *Md State Med J* 1960;9:66–68.
*162. McDivitt RW, Urban JA, Farrow JH: Cystosarcoma phyllodes. *Johns Hopkins Med J* 1967;120:33–45.
163. McDonald JR, Harrington SW: Giant fibro-adenoma of the breast—"cystosarcoma phyllodes." *Ann Surg* 1950;131:243–251.
164. Mentzel T, Kosmehl H, Katenkamp D: Metastasizing phyllodes tumour with malignant fibrous histiocytoma-like areas. *Histopathology* 1991;19:557–560.
*165. Minkowitz S, Zeichner M, Di Maio V, et al: Cystosarcoma phyllodes: A unique case with multiple unilateral lesions and ipsilateral axillary metastais. *J Pathol Bacteriol* 1986;96: 514–517.
*166. Mueller J: *Ueber den feinern Bau und die Formen der krankhaften Geschwuelste*. Berlin, G. Reimer, 1838, p 56.
167. Nambiar R, Kutty MK: Giant fibro-adenoma (cystosarcoma phyllodes) in adolescent females—a clinicopathological study. *Br J Surg* 1974;61:113–117.

*168. Norris HJ, Taylor HB: Relationship of histologic features to behavior of cystosarcoma phyllodes. *Cancer* 1967;20:2090–2099.

169. Notley RG, Griffiths HJL: Bilateral malignant cystosarcoma phyllodes. *Br J Surg* 1965;52:360–362.

*170. Oberman HA: Cystosarcoma phyllodes. A clinicopathologic study of hypercellular periductal stromal tumors of the breast. *Cancer* 1965;18:697–710.

*171. Oberman HA, Nosanchuk JS, Finger JE: Periductal stromal tumors of the breast with adipose metaplasia. *Arch Surg* 1969;98:384–387.

172. Pantoja E, Llobet RE, Lopez E: Gigantic cystosarcoma phyllodes in a man with gynecomastia. *Arch Surg* 1976; 1974–1983.

*173. Pietruszka M, Barnes L: Cystosarcoma phyllodes: A clinicopathologic analysis of 42 cases. *Cancer* 1978;1974–1983.

*174. Qizilbash AH: Cystosarcoma phyllodes with liposarcomatous stroma. *Am J Clin Pathol* 1976;65:321–327.

*175. Rao BR, Meyer JS, Fry G: Most cystosarcoma phyllodes and fibroadenomas have progesterone receptors but lack estrogen receptor. Stromal localization of progesterone receptors. *Cancer* 1981;47:2016–2921.

*176. Reich T, Solomon C: Bilateral cystosarcoma phyllodes, malignant variant, with a 14 year follow-up. A case report. *Ann Surg* 1958;147:39–43.

*177. Reingold IM, Ascher GS: Cystosarcoma phyllodes in a man with gynecomastia. *Am J Clin Pathol* 1970;53:852–856.

178. Rhodes RH, Frankel KA, Davis RL, et al: Metastatic cystosarcoma phyllodes: A report of two cases presenting with neurological symptoms. *Cancer* 1978;41:1179–1187.

179. Rix DB, Tredwell JJ, Forward AD: Cystosarcoma phyllodes (cellular intracanalicular fibroadenoma): Clinicopathological relationship. *Can J Surg* 1971;14:31–37.

180. Rosen PP, Urban JA: Coexistant mammary carcinoma and cystosarcoma phyllodes. *Breast* 1975;1:9–15.

*181. Salvadori B, Cosumano F, Del Bo R, et al: Surgical treatment of phyllodes tumors of the breast. *Cancer* 1989;63: 2532–2536.

182. Simpson TE, Vandervoort RL Jr, Lynn HB: Giant fibroadenoma (benign cystosarcoma phyllodes): Report of a case in a 13-year-old girl. *Surgery* 1969;65:341–342.

*183. Smith BH, Taylor HB: The occurrence of bone and cartilage in mammary tumors. *Am J Clin Pathol* 1969;51:610–618.

184. Toker C: Cystosarcoma phyllodes: An ultrastructural study. *Cancer* 1968;21:1171–1179.

*185. Treves N: A study of cystosarcoma phyllodes. *Ann NY Acad Sci* 1964;114:922–936.

*186. Treves N, Sunderland DA: Cystosarcoma phyllodes of the breast: A malignant and a benign tumor. *Cancer* 1951;4: 1286–1332.

*187. Velpeu A: *Traite des Maladies du Sein et de la Region Mammaire*. Paris, V Mason, 1854, p 338.

*188. Ward RM, Evans HL: Cystosarcoma phyllodes. A clinicopathologic study of 26 cases. *Cancer* 1986;58:2282–2289.

189. West TL, Weiland LH, Claggett OT: Cystosarcoma phyllodes. *Ann Surg* 1971;173:520–528.

190. White JW: Malignant variant of cystosarcoma phyllodes. *Am J Cancer* 1940;40:458–464.

*191. World Health Organization: Histological Typing of Breast Tumors, in *International Histological Classification of Tumors*, ed 2, no. 2. Geneva, WHO, 1981.

192. Williams WR: *Diseases of the Breast*. London, John Bole & Sons, 1894, p 417.

193. Wulsin JH: Large breast tumors in adolescent females. *Ann Surg* 1960;152:151–159.


### Carcinoma in CP


*194. Azzopardi JG: *Problems in Breast Pathology*. Philadelphia, WB Saunders, 1979, pp 354–355.

195. Cornog JL, Mobini J, Steiger E, et al: Squamous carcinoma of the breast. *Am J Clin Pathol* 1971;55:410–417.

*196. Gilks B, Tavassoli FA: Coexistence of intracytoplasmic lumens and membrane bound vesicles in an invasive carcinoma arising in a cystosarcoma phyllodes. *Ultrastruct Pathol* 1988;12:631–642.

*197. Harris M, Persaud V: Carcinosarcoma of the breast. *J Pathol* 1974;112:99–105.

198. Ishida T, Izuo M, Kawai T: Breast carcinoma arising in cystosarcoma phyllodes: Report of a case with a review of the literature. *Jpn J Clin Oncol* 1984;14:99–106.

199. Leong AS-Y, Meredith DJ: Tubular carcinoma developing within a recurring cystosarcoma phyllodes of the breast. *Cancer* 1980;46:1863–1967.

200. Knudsen PJT, Ostergaard J: Cystosarcoma phylloides with lobular and ductal carcinoma in situ. *Arch Pathol Lab Med* 1987;111:873–875.

201. Rosen PP, Urban JA: Coexistent mammary carcinoma and cystosarcoma phyllodes. *Breast* 1975;1:9–15.

202. Ross DE: Malignancy occurring in cystosarcoma phyllodes. *Am J Surg* 1954;88:243–247.


### Carcinosarcoma


*203. Abenoza P, Manivel JC, Swanson PE, et al: Synovial sarcoma: Ultrastructural study and immunohistochemical analysis by a combined peroxidase-antiperoxidase/avidin-biotin-peroxidase complex procedure. *Hum Pathol* 1986;17: 1107–1115.

*204. Azzopardi JG: *Problems in Breast Pathology*. Philadelphia, WB Saunders Co, 1979, pp 297–301.

*205. Cameron HM, Hamperl H, Warembo W: Leiomyosarcoma of the breast originating from myothelium (myoepithelium). *J Pathol* 1974;114:89–92.

*206. Carstens PHB, Cooke JL: Mammary carcinosarcoma presenting as rhabdomyosarcoma: An ultrastructural and immunocytochemical study. *Ultrastruct Pathol* 1990;14:537–544.

207. Cornog JL, Mobini J, Steiger E, et al: Squamous carcinoma of the breast. *Am J Clin Pathol* 1971;55:410–417.

208. Gersell DJ, Katzenstein A-LA: Spindle cell carcinoma of the breast. A clinicopathologic and ultrastructural study. *Hum Pathol* 1981;12:550–561.

* 209. Ghadially F: Is synovial sarcoma a carcinosarcoma of connective tissue? *Ultrastruct Pathol* 1987;11:147–151.

210. Gonzalez-Licea A, Yardley JH, Hartmann WH: Malignant tumor of the breast with bone formation. *Cancer* 1967;20:1234–1247.

* 211. Huvos AG, Lucas JC, Foote FW: Metaplastic breast carcinoma. A rare form of mammary cancer. *NY State J Med* 1973;73:1078–1082.

212. Jones EL: Primary squamous-cell carcinoma of breast with pseudosarcomatous stroma. *J Pathol* 1969;97:383–385.

* 213. Kahn LB, Uys CJ, Dale J, et al: Carcinoma of the breast with metaplasia to chondrosarcoma: A light and electron microscopic study. *Histopathology* 1978;2:93–106.

214. Kaufman MW, Marti JR, Gallager HS, et al: Carcinoma of the breast with pseudosarcomatous metaplasia. *Cancer* 1984;53:1908–1917.

* 215. Krall RA, Kostianovsky M, Patchefsky AS: Synovial sarcoma. A clinical, pathological, and ultrastructural study of 26 cases supporting the recognition of a monophasic variant. *Am J Surg Pathol* 1981;5:137–151.

216. Leader M, Patel J, Collins M, et al: Synovial sarcomas. True carcinosarcoma? *Cancer* 1987;59:2096–2098.

* 217. Miettinen M, Virtanen I: Synovial sarcoma—A misnome. *Am J Pathol* 1984;117:18–25.

* 218. Salisbury JR, Isaacson JR: Synovial sarcoma: An immunohistochemical study. *J Pathol* 1985;147:49–57.

* 219. Stewart FW: *Tumors of the Breast*, Fasc 34. Atlas of Tumor Pathology, section a, Washington DC, Armed Forces Institute of Pathology, 1950, pp 75–87.

* 220. Tavassoli FA: Classification of metaplastic carcinomas of the breast in Rosen PP, Fechner RD (eds): *Pathology Annual* 1992;27(pt 2):89–119. Norwalk CT, Appleton & Lange.

221. Wargotz ES, Norris HJ: Metaplastic carcinomas of the breast. III. Carcinosarcoma. *Cancer* 1989;64:1490–1499.

* 222. Willis RA: Squamous-cell carcinoma of predominantly fibrosarcoma-like structure. *J Pathol Bacteriol* 1958;76:511–515.

# 12

# Vascular Lesions



A variety of vascular lesions occur in the breast. Among these, intramammary and postmastectomy angiosarcomas account for the largest group of reported vascular tumors. Recently, attention has been directed toward a variety of benign vascular lesions and pseudoangiomatous alterations which should be distinguished from angiosarcoma.

The mammary vascular lesions can be divided into three major categories. The first category is comprised of the malignant vascular tumors, all reported examples of which have been angiosarcomas (17,20,21,24,32,38,47,63). The second group consists of the microscopic, perilobular and periductal hemangiomas (55,74,75); these are all benign. Clinically palpable benign vascular lesions such as hemangiomas, angiomatosis, hemangiopericytoma, and intravascular papillary endothelial hyperplasias constitute the third group (20,86,92,96).

## ANGIOSARCOMA

Angiosarcoma, first described by Schmidt in 1887 (59) and subsequently by Borrmann in 1907 (10), is a highly lethal and a rather rare neoplasm accounting for less than 0.05% of primary mammary cancers. While it is most commonly known as angiosarcoma (45), it has also been referred to as hemangiosarcoma (43,63,68), hemangio-endothelioma (14,66), hemangioblastoma (7), angioblastoma (25), and benign metastasizing hemangioma (54,67). It is generally present in its pure form; unlike some other sarcomas, it would be most unusual to find angiosarcoma as a component of cystosarcoma phyllodes though we have seen one such case at AFIP. Stewart (64) reported one angiosarcoma for every 2,000 to 3,500 breast cancers. A variety of reports ranging from description of a single case to discussion of a large series of cases of angiosarcoma are abundant in the literature (30,44,46,49). Occurring almost exclusively in the female breast, angiosarcoma often presents during the third or fourth decade of life; the age at presentation ranges from 14 to 82 years with a mean of 35 years (17). Angiosarcoma rarely develops in the male breast, with only five cases reported in the literature (52,53,70). Rosen has questioned the case reported by Yadev et al because of the clinical evidence of bone metastases two years prior to the presentation of the breast lesion.

Bilateral synchronous and metachronous tumors have been reported (6) including several cases diagnosed during pregnancy (7,20,25,39,63,67) and in postmenopausal women.

## Clinical Presentation

Angiosarcomas may have an insidious clinical onset presenting as a painless, often discrete, mass which rapidly grows and may assume massive proportions on rare occasions. In young women, the discrete nature of the lesion has led to an erroneous clinical impression of fibroadenoma.

Approximately 12% of patients present with diffuse enlargement of the breast. A bluish-red discoloration of the overlying skin may ensue. There is a report of a patient whose tumor presented as a pulsatile mass associated with bruit (51). Nipple retraction, discharge, or axillary node enlargement are generally absent despite the large size of some lesions. Xeromammographically, angiosarcoma presents as a lobulated mass with poorly defined borders; sonographically, it appears well-defined and lobulated, with both hyper- and hypoechoic appearance and no acoustic shadowing (30).

## Gross Appearance

All tumors are grossly evident with poorly-defined margins. They vary in size from 1.5 to 12 cm with a spongy or friable consistency and hemorrhagic areas. The tumors are located within the substance of the breast. A rim of congested, thin-walled vessels surrounds the main mass. While the tumor may involve the skin, extension to the pectoral fascia is quite rare.

## Microscopic Features

Microscopically, angiosarcoma is composed of irregular, anastomosing vascular channels lined by one or more layers of endothelial cells, papillae, and solid nests of spindle cells in variable proportions (Fig. 12.1). Typically, angiosarcomas proliferate into the lobular stroma resulting in eventual distortion of the lobular architecture (Fig. 12.2), and advance into the surrounding tissue displaying highly irregular margins and significant infiltration of adipose tissue. The endothelial cells are plump and hyperchromatic. Atypism is mild and mitotic activity is variable. The proportion and distribution of well-formed vascular spaces, papillary, and solid areas vary significantly in different tumors and within a given tumor and serve as the basis for grading angiosarcomas. Solid areas composed of spindle cells, blood lakes, and necrosis—features readily apparent in poorly-differentiated (high grade) angiosarcomas—are absent in the well-differentiated lesion. Conversely, deceptively benign areas may be found, particularly in the periphery of the lesion, even in the most poorly-differentiated tumor; this feature had led to the designation of almost one third of the angiosarcomas reported up to 1980 (17) by the misleading term of "metastasizing hemangioma." Therefore, to avoid undercalling angiosarcomas, generous sampling of large lesions and processing of small ones in their entirety are crucial. A myxoid change occurs in some cases, and occasionally it may be prominent enough to cause misinterpretation of the lesion on needle aspiration biopsy samples (Fig. 12.3).

## Grading Angiosarcomas and Its Prognostic Significance

While formerly thought to be inevitably fatal regardless of their histologic appearance (17), useful criteria for grading of angiosarcomas have been developed over the past decade. According to these studies, approximately one third of angiosarcomas are well-differentiated (Fig. 12.4), and patients with such tumors have a favorable prognosis (20,47,55). In contrast, poorly-differentiated neoplasms (Figs. 12.5–12.6) have an unfavorable prognosis. An intermediate histologic grade (Fig. 12.7) has also been described, but the behavior of tumors in this group has been variable, and a more precise definition for this group is needed to better establish their prognostic significance. The stratification of angiosarcomas into separate prognostic categories relies mainly on histologic features. Based on the degree of endothelial cell atypia, proliferation, and formation of papillary tufting, and solid spindle cell areas, angiosarcomas can be stratified into three groups, designated as types I, II, and III (20) (see Table 12.1); alternately, they may also be divided into well-differentiated, moderately-differentiated and poorly-differentiated tumors based on the quantity of the solid spindle cell areas and tufting of atypical endothelial cells in the lesion (47) (see Table 12.2). All groups exhibit hyperchromatic endothelial cells and anastomosing vascular channels irregularly permeating the breast parenchyma. In both systems of classification, tufting and papillae are absent or minimal in group I, but they constitute the major distinctive feature of the second group (type II or moderately-differentiated tumors). In the third group (type III or poorly-differentiated lesions) there are solid areas of spindle cell proliferation, hemorrhage, necrosis, and numerous mitotic figures often in addition to features present in the first two groups. While the type I of Donnell et al (20) and the well-differentiated group of Merino et al (47) are basically identical, the quantitative approach of Merino et al can be applied with greater ease for further separation of the more advanced lesions.

Another feature of possible prognostic significance is tumor size. In a study of ten cases, tumor size larger than 3 cm, high mitotic count, and long pretreatment duration of lesion were suggested as evidence of poor prognosis (63). In Donnell et al's series (20), no patient with a tumor less than 3 cm died from the disease. But even 1.5 cm angiosarcomas are known to have metastasized, therefore, while size is an important factor, it cannot be relied upon as the sole factor for the purpose of prognostication. It is important to remember, however, that there are no known examples of minute angiosarcomas that have been recognized only microscopically. In a more recent study, duration of the lesion prior to treatment and tumor size did not appear to be significant risk factors relative to recurrence and survival (55).

## Behavior and Treatment

Angiosarcoma is a highly aggressive neoplasm. Close to 90% of the women reported in the literature died from their disease, generally within two years of diagnosis (26). Metastases develop shortly after the primary lesion, and most frequently involve lungs, liver, skin, bone, and contralateral breast. Only in rare exceptions have patients survived 7, 11, 14, and 18 years postoperatively (36,55,56,63). The three-year disease-free interval among 87 patients reported in the literature prior to 1980 was 14% (17), and three of five patients with five-year disease-free survival had type I or II lesions (20).

The degree of tumor differentiation appears to be important in predicting the behavior of angiosarcomas. The probability of disease-free five-year survival after initial treatment was estimated to be 76% for type I (well-differentiated) tumors, 70% for type II (moderately-differentiated), and 15% for the type III (poorly-differentiated) lesions. The median length of disease-free survival was also related to tumor type, being more than 15 years for type I, more than 12 years for type II, but only 15 months for type III tumors. Obviously, there is a significant difference in the behavior of the well-differentiated and the poorly-differentiated groups. The moderately-differentiated tumors do not seem to behave much differently from the well-differentiated ones; perhaps a better definition and different criteria are needed to more optimally stratify the three groups. Complete excision and generous sampling of the lesion is necessary for accurate grading or typing of the tumor.

Only a few other documented cases of axillary node metastases have been reported in the literature (24,32), but a rare angiosarcoma with metastases to 20 of 20 nodes has been encountered (1).

Metastases may resemble the primary tumor or appear less differentiated. A rare example of extramedullary hematopoeisis has been reported in the metastatic tumor despite its absence in the primary tumor (63). The contralateral breast is involved in 21% of cases (17), and in half of the cases, the contralateral breast lesion presents before dissemination of the disease. Death occurs as a result of disseminated angiosarcoma.

Despite rare instances of axillary node metastases, the treatment of choice remains simple mastectomy unless the axillary nodes are enlarged or axillary dissection is necessary to obtain a satisfactory resection margin. Judging from the available information, there is very little chance of cure by surgery alone in patients with type III (poorly-differentiated) angiosarcoma. It has been suggested that Actinomycin D (dactinomycin) may be effective in limiting the chances of recurrence (20). Recurrences are less frequent among women treated with adjuvant chemotherapy, but there appear to be no statistically signif-

A

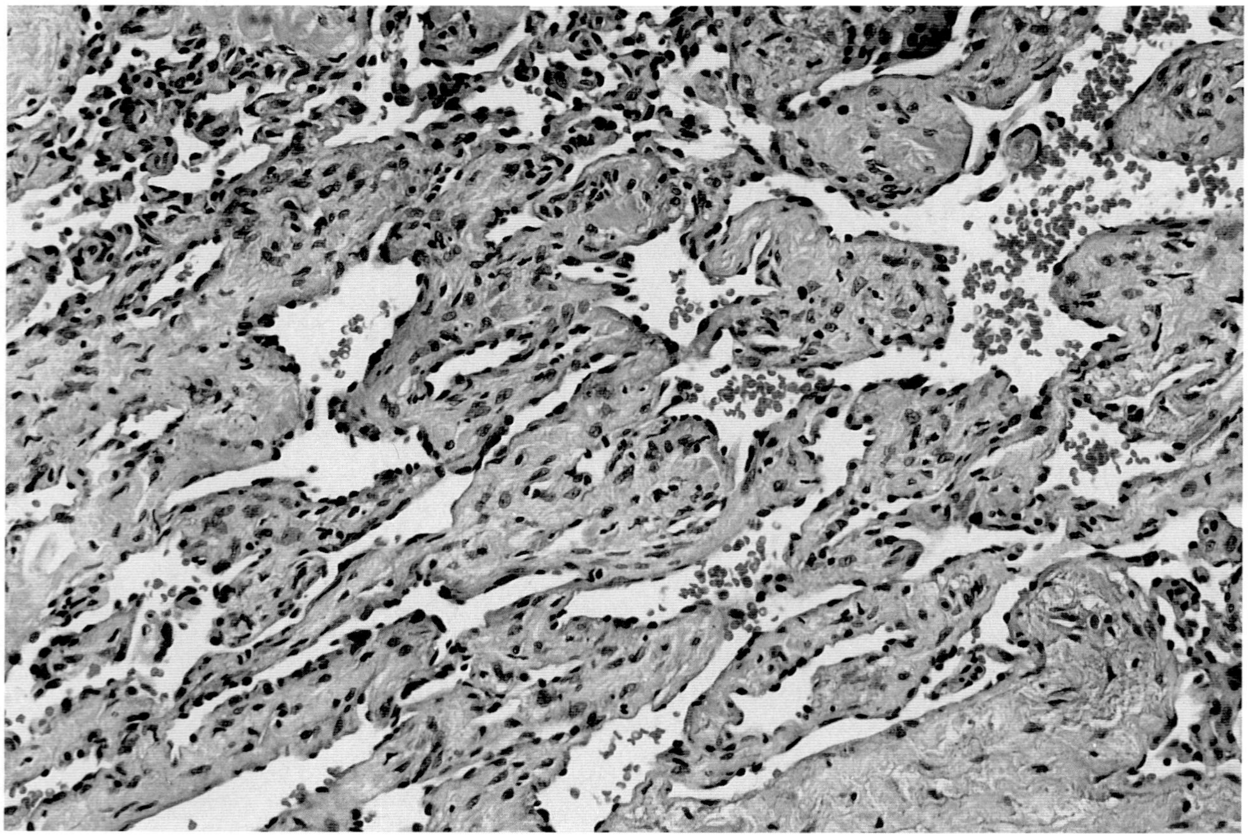

B

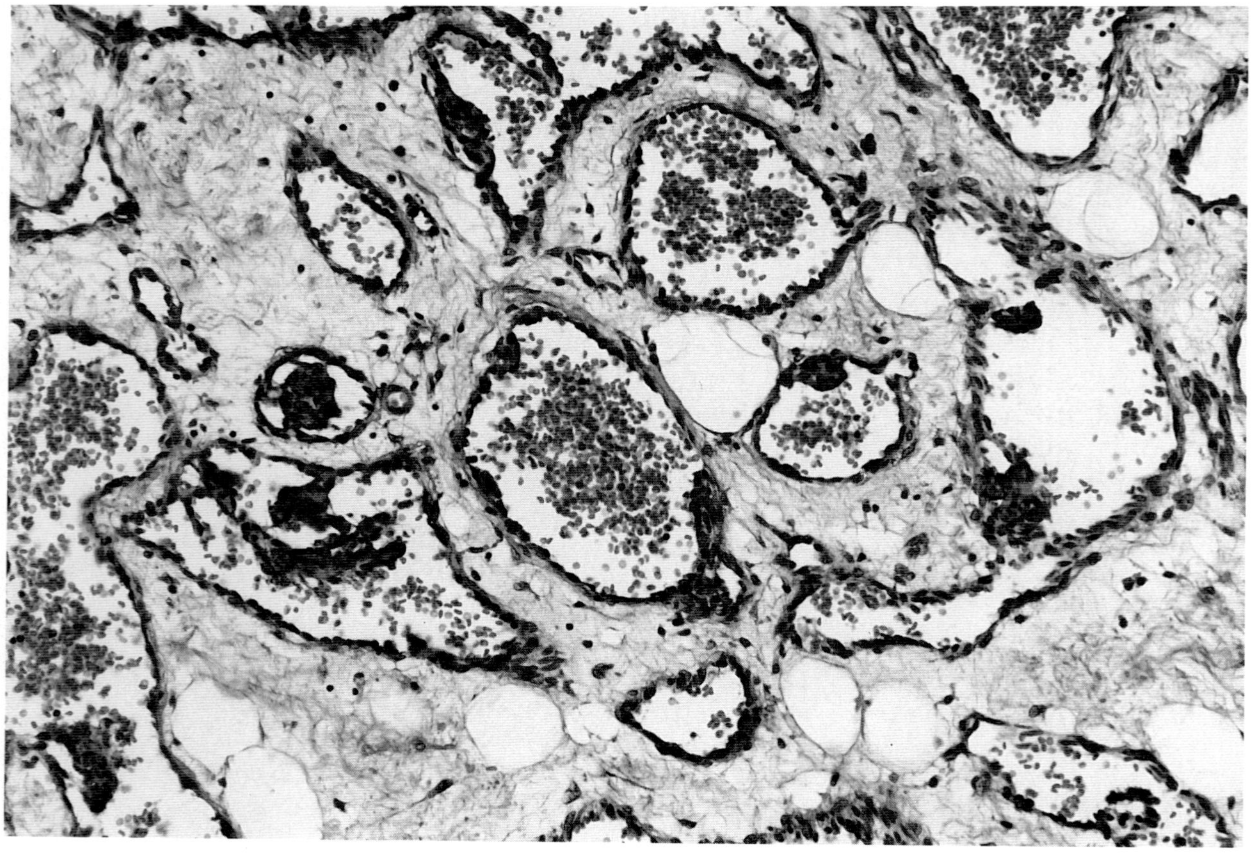

**Figure 12.1** Angiosarcoma. Various patterns of angiosarcoma with increasing density of endothelial proliferation (a) anastomosing channels, (b) anastomosing channels and early endothelial tufting, (c) relatively compact proliferation of small caliber vascular channels, endothelial tufts and papillae, and (d) solid spindle cell growth. (H&E (a) X200; (b) 300; (c) X240; (d) X200)

C

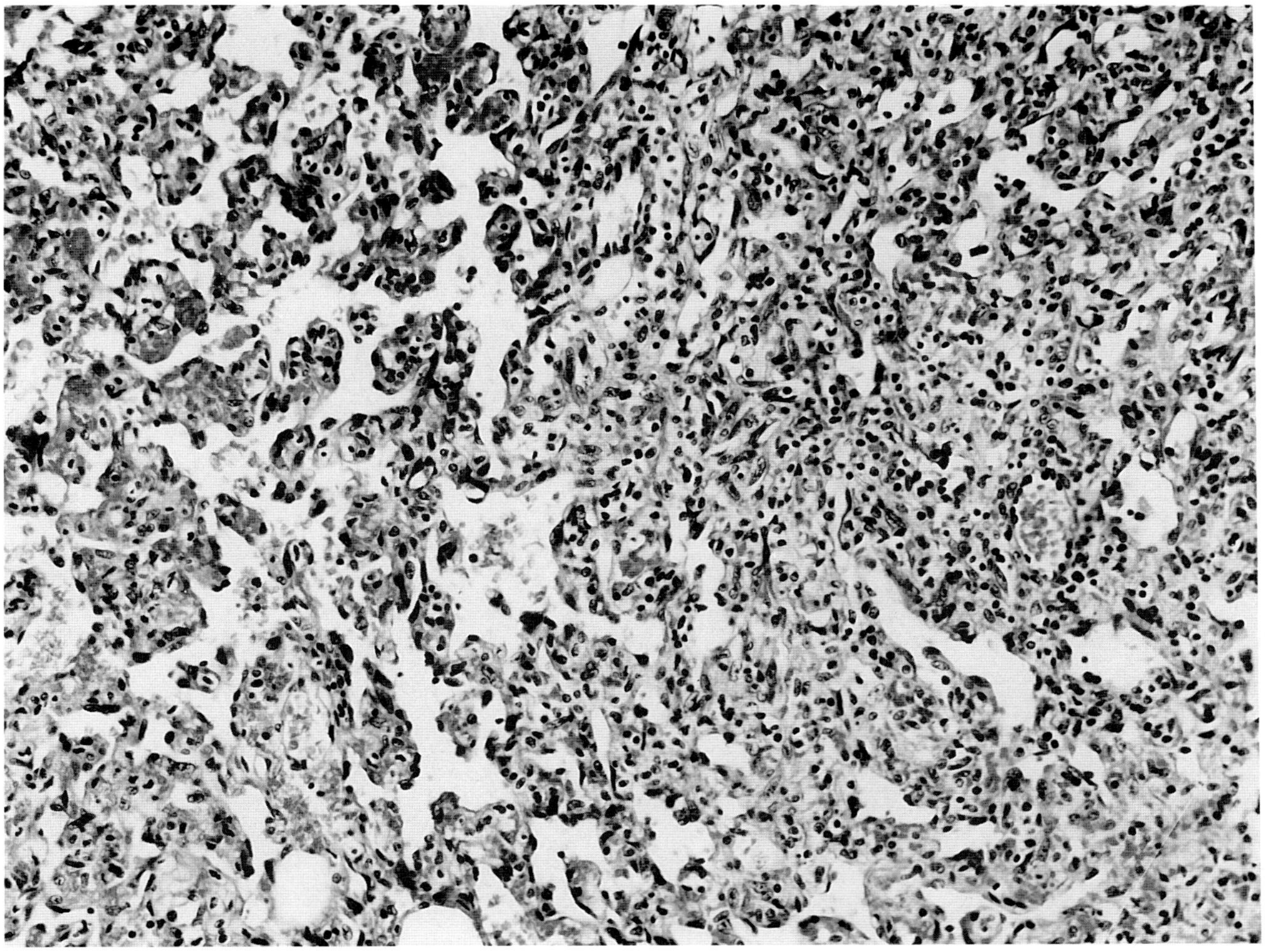

D

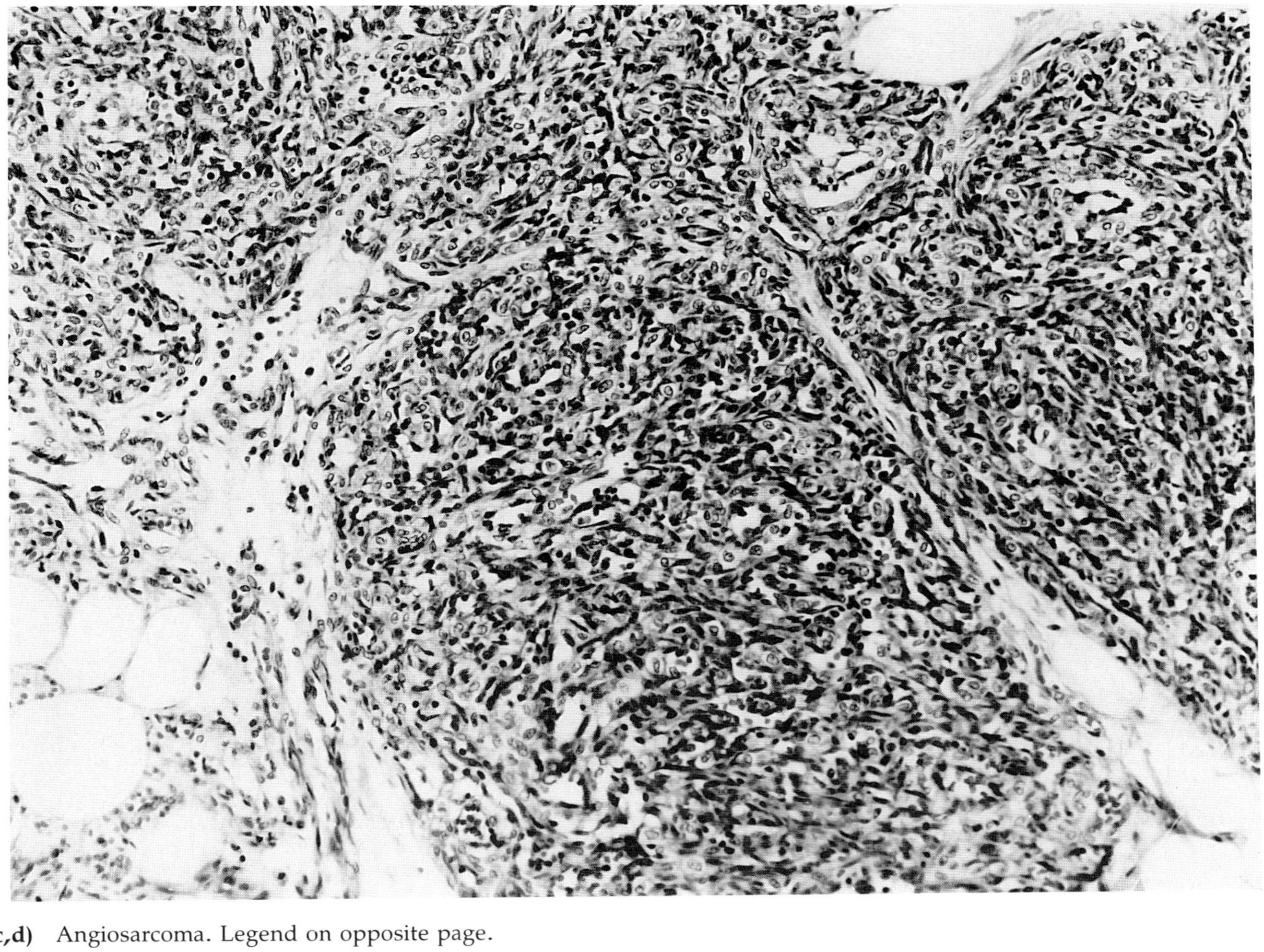

**Figure 12.1(c,d)** Angiosarcoma. Legend on opposite page.

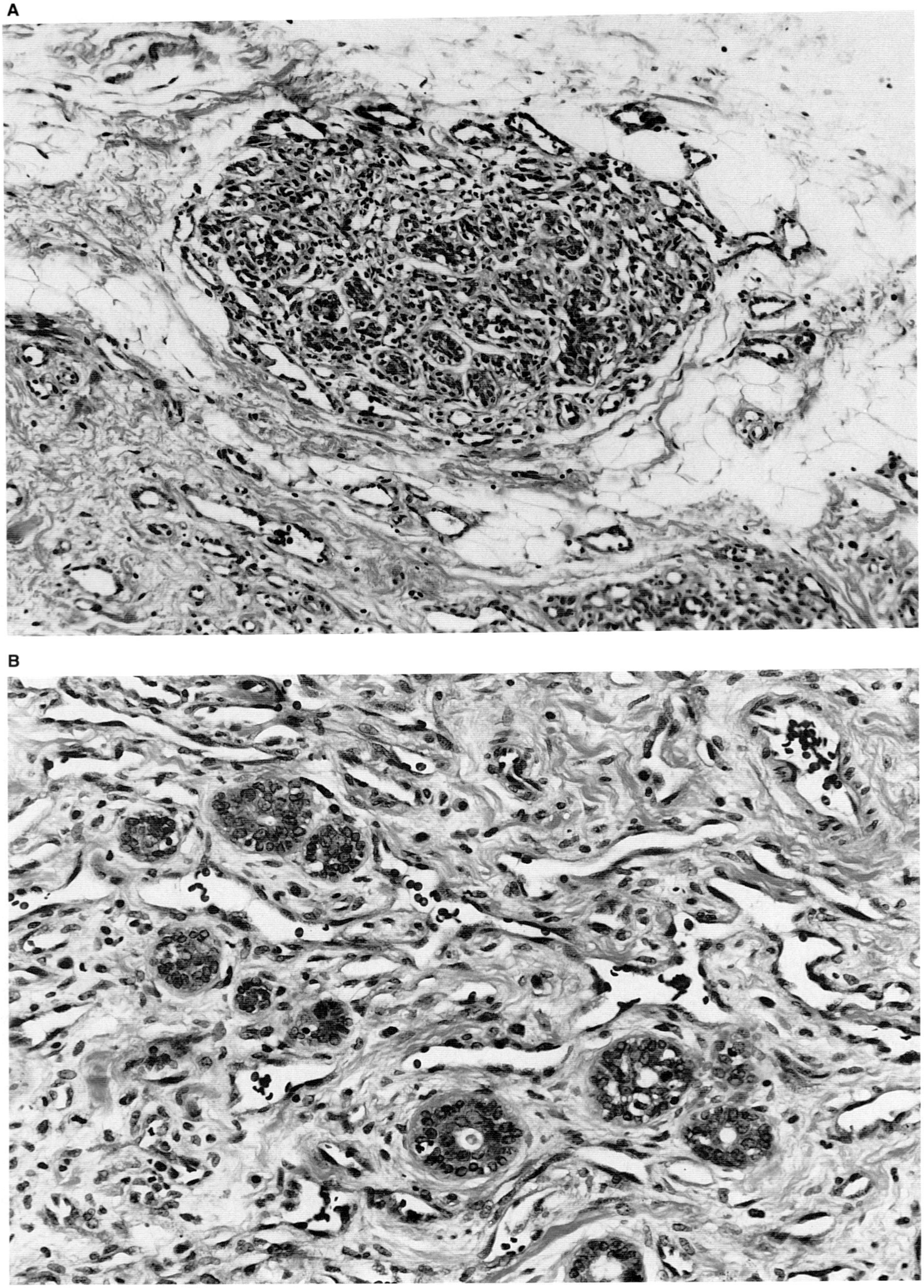

**Figure 12.2** Angiosarcoma (a) invading and (b) disrupting the lobular architecture by piercing in between acini (ductules). (H&E, (a) X120; (b) X300)

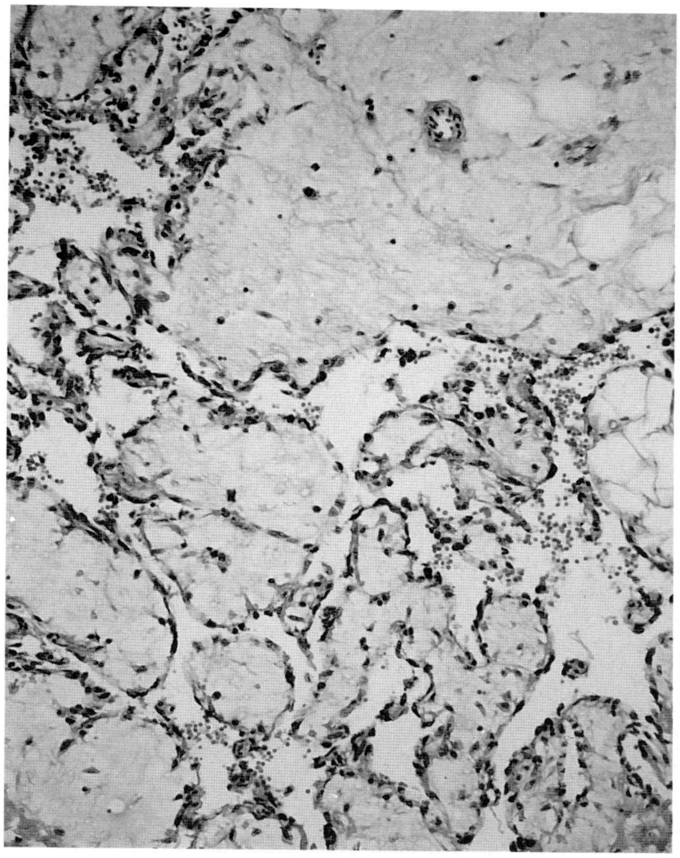

**Figure 12.3** Angiosarcoma with prominent myxoid stromal change. The discrete nature of this lesion clinically, coupled with the needle aspiration of the myxoid areas of this lesion had led to an initial, erroneous interpretation of this angiosarcoma. (H&E, X160)

icant effects on prognosis (55). While a multimodality approach to treatment has already been initiated (47) and will be considered with increasing frequency in the case of high grade angiosarcomas, additional studies are needed to determine the most effective treatment for the various grades or types of angiosarcoma.

## Hormone Receptors, Immunohistochemical, and Ultrastructural Features

Estrogen and glucocorticoid receptors have been demonstrated in some angiosarcomas, but the receptor levels have been low, and there is no good evidence that these tumors are hormone-dependent even though the young age of many patients affected may suggest a hormonal relationship (4,13,37). Others have been totally unable to detect receptors for either estrogen, progesterone, or testosterone in one case of angiosarcoma (11).

Factor VIII antigen can be demonstrated in most well-differentiated lesions, but the poorly-differentiated tumors fail to elaborate this antigen uniformly or at all. The endothelial cells may also elaborate a positive reaction for Ulex europaeus particularly in the better-differentiated lesions. Neither of these markers label angiosarcomas consistently, however. Alles and Bosslet (2) found BMA 120, an endothelial-cell-specific monoclonal antibody detecting an epitope of a formalin-resistant antigen, the most sensitive immunohistochemical method to study and diagnose angiosarcomas adequately.

At the ultrastructural level, Weibel-Palade bodies (Fig. 12.4d) have been identified in well-differentiated angiosarcomas (3), but these structures are practically absent in poorly-differentiated areas.

## Differential Diagnosis

Angiosarcoma should be distinguished from benign hemangiomas and angiolipoma. Angiosarcomas are ill-defined with diffuse and irregular infiltration of breast parenchyma and adipose tissue. Hemangiomas and angiolipomas, in contrast, are usually sharply-demarcated from the surrounding breast tissue. The vessels in hemangiomas are more uniform in shape and there is no endothelial atypia, while those in angiolipomas have typical microthrombi. Furthermore, in contrast to angiosarcomas, which permeate lobules and surround ducts, angiolipomas displace the normal breast parenchyma. Stewart (64) and Azzopardi (5) have stressed that "a benign angioma has never to date constituted a palpable or symptom-producing mass." In light of a number of recent reports (74,81) and our observations at AFIP, this statement is no longer valid.

# ANGIOSARCOMA ASSOCIATED WITH LYMPHEDEMA

Postmastectomy lymphangiosarcoma resulting as a complication of chronic lymphedema is a rare but devastating lesion. Though the clinical setting indi-

A

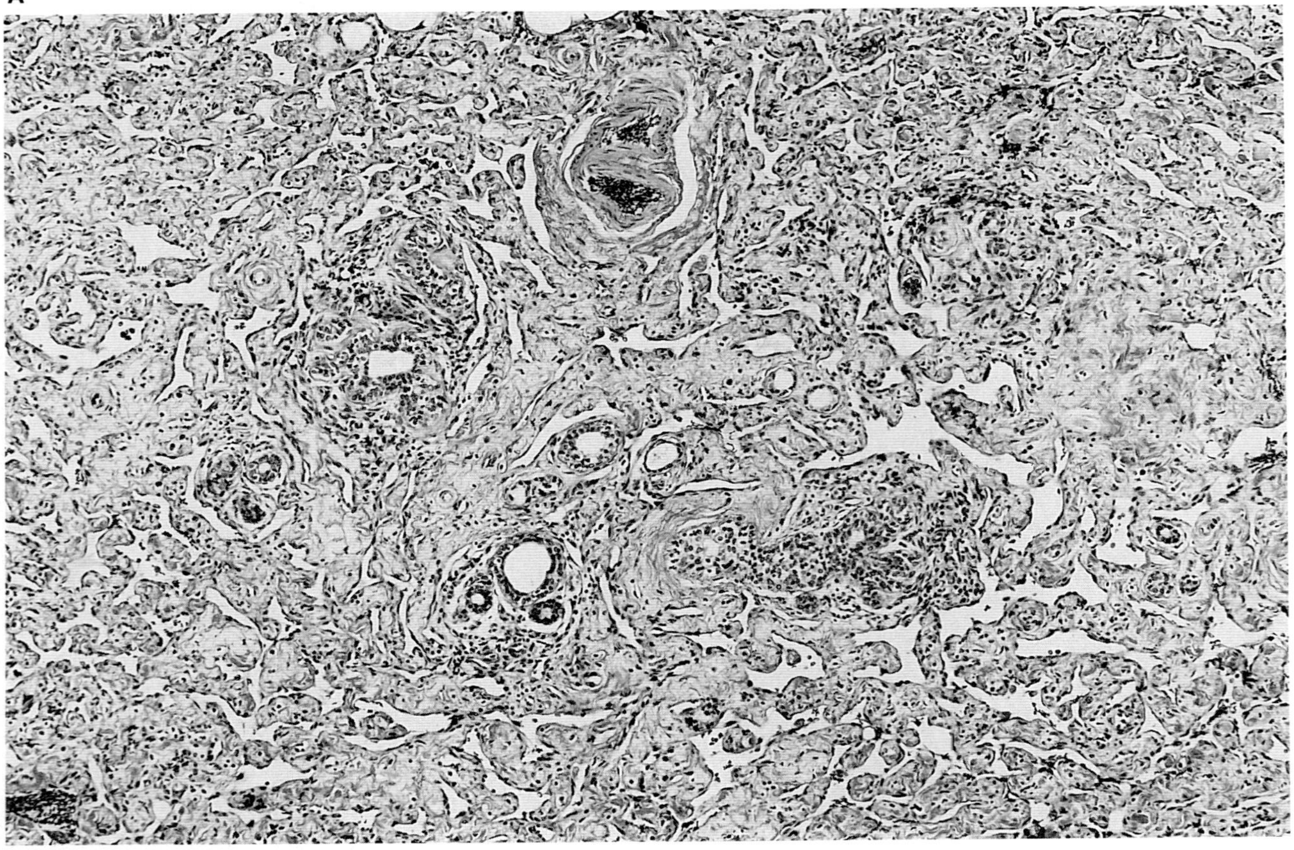

**Figure 12.4** Well-differentiated angiosarcoma, type I. This low grade lesion is characterized by an invasive growth of (a) anastomosing channels and (b) lack of significant endothelial atypia. (H&E, (a) X300; (b) X800) At the ultrastructural level, (c) the vascular channels are lined by plump endothelial cells. (Uranyl acetate-lead citrate, X4,990)

cates origin in the endothelial lining of lymphatic channels, morphologically these tumors are indistinguishable from other angiosarcomas; therefore, they are discussed in this section on angiosarcomas. Stewart and Treves (65) were the first to describe six patients who developed angiosarcomas following radical mastectomy and axillary node dissection for mammary carcinoma. Chronic lymphedema, supervening shortly after mastectomy, was the common denominator of these cases. While a majority (90%) of these angiosarcomas have occurred in postmastectomy women with or without irradiation (9,27,29,61, 69), they may develop in any chronic lymphedematous extremity following excision of other types of tumors such as melanoma (31) or even in the absence of any previous tumors (69), as well as in limbs affected by congenital lymphedema (18).

A majority of these angiosarcomas become evident about ten years following mastectomy for breast carcinoma; some appear within only three to four years, or as late as three decades after the diagnosis (26), however. The initial lesion may cause nothing more than a focal purple discoloration of the skin. This subtle change rapidly evolves into plaques and nodules which may ulcerate and bleed easily. Postmastectomy angiosarcoma almost invariably develops in the ipsilateral arm (69), but three cases have been reported in the irradiated chest wall and the residual breast after segmental or complete mastectomy without any tumor in the arm (8,19,28,42).

Doubts had been expressed regarding the vascular nature of Stewart-Treves (post-radiation) angiosarcoma with a suggestion that it may reflect a recurrent, metaplastic variant of the original mammary carcinoma (57,58). This concept has been refuted, however, by the application of electron microscopic and immunohistochemical techniques. At the ultrastructural level, angiosarcomas arising in lymphedematous extremities show endothelial type cells with pinocytotic vesicles, desmosomal-type attachments, and occasional paranuclear filamentous aggregates in the well-differentiated lesions (21,48). In

B

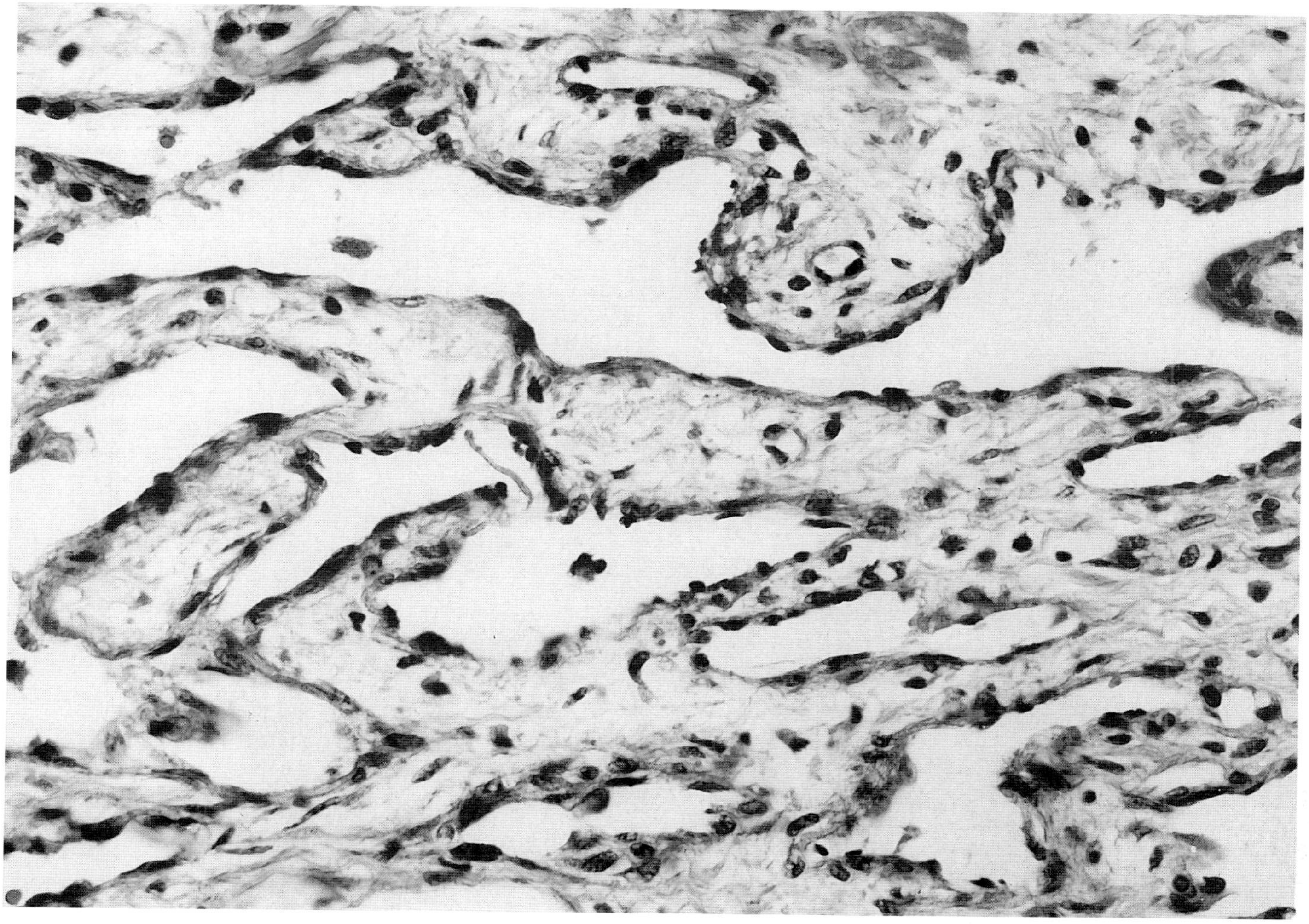

C

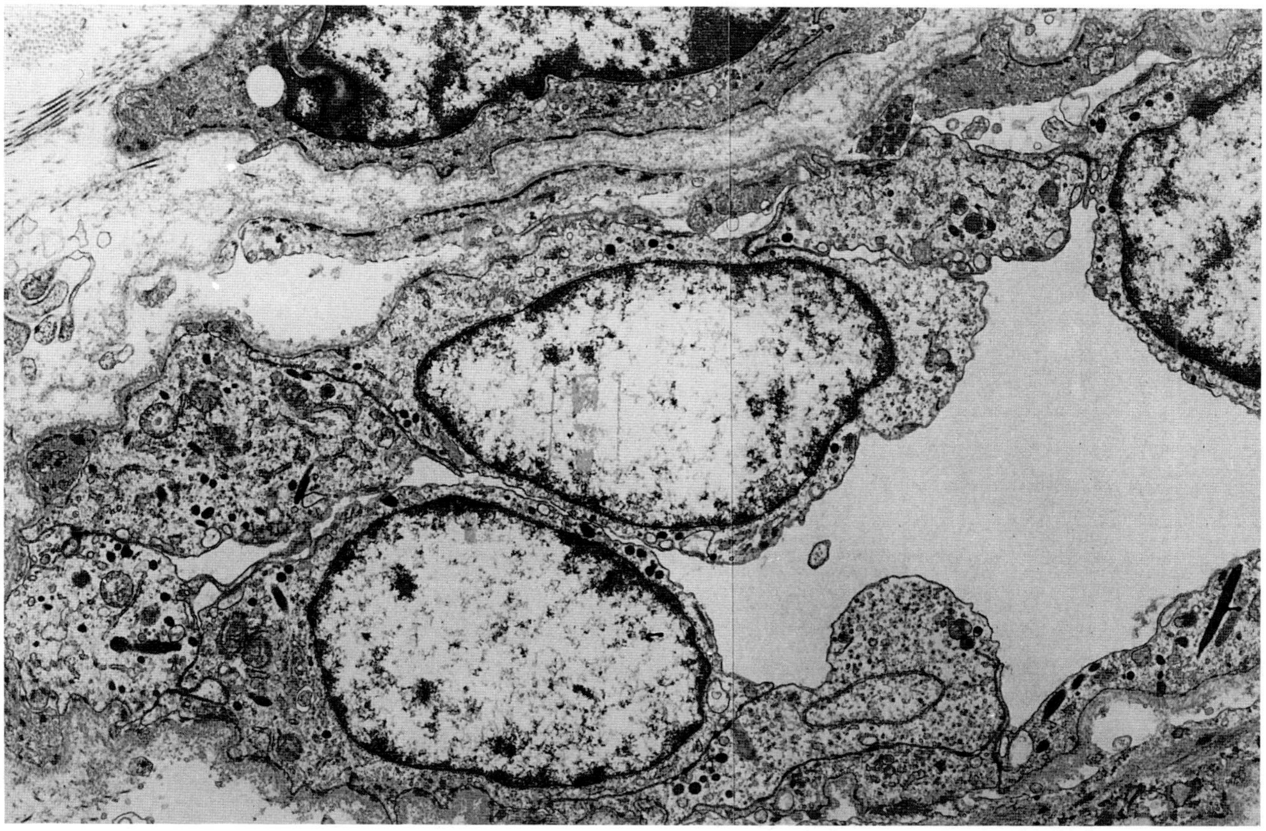

**Figure 12.4(b,c)** Well-differentiated angiosarcoma. Legend on opposite page.

D

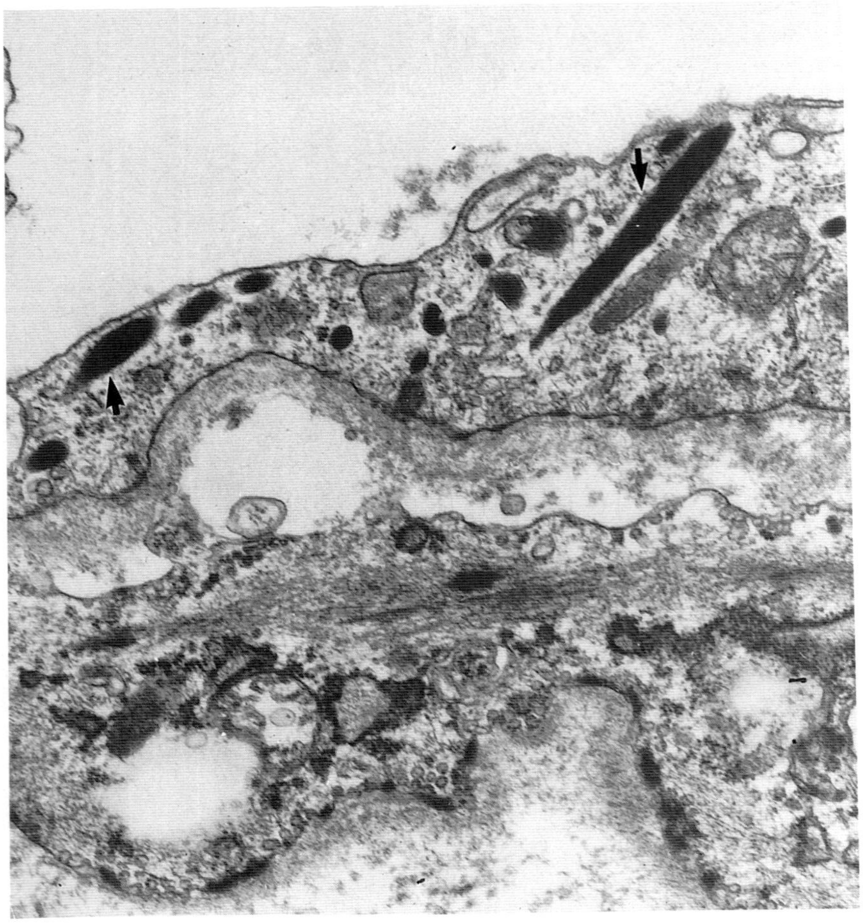

**Figure 12.4(d)** Well-differentiated angiosarcoma, type I. Weibel-Palade bodies (arrow) are present in the cytoplasm of the endothelial cells. (Uranyl acetate-lead citrate, X11,620)

the poorly-differentiated tumors, there are basically primitive mesenchymal cells with a few tight junctions (61). Immunohistochemical stains of four such tumors (19,28,34,48) has confirmed the endothelial nature of the cells by their positive reaction for Factor VIII. It is noteworthy that immunohistochemistry is more helpful than electron microscopy in differentiating an angiosarcoma from a carcinoma. This is due to the fact that desmosomes and tight junctions, features generally used to separate epithelial tumors from mesenchymal lesions, are normally present in the endothelial cell population.

## Pathogenesis

Chronic lymphedema, generally of several years duration, is a recognized risk factor predisposing the patient to the development of angiosarcoma (23,35). It has been suggested that chronic lymphatic obstruction leads to collateralization and neovascularization which at some point may escape tissue control mechanisms (27). Furthermore, it has been proposed that the loss of afferent lymphatic circulation in the lymphedematous sites results in the absence of immunologic surveillance of mutant cell populations which would proliferate into angiosarcoma (60). The survival of skin grafts for longer periods in lymphedematous areas compared to those transplanted in normal extremities supports this notion (60).

Radiation therapy may also contribute to the development of angiosarcoma (16,50). Several examples of radiation-associated angiosarcoma have been reported (19,28,33,40). These generally develop in the cutaneous or subcutaneous chest wall after postmastectomy irradiation of the chest wall. The magnitude of the influence of radiation on the development of

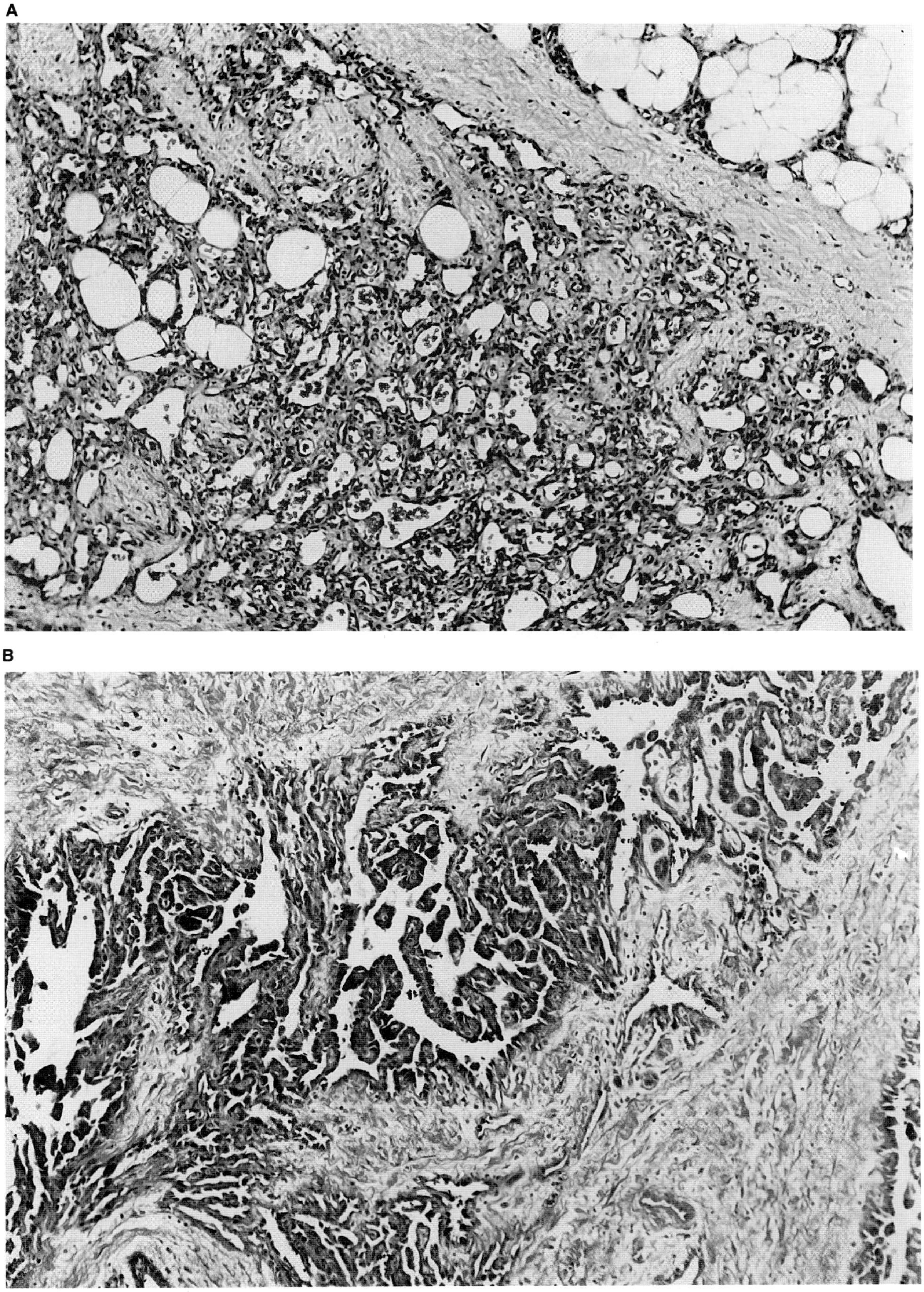


**Figure 12.5** Poorly-differentiated angiosarcoma, type III. (a) A relatively compact proliferation of small caliber vascular channels and spindle cells. (b) A papillary growth pattern dominates in this tumor. (H&E, (a) X240; (b) X300)

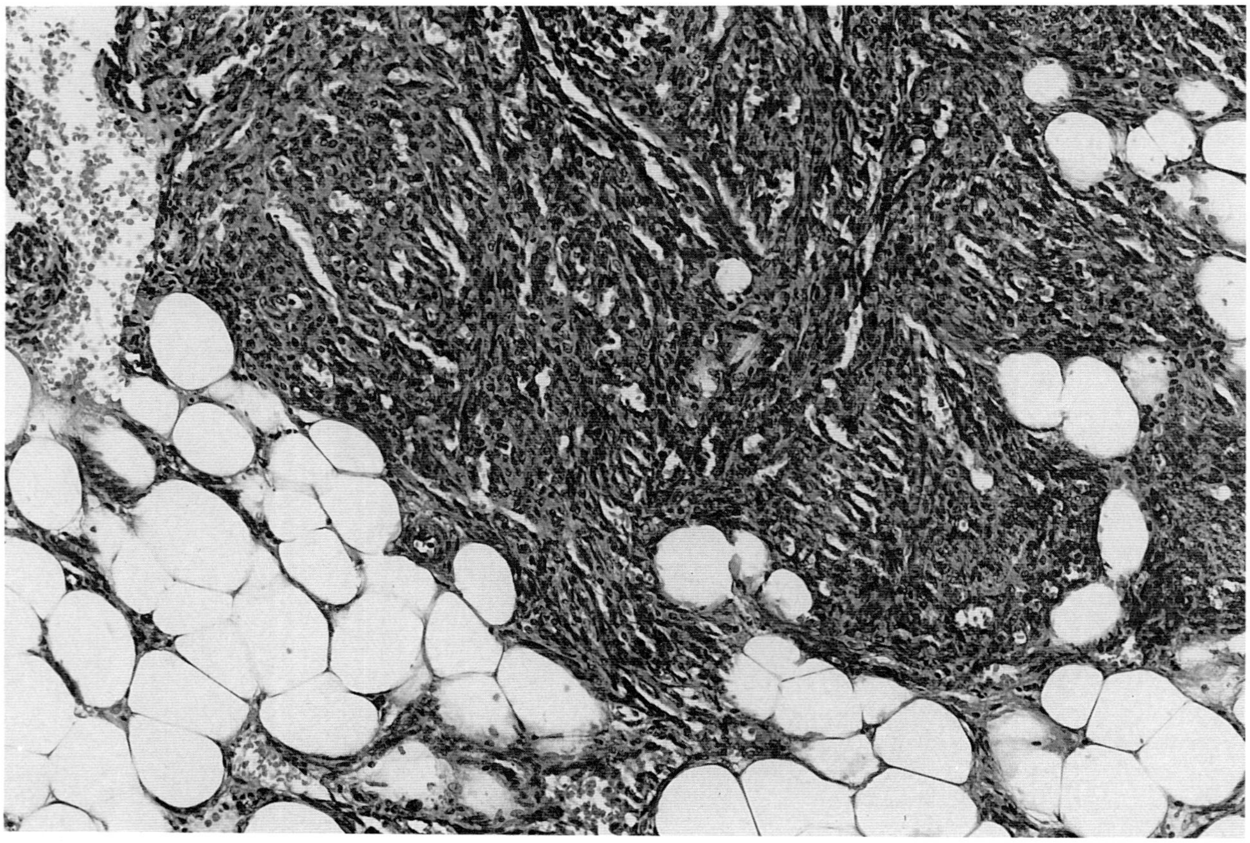

**Figure 12.6(a)** Poorly-differentiated angiosarcoma, type III. In another variant, spindled endothelial cells proliferate as solid nodules. (H&E, X80)

angiosarcoma is difficult to assess since many such patients who have received radiation for tumors may also have had lymphedema. It is important to emphasize that a direct causal relationship between breast irradiation and the development of angiosarcoma has not been firmly established. The possible role of other factors, unknown at this time, cannot be excluded.

## Microscopic Features

Microscopically, post-radiation angiosarcoma is highly variable in appearance even within a single case. It often shows well-formed small capillary-sized vessels lined by obviously malignant endothelial cells, anastomosing vascular channels and papillary endothelial tufts. The association of these changes with lymphangiomatosis in some cases is the only feature distinguishing "lymphangiosarcoma" from conventional angiosarcomas (69). Not infrequently, tufts or relatively solid morules of rounded, epithelioid endothelial cells protrude into vascular channels (Fig. 12.8), and irregular nests of epithelioid endothelial cells invade the soft tissue and any residual breast tissue underlying the skin; these are easily confused with a recurrent breast carcinoma. The content of the vascular channels varies from clear fluid to erythrocytes, or the vessels may be empty.

## Treatment

There is no treatment for this lesion that has produced consistent results. Wide excision can provide local control for a limited period of time. Complete surgical resection has been the treatment of all patients cured of chest wall or primary breast angiosarcoma (28). Tumor grade and size should be assessed because of their proven prognostic significance in mammary angiosarcomas (37,42,47,55). Very few patients survive more than five years (15,62). A majority of these five-year survivors were treated by amputation alone or in combination with chemotherapy and radiation therapy.

B

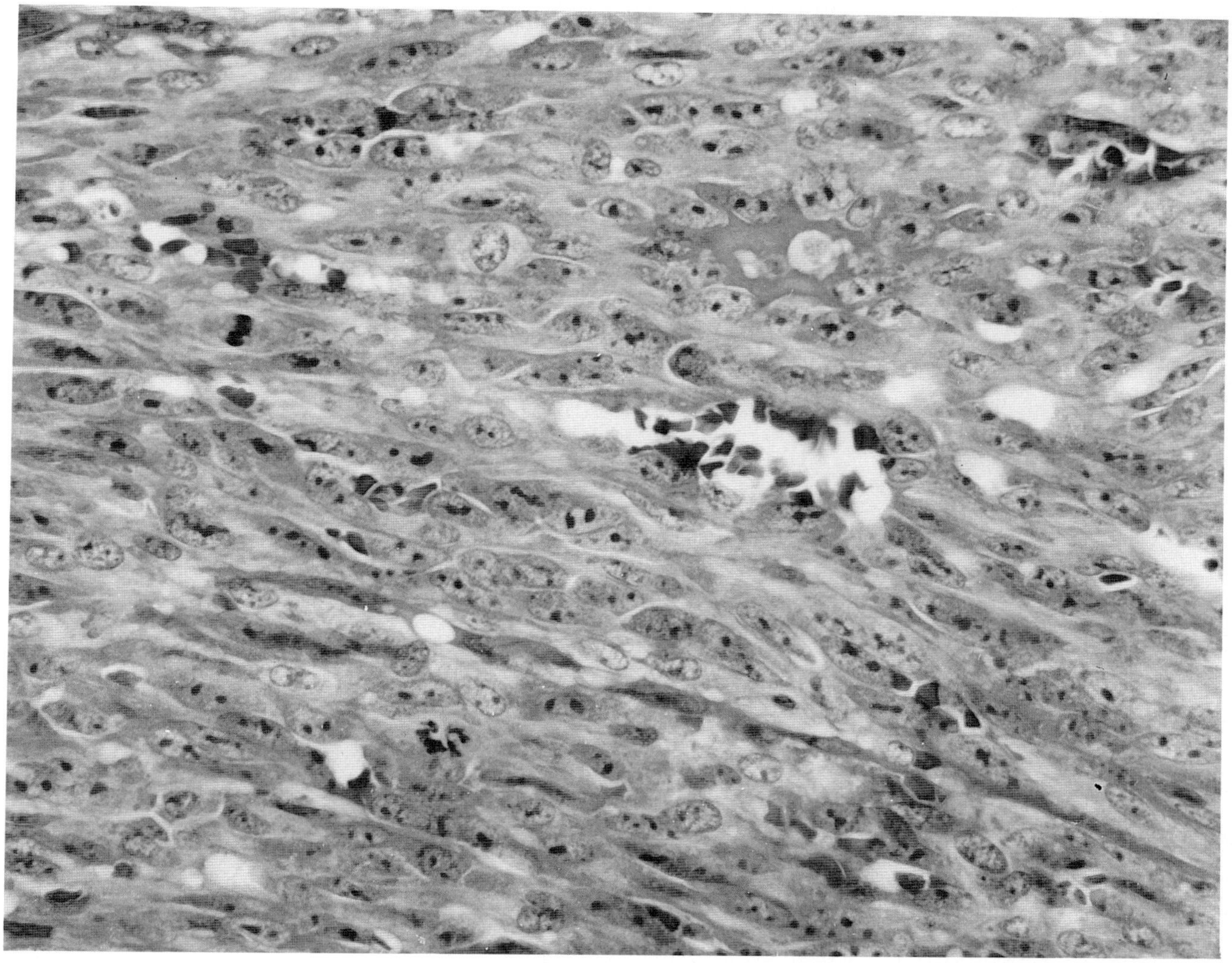

**Figure 12.6(b)** Poorly-differentiated angiosarcoma. A more primitive population of spindled endothelial cells display formation of small vascular channels. (H&E, X800)

## BENIGN VASCULAR TUMORS

## MICROSCOPIC HEMANGIOMAS

While Hamperl drew attention to the occurrence of benign vascular lesions in the breast in 1973 (72), only recently have a number of reports confirmed the existence of a variety of these benign lesions in the breast. The benign vascular lesions may be microscopic or palpable lesions. The most common microscopic hemangioma is the perilobular hemangioma. In a review of 555 mastectomy specimen performed during a 12-month period, Rosen and Ridolfi (84) identified seven perilobular hemangiomas, a 1.2% incidence. Among 210 postmortem cases evaluated by Lesueur et al (75), the incidence was 11%. The mean age of the patients was 56 years.

Twenty-two examples of microscopic hemangiomas (19 perilobular and three periductal) were diagnosed at AFIP from January 1, 1978 to January 1, 1988. One of the 22 patients was a 22-year-old male with gynecomastia, the remaining 21 patients were female and ranged in age from 21 to 66 years with a median of 40 years. Two patients had bilateral perilobular hemangiomas, and four were multiple. All of these lesions were microscopic in size and grossly inapparent to the prosectors. Two of the 22 patients had mastectomy for infiltrating duct carcinomas, all remaining 20 cases were incidental findings in biop-

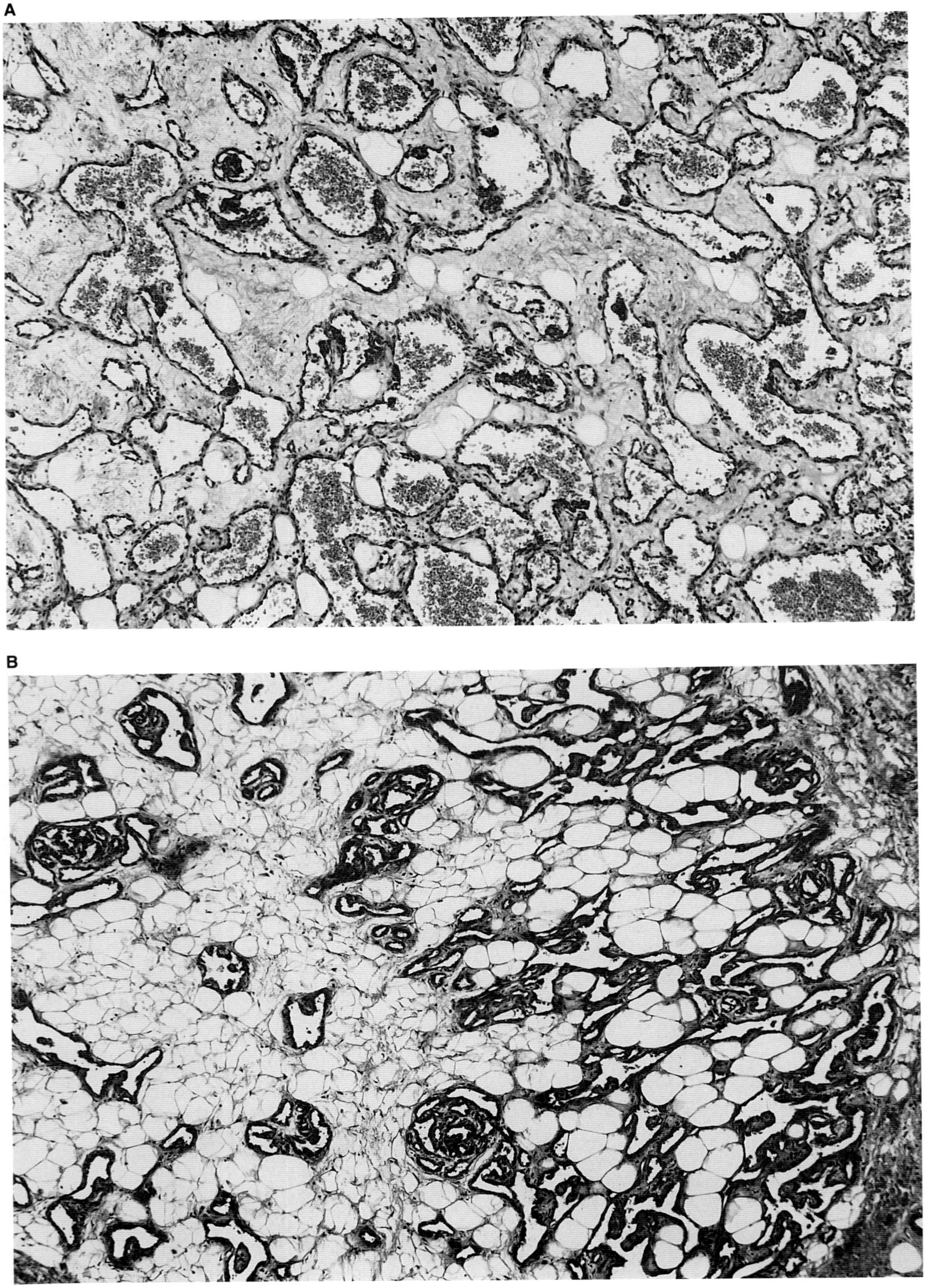


**Figure 12.7** Moderately-differentiated angiosarcoma, type II. (a) Anastomosing vascular channels are distended by red blood cells and show focal endothelial tufting. (b&c) This case shows more abundant tufting and a papillary arrangement of the neoplastic endothelial cells. (H&E, (a) X120; (b) X200; (c) X400)

c

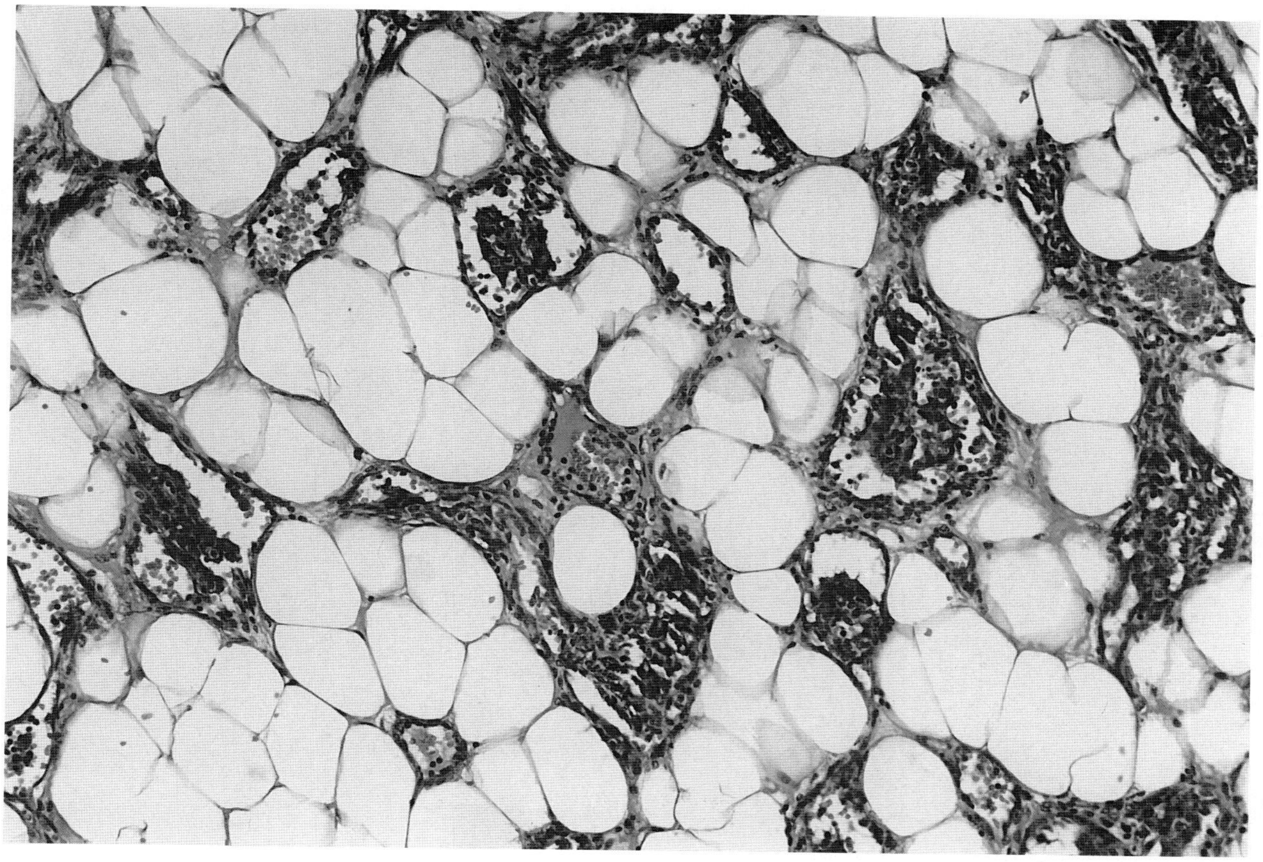

**Figure 12.7(c)** Legend on opposite page.

sies removed for a variety of benign diseases. One of the patients with bilateral hemangiomas also had an angiolipoma.

## Microscopic Features

Perilobular hemangiomas may be solitary or multiple and range in size from 0.5 to 4.0 mm. These minuscule hemangiomas are composed of a delicate meshwork of small vascular channels which proliferate into and around the lobular stroma, or in the interlobular and periductal stroma (Figs. 12.9–12.10); the margins are generally ill-defined. The endothelial-lined spaces do not exhibit a muscle layer and contain erythrocytes or lymph. Atypia or pleomorphism is absent in the endothelial cells. Because of their small size, they are easily overlooked.

**Table 12.1** Major Features of the Three Types of Angiosarcoma Described by Donnell et al (19)

*Type I:* Anastomosing vascular channels lined by inconspicuous endothelial cells and occasional endothelial tufting.
*Type II:* Scattered foci of papillary endothelial proliferation (with occasional mitotic figures) and solid spindle cell areas in a lesion composed largely of type I angiosarcoma.
*Type III:* Spindle sarcomatous areas with necrosis with or without features described for types I and II.

**Table 12.2** Features of the Three Grades of Angiosarcoma Described by Merino et al (43)

*Well-differentiated:* Well-formed vascular channels lined by 1 or 2 layers of endothelial cells with rare mitotic figures; no hemorrhage, necrosis, pleomorphism or anaplasia.
*Moderately-differentiated:* Foci of solid tumor comprising less than 20% of total tumor mass present in a patchy fashion throughout the neoplasm.
*Poorly-differentiated:* Composed predominantly of solid, spindle cell areas with few well-formed vascular areas. Mitotic figures, hemorrhage, necrosis and marked pleomorphism are present.

A

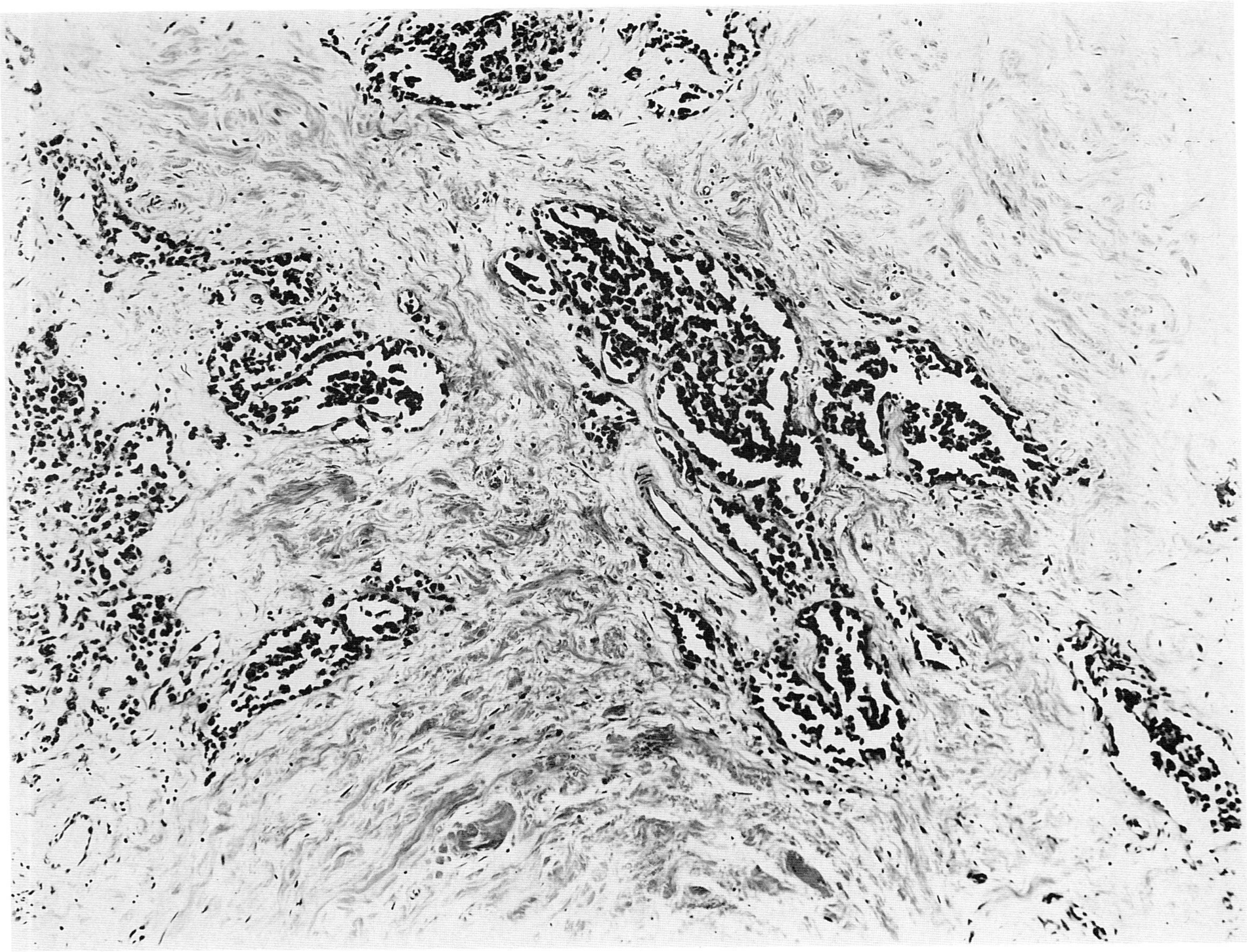

**Figure 12.8(a)** Post-radiation angiosarcoma (Stewart-Treves angiosarcoma). The patient was treated by radiation following lumpectomy for an infiltrating duct carcinoma. At low magnification the lesion simulates a papillary intraductal carcinoma of the peripheral type. (H&E, X240)

## PALPABLE HEMANGIOMAS (CAVERNOUS, CAPILLARY, JUVENILE AND VENOUS TYPES)

As a rule, mammary lesions designated as any of the above subtypes of hemangioma exceed 5 mm in size. These may be located either at some distance from both ducts and lobules or adjacent to them within the stroma. Hemangiomas occur most frequently in the female breast, but there are sporadic reports of palpable vascular lesions in the male breast as well (52,85). During the same ten-year period when 22 perilobular and periductal hemangiomas were diagnosed at AFIP, there were 21 cavernous hemangiomas, 11 capillary hemangiomas, two juvenile hemangiomas, and 38 hemangiomas, not otherwise specified. All of these tumors were within the breast parenchyma; subcutaneous vascular lesions were excluded. The patients with hemangioma ranged in age from 8 to 85 years with a median of 54 years; 28 patients were caucasian, one was black and one was

B

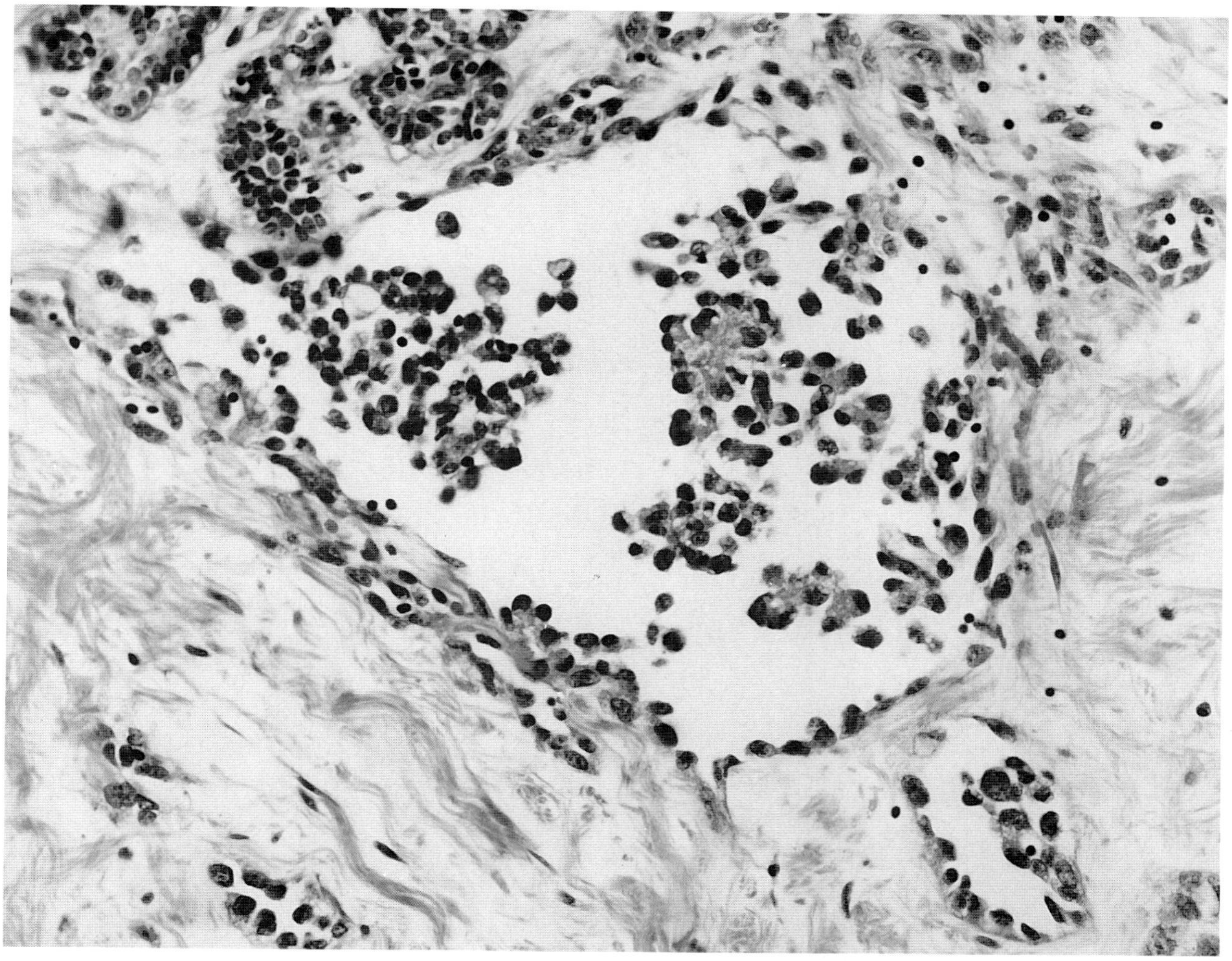

**Figure 12.8(b)** Post-radiation angiosarcoma (Stewart-Treves angiosarcoma). Proliferating atypical endothelial cells protrude into irregular spaces. The proliferating cells failed to react with cytokeratin but displayed positivity with Factor VIII. (H&E, X600)

oriental. Two of the 38 patients were male. Three of the 21 patients with cavernous hemangiomas were male. The 21 patients with cavernous hemangioma ranged in age from 18 to 74 years with a median of 60. The racial origin was known in 16 cases, and all were caucasians. All 11 patients with capillary hemangiomas were female. Their ages ranged from 18 to 70 with a median of 48 years. The racial origin was known for five women and they were all caucasians. The two patients with juvenile hemangioma were both five years of age, female, and caucasian. Two examples of venous, as well as one of arteriovenous hemangioma (83) have also been seen recently at the AFIP.

Microscopically, in contrast to the invasive margins of angiosarcomas, hemangiomas generally exhibit well-defined margins. The cavernous hemangiomas consist of dilated, blood-filled vessels lined by flattened endothelium and arranged in a lobular pattern (Fig. 12.11). Focally, the presence of valve-like structures in the vascular spaces gives the appearance of anastomosing channels, but endothelial atypia and mitotic activity are generally absent. The capillary hemangiomas are composed of capillary-sized vessels lined by flattened endothelium (Fig. 12.12). The juvenile hemangioma, an immature form of capillary hemangioma, shows a combination of vascular spaces with inconspicuous lumens lined by plump endothelial cells and spaces lined by flattened endothelial cells; a moderate number of mitotic figures may be present. With maturation, the lesion will resemble adult capillary hemangioma. The venous (Fig. 12.13) and arteriovenous hemangiomas consist of a cluster of thick-walled, muscular vessels with an elastic layer in the vessel wall of those with an arterial component.

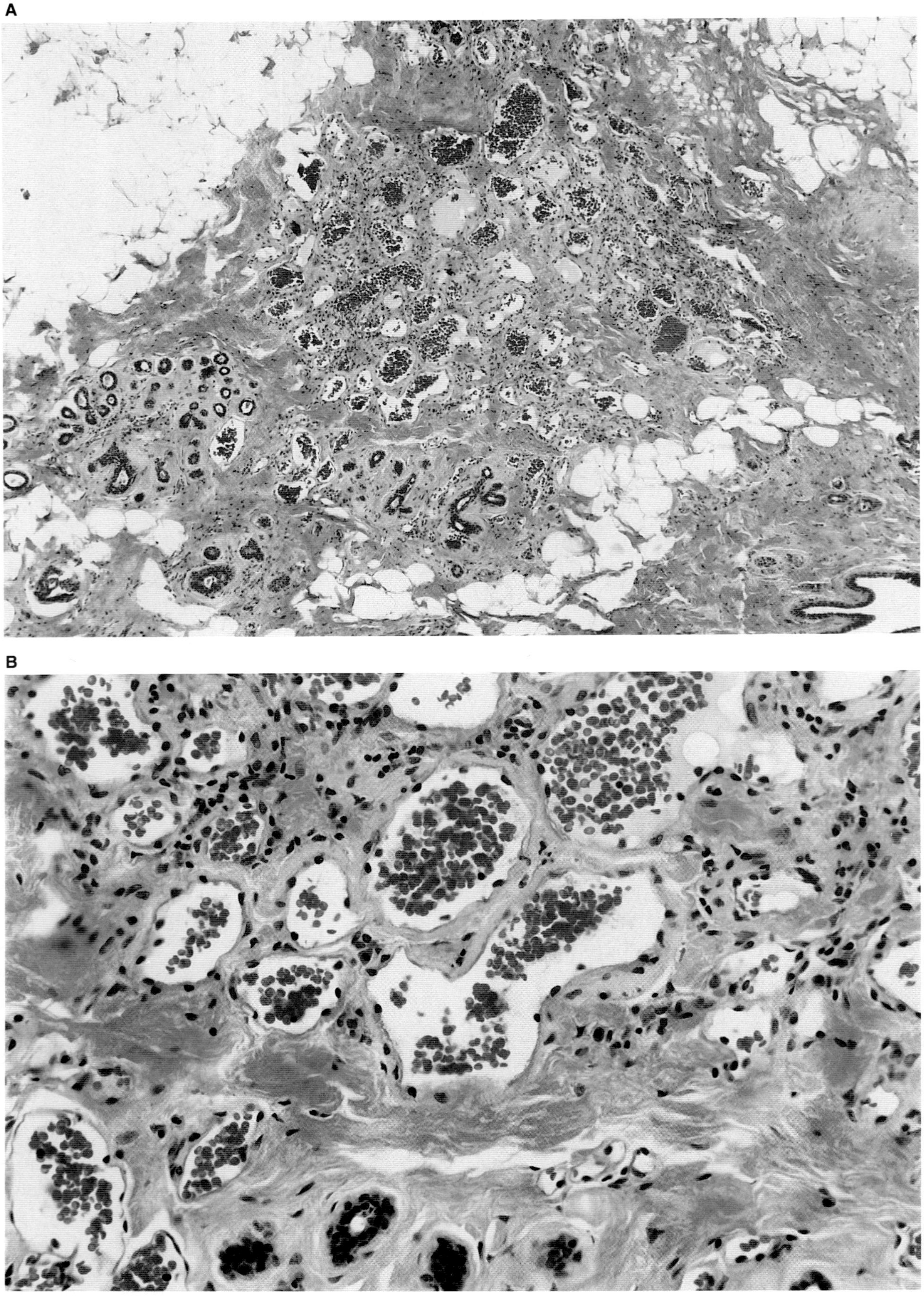


**Figure 12.9** Perilobular hemangioma. (a) A small, microscopic cluster of dilated vascular channels is evident adjacent to several lobules. (b) The endothelial cells lack atypia, and the vascular channels are filled with red blood cells in this case. (H&E, (a) X100; (b) X400)

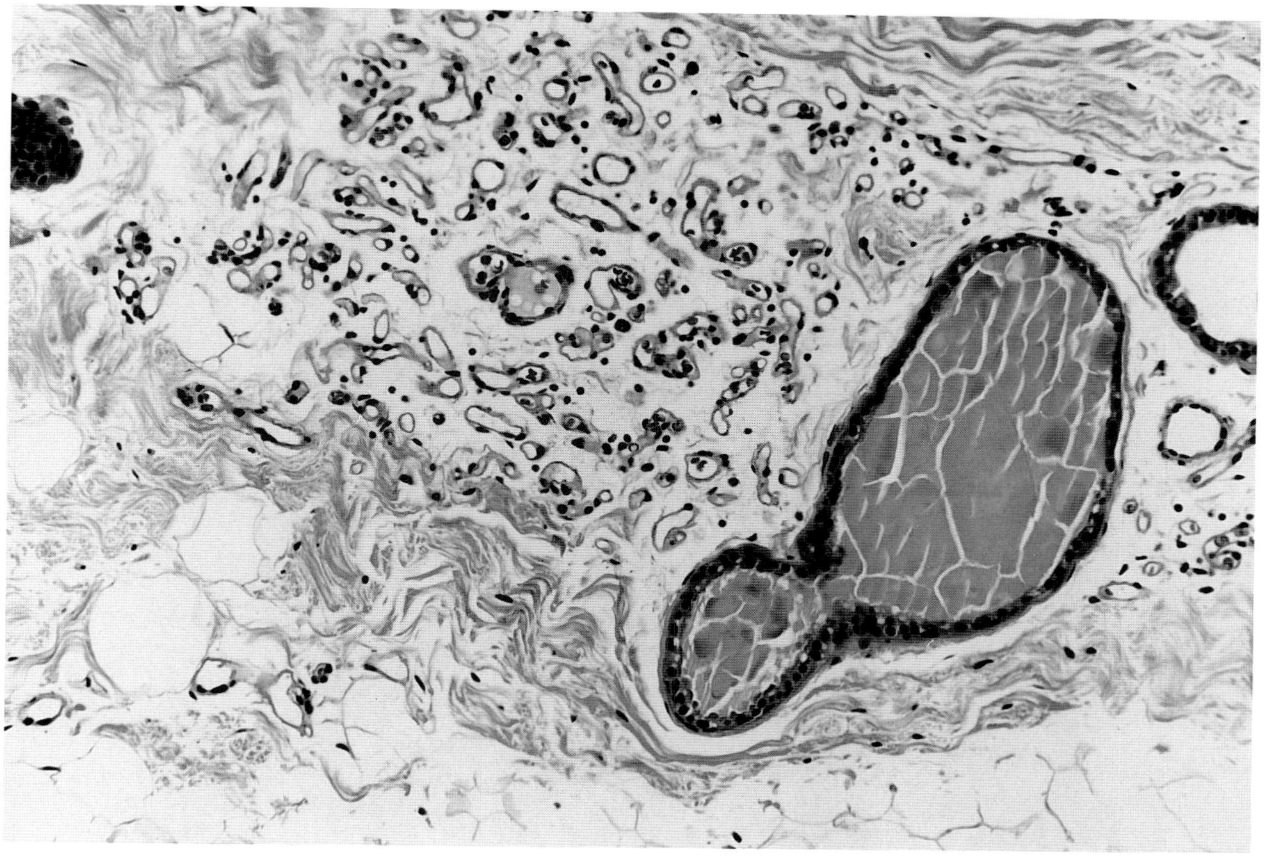

**Figure 12.10** Periductal hemangioma. The mostly empty vascular channels in this case are distributed adjacent to a duct. (H&E, X200) (Photo courtesy of Dr. Mark A. Ashton)

Occasionally, any of these hemangiomas may display irregularities in their margin of growth, focal anastomosing pattern, sclerosis, variation in the caliber of the vascular channels, and plump endothelial cells; the term atypical hemangioma may be applied when these changes are notable.

## Relationship to Angiosarcoma

While it is possible that some of these hemangiomas serve as precursors of angiosarcoma, an undisputable transition from benign angioma to an angiosarcoma has not been documented. None of the studies on angiosarcomas have linked the so-called "perilobular hemangioma" to malignant vascular tumors (41,46, 63). One of the angiosarcomas reported by Breitfellner (12) was preceded by lobular angiomatosis, however; the interval between the angiomatosis and the sarcoma was one year.

## ATYPICAL HEMANGIOMA

The variable presence of relative circumscription, anastomosing channels, and focal endothelial hyperplasia in hemangiomas 2 cm or smaller in size has been proposed as indicative of atypia (73). Approximately 60% of these lesions have been detected mammographically. There were no local recurrences or metastases among 18 patients even though the diagnostic biopsy was the only treatment in nine cases.

## ANGIOMATOSIS

Angiomatosis is one of the least common benign vascular lesions of the breast, but one of the most difficult to diagnose accurately. It may be congenital

A

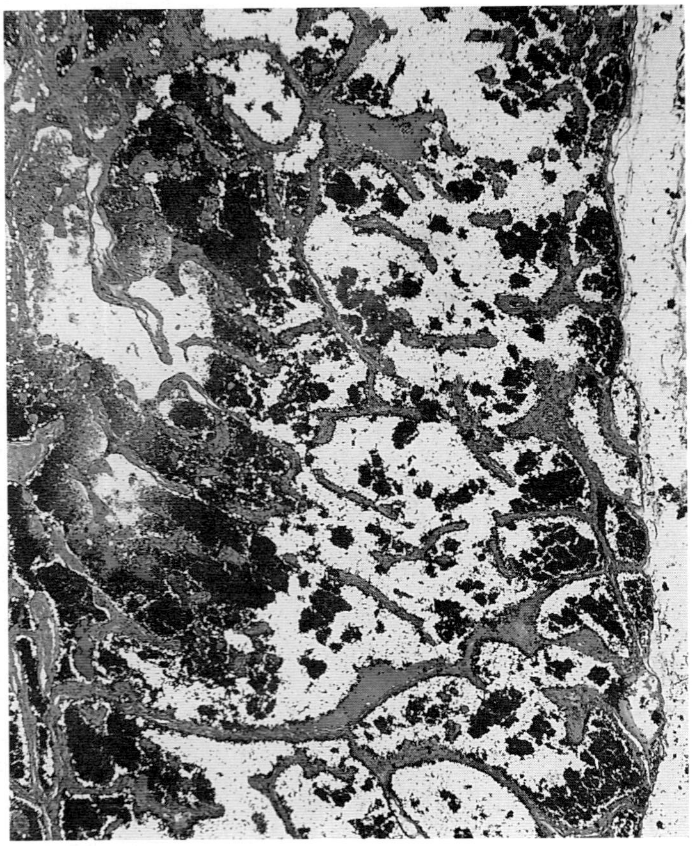

B

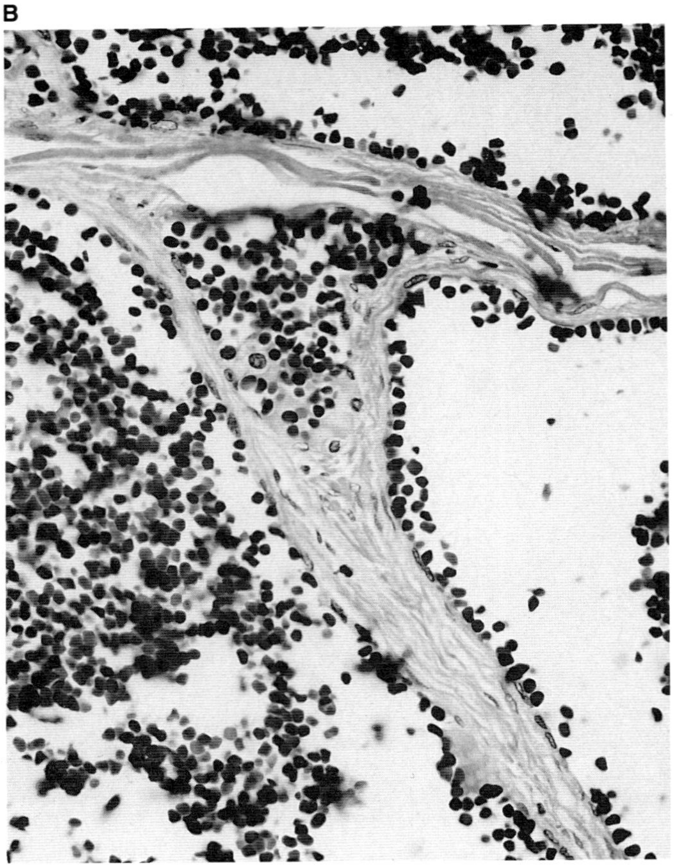

C

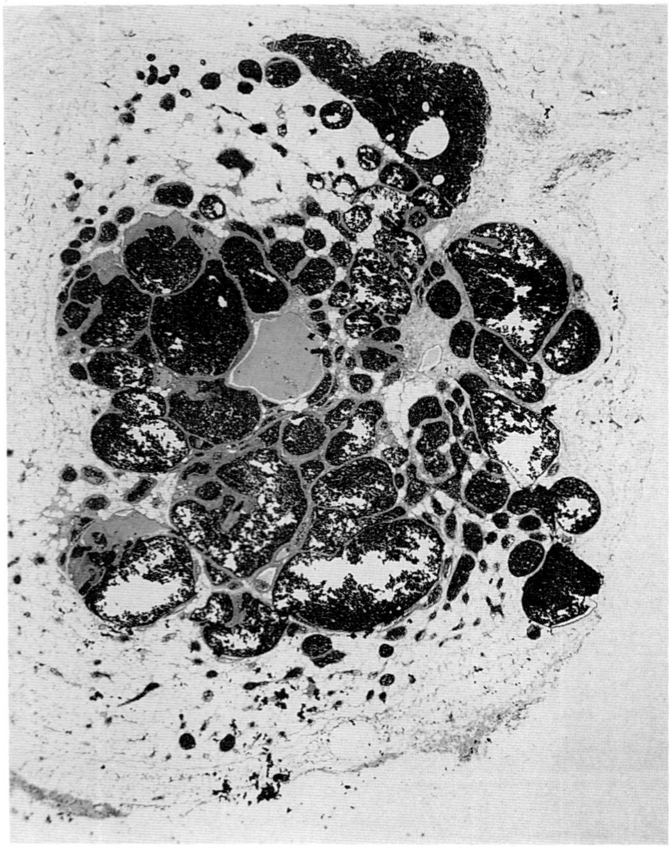

**Figure 12.11** Cavernous hemangioma. Both of the lesions illustrated here presented as a palpable mass. (a) In one lesion, the margins are sharply circumscribed and the lesion is composed of large, irregular vascular spaces filled by RBC's. (b) The endothelial cells, when apparent, lack atypia. (c) The second lesion displays a more irregular outline. (H&E, (a) X40; (b) X400; (c) X15)

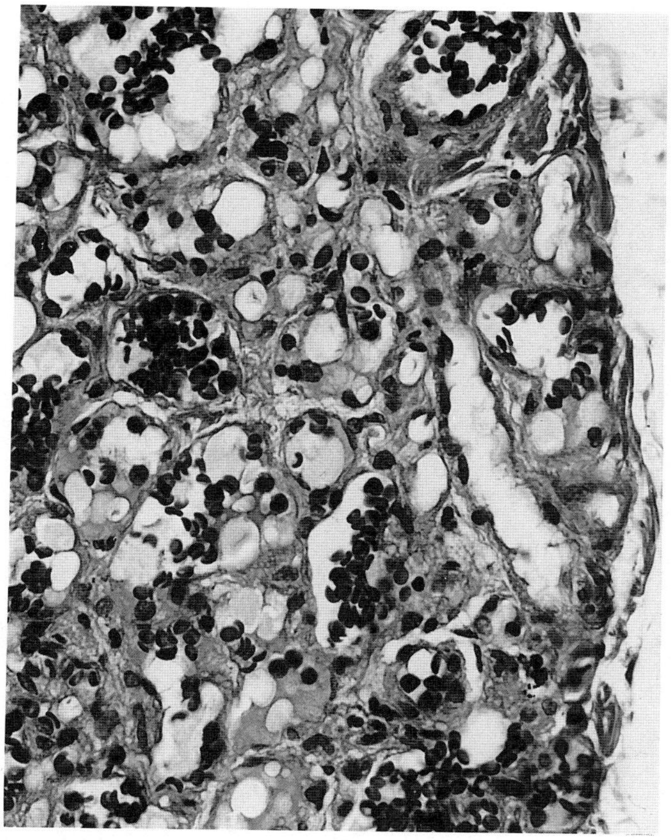

**Figure 12.12** Capillary hemangioma. This palpable nodule consisted of a compact proliferation of small, rounded vascular spaces filled by RBC's; the margins are sharply delineated. (H&E, X120)

and affects young women with a mean age of 33 years for the first four reported cases (77,81). A cystic variant of angiomatosis has also been described (93). Dramatic tumor growth observed during pregnancy in a 21-year-old woman (71) suggests hormonal dependence, but estrogen (8 fmol/mg) and progesterone (<5 fmol/mg) levels were negative in the tumor. There are four examples of this lesion in the AFIP files. The patients were 20, 31, 57, and 61 years of age. The 57-year-old patient was a caucasian male. The lesions are generally large, ranging in size from 9 to 22 cm, but one of the cases reviewed at AFIP was only 2.5 cm in maximum diameter. One case was cystic and two had extended to the axilla.

Microscopically, angiomatosis is characterized by an irregular proliferation of benign, small caliber, rounded vascular channels in the breast (Fig. 12.14). The marginal irregularity and permeation around ducts and lobules is a feature that can cause tremendous difficulty in separating this lesion from a well-differentiated angiosarcoma. The lack of endothelial cell atypia or hyperchromasia, disruption of lobules, and anastomosing channels help distinguish this lesion from angiosarcoma.

Two of the reported cases developed recurrences. Because of the difficulty in distinguishing angiomatosis from well-differentiated angiosarcoma and its propensity for local recurrence, wide local excision of the lesion is required. Considering the large size of most lesions, this approach may require simple mastectomy in some cases. Follow-up of all patients with limited surgery is necessary because of our limited experience with this rare lesion.

## INTRAVASCULAR PAPILLARY ENDOTHELIAL HYPERPLASIA

This lesion characterized by an exuberant intravascular papillary endothelial hyperplasia (Figs. 12.15–12.16) is easily mistaken for an angiosarcoma. When first described by Masson (76) in 1923, it was designated as vegetant intravascular hemangioendothelioma. Three examples of this lesion in the breast or the subcutaneous tissue of the breast have been reported (78,80,82). The case reported by Rosen (82) occurred in a 76-year-old female and there was no breast tissue around it; the case reported by Murao et al (78) occurred in a 76-year-old Japanese woman. At least four examples of this lesion are in the AFIP files. One of these tumors occurred in a 12-year-old boy; it became apparent shortly after a sports injury to the breast area. Because of the complex papillary growth pattern, three of the four cases were sent in with a diagnosis or suspicion of angiosarcoma. The presence of a fibrous pseudocapsule and demonstration of elastic tissue and muscle in the vessel wall often unmasks the true nature of the lesion. In some cases, neither muscle nor elastic tissue may be easily demonstrable in the pseudocapsule, but the circumscription of the lesion and the intimate association with thrombotic material are important clues to the diagnosis. The lesion is cured by simple excision.

## HEMANGIOPERICYTOMA

Fifteen examples of hemangiopericytoma have been reported in the breast (86,87,90–92,95,96). The patients have ranged in age from 5 to 67 years. The youngest patient was a boy. The tumors were 1.0 to

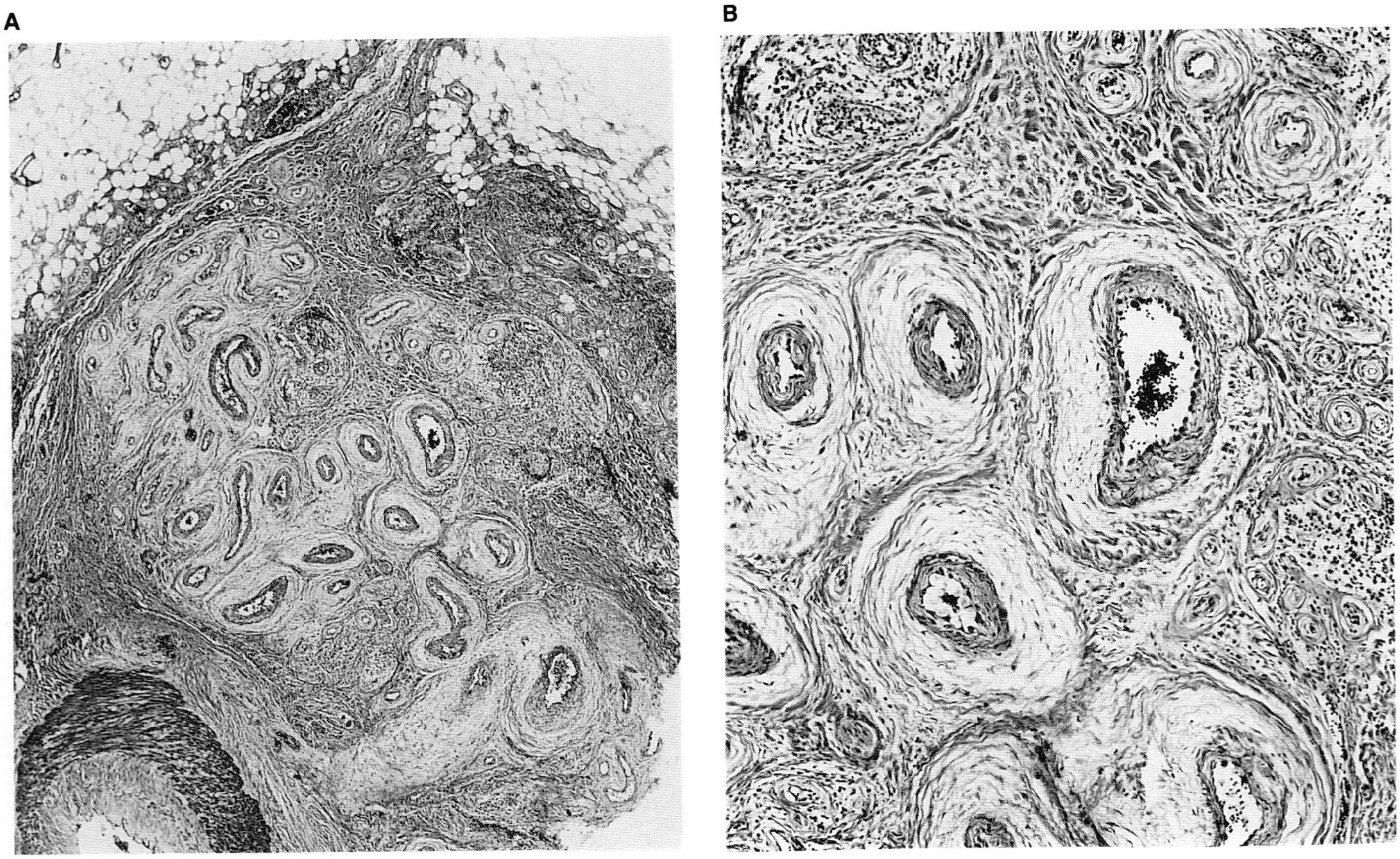

**Figure 12.13** Venous hemangioma. (a&b) This lesion is composed of thick walled vessels aggregating in the breast. (H&E (a) X30; (b) X75)

20 cm in size with a mean of 3.2 cm. Grossly, the tumors are generally well-circumscribed, round to ovoid. The cut surface varies from tan to pinkish-white. Myxoid areas and cystic foci filled with watery fluid are seen in some tumors.

Microscopically, the tumors may have a partial capsule. They are highly cellular, composed of round, oval, or elongated spindle cells packed between endothelial-lined spaces. Areas of edema and myxoid change interrupt the cellular areas. The vascular channels vary from irregular branching vessels to slit-like lumens lined by flat endothelial cells and typical staghorn vascular spaces (Fig. 12.17). Hyaline bands surround some vessels. Reticulin sheath is present around capillaries and individual cells. Pleomorphism is mild and mitotic figures are infrequent. The endothelial cells show a positive reaction for factor VIII while other cells stain positively with vimentin. Features indicating possible aggressive potential include a mitotic rate of more than five per ten high power fields, cellular atypia, and necrosis.

At the ultrastructural level, the presence in the lesion of both endothelial cells and pericytes has been confirmed (95) (Fig. 12.18).

Local excision, preferably with a margin of normal breast tissue, particularly for tumors exhibiting aggressive features, is adequate therapy. The 15 reported patients had no evidence of recurrence from 0.5 to 23 years after excision of the mass.

## Treatment and Behavior

Complete excision of all benign vascular lesions of the breast is necessary with careful evaluation of the lesion to exclude the possibility of an angiosarcoma. Hemangiomas are benign, but rarely they may recur. Two of the hemangiomas reviewed at AFIP reflected recurrences. Wide local excision would be prudent in such recurrent cases again to avoid undercalling an angiosarcoma. The absence of endothelial atypia, proliferation, anastomosing channels, and spindle cell areas coupled with a generally pushing or lobu-

A

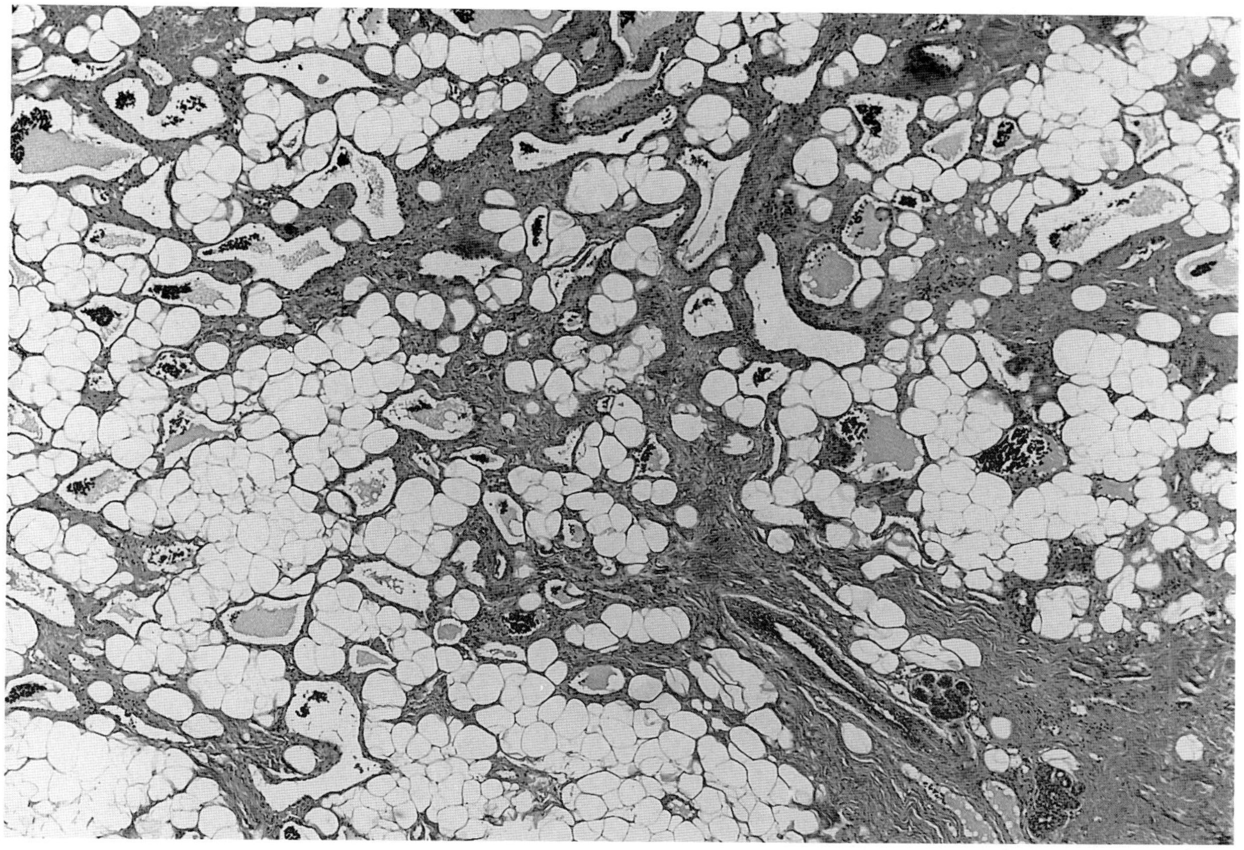

B

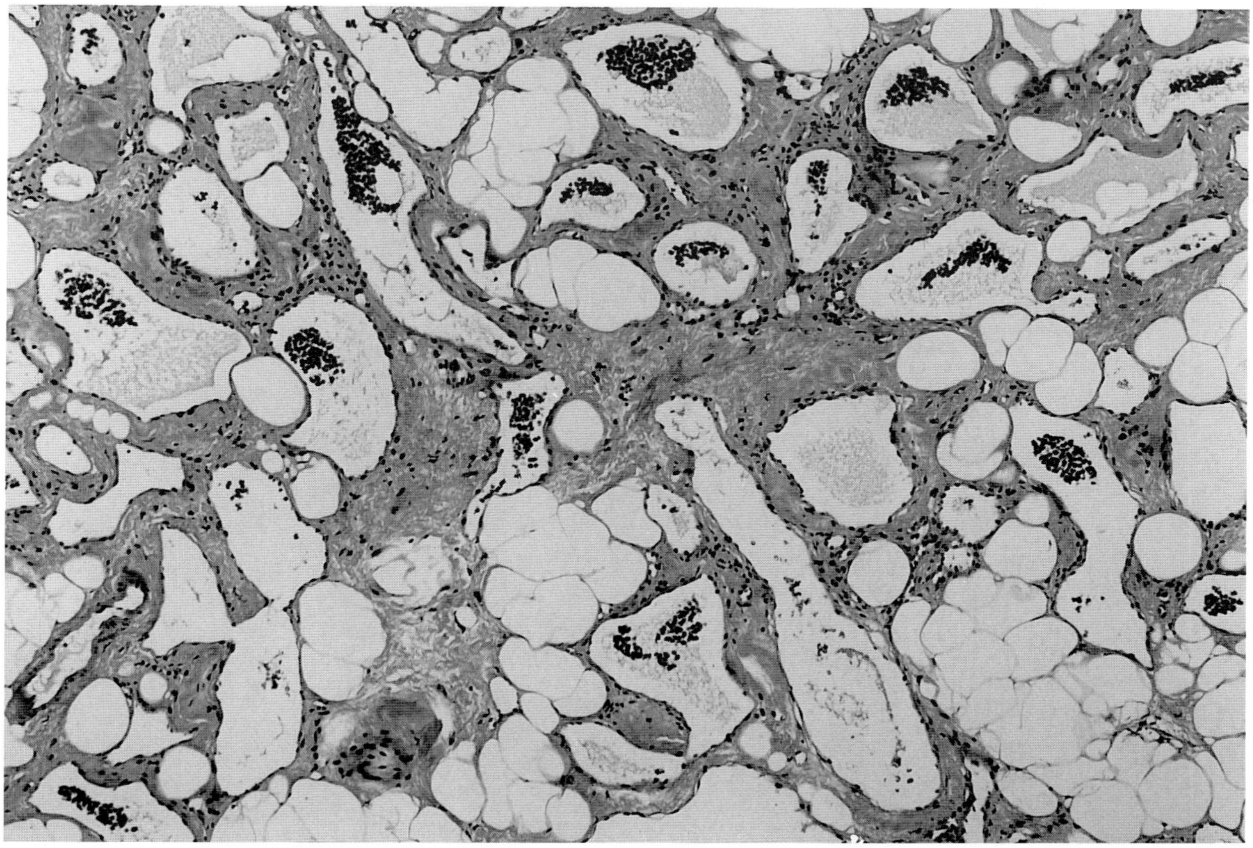

**Figure 12.14** Angiomatosis. (a) Numerous irregularly-shaped vascular channels are infiltrating the adipose tissue and proliferating around ducts and lobules. (b) While the vascular spaces are irregularly shaped and invasive in appearance, there are no anastomosing channels and there is no endothelial atypia. (H&E (a) X30; (b) X60)

A

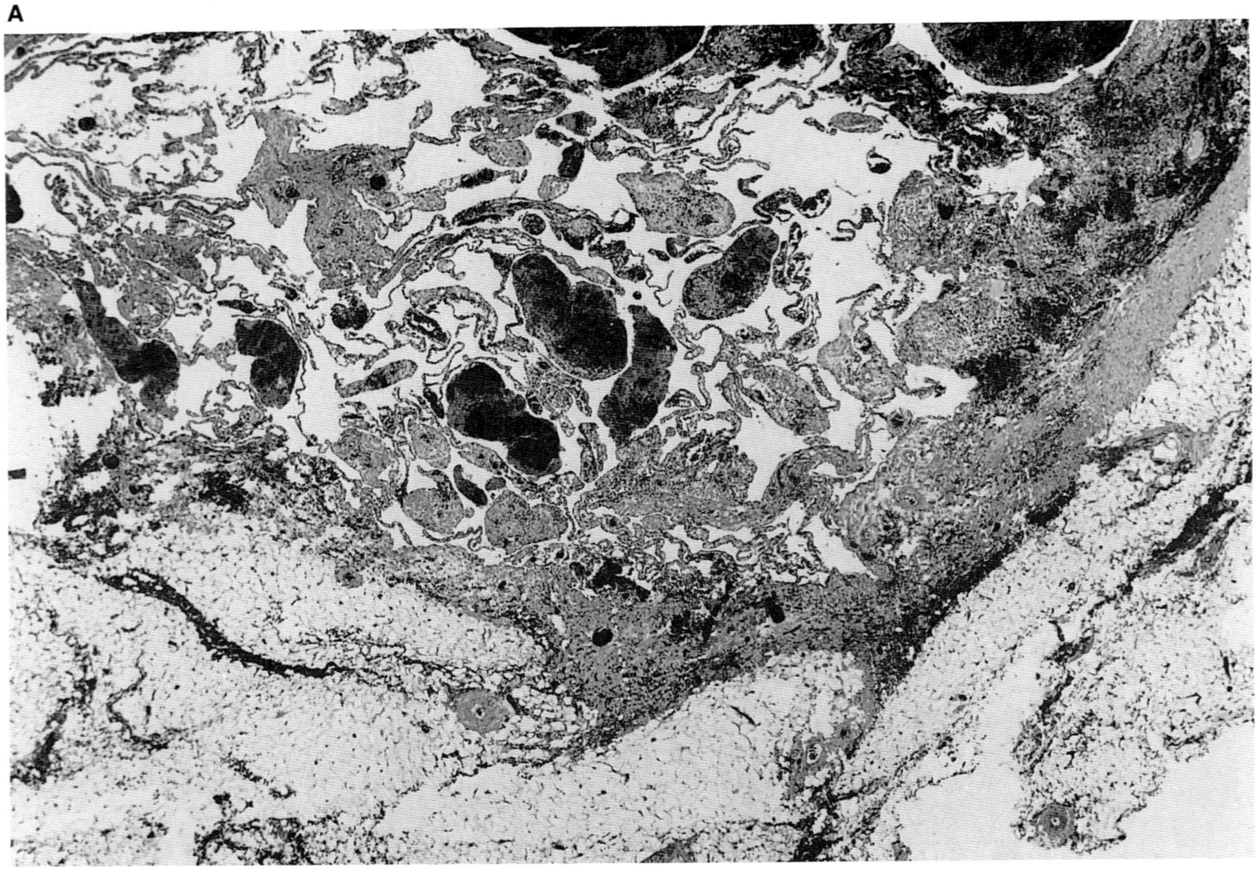

B

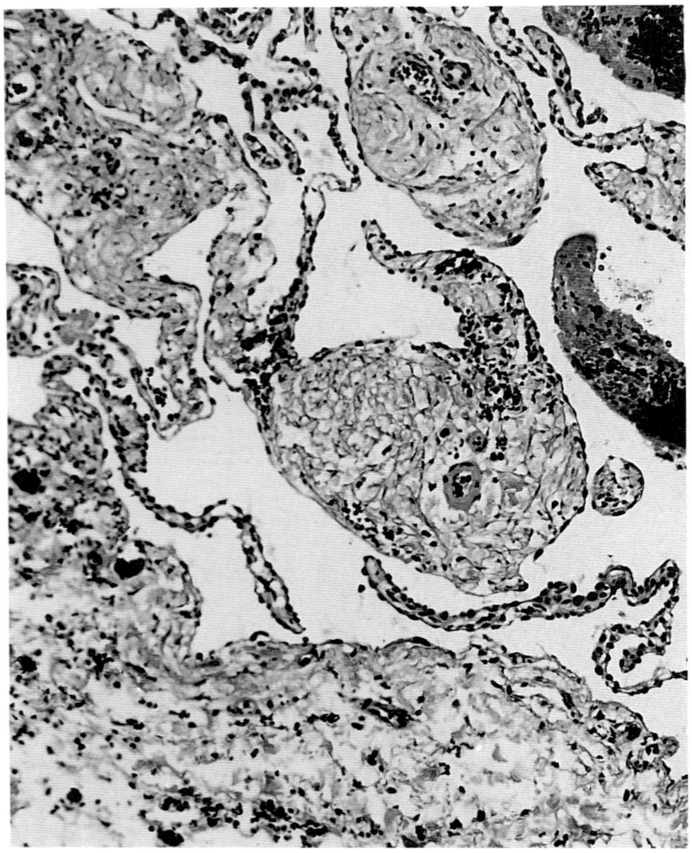

**Figure 12.15** Intravascular, papillary endothelial hyperplasia. (a) The lesion is sharply demarcated by the wall of the vessel; a prominent papillary proliferation and thrombi in vascular spaces are evident. (b) Delicate and broad papillae lined by endothelial cells alternate. (H&E, (a) X40; (b) X300)

A

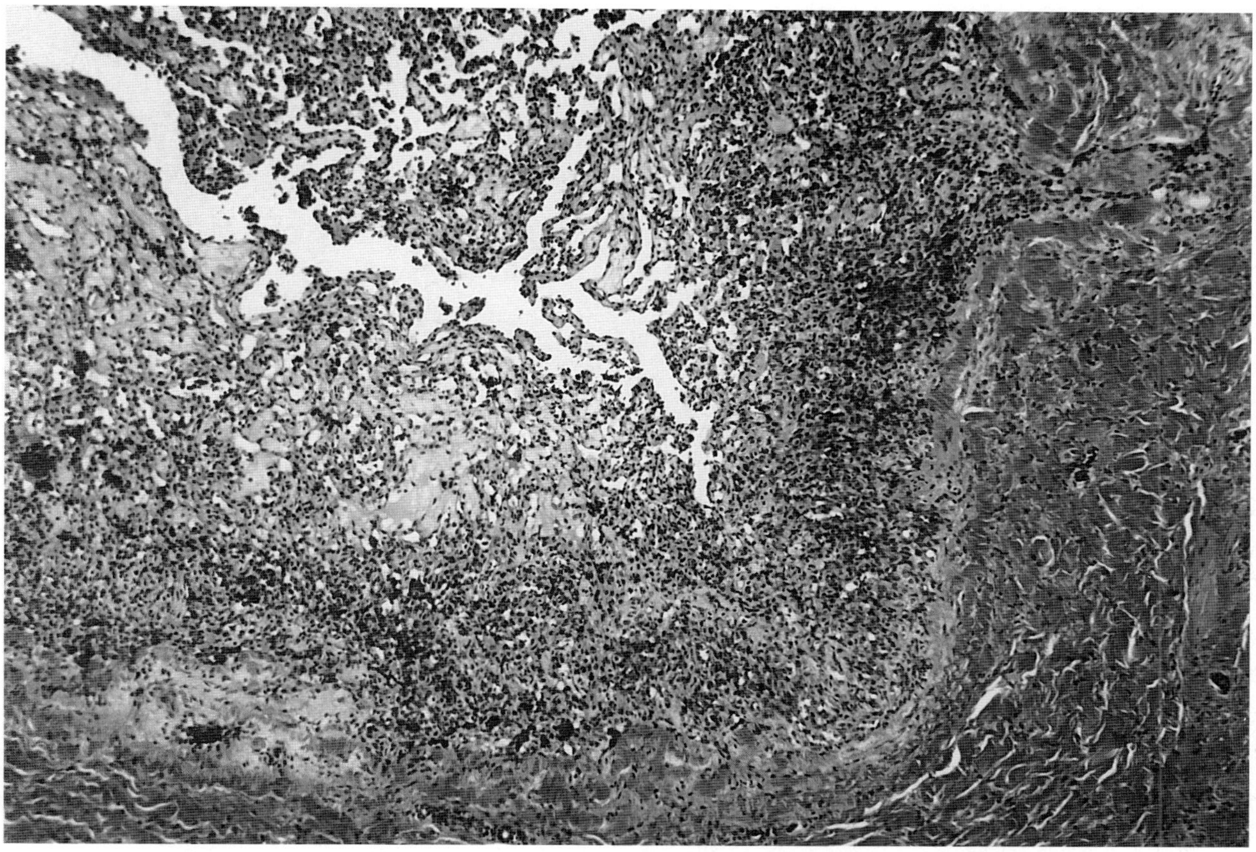

**Figure 12.16(a)** Post-traumatic, intravascular, papillary endothelial hyperplasia. This lesion presented in a 12-year-old boy shortly following chest trauma during a ball game. The margin is sharply defined and part of the vessel wall with its undulating elastica is apparent. (H&E, X15)

lated growth margin would help exclude an angiosarcoma. Nonetheless, every case should be scrutinized carefully.

## PSEUDOANGIOMATOUS HYPERPLASIA OF THE MAMMARY STROMA

Characterized by interanastomosing, angulated, and slit-like channels lined by slender spindle cells in a dense collagenous stroma (Fig. 12.19), pseudoangiomatous hyperplasia may be mistaken for a true vascular lesion. The pseudoangiomatous spaces are caused by separation of stromal cells in a densely collagenized background. Although the nine initially reported cases (98) were all in premenopausal women ranging in age from 22 to 52 years, we have observed the asymptomatic, microscopic variant of this change in elderly women, some of whom were on estrogen replacement therapy. In a review of 200 consecutive breast specimen, Ibrahim et al (89) found pseudoangiomatous hyperplasia in 23% of cases. The patients ranged in age from 17 to 76 years, with a mean age of 40 years. Five patients were older than 50, and two were male. The change was seen in the stroma associated with a variety of benign and malignant lesions, but 51% of the patients had proliferative fibrocystic changes. In the original report on this stromal change, the patients presented with a discrete painless mass ranging from 2 to 7 cm in size; the lesions were firm and rubbery.

Microscopically, the low power impression is that of a complex vascular proliferation in a densely collagenized background. The lesion may be well-circumscribed or irregular in outline but it is generally discrete. The changes are confined to one solitary focus in 40% of cases, but are multifocal in the remainder (89). There are no mitotic figures or anastomosing channels in the lesion.

B

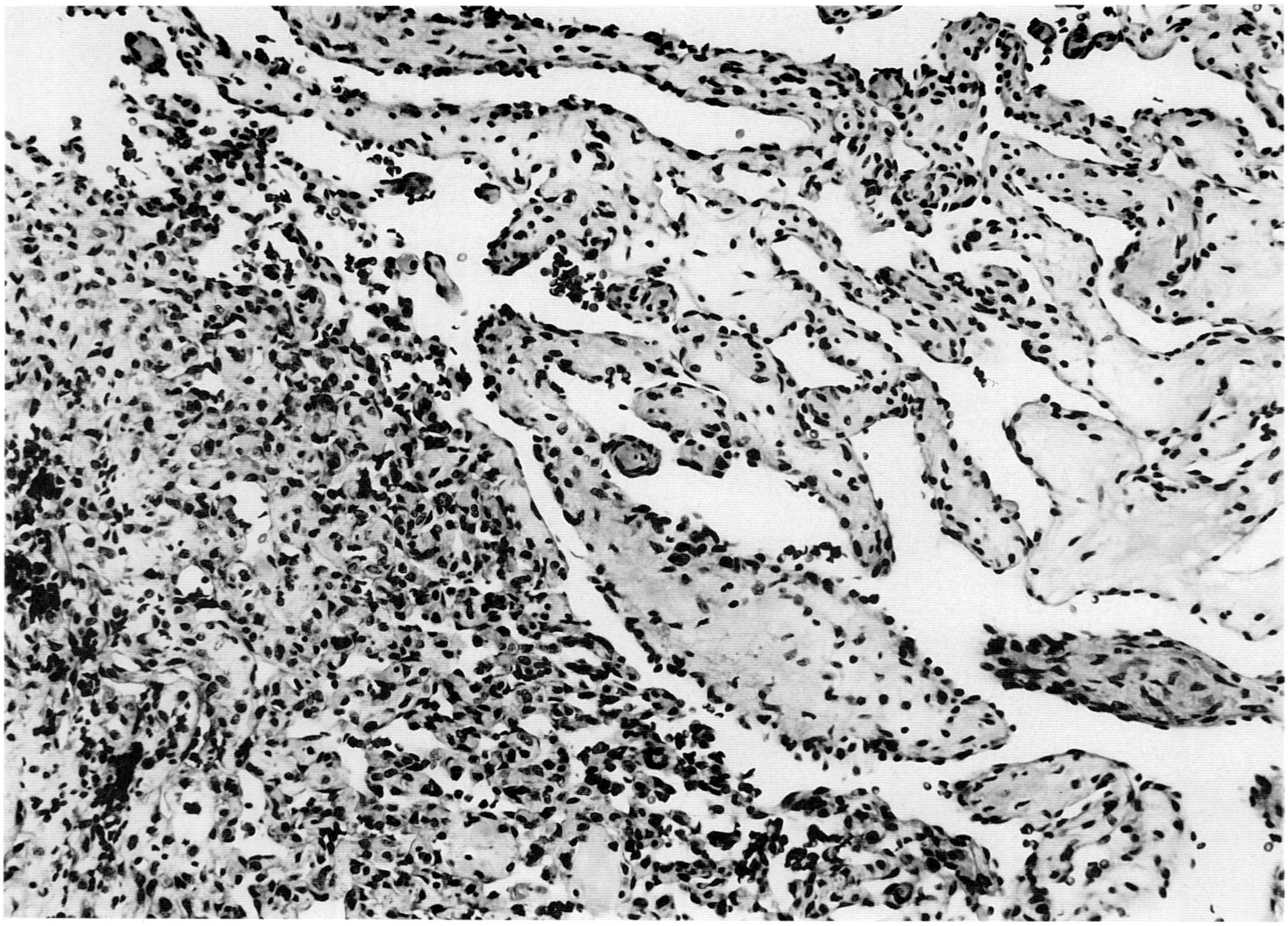

**Figure 12.16(b)** Intravascular, papillary endothelial hyperplasia. The complex proliferation in the vascular lumen can be misinterpreted as angiosarcoma if location of the process at low magnification is overlooked. (H&E, X350)

Pseudoangiomatous hyperplasia appears to reflect an unusual or exaggerated stromal response to hormonal stimulus judging from the young age of many patients and its occurrence in some older women who have been on estrogen replacement therapy. The intensely positive reaction of these stromal cells for progesterone receptors (PR) (86) supports a hormonal etiology for this process. In contrast, the mammary stroma fails to immunoreact with PR except during gestation. The stromal cells show a more variable and faint positivity for estrogen receptors.

At the ultrastructural level, the slit-like empty spaces are lined by the elongated processes of stromal fibroblastic cells (89).

## CYSTIC HYGROMA

Two cases of cystic hygroma have been reported in the breast (88,94). One of these was a 49-year-old woman (88,94). The lesions consist of multiple dilated vascular channels with aggregates of lymphocytes which may be detected mammographically as a cystic lesion.

## MONDOR'S DISEASE

The clinical findings of superficial thrombophlebitis of the veins of the anterior chest and breast was first

A

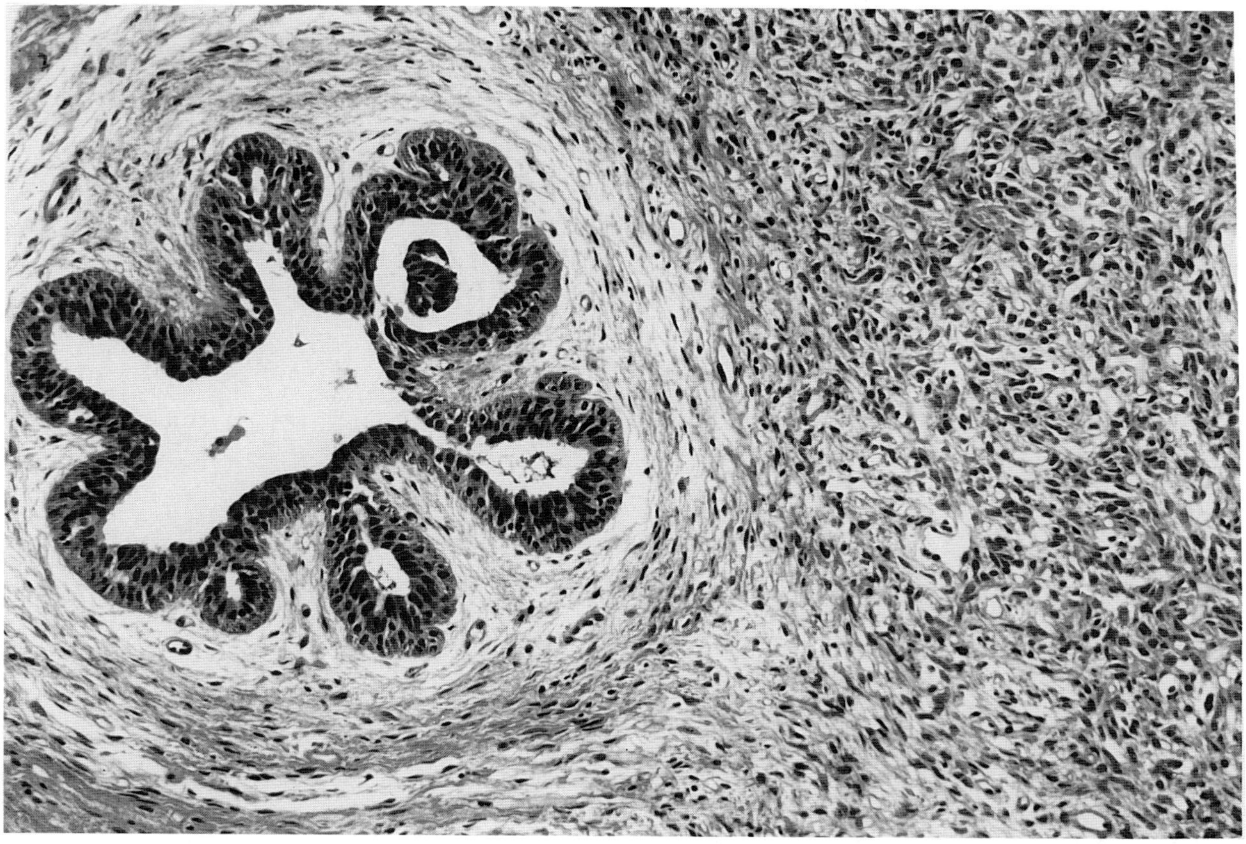

B

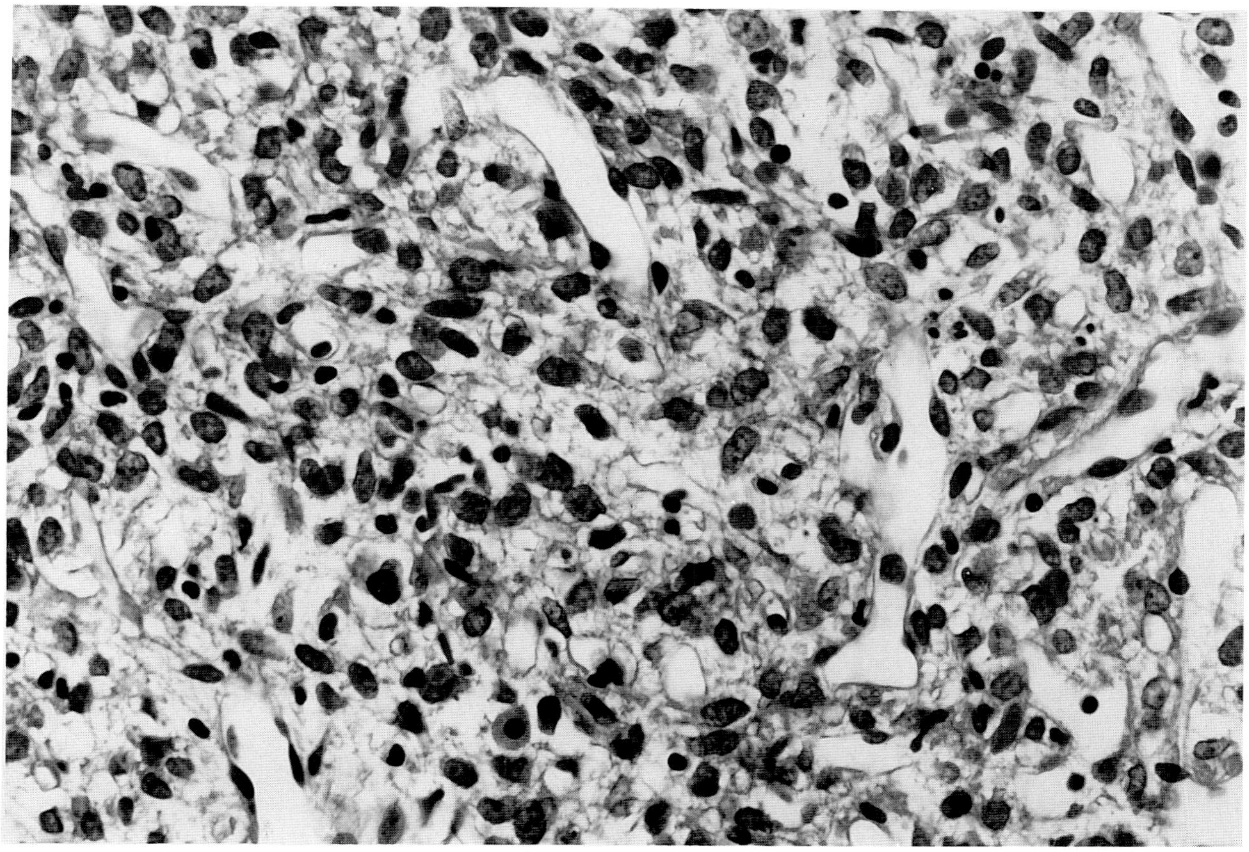

**Figure 12.17(a,b)** Hemangiopericytoma. (a) The tumor is proliferating adjacent to a lactiferous duct. (b) The tumor cells with ill-defined margins and plump, ovoid nuclei surround irregularly-shaped vascular spaces. (H&E (a) X60; (b) X250) (Figs. 12.17a–c from Tavassoli FA, Weiss S: *Am J Surg Pathol* 1981;5:745–752, with permission)

c

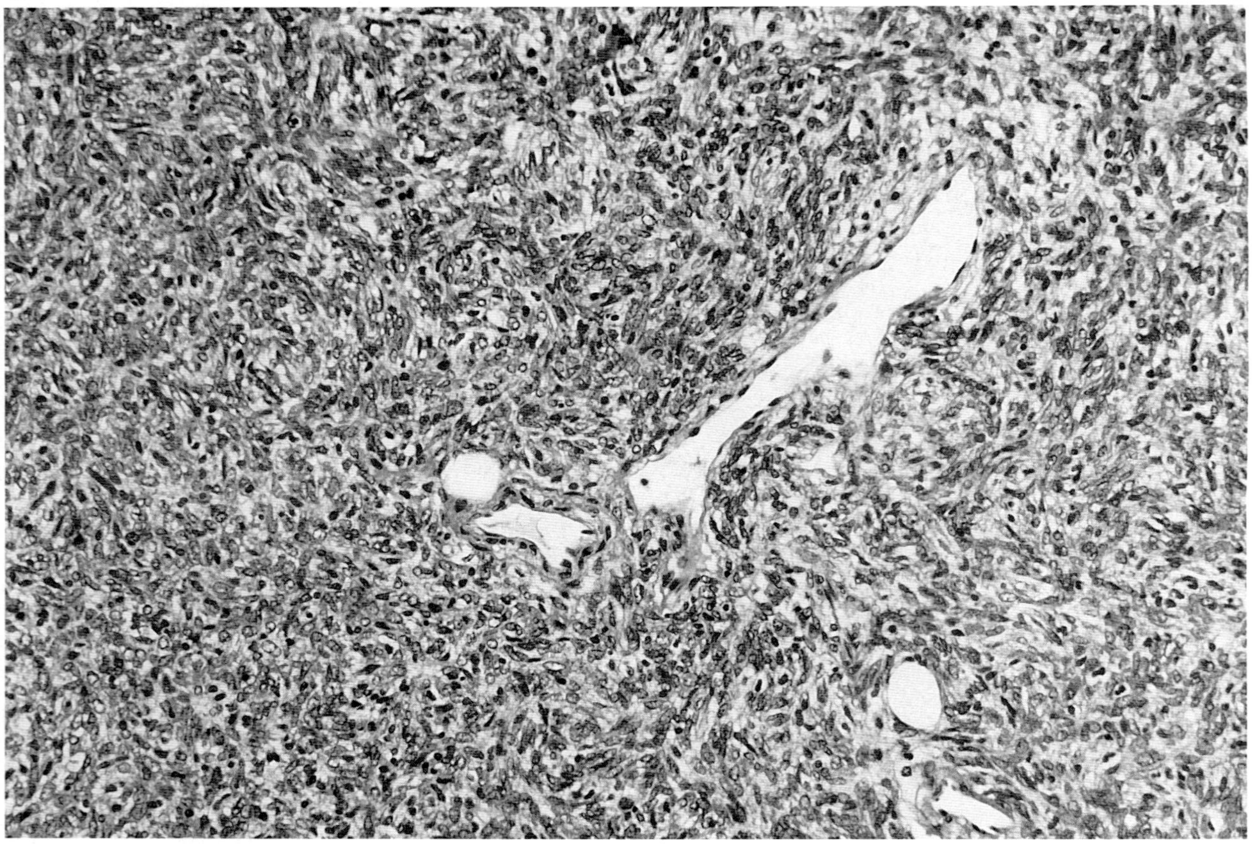

**Figure 12.17(c)** Hemangiopericytoma. A more spindled cell population around stag-horn shaped vessels. (H&E, X160)

noted by Fagge in 1869 (106) but the changes were mistakenly attributed to scleroderma. It was not until 1922 that a detailed clinical description of the lesion was provided by French investigators Feissinger and Mathieu (107). Three additional examples of this lesion were described (102,109,127) before the first histologic proof of the inflammatory nature of the lesion was provided by the French surgeon Henri Mondor (119). Following Mondor's 1939 report, superficial phlebitis of the veins of the chest wall became widely recognized as Mondor's disease. Approximately 300 examples of this lesion have been reported in the world literature and the majority of these reports appeared prior to 1970s (99,105,108,111–117,126).

Mondor's disease occurs in both men and women, but more frequently in the latter. It generally affects patients between ages of 30 to 78. In most cases, no specific etiology has been identified. Traumatic injury to the chest wall and breast surgery including plastic surgical procedures for augmentation or reduction (110) and excisional biopsies have been the preceding events in selected cases. In one patient Mondor's disease became apparent in association with recurrent axillary metastasis from mammary carcinoma (118). Three cases have been reported in pregnant women (98,104,111), and two in the postpartum period (99,112).

## Clinical Features

There is a sudden onset of pain in the breast or anterior chest wall followed by the appearance of a tender cord-like lesion of varying length (124) which provokes retraction of the overlying skin. This retraction may be mistaken for the peau d'orange of carcinoma. The lesions are located along the distribution of one of the three major superficial veins of the chest. There is associated erythema. The lesion is generally unilateral, but bilateral lesions have been

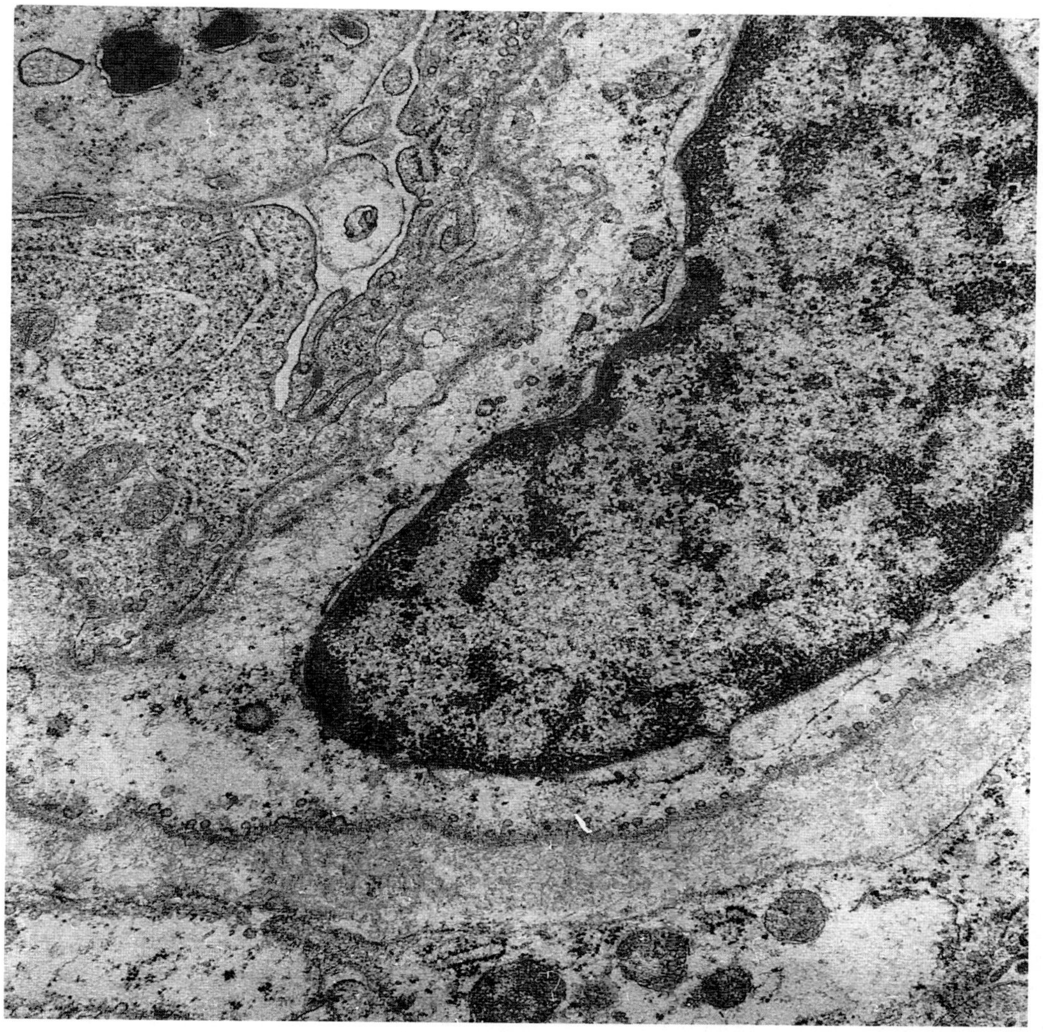

**Figure 12.18** Hemangiopericytoma. At the ultrastructural level, the pericyte displays basal laminar investiture and prominent pinocytotic vesicles. (Uranyl acetate-lead citrate, X14,970) (From Tavassoli FA, Weiss S: *Am J Surg Pathol* 1981;5:745–752, with permission)

reported (108,112). Most patients have no other evidence of thrombophlebitis. Rarely, the lesion has been associated with systemic disorders such as rheumatoid arthritis (119,114) and overt deep vein thrombosis in the legs (111).

## Microscopic Features

Johnson et al (114) described four stages in the evolution of the disease. The first stage involves formation of a thrombus within the lumen of the vein with surrounding inflammatory infiltrate composed of polymorphonuclear leukocytes. In the second stage, the thrombus organizes and except for rare areas of recanalization, the lesion consists of a solid cord. In the third stage, recanalization is in progress with gradual coalescence to form a single lumen. In the final stage, the vein has become completely recanalized with a thickened fibrous wall and minimal perivascular inflammatory infiltrate. This process evolves over two to 24 weeks.

## Behavior and Treatment

Symptoms last only a few weeks and all signs of the disease usually resolve without any treatment within two months. In isolated cases, the lesion has recurred (115,116). Treatment consists of the use of salicylates and warm compresses for the relief of pain along with avoidance of overly restrictive breast support.

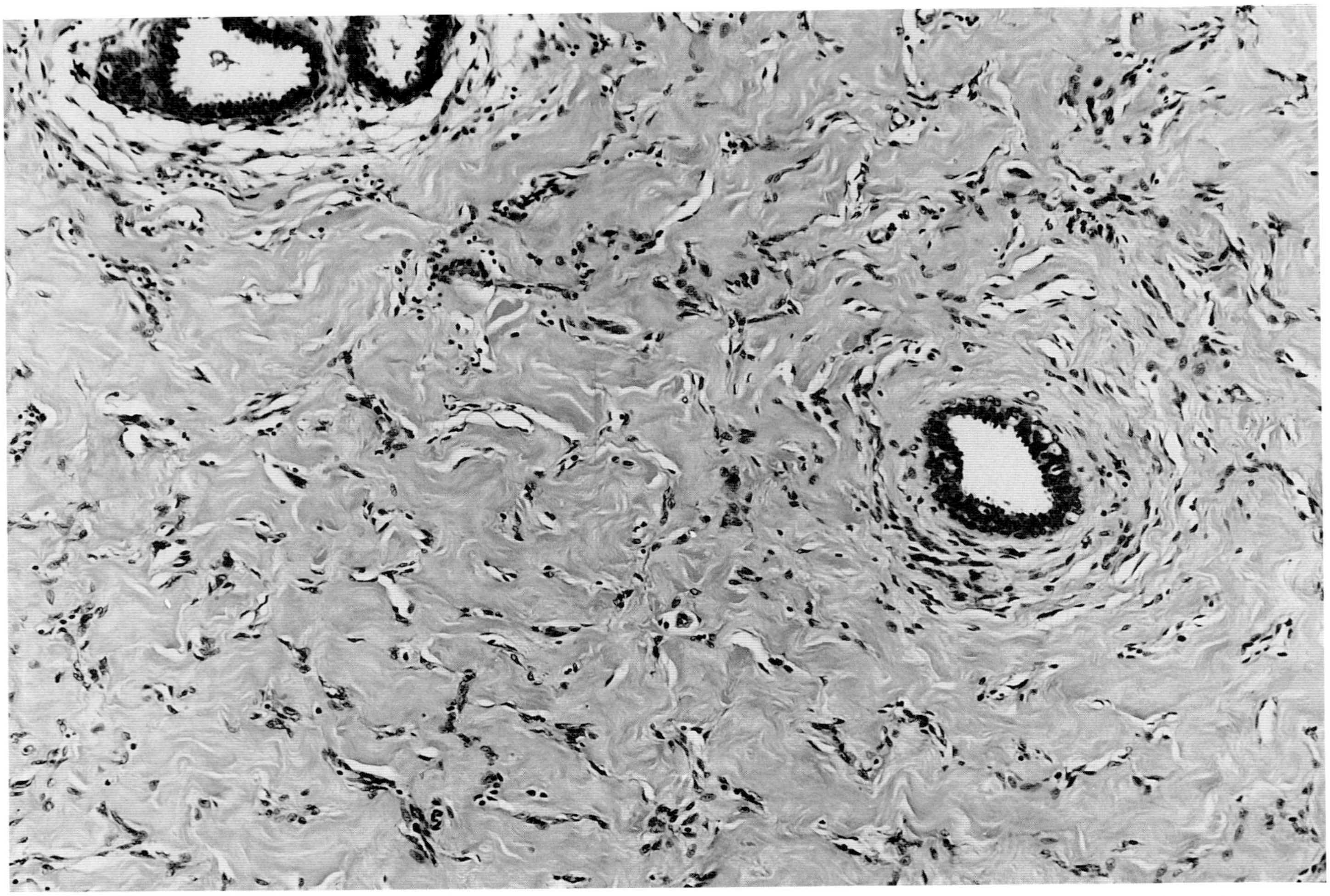

**Figure 12.19** Pseudoangiomatous stromal change. A densely collagenous stroma displays irregular, slit-like spaces. The collagen has a wavy characteristic and the spaces appear to be lined by spindle cells. (H&E, X300)

## VASCULITIS

Various forms of vasculitis occur in the breast. Giant cell arteritis most frequently affects the temporal arteries. Rarely, giant cell arteritis affects other sites including the breast. Eight examples of this lesion have been reported in the literature (100,101,103,121–123,125,126). The patients were all elderly women, 54 to 72 years of age. Typically, the women exhibit elevated erythrocyte sedimentation rate (ESR) ranging between 40 to 124 mm/h. The patients may present with unilateral or bilateral breast masses; the bilaterality may be synchronous or metachronous. The masses are 0.2 to 4 cm in size, firm, tender, and occasionally adherent to the overlying skin. The presence of nipple retraction and palpable axillary nodes in some cases may lead to the erroneous clinical impression of carcinoma. Malaise, fever, anorexia, weight loss, muscle weakness, and joint pain and stiffness are present in half of the reported cases at the time of presentation.

Microscopically, the changes involve small and medium-sized arteries. The media of the arteries is infiltrated by numerous inflammatory cells, histiocytes, and giant cells. The lumen is narrowed due to intimal fibrosis. Nonspecific inflammation and fibrosis may be present in the surrounding breast tissue. The lesion should be distinguished from other types of vasculitidis including polyarteritis, four examples of which have been described in the breast (105,117, 120). The latter exhibits panarteritis with prominent fibrinoid necrosis and a mixed inflammatory infiltrate, including eosinophils, but giant cells are absent. Necrotizing arteritis (Fig. 12.20) also occurs in the breast; a specific etiology has not been established for this lesion in the breast.

Postoperative treatment with steroids alleviates

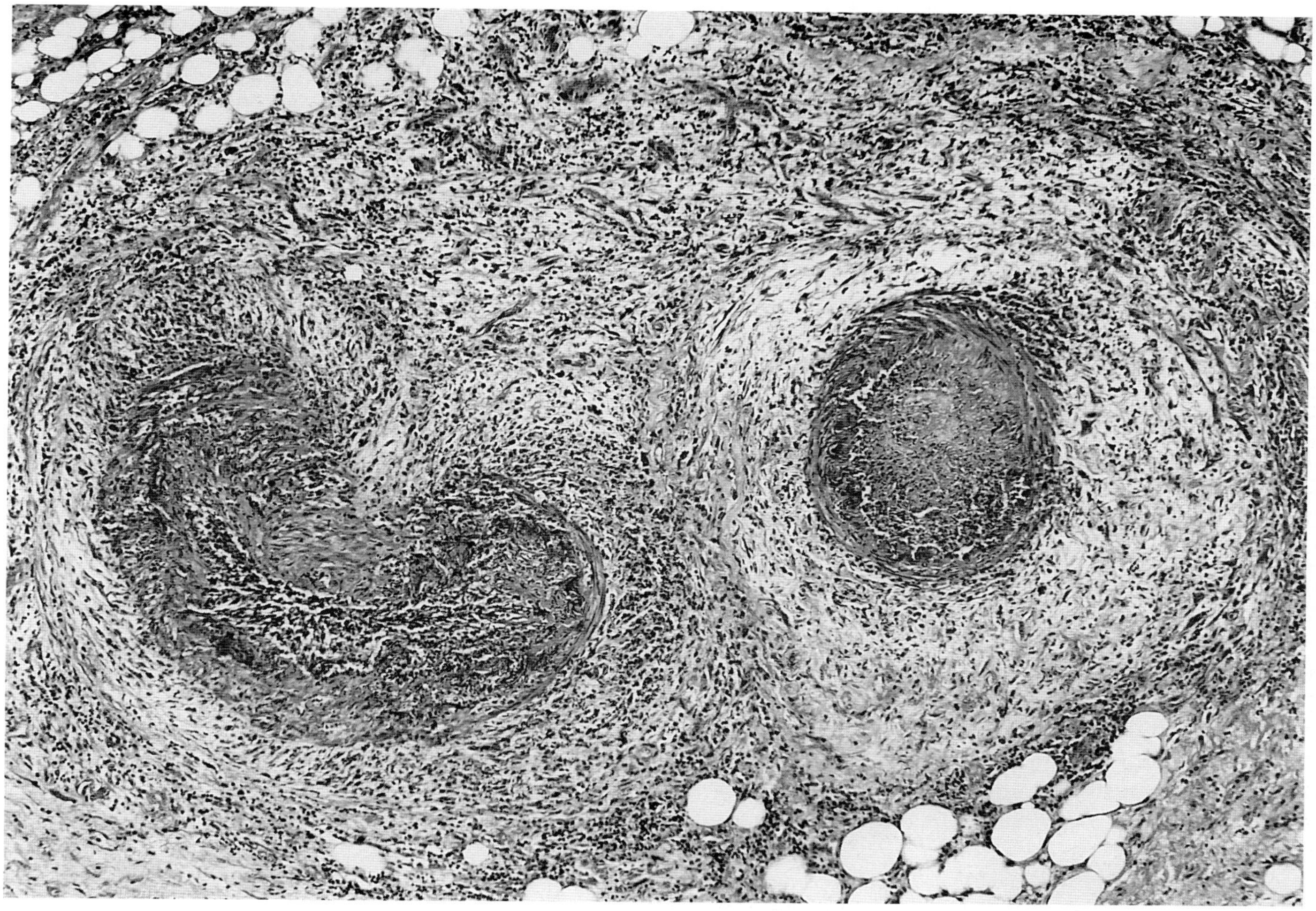

**Figure 12.20** Necrotizing vasculitis. Two vessels show necrosis and inflammatory infiltrate in the wall. (H&E, X150)

symptoms and prevents further complications (101). Occasionally a patient may exhibit spontaneous regression of the disease; longer follow-up of these patients is necessary, however.

## REFERENCES


### Angiosarcoma

1. Ackerman LV, Taylor HB: in Hartman WH (ed) Proceedings of the Thirty-fifth Seminars of the American Society of Clinical Pathologists. 1969, p 14.
* 2. Alles JU, Bosslet K: Immunocytochemistry of angiosarcoma: A study of 19 cases with special emphasis on the applicability of endothelial cell specific markers to routinely prepared tissues. *Am J Clin Pathol* 1988;89:463–471.
* 3. Alvarez-Fernandez E, Salinero-Paniagua E: Vascular tumors of the mammary gland. *Virchows Arch (Pathol Anat)* 1981;394:31–47.
* 4. Antman KH, Corson J, Greenberger J, et al: Multimodality therapy in the management of angiosarcoma of the breast. *Cancer* 1982;20:2000–2003.
5. Azzopardi JG: *Problems in Breast Pathology*. Philadelphia, WB Saunders, 1979, pp 368–371.
6. Barber KW, Harrison EG, Clagget OT, et al: Angiosarcoma of the breast. *Surgery* 1960;48:869–887.
7. Batchelor GB: Hemangioblastoma of the breast associated with pregnancy. *Br J Surg* 1958;46:647–649.
* 8. Benda JA, Al Jurf AS, Benson AB: Angiosarcoma of the breast following segmental mastectomy complicated by lymphedema. *Am J Clin Pathol* 1987;87:651–655.
* 9. Body G, Sauvant E, Calais G, et al: Angiosarcome cutane du sein apres adenocarcinome mammaire opere et irradie. *J Gynecol Obstet Biol Reprod* (Paris) 1987;16:479–483.
* 10. Borrmann R: Metastasenbilding bei Histologisch Gutartigen Geschwulsten: Fall von Metastasierendem Angiom. *Beitr Path Anat* 1907;40:372–393.
11. Bracaglia R, Seccia A, Farralo E, et al: Steroid hormone receptors in female breast angiosarcomas. *Ann Plast Surg* 1982;9:61–64.
* 12. Breitfellner G: Zur Frage des Zusammenhanges zwischen

lobularer Angiomatose und multiplen Angiosarkomen der Mamma. *Z Krebsforsch* 1975;84:345–350.

13. Brentani MM, Pacheco MM, Oshima CTF, et al: Steroid receptors in breast angiosarcoma. *Cancer* 1983;51:2105–2111.
14. Cabanne F, Michiels R, Dusserre P, et al: Hemangioendotheliomes du sein. Etude antomo-clinique de deux cas. *Laval Med* 1966;37:579–583.
15. * Capo V, Ozzelo L, Fenoglio CM, et al: Angiosarcomas arising in edematous extremities: Immunostaining for factor VIII-related antigen and ultrastructural features. *Hum Pathol* 1985;16:144–150.
16. Chen KT, Hoffman KD, Hendricks EJ: Angiosarcoma following therapeutic irradiation. *Cancer* 1979;44:2044–2048.
17. * Chen KTK, Kirkegaard D, Bocian J: Angiosarcoma of the breast. *Cancer* 1980;46:368–371.
18. Danese CA, Grishman E, Oh C, et al: Malignant vascular tumors of the lymphedematous extremity. *Ann Surg* 1967;166:245–253.
19. * Davies JD, Rees GJG, Mera SL: Angiosarcoma in irradiated postmastectomy chest wall. *Histopathology* 1983;7:947–956.
20. * Donnell RM, Rosen PP, Lieberman PH, et al: Angiosarcoma and other vascular tumors of the breast: Pathologic analysis as a guide to prognosis. *Am J Surg Pathol* 1981;5:629–642.
21. Dubin HU, Creehan EP, Headington JT: Lymphangiosarcoma and congenital lymphedema of the extremity. *Arch Dermatol* 1974;110:608–614.
22. * Dunegan LJ, Tobon H, Watson CG: Angiosarcoma of the breast: A report of two cases and a review of the literature. *Surgery* 1976;79:57–59.
23. Eby CS, Brennan MJ, Fine G: Lymphangiosarcoma: A lethal complication of chronic lymphedema. *Arch Surg* 1967;94:223–230.
24. Edwards AT, Kellett HS: Hemangiosarcoma of breast. *J Pathol Bacteriol* 1968;95:457–459.
25. Enticknap JB: Angioblastoma of the breast complicating pregnancy. *Br J Med* 1946;2:51–55.
26. * Enzinger FM, Weiss SW: *Soft Tissue Tumors*, ed 2. St. Louis, CV Mosby, 1988, pp 554–561.
27. Friederici HHR, Roberts SS: The fine structure of two postmastectomy angiosarcomas (abstract). *Lab Invest* 1967;16:644.
28. * Givens SS, Ellerbroek NA, Butler JJ, et al: Angiosarcoma arising in an irradiated breast. A case report and review of the literature. *Cancer* 1989;64:2214–2216.
29. Govoni E, Pileri S, Bazzocchi F, et al: Postmastectomy angiosarcoma: Ultrastructural study of a case. *Tumori* 1981;67:79–86.
30. Grant EG, Holt RW, Chun B, et al: Angiosarcoma of the breast. Sonographic, xeromammographic, and pathologic appearance. *AJR* 1983;141:691–692.
31. Gray GF Jr, Gonzales-Licea A, Hartmann WH, et al: Angiosarcoma in lymphedema—an unusual case of Stewart-Treves syndrome. *Bull John Hopkins Hosp* 1966;119:117–128.
32. Gulesserian HP, Lawton RL: Angiosarcoma of the breast. *Cancer* 1969;24:1021–1026.
33. Hamels J, Blondiau P, Mirgaux M: Cutaneous angiosarcoma arising in a mastectomy scar after therapeutic irradiation. *Bull Cancer* (Paris) 1981;68:353–356.
34. * Hashimoto K, Matsumoto M, Eto H, et al: Differentiation of metastatic breast carcinoma from Stewart-Treves angiosarcoma. Use of anti-keratin and anti-desmosome monoclonal antibodies and factor VIII-related antibodies. *Arch Dermatol* 1985;121:742–746.
35. Hilfinger MF, Eberle RD: Lymphangiosarcoma in postmastectomy lymphedema. *Cancer* 1953;6:1192–1199.
36. Horne WI, Percival WL: Hemangiosarcoma of the breast. *Can J Surg* 1975;18:81–84.
37. Hunter TB, Martin PC, Dietzen CD, et al: Angiosarcoma of the breast: Two case reports and a review of the literature. *Cancer* 1985;56:2099–2106.
38. Kessler E, Kozenitzky IL: Hemangiosarcoma of the breast. *J Clin Pathol* 1971;24:530–532.
39. Khanna SD, Manchester RL, Saigal RK, et al: Hemangioendothelioma (angiosarcoma) of the breast. *Arch Surg* 1964;88:807–809.
40. Kuten A, Sapir D, Cohen Y, et al: Postirradiation soft tissue sarcoma occurring in breast cancer patients: Report of seven cases and results of combination chemotherapy. *J Surg Oncol* 1985;28:168–171.
41. Lattes R: Sarcomas of the breast. *JAMA* 1967;201:531–532.
42. Maddox JC, Evans HL: Angiosarcoma of skin and soft tissue. A study of forty-four cases. *Cancer* 1981;48:1907–1921.
43. Mallory TB, Castleman B, Parris EE: Hemangiosarcoma of the breast. *N Engl J Med* 1949;241:241–243.
44. * Masse SR, Mongeau CJ, Rioux A: Angiosarcoma of the breast. *Cancer* 1980;46:368–371.
45. McCarthy WD, Pack GT: Malignant blood vessel tumors: A report of 56 cases of angiosarcoma and Kaposi's sarcoma. *Surg Gynecol Obstet* 1959;9:465–482.
46. McClanahan BJ, Hogg L Jr: Angiosarcoma of the breast. *Cancer* 1954;7:586–594.
47. * Merino M, Carter D, Berman M: Angiosarcoma of the breast: A clinicopathologic study. *Am J Surg Pathol* 1983;7:53–60.
48. * Miettinen M, Lehto V, Virtanen I: Postmastectomy angiosarcoma (Stewart-Treves syndrome): Light microscopic, immunohistological, and ultrastructural characteristics of two cases. *Am J Surg Pathol* 1983;7:329–339.
49. Myerowitz RL, Pietruszka M, Barnes EL: Primary angiosarcoma of the breast. *JAMA* 1978;239:403.
50. Otis CN, Peschel R, McKhann C, et al: The rapid onset of cutaneous angiosarcoma after radiotherapy for breast carcinoma. *Cancer* 1986;57:2130–2134.
51. Polo IM: Sarcomi primitivo della mammella. Arch Ital Anat Patol Clin. *Tumori* 1970;44:215–243.
52. Procter DSC: Angioma of a male breast with malignant characteristics. *Afr Med J* 1958;32:407–409.

53. Rainwater LM, Martin K Jr, Gaffey TA, et al: Angiosarcoma of the breast. *Arch Surg* 1986;121:669–672.

54. Robinson JM, Castleman B: Benign metastasizing hemangioma. *Ann Surg* 1936;104:453–459.

* 55. Rosen PP, Kimmel M, Ernsberger D: Mammary Angiosarcoma. The prognostic significance of tumor differentiation. *Cancer* 1988;62:2145–2151.

56. Ryan JF, Keally WF: Concommitant angiosarcoma and carcinoma of the breast: A case report. *Histopathology* 1985; 9:893–899.

57. Salm R: The nature of the so-called postmastectomy lymphangiosarcoma. *J Pathol Bacteriol* 1968;85:445–446.

58. Schafler K, McKenzie CG, Salm R: Post mastectomy lymphangiosarcoma: A reappraisal of the concept, a critical review of an illustrative case. *Histopathology* 1979;3:131–152.

59. Schmidt GB: Ueber das Angiosarkom der Mamma. *Arch Klin Chir* 1887;26:121–127.

60. Schreiber H, Barry FM, Russell WL, et al: Stewart-Treves syndrome. *Arch Surg* 1979;114:82–85.

61. Silverberg SG, Kay S, Koss LG: Postmastectomy lymphangiosarcoma: Ultrastructural observations. *Cancer* 1971;27: 100.

62. Sordello PP, Magill GB, Brenner J, et al: Cisplatin. A phase II evaluation in previously untreated patients with soft tissue sarcomas. *Cancer* 1987;59:884–886.

* 63. Steingaszner LC, Enzinger FM, Taylor HB: Hemangiosarcoma of the breast. *Cancer* 1965;18:352–361.

64. Stewart FW: *Tumors of the Breast*, Fasc 34. Atlas of Tumor Pathology, section a, Washington DC, Armed Forces Institute of Pathology, 1950, pp 70–87.

* 65. Stewart FW, Treves N: Lymphangiosarcoma in postmastectomy lymphedema: A report of six cases on elephantiasis chirurgica. *Cancer* 1948;1:64–81.

66. Stout AP: Hemangioendothelioma—a tumor of blood vessels featuring vascular endothelial cells. *Ann Surg* 1943;118: 445–464.

67. Tibbs D: Metastasizing hemangiomata: A case of malignant hemangioendothelioma. *Br J Surg* 1953;40:465–470.

68. Van Zyl JA, Van Der Walt JJ, Van Zyl JJW: Hemangiosarkom van der Bros. *S Afr Med J* 1975;49:525–527.

69. Woodward AH, Ivins JC, Soule EH: Lymphangiosarcoma arising in chronic lymphedematous extremities. *Cancer* 1972;30:562–572.

70. Yadav RVS, Sahariah S, Mittal VK, et al: Angiosarcoma of the male breast. *Int Surg* 1976;61:463–464.


## Hemangiomas


* 71. Alvarez-Fernandez E, Salinero-Paniagua E: Vascular tumors of the mammary gland. A histochemical and ultrastructural study. *Virchows Arch* (*Pathol Anat*) 1981;394:31–47.

72. Hamperl H: Hamangiome der menschlichen Mamma. *Geburtshilfe un Frauenheilkund* 1973;33:13–17.

* 73. Hoda SA, Cranor ML, Rosen PP: Hemangiomas of the breast with atypical histological features. Further analysis of histological subtypes confirming their benign character. *Am J Surg Pathol* 1992;16:553–560.

* 74. Jozefczyk MA, Rosen PP: Vascular tumors of the breast. II. Perilobular hemangiomas and hemangiomas. *Am J Surg Pathol* 1985;9:491–503.

75. Lesueur GC, Brown RW, Bhathal DS: Incidence of perilobular hemangioma in the female breast. *Arch Pathol Lab Med* 1983;107:308–310.

76. Masson P: Hemengioendotheliome vegetant intravasculaire. *Bull Soc Anat* (Paris) 1923;93:517–524.

* 77. Morrow M, Berger D, Thelmo W: Diffuse cystic angiomatosis of the breast. *Cancer* 1988;62:2392–2396.

78. Murao T, Nakai M, Hamad E: Intravascular endothelial hyperplasia of the breast—report of a case with scanning electron microscopic observations. *Gan No Rinsho* 1986;32: 1471–1474.

* 79. Nielsen B: Hemangiomas of the breast. *Pathol Res Pract* 1983;176:253–257.

80. Rosai J: Ackerman's Surgical Pathology, ed 7. St. Louis, CV Mosby, 1989, vol 2, p 1250.

* 81. Rosen PP: Vascular tumors of the breast. III. Angiomatosis. *Am J Surg Pathol* 1985;9:652–658.

* 82. Rosen PP: Vascular tumors of the breast. V. Nonparenchymal vascular tumors of the mammary subcutaneous tissues. *Am J Surg Pathol* 1985;9:723–729.

* 83. Rosen PP, Jozefczyk MA, Boram LH: Vascular tumors of the breast. 1V. The venous hemangioma. *Am J Surg Pathol* 1985;9:659–665.

* 84. Rosen PP, Ridolfi RL: The perilobular hemangioma. A benign microscopic vascular lesion of the breast. *Am J Clin Pathol* 1977;68:21–23.

85. Shousha S, Theodorou NA, Bull TB: Cavernous hemangioma of breast in a man with contralateral gynaecomastia and a family history of breast carcinoma. *Histopathology* 1988;13:221–236.


## Hemangiopericytoma, Cystic Hygroma, Pseudoangiomatous Hyperplasia


86. Anderson C, Ricci A Jr, Pedersen CA, et al: Immunocytochemical analysis of estrogen and progesterone receptors in benign stromal lesions of the breast. Evidence for hormonal etiology in pseudoangiomatous hyperplasia of mammary stroma. *Am J Surg Pathol* 1991;15:145–149.

87. Arias-Stella J Jr, Rosen PP: Hemangiopericytoma of the breast. *Mod Pathol* 1988;1:98–103.

88. Hessler C: Cystic lymphangioma of the breast. *Radiology* 1967;88:135–137.

89. Ibrahim RE, Schiotto CG, Weidner N: Pseudoangiomatous hyperplasia of mammary stroma. Some observations regarding its clinicopathologic spectrum. *Cancer* 1989;63: 1154–1160.

90. Kaufman SL, Stout AP: Hemangiopericytoma in children. *Cancer* 1960;13:695–710.

91. Khushbakhat R, Mittal R, Gerald W, et al: Hemangiopericytoma of breast: Report of a case with ultrastructural and

immunohistochemical findings. *Hum Pathol* 1986;17:1181–1183.

92. Mittal KR, Gerald W, True LD: Hemangiopericytoma of breast: Report of a case with ultrastructural and immunohistochemical findings. *Hum Pathol* 1986;17:1181–1183.
93. Morrow M, Berger D, Thelmo W: Diffuse cystic angiomatosis of the breast. *Cancer* 1988;62:2392–2396.
94. Sieber PR, Sharkey FE: Cystic hygroma of the breast. *Arch Pathol Lab Med* 1986;110:353.
95. Tavassoli FA, Weiss S: Hemangiopericytoma of the breast. *Am J Surg Pathol* 1981;5:745–752.
96. Torino L: In tema di neoplasie della mammella maschile. *Rass Int Clin Ter* 1972;52:675–680.
97. Volmer J, Pickarz H, Javtzke G: Vascular tumor in the region of the breast. *Virchows Arch* (A) 1980;385:201–214.
98. Vuitch MF, Rosen PP, Erlandson RA: Pseudoangiomatous hyperplasia of mammary stroma. *Hum Pathol* 1986;17:185–191.

**Vasculitis**

99. Abramson DJ: Mondor's disease and string phlebitis. *JAMA* 1966;196:1087–1089.
100. Chaitin B, Kohout ND, Goldman RL: Focal arteritis of the breast. *Angiology* 1981;32:334–337.
101. Clement PB, Senges H, How AR: Giant cell arteritis of the breast: Case report and literature review. *Hum Pathol* 1987;18:1189–1187.
102. Daniels WB: Superficial Thrombophlebitis: A new cause of chest pain. *Am J Med Sci* 1932;183:398–401.
103. Dega FJ, Hunder GG: Vasculitis of the breast. *Arthritis Rheum* 1974;17:973–976.
104. Duff P: Mondor's disease in pregnancy. *Obstet Gynecol* 1981;58:117–119.
105. Elsner B: Vasculitis Mamaria primitiva. *Prensa Med Argent* 1970;57:451–453.
106. Fagge CH: Remarks on certain cutaneous affections, with cases. *Guy's Hosp Rep* 1869–1870;15(3rd series):302–363.
107. Feissinger N, Mathieu P: Thrombo-phlebites des veines de la paroi thoraco-abdominale. *Bull Mem Soc Med Hop Paris* 1920;46:352–354.
108. Farrow JH: Thrombophlebitis of the superficial veins of the breast and anterior chest wall (Mondor's disease). *Surg Gynecol Obstet* 1955;101:63–68.
109. Favre M, Sedallian P: Sur deux formes anatomopathologiques d'alteration des vaisseaux superficiels chez les tuberculeux; angeites segmentaires resulutives; vascularites "fils de fer" des tuberculeux. *J Med Lyon* 1929;10:779–788.
110. Fischl RA, Kahn S, Simon BE: Mondor's disease. An unusual complication of mammaplasty. *Plast Reconstruct Surg* 1975;56:319–322.
111. Grow JL, Lewison EF: Superficial thrombophlebitis of the breast. *Surg Gynecol Obstet* 1963;116:180–182.
112. Hogan GF: Mondor's disease. *Arch Intern Med* 1964;113:881–885.
113. Honig C, Rado R: Mondor's disease—superficial thrombophlebitis of the chest wall. *Ann Surg* 1961;153:589–591.
114. Johnson WC, Wallrich R, Helwig EB: Superficial thrombophlebitis of chest wall. *JAMA* 1962;180:103–108.
115. Kaufman PA: Subcutaneous phlebitis of the breast and chest wall. *Ann Surg* 1956;144:847–853.
116. Lunn GM, Potter JM: Mondor's disease (Subcutaneous phlebitis of the breast region). *Br J Med* 1954;1:1074–1076.
117. McCarthy DJ, Imbriglia J, Hung JK: Vasculitis of the breasts. *Arthritis Rheum* 1968 11:796–803.
118. Miller DR, Cesario TC, Slater LM: Mondor's disease associated with metastatic axillary nodes. *Cancer* 1985;56:903–904.
119. Mondor H: Tronculite sous-cutanee subaigue de la paroi thoracique antero-laterale. *Mem Acad Chir* (Paris). 1939;65:1271–1278.
120. Nielsen BB, Lorentzen M: Arteritis i brystet. *Ugeskr Laeger* 1985;147:2230–2232.
121. Nirodi NS, Stirling WJ, White MF: Giant cell arteritis presenting as a breast lump. *Br J Clin Pract* 1985;39:84–86.
122. Potter BT, Housley E, Thomson D: Giant cell arteritis mimicking carcinoma of the breast. *Br J Med* 1981;282:1665–1666.
123. Stephenson TJ, Underwood JCE: Giant cell arteritis: An unusual cause of palpable masses in the breast. *Br J Surg* 1986;73:105.
124. Tabar L, Dean PB: Mondor's disease: Clinical, mammographic, and pathologic features. *Breast* 1982;7:18–20.
125. Thaell JF, Saue GL: Giant cell arteritis involving the breast. *J Rheumatol* 1983;10:329–331.
126. Waugh TR: Bilateral mammary arteritis: Report of a case. *Am J Pathol* 1950;26:851–861.
127. Williams GA: Thoraco-epigastric phelebitis producing dyspnea. *JAMA* 1931;96:2196–2197.

# 13

# Mesenchymal Lesions



The breast stroma consists of fibroblasts, myofibroblasts, fat cells, nerve fibers, as well as the endothelial and smooth muscle cells of the vasculature. Any of these cells can and do give rise to a variety of benign and malignant tumors. The myofibroblast not only forms a variety of tumors, but participates in the formation of many others as a component of their supporting stroma. The many facets of the myofibroblast and its role in a variety of breast lesions has been discussed by Ahmed (2). Furthermore, a variety of non-neoplastic alterations in these stromal cells is occasionally encountered that may be misinterpreted as a malignant process, while changes such as elastosis—a reflection of varied functional states of the fibroblast—are commonly observed in association with, but are not exclusive to, malignancy. This chapter addresses the variety of stromal lesions exclusive of vascular lesions and lymphomas.

## NON-NEOPLASTIC STROMAL ALTERATIONS

### Stromal Giant Cells

Multinucleated giant cells are sometimes present in the interlobular stroma either in one small focus or in multiple foci. These giant cells are seen in 4.5% of mastectomy specimen removed for carcinoma but also occur in the stroma of benign lesions and are not a component of fat necrosis. Stromal giant cells have scant cytoplasm and hyperchromatic nuclei. The number of nuclei per cell is highly variable and often the nuclei display a florette arrangement within the giant cell (Fig. 13.1a). Most patients with stromal giant cells are between 40 and 50 years of age (18). Similar cells are also seen in fibroadenomas that generally occur in a younger age group, as well as in fibromatosis.

A

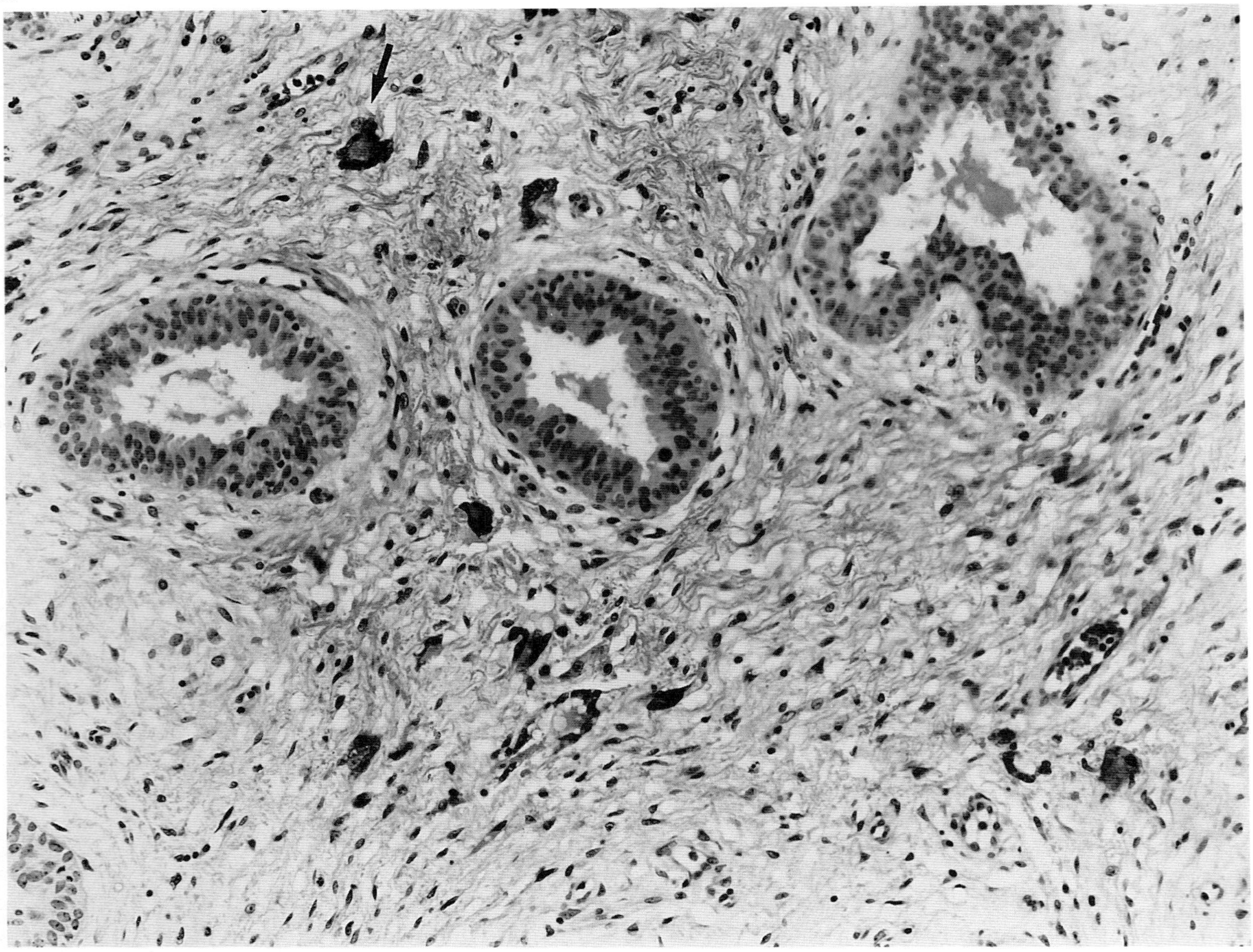

**Figure 13.1(a)** Stromal giant cells in a juvenile fibroadenoma display florette-like arrangement of the nuclei (arrow). (H&E, X240)

Ultrastructurally, the cells may show a complex lobulated nucleus or multiple nuclei (Fig. 13.1b). The precise nature of this finding is not known. Whether it is a reactive, degenerative, or hormonally-induced change has not been established. The significance, if any, of this change for subsequent development of a malignancy has not been determined either, but it is doubtful that it would constitute a risk factor.

## Stromal Metachromasia

Stromal metachromasia is a common finding at the infiltrating edge of breast carcinomas (10). It is also evident as a halo surrounding some of the ducts containing intraductal carcinoma. The metachromasia reflects an increase in the spaces between the strands of connective tissue. The spaces may become filled with a fibrillar metachromatic substance. The separation of connective tissue may cause disruption of the duct wall and facilitate invasion (19). In other words, the disruption of the duct wall resulting in invasion may reflect an extension of the stromal disruptive changes rather than resulting from the expansile force of the proliferating intraductal cancer cells.

## Stromal Elastosis

Stromal elastosis is seen in normal breasts as well as in both benign and malignant lesions (Fig. 13.2).

B

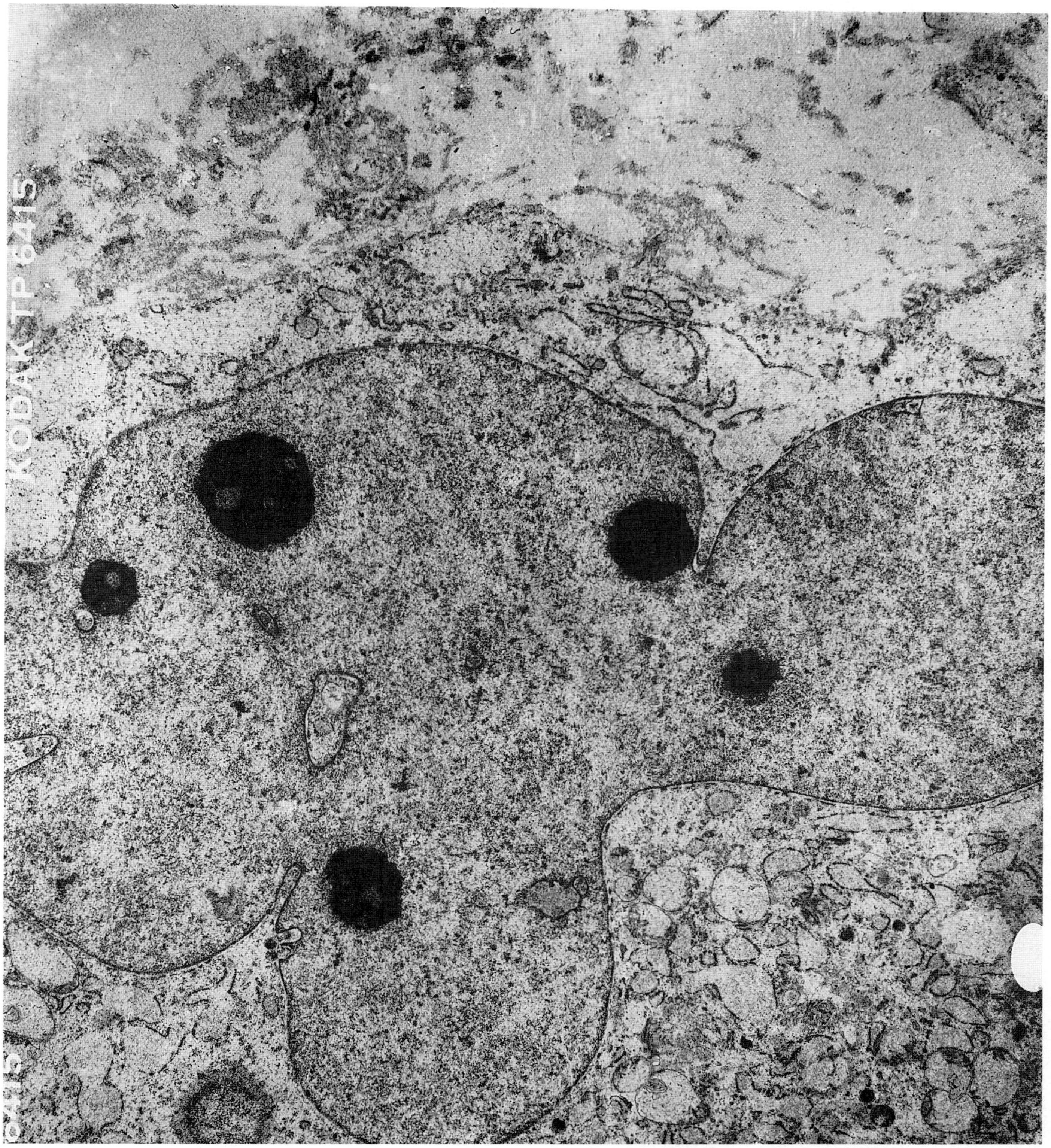

**Figure 13.1(b)** Stromal giant cells. At the ultrastructural level, the giant cells show multilobulated nuclei. (Uranyl acetate-lead citrate, X3,560)

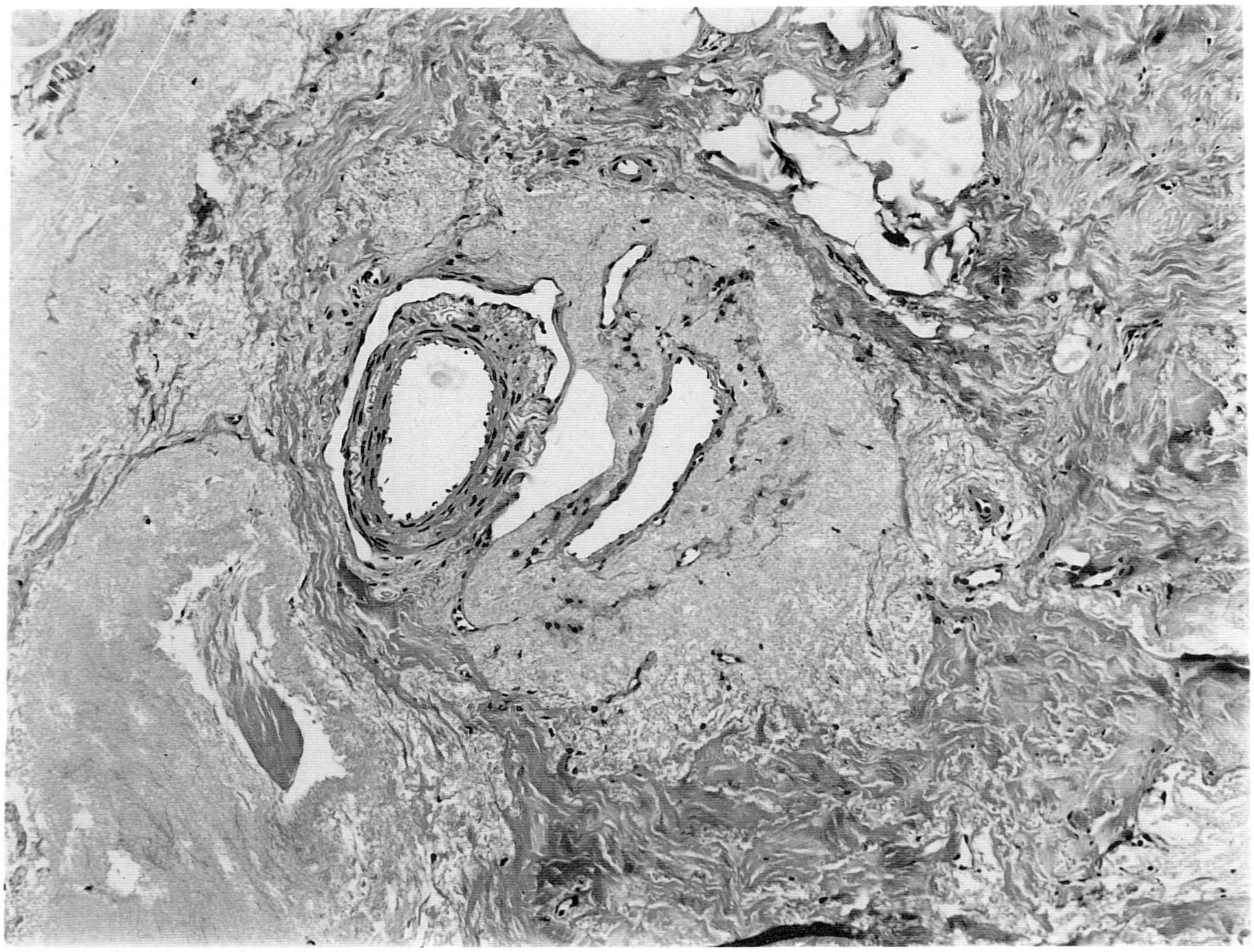

**Figure 13.2** Elastosis. Extensive elastosis around vessels. (H&E, X120)

In the normal breast, elastosis is found focally in the stroma, around ducts, and less commonly around vessels. Periductal elastosis appears to progressively accumulate until around 50 years of age and may be related to parity (6). There is a high incidence of elastosis in breast carcinomas with reports of its occurrence in up to 88.2% to 95% of the infiltrating tumors (1,7). Opinions regarding the significance of elastosis as a prognostic factor vary. Some investigators have considered marked elastosis a favorable prognostic feature (21), while others have noted that abundant elastosis has an unfavorable influence on prognosis (3,9) and a third group has concluded that elastosis does not correlate with the clinical behavior of the lesion (11,15). Florid elastosis is associated with estrogen receptor positivity (11,14,15). The extent of elastosis varies in different tumors but it may be marked enough to be grossly apparent and it occurs in a variety of invasive carcinomas. The yellow, chalky streaks observed on cut surface of scirrhous carcinoma reflect periductal and stromal elastosis (4,12). Elastosis was referred to as an amyloid-like material by some investigators; its true nature was clarified by enzymatic and ultrastructural studies (20,22). While most investigators believe fibroblasts in the area synthesize the elastic fibers (1,7,20,22), others believe that the carcinoma cells play a significant role in the production of the elastic fibers (8). Both groups have based their conclusion on the finding of elastic fibers inside and around the respective cells.

In addition to its association with carcinomas, elastosis is seen in a variety of benign lesions as well (5,16,17,22) and it is particularly conspicuous in some radial scars.

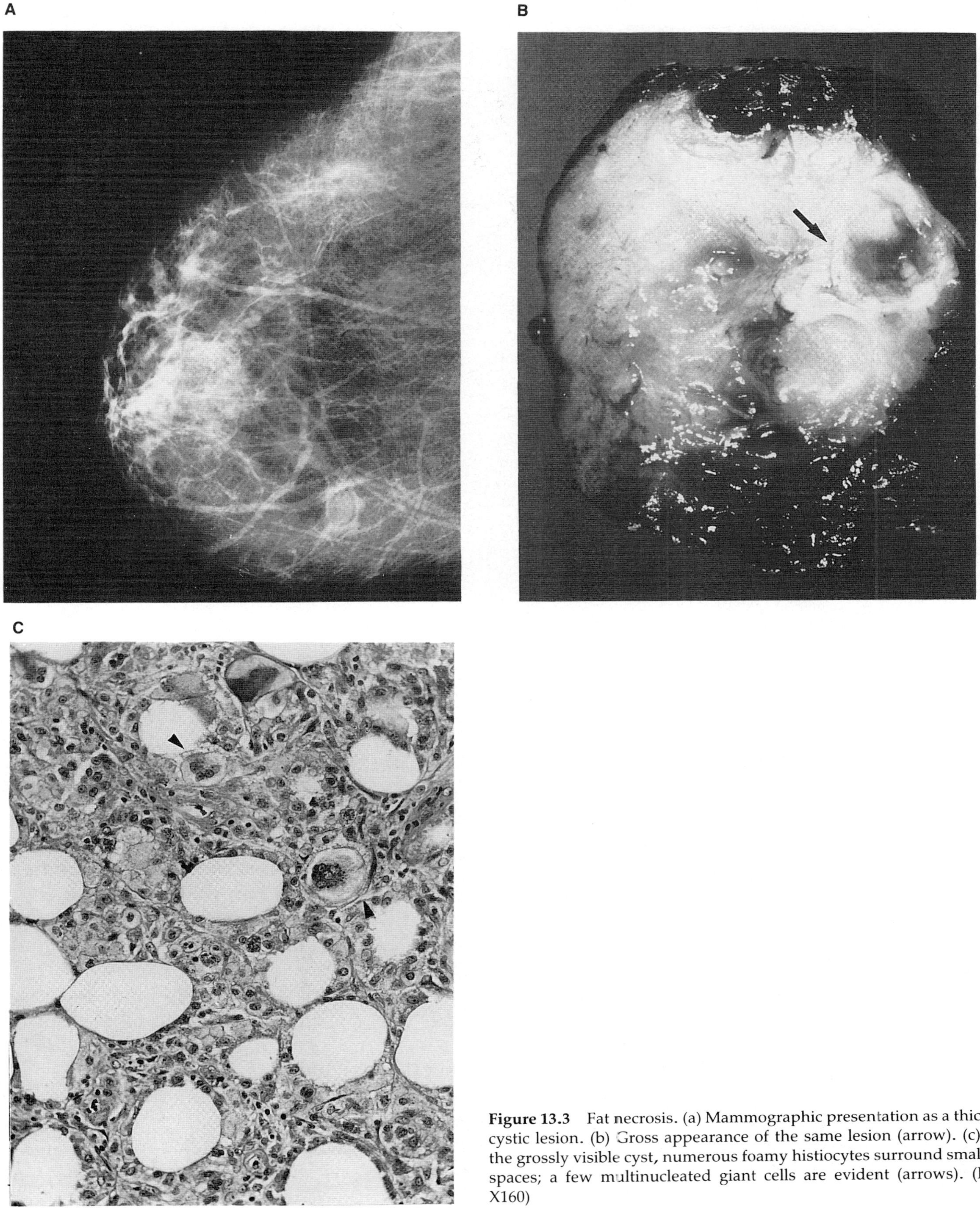


**Figure 13.3** Fat necrosis. (a) Mammographic presentation as a thick-walled cystic lesion. (b) Gross appearance of the same lesion (arrow). (c) Around the grossly visible cyst, numerous foamy histiocytes surround smaller cystic spaces; a few multinucleated giant cells are evident (arrows). (H&E, (c) X160)

A

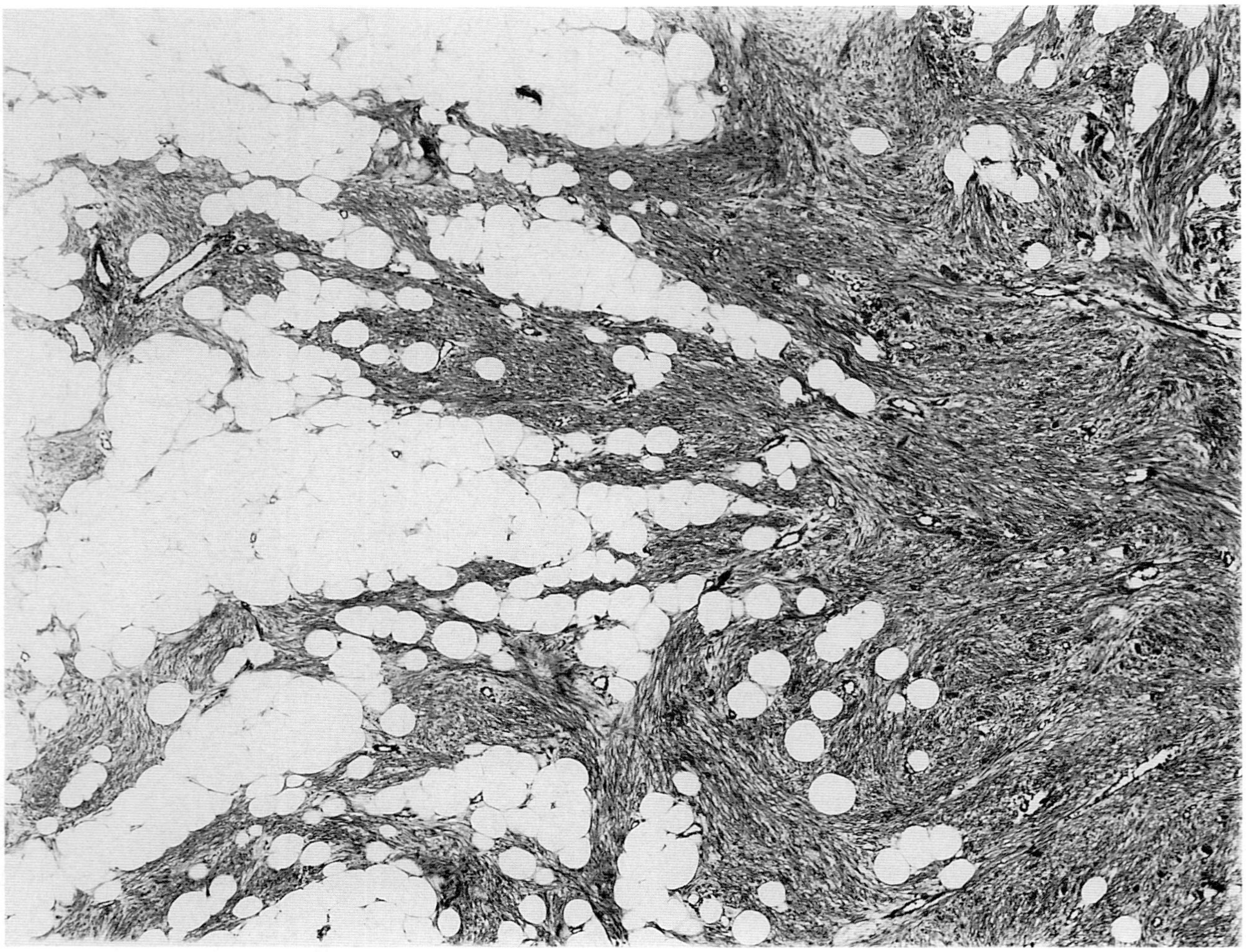

**Figure 13.4(a)** Fibromatosis. The margin is characteristically infiltrating. (H&E, X50)

## Fat Necrosis

Fat necrosis, manifesting as a clinically detectable mass, is uncommon. Over a 37-year period, Haagensen (24) encountered 54 such lesions and noted that breast carcinoma was 40 times as frequent during the same period in his practice. It is believed that most cases have a traumatic origin (26) although a history of trauma is obtained in only 32% to 44% of the women (23,24).

The patients range in age from 14 to 80 years of age with a mean age of 52 years (23,24). Characteristically, fat necrosis is located superficially in the breast. It occurs most frequently in the areolar region, but it may occur anywhere in the breast. The tumor is palpable in all cases, and it often enlarges gradually after it is discovered. About one third of the patients complain of pain and tenderness, and in approximately a quarter of the cases, echymosis is evident in the overlying skin.

Fat necrosis may clinically simulate a carcinoma particularly when fixed to the skin and associated with retraction. Skin retraction occurs in 41% to 58% of the women (23,24). When the skin overlying the tumor appears red and warm, the tumor simulates an abscess clinically.

The average size of the lesion is less than 2 cm. The tumor is firm and fixed to the surrounding tissues. The cut surface shows a well-delineated, round mass unlike the irregular outlines of carcinoma. In early lesions, hemorrhage is characteristically present. As the lesion ages, the cut surface develops a variegated appearance with areas of necrosis and cavitation. The end stage of the lesion may manifest as a dense scar or the lesion may transform

B

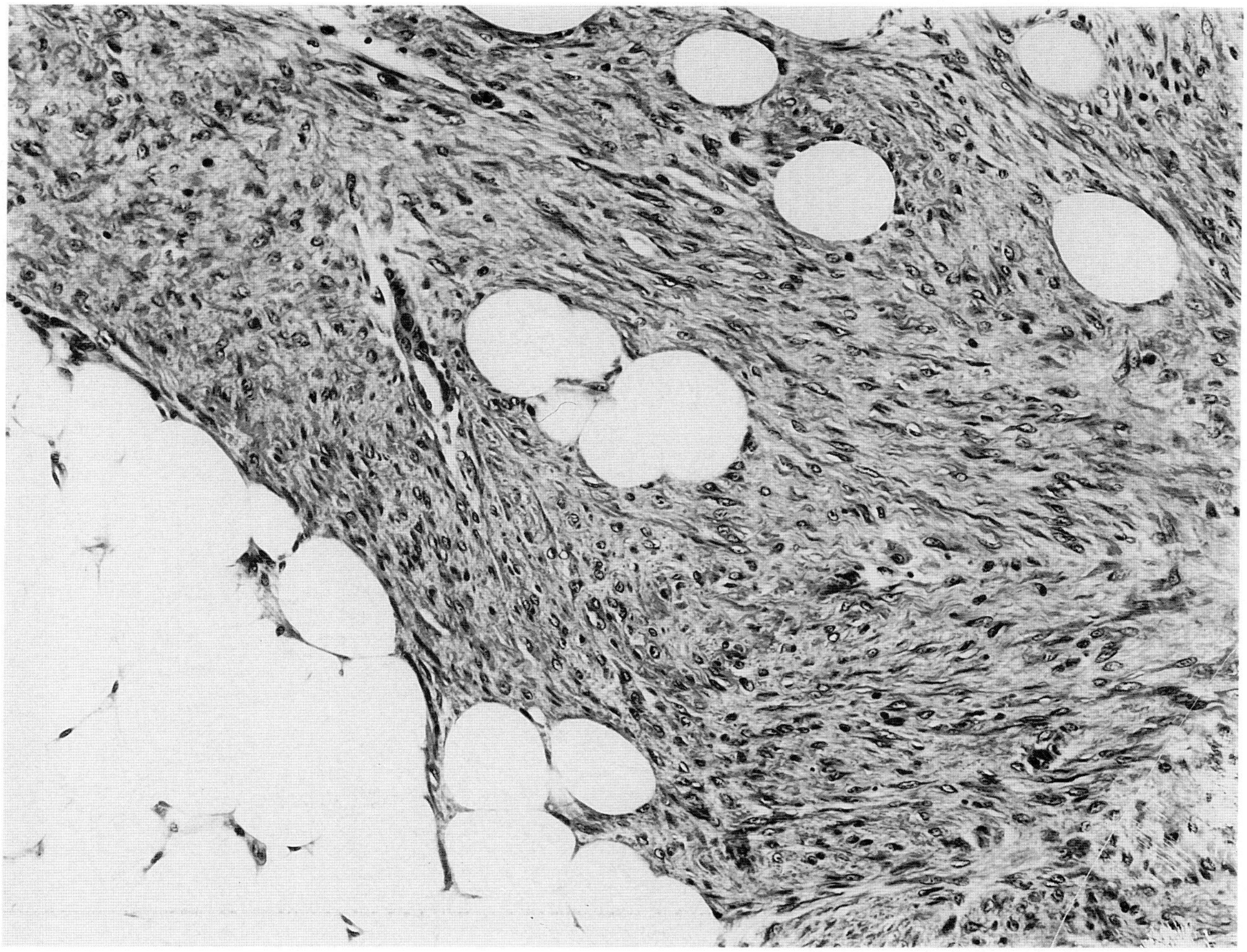

**Figure 13.4(b)** Fibromatosis. The cellularity of fibromatosis is generally of a mild to moderate degree, and the cells lack atypia or notable mitotic activity. (H&E, X120)

into a cyst with calcified (25) or thick, radio-opaque walls that can be picked up mammographically (Fig. 13.3).

Microscopically, small cysts resulting from the dissolution and fusion of necrotic fat cells are surrounded by lipid-laden, foamy histiocytes, foreign-body-type giant cells with or without acute inflammatory cells (Fig. 13.3c). Gradually, fibroblasts move in the peripheral areas and begin depositing collagen. Eventually, the entire area is replaced by dense fibrous tissue.

As mentioned before, trauma is thought to be the major etiology of fat necrosis even though a history of trauma is obtained in less than 50% of the patients. Fat necrosis also occurs after surgical trauma as well as following radiation therapy for carcinoma.

## Metaplasias

A variety of metaplastic changes many develop in the stroma. Smooth muscle metaplasia occurs occasionally in the stroma of fibroadenomas and cystosarcoma phyllodes but it is not common (27,29,30). When present, smooth muscle metaplasia is usually confined to a few small areas within the biphasic tumor. Occasionally, however, it can become quite prominent and even assume dominance in some fibroadenomas. The origin of smooth muscle cells has been attributed to a metaplastic process in the stroma (28).

Osseous and cartilagenous metaplasia are rare but occur most frequently in cystosarcoma phyllodes through metaplastic changes in the stromal cells (30,31,33). The development of liposarcoma and

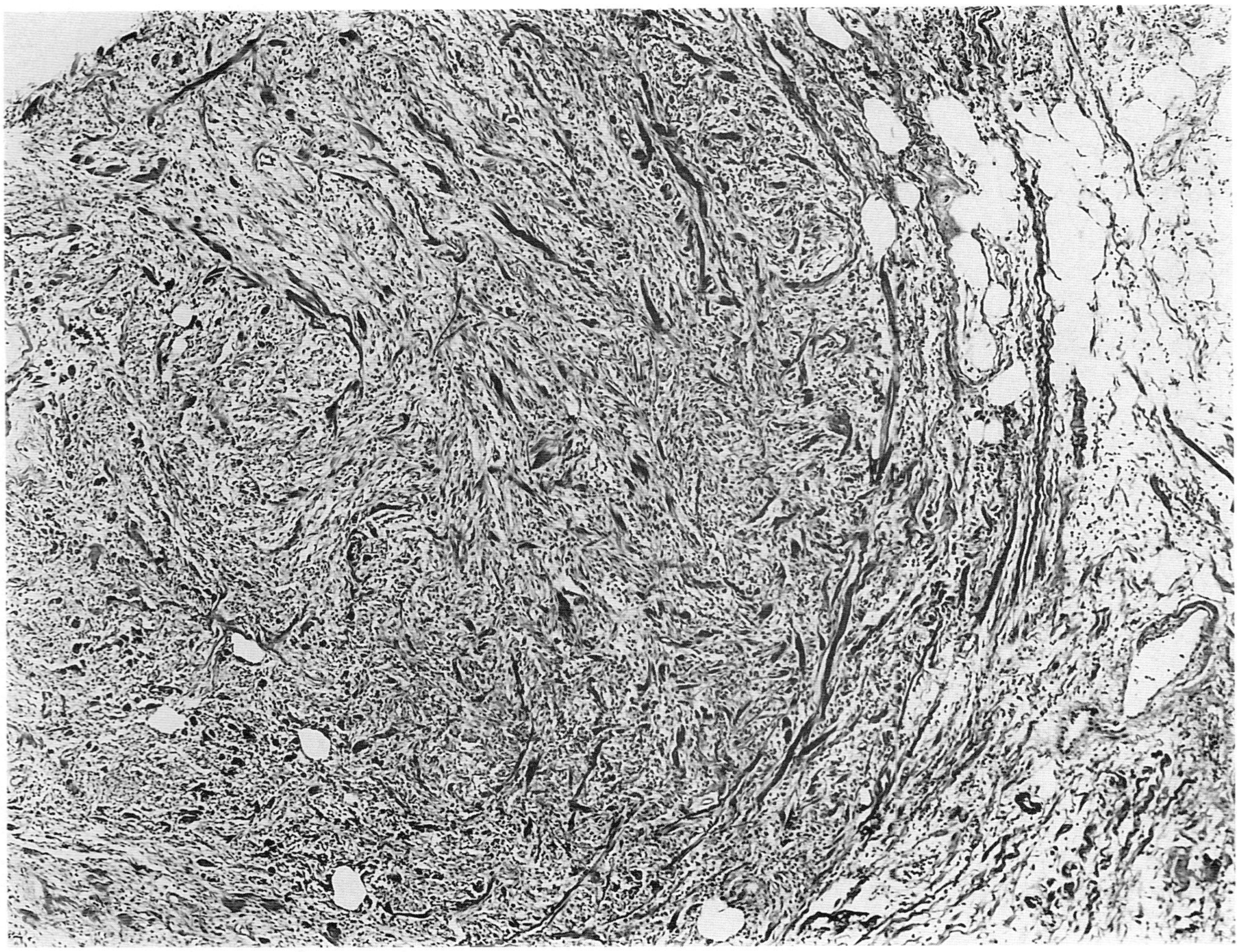


**Figure 13.5(a)** Myofibroblastoma. The tumor has a well-defined margin with dense cellularity and interspersed ribbons of collagen. (H&E, X150)

rhabdomyosarcoma in cystosarcoma has also been ascribed to a metaplastic process (31,32).

## Ochronosis

The presence of a simple autosomal recessive allele resulting in homogentisic acid oxidase deficiency is the cause of a clinical syndrome characterized by alcaptonurea (homogentisic acid in the urine) and ochronosis (pigment deposition in the soft tissues). The only reported case of ochronosis involving the breast occurred in a 67-year-old woman with the clinical syndrome (13). She presented with a breast mass. Two nodules were discovered in the breast. The larger one was 4 cm, firm and lobulated. It was brownish-black on the cut surface. The pigment appeared as yellow-brown, finely particulate deposits both intracellular and extracellular in location between and within the stromal cells, smooth muscle, and endothelial cells. There was an associated fibroblastic proliferation which resulted in formation of hard nodules. The pigment, which was probably a product of cellular tyrosine metabolism (13), resembled melanin. Special stains cannot reliably differentiate melanin from ochronotic pigment, however. The presence of other clinical features of the syndrome (darkening of ears, nose, and nails) or symptomatic family members serve as important clues to the nature of the pigment deposits in the breast.

B

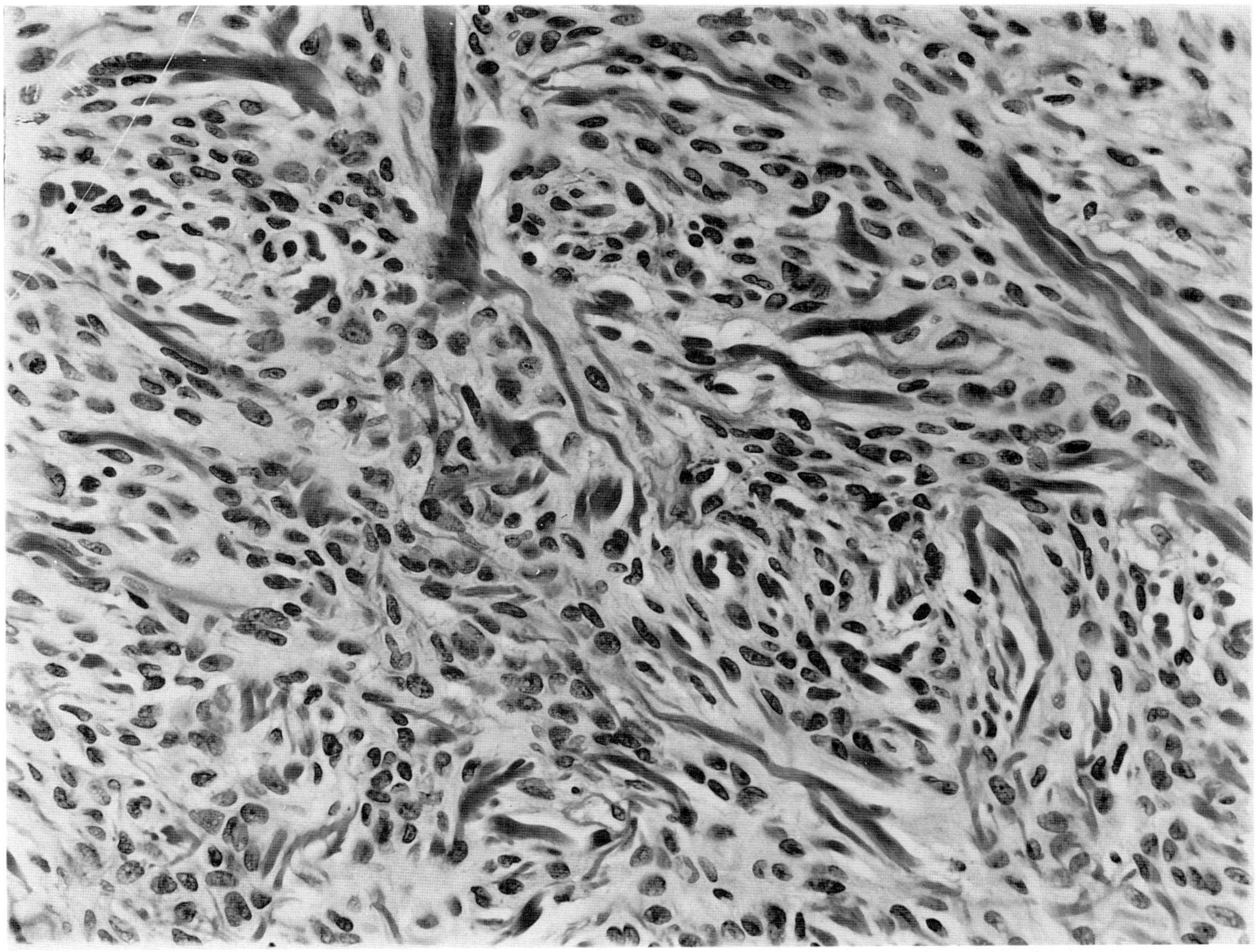

**Figure 13.5(b)** Myofibroblastoma. The proliferating spindle cells lack atypia or mitotic activity; the ribbons of collagen are characteristic. (H&E, X500)

## Pseudoangiomatous Change

This type of stromal alteration is described in Chapter 12, Vascular Lesions.

# BENIGN TUMORS

## Fibromatosis

A locally aggressive lesion, fibromatosis is most commonly encountered in the abdominal wall and less frequently in the breast.

Unlike abdominal desmoid, fibromatosis of the breast has not been associated with pregnancy and has been observed even in nulliparous women.

The first case involving the breast was reported by Nichols (48). Subsequently, sporadic cases were reported (34,37,39,40,44) with the first of several series appearing in 1981 (42,50,52).

### *Clinical Features*

Patients range in age from 14 to 80 with a median age of about 40 years. In the three reported series, all patients whose gender was known were women. A majority of cases are unilateral but both synchronous and asynchronous bilaterality occurs (50). A rare example of bilateral fibromatosis has been reported in a patient with Gardner's syndrome (43). Fibromatosis manifests as a painless, palpable, discrete mass that is firm and suggestive of carcinoma clinically. Skin dimpling, nipple retraction and a stellate mammographic appearance may be present (42,50), further complicating the clinical assessment of the lesion.

A

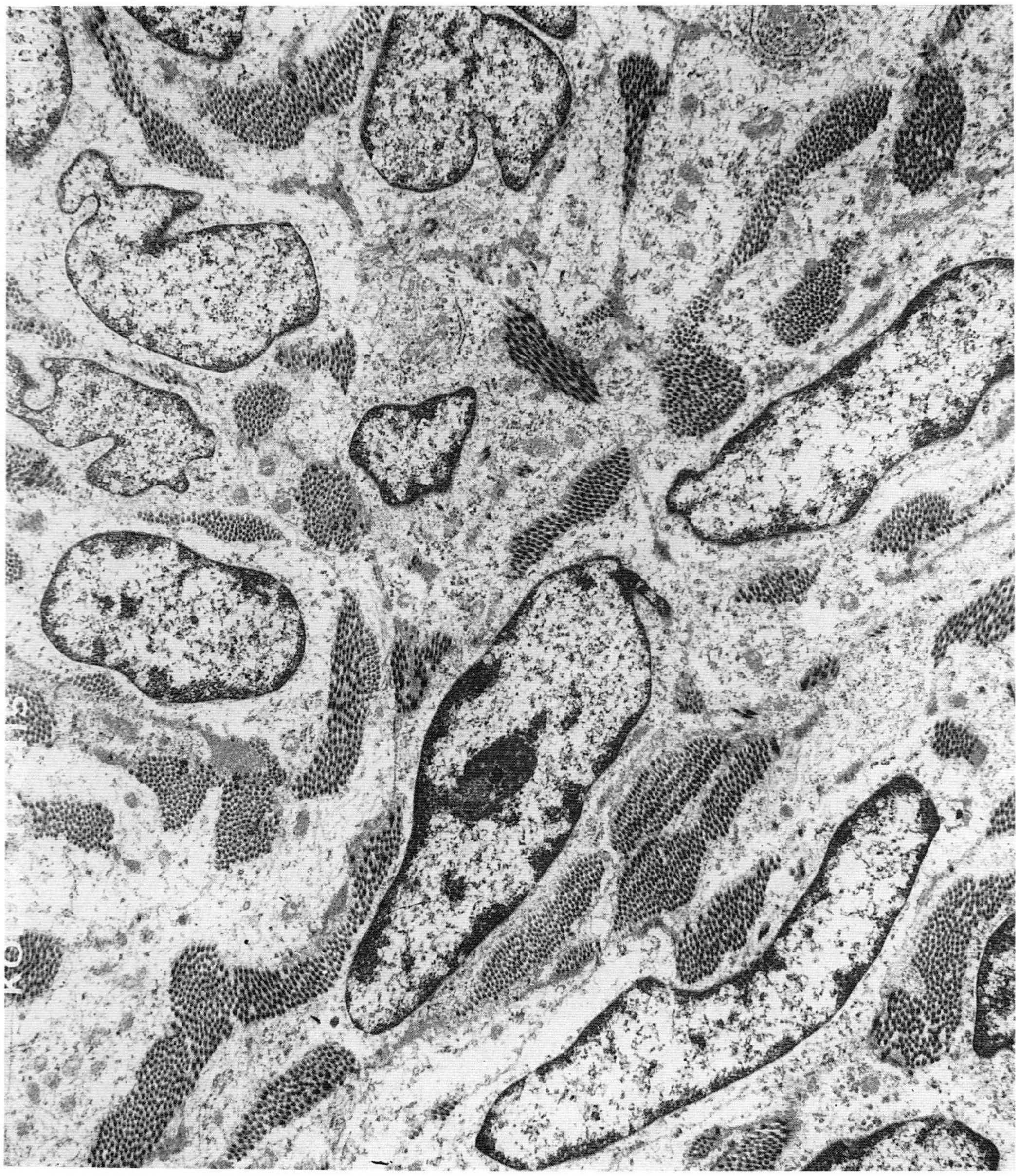

**Figure 13.6(a)** Ultrastructure of myofibroblastoma. Numerous spindle cells in this field are separated by collagen bands seen in cross section. (Uranyl acetate-lead citrate, X8,900)

B

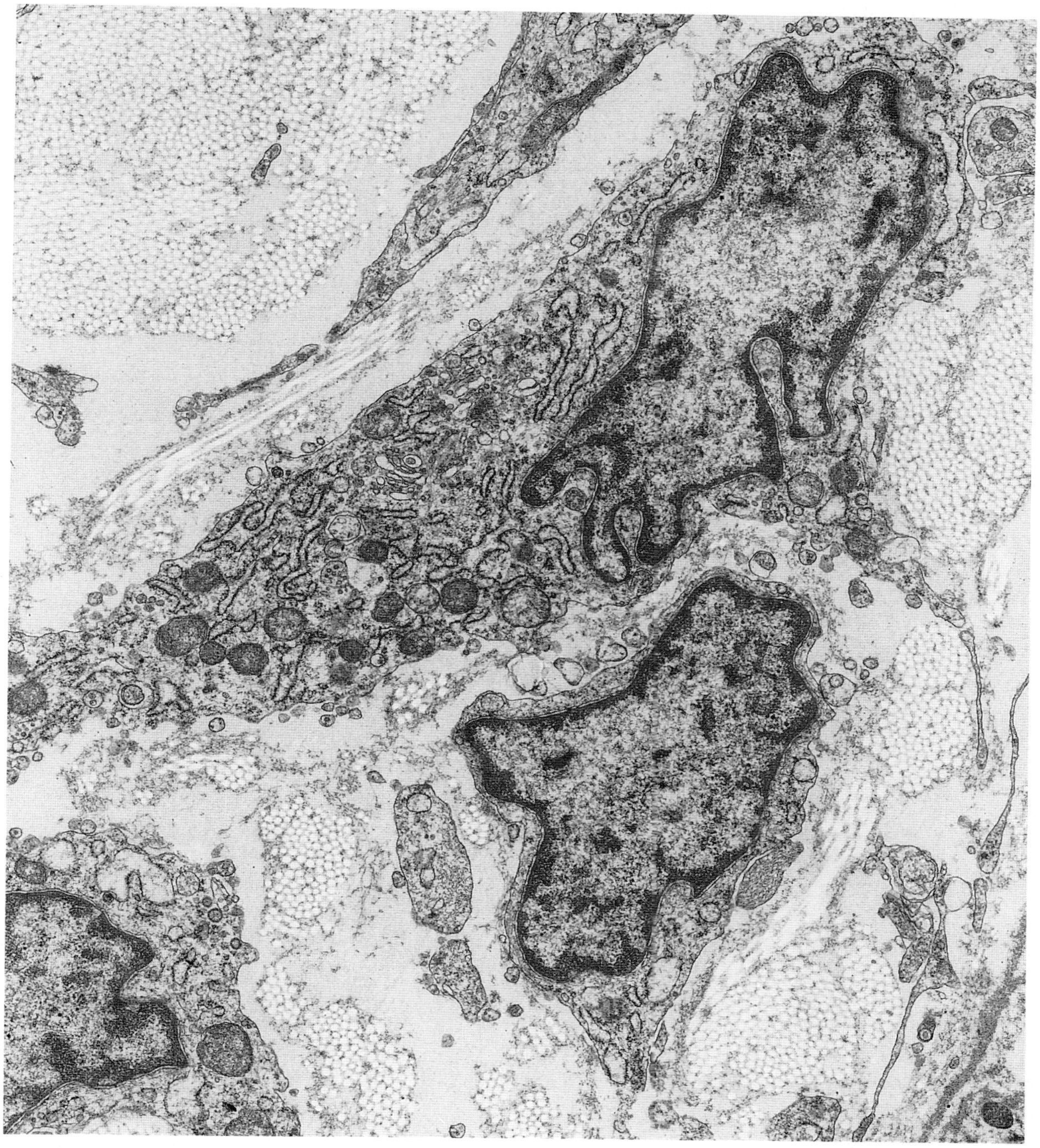

**Figure 13.6(b)** Ultrastructure of myofibroblastoma. The cell displayed is a typical fibroblast with abundant rough endoplasmic reticulum, but lacking pinocytotic vesicles and myofibrils with dense bodies. (Uranyl acetate-lead citrate, X4,400)

c

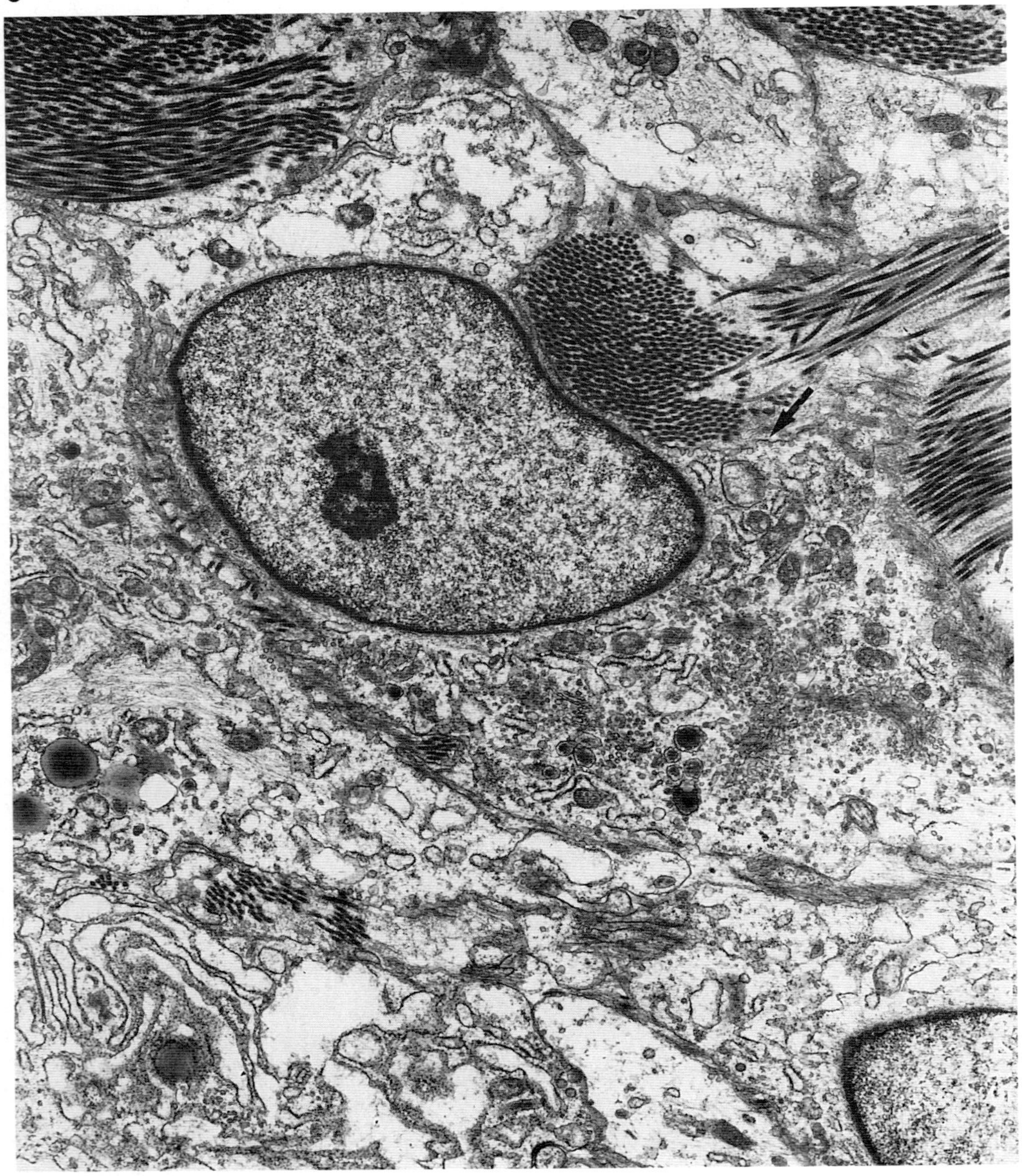

**Figure 13.6(c)** Ultrastructure of myofibroblastoma. This cell has pinocytotic vesicles (arrow) and a prominent Golgi apparatus, but lacks myofibrils and dense bodies or basal laminar investment. (Uranyl acetate-lead citrate, X11,000)

A

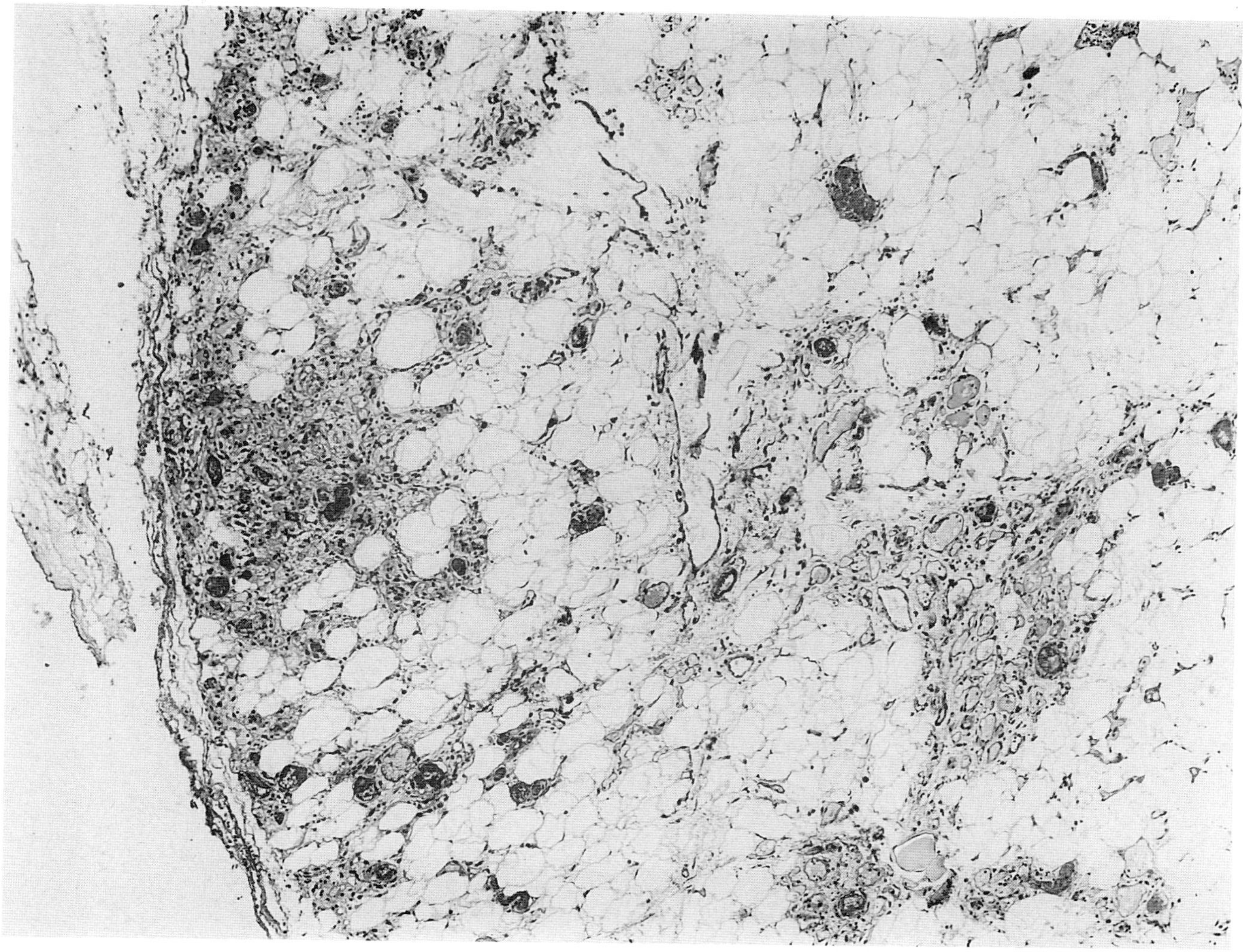

**Figure 13.7(a)** Angiolipoma. Note the delicate capsule and the relative abundance of the vascular component in this tumor. (H&E, X75)

Mammographically, it may mimic carcinoma (38,46). The duration of symptoms varies from several weeks to five years. One patient has developed fibromatosis from the capsule around a silicone breast implant (45). A case of fibromatosis with positive cytosol assays for estradiol and progesterone receptors has been described (49).

## *Macroscopic Features*

The lesions vary from 0.7 to 10 cm with a median of 2.5 to 3.0 cm. In contrast to the clinical features which suggest carcinoma, cross section of the lesion may be almost indistinguishable from normal breast tissue as it lacks the hardness of carcinoma or the fleshy consistency of some other cellular lesions. Most often, however, it is ill-defined. The color of the lesion varies from gray-yellow to gray-white depending on the amount of its collagen content. The gross appearance is far less impressive than the associated skin retraction.

## *Microscopic Features*

The lesion has irregular, infiltrating margins. It is composed of uniform, plump, spindle-shaped fibroblasts arranged in fascicles and interlacing bundles entrapping ducts and lobules (Fig. 13.4). The cells are intimately admixed with various amounts of fine collagen, and focally some display a myxoid matrix. The degree of cellularity varies ranging from relatively cellular lesions to predominantly collagenized tumors. If present at all, mitotic figures rarely exceed three to four per ten high power fields. Calcification and necrosis are absent. Finger-like projections into the surrounding adipose tissue are common but an

B

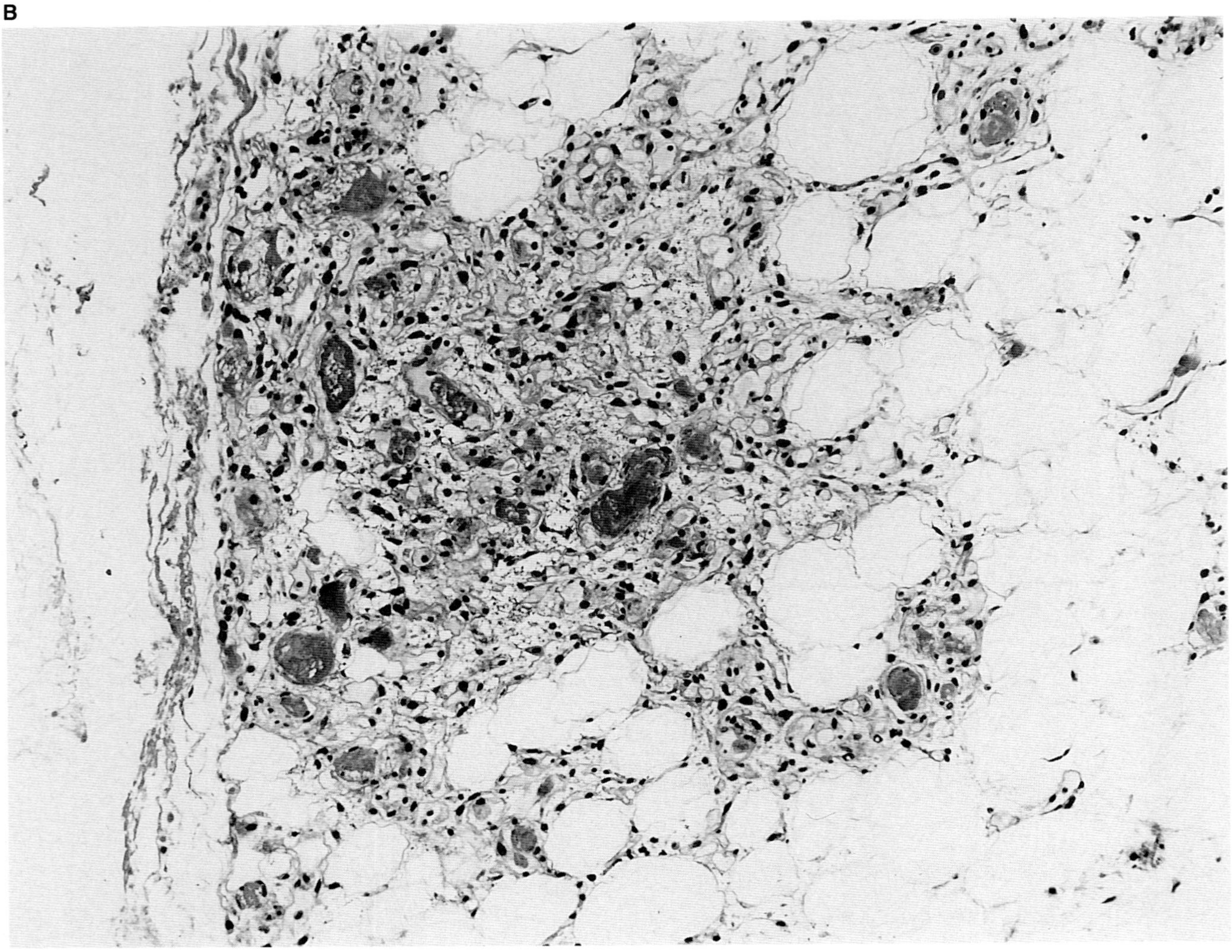

**Figure 13.7(b)** Angiolipoma. The vascular islands are composed of compact arrangements of small caliber vessels and capillaries packed with red blood cells (RBC) and fibrin thrombi. (H&E, X120)

occasional case is nodular with only minor irregularities in the margin.

## *Ultrastructural Features*

Fibromatosis consists of an admixture of fibroblasts and myofibroblasts. Gabbiani and Majno (41) have suggested that myofibroblasts are responsible for the contraction phase of palmar fibromatosis (Dupuytren's) contracture. They may also be responsible for the nipple retraction and the skin dimpling observed in mammary fibromatosis.

## *Differential Diagnosis*

Fibromatosis should be distinguished from fibrosarcoma. In general, sarcomas are richly cellular and display more cytologic atypia and pleomorphism, as well as more numerous mitotic figures. The proliferating cells in fibrosarcoma form long fascicles, herringbone patterns, and focal necrosis. These features are generally sufficient to make the accurate diagnosis.

## *Treatment*

Wide (total) local excision of this ill-defined lesion is the initial step in its management. Very large tumors may necessitate mastectomy to insure complete excision. Because of the benign nature of fibromatosis, every effort should be made to prevent undue deformity of the breast as a result of an excessive surgical procedure. Antiestrogen therapy (tamoxifen) has been reported to induce remission in cases of recurrent or locally aggressive fibromatosis not amenable

C

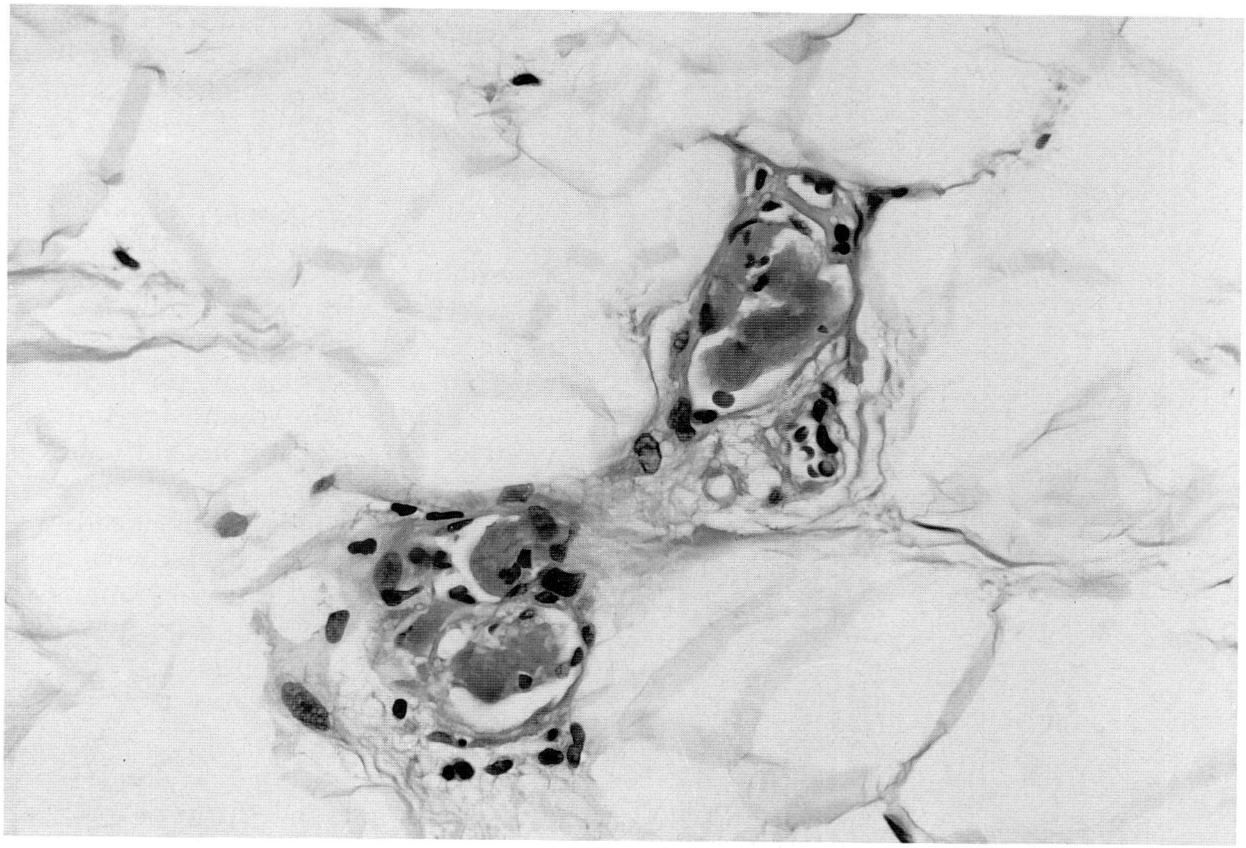

**Figure 13.7(c)** Angiolipoma. Typical microthrombi in multiple small vessels. (H&E, X240)

to wide local excision in other parts of the body (47,51).

As mentioned earlier, since this lesion may be grossly indistinguishable from relatively normal breast, surgeons face a difficult task of determining the precise extent of the lesion. Careful assessment of the margins of resection is particularly important for this lesion and may require multiple frozen sections of the margins intraoperatively.

### *Recurrence*

When recurrences develop, a majority do so within five years of the initial diagnosis (42). About 20% of cases with follow-up recur. Multiple recurrences are not uncommon. Therefore, continued follow-up is required. The morphology of the recurrent tumor is generally similar to that of the original lesion.

## Myofibroblastoma

A lesion that is seen predominantly in the male breast, myofibroblastoma is characterized by a nodular proliferation of plump spindle cells, punctated by wide ribbons of collagen (53).

### *Clinical Features*

Myofibroblastoma is a solitary, palpable, firm mass that is freely moveable, predominantly affecting men. Patients range in age from 41 to 85 years with a median of 63. Duration of symptoms ranges from one to six months. All but one of the reported cases have been painless. Patients have no history of prior trauma and no evidence of nipple retraction.

A

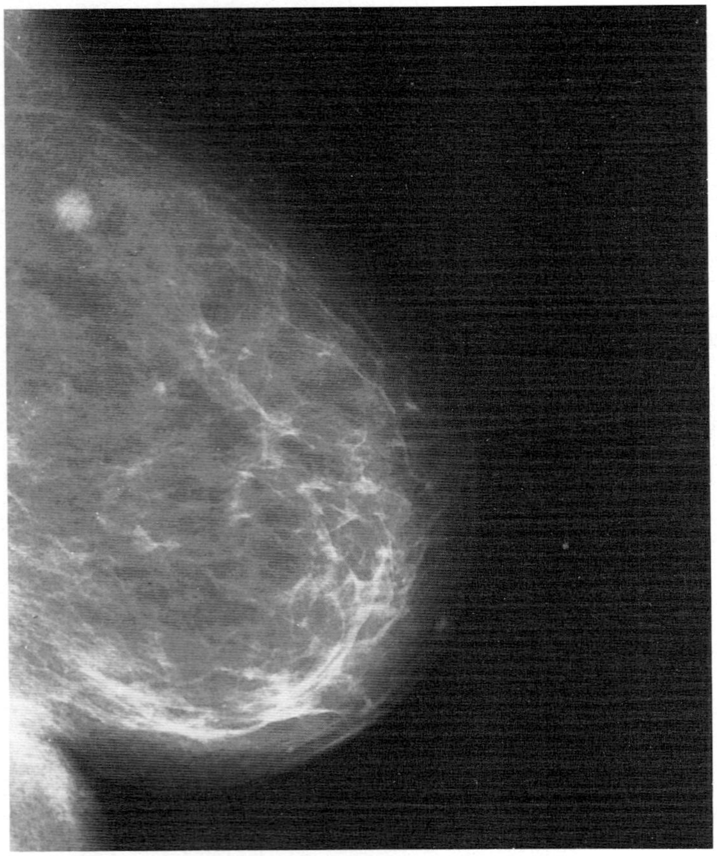

**Figure 13.8(a)** Granular cell tumor. Mammographically, the lesion often forms a discrete nodule.

### *Macroscopic Features*

All lesions are located in the breast parenchyma and range in size from 1 to 5 cm. Myofibroblastomas tend to be nodular, round, slightly lobulated and well circumscribed. Cut surface of the lesions appears dull, gray-pink to tan-white. Cysts and hemorrhage are absent.

### *Microscopic Features*

Some myofibroblastomas have a delicate fibrous capsule, while others are simply well-defined and circumscribed, often compressing the surrounding mammary stroma (Fig. 13.5a). The tumor is generally moderately cellular and composed of uniform, bipolar, ovoid to spindle cells arranged diffusely or in clusters and interspersed by broad ribbons and bands of collagen. Mitotic figures are rare and around 0 to 1 per 10 HPF. About 15% display diffuse increased cellularity but even these lack atypia or significant mitotic activity (Fig. 13.5b). Mast cells are seen in many cases. Occasionally, cartilagenous metaplasia is seen in myofibroblastoma (53), but this feature does not seem to significantly influence the clinical behavior. Focal or diffuse prominent vascularity is noted in some cases.

### *Immunohistochemistry*

Depending on the myofibroblastic content of the tumor, the reaction for actin varies considerably. Some cases display minimal if any positivity with actin while others show positivity in up to three quarters of the cells. Interestingly, six of seven cases evaluated for vimentin at AFIP showed diffuse and strongly positive reaction and the seventh case had focal positivity. But then, practically all mesenchymal lesions and even some epithelial tumors have displayed positive reaction for vimentin in my experience at AFIP. The tumor cells do not react with either desmin or S-100 protein.

### *Ultrastructural Features*

In my personal evaluation of four examples of this lesion at the ultrastructural level, the lesion displayed great variation in its cellular composition—from those having a preponderance of either fibroblasts or myofibroblasts to those composed of an almost equal admixture of the two. A case with abundant fibroblasts and occasional smooth muscle cells has also been described (35). Thick bundles of collagen, corresponding to the collagen bands seen on H&E sections, are interspersed between the cells (Fig. 13.6). A previously described benign spindle cell tumor of the male breast was also composed of myofibroblasts at the ultrastructural level and judging from the light microscopic illustration would qualify as a myofibroblastoma (36).

### *Treatment*

Local excision is adequate treatment for myofibroblastomas. Recurrences have not been reported.

## Lipoma

A relatively common benign lesion, lipoma also occurs in the breast (54,56,57). The typical patient with

B

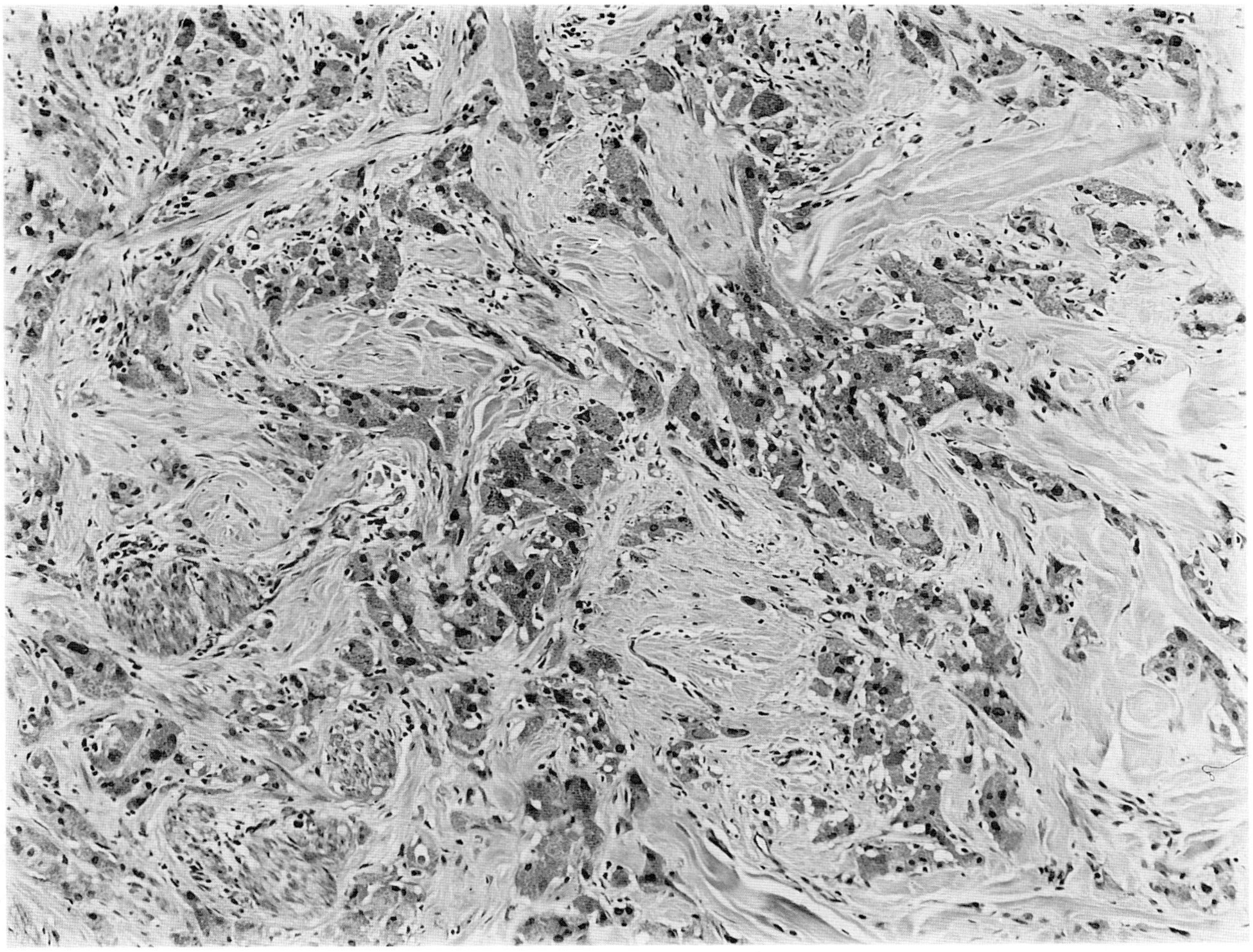

**Figure 13.8(b)** Granular cell tumor. Microscopically, some infiltrate the breast in small irregular islands and cords separated by dense stroma. (H&E, X60)

lipoma is in her late forties or early fifties. The tumor presents as a solitary, unilateral mass in the majority of patients but in about 3% of the patients, bilateral tumors are identified. Lipoma is soft, freely moveable and well delineated. The average size of the tumor is around 2.5 cm but they can be larger than 10 cm (55). Cross section of lipoma reveals a well-circumscribed, lobulated, yellow mass.

Microscopically, the majority are composed of typical round, mature lipocytes. Because of the abundance of adipose tissue in the breast, the presence of at least a delicate capsule around the tumor is required for diagnosing a lipoma. Lipoblasts and nuclear atypia are absent. Rarely, uniform spindle cells associated with a mucoid matrix and bundles of mature collagen are present; this finding would qualify the tumor as a spindle cell lipoma.

## Angiolipoma

Clinically and grossly, angiolipomas very much resemble lipomas. More than 75% of the patients reported in the literature have been older than 50 years; the youngest patient was 26 years of age (58,60–62). Fifty-six mammary angiolipomas were diagnosed at AFIP between 1970 and 1989. The youngest patient was a 1-year-old black female and the oldest patient was an 82-year-old caucasian male. The median age was 59 years. Fifteen of the 56 patients were male. One patient, a 71-year-old man, had bilateral angiolipomas, and another patient had a simultaneous angiolipomas on the shoulder. Computed tomography has pointed to subtle differences which can distinguish angiolipomas from carcinoma (62).

C

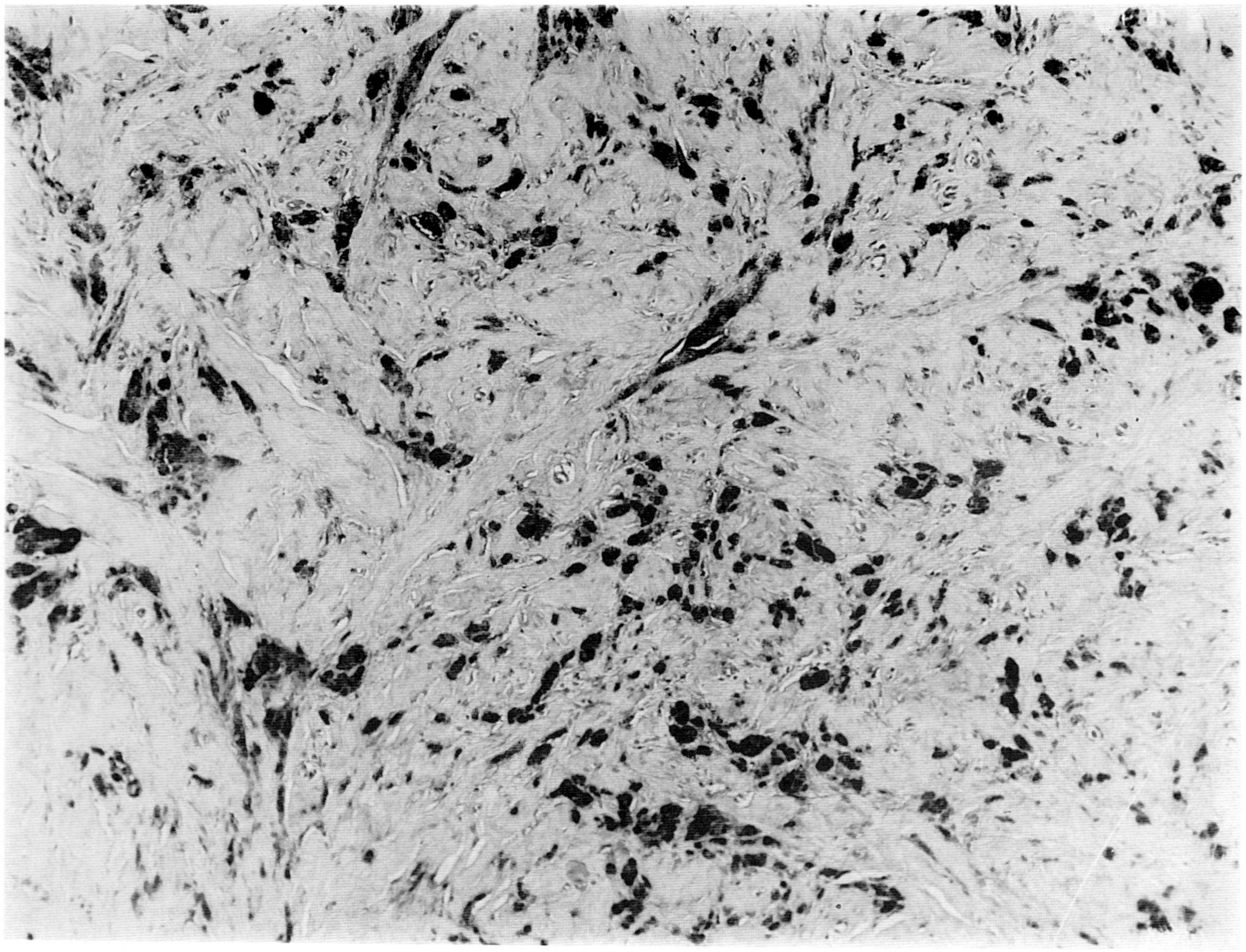

**Figure 13.8(c)** Granular cell tumor. The cells show a positive reaction for S-100 protein. (S-100, X60)

Angiolipoma presents as a solitary, unilateral, multiple synchronous or metasynchronous bilateral tumor mass(es), (58). While more than half of angiolipomas occurring in other sites present with pain, particularly on palpation, mammary angiolipomas are notoriously painless. Rarely exceeding 2 cm in size, angiolipomas are encapsulated, yellow nodules with focal gray or reddish areas.

Microscopically, a conspicuous vascularity is a distinctive feature of angiolipomas (58,62). The branching vascular network is generally distributed diffusely among the mature lipocytes but clustering in the subcapsular region is common (Fig. 13.7). Some of the congested vessels may simulate a cavernous hemangioma. The hallmark of this lesion is the presence of scattered microthrombi in small vessels (Fig. 13.7c). Mature lipocytes are the dominant component of the lesion in most cases. We have not seen any infiltrating angiolipomas among the 56 mammary angiolipomas reviewed at AFIP. The richly vascular intramuscular tumor diagnosed as angiolipoma by Franzini et al (61) probably reflects an intramuscular hemangioma in which portions of the muscle have been replaced by fat. Enzinger and Weiss (59) did not describe any examples of infiltrating angiolipoma in their discussion of soft tissue angiolipomas. They suggested that tumors previously described as infiltrating angiolipoma represent either examples of intravascular hemangiomas or angiomatosis.

The etiologic factors in the development of angiolipoma remain uncertain. Some have raised the possibility that it results from alterations within preexisting lipomas triggered by repeated mild trauma, but a direct relationship to trauma does not exist in most cases. The possible role of hormonal factors

D

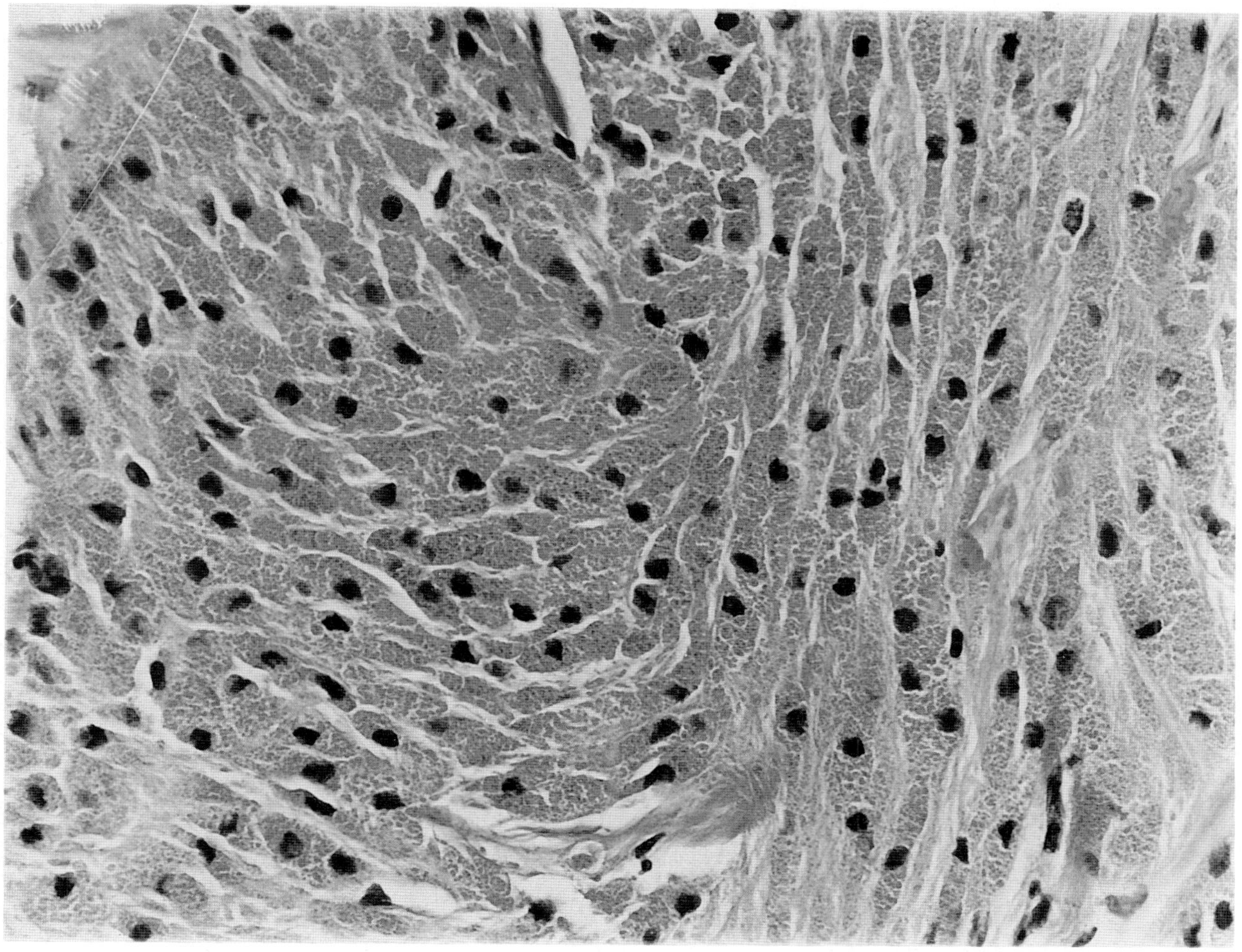

**Figure 13.8(d)** Granular cell tumor. Other tumors form solid nests of cells without intervening stroma; the proliferating cells have finely granular eosinophilic cytoplasm. (H&E, X400)

elaborated by the tumor (angiogenesis factor) has also been implicated (63). Angiolipomas are benign and simple excision is adequate treatment.

## Granular Cell Tumor

Granular cell tumor is a well-recognized lesion which occurs in a wide variety of visceral and cutaneous sites. Until recently, the nature and histogenesis of this tumor has been controversial resulting in the noncommital designation of granular cell tumor. The positive immunoreaction of the tumor cells with S-100 protein has established the neural origin of granular cell tumor (63,70,72).

The predilection for women demonstrated by these tumors suggests a hormonal relationship. None of the four mammary granular cell tumors evaluated demonstrated significant estrogen or progestin binding, however (68). A positive reaction for carcinoembryonic antigen (CEA) has been observed in granular cell tumors (68,71).

About 6% of these tumors have been reported in the breast (63,64,68,69,73). Haagensen and Stout (67) provided one of the earlier descriptions of granular cell tumor in the mammary glands reporting five cases in 1946. Granular cell tumors are far less common than breast carcinomas; there are about 1,000 cases of breast carcinoma for every case of mammary granular cell tumor (66). Mammary granular cell tumor occurs in a wide age range (21 to 75 years), the average being in the 30s (65). While the majority of patients are female, occasionally the lesion does develop in the male breast. Clinically the lesion can simulate carcinoma because of its fibrous consistency,

A

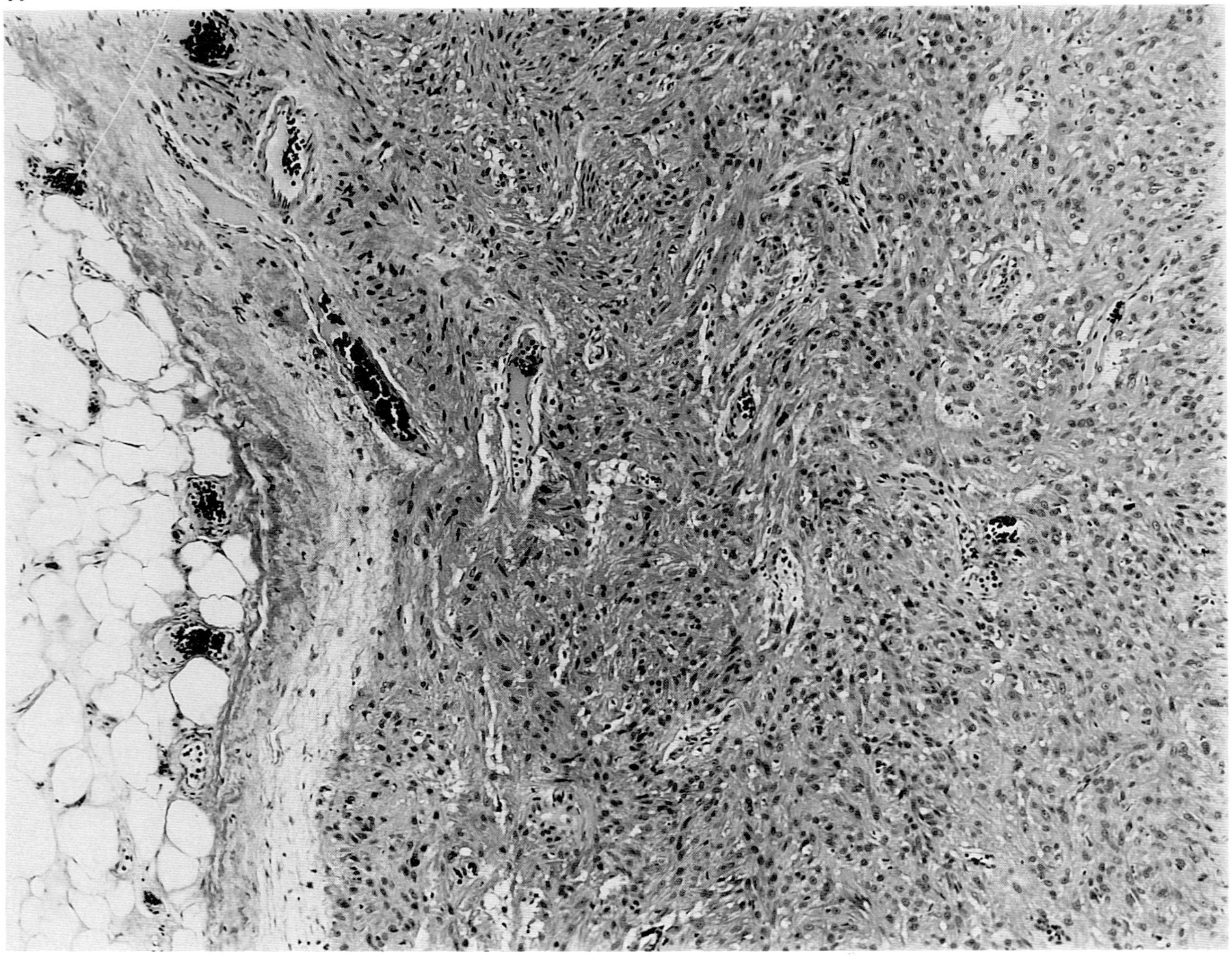

**Figure 13.9** Leiomyoma. (a) The margin is encapsulated. (b) Typical interlacing bundles of smooth muscle lacking atypia or mitotic activity with entrapped ductules. (H&E, (a) X175; (b) X100)

fixation to pectoral fascia, and skin retraction. While some granular cell tumors manifest as discrete rounded nodules mammographically (Fig. 13.8), others tend to present as stellate lesions on mammogram which strengthens the clinical impression of carcinoma.

A majority of these tumors are located within the breast parenchyma but they may involve the nipple enlarging it "massively" (4.5 cm). Most tumors are less than 2 cm in size, however. Cross section of the lesion is generally more sharply circumscribed and more uniform than the typical carcinoma but some are endurated and irregular enough in their outline that carcinoma cannot be excluded without microscopic inspection (74).

## *Microscopic Features*

Microscopically, granular cell tumors display either a well-defined, lobulated, pushing margin, or a stellate, infiltrating pattern. The latter can easily be confused with carcinoma especially when associated with marked desmoplasia or when tissue preparation is suboptimal. Needle biopsies can be particularly problematic. Granular cell tumor is composed of infiltrating cords and clusters or solid nests of uniformly rounded or polygonal cells with coarsely granular cytoplasm and small centrally-located round nuclei (Figs. 13.8b, 13.8d). Some tumors display mild nuclear pleomorphism. The cytoplasmic granules do not reflect glycogen as they stain with PAS both before and after diastase predigestion. A positive

B

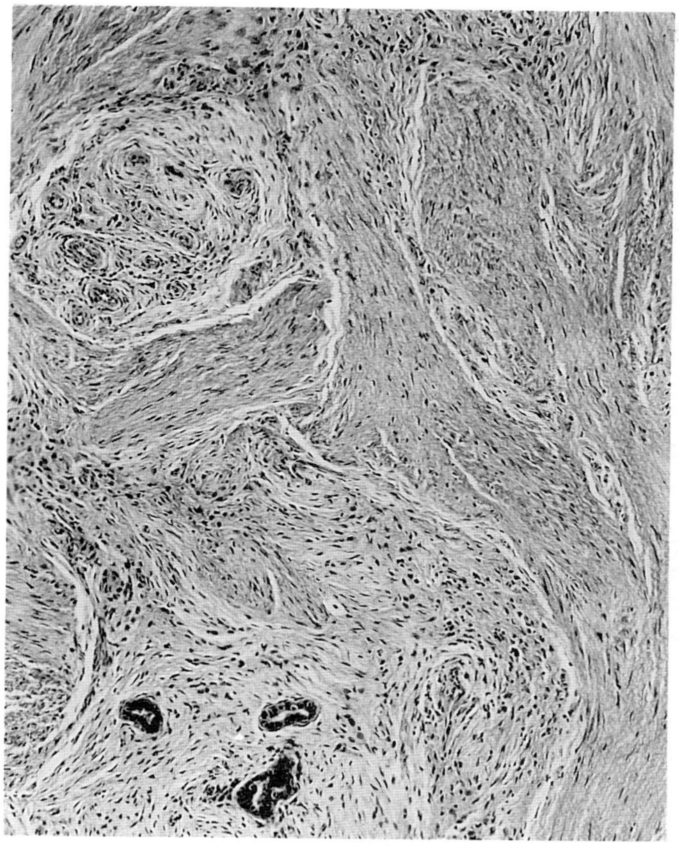

**Figure 13.9(b)** Leiomyoma. Legend on opposite page.

immunoreaction for S-100 protein confirms the diagnosis (Fig. 13.8c). To avoid missing a carcinoma, special stains are recommended for confirmation of the diagnosis for tumors that deviate from the classic appearance, in particular those simulating a carcinoma.

On very rare occasions, granular cell tumor may metastasize to axillary lymph nodes. Only one such case has been reported in the literature (65) and we recently reviewed a granular cell tumor with axillary node metastases at AFIP. The metastasis was in the contralateral axillary nodes in a patient who also had asynchronous bilateral breast carcinoma. In contrast to malignant granular cell tumors that are generally large with local invasion, pleomorphism and mitotic activity, the tumor with nodal metastases reviewed at AFIP lacked atypia or mitotic figures. The precise aggressive potential of granular cell tumors that metastasize to axillary nodes has not been established. Local excision of the tumor is curative in almost all cases.

## Myoid Lesions

Benign smooth muscle tumors and lesions with rhabdomyoblastic differentiation are particularly rare in the breast. A few cases of benign leiomyoma have been reported (77,78,84,86). The three cases I have seen over a five-year period displayed either irregular proliferation of bundles of smooth muscle in the nipple and beneath the areola or actually formed a discrete nodule in the subareolar region (Fig. 13.9). Mitotic activity and atypia are absent in these benign smooth muscle proliferations. There are no mammary rhabdomyomas in the AFIP files.

## Neurofibroma and Neurilemoma

Neurofibromas and neurilemomas have rarely been reported in the breast (85). Excluding all unequivocally subcutaneous lesions in the region of the breast, there are 50 mammary neurofibromas in the AFIP files. The 50 patients ranged in age from 14 to 73 with a median of 36 years. Seventeen of the patients were known to have von Recklinghausen's disease. It is quite possible that an additional number may have had neurofibromatosis, but the information was not provided to reviewers at AFIP.

Fifteen neurilemomas have been diagnosed in the breast at AFIP. Eight of the patients were men. Patients ranged in age from 20 to 90 years with a median of 30 years.

Grossly and microscopically, neurilemomas and neurofibromas occurring in the breast are identical to those occurring in soft tissues elsewhere in the body.

The neurilemomas and neurofibromas are benign and local excision is adequate treatment.

During the same period of time, two cases of malignant schwannoma and one case of neurofibrosarcoma were diagnosed at AFIP.

## Miscellaneous Benign Tumors

In addition to the tumors listed already, chondroma (80), chondrolipoma (76,79,81,83), chondromyoli-

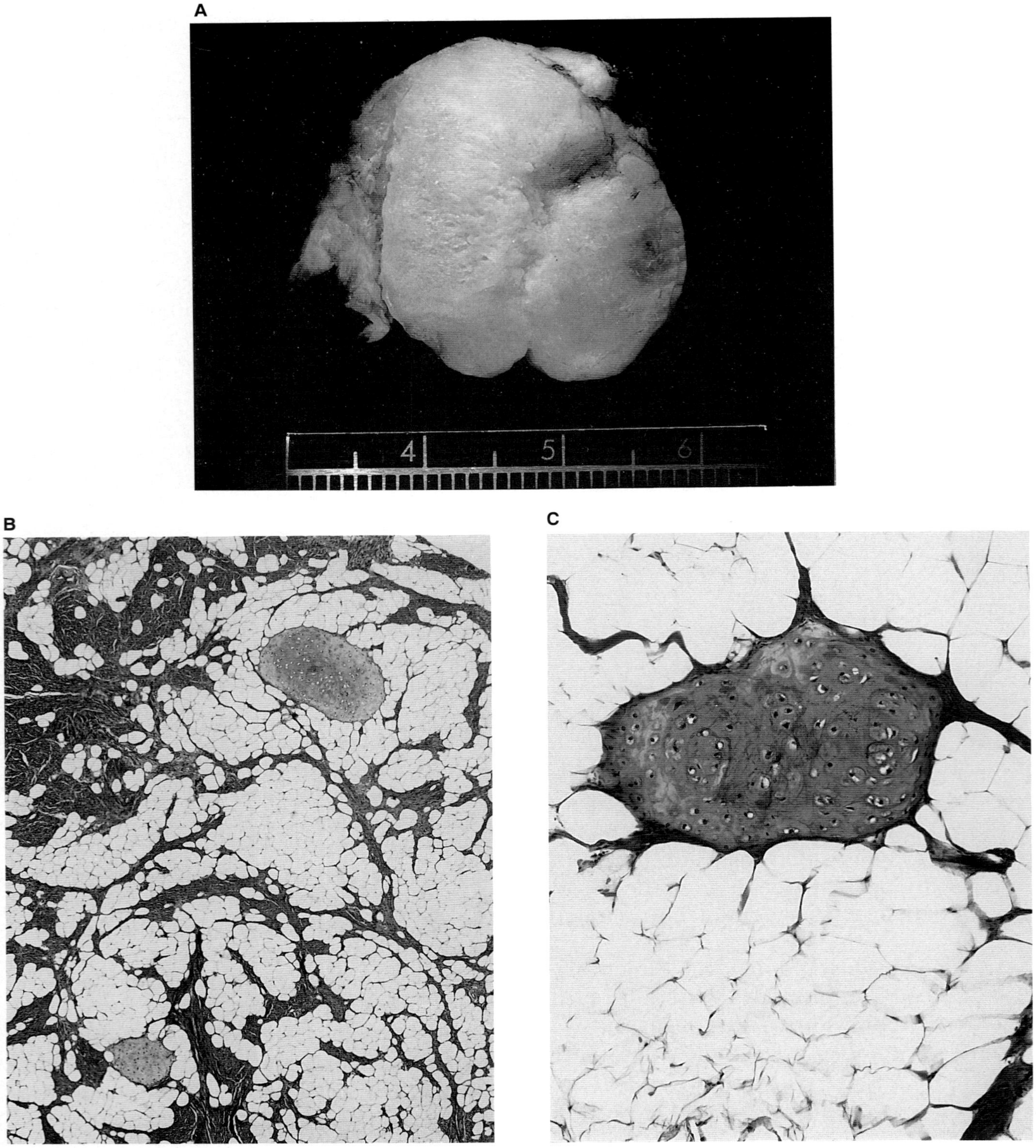


**Figure 13.10** Chondromyolipoma. (a) Grossly, the tumor is well circumscribed and solid, with a relatively uniform appearance on its cut surface. (b) Islands of fat cells are separated by bands of smooth muscle with small nodules of cartilage dispersed in between. (c) The cartilage is mature and lacks atypia. (H&E, (b) X12; (c) X24)

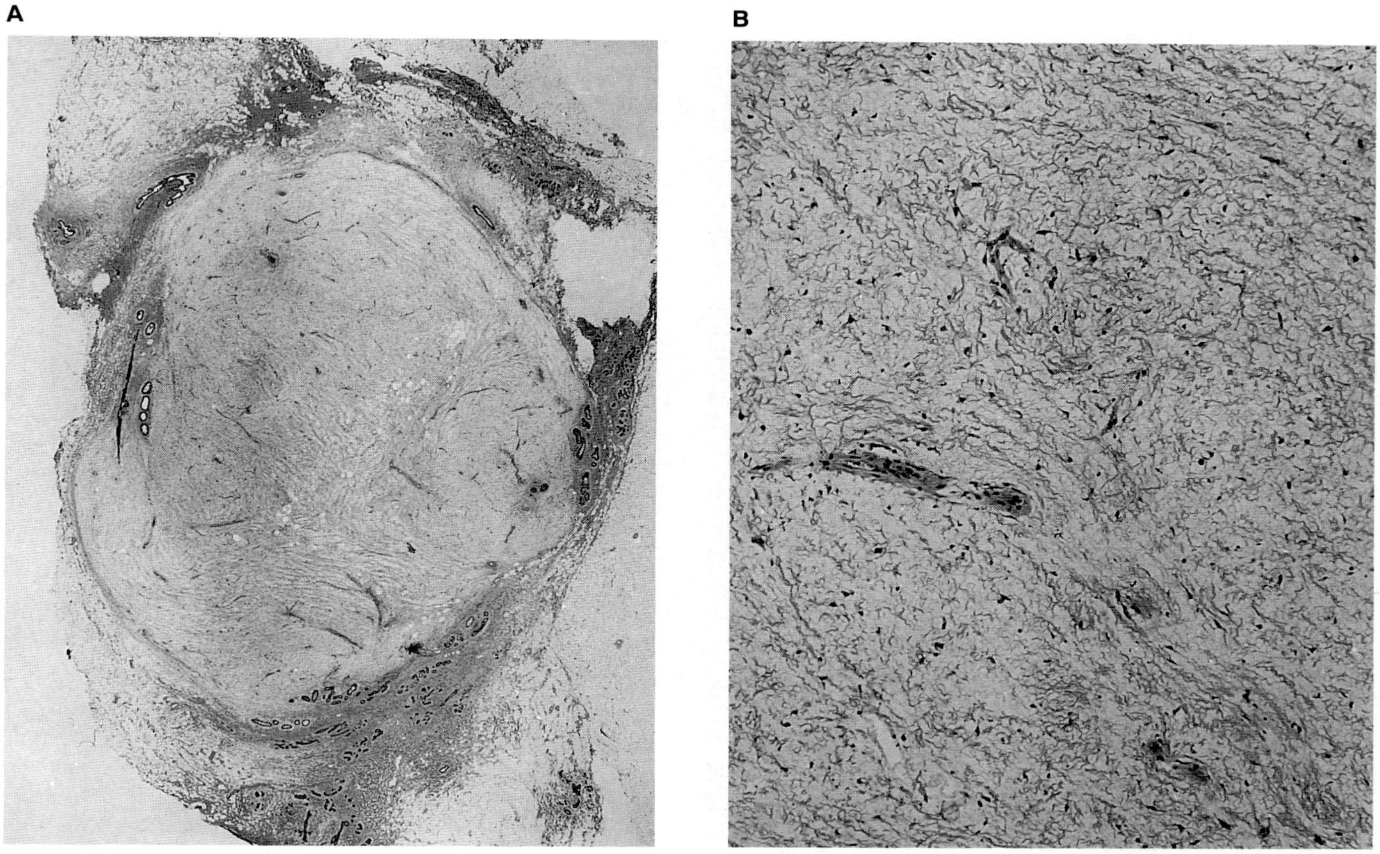


**Figure 13.11** Myxoma. (a) The lesion is well circumscribed and appears hypocellular at low magnification. (b) Small pyknotic nuclei are dispersed in a myxedematous-appearing background. (H&E, (a) X7.5; (b), X100)

poma (Fig. 13.10), myxoma (Fig. 13.11) (75), fibromyoma (83), and nodular fasciitis also occur in the breast.

## SARCOMAS

Malignant mesenchymal tumors (sarcomas) constitute less than 1% of all malignant neoplasms of the breast. Most studies using the designation of mammary sarcoma describe a variety of lesions including cystosarcoma phyllodes and angiosarcoma (88,89,92, 93,95). Some have proposed the term stromal sarcoma for pure spindle cell sarcomas developing from the "specialized" breast stroma. Most breast sarcomas can and should be classified histogenetically; the spindle cell sarcomas that cannot be subclassified should be designated as spindle cell sarcoma, not otherwise specified (NOS), rather than stromal sarcoma (Fig. 13.12). Many of these spindle cell sarcomas are composed of fibroblasts variably admixed with myofibroblasts. Among other sarcomas, malignant fibrous histiocytoma, chondrosarcoma, and rhabdomyosarcoma are seen with greater frequency than leiomyosarcoma and alveolar soft part sarcoma which are particularly rare. When they occur, chondrosarcoma and rhabdomyosarcoma are encountered more often as a component of a biphasic tumor (cystosarcoma phyllodes or carcinosarcoma) than in pure form.

Following histogenetic classification, the sarcomas should be graded noting the number of mitotic figures per ten high power fields (10 HPF), cellularity, pleomorphism (atypia), and presence or absence of necrosis (91). The mammary sarcomas can be divided into low, intermediate, or high grade on the basis of these features and the type of margin (Table 13.1). Necrosis has been found to be the best histopathologic parameter in predicting the time interval to recurrence and the overall survival of the patients with soft tissue sarcomas (87). The presence of either a focally invasive margin or focal necrosis in an otherwise low grade tumor would qualify it as an

A B

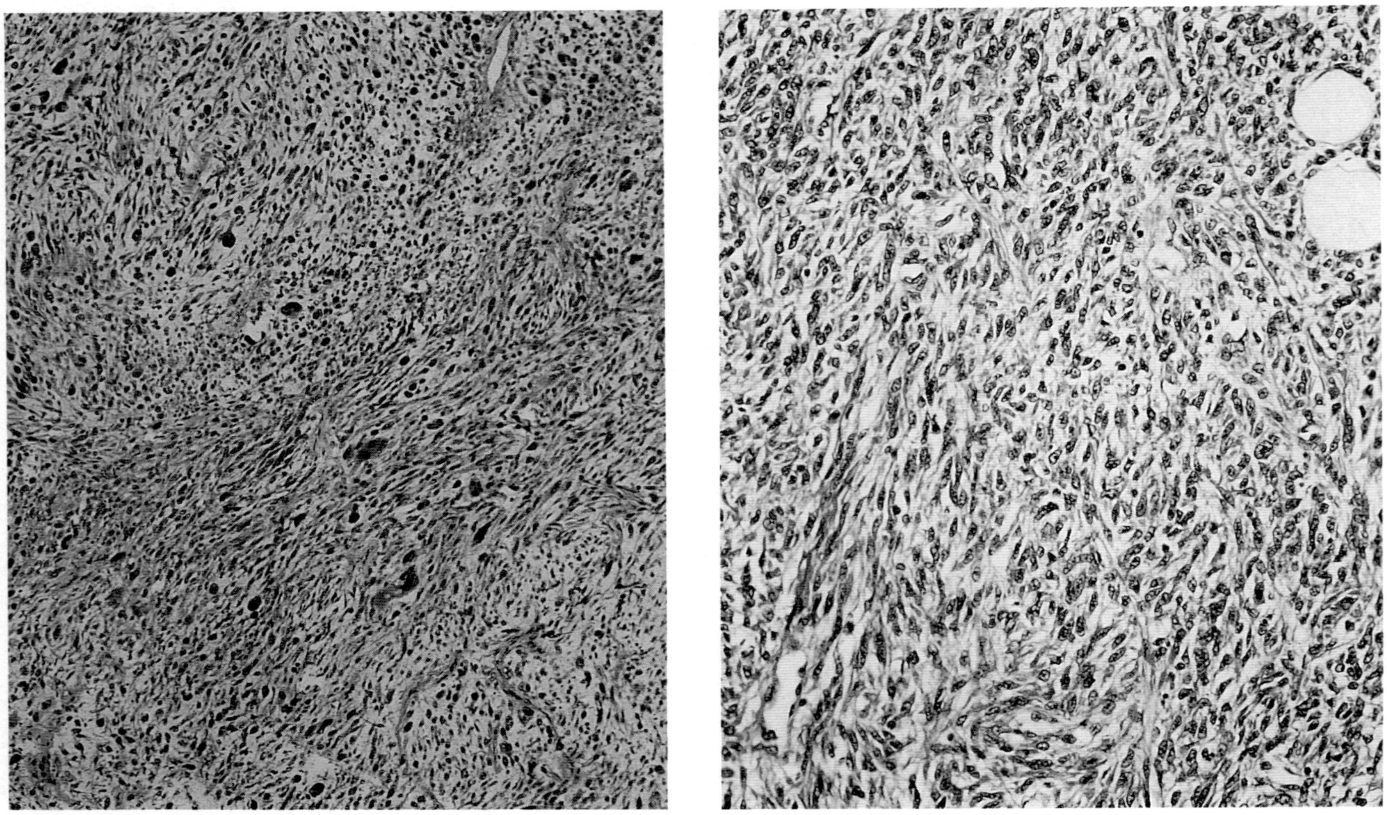

**Figure 13.12** Low grade spindle cell sarcoma, "stromal sarcoma." (a&b) A densely cellular spindle cell tumor with occasional atypical and multinucleated cells, which lack significant pleomorphism and mitotic activity. Necrosis is absent. (H&E, (a) X75; (b) X100)

**Table 13.1** Microscopic Features of Low-Grade vs High-Grade Sarcoma

| |
|---|
| **Low-grade sarcoma** |
| <5 mitotic figures/10 HPF |
| absent to mild atypia |
| moderate cellularity |
| pushing margins |
| necrosis absent |
| **High-grade sarcoma** |
| ≥5 mitotic figures/10 HPF |
| moderate to severe atypia |
| dense cellularity |
| irregular or invasive margins |
| necrosis may be present |
| **Intermediate-grade sarcoma** |
| A low grade sarcoma with either focal necrosis or focally infiltrating margins |

intermediate grade lesion. The significance of necrosis as a prognostic factor has not been systematically assessed in mammary sarcomas.

Factors that have been noted as having an adverse effect on prognosis of mammary sarcomas include histologic grade, high mitotic rate, and infiltrating margins (Fig. 13.13) (87,94). The guidelines recommended for separating low grade from high grade sarcomas are listed in Table 13.1.

Tumor size was included among adverse prognostic factors by Norris and Taylor (94), but two subsequent studies did not find a correlation between tumor size and outcome (87,96).

When sarcomas metastasize, they do so through the bloodstream and most frequently go to the lungs. Axillary node metastasis is extremely rare and involvement is often by contiguous spread rather than through metastasis.

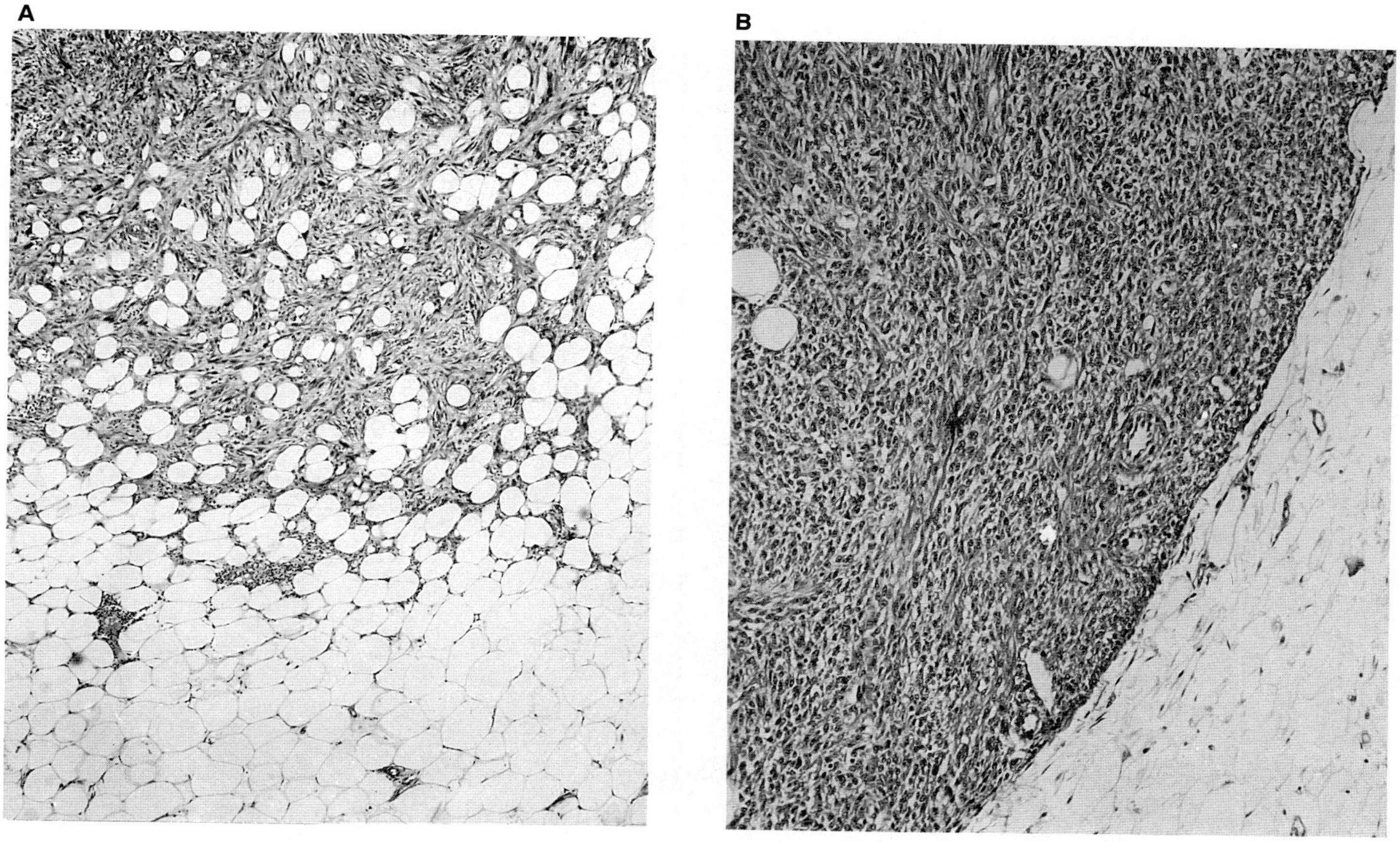


**Figure 13.13** Spindle cell sarcoma. (a) Some tumors display a deeply invasive margin extending into adipose tissue. (b) In contrast, others show a pushing margin. (H&E, (a) X50; (b) X160)

## *Treatment*

Recommendations for treatment of mammary sarcomas have varied from total excision to mastectomy with adjuvant therapy. Callery et al (90) consider simple mastectomy adequate treatment as it affords excellent local control. Total excision is probably sufficient for small, circumscribed, low grade sarcomas. Wide local excision has been recommended for treatment of sarcomas in general in some of the older studies (94). For high grade sarcomas, longer disease-free intervals are obtained in patients with adjuvant chemotherapy. Excision of axillary nodes is not warranted considering the rarity of their involvement.

## *Differential Diagnosis*

Spindle cell sarcomas should be distinguished from fibromatosis, metaplastic carcinomas, malignant myoepitheliomas, and sarcomatous overgrowth in a cystosarcoma phyllodes. Adequate sampling is important particularly in identifying the epithelial component of cystosarcomas and of those metaplastic carcinomas containing recognizable epithelial elements. Evaluation of one tissue block per 1 cm of maximum tumor diameter would ensure adequate sampling in solid tumors. Fibromatosis is less cellular, lacks atypia, and its mitotic activity does not exceed 0 to 1 per 10 HPF; nonetheless, it can be

**Table 13.2** Dominant Immunohistochemical and Ultrastructural Features of the Neoplastic Cells in Stromal Sarcoma, Spindle Cell Carcinoma, and Malignant Myoepithelioma

| | **Stromal sarcoma** | **Spindle cell ca** | **Malignant ME** |
|---|---|---|---|
| Kermix | − | + | ± |
| Actin | ±* | − | + |
| S-100 | − | − | ± |
| Tonofilaments | − | + | ± |
| Desmosomes | − | + | ± |
| Myofibrils with dense bodies | − | − | + |
| Pinocytotic vesicles | − | − | + |
| Basal lamina | ± | − | + |

Abbreviations: ME = myoepithelioma; + = generally present in a diffuse manner; ± = present in some cells; ±* = present in some cases; − = Generally absent

A

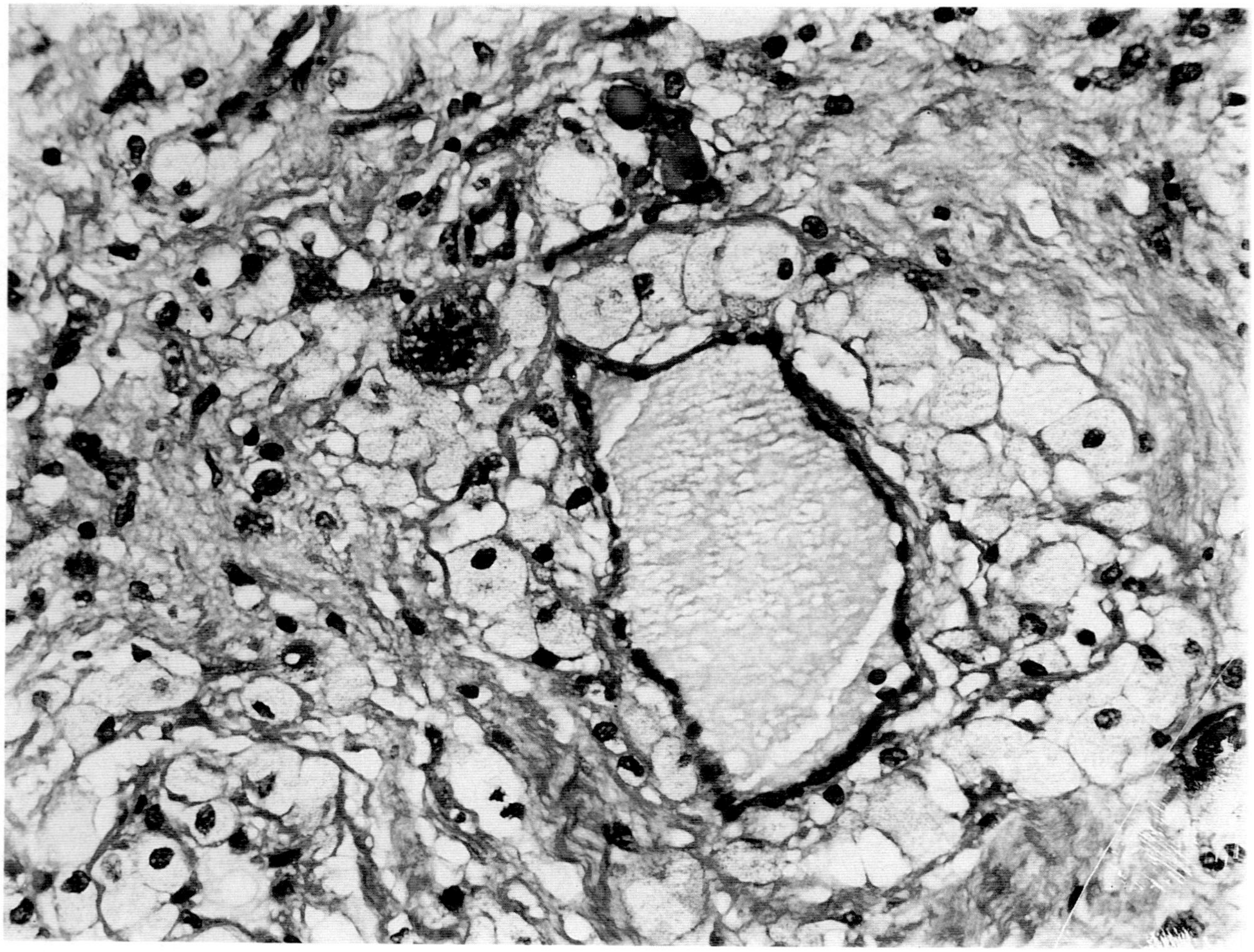

**Figure 13.14(a)** Liposarcoma. Other than an abnormal mitotic figure, there is little evidence of atypia in most cells in this field. (H&E, X700)

B

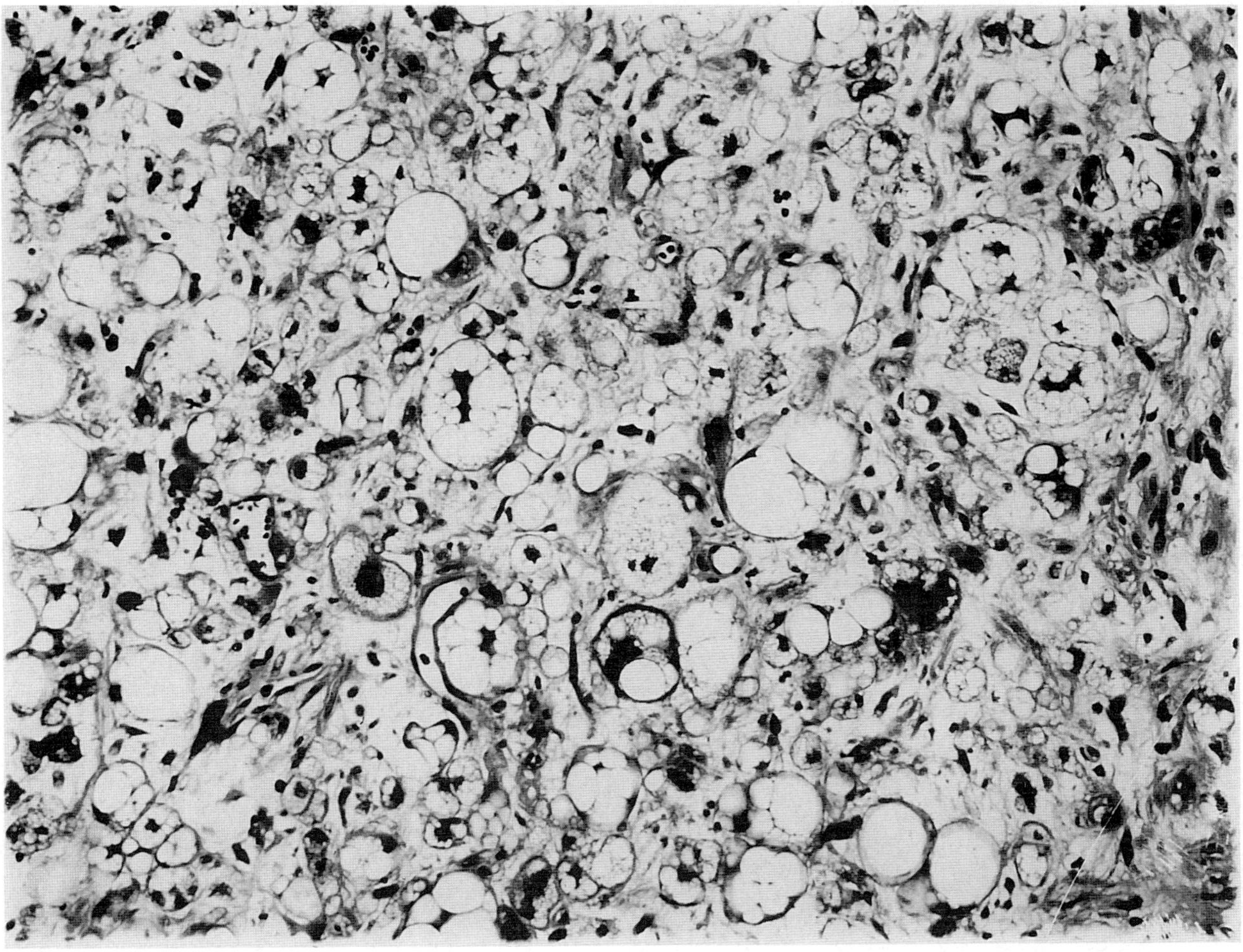

**Figure 13.14(b)** Liposarcoma. Lipoblasts with vacuolated cytoplasm and typical scalloped nuclear margin are readily recognizable. (H&E, X450)

A

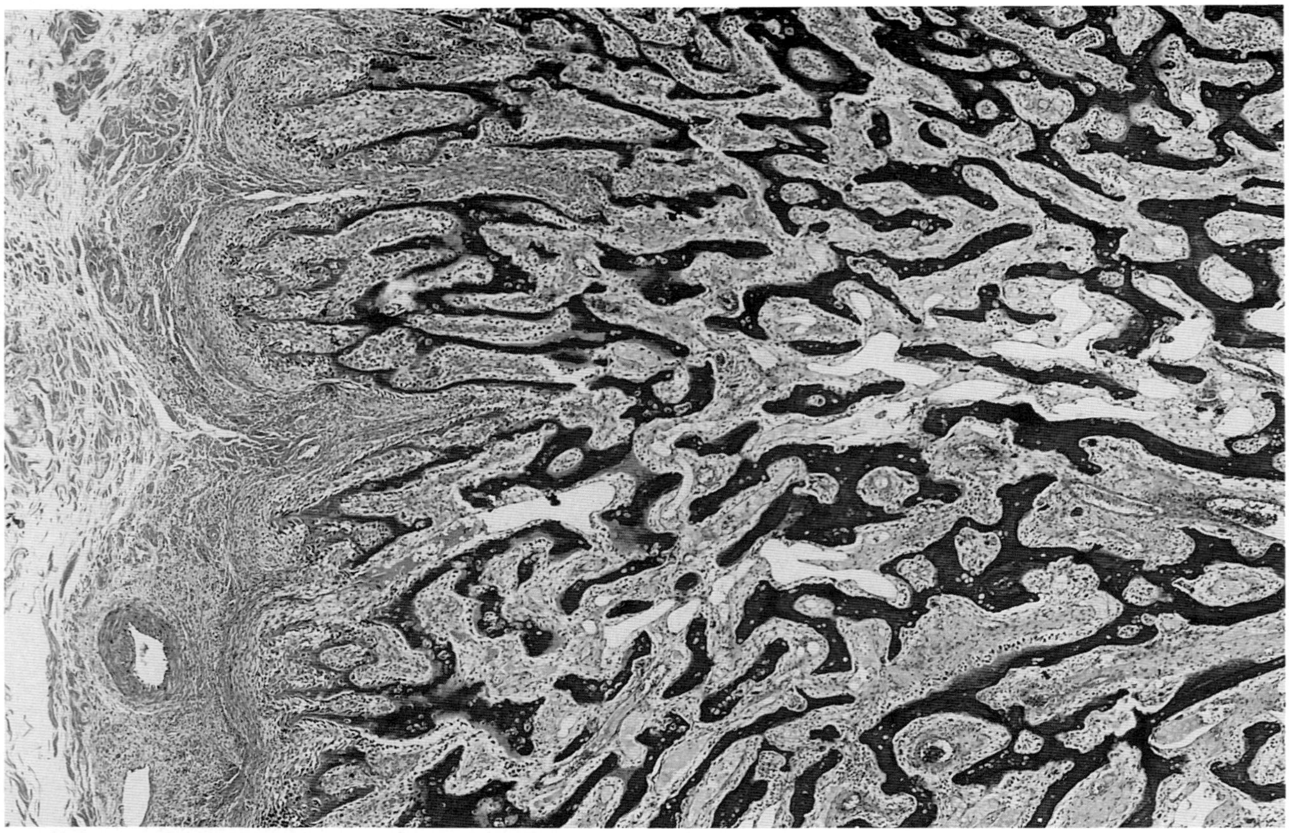

B

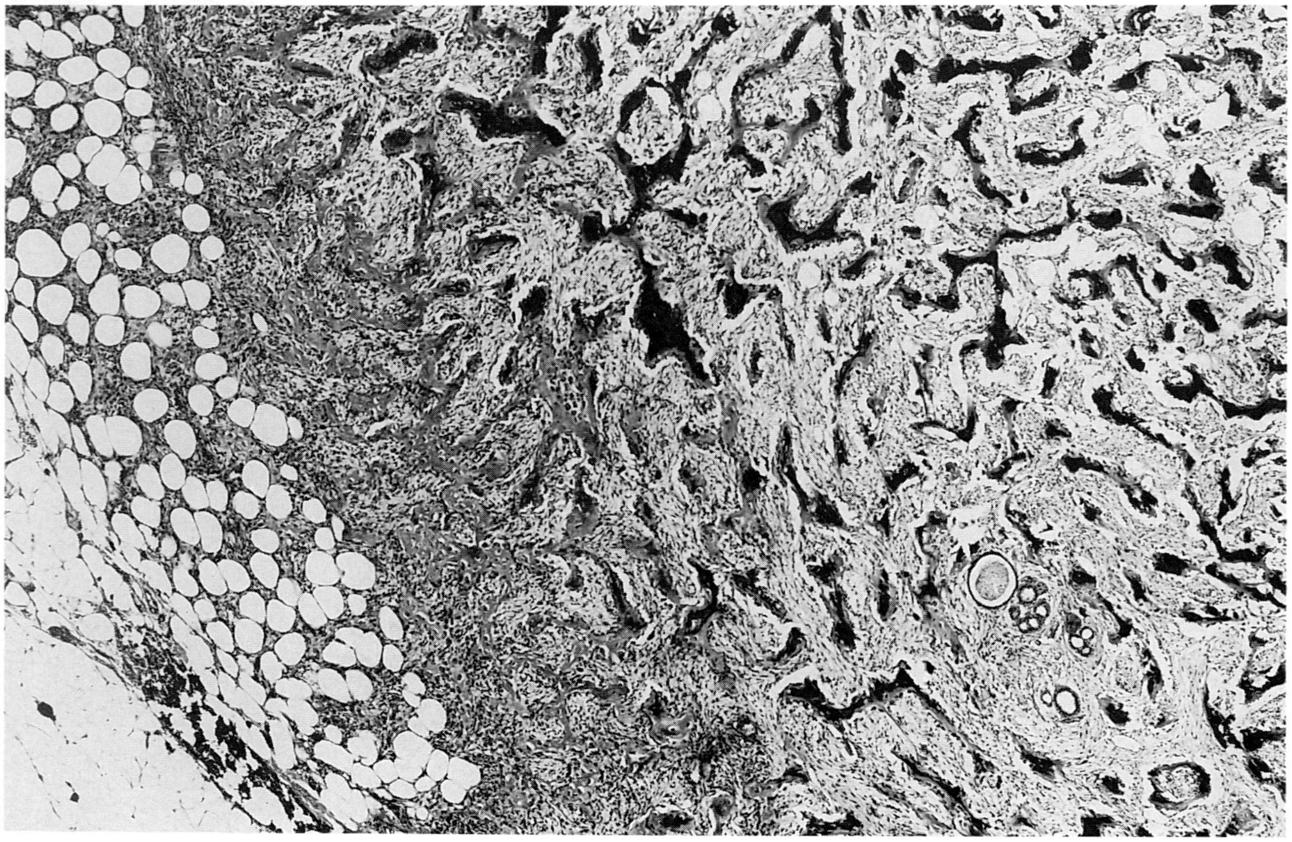

**Figure 13.15** Osteogenic sarcoma. (a) The central, more mature portion of the tumor showing a lace-like arrangement of calcified osteoid trabeculae; note the pushing margin at the periphery. (b) Focal marginal irregularity and non-calcified trabeculae of osteoid at the periphery. (c) A spindle cell sarcoma with mitotic figures (arrow) occupies the spaces between the trabecular network of osseous material. (H&E, (a) X60; (b) X60; (c) X75)

C

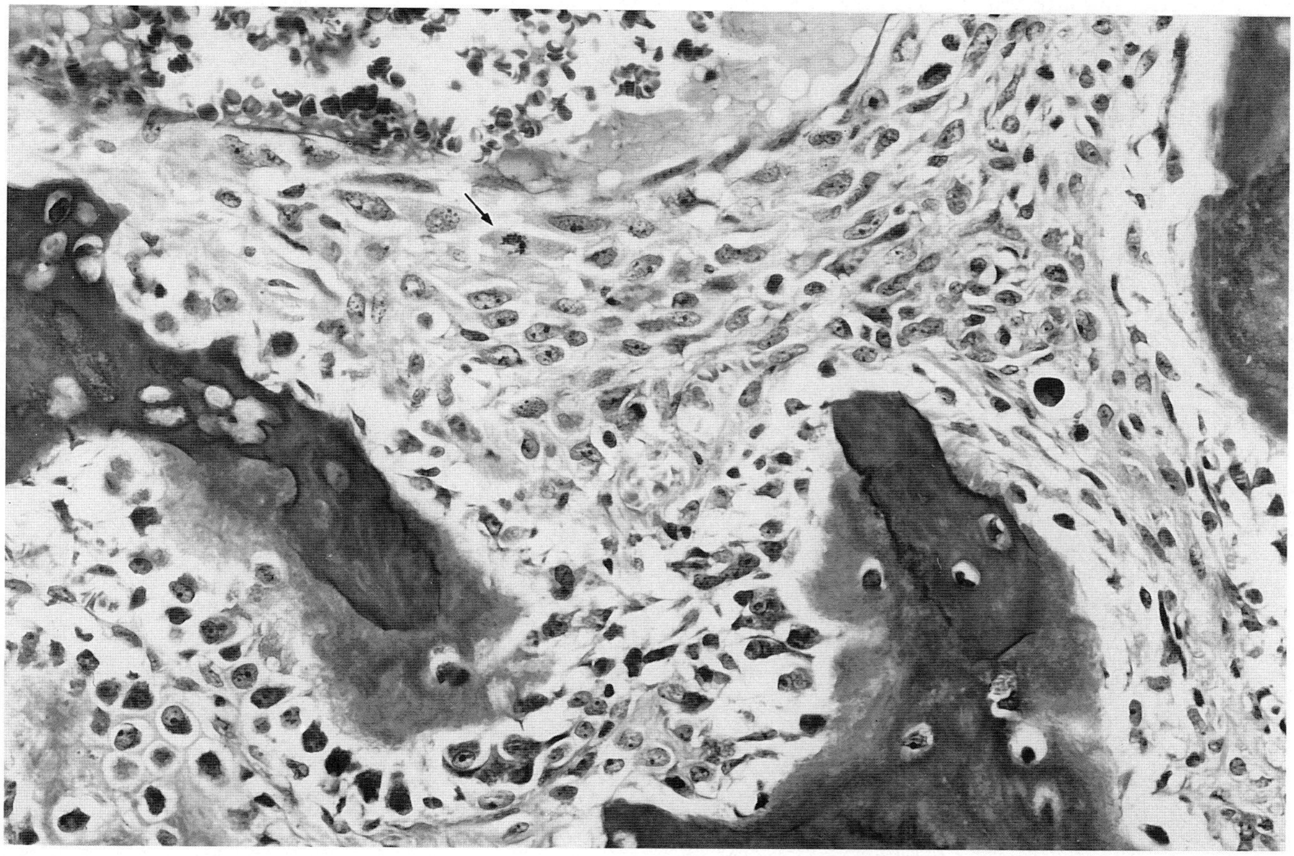

**Figure 13.15(c)** Osteogenic sarcoma. Legend on opposite page.

difficult to separate fibromatosis from a low grade fibrosarcoma. Branching, broad bundles of spindle cells dissecting between normal breast structures is more typical of fibromatosis.

Distinguishing pure spindle cell carcinoma and malignant myoepithelioma from spindle cell sarcoma requires a number of special studies. Immunoreaction for cytokeratin, S-100 protein, and actin can resolve the problem in about 80% to 85% of cases but ultrastructural analysis is necessary in the remaining cases. It is quite possible that the series of spindle cell sarcomas reported in some of the older studies (prior to the utilization of either immunohistochemistry or electron microscopy) were contaminated by spindle cell carcinomas and myoepithelial carcinomas. As a general rule, sarcomas do not show a positive reaction for cytokeratin. Exceptions occur particularly in leiomyomas and post-radiation sarcomas which may show a positive reaction for cytokeratin. In general, in these situations rare cells may show a positive reaction for cytokeratin or epithelial membrane antigen but such cells constitute less than 5% of the cell population. On the other hand, spindle cell carcinoma shows a uniform and diffuse positivity. Some spindle cell carcinomas have a prominent fibroblastic/myofibroblastic stroma; in these tumors, immunoreactions for cytokeratin unmasks a more recognizable epithelial pattern. Myoepithelial carcinomas display a positive reaction for both actin and S-100 protein but generally not to the same degree. It should be kept in mind that immunoreactions do not always provide the answer.

Ultrastructural analysis may be needed to more precisely determine the nature of some pure spindle cell tumors. Ultrastructurally, myoepithelial cells have myofibrils with dense bodies, pinocytotic vesicles, patchy to complete basal lamina reflecting the myoid aspect of their differentiation, and tonofilaments as well as occasional tight junctions representing their epithelial features. Unfortunately, a number of recent reports have illustrated what is claimed to be a myoepithelial cell when hardly more than a few bundles of intermediate filaments are demonstrated in the cytoplasm. Based on such erroneous interpretations, conclusions have been made which are not justified. Rare tight junctions and desmosomes have been observed in a variety of sarcomas. Therefore, the ultimate diagnosis in difficult cases should be

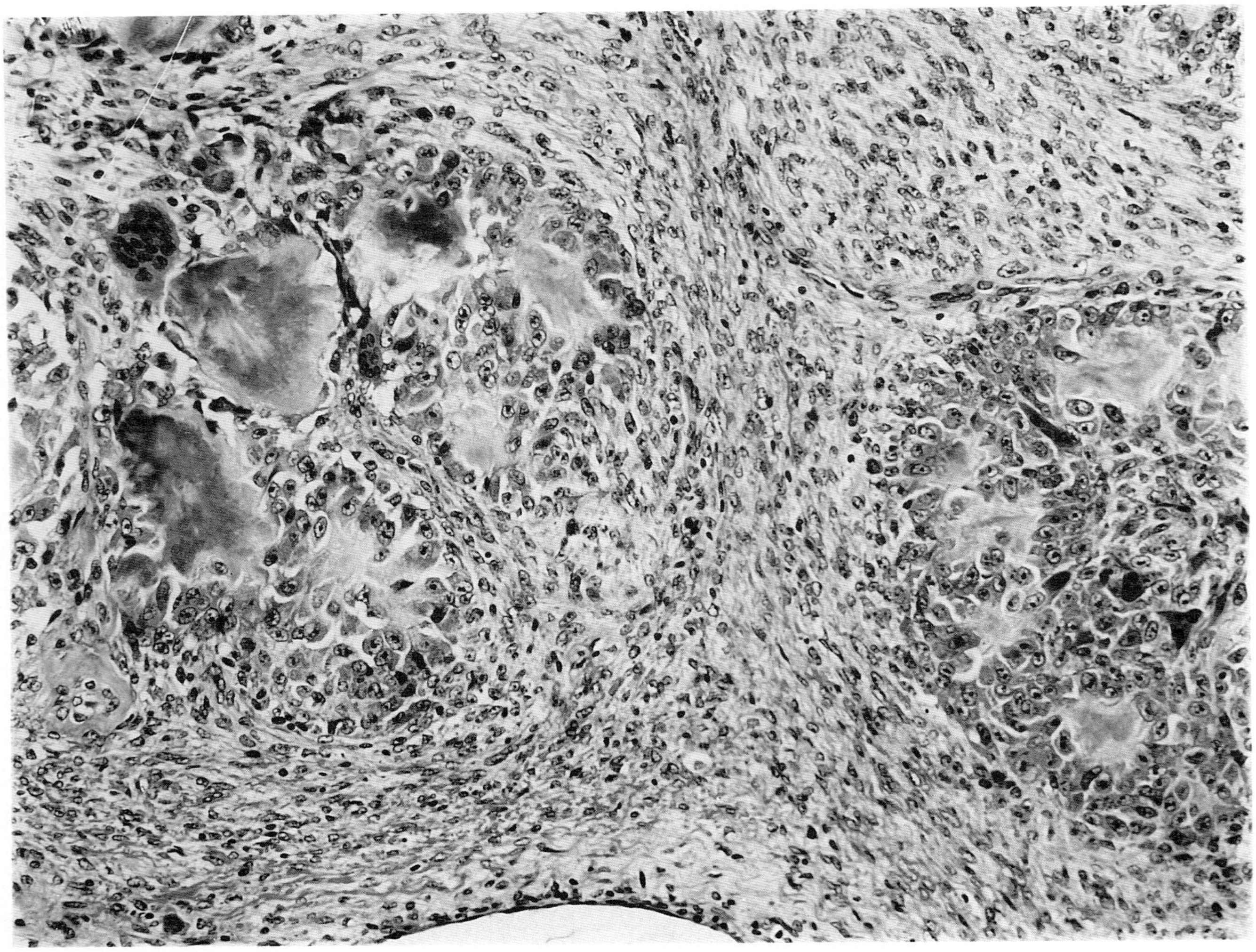

**Figure 13.16** Osteogenic sarcoma. A fibrosarcomatous spindle cell background with aggregates of osteoid undergoing mineralization; numerous osteoblasts and a few osteoclasts surround the osteoid material. (H&E, X200)

based on a combination of morphology on light microscopic evaluations, immunohistochemical profile, and the dominant cell population ultrastructurally (Table 13.2).

## Liposarcoma

Liposarcoma is among the rarest of malignant breast tumors (98,99,102,105,109,112,113). It may arise directly from the mammary adipose tissue or it may develop as a component of a cystosarcoma phyllodes. Around one hundred cases of mammary liposarcoma have been reported with detailed pathologic description and follow-up information available on about 40% of these cases (97,98,103,104,106). Rarely, liposarcoma develops following radiation therapy for breast carcinoma (97).

### *Clinical Features*

Patients with pure liposarcoma range in age from 26 to 76 with a median of 47. While a majority of patients have been female, two of the 13 patients in the most recent series (98,100) were male. Most tumors manifest as slowly enlarging, painful breast masses that have been present from several months to several years. While liposarcoma is characteristically unilateral at presentation, bilateral mammary involvement has been reported (107). Generally, skin changes and axillary node enlargement do not occur.

### *Gross Pathology*

While the median size of liposarcomas is large at 8 cm in greatest diameter, some reach an enormous size measuring 19 cm in diameter. Many are well circumscribed or encapsulated but about one third of the tumors are irregular, infiltrative, or lobulated. The cut

A

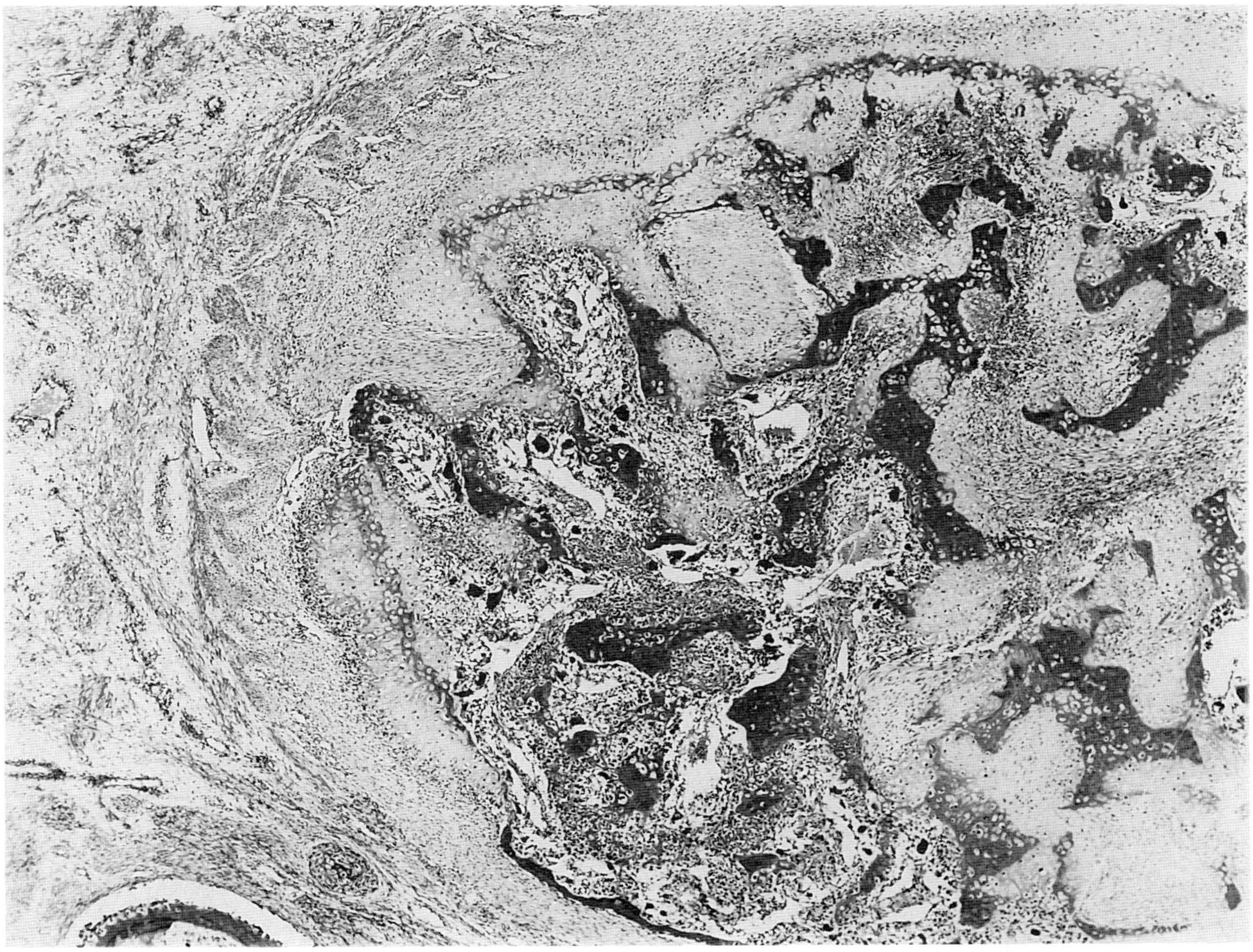

**Figure 13.17(a)** Osteogenic sarcoma. A sharply-circumscribed tumor nodule showing alternating zones of enchondrol ossification surrounded by spindle cells. (H&E, X100)

surface appearance varies depending on the histologic types. Some are soft and gelatinous reflecting the myxoid component of the tumor. Others are more firm and yellow to tan in color. Necrosis and hemorrhage are present in some of the larger tumors.

### *Microscopic Features*

Three variants of liposarcoma have been seen in the breast. These include myxoid, well differentiated and pleomorphic liposarcoma (Fig. 13.14). The myxoid variant is characterized by a myxoid matrix and a delicate capillary pattern providing background support for the proliferating lipoblasts in various stages of differentiation. The well-differentiated liposarcoma closely resembles a lipoma except for the presence of scattered lipoblasts along fibrous septae. A lymphoplasmacytic infiltrate is present in some. The pleomorphic liposarcoma is composed of a highly pleomorphic cell population and giant cells containing lobulated aggregates of chromatin. Mitotic figures are readily identifiable in pleomorphic liposarcoma.

### *Differential Diagnosis*

Vacuolated cells occur in a variety of other lesions that may be confused with lipoblast. Lipoblasts have scalloped, irregular nuclei with sharply-defined intracytoplasmic vacuoles in contrast to ill-defined vacuoles and round, regular nuclei of other vacuolated cells. Furthermore, the vacuoles contain lipid rather than mucin or glycogen.

### *Behavior*

Of the mammary liposarcomas associated with recurrence, the majority have been of the pleomorphic and myxoid types. Well-differentiated liposarcoma may

B

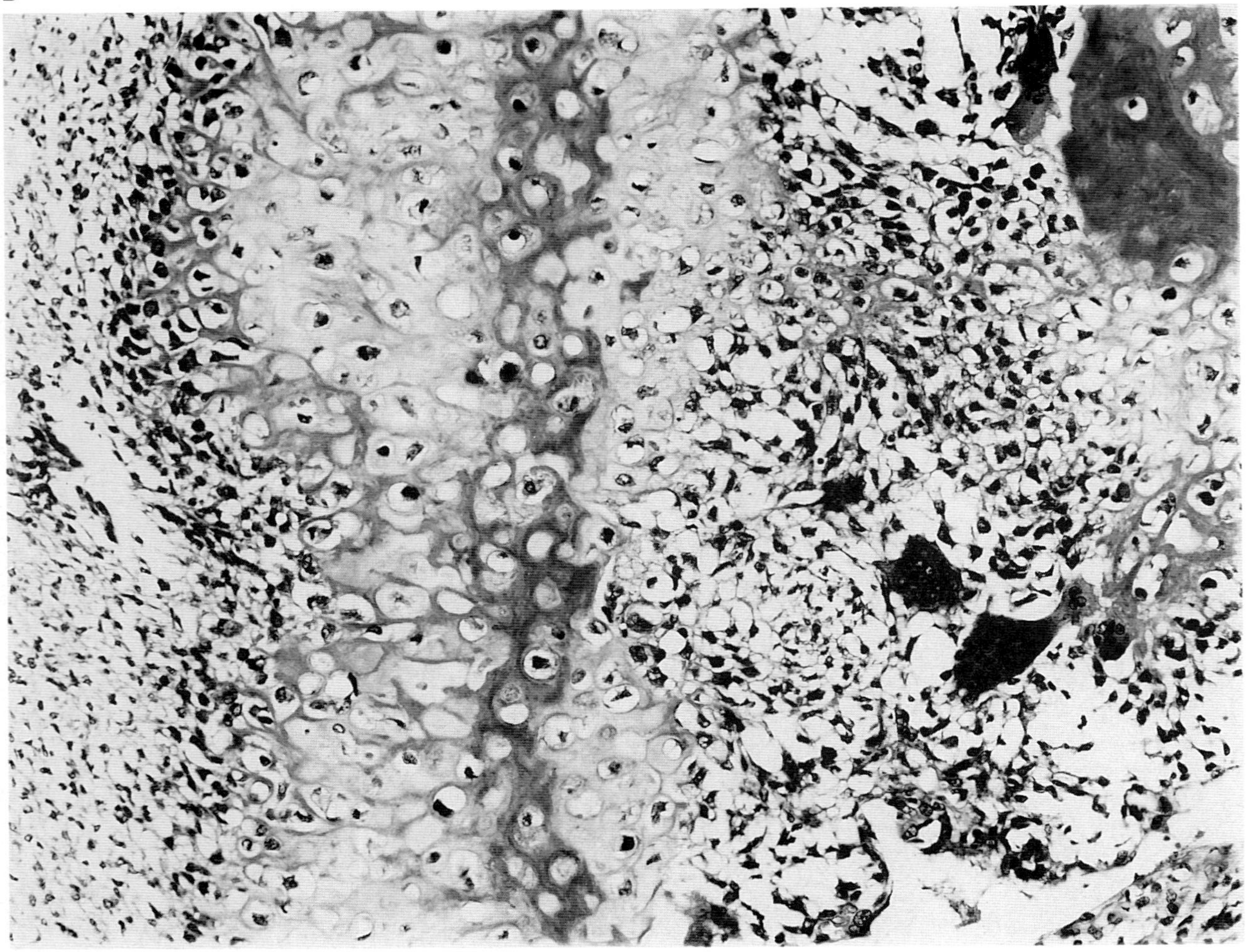

**Figure 13.17(b)** Osteogenic sarcoma. Spindle cells with osteoclastic giant cells separate aggregates of ossifying cartilage. (H&E, X500)

recur locally (101), but rarely, if ever, does it metastasize. Axillary node metastasis is exceptional but has been reported (111). Of the five reported fatal cases for which the type of liposarcoma was known, three were of the myxoid, and two of the pleomorphic type (98,108,110).

Liposarcoma appears to be particularly aggressive when associated with pregnancy. Two cases that were diagnosed during pregnancy were rapidly fatal (98,108). Another rapidly progressive bilateral liposarcoma was first detected during lactation (110). Vascularity associated with gestation may facilitate hematogenous spread.

Recurrences that develop do so within a year after the diagnosis and patients who die from the disease do so within 18 months.

It is important to determine the type and grade of these tumors. An infiltrating margin has been suggested as a factor influencing behavior (98), but a majority of liposarcomas are infiltrative. Considering the frequency of infiltrating margins, a wide rim of uninvolved breast tissue should be excised if a mastectomy is not elected. The efficacy of chemotherapy has not been established in view of the rarity of these tumors.

## Osteogenic Sarcoma

Pure osteogenic sarcomas of the breast, without attachment to the skeleton as determined by roentgenographic studies are rare, with less than 50 cases reported in the literature (87,94,95,115,120,124,126,127,130,131). It is much more common than other heterologous sarcomas, however.

A

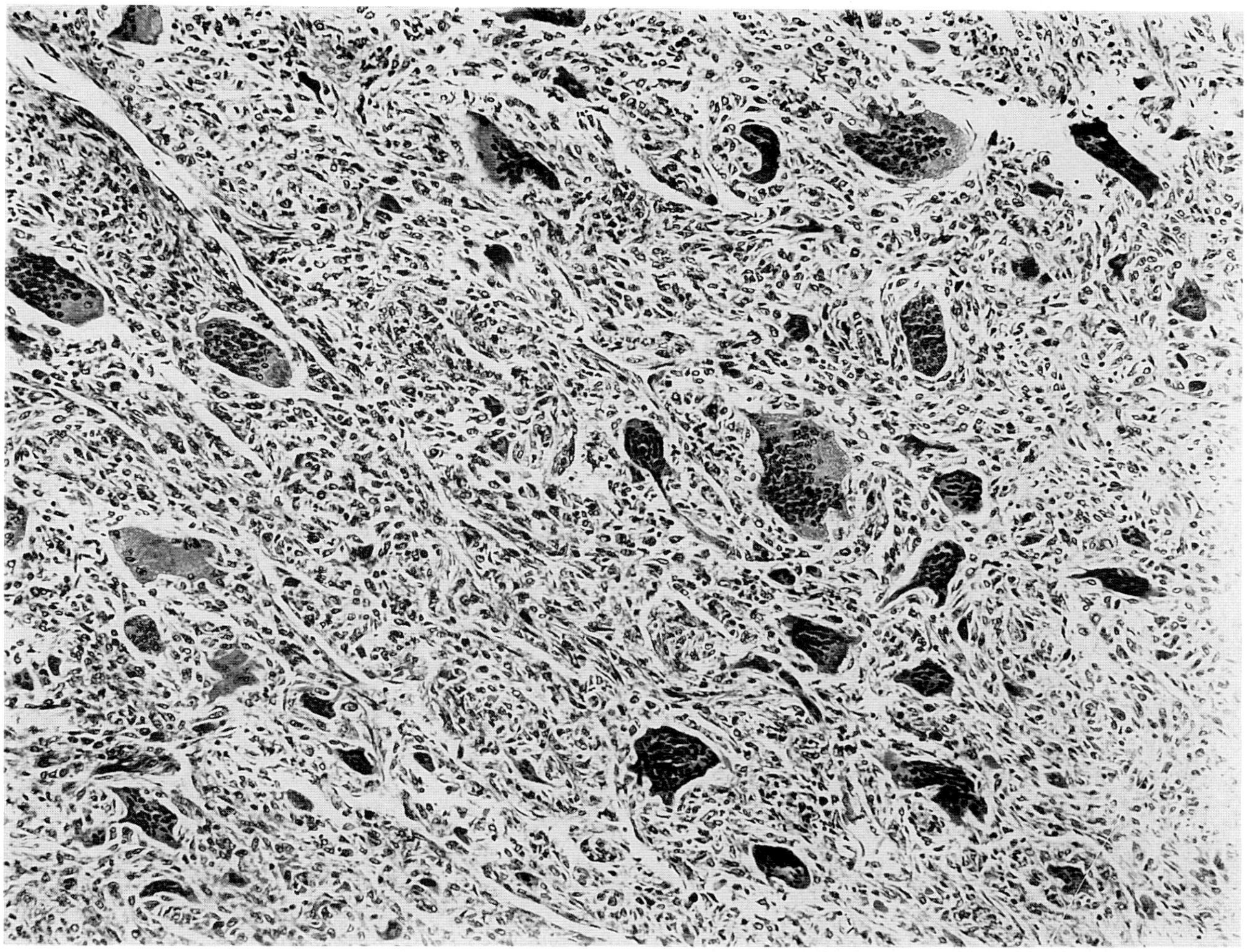

**Figure 13.18** Osteogenic sarcoma, osteoclastic type (osteoclastoma). (a) Multinucleated osteoclastic giant cells are scattered in a background of irregularly-bundled spindle cells. (H&E, X120)

## *Clinical Features*

Osteosarcomas occur predominantly in older women and are rarely encountered in women less than 40 years of age. The 35 patients with mammary osteosarcoma in the AFIP files ranged in age from 36 to 89 with a median age of 65 years. All but one of the patients were female. The only male patient was 77 years of age. Two of the 17 patients whose racial origin was known were black; the others were caucasians. The patients often presented with a progressively enlarging mass associated with pain in a fifth of the cases. Two patients noted the tumor following trauma to the breast. A bloody nipple discharge was noted in one patient three years prior to the detection of a 6 cm subareolar mass. Nipple retraction was present in two of the 35 cases. The smaller tumors are firm to stony hard on palpation and most are freely moveable. The larger tumors may adhere to the skin and eventually ulcerate. Mammographically, they manifest as a soft tissue mass with speckled, coarse calcification. Extensive calcification is observed in some cases.

A prior history of radiotherapy has been present in some patients. In one case, the patient had received 4,800 rads of radiation following removal of an infiltrating duct carcinoma. Eight years later, she developed an osteosarcoma that extended to the pectoralis muscle (114). The presence of radiation-induced dermatitis in the overlying skin is a helpful feature in the radiation-induced sarcomas (118).

## *Pathologic Features*

Mammary osteosarcomas range in size from 1.7 to 12 cm. Most are between 5 to 7 cm in size. They are generally sharply circumscribed and often lobulated. Less frequently, part or all of the tumor blends with

B

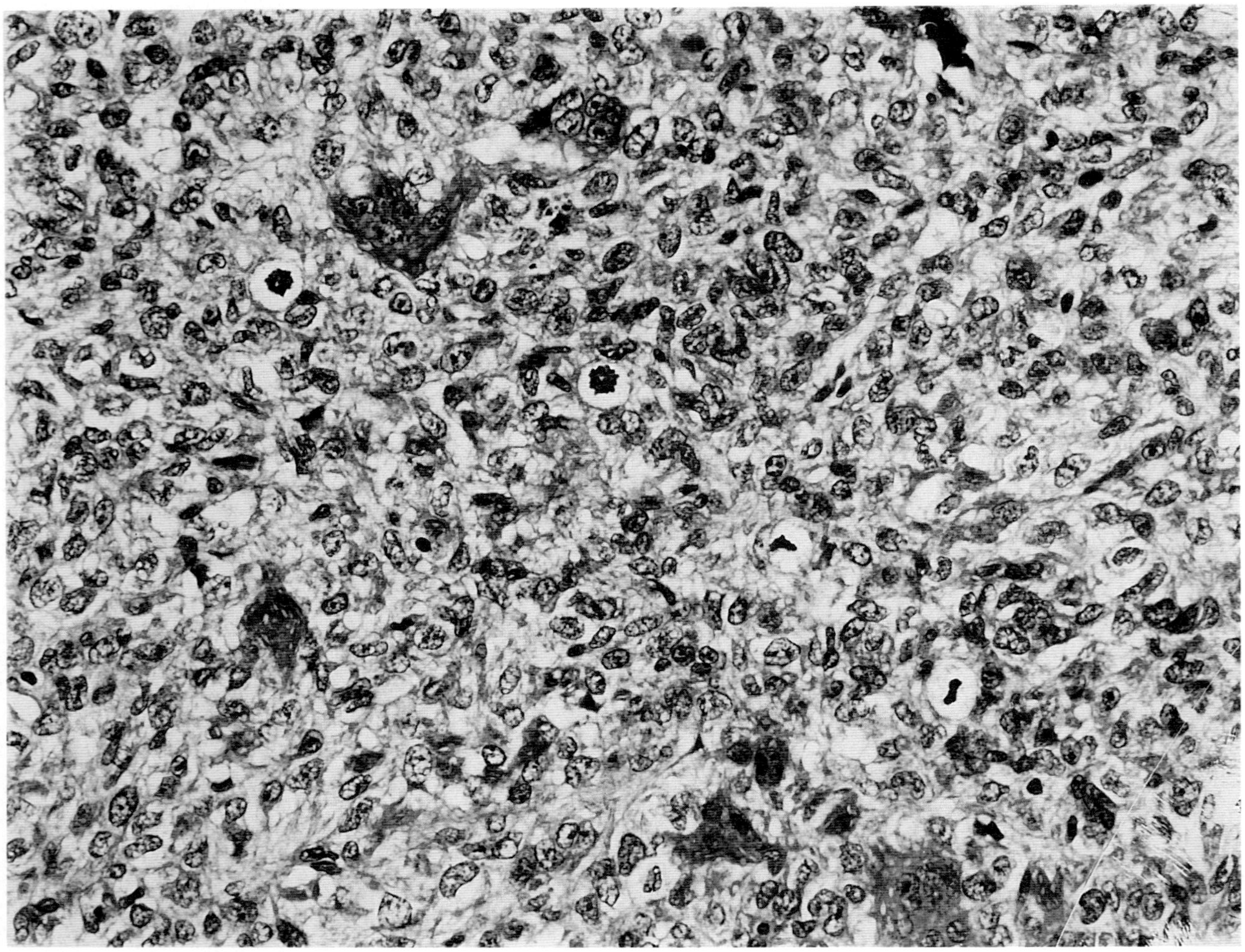

**Figure 13.18(b)** Osteogenic sarcoma. Numerous mitotic figures are readily apparent. (H&E, X400)

c

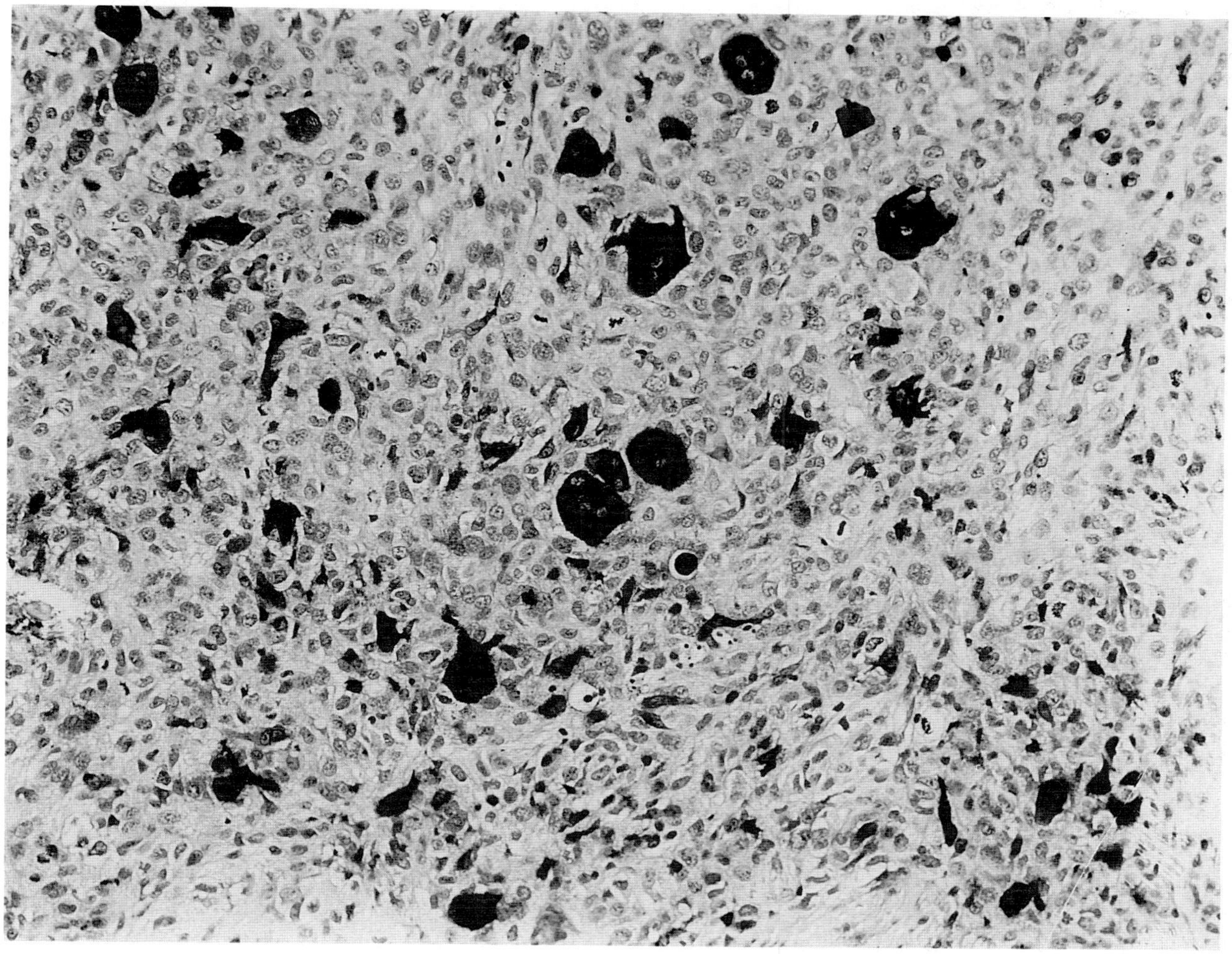

**Figure 13.18(c)** Osteogenic sarcoma. Acid phosphatase stain enhances the osteoclastic giant cells. (acid phosphatase, X340)

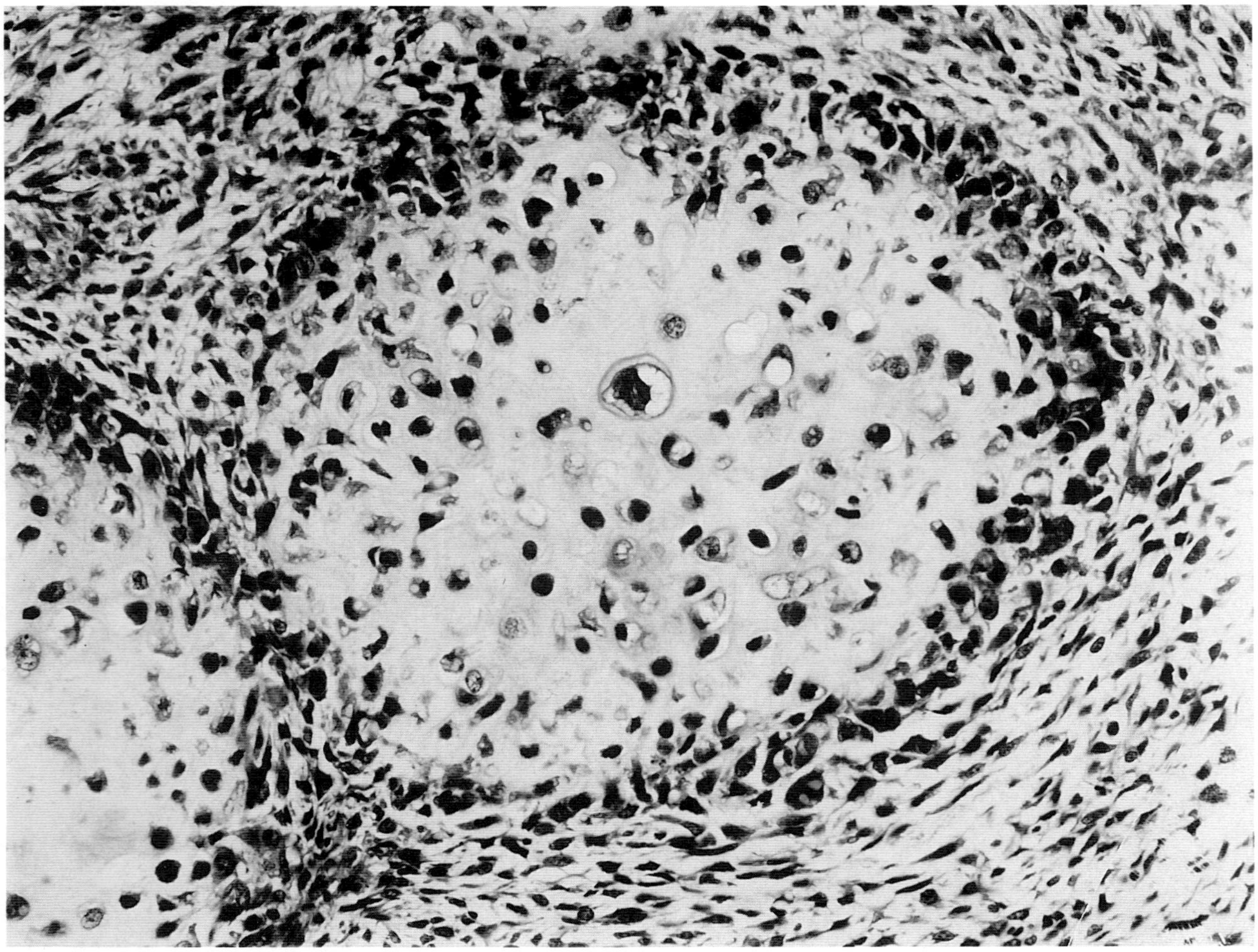

**Figure 13.19** Chondrosarcoma. A hypercellular spindle cell background with a nodule of atypical, pleomorphic chondrocytes occupying the lacunar spaces. (H&E, X600)

the surrounding tissues. With few exceptions, the tumors are described as gritty under the knife. Depending on the degree of osseous differentiation, the consistency of the tumor varies from firm to stony hard. The cut surface appears highly variable. Some are described as fleshy with a few glistening, pearly nodules while others have abundant chondroosseous differentiation apparent on macroscopic examination. Central cavitation with a bloody fluid content has been noted in several of the larger tumors. Necrosis may be present particularly in tumors larger than 6 cm.

Microscopically, mammary osteosarcomas are highly variable but are characterized by the presence of neoplastic osteoid and bone in a background of spindle to plump ovoid cells. In a good proportion of cases, there is also neoplastic cartilage. The actual appearance of the tumor varies depending on the proportion of the constituent cells and matrix (Figs. 13.15–13.17).

Some are composed predominantly of spindle, fibroblastic-type cells with areas of osteoid formation. Others show predominance of osteoblastic cells proliferating among branching trabeculae of bone and osteoid material. A surprising number appear extremely bland with layers of osseous tissue alternating with spindle cells, a zoning effect that may be mistaken for myositis ossificans, but then the spindle cells are peripheral in location and at least focally invade the surrounding tissues. Others show round nodules of osteoclastic giant cells admixed with mitotically active, atypical plump cells; these areas are generally hemorrhagic and may cavitate corresponding to the grossly visible cavitations filled by bloody fluid.

A

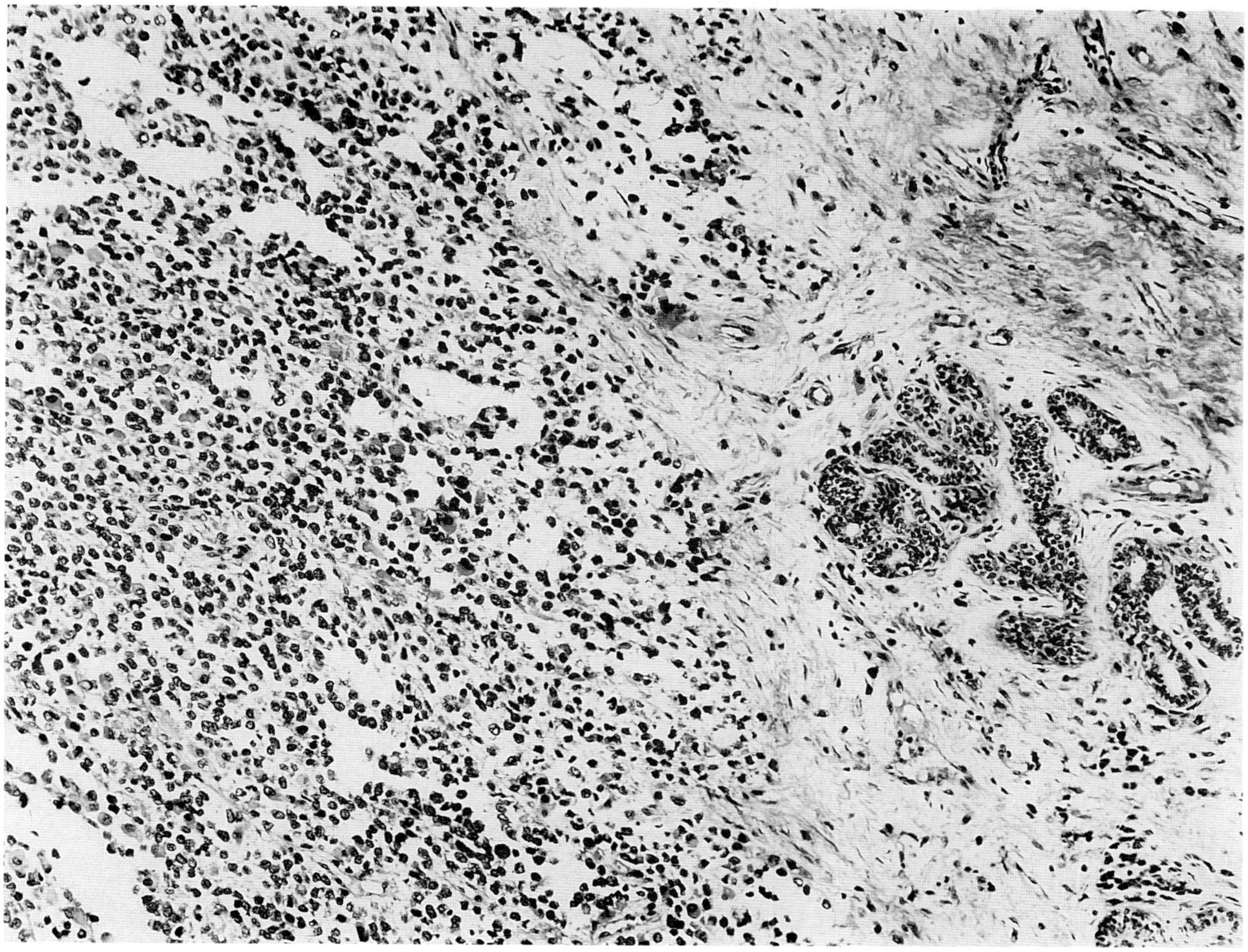

**Figure 13.20(a)** Rhabdomyosarcoma, alveolar type. The rounded rhabdomyoblasts with sparse cytoplasm are admixed with pyknotic nuclei of degenerated tumor cells. (H&E, X300)

### *Behavior*

Mammary osteosarcomas are highly aggressive lesions even when they appear bland morphologically. Recurrences develop at the biopsy or mastectomy site within weeks or a few months after the diagnosis. Recurrent tumors often show more osseous differentiation. Most patients either develop metastasis or die from the disease within two years despite performance of radical mastectomy in many cases. The absence of axillary node metastasis and frequent metastases to the lungs are characteristic of osteogenic sarcomas. Rarely, however, actual axillary node metastasis occurs. Most aggressive tumors are characterized by large size at presentation, infiltrating margins, and necrosis. Otherwise, the morphology of the tumor does not correlate well with the behavior. At least two of the cases reviewed at AFIP were extremely bland with mature bone and had been originally interpreted as a benign change or myositis ossificans by a number of bone pathologists, but both cases developed distant metastases shortly after the diagnosis. Both of these cases were predominantly well circumscribed but had mitotically active spindle cells focally invading the surrounding breast tissue.

As with all other sarcomas, adequate sampling of the specimen is required to exclude the presence of epithelial elements and origin in a cystosarcoma phyllodes. The presence of a malignant epithelial component would qualify the lesion as a carcinosarcoma.

B

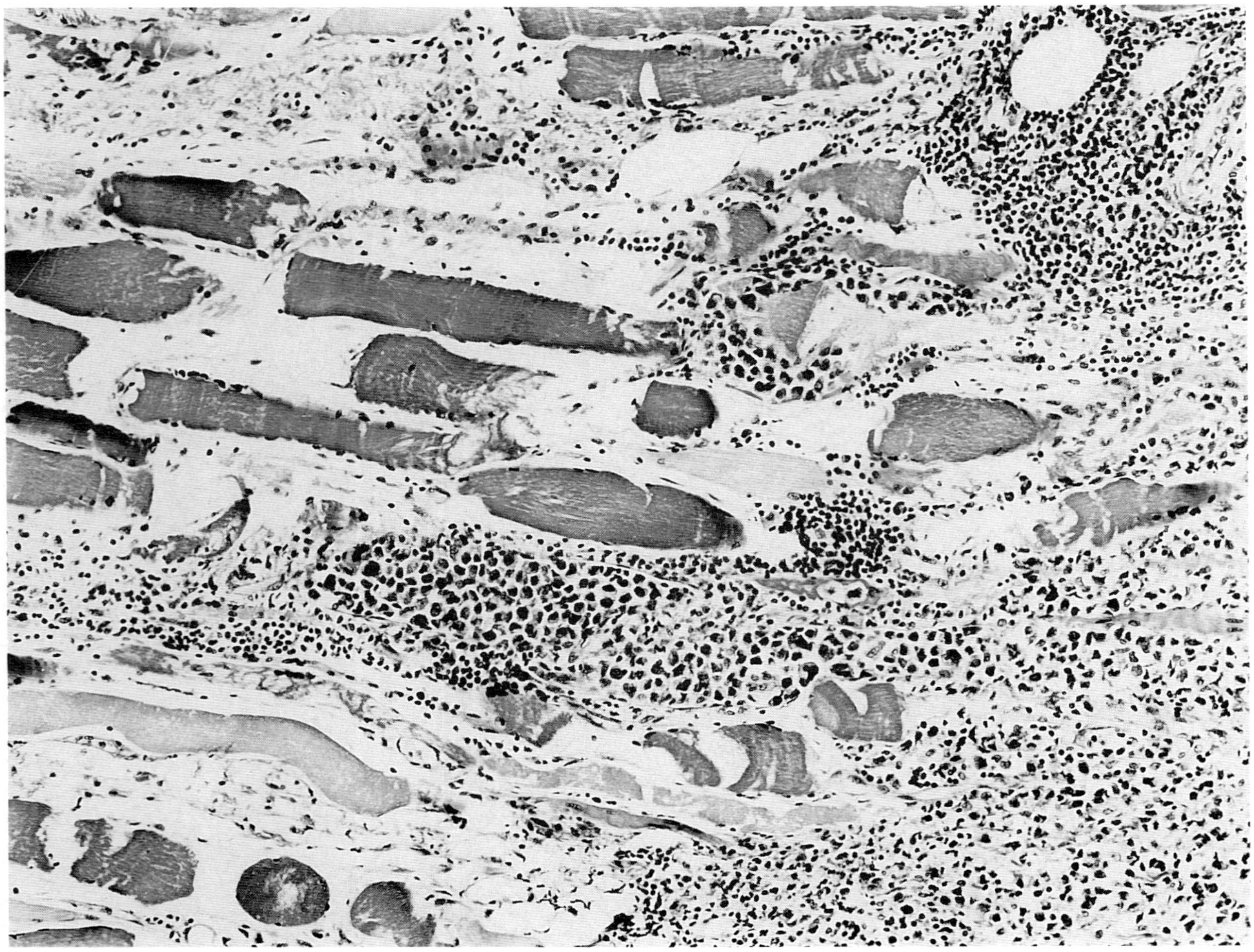

**Figure 13.20(b)** Rhabdomyosarcoma, aveolar type. Small round cells extending into the pectoralis muscle. (H&E, X340)

## Osteoclastoma

Either a variant of osteosarcoma with minimal osteoid production or a malignant fibrous histiocytoma of the giant cell variety, these tumors are characterized by the presence of a large number of osteoclastic giant cells distributed in a background of spindle cells or a rather pleomorphic sarcoma. Osteoclastoma is also seen as a component of cystosarcoma phyllodes and carcinosarcomas.

In a recent review of this tumor Mufarrij and Feiner (128) collected eight cases that were described in detail from the English literature and added one of their own. Another case has been reported by Going et al (123). The patients ranged in age from 23 to 69 years with a median of 52. All patients presented with a breast mass, half of which had manifested recent rapid growth. All were freely moveable except for one that was fixed and ulcerated.

The tumors ranged in size from 2 to 12 cm with a median of 4 cm. Half of the tumors appeared well delineated and firm. Hemorrhage and necrosis was described in half of the cases. About a third felt gritty upon cutting.

Morphologically, the typical lesion contains numerous osteoclastic giant cells admixed with malignant spindle cells with focal osteoid production (Fig. 13.18). Bone and cartilage may be present as well, but the latter is particularly rare. There should be absolutely no neoplastic epithelial component in the lesion to qualify as a pure sarcoma. The giant cells display a positive reaction for acid phosphatase and a negative reaction for cytokeratin and vimentin supporting their osteoclastic nature. Those tumors without any osteoid or osseous differentiation probably

c

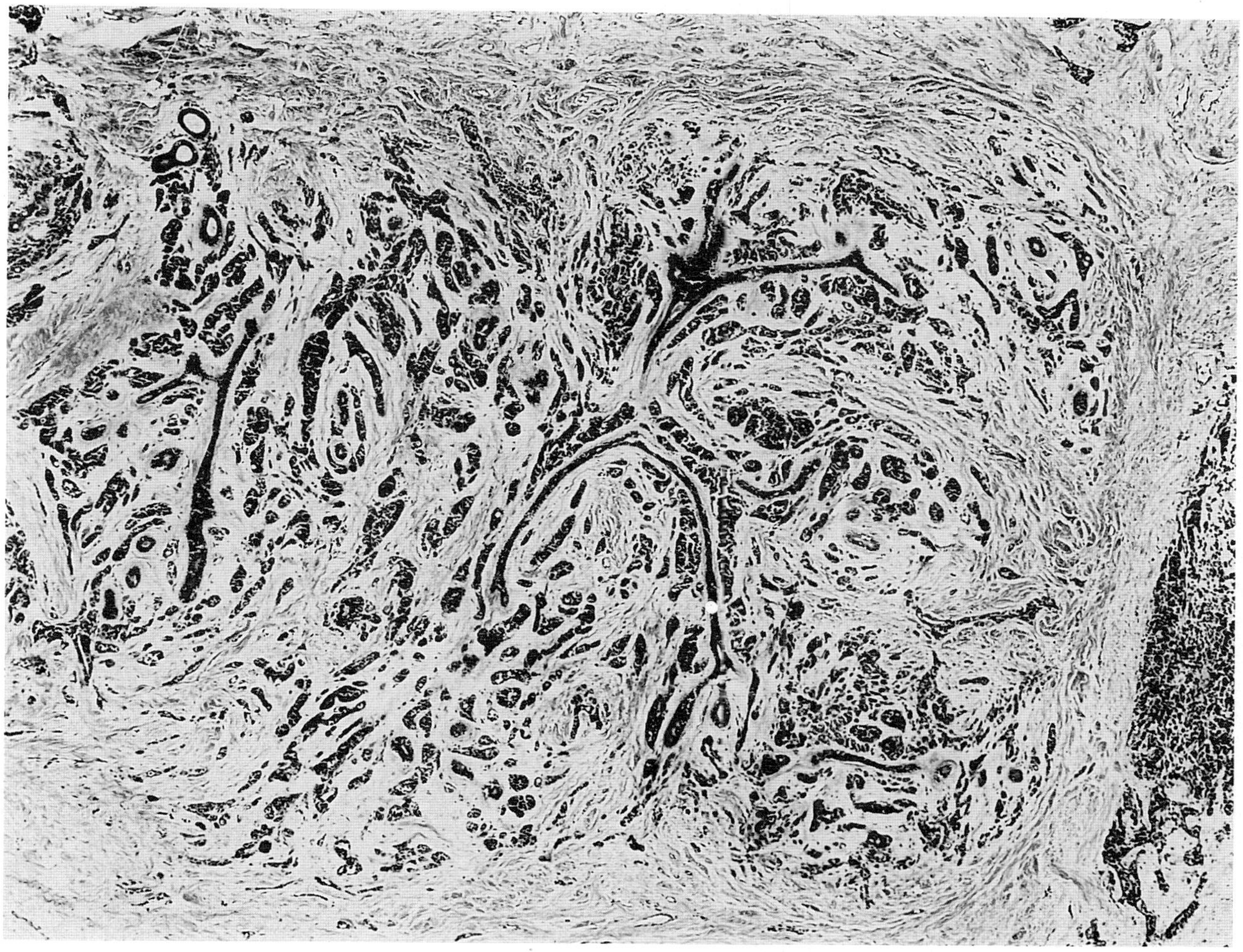

**Figure 13.20(c)** Rhabdomyosarcoma, aveolar type. Rhabdomyosarcoma extending into and distorting lobules; in sections where this feature is evident, tumor cells mimic an invasive carcinoma. (H&E, X240)

reflect the giant cell variant of malignant fibrous histiocytoma.

### *Treatment and Follow-up*

With rare exceptions, various forms of mastectomy have been performed for mammary osteosarcomas and osteoclastomas. A majority of patients have died within a few months generally after development of pulmonary metastases (116,117,119,121,122,128–130), and rarely with bone metastases (122). Considering the poor outcome in these patients, a wide local excision for the low grade and smaller tumors (relative to the overall size of the breast) could be adequate as initial therapy. A mastectomy is often necessary to ensure complete excision of the large and high grade lesions with infiltrating margins. A more individualized approach to the treatment of the high grade lesions is warranted; combination therapy (multimodality) may provide the best hope for alleviation of symptoms and prolonging survival.

## Chondrosarcoma

Pure mammary chondrosarcoma is extremely rare (128–130). Only seven cases of chondrosarcoma have been diagnosed at AFIP. The patients were all women ranging in age from 46 to 75 years with a median of 54 years. The tumors are generally well delineated and often lobulated. Some have a distinct chondromyxoid matrix with a rim of cellularity in the peripheral margin of the lesion. Others are densely cellular sarcomas composed of spindle or round cells with nodular islands of well-differentiated cartilage (Fig. 13.19). These should be distinguished from

A

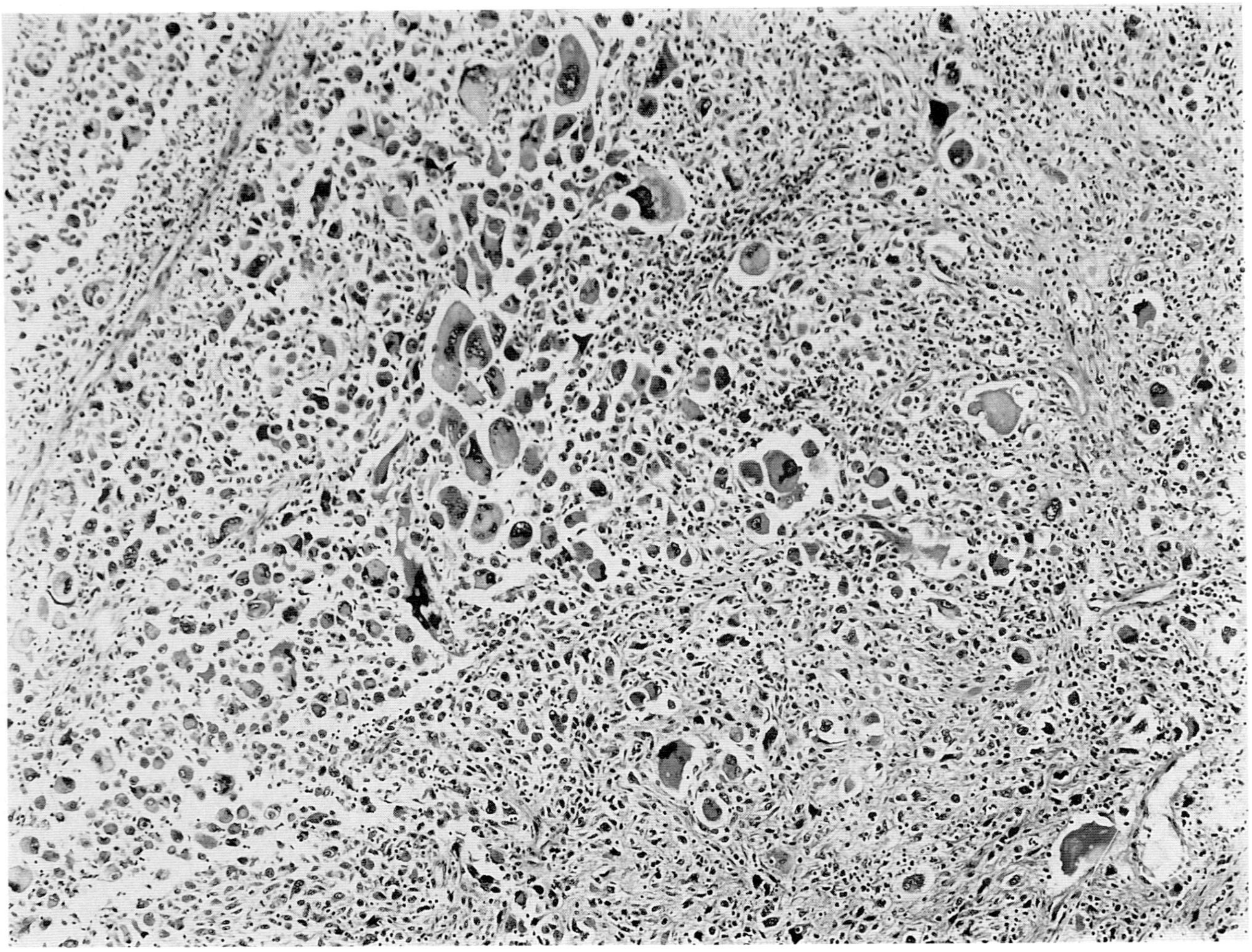

**Figure 13.21(a)** Rhabdomyosarcoma, pleomorphic type. A background of small and spindle cells is dispersed by aggregates of round and giant cells with abundant pink cytoplasm (rhabdomyoblasts). (H&E, X340)

cartilage-producing metaplastic carcinomas which should have cells that show a positive reaction for cytokeratin admixed with benign chondroid elements.

## Leiomyosarcoma

Leiomyosarcoma is one of the rarest of the breast sarcomas with less than 10 cases reported in the literature (87,135–137,139–141,148). Most patients are about 50 years of age or older but one case was reported in a 24-year-old woman. At least two of the reported cases occurred in the male breast.

Unlike the highly aggressive osteosarcomas, only two of the reported leiomyosarcomas developed recurrences and metastasis 14 and 15 years after the initial excision (136,140). One of these patients died with metastatic tumor in kidney, lungs, brain, and the dermis; the other was alive with liver metastasis at the time of the report. Chen et al (135) suggested that the presence of three mitotic figures per 10 HPF is sufficient to designate a mammary smooth muscle tumor as a sarcoma. Nielsen (139) has proposed that all tumors that recur and have two mitotic figures per 10 HPF should be considered as leiomyosarcoma, while tumors without mitotic figures, necrosis, or atypia would qualify as leiomyoma. Benign leiomyomas are completely devoid of mitotic activity. Origin from myoepithelium, blood vessels, and nipple musculature has been suggested. Since spindle cell myoepitheliomas look identical to smooth muscle tumors, the presence of positive reaction for S-100 protein and

B

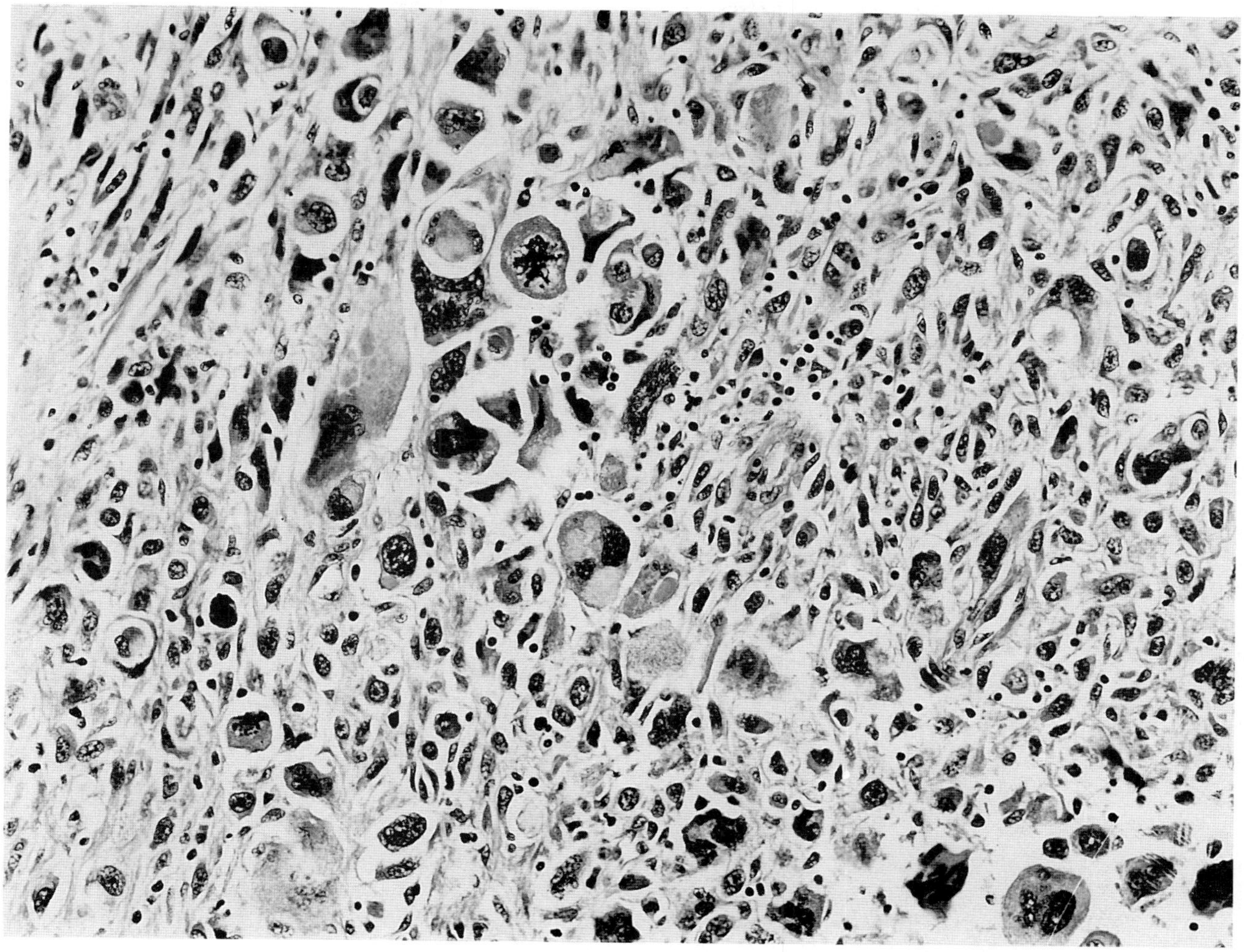

**Figure 13.21(b)** Rhabdomyosarcoma, pleomorphic type. The rhabdomyoblasts are highly pleomorphic with bizarre mitotic figures. (H&E, X600)

focal positivity for cytoketatin would favor a myoepithelial lesion; both lesions will show a positive reaction to actin.

## Rhabdomyosarcoma

Primary mammary rhabdomyosarcoma occurs more frequently as a component of a biphasic tumor (carcinosarcoma and cystosarcoma phyllodes) rather than in pure form. In the biphasic tumors, rhabdomyosarcoma may represent the dominant or sole sarcomatous element. In one such case reviewed at AFIP, the patient developed liver metastasis shortly after a diagnosis of mammary carcinosarcoma, and the metastasis was composed purely of rhabdomyosarcoma.

In its pure form, mammary rhabdomyosarcoma is indeed rare (138), but occurs either as a primary or metastatic tumor. Of 22 rhabdomyosarcomas diagnosed at AFIP, only four were in women older than 40 years; the age range was from 11 to 70 years and the median age was 24 years. Almost all patients less than 40, however, were either known to have disseminated rhabdomyosarcoma or a primary site elsewhere in the body. Only four of the 22 rhabdomyosarcomas could be considered as primary in the breast; all four patients were older than 40 years, and one of these tumors was predominantly in the pectoralis muscle.

Microscopically, rhabdomyosarcomas of the alveolar and embryonal type are the two most common variants seen in young girls and women with metastatic rhabdomyosarcoma to the breast (Fig. 13.20). Primary rhabdomyosarcoma is characterized by a highly cellular spindle to round cell population with numerous mitotic figures. Rhabdomyoblasts are dis-

c

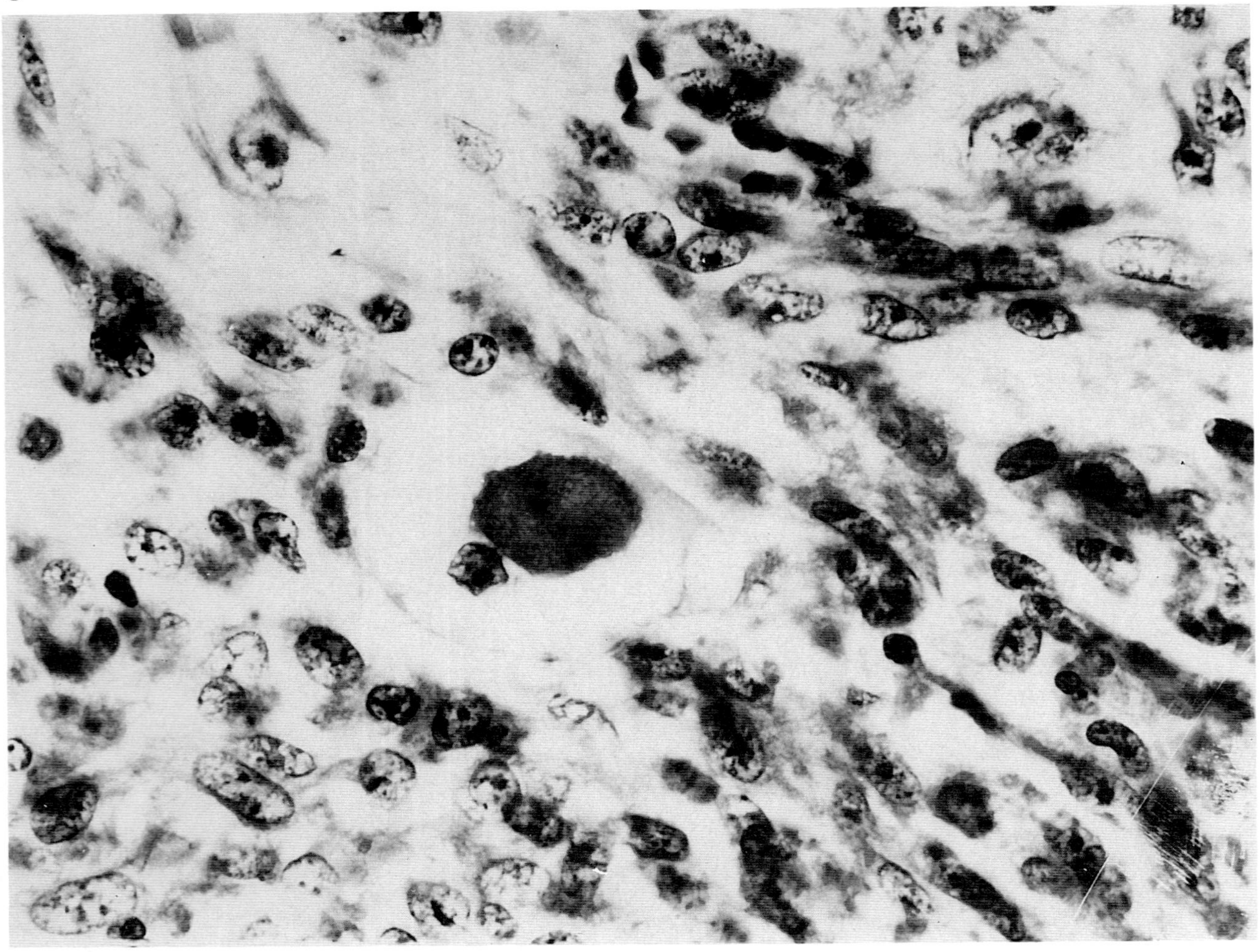

**Figure 13.21(c)** Rhabdomyosarcoma, pleomorphic type. Cross striations at the periphery of a cell. (H&E, (c) X1500)

persed throughout the lesion but tend to concentrate in some areas (Fig. 13.21).

The rhabdomyoblasts may be quite large and bizarre with multinucleation. Characteristically, a round, tangled, fibrillar mass is present within these cells. Cross-striations are found with difficulty in the periphery of the tangled fibrillar masses. Many of the rhabdomyoblasts appear to have a halo around the fibrillar tangle probably secondary to removal of glycogen. Strap cells are present but are few in number and rarely display cross-striation.

Rhabdomyosarcomas are highly aggressive and are generally disseminated by the time the breast lesion manifests itself. Of the four primary mammary tumors reviewed at AFIP, one patient developed pulmonary metastases within a year after mastectomy and died shortly thereafter from other causes. Another patient developed a recurrent mass three months following mastectomy under the scar as well as pulmonary metastases. She died seven months after the initial diagnosis despite multiagent chemotherapy (cytoxin, nitrogen mustard and actinomycin D). The third patient was well without evidence of a recurrence or metastasis one year after shelling out a 4 cm tumor. The last patient's tumor was mainly in the pectoralis muscle; no follow-up is available on her.

## Malignant Fibrous Histiocytoma

Malignant fibrous histiocytoma (MFH) occurs occasionally as a primary breast tumor (144). Two of the reported cases developed two and 16 years following radiation therapy for breast carcinoma (146,149). In a recent review of 25 mammary sarcomas, 11 had been

A

B

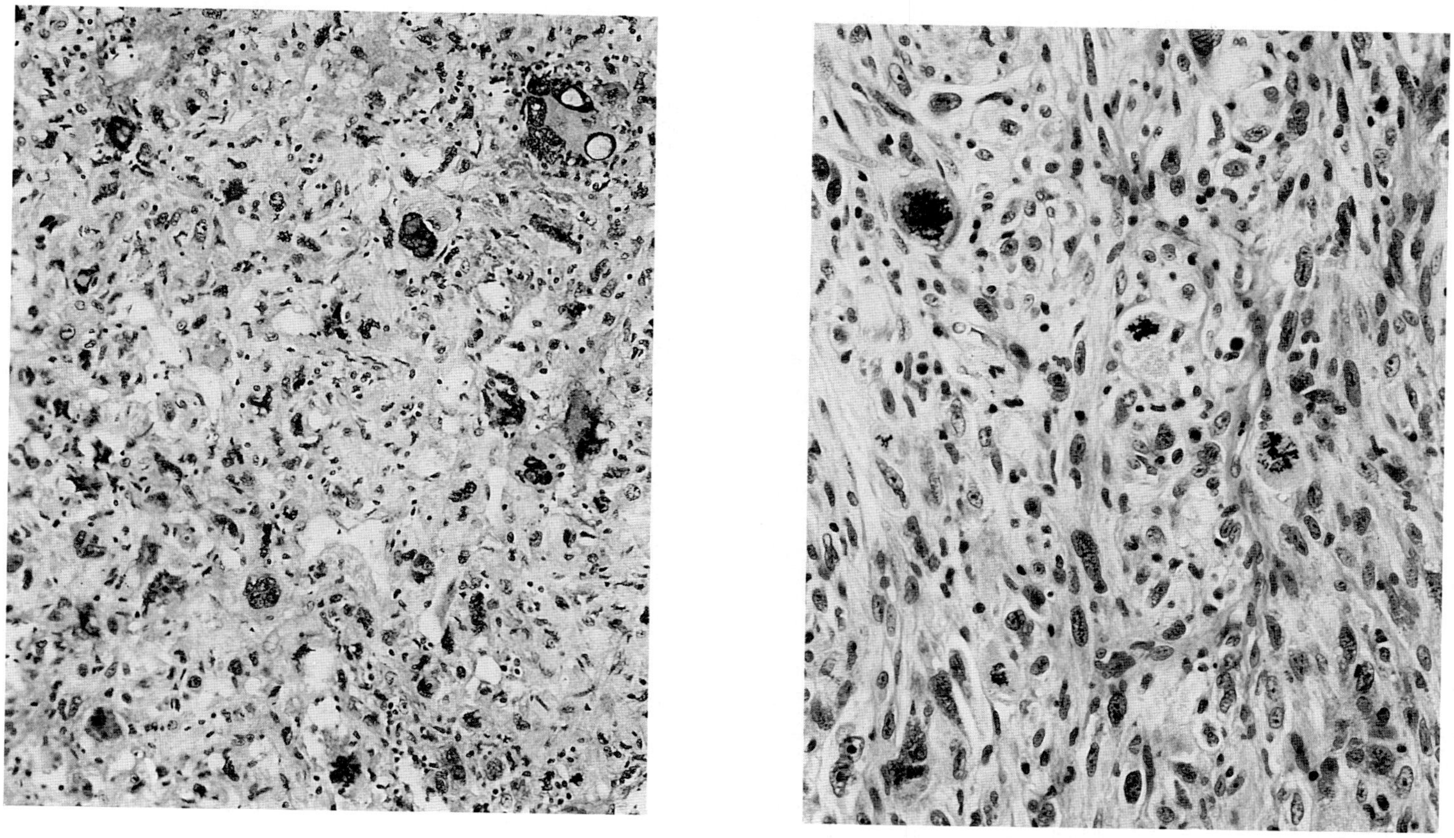

**Figure 13.22** Malignant fibrous histiocytoma, pleomorphic type. (a) Bizarre cells with abundant, irregular and eosinophilic cytoplasm are admixed with smaller neoplastic and inflammatory cells. (b) Mitotic figures are readily apparent. (H&E, (a) X160; (b) X250)

interpreted as malignant fibrous histiocytoma (148). Of 27 mammary tumors diagnosed as MFH in the AFIP files, three were metastatic. Five of the remaining 24 patients were men. Of 16 patients whose racial origin was known, two were black, the remainder were caucasian. The patients ranged in age from 19 to 94 with a median of 58 years. One of the cases occurred in a 63-year-old woman who had received radiation in the same breast for breast carcinoma. The patients generally presented with a palpable breast mass. Cut surface of the tumors appeared gray to tan with foci of hemorrhage and necrosis in several cases. A translucent mucoid appearance is typical of the myxoid variant. Microscopically, all varieties of MFH occur in the breast including the myxoid, inflammatory, giant cell, and pleomorphic types. The most common lesion is composed of plump spindle cells with numerous mitotic figures and bizarre, giant cells and inflammatory cells (Fig. 13.22). Aggregates of bizarre cells with abundant eosinophilic cytoplasm are present focally in most tumors. A storiform pattern may be seen in the spindle cell areas. The myxoid variant lacks any specific orientation of proliferating cells. The osteoclastoma-like lesions lacking osteoid or osseous differentiation probably reflect a giant cell variant of malignant fibrous histiocytomas.

Ultrastructurally, the large eosinophilic tumor cells contain abundant intracytoplasmic microfibrils. Immunohistochemically, the cells show a positive reaction for lysozyme and alpha-1-anti-trypsin (142).

In the breast, malignant fibrous histiocytomas behave aggressively with a high rate of local recurrence (142). Cutaneous involvement has been reported in several cases (147,150). Metastases are found most often in the lungs, but a single case of metastatic MFH to the axillary nodes has been reported (150). In Pollard et al's (148) study of mammary sarcomas, nine of the 11 patients with malignant fibrous histiocytoma died from disseminated disease; the average survival of the 14 patients who died from their sarcoma was 18.7 months from diagnosis. Excision of the tumor with a margin of uninvolved breast tissue is necessary particularly for those displaying an infiltrating margin. Some have advocated total mastectomy for most patients, with postoperative radiation therapy when the adequacy of the margins is in doubt (141). The value of chemotherapy in the treatment of disseminated disease has not been established.

MFH also occurs as a component of cystosarcoma phyllodes.

## Miscellaneous Sarcomas

A variety of other sarcomas also develop in the breast with extreme rarity. There are two examples of malignant schwannoma, one of neurofibrosarcoma, one alveolar soft part sarcoma, as well as several cases of dermatofibrosarcoma protuberans in the AFIP files. A case of synovial sarcoma occurring in the breast has been discussed in Chapter 11, Biphasic Tumors.

### REFERENCES


**Stromal Giant Cells, Elastosis, and Metachromasia**

1. Adnet JJ, Pinteaux A, Caulet T, et al: L'elastose dans les cancers du sein. Etude anatomo-clinique, histochimique et ultrastructurale. Annales de Medicine de Reims 1976;13: 147–153.
* 2. Ahmed A: The myofibroblast in breast disease. *Pathol Annu* 1990;25(Pt 2):237–286.
3. Anastassiades OT, Bouropoulou V, Kontogeorgos G, et al: Duct elastosis in infiltrating carcinoma of the breast. *Pathol Res Pract* 1979;165:411–421.
* 4. Azzopardi JG, Laurini RN: Elastosis in breast cancer. *Cancer* 1974;33:174–183.
* 5. Davies JD: Hyperelastosis, obliteration and fibrous plaques in major ducts of the human breast. *J Pathol* 1973;110:13–26.
6. Farahmand S, Cowan DF: Elastosis in the normal aging breast. A histopathologic study of 140 cases. *Arch Pathol Lab Med* 1991;115:1241–1246.
7. Fisher ER, Gregorio RM, Fisher B, et al: The pathology of invasive breast cancer. A syllabus derived from findings of the National Surgical Adjuvant Breast Project (No. 4). *Cancer* 1975;36:1–85.
8. Ghosh L, Ghosh BC, Das Gupta TK: Ultrastructural study of stroma in human mammary carcinoma. *Am J Surg* 1980; 139:229–232.
9. Glaubitz LC, Bowen LH, Cox ED, et al: Elastosis in human breast cancer. Correlation with sex steroid receptors and comparison with clinical outcome. *Arch Pathol Lab Med* 1984;108:27–30.
* 10. Hartveit F: Mast cells and metachromasia in human breast cancer: their occurrence, significance and consequence: A preliminary report. *J Pathol* 1981;134:7–11.
* 11. Humeniuk V, Forest APM, Hawkins RA, et al: Elastosis and primary breast cancer. *Cancer* 1983;52:1448–1452.
* 12. Jackson JG, Orr JW: The ducts of carcinomatous breasts, with particular reference to connective tissue changes. *J Pathol Bacteriol* 1957;74:265–273.
* 13. Lefer LG, Rosier RP: Ochronosis in the breast. *Am J Clin Pathol* 1979;71;349–352.
14. Masters JRW, Sangster K, Hawkins RA, et al: Elastosis and estrogen receptors in human breast cancer. *Br J Cancer* 1976;33:342–343.
* 15. Rasmussen BB, Pedersen BV, Thorpe SM, et al: Elastosis in relation to prognosis in primary breast carcinoma. *Cancer Res* 1985;45:1428.
16. Reyes MG, Bazile DB, Tosch T, et al: Periductal elastic tissue of breast cancer. *Arch Pathol Lab Med* 1982;106:610.
17. Rickert RR, Kalisher L, Hutter RVP: Indurative mastopathy: A benign sclerosing lesion of breast with elastosis which may simulate carcinoma. *Cancer* 1981;47:561–571.
* 18. Rosen PP: Multinucleated mammary stromal giant cells. A benign lesion that simulates invasive carcinoma. *Cancer* 1979;44:1305–1308.
* 19. Sandstad E, Hartveit F: Stromal metachromasia: A marker for areas of incipient invasion in ductal carcinoma of the breast? *Histopathology* 1987;11:73–80.
* 20. Schiodt T, Jensen H, Nielsen M, et al: On the nature of amyloid-like duct wall changes in carcinoma of the breast. *Acta Pathol Microbiol Scand.* (A) 1972;80(Suppl 233):151–157.
21. Shivas AA, Douglas JG: The prognostic significance of elastosis in breast carcinoma. *J R Coll Surg Endinb* 1972;17: 315–320.
22. Tremblay G, Buell RH, Seemayer TA: Elastosis in benign sclerosing ductal proliferations of the female breast. *Am J Surg Pathol* 1977;1:1155–1158.

**Fat Necrosis**

* 23. Adair FE, Munger JT: Fat necrosis of the female breast: Report of 110 cases. *Am J Surg* 1947;74:117–128.
24. Haagensen CD: *Diseases of the Breast*, ed 3. Philadelphia, WB Saunders, 1986, pp 369–377.
25. Laborgne R: Esteatonecrosis quistica calcificada de la mamma. *Torax* 1967;16:172.
* 26. Lee BJ, Adair FE: Traumatic fat necrosis and its differentiation from carcinoma. *Ann Surg* 1920;37:189.

**Metaplasias**

* 27. Davies JD, Riddle RH: Muscular hamartomas of the breast. *J Pathol* 1973;111:209–211.
* 28. Eusebi V, Cunsolo A, Fedeli F, et al: Benign smooth muscle metaplasia in breast. *Tumori* 1980;66:643–653.
29. Mackenzie DH: A fibroadenoma of the breast with smooth muscle. *J Pathol Bacteriol* 1968;96:231–232.
30. Norris HJ, Taylor HB: Relationship of histologic features to behavior of cystosarcoma phyllodes. *Cancer* 1967;20:2090–2099.
31. Pietruszka M, Barnes L: Cystosarcoma phyllodes: A clinicopathologic analysis of 42 cases. *Cancer* 1978;1974–1983.

32. Qizilbash AH: Cystosarcoma phyllodes with liposarcomatous stroma. *Am J Clin Pathol* 1976;65:321–327.

* 33. Smith BH, Taylor HB: The occurrence of bone and cartilage in mammary tumors. *Am J Clin Pathol* 1969;51:610–618.


## Fibromatosis and Myofibroblastoma


* 34. Ali M, Fayemi AO, Braun EV, et al: Fibromatosis of the breast. *Am J Surg Pathol* 1979;3:501–505.

35. Begin LR: Myogenic stromal tumor of the male breast (so-called myofibroblastoma). *Ultrastruc Pathol* 1991;15:613–622.

36. Boger A: Benign spindle cell tumor of the male breast. *Path Res Pract* 1984;178:395–398.

37. Bogomoletz WV, Boulenger E, Simatos A: Infiltrating fibromatosis of the breast. *J Clin Pathol* 1981;34:30–34.

38. Cederlun C-G, Gustavsson S, Linell F, et al: Fibromatosis of the breast mimicking carcinoma at mammography. *Br J Radiol* 1984;57:98–101.

39. Chen KTK: Fibromatosis of the breast. *Breast* 1984;10:25–26.

40. El-Naggar A, Abdul-Karim FW, Marshalleck JJ, et al: Fine needle aspiration of fibromatosis of the breast. *Diagn Cytopathol* 1987;3:320–322.

41. Gabbiani G, Majno G: Dupuytren's contracture: Fibroblast contraction? *Am J Pathol* 1972;66:131–146.

42. Gump FE, Sternschein MJ, Wolff M: Fibromatosis of the breast. *Surg Gynecol Obstet* 1981;15:57–60.

43. Haggitt RC, Booth JF: Bilateral fibromatosis of the breast in Gardner's syndrome. *Cancer* 1970;25:161–166.

44. Hanna WM, Jambrostic J, Fish E: Aggressive fibromatosis of the breast. *Arch Pathol Lab Med* 1985;109:260–262.

45. Jewett ST Jr, Mead JH: Extra-abdominal desmoid arising from a capsule around a silicone breast implant. *Plast Recontr Surg* 1979;63:577–579.

46. Kalisher L, Long JA, Peyster RG: Extraabdominal desmoid of the axillary tail mimicking breast carcinoma. *Am J Roentgenol* 1976;126:903–906.

* 47. Kinzbrunner B, Ritter S, Domingo J, et al: Remission of rapidly growing desmoid tumors after tamoxifen therapy. *Cancer* 1983;52:2201–2204.

* 48. Nichols RW: Desmoid tumors: A report of 31 cases. *Arch Surg* 1923;7:227–236.

49. Pierce VE Jr, Rives DA, Sisley JF, et al: Estradiol and progesterone receptors in a case of fibromatosis of the breast. *Arch Pathol Lab Med* 1987;111:870–872.

* 50. Rosen PP, Ernsberger D: Mammary Fibromatosis. A benign spindle-cell tumor with significant risk for local recurrence. *Cancer* 1989;63:1363–1369.

51. Waddell WR, Gerner RE, Reich MP: Nonsteroid anti-inflammatory drugs and tamoxifen for desmoid tumors and carcinoma of the stomach. *J Surg Oncol* 1983;22:197–211.

52. Wargotz ES, Norris HJ, Austin RM, et al: Fibromatosis of the breast: A clinical and pathological study of 28 cases. *Am J Surg Pathol* 1987;11:38–45.

* 53. Wargotz ES, Weiss S, Norris HJ: Myofibroblastoma of the breast. Sixteen cases of a distinctive benign mesenchymal tumor. *Am J Surg Pathol* 1987;11:493–502.


## Lipoma


54. Brebner DM, Cosman B, Shapiro J: Lipomata of the breast diagnosed by film and xeromammography. *S Afr Med J* 1976;50:685–688.

55. Haagensen CD: *Diseases of the Breast*, ed 3. Philadelphia, WB Saunders, 1986, pp 333–335.

* 56. Spalding JE: Adenolipoma and lipoma of the breast. *Guys Hosp Rep* 1945;94:80–84.

* 57. Tedeschi CG: Mammary lipoma. *Arch Pathol Lab Med* 1948; 46:386–397.


## Angiolipoma


58. Brown RW, Bhathal PS, Scott PR: Multiple bilateral angiolipomas of the breast. *Aust NZ J Surg* 1982;52:614–616.

* 59. Enzinger FM, Weiss SW: *Soft Tissue Pathology*. St. Louis, CV Mosby Co., 1988, pp 405–407.

* 60. Fleishman JS, Schwartz RA: Angiolipoma presenting as a breast mass. *Ariz Med* 1980;37:403–404.

* 61. Franzini M, Castigliuni G, Martinelli R: Angiolipoma of the breast. *Pathologica* 1981;73:823–826.

62. Sibala JL, Chang CH, Lin F, et al: Computer tomography of angiolipoma of the breast. *AJR* 1980;134:840–841.


## Granular Cell Tumor


63. Armin A, Connelly EM, Rowden G: An immunoperoxidase investigation of S-100 protein in granular cell myoblastoma: Evidence for Schwann cell derivation. *Am J Clin Pathol* 1983;79:37–44.

64. Bassett LW, Cove HC: Myoblastoma of the breast. *AJR* 1979;132:122–123.

* 65. Demay RM, Kay S: Granular cell tumor of the breast. *Pathol Annu* 1984;19(pt 2):121–148.

* 66. Gordon AB, Fisher C, Palmer B, et al: Granular cell tumors of the breast. *Br J Surg Oncol* 1985;11:269–273.

* 67. Haagensen CD, Stout AT: Granular cell myoblastoma of the mammary gland. *Ann Surg* 1946;124:218–227.

* 68. Ingram DL, Mossler JA, Snowhite J, et al: Granular cell tumors of the breast. Steroid receptor analysis and localization of carcinoembryonic antigen, myoglobin, and S-100 protein. *Arch Pathol Lab Med* 1984;108:897–901.

69. Mulcare R: Granular cell myofibroblastoma of the breast. *Ann Surg* 1968;168:262–268.

70. Raju GC, O'Reilly AP: Immunohistochemical study of granular cell tumour. *Pathology* 1987;19:402–406.

71. Shousha S, Lyssiotis T: Granular cell myoblastoma: Positive staining for carcinoembryonic antigen. *J Clin Pathol* 1979;32:219–224.

72. Stefansson K, Wollmann RL: S-100 protein in granular cell tumours (granular cell myoblastomas). *Cancer* 1982;49: 1834–1838.

* 73. Umansky C, Bullock WK: Granular cell myoblastoma of the breast. 1968;168:810–817.

* 74. Zemoura L, Contesso G, Caillou B, et al: Myoblastomes

granuleux du sein. A propos de sept observations. *Ann Pathol* 1984;4:151–156.

### Leiomyoma, Neurilemomma, Chondrolipoma

75. Chan YF, Yeung HY, Ma L: Myxoma of the breast: Report of a case and ultrastructural study. *Pathology* 1986;18:153–157.
76. Dharkar DD, Kraft JR: Benign chondrolipomatous tumour of the breast. *Postgrad Med J* 1981;7:129–131.
* 77. Diaz-Arias AA, Jurt MA, Loy TS, et al: Leiomyoma of the breast. *Hum Pathol* 1989;20:396–399.
78. Huntrakoon M, Lin F: Muscular hamartoma of the breast. An electron microscopic study. *Virchows Archiv (Pathol Anat)* 1984;403:307–312.
79. Kaplan L, Walts AE: Benign chondrolipomatous tumor of the human female breast. *Arch Pathol Lab Med* 1977;101:149–151.
80. Koischowitz D, Helpap B: Chondroma of the breast. *Fortschr Geb Roentgenstr Nuklearmed* 1976;125:190–191.
81. Lugo M, Reyes JM, Putong PB: Benign chondrolipomatous tumors of the breast. *Arch Pathol Lab Med* 1982;102:691–692.
* 82. Marsh WL, Lucas JG, Olsen J: Chondrolipoma of the breast. *Arch Pathol Lab Med* 1989;113:369–371.
83. Melnick PJ: Fibromyoma of the breast. *Arch Pathol* 1932;14:794–798.
* 84. Nascimento AE, Rosen PP, Karas M, et al: Leiomyoma of the nipple. *Am J Surg Pathol* 1979;3:151–154.
* 85. Van der Walt JD, Reid HAS, Shaw JHF: Neurilemoma appearing as a lump in the breast. *Arch Pathol Lab Med* 1982;106:539–540.
86. Webber B: Leiomyoma of the nipple. *S Afr J Surg* 1975;13:117–120.

### Stromal Sarcoma

* 87. Barnes L, Pietruszka M: Sarcomas of the breast. A clinicopathologic analysis of ten cases. *Cancer* 1977;40:1577–1585.
88. Berg JW, De Cosse JJ, Fracchia AA, et al: Stromal sarcoma of the breast. *Cancer* 1962;15:418–424.
* 89. Botham RJ, McDonald JR, Claggett OT: Sarcoma of mammary gland. *Surg Gynecol Obstet* 1958;107:55–61.
* 90. Callery CD, Rosen PP, Kinne DW: Sarcoma of the breast. A study of 32 patients with reappraisal of classification and therapy. *Ann Surg* 1985;201:527–532.
91. Costa J, Wesley RA, Glatstein E, et al: The grading of soft tissue sarcomas. Results of a clinicopathologic correlation in a series of 163 cases. *Cancer* 1984;53:530–541.
92. Curran RC, Dodge DG: Sarcoma of breast with particular reference to its origin in fibroadenoma. *J Clin Pathol* 1962;15:1–16.
93. Hill RP, Stout AP: Sarcoma of the breast. *Arch Surg* 1965;44:1233–1243.
* 94. Norris HJ, Taylor HB: Sarcoma and related mesenchymal tumors of the breast. *Cancer* 1968;22:22–28.
* 95. Oberman HA: Sarcomas of the breast. *Cancer* 1965;18:1233–1243.
* 96. Salvadori B, Greco M, Galluzzo D, et al: Surgery for malignant mesenchymal tumors of the breast: A series of 31 cases. *Tumor* 1982;68:325–329.

### Liposarcoma

* 97. Arbabi L, Warhol MJ: Pleomorphic liposarcoma following radiotherapy for breast carcinoma. *Cancer* 1982;49:878–880.
* 98. Austin RM, Dupree WB: Liposarcoma of the breast: A clinicopathologic study of 20 cases. *Hum Pathol* 1986;17:906–913.
99. Breckenridge RL: Liposarcoma of the breast: Report of a case. *Am J Clin Pathol* 1954;24:954–956.
100. Carpanelli JB, Lempel G, Gatta C: Sobre un cao de liposarcoma de a glandula mamaria. *Semana Medica* 1963;123:321–322.
* 101. Delage J, Massabeau: Les lipomes du sein: et de la region mammaire. *Rev Chir* (Paris) 1904;30:484–506.
102. DeNavosquez S, Horton RE: Liposarcoma of the breast. *Guys Hosp Rep* 1947;96:57.
* 103. Enterline HT, Culberson JD, Rochlin DB, et al: Liposarcoma: A clinical and pathologic study of 53 cases. *Cancer* 1960;13:932–950.
104. Haagensen CD: *Diseases of the Breast*, ed 3. Philadelphia, WB Saunders, 1986, pp 336–338.
105. Hamazaki M, Hamaya K, Fujita H: Liposarcoma of the breast. *J Karyopath* 1968;12:73–82.
106. Huebert HT: Liposarcoma: The Manitoba experience. *Can J Surg* 1981;24:391–396.
107. Hummer CD, Burkart TJ: Liposarcoma of the breast: A case of bilateral involvement. *Am J Surg* 1967;113:558–561.
108. Ii K, Hizawa K, Okazaki K, et al: Liposarcoma of the breast: Fine structural and histochemical study of a case. *Tokushima J Exp Med* 1980;27:45–56.
109. Lederer M, Livingstone S: Liposarcoma, intracanalicular fibroma, pericanalicular fibroma, and cystic change of the breast. *Arch Pathol* 1933;16:171–174.
110. Lifvendahl RA: Liposarcoma of the mammary gland. *Surg Gynecol Obstet* 1930;50:81–84.
111. Millo L: Liposarcoma della mammela. *Arch Ital Patol Clin Tumor* 1958;2:610–622.
* 112. Rasmussen J, Jensen H: Liposarcoma of the breast: A case report and review of the literature. *Virchows Arch (A)* 1979;385:117–124.
* 113. Stout AP, Bernanke M: Liposarcoma of the female mammary gland. *Surg Gynecol Obstet* 1946;83:216–218.

### Osteosarcoma

114. Alpert LI, Abaci IF, Werthamer S: Radiation-induced extraskeletal osteosarcoma. *Cancer* 1973;31:1359–1363.
* 115. Altavilla G, Cavazzini L, Rossi S: Osteogenic sarcoma of the breast. A case report and review of the literature. *Pathologica* 1985;77:101–106.
116. Annani PA, Baumann RP: Osteosarcoma of the breast. *Virchows Arch (A)* 1972;347:212–218.
* 117. Aubrey DA, Andrews GS: Mammary osteogenic sarcoma. *Br J Surg* 1971;58:472–474.

118. Boyer CW, Navin JJ: Extraskeletal osteogenic sarcoma. A late complication of radiation therapy. *Cancer* 1965;18:628–633.

119. Carlucci GA, Wagner RF: Osteochondrofibrosarcoma of the breast. *Am J Surg* 1943;61:271–276.

120. Curran RC, Dodge RC: Sarcoma of breast, with particular reference to its origin from fibroadenoma. *J Clin Pathol* 1962;15:1–16.

121. Fry HJB: Osteoclastoma (myeloid sarcoma) of the human female breast. *J Pathol Bacteriol* 1927;30:529–536.

*122. Gonzalez-Licea A, Yardley JH, Hartman WH: Malignant tumor of the breast with bone formation. Studies by light and electron microscopy. *Cancer* 1967;20:1234–1247.

*123. Going JJ, Lumsden AB, Anderson TJ: A classical osteogenic sarcoma of the breast: Histology, immunohistochemistry, and ultrastructure. *Histopathology* 1986;10:631–641.

124. Haagensen CD: *Diseases of the Breast*, ed 3. Philadelphia, WB Saunders, 1986, 318–349, 843–850.

125. Jernstrom P, Lindberg AL, Meland ON: Osteogenic sarcoma of the mammary gland. *Am J Clin Pathol* 1963;40:521–526.

126. Llombart-Bosch A, Peydro A: Malignant mixed osteogenic tumours of the breast. An ultrastructural study of two cases. *Virchows Arch A Path Anat and Histol* 1975;366:1–14.

127. Mertens HH, Langnickel D, Staedler F: Primary osteogenic sarcoma of the breast. *Acta Cytol* 1981;26:512–516.

*128. Mufarrij AA, Feiner HD: Breast sarcoma with giant cells and osteoid. A case report and review of the literature. *Am J Surg Pathol* 1987;11:225–230.

129. Rottino A, Howley CP: Osteoid sarcoma of the breast: A complication of fibroadenoma. *Arch Pathol* 1945;40:44–50.

130. Smith BH, Taylor HB: The occurrence of bone and cartilage in mammary tumors. *Am J Clin Pathol* 1969;51:610–618.

## Chondrosarcoma

131. Beltaos E, Banerjee TK: Chondrosarcoma of the breast. Report of 2 cases. *Am J Clin Pathol* 1979;71:345–349.

132. Kennedy T, Biggart JD: Sarcoma of the breast. *Br J Cancer* 1967;21:635–644.

133. Schottenfeld L: Sarcoma of the breast. Review of the literature with a report of 14 cases. *Am J Surg* 1954;88:229–246.

## Myosarcoma

*134. Cameron HM, Hamperl H, Warambo W: Leiomyosarcoma of the breast originating from myoepithelium. *J Pathol* 1974;114:89–92.

135. Chen KTK, Kuo TT, Hoffman KD: Leiomyosarcoma of the breast. *Cancer* 1981;47:1883–1886.

136. Crocer FJ, Murad TM: Ultrastructure of fibrosarcoma in a male breast. *Cancer* 1969;23:891–899.

137. Elhence IP, Mital VP, Upadhayaya SC, et al: Rhabdomyosarcoma of breast. *Ind J Cancer* 1972;9:171–174.

*138. Hernandez FJ: Leiomyosarcoma of male breast originating in the nipple. *Am J Surg Pathol* 1978;2:299–304.

*139. Nielsen BB: Leiomyosarcoma of the breast with late dissemination. *Virchows Archiv (Pathol Anat)* 1984;403:241–245.

*140. Pardo-Mindan J, Garcia-Julian G, Eizaguirre AM, et al: Leiomyosarcoma of the breast. *Am J Clin Pathol* 1974;62:477–480.

## Malignant Fibrous Histiocytoma

141. Callery CD, Rosen PP, Kinne DW: Sarcoma of the breast. A study of 32 patients with reappraisal of classification and therapy. *Ann Surg* 1984;201:527–532.

142. Iellin A, Waizbard E, Levine T, et al: Malignant fibrous histiocytoma of the breast. *Int Surg* 1990;75:63–66.

143. Kobayashi Y, Kitamura T, Yaso K, et al: A case of primary malignant fibrous histiocytoma of the breast. *Gann No Rinsho* 1977;23:1085–1089.

*144. Langham MR Jr: Malignant fibrous histiocytoma of the breast. A case report and review of the literature. *Cancer* 1984;54:558–563.

145. Liebert CW, Edwards OK: Malignant fibrous histiocytoma of the breast. *South Med J* 1982;33:1718–1725.

*146. Luzzatto R, Grossman S, Scholl JG, et al: Postradiation pleomorphic malignant fibrous histiocytoma of the breast. *Acta Cytol* 1986;30:48–50.

147. Osryn C, Spector I, Brenner CG: Malignant fibrous histiocytoma of the breast. A case report. *S Afr Med J* 1987;71:665–666.

148. Pollard SG, Marks PV, Temple IN, et al: Breast sarcoma. A clinicopathologic review of 25 cases. *Cancer* 1990;66:941–944.

149. Tsuneyoshi M, Enjoji M: Post-irradiation sarcoma (malignant fibrous histiocytoma) following breast carcinoma—an ultrastructural study of a case. *Cancer* 1979;45:1419–1423.

*150. Van Niecker JLM, Wobbes TH, Holland R, et al: Malignant fibrous histiocytoma of the breast with axillary node involvement. *J Surg Oncol* 1987;34:32–35.

*151. Vera-Sampere F, Llombart-Bosch A: Malignant fibrohistiocytoma of the breast. Primary and post-irradiation variant: An ultrastructural study. *Pathol Res Pract* 1984;178:289–296.

152. Ushijima S, Minagawa M, Kiyohara K, et al: Malignant fibrous histiocytoma of the breast. Report of a case. *Nippon Geka Gakkai Zasshi* 1987;88:119–122.

# 14

# Diseases of the Nipple



There are two major primary lesions and a number of less common alterations that affect the nipple. The two most notable lesions of the nipple are Paget's disease and adenoma of the nipple. Clinically, these two lesions can be confused because both can cause erosion, ulceration, and enlargement of the nipple. Microscopically, however, each is quite distinctive.

## PAGET'S DISEASE

Described in 1874 by Sir James Paget (33), this lesion constitutes 1% to 5% of all breast carcinomas and is characterized by the presence of large cells with abundant, pale cytoplasm and large nuclei with prominent nucleoli in the surface epithelium of the nipple. These cells are generally referred to as Paget's cells, though Treves (47) questioned this practice since Paget did not actually describe the histologic features or the cellular morphology of the lesion. One of the earliest clinical descriptions of Paget's disease has been attributed to John of Arderne (11) who recorded the development of a sore in the nipple of a priest in the early fourteenth century (1307); within two years, the cancerous change extended into the underlying breast and was associated with livid changes in the overlying skin.

Velpeau (48) also discussed the dermatitis-like changes of the nipple and areola that precede cancer of the breast in women in 1841. But it is Sir James Paget (32) who has been credited with recognition of the lesion as a clinical entity. As he did not provide a histologic description of the lesions that he observed, some confusion followed regarding which cases should be designated as Paget's disease. This designation would be appropriate upon identification of Paget's cells in the surface epithelium of the nipple or areola, regardless of the mode or mechanism of arrival or development of these cells at these foci. Interestingly, Darier designated Paget cells with dyskeratotic features as "psorosperms," and referred to Paget's disease as a new form of cutaneous psorospermosis (8).

## Histogenesis

Over the years, a variety of viewpoints have been offered in an attempt to explain the nature of the Paget cells. Orr and Parrish (31) suggested that Paget cells represent altered melanocytes. Derived in part from the finding of melanin pigment within some Paget cells, this viewpoint is no longer tenable since the cells fail to show a positive reaction to S-100 protein or HMB-45, but do show a positive reaction to cytokeratin and polyclonal CEA (27,47). Furthermore, at the ultrastructural level, Paget cells show microvilli along the plasma membrane, intracellular and extracellular lumen formation, as well as desmosomal attachment to adjacent keratinocytes and other Paget cells; well-developed desmosomal junctions are almost never identified in melanocytic cells (41). It is now accepted that Paget cells are capable of phagocytizing melanin, as melanin can be identified within these cells by light microscopy (7,35) and both free and membrane-bound melanosomes have been identified within Paget cells at the ultrastructural level just as they have been found occasionally in keratinocytes.

Another viewpoint is that Paget cells are derived through an in situ alteration in the keratinocyte (34,50). This type of transformation would account for the 4% to 5% of cases of Paget's disease in which no underlying carcinoma can be identified in the mastectomy specimen despite exhaustive sampling. The presence of cells with morphologic features intermediate between Paget cells and keratinocytes, as well as the occasional "dyskeratotic" appearance of Paget cells as they migrate into the stratum corneum support this possibility. Sagami (40) and Sagebiel (41) independently provided substantial evidence in support of an in situ transformation in the development of Paget's disease. Both demonstrated desmosomal junctions between Paget's cells and adjacent keratinocytes. Sagebiel's (41) description of keratinocytes that exhibited a paucity of desmosomes and separation of tonofibrils by a clear peripheral zone of cytoplasm adjacent to Paget cells may reflect early stages of transformation of keratinocytes to Paget cells at the ultrastructural level.

A

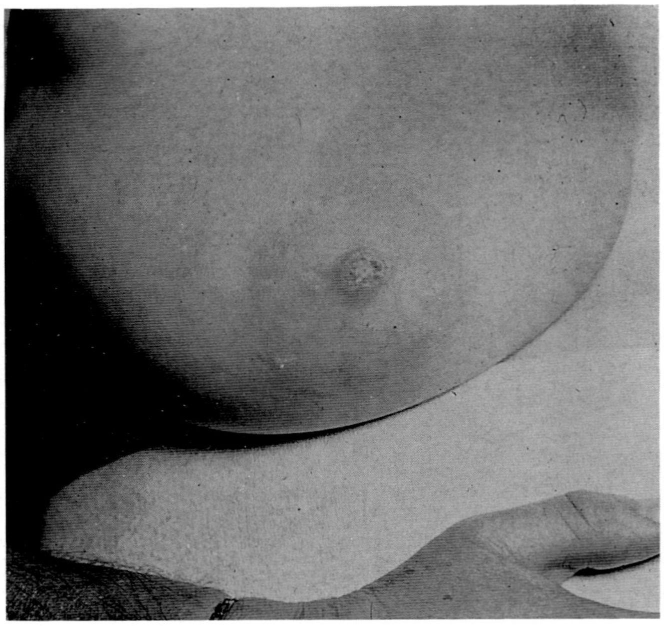

**Figure 14.1** Paget's disease. The clinical appearance varies from those showing subtle irregularities in the areolar margin (a), to development of eczematoid change and distortion of the nipple (b), and those showing such massive underlying carcinoma that the tumor distorts the overlying skin along with retraction and focal erosion of the nipple (c).

The current and most widely accepted viewpoint is that Paget cells are adenocarcinoma cells. While some believe that these cells arrive in the nipple through an epidermotropic migration of an underlying carcinoma (13,14,45,46), others have held the opinion that, in some cases, the underlying cancer is an independent lesion (26,27). The presence of microvilli along the plasma membrane, and formation of intracellular and extracellular lumens or canaliculi at the ultrastructural level (41) support the interpretation of these cells as glandular in nature. Toker (45) identified clear and dark Paget cells which he interpreted as the neoplastic counterpart of the luminal epithelial clear and dark cells respectively. Furthermore, Bussolati and Pich (4) demonstrated casein in 14 of 16 cases of both mammary and extramammary Paget's disease. Kirkham et al (17) demonstrated milk fat globule membrane antigens (HMFG-1 and HMFG-2) in 12 cases of mammary Paget's disease; the staining pattern of the Paget cells was similar to that of the underlying intraductal and invasive ductal carcinomas supporting ductal origin of the Paget

B

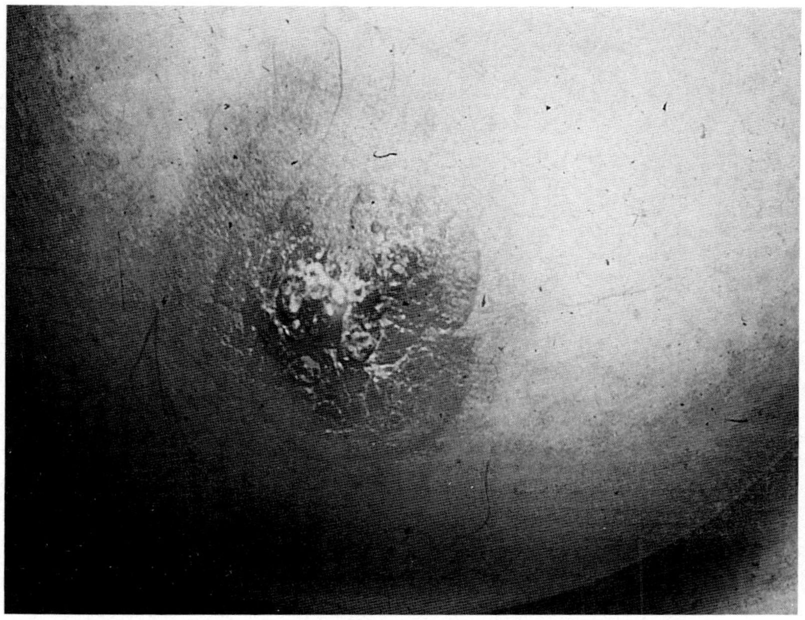

C

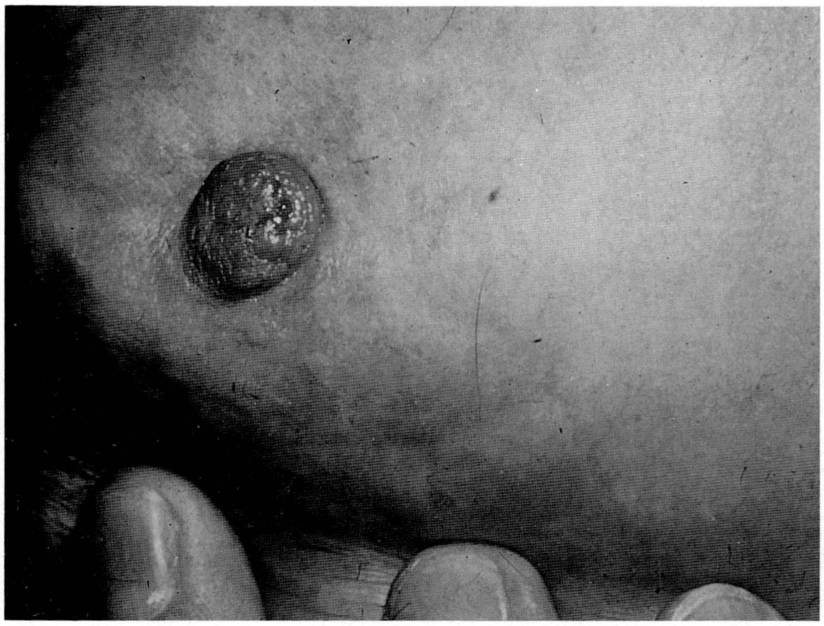

**Figure 14.1(b,c)** Paget's disease. Legend on opposite page.

cells. The identification of CEA in Paget cells further supports their glandular nature (28,48).

## Clinical Features

Paget's disease accounts for 1% to 4.3% of mammary carcinomas (16,18,22). The appearance of the involved nipple varies depending on the extent and stage of progression of the disease (Fig. 14.1). It initially causes simple reddening of the nipple and areola associated with pruritis. This progresses to a scaling, eczematoid change which is moist with eventual erosion and ulceration. A painless mass is palpable in the underlying breast tissue in about 50% of cases. Paget's disease is generally unilateral, but bilateral lesions have been reported (1). Paget's disease is seen in both female and male (2,39,43,47) breasts. In one series of male breast carcinomas (31), 12% had Paget's disease. Paget's disease has also been reported in patients with Klinefelter's syndrome

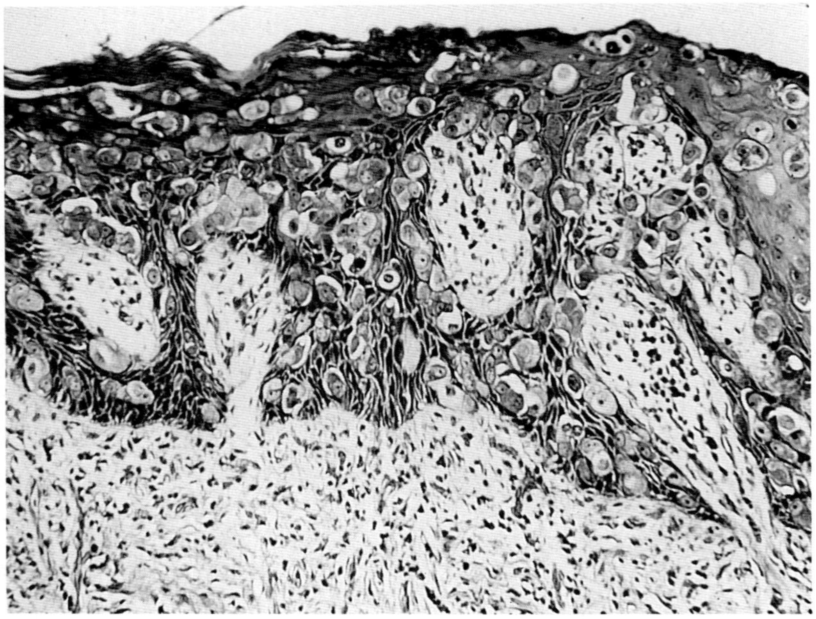

**Figure 14.2** Paget's disease is characterized by the presence of large cells with abundant pale cytoplasm infiltrating the epidermis. (H&E, X160)

(25). It has also developed in the nipple after conservative management of early breast cancer (23).

## Microscopic Features

The salient feature of the disease is the presence of Paget cells singly or in clusters within the surface epithelium of the nipple, the areola, or both (Fig. 14.2). Occasionally, the neoplastic cells form acini (Fig. 14.3). In approximately 95% of cases, there is an underlying carcinoma, and many of these are simply an intraductal carcinoma within the lactiferous ducts (Fig. 14.4). When invasive, the underlying carcinomas are of various types with a majority being ductal, but in situ and invasive lobular, medullary, and papillary carcinomas are also observed (3). The underlying invasive carcinoma is often mammographically detectable (Fig. 14.5). Since the cells in the

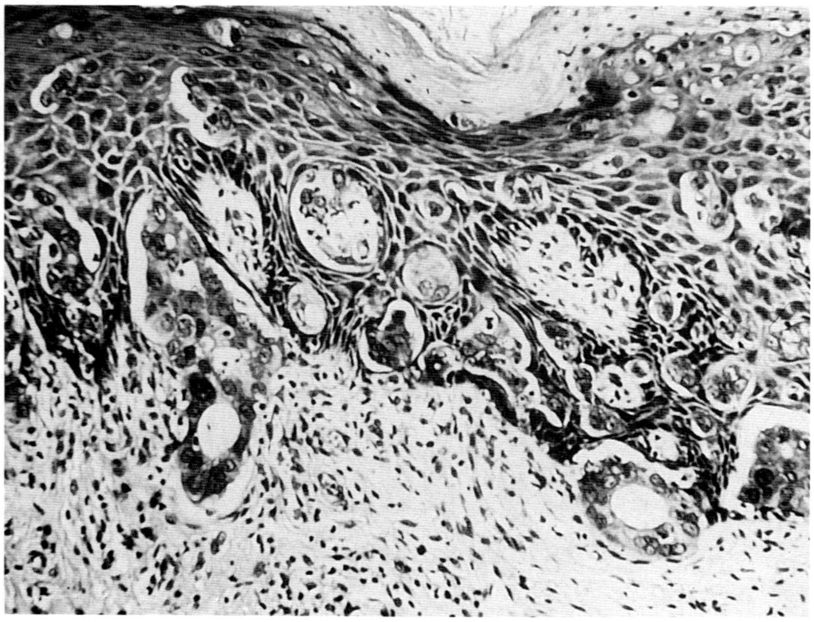

**Figure 14.3** Rarely, Paget's cells may form acini within the epithelium, particularly at the dermal-epidermal junction. (H&E, X160)

A

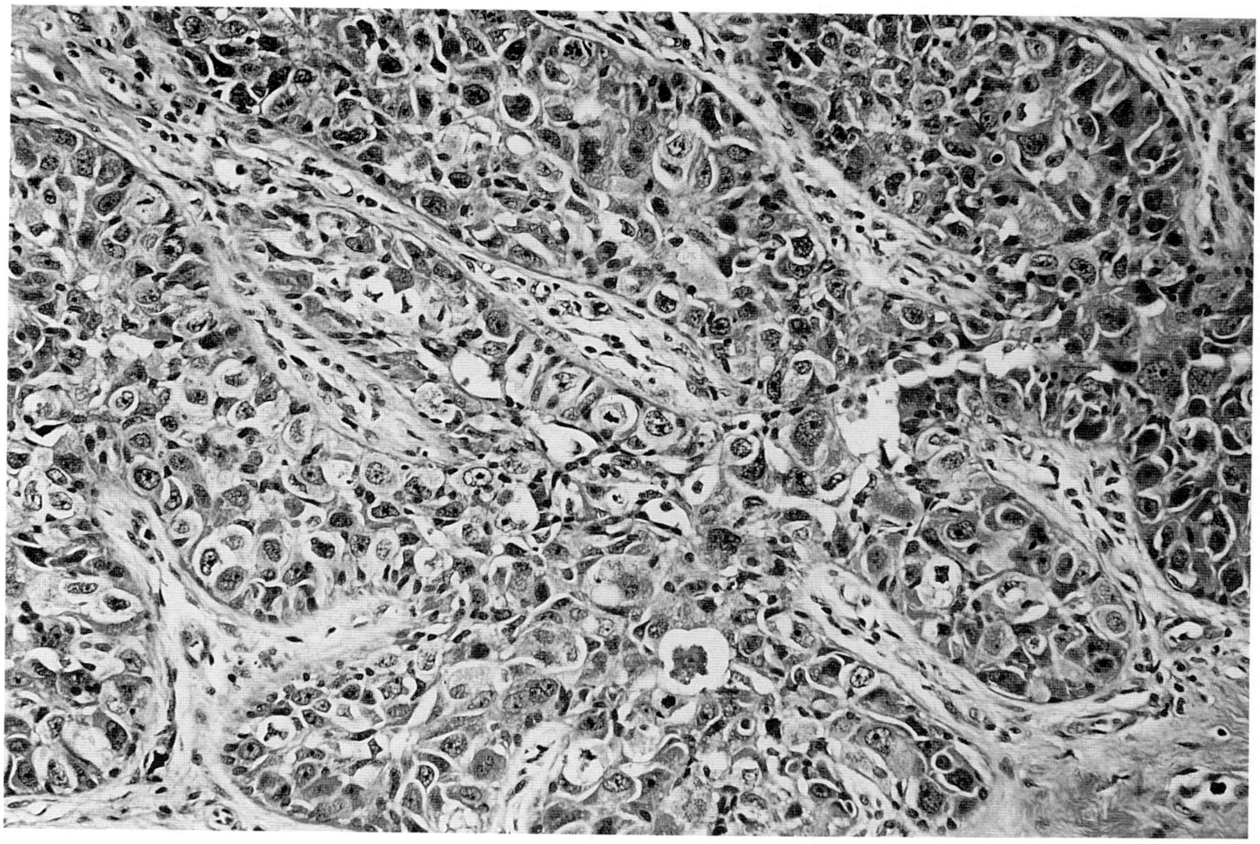

B

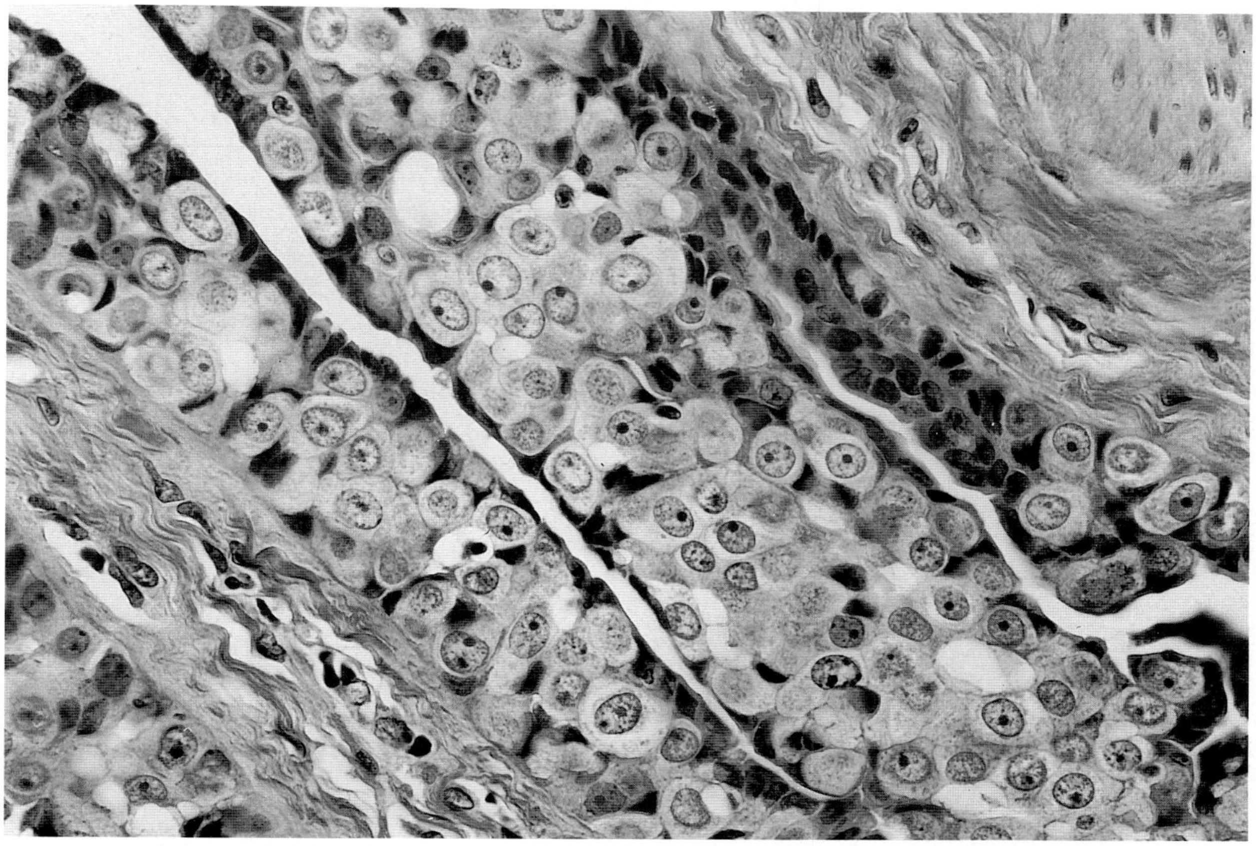

**Figure 14.4** (a) The underlying intraductal carcinoma is composed of large cells with abundant cytoplasm and prominent nucleoli. (H&E, X160) (b) Note the pagetoid growth pattern under the native epithelial cell layer. (H&E, X400)

C

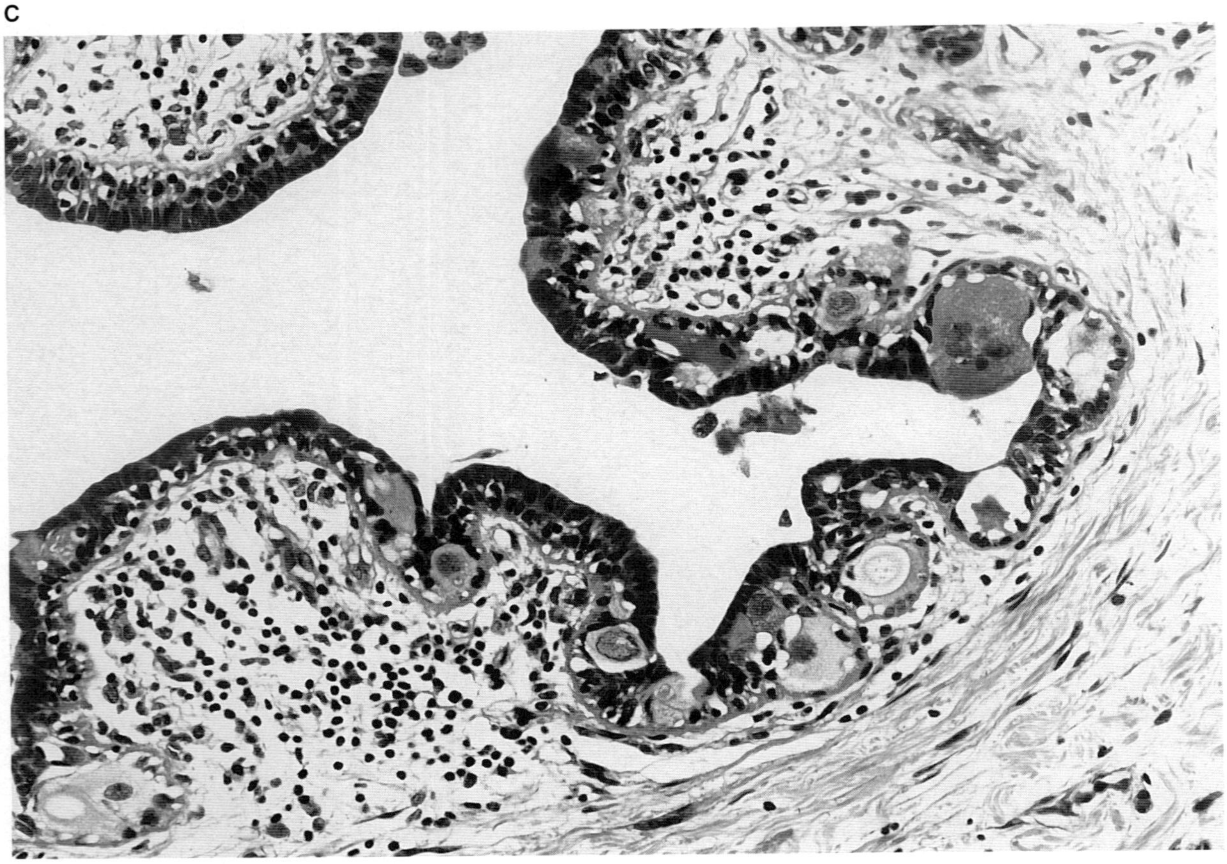

**Figure 14.4(c)** Paget's cell in a lactiferous duct. Farther away from the major area of involvement isolated cells can be found in a pagetoid fashion in the lactiferous ducts. (H&E, X400)

epidermis reflect a variety of underlying breast carcinomas, a certain degree of variation in their appearance is clearly anticipated. It is this variation from the classic Paget's cell appearance that causes diagnostic problems in some cases. Only about 50% to 60% of Paget cells will be mucin and PAS-positive (Fig. 14.6) since approximately a similar percentage of breast carcinomas will have a notable degree of stainable mucin in their cytoplasm.

In situ lesions predominate among patients without a palpable mass, while invasive carcinomas are preponderant among those with a palpable mass. In Ashikari et al's (3) series, of the 96 patients without a palpable mass at presentation, 63 had non-invasive carcinomas and 33 had invasive tumors; of the 113 patients with a palpable mass, 106 had invasive carcinomas and only seven had in situ lesions. In Salvadori et al's (42) series of 41 women without a palpable mass, eight had an in situ carcinoma, while 33 had an invasive carcinoma; of the 50 women with a palpable nodule, all had invasive carcinomas. Clearly, the clinical finding of a palpable mass associated with the nipple changes of Paget's disease is an ominous sign.

## Immunohistochemical Characteristics

Mammary Paget's cells have shown a positive reaction for CEA in all 12 cases evaluated in two separate studies (28,48). A positive immunoreaction for antibody 21N, a peptide component of c-erbB-2 protein, has been observed in 91% to 100% of cases of Paget's disease (12,20). Meissner et al (24) have shown expression of neu-protein by Paget cells. The cells are also positive for cytokeratin (CAM 5.2), (12). Paget cells express a keratin phenotype characteristic of simple epithelial cells as seen in glandular epithelium according to Chaudary et al (5). Paget cells do not react with S-100 protein or HMB-45.

## Differential Diagnosis

Diagnostic problems arise particularly when fixation and tissue preparation are not optimal (Fig. 14.7), when the biopsy is taken from degenerating areas,

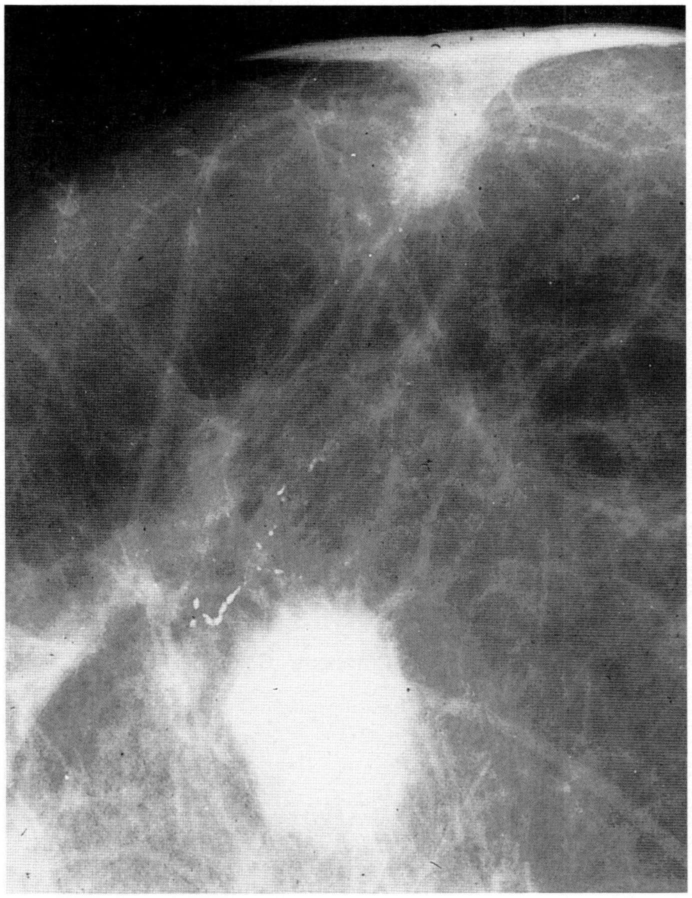

**Figure 14.5** Mammographically, a large mass is apparent in the underlying breast along with nipple retraction and extensive alterations in the lactiferous ducts.

when only a few atypical cells are present, and when the cells contain melanin pigment. Morphologically, these less than ideal situations raise the possibility of a melanocytic lesion and dysplastic squamous changes.

Paget's cells involving the nipple can phagocytize melanin and mimic melanoma (7,36,107). Fortunately for the pathologists, dysplastic lesions of the squamous epithelium and melanocytic lesions occur with such a low frequency in the nipple and areola that, for practical purposes, these diagnoses should be made only after excluding the possibility of Paget's disease. A positive mucin stain will resolve the problem in a good proportion of cases since about 50% to 60% of cases of Paget's disease will display mucin positivity in the neoplastic cells. A negative reaction does not exclude Paget's disease, however (30). Immunostains are the next step to be taken in such a situation. A positive CEA (Fig. 14.8) would confirm a diagnosis of Paget's disease, while a negative reaction for S-100 protein or HMB-45 along with a positive reaction for an epithelial marker would exclude melanoma. If these steps do not resolve the problem or the questionable cells disappear from the section before completion of special studies, it is best to request a rebiopsy from viable areas rather than make a definitive diagnosis on questionable material, particularly if a diagnosis of melanoma is being considered.

Assuming that one comes across a case in

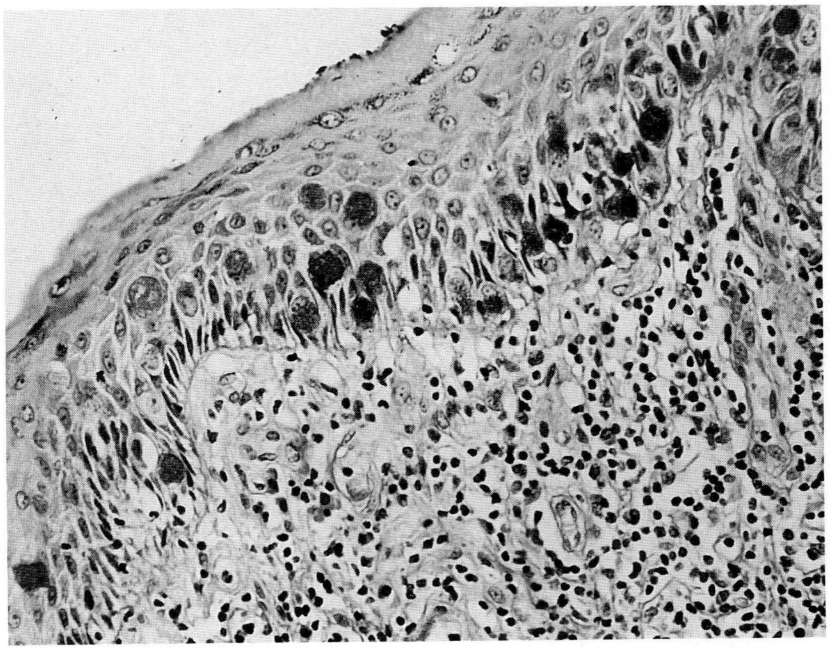

**Figure 14.6** The cytoplasm of Paget's cells shows a positive reaction for PAS. (X160)

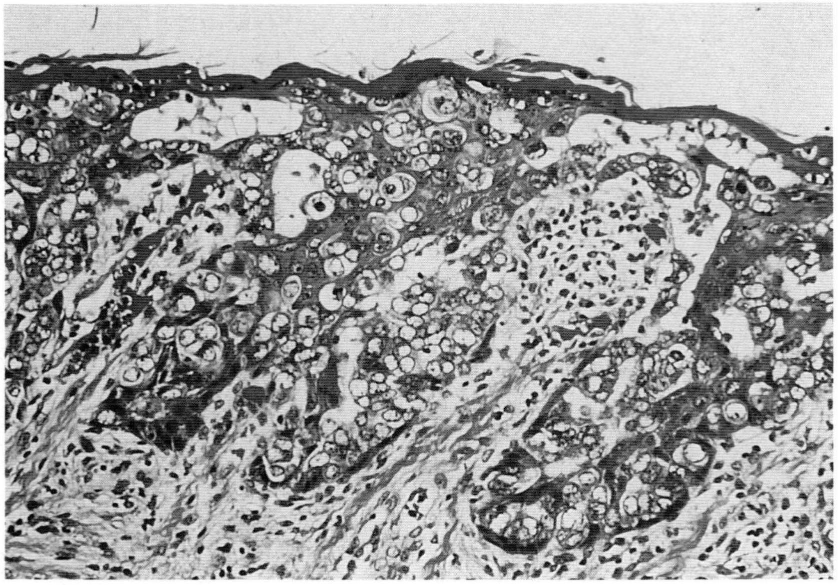

**Figure 14.7** Poor fixation of the tissue makes distinction of Paget's cells from a melanocytic cell population difficult. (H&E, X160)

which the cells are mucin negative but have phagocytized melanin, immunostains should be the first step in the diagnostic process if there are cells that lack phagocytized melanin. In general, it would be a rare event for every cell to contain melanin. Immunohistochemical evaluation of the non-pigmented cells in these cases generally resolves the problem. If there are no cells free of melanin, electron microscopy would be the only way to unequivocally establish the nature of these cells. Paget cells phagocytizing melanin lack melanosomes, and display well-developed desmosomes; melanocytic cells contain melanosomes and only rarely would display tight junctions or desmosomes. Before resorting to electron microscopy, however, a rebiopsy should be attempted; additional tissue often provides the answer.

Other cutaneous lesions such as pemphigus vulgaris rarely coexist with Paget's disease of the nipple (37) and can complicate the diagnosis.

Occasionally, normal squamous epithelium of the nipple contains clear cells (see Chapter 1, Normal Breast) which lack nuclear atypia and are smaller and far more uniform in size than Paget cells. Toker (44) described clear cells in 9% of mastectomy specimen of cancer patients and 12% of nipples in autopsy cases. The precise nature of these clear cells is not well established and requires further evaluation.

## Treatment

Mastectomy has remained the preferred treatment for Paget's disease regardless of the presence or absence of a palpable underlying mass. The presence of a clinically palpable nodule has been used as a discriminating factor in the selection of the type of surgical approach. Partial or complete excision of the nipple and areolar complex has been used in five patients (19). One of the patients developed recurrence 12 months after partial excision of the nipple-areolar complex; the remaining four patients were free of tumor 30 to 69 months after complete excision of the nipple-areolar complex. For patients presenting with a cutaneous lesion and an underlying mass, treatment has generally consisted of radical or modified radical mastectomy. A simple or total mastectomy has been recommended for women without a palpable nodule (6,16,22,38). Considering the central location of Paget's disease in the breast, Salvadori et al (42) suggested dissection of the chain of internal mammary lymph nodes for these patients.

A conservative approach consisting of either wide local excision followed by axillary node dissection, with or without radiation therapy, or radiation therapy alone has been used in a few patients. The subjects of conservative therapy have been women without a palpable mass, those with lesions confined

A

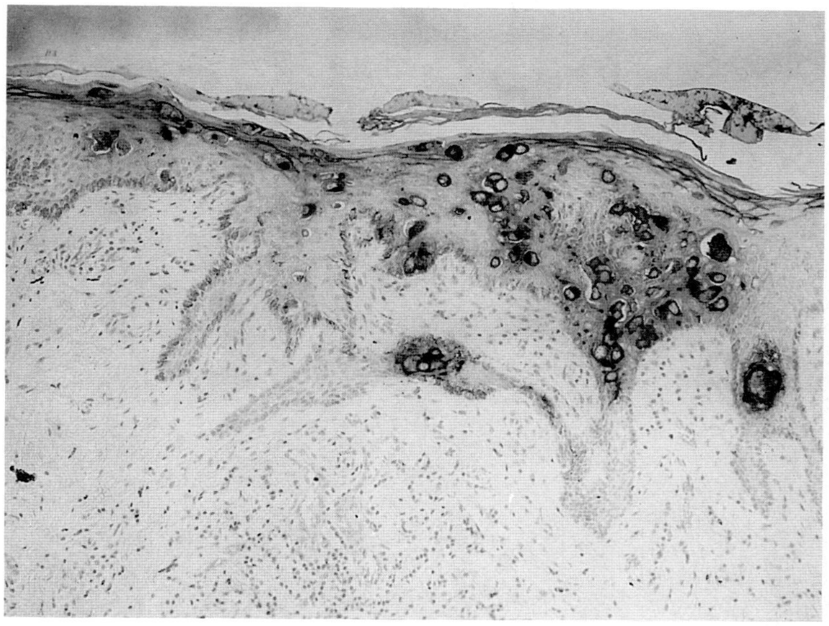

B

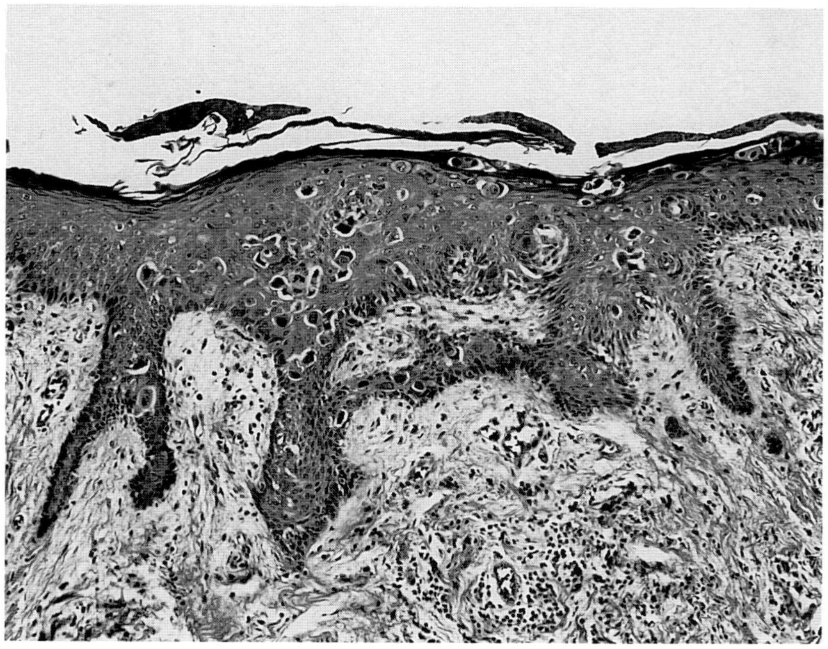

**Figure 14.8** (a) Paget's cells show a positive reaction for CEA. (X120) (b) The same lesion stained with H&E. (X120)

**Table 14.1** Paget's Disease: Clinical Features

| Reference | No. of Cases | No. of Inv (%) | % LN Mets | 5-Yr Surv | 10-Yr Surv |
|---|---|---|---|---|---|
| | | **Paget's, WOPT** | | | |
| 3 | 96 | 33 (34) | 13 | 92% | 87% |
| 41 | 41 | 33 (80) | 0 | 92% | 82% |
| | | **Paget's, WPT** | | | |
| 3 | 113 | 103 (91%) | 65 | 45% | 38% |
| 41 | 50 | 50 (100%) | 84 | 38% | 22% |

*Abbreviations*: WOPT = without palpable tumor; WPT = with palpable tumor; Inv = invasive; LN = lymph node; Mets = metastasis; Surv = survival

to the nipple without an underlying breast carcinoma, those with only a minimal intraductal carcinoma in the lactiferous ducts, and all those reluctant to have mastectomy. It is difficult to ascertain absence of an underlying carcinoma without a mastectomy, however. But if this could be accomplished with clinical and mammographic studies, conservative treatment would be an option for women with limited lesions considering the good results that have been obtained in the small number of reported cases (9,10,19,21).

It should be emphasized, however, that a palpa-

A

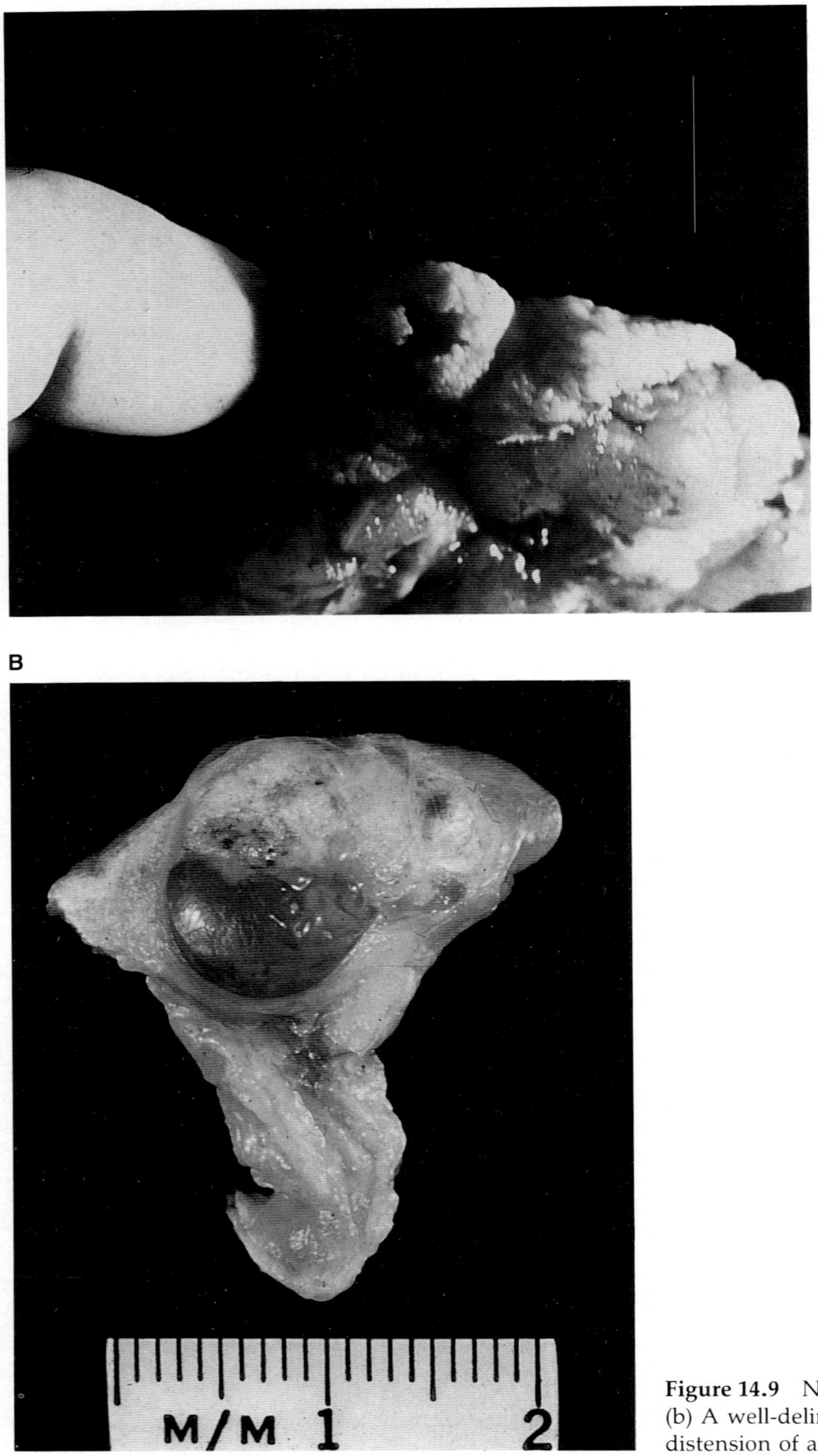


**Figure 14.9** Nipple duct adenoma. (a) The nipple is enlarged, irregular and fissured. (b) A well-delineated mass has replaced the nipple, compressing and causing cystic distension of an underlying duct.

A

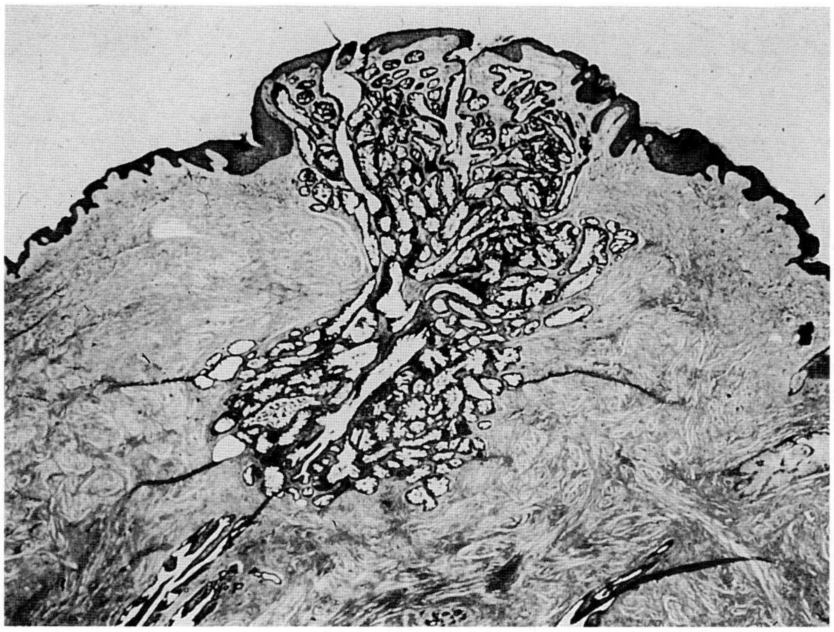

B

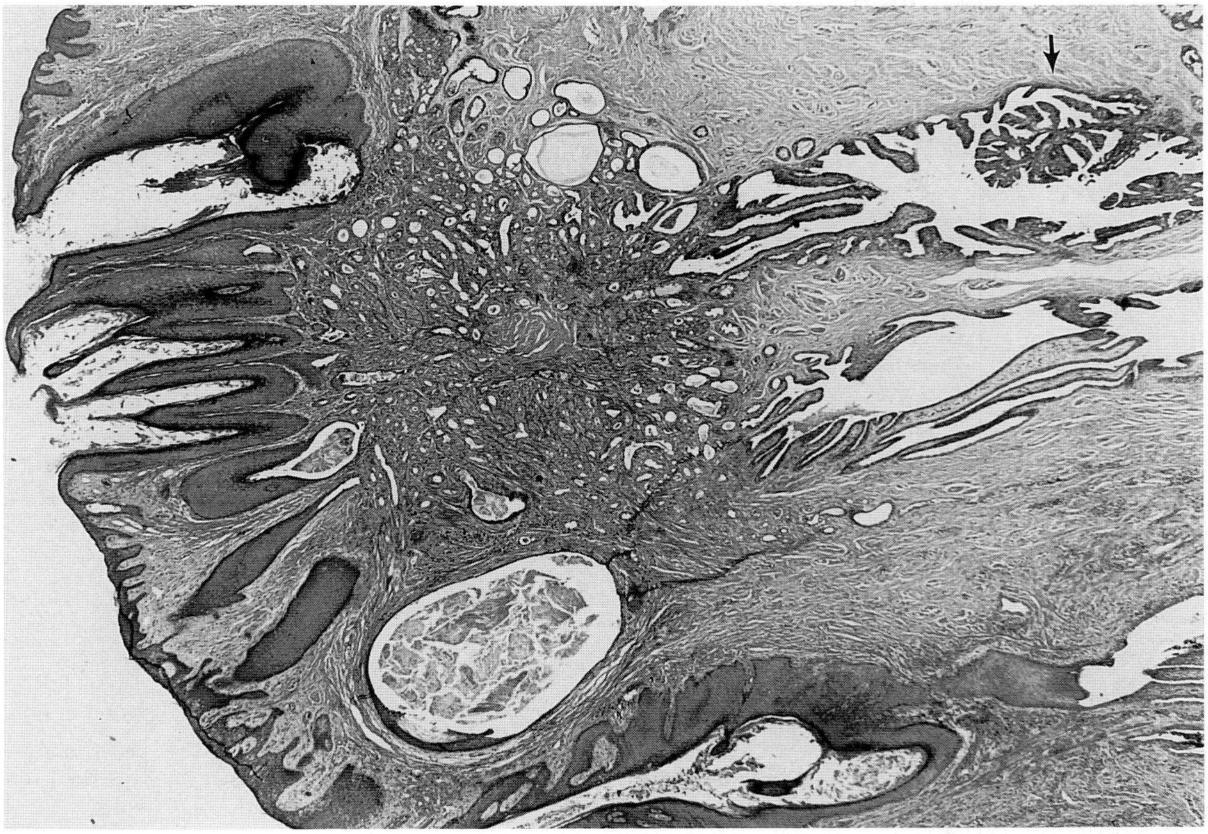

**Figure 14.10** Asymptomatic nipple duct adenoma. (a) Proliferating tubules have clustered around a lactiferous duct in the nipple. (b) Another case showing a small NDA associated with a papillary hyperplasia in the underlying lactiferous duct (arrow). (H&E, (a) X12; (b) X30)

ble nodule is a clinical parameter, and its absence is not always synonymous with the absence of an invasive tumor. It is quite possible to have an invasive carcinoma with positive axillary nodes even when there is no evidence of a palpable mass; axillary node metastases were found in 13% of the 96 women without an underlying palpable mass in Ashikari et al's series (3).

A

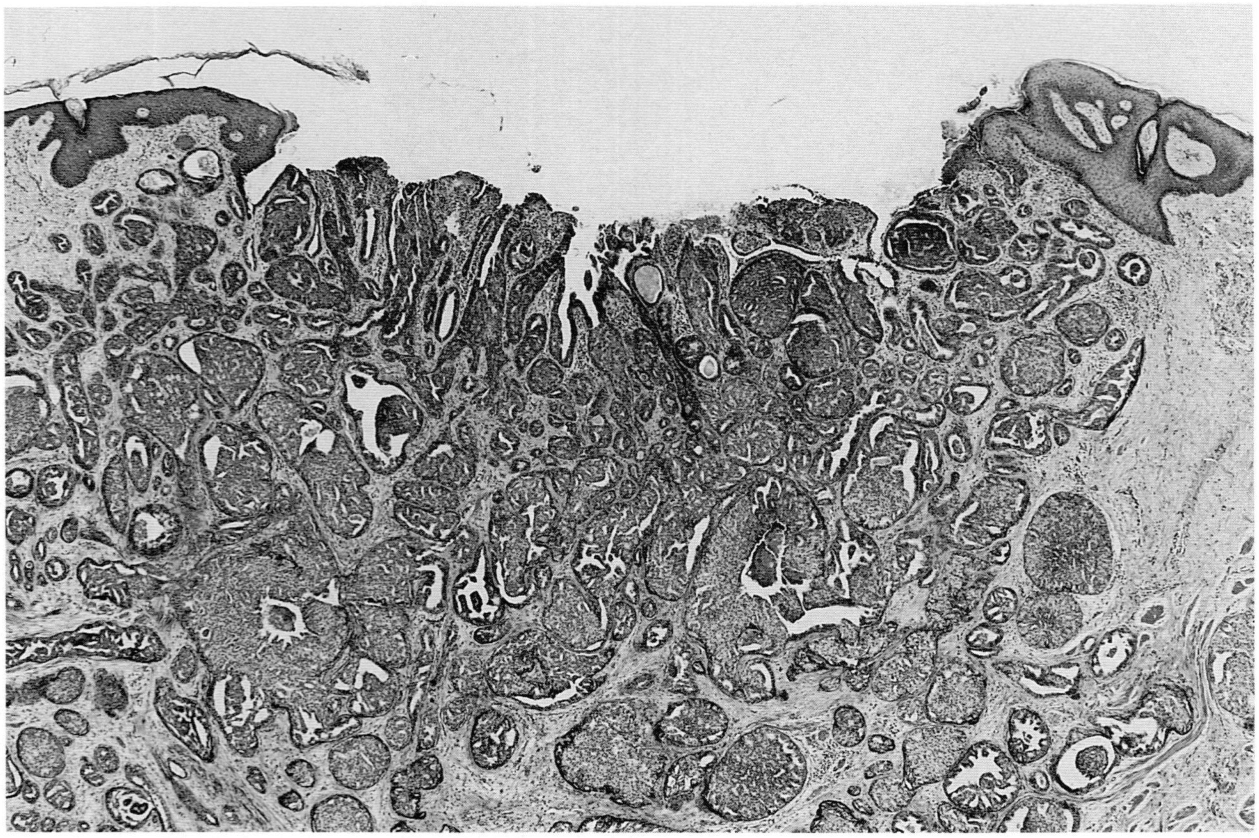

B

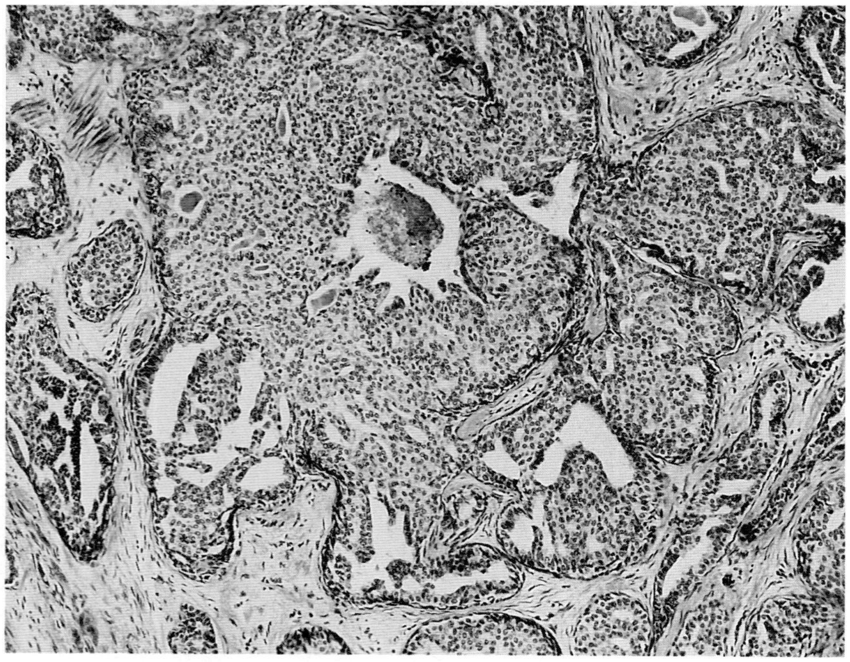

**Figure 14.11** (a) Nipple duct adenoma eroding the surface epithelium and associated with epithelial hyperplasia; (b) Note the presence of central necrosis within one of the ducts. The presence of epithelial and ME cells within this proliferation pointed against a diagnosis of IDCA. (H&E, (a) X25; (b) X100)

## Prognosis

The prognosis of the disease depends on the presence of an underlying carcinoma, size of the tumor, and the status of the axillary lymph nodes. Since the presence of a palpable mass is one reflection of the larger size of these tumor compared to the nonpalpable lesions, patients with a palpable mass at presentation have a worse prognosis compared to

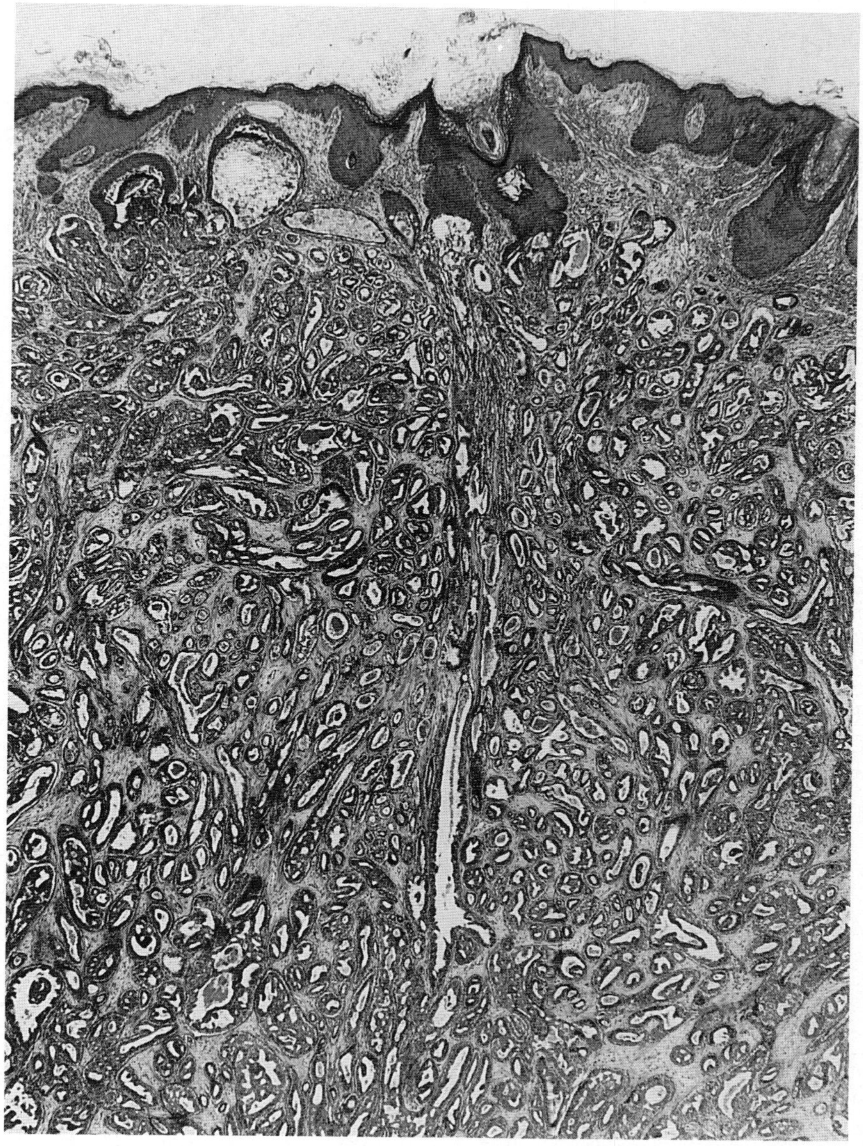

**Figure 14.12** Nipple duct adenoma showing extensive replacement of the nipple stroma by an adenomatous proliferation of tubules without significant intervening stroma. (H&E, X10)

those without a mass (Table 14.1). In Ashikari et al's series (3), patients without a palpable mass and negative axillary nodes had a five-year survival of 97% which dropped to 95% at ten years. Axillary lymph node metastases were found in 13% of the women without an underlying palpable mass. The overall survival for those without a palpable mass was 92% at five years and 87% at ten years. In contrast, the five-year survival for the 113 patients with a palpable mass was 40% at five years and 38% at ten years. For patients with a palpable mass but with negative nodes, the five-year survival was 73%. This classic study clearly demonstrated the influence of tumor size and axillary node metastases on prognosis and survival; unfortunately, it is not clear whether the survival rates are actuarial or absolute. In Salvadori et al's (42) series, which provides actuarial survival rates, 41 patients presented without a palpable nodule. The five-year survival for these patients was 92% and dropped to 82% at ten years; the median survival of these patients was 16.4 years. Of these, 34 had histologic assessment of the lymph nodes and none had evidence of nodal involvement. Of the 50 women with a palpable nodule, survival was 38% at five years and it dropped to 22% at ten years. Forty-eight of these patients had histologic

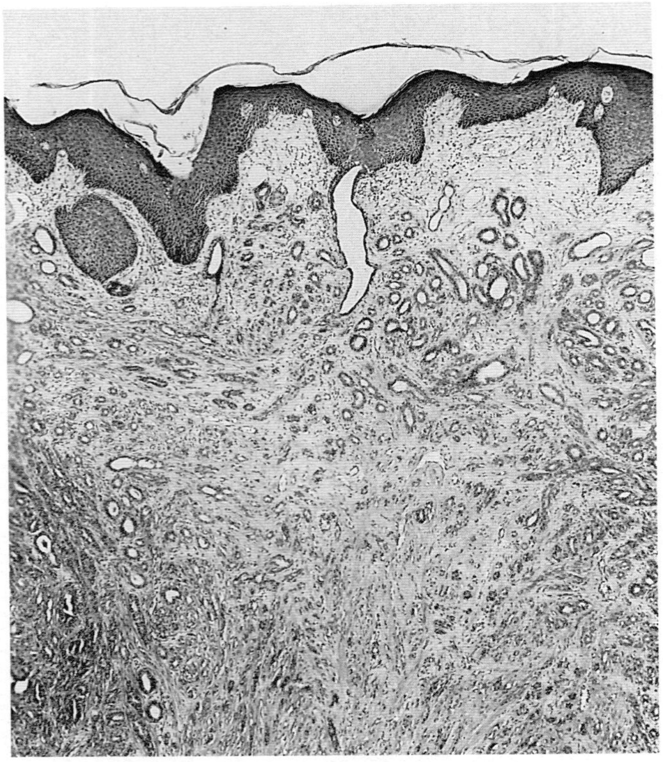

**Figure 14.13** Nipple duct adenoma showing focal sclerosis of the stroma. (H&E, X40)

assessment of their lymph nodes, and of these, 42 (84%) had positive nodes.

In a subsequent but comparatively smaller study of 50 patients, Paone and Baker (34) found that the actuarial survival rates for patients with a palpable breast mass were similar to those of patients with infiltrating duct carcinoma with five- and ten-year actuarial survival rates of 22% and 9.9% respectively for those with positive nodes. In contrast, none of the 19 patients with Paget's disease confined to the nipple and without a palpable mass developed recurrent carcinoma.

## NIPPLE DUCT ADENOMA

This uncommon lesion, which can be mistaken for Paget's disease clinically and misinterpreted as carcinoma microscopically, has been variably referred to as adenoma of the nipple (56,57,59), erosive adenosis (60,65), erosive adenomatosis (66,67,74,75), papillary adenoma (54,69), and florid papillomatosis, or simply papillomatosis (70,72,77). It was first described in 1955 when Jones (64) reported five examples of the tumor to underscore the benign nature of the lesion which he designated as florid papillomatosis of the nipple duct to distinguish it from carcinomas. This designation is somewhat curious since none of the lesions had true papillomas; they consisted of an adenomatous proliferation of tubular glands some of which had epithelial hyperplasia. In a subsequent report (68), 13 of the 16 cases had been diagnosed as carcinoma and mastectomies had been performed on 15 cases. Eleven of the 16 were followed for eight to 20 years; none developed a recurrence, indicating the benign nature of this lesion. Handley and Thackray (63) questioned the designation of papillomatosis and suggested the term "adenoma of the nipple," since the salient feature of the lesion is the adenomatous proliferation of tubules in the nipple stroma, and the epithelial proliferation within these tubules is frequently a secondary feature. Taylor and Robertson (76) also preferred to designate this lesion as an adenoma. They described 29 additional cases; ten of the patients had radical mastectomies because of a diagnosis of carcinoma, while the remaining 19 patients had local excisions. Perzin and Lattes (69) designated these tumors as papillary adenomas because 12 of their 65 cases had papillary intraductal proliferation found after reviewing serial sections of the cases. None of the patients with axillary node dissection in any of the reports had axillary node metastases confirming the benign nature of the lesion. While at AFIP the term nipple duct adenoma is used only for lesions that have an adenomatous tubular component, Rosen and Caicco (72) include pure papillomas (including the sclerosing variant) of the lactiferous ducts, along with lesions having either an exclusive adenosis pattern or adenosis admixed with a papilloma or papillomatosis under the designation of florid papillomatosis of the nipple.

### Definition

The term nipple duct adenoma (NDA) is used in this chapter to refer to a lesion within the nipple that consists of an adenomatous proliferation of small tubules, with or without any pattern of epithelial proliferation (including papillary growth) within these tubules or within the native lactiferous ducts of the region.

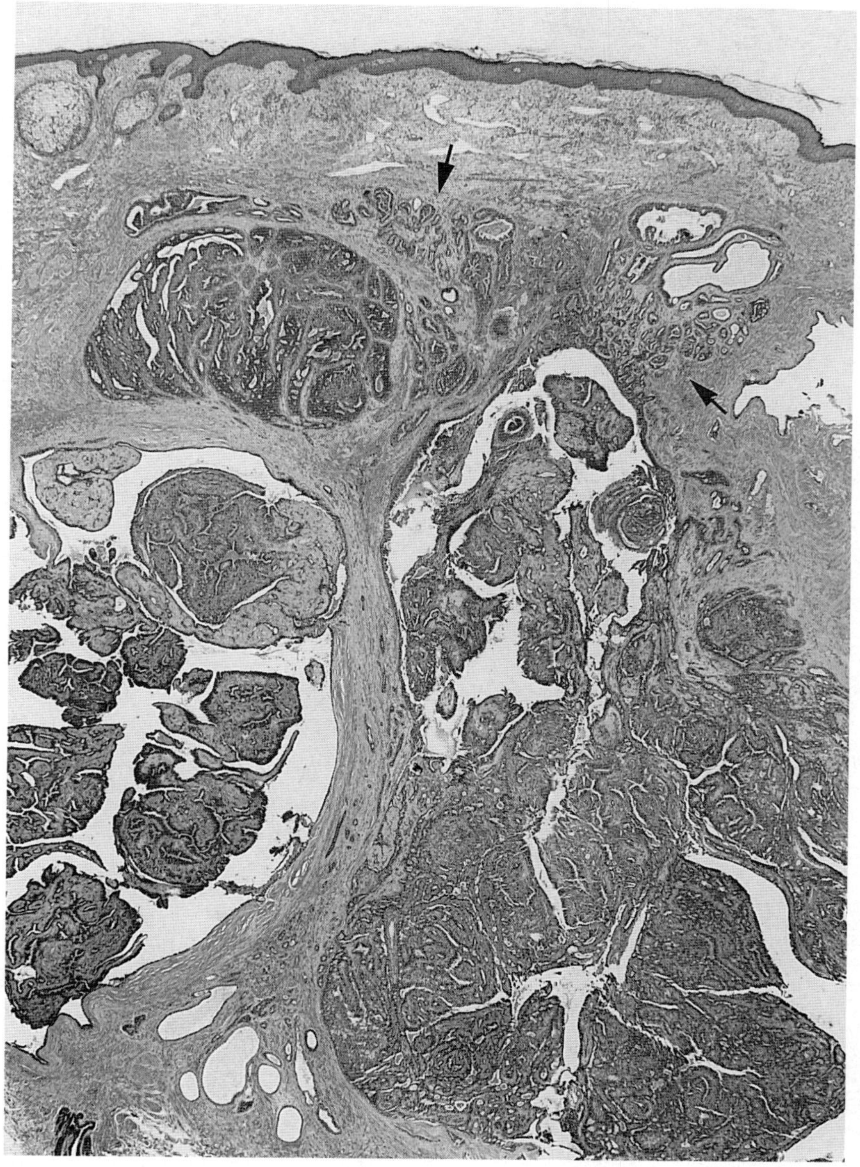

**Figure 14.14** Nipple duct adenoma with minimal adenosis (arrows) and associated with prominent papillomas within the lactiferous ducts. (H&E, X10)

When changes identical to NDA are found in the subareolar region without involvement of the substance of the nipple, the term subareolar sclerosing duct hyperplasia has been used (71).

## Clinical Features

Nipple duct adenoma occurs predominantly in the female breast, but it also occurs occasionally in the male breast (73,77). Two of the 51 cases in Rosen and Caicco's series (72) and three of the 29 in Taylor and Robertson's study (76) were men. Waldo et al (77) reported a case of florid papillomatosis of the nipple after diethystilbestrol therapy. It has been reported in caucasians, blacks and oriental women. The patients range in age from newborn to 89 years, with the average age reported between 43 and 45 years in the larger series. The duration of symptoms varies from a month to 15 years; the average in a majority of cases is less than a year. The lesion is generally unilateral, but rarely bilateral lesions have been reported (52,63). Nipple discharge is the most common complaint, present in 65% to 70% of the patients (69,76), followed by enlargement and induration of the nipple associated with ulceration. Sometimes the lesion presents through the distended orifice of a duct as a

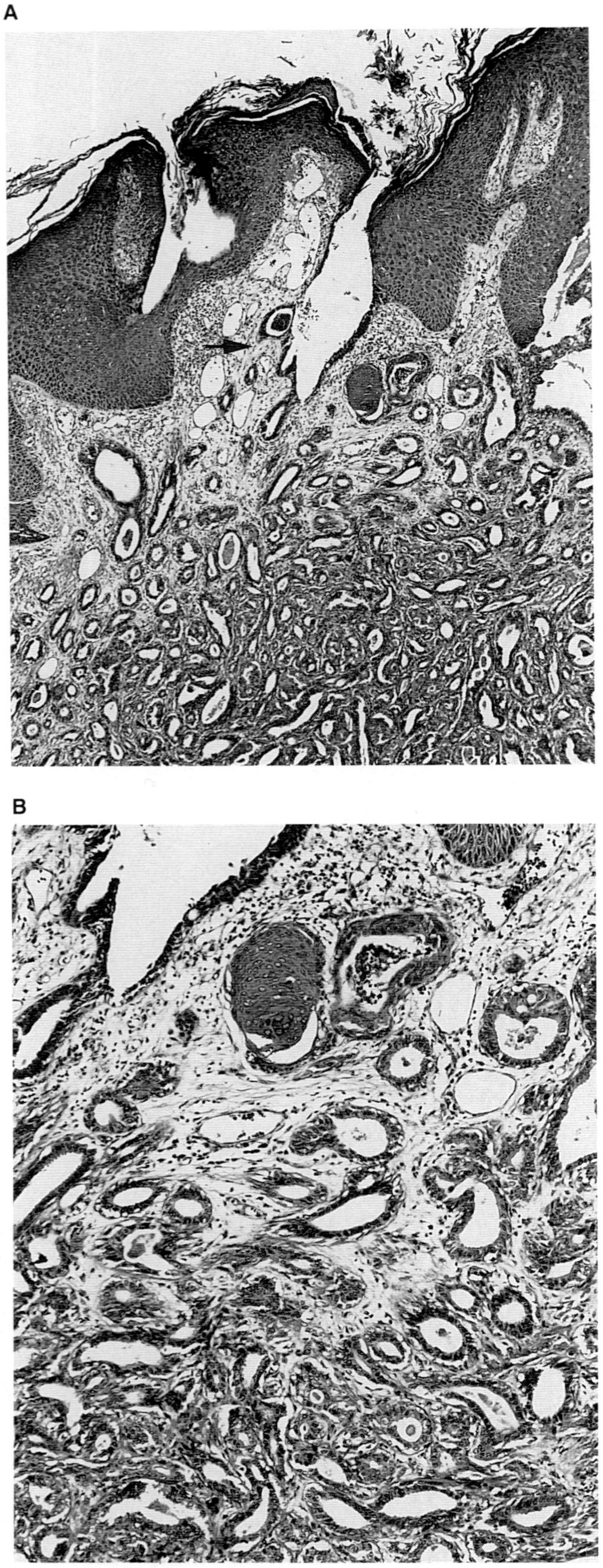

**Figure 14.15** (a) Nipple duct adenoma showing extension to the surface (arrow), and (b) squamous metaplasia in a tubule close to the surface. (H&E, (a) X100; (b) X150)

friable, granulating mass (62). These changes may be accompanied by pain, itching, or burning. These characteristics often lead to confusion with Paget's disease clinically. About a quarter of the cases in the AFIP series (76) were asymptomatic and incidental findings.

## Macroscopic Features

The fully-developed lesion has a well-delineated margin and can cause cystic dilatation of the underlying ducts (Fig. 14.9).

## Microscopic Features

While the asymptomatic lesion consists of only a small number of ductules clustered around a major duct (Fig. 14.10), the more advanced lesion can replace part or all of the nipple stroma. It can also expand and enlarge the nipple and erode the surface epithelium by direct extension, replacing it partially and giving the appearance of an ulcer or erosion. The eroded area generally reflects exposed tumor, but true ulcers may also develop (Fig. 14.11). While grossly the lesion appears well-delineated, microscopically the margins are often ill defined. Basically, the lesion is composed of a compact aggregation of tubules proliferating within and replacing the nipple stroma (Fig. 14.12). The residual stroma, when notable, often becomes sclerotic and causes distortion of the tubules, simulating sclerosing adenosis (Fig. 14.13). Epithelial hyperplasia, papillomas and papillomatosis may be present within the proliferating tubules, or within the lactiferous ducts in the region; the papillary component can be quite prominent (Fig. 14.14). Apocrine metaplasia is present in approximately 15% of the cases and squamous metaplasia is observed in around 50% of the lesions. The metaplasia is often located within tubules close to the surface (Fig. 14.15), some of which may become cystically dilated. The epithelial proliferation may show atypia and necrosis (see Fig. 14.11), a finding which leads to frequent misinterpretation of the changes as carcinoma. Mitotic figures are seen in more than 50% of the lesions. The presence of both epithelial and

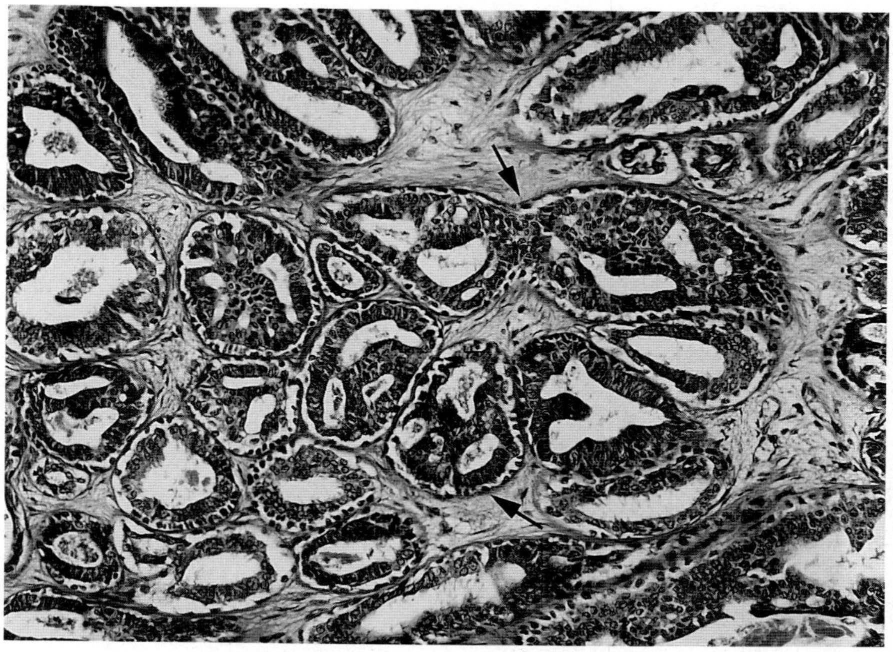

**Figure 14.16** Nipple duct adenoma. The presence of a distinct myoepithelial cell layer around the tubules (arrows) confirms the benign nature of this often florid and complex tubular proliferation. (H&E, X150)

A

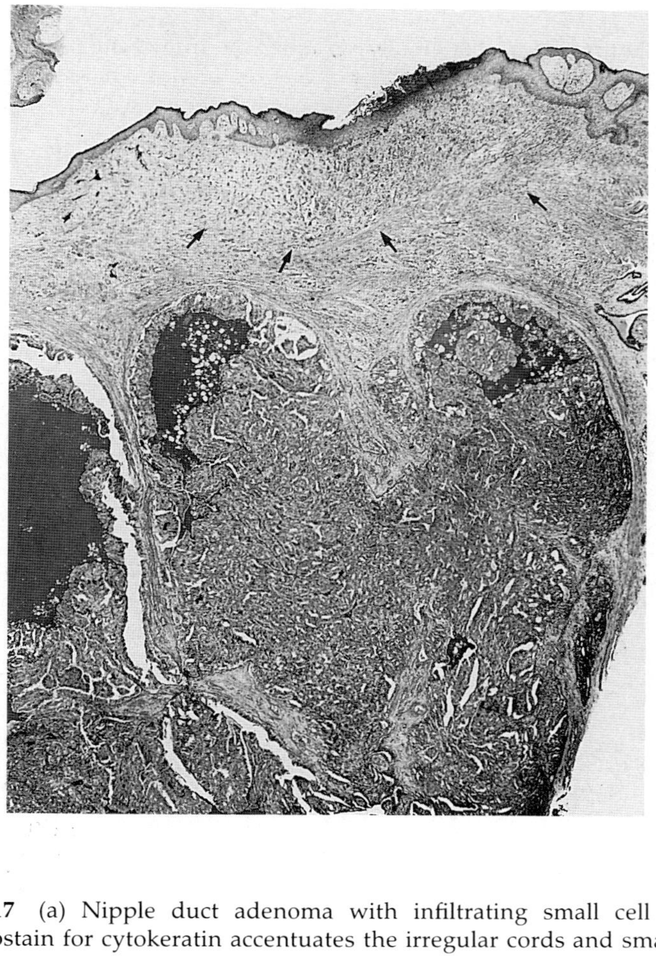

B

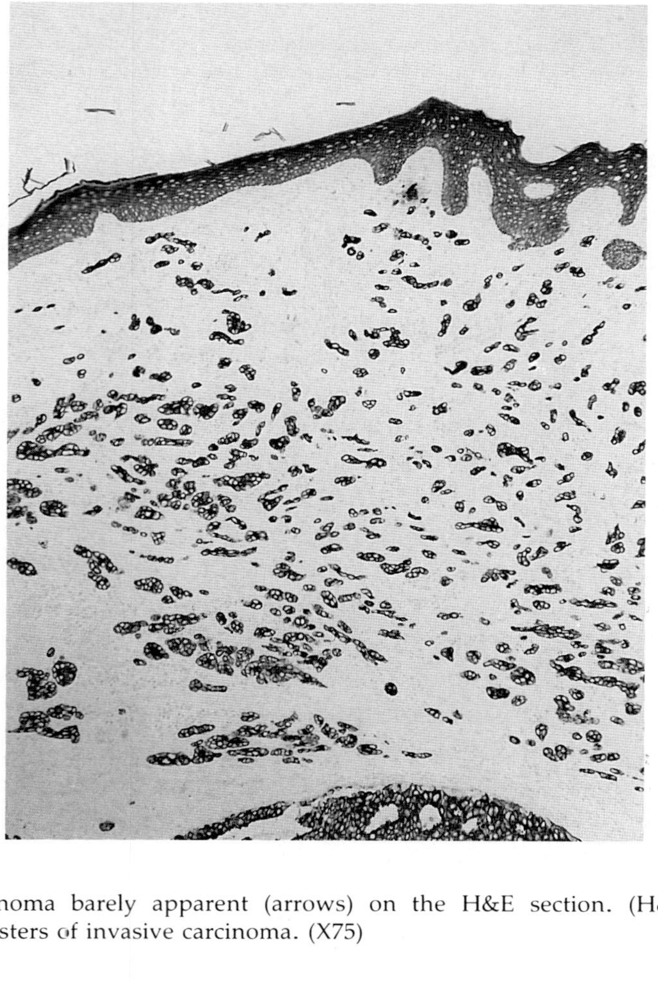

**Figure 14.17** (a) Nipple duct adenoma with infiltrating small cell carcinoma barely apparent (arrows) on the H&E section. (H&E, X20) (b) Immunostain for cytokeratin accentuates the irregular cords and small clusters of invasive carcinoma. (X75)

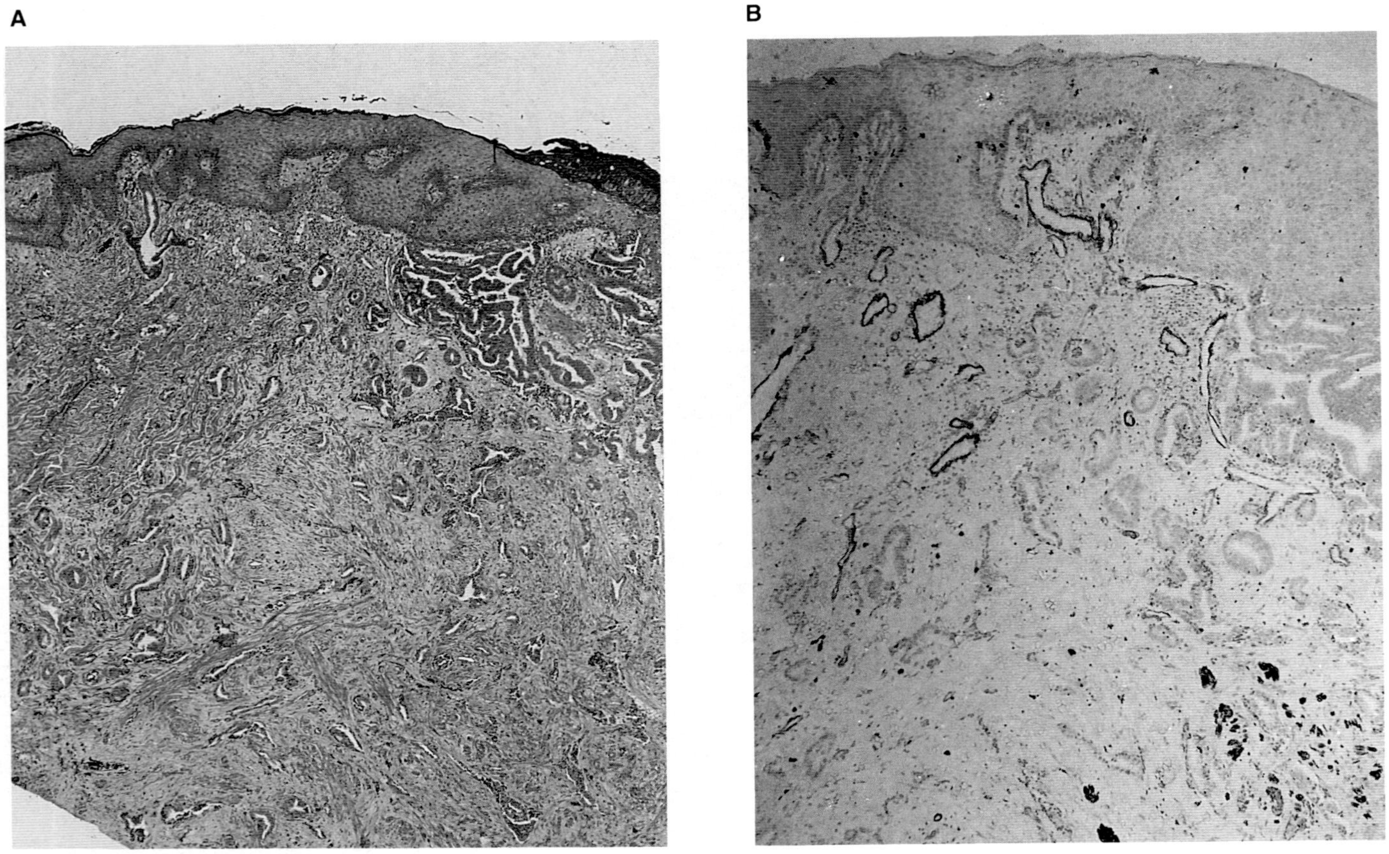


**Figure 14.18** Tubular carcinoma in the nipple. (a) There is a haphazard distribution of irregular tubules separated by stroma within the nipple. (H&E, X40) (b) Immunoreaction for actin decorates the vessels and muscle bundles, but fails to show a myoepithelial cell layer around the tubules. (X100)

myoepithelial cell layers lining the tubules (Fig. 14.16) provides morphologic proof of their benign nature.

## Malignant Changes

Malignant change in nipple duct adenoma, though rare, has been well-documented in four patients; one was a 53-year-old man, the others were women 43, 56 and 67 years of age (53,55,61). The 56-year-old woman reported by Gudjonsdottir et al (61) presented with disseminated carcinoma with involvement of axillary nodes, bones, and liver, and she died shortly thereafter. None of the other three patients had any evidence of axillary node metastases, but no follow-up was provided on any of them. I recently reviewed two examples of invasive carcinoma within the nipple along with nipple duct adenomas. Curiously, in one case, the intraductal proliferative changes and the carcinoma were present in half of the NDA, while the other half had very little proliferative activity. In one case, the infiltrating cells were rather pale and blended with the stromal cells immediately beneath the surface epithelium; an immunostain for cytokeratin enhanced the invasive nature of these cells (Fig. 14.17). In the second case, the invasive tumor was a tubular carcinoma replacing most of the nipple stroma. An immunostain for actin was performed to ascertain absence of the myoepithelial cell layer prior to interpreting the lesion and an invasive carcinoma (Fig. 14.18). It is always best to be conservative when there is any doubt regarding the diagnosis of malignancy, particularly intraductal carcinoma, arising in NDA.

The proportion of breast carcinomas associated with, but independent of NDA varies from 1.2% to 5%. In a series of 967 patients whose carcinoma was treated by mastectomy, "florid papillomatosis" was present in 12 (1.2%) of the nipples examined (58). Azzopardi (51) stated that the incidence is about 5%. Rosen and Caicco (72) reviewed the literature and found 173 cases of NDA reported prior to their own study. Carcinoma was described in 24 (14%) of them compared to ten of the 51 (19.6%) cases that they reported themselves. The 24 cases included the four carcinomas arising in NDA; the remaining 20 cases and the ten in Rosen and Caicco's report were separate lesions discovered either concurrent with, prior to, or following the NDA.

## Differential Diagnosis

Clinically, NDA is often misinterpreted as Paget's disease. The microscopic picture, however, is distinctive enough that it is easily recognized as different from Paget's disease.

At the microscopic level, nipple duct adenoma should be distinguished from pure papillomas and sclerosing papillomas which may occur as solitary or multiple lesions in the major lactiferous ducts of the nipple (see Chapter 6, Papillary Lesions). These papillary lesions lack the adenomatous proliferation of tubules outside the lactiferous ducts and within the stroma of the nipple which is characteristic of nipple duct adenomas. Another lesion that can be confused with NDA is infiltrating syringomatous adenoma which also occurs in the nipple, though rarely. In contrast to NDA, which replaces the nipple stroma, syringomatous adenoma either permeates the nerve and muscle bundles of the nipple stroma or is associated with a distinct reactive-appearing stroma which separates the proliferating tubules. In either case, the tubules are separated by abundant stroma, whereas there is negligible intervening stroma between tubules of NDA.

## Treatment

Complete excision with a narrow rim of uninvolved breast tissue is adequate treatment. A margin of grossly normal appearing breast tissue should be excised since many of these tumors extend beyond the grossly apparent margins. Recurrences may develop if the lesion is incompletely excised. Only one of the 18 patients reported by Taylor and Robertson (76) developed recurrence following local excision, and this was due to incomplete excision of the lesion.

# SYRINGOMATOUS ADENOMA

Syringomatous adenoma of the nipple is quite rare with only a small number of cases reported in the literature (79,82–84). Four examples of a similar lesion under the designation of "syringomatous squamous tumor of the breast" have been reported deep within the breast (84). Patients with syringomatous adenoma of the nipple range in age from 11 to 76 years, with an average age of around 40 years. A majority of the patients are women, but one of the five cases reported by Rosen (71) occurred in a man. Clinically, there is a discrete, firm mass in the nipple with induration of the subareolar region. The overlying skin may be focally hyperkeratotic. Nipple discharge occurs occasionally but is not common; pain, itching, and tenderness occur only with slightly higher frequency. Duration of symptoms ranges from three months to several years. All reported lesions have been unilateral and none has been associated with axillary lymph node enlargement.

## Macroscopic Features

Syringomatous adenomas range in size from 1 to 3 cm with a mean of 1.6 cm. They are generally ill-defined, irregular masses with a gray or tan cut surface, but

**Table 14.2** Distinctive Features of Nipple Duct Adenoma, Tubular Carcinoma, and Syringomatous Adenoma

| | **Nipple Duct Adenoma (NDA)** | **Tubular Carcinoma (TC)** | **Syringomatous Adenoma (SYAD)** |
|---|---|---|---|
| Squamous Metaplasia | +, Superficial | – | +, Diffuse |
| Myoepithelial Cell Layer | + | – | + |
| Intervening Stroma | Sparse | Abundant, Reactive | Abundant, Reactive |
| Nipple Involvement | 100% | Rare | 80% |

A

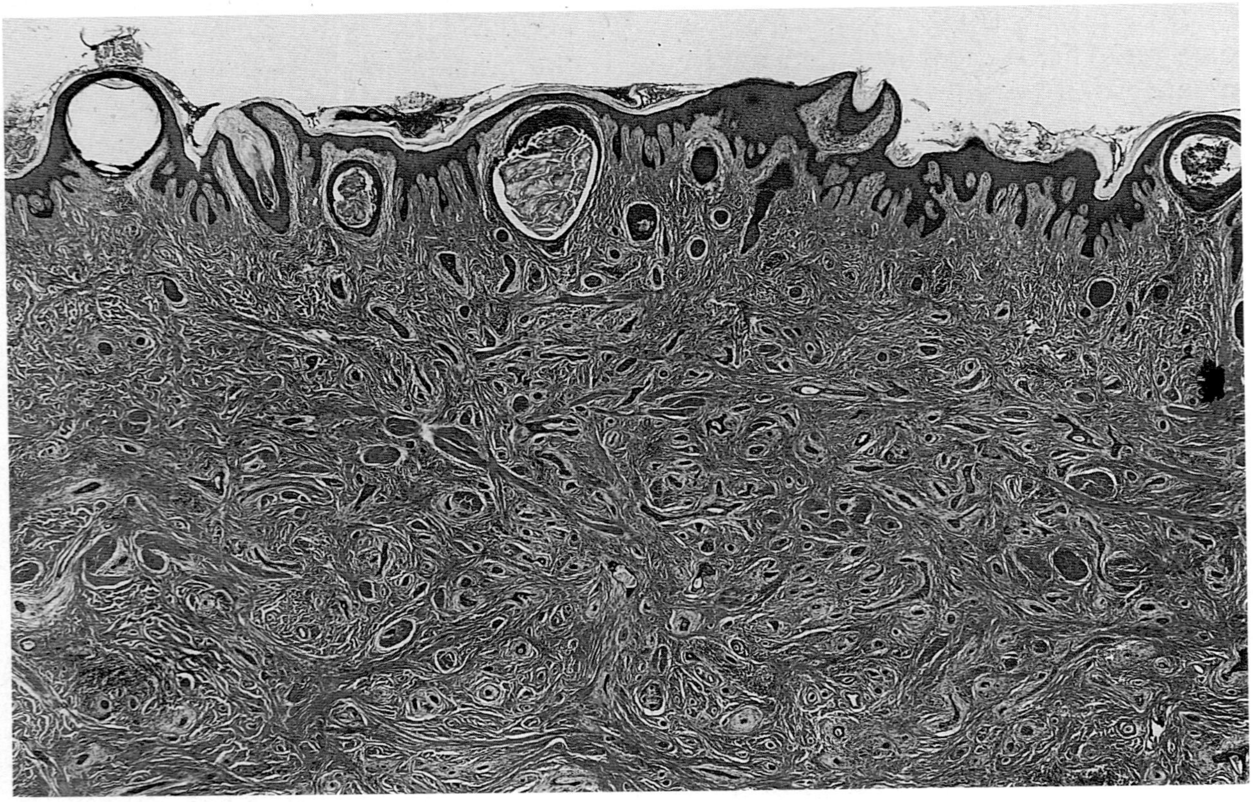

**Figure 14.19** (a) Infiltrating syringomatous adenoma shows subtle permeation of the nipple stroma by small tubules. The tubules vary from small structures with obliterated lumens (b), to some irregularly shaped and branching structures with open lumens (c). Two cell populations, epithelial and myoepithelial, are readily apparent in the larger tubules (d). (H&E, (a) X40; (b) X120; (c) X75; (d) X200)

occasionally they present as well-defined nodules. Small cystic areas may be evident on the cut surface.

## Microscopic Features

The typical syringomatous adenoma is composed of small, curved, angulated, and compressed, cord-like tubules haphazardly permeating the nipple stroma with rare connections to the surface epidermis. The tubules are generally separated by abundant fibrous stroma. Only occasionally and focally do these ducts aggregate in clusters. At low power, some of the tumors may be missed because of the small size of the proliferating tubules which appear to permeate rather than displace the normal nipple structures (Fig. 14.19). The ducts are lined by two cell layers, a luminal layer of epithelial cells and a peripheral myoepithelial cell layer. Epithelial hyperplasia of an occlusive type occurs in some ducts. Mitotic figures are infrequent. As a rule, the proliferating cells within the tubules are squamous with keratinization or squamoid, though ordinary epithelial hyperplasia may also occur less commonly. Squamous cysts may develop. The surrounding stroma is either the unaltered nipple stroma, or in some cases a reactive, cellular or edematous stroma forming a distinctive background for the proliferating tubules (Fig. 14.20). A myxochondroid stromal change may develop in some cases. When this occurs, the term chondroid syringomatous adenoma would be appropriate. Perineural invasion has been observed in some lesions (85). A positive reaction for carcinoembryonic antigen has been noted in the luminal contents and periluminal cytoplasm (85). Immunostain for actin displays positivity in the ME cells; Langerhans' cells have been identified within neoplastic cell aggregates by their positive reaction to S-100 protein (85).

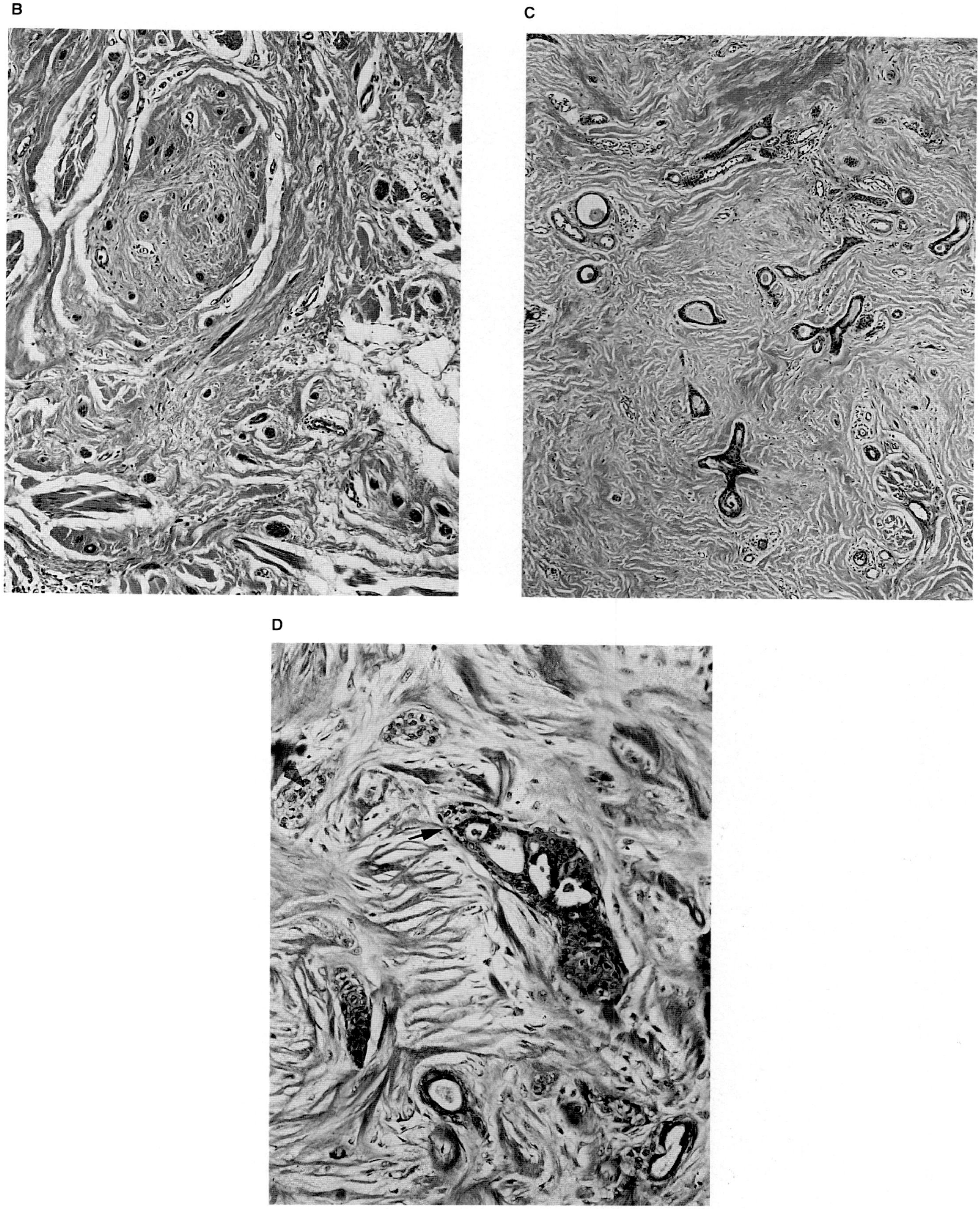


**Figure 14.19(b–d)** Infiltrating syringomatous adenoma. Legend on opposite page.

A

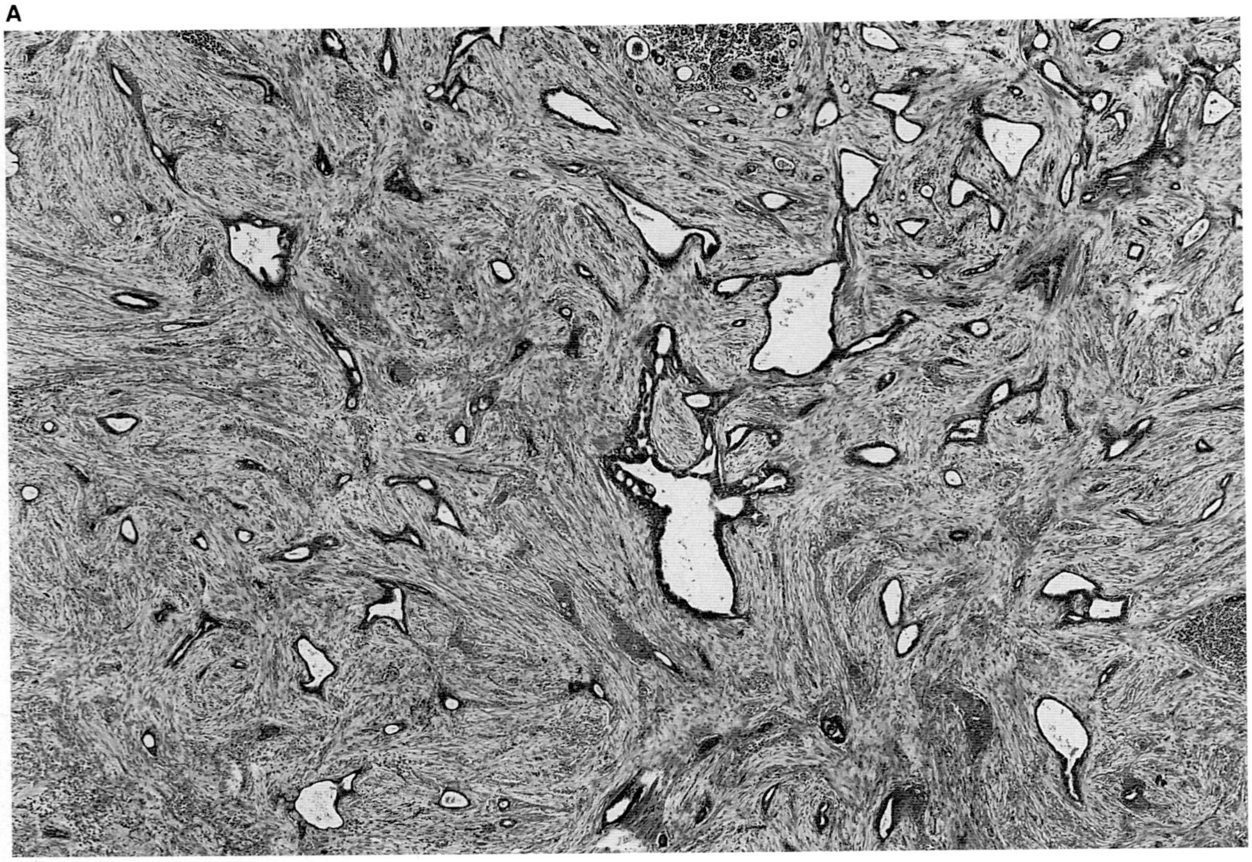

B

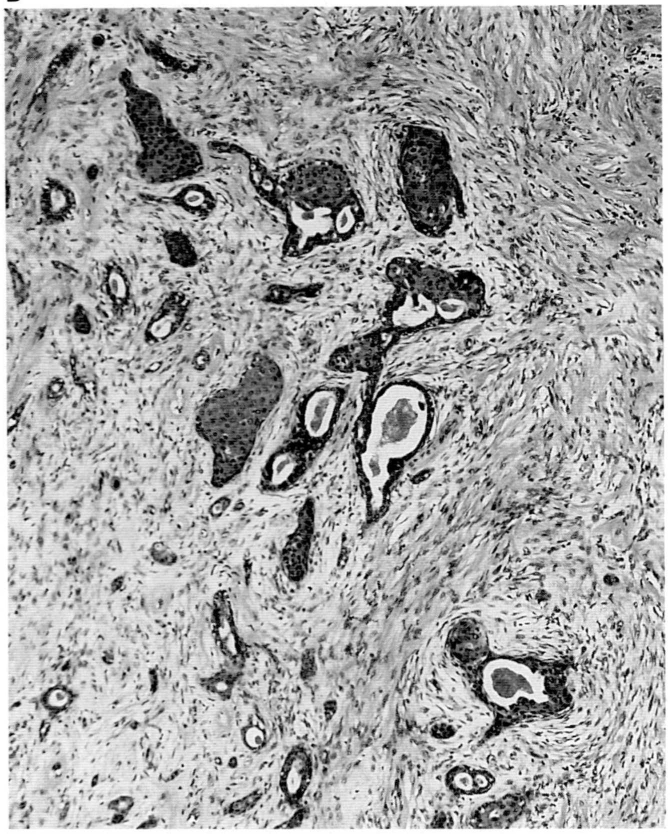

**Figure 14.20** (a) Infiltrating syringomatous adenoma showing widely dispersed tubules within the nipple separated by abundant reactive-appearing stroma. (b) The tubules form focal clusters, with some of the tubules obliterated by proliferating metaplastic squamous cells. (c) A complex branching tubule with squamous metaplasia (long arrow) and a cuticular-like luminal cell layer. (H&E, (a) X40; (b) X75; (c) X240)

C

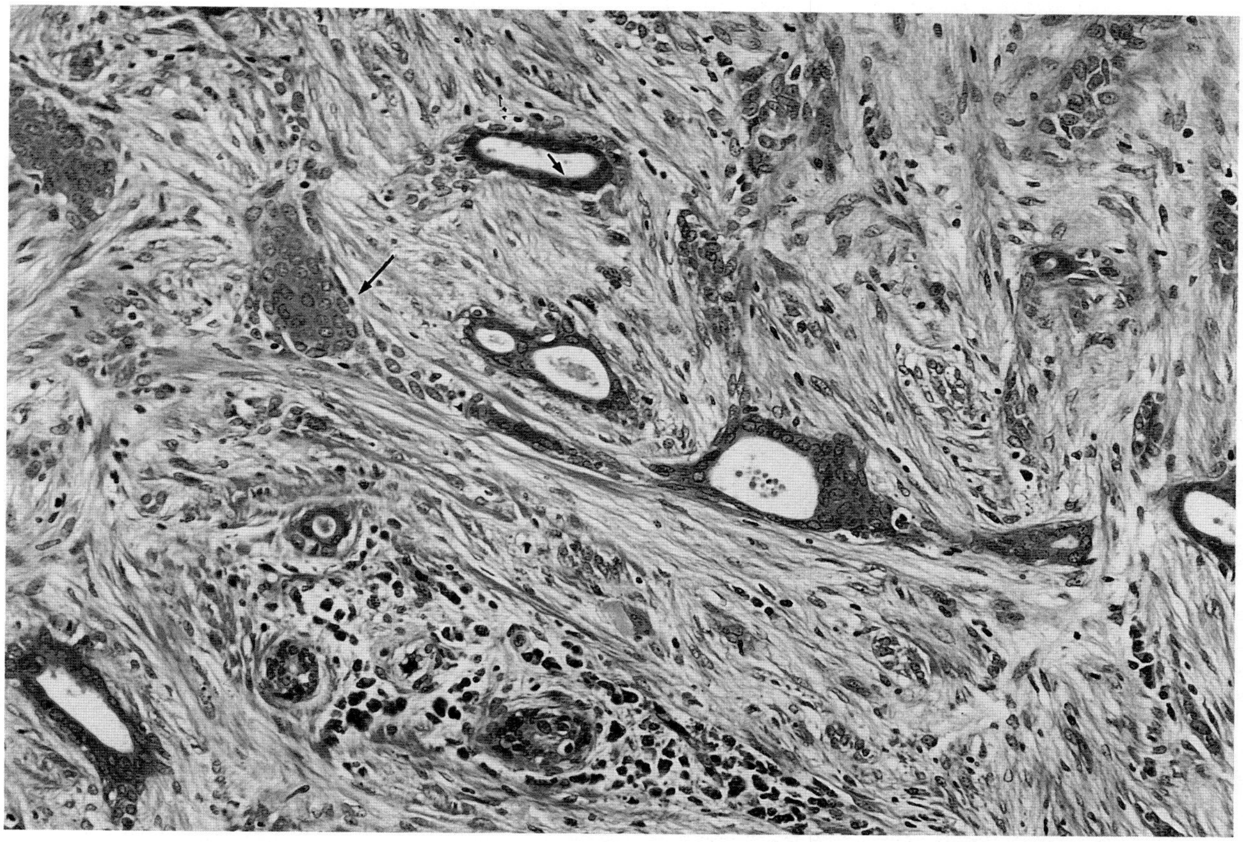

**Figure 14.20(c)** Infiltrating syringomatous adenoma. Legend on opposite page.

## Treatment

Local excision is sufficient treatment. The five cases that recurred in the study from AFIP (80) had been incompletely excised.

## Differential Diagnosis

Syringomatous adenoma should be distinguished from nipple duct adenoma and tubular carcinoma. The distinctive features of these three lesions are listed in Table 14.2. Nipple duct adenoma forms a distinct lesion displacing the nipple stroma, whereas, syringoma permeates the nipple and areolar stroma or shows a distinctive, reactive stroma. The ducts in NDA are clustered together with little intervening stroma; in contrast, the ducts in syringomatous adenoma are separated by abundant stroma. Epithelial hyperplasia is commonly observed in NDA where it assumes a variety of patterns showing solid clusters with or without secondary lumens and tufting; the

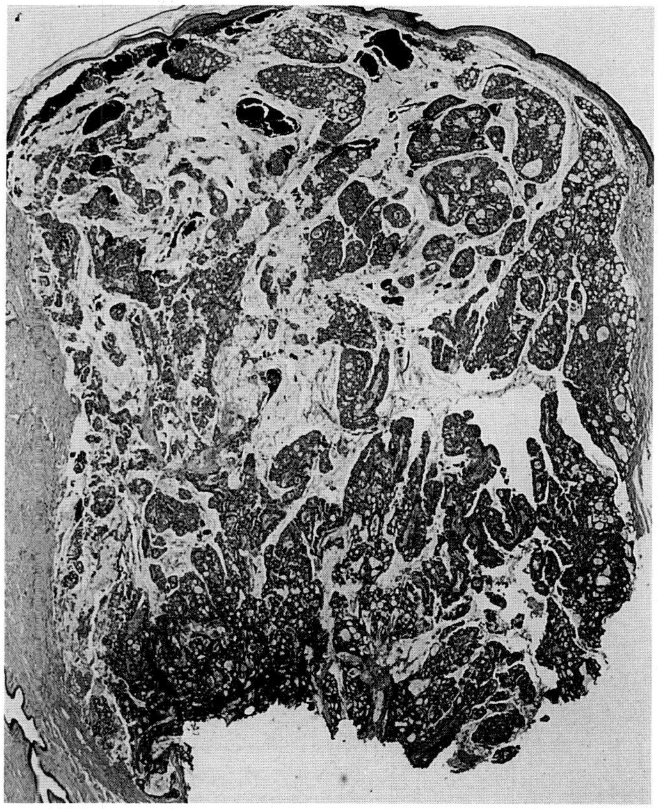

**Figure 14.21** Replacement of the nipple by an infiltrating duct carcinoma. (H&E, X15)

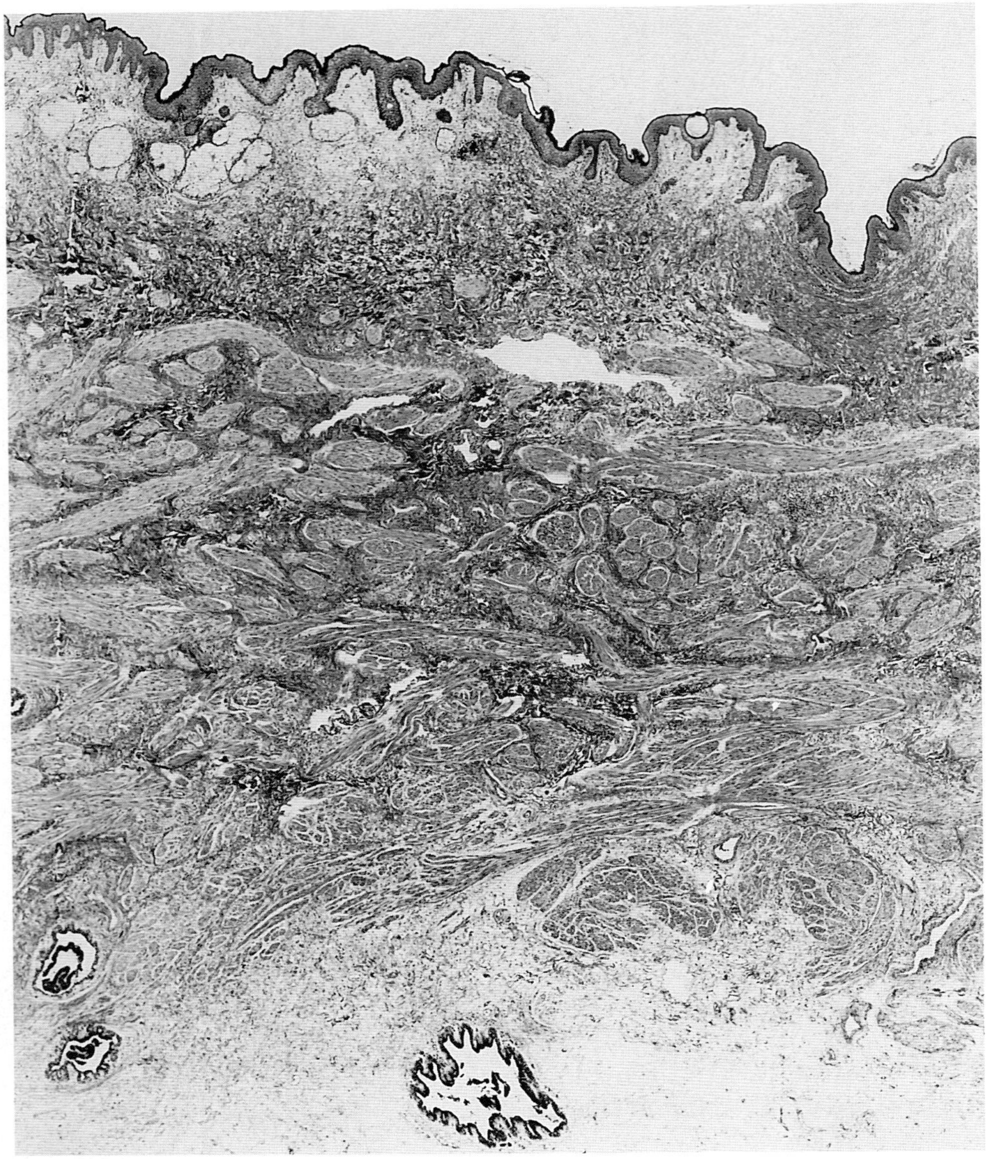

**Figure 14.22** Hyperplasia of muscle in the areolar regions of the nipple. (H&E, X120)

proliferating cells are generally epithelial or metaplastic apocrine cells with squamous metaplasia confined to areas close to the surface only. The proliferating cells protruding into the lumen of the tubules in syringomatous adenoma are always squamous or squamoid and form solid morules with an occlusive tendency. The squamous cells are present even in deep-seated ducts and ductules and are not confined to those close to the surface. Erosion of the surface epithelium is common in advanced NDA, but would be most unusual in syringomatous adenoma. The most important feature that helps distinguish syringomatous adenoma from a well-differentiated (tubular) carcinoma is the presence of two cell layers (epithelial and myoepithelial) in the widespread ducts of syringoma in contrast to the single layer of epithelial cells in well-differentiated carcinoma. The presence of squamous differentiation in practically all syringomatous adenomas is another distinctive feature not observed in well-differentiated carcinomas.

## Histogenesis

Morphologically, lesions designated as syringomatous adenoma of the nipple encompass the variety of changes observed in the group of skin adnexal lesions designated as microcystic adnexal carcinoma (79,81,

82) and sclerosing sweat duct (syringomatous) carcinoma (78). There are some syringomatous adenomas that lack significant cyst formation, stromal sclerosis, or both. In a good number of the mammary lesions, the stroma is reactive and fibroblastic in nature. While the reason for designating one of the cutaneous variants (the microcystic adnexal carcinoma) as carcinoma is that some of the cases have recurred, metastases have not been reported in any cases. It is quite possible that the recurrences have been due to incomplete excision of this occasionally ill-defined lesion which often extends beyond the grossly apparent margins rather than a reflection of an aggressive tumor.

The syrinogmatous adenomas seen in the nipple appear to be skin adnexal in origin and differentiation. The tubular structures in syringomatous adenoma bear a close resemblance to the sweat gland ducts that are occasionally seen in the nipple. Therefore, the histogenesis would be similar to that speculated for microcystic adnexal carcinomas and sclerosing duct (syringomatous) carcinoma.

## BASAL CELL CARCINOMA

About 13 examples of basal cell carcinoma (86–96) have been reported in the nipple, and actually in one case, the carcinoma was associated with axillary node metastasis (94). The youngest patient whose age has been recorded was 43 and the oldest was 75; seven of the patients were male, while six were female. Only two patients (both male) had mastectomy for their lesions; one patient had a simple mastectomy, the other had radical mastectomy after axillary node biopsy demonstrated metastatic carcinoma.

## MISCELLANEOUS LESIONS

The nipple may be involved by direct extension of a variety of underlying carcinomas (Fig. 14.21), (97,98, 108). Occasionally, intraductal carcinomas confined to the major lactiferous ducts and not associated with Paget's disease also occur.

Melanomas occur so rarely in the nipple, that special effort should be made to exclude the possibility of Paget's disease with phagocytosis of melanin (101,105), or direct extension to the nipple of a carcinoma with subsequent melanocytic colonization of the tumor resulting in a pigmented lesion (99,103,106, 107) before making a diagnosis of melanoma. In the latter situation, the melanin pigment is transferred or phagocytized by the neoplastic cells. While metastatic melanomas in the breast proper have been reported (100) and also seen at the AFIP, there are no examples of primary melanomas of the nipple in the AFIP files.

Aside from epithelial lesions, occasionally the smooth muscle bundles in the nipple show hyperplasia (Fig. 14.22) or actually give rise to leiomyomas (104,109), or leiomyosarcoma (102).

A myxoid and mucinous alteration is also observed occasionally. Designated as mucinosis (Fig. 14.23), it is characterized by accumulation of multiple degenerative-appearing myxoid and mucinous material in the stroma of the nipple separating the stromal cells. Care should be taken to search carefully for the presence of epithelial islands in the lakes of mucin on multiple levels to exclude the possibility of mucinous carcinoma before designating such lesions as mucinosis.

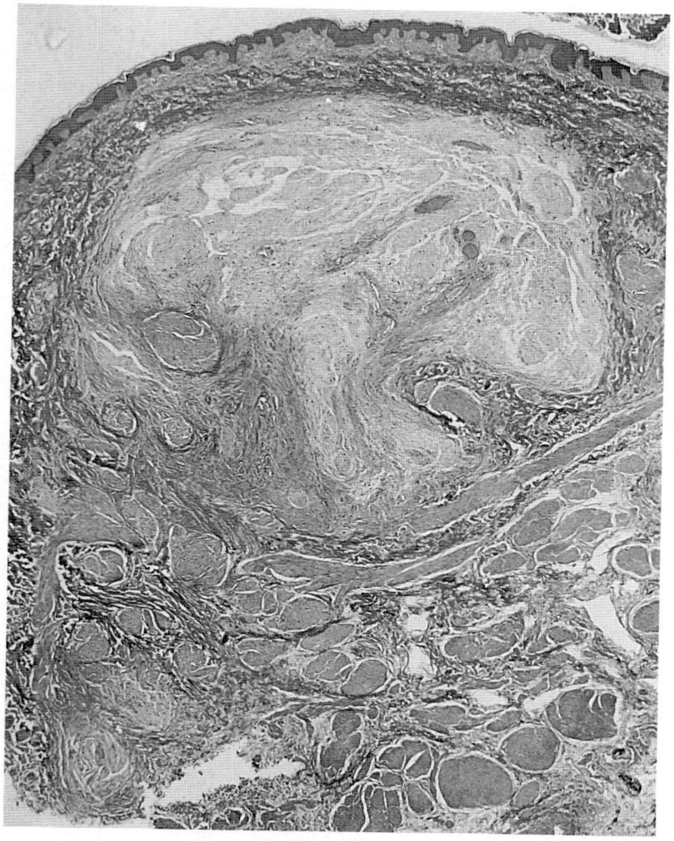

**Figure 14.23** Mucinosis is characterized by myxoid and mucinous degeneration in the stroma; the absence of epithelial cells within these areas helps distinguish them from a mucinous carcinoma. (H&E, X15)

## REFERENCES

### Paget's Disease


1. Anderson WR: Bilateral Paget's disease of the nipple: Case report. *Am J Obstet Gynecol* 1979;134:877–878.
2. Archibald RG: A case of Paget's disease associated with carcinomatous infiltration of the breast of a male native of the Sudan. *Am J Trop Med* 1922;2:133–137.
3. * Ashikari R, Park K, Huvos AG, et al: Paget's disease of the breast. *Cancer* 1970;26:680–685.
4. * Bussolati G, Pich A: Mammary and extramammary Paget's disease: An immunohistochemical study. *Am J Pathol* 1975; 80:117–128.
5. * Chaudary MA, Millis RR, Lane EB, et al: Paget's disease of the nipple: A ten year review including clinical, pathological, and immunohistochemical findings. *Breast Cancer Res Treat* 1986;8:139–146.
6. Colcock BP, Sommers SC: Prognosis in Paget's disease of the breast. *Surg Clin N Am* 1954;34:773–783.
7. * Culberson JD, Horn RC: Paget's disease of the nipple: Review of 25 cases with special reference to melanin pigmentation of "Paget cells." *Arch Surg* 1956;72:224–231.
8. * Darier J: Sur une nouvelle forme de psorospermose cutanee: la maladie de Paget du mamelon. *C R Soc Biol* 1889;1:294–297.
9. du Toit RS, van Rensburg PS, Goedhals L: Paget's disease of the breast. *S Afr Med J* 1988;73:95–97.
10. * Fourquet A, Campana F, Viehl P, et al: Paget's disease of the nipple without detectable breast tumor: Conservative management with radiation therapy. *Int J Radiat Oncol Biol Phys* 1987;13:1463–1465.
11. Graham H: *The Story of Surgery*. New York, Doubleday, Doran & Co, Inc, 1939.
12. Hitchcock A, Topham S, Bell J, et al: Routine diagnosis of mammary Paget's disease. A modern approach. *Am J Surg Pathol* 1992;16:58–61.
13. * Inglis K: Paget's disease of the nipple: With special reference to the changes in the ducts. *Am J Pathol* 1946;22:1–33.
14. * Inglis K: The essential difference between the epidermal changes in Paget's disease of the nipple and those in Bowen's "precancerous dermatosis." *J Pathol Bacteriol* 1952; 64:637–643.
15. * Jones RR, Saul J, Gusterson B: The histogenesis of mammary and extramammary Paget's disease. Histopathology 1989;14:409–416.
16. Kay S: Paget's disease of the nipple. *Surg Gynecol Obstet* 1966;123:1010–1014.
17. Kirkham N, Berry N, Jones DB, et al: Paget's disease of the nipple. Immunohistochemical localization of milk fat globule membrane antigens. *Cancer* 1985;55:1510–1512.
18. * Kister SJ, Haagensen CD: Paget's disease of the breast. *Am J Surg* 1970;119:606–609.
19. * Lagios MD, Westdahl PR, Rose MR, et al: Paget's disease of the nipple. Alternative management in cases without or with minimal extent of underlying breast carcinoma. *Cancer* 1984;54:545–551.
20. Lammie GA, Barnes DM, Millis RR, et al: An immunohistochemical study of the presence of c-erbB-2 protein in Paget's disease of the nipple. *Histopathology* 1989;15:505–514.
21. * Lichter AS, Lippman ME: Special situations in the treatment of breast cancer, in Lippman ME, Lichter AS, Danforth DN (eds): *Diagnosis and Management of Breast Cancer*. Philadelphia, WB Saunders Co, 1988, pp 422–423.
22. Maier WP, Rosemont GP, Harasym EL, et al: Paget's disease of the female breast. *Surg Gynecol Obstet* 1969;128: 1253–1263.
23. * Markopoulos C, Gazet JC: Paget's disease of the nipple occurring after conservative management of early breast cancer. *Eur J Surg Oncol* 1988;14:77–78.
24. Meissner K, Riviere A, Haupt G, et al: A study of neu-protein expression in mammary Paget's disease with and without underlying breast carcinoma and in extramammary Paget's disease. *Am J Pathol* 1990;137:1305–1309.
25. Moshakis V, Fordysce MJ, Griffiths JD: Klinefelter's syndrome associated with breast carcinoma and Paget's disease of the nipple. *Clin Oncol* 1983;9:257–261.
26. * Muir R: Further observations on Paget's disease of the nipple. *J Pathol Bacteriol* 1939;49:299–312.
27. * Muir R: The pathogenesis of Paget's disease of the nipple and associated lesions. *Br J Surg* 1935;22:728–237.
28. * Nadji M, Morales AR, Girtanner RE, et al: Paget's disease of the skin. A unifying concept of histogenesis. *Cancer* 1982;50:2203–2206.
29. Nagel RB, Lucas DO, McDaniel KM, et al: Paget's cells. New evidence linking mammary and extramammary Paget's cells to a common cell phenotype. *Am J Clin Pathol* 1985;83:431–438.
30. * Neubecker RD, Bradshaw RP: Mucin, melanin, and glycogen in Paget's disease of the breast. *Am J Clin Pathol* 1961;36:49–53.
31. Norris HJ, Taylor HB: Carcinoma of the male breast. *Cancer* 1969;23:1428–1435.
32. Orr JW, Parrish DJ: The nature of the nipple changes in Paget's disease. *J Pathol Bacteriol* 1962;84:201–208.
33. * Paget J: On disease of mammary areola preceding cancer of the mammary gland. *St Barth Hosp Rep* 1874;10:87–89.
34. * Paone JF, Baker RR: Pathogenesis and treatment of Paget's disease of the breast. *Cancer* 1981;48:825–829.
35. Peison B, Benisch B: Paget's disease of the nipple simulating malignant melanoma in a black woman. *Am J Dermatopathol* 1985;7:165–169.
36. Poires-Baptista A, Abreu de Vasconcelos A: Cutaneous pigmented metastasis from breast carcinoma simulating malignant melanoma. *Int J Dermatol* 1988;27:124–125.
37. Rae V, Gould E, Ibe MJ, et al: Coexistent pemphigus vulgaris and Paget's disease of the nipple. An immunohistochemical study. *J Am Acad Dermatol* 1987;16:235–237.
38. Rissanen PM, Holsti P: Paget's disease of the breast. *Oncology* 1969;23:209–216.

39. Rubenstein MW: Paget's disease of the male nipple and areola. *Arch Dermatol Syph* 1930;22:281–300.

* 40. Sagami S: Electron microscopic observations in Paget's disease. *Med J Osaka Univ* 1963;14:173–187.

* 41. Sagebiel RW: Ultrastructural observations on epidermal cells in Paget's disease of the breast. *Am J Pathol* 1969;57: 49–64.

* 42. Salvadori B, Fariselli G, Saccozzi R: Analysis of 100 cases of Paget's disease of the breast. *Tumori* 1976;62:529–536.

43. Sarason EL, Prior JT: Paget's disease of the male breast. *Ann Surg* 1952;135:253–261.

* 44. Toker C: Clear cells of the nipple epidermis. *Cancer* 1970; 25:601–610.

45. Toker C: Further observations on Paget's disease of the nipple. *J Natl Cancer Inst* 1967;38:79–92.

46. Toker C: Some observations on Paget's disease of the nipple. *Cancer* 1961;14:653–672.

* 47. Treves N: Paget's disease of the male mamma. A report of two cases. *Cancer* 1954;7:325–330.

* 48. VanStapel M-J, Gatter KC, De Wolf-Peeters C, et al: Immunohistochemical study of mammary and extra-mammary Paget's disease. *Histopathology* 1984;8:1013–1023.

* 49. Velpeau AALM: Lecons orales de clinique chirurgicale faites a l'Hopital de la Charite, recuillies et publiees par Gustave Jeanselme, Vol 2. Paris, Germer-Bailliere, 1841.

50. Willis RA: *Pathology of Tumors*, ed 3. Washington, Butterworth Inc, 1960, p 247.


### Nipple Duct Adenoma


51. Azzopardi JG: *Problems in Breast Pathology*. Philadelphia, WB Saunders Co, 1979.

52. Bergdahl L, Bergman F, Rais 0, et al: Bilateral adenoma of the nipple. Report of a case. *Acta Chir Scand* 1971;137:583–586.

53. Bhagavan BS, Patchefsky A, Koss LG: Florid subareolar duct papillomatosis (nipple adenoma) and mammary carcinoma: Report of three cases. *Hum Pathol* 1973;4:289–295.

54. Brownstein MH, Phelps RG, Magnin PH: Papillary adenoma of the nipple: Analysis of fifteen new cases. *J Am Acad Dermatol* 1985;12:707–715.

55. Burdick C, Reinhart RM, Matsumoto T, et al: Nipple adenoma and Paget's disease in a man. *Arch Surg* 1965;91: 835–838.

56. Doctor VM, Sirsat MV: Florid papillomatosis (adenoma) and other benign tumors of the nipple and areola. *Br J Cancer* 1971;25:1–9.

57. Evans DDE, Woodward W: Adenoma of a nipple. *Med J Aust* 1964;2:712.

58. Fisher ER, Gregorio RM, Fisher B, et al: The pathology of invasive breast cancer. A syllabus derived from findings of the National Surgical Adjuvant Breast Project. (Protocol No. 4). *Cancer* 1975;36:1–84.

59. Goldman RL, Cooperman H: Adenoma of the nipple. A benign lesion simulating carcinoma clinically and pathologically. *Am J Surg* 1970;119:322–325.

* 60. Gros C-M, LeGal Y, Bader P: L'adenomatose erosive du mamelon. *Presse Med* 1959;67:615–616.

* 61. Gudjonsdottir A, Hagerstrand I, Ostberg G: Adenoma of the nipple with carcinomatous development. *Acta Pathol Microbiol Scand (A)* 1971;79:676–680.

62. Haagensen CD, Stout AP, Phillips JS: The papillary neoplasms of the breast. I. Benign intraductal papilloma. *Ann Surg* 1951;133:18–36.

* 63. Handley RS, Thackray AC: Adenoma of nipple. *Br J Cancer* 1962;16:187–194.

* 64. Jones DB: Florid papillomatosis of the nipple ducts. *Cancer* 1955;8:315–319.

* 65. LeGal Y, Gros CM, Bader P: L'adenomatose erosive du mamelon. *Ann Anat Pathol* 1959;4:292–304.

66. Lewis HM, Ovitz ML, Golitz LE: Erosive adenomatosis of the nipple. *Arch Dermatol* 1977;2:79–83.

67. Miller G, Bernier L: Adenomatose erosive du mamelon. *Can J Surg* 1965;8:261–266.

68. Nichols FC, Dockerty MD, Judd ES: Florid papillomatosis of the nipple. *Surg Gynecol Obstet* 1958;107:474–480.

* 69. Perzin KH, Lattes R: Papillary adenoma of the nipple (florid papillomatosis, adenoma, adenomatosis). A clinicopathologic study. *Cancer* 1972;29:996–1009.

70. Robert H, DeBrux J, Winaver D: La papillomatose benigne du mamelon. *Presse Med* 1963;71:2713–2715.

71. Rosen PP: Subareolar sclerosing duct hyperplasia of the breast. *Cancer* 1987;59:1927–1930.

* 72. Rosen PP, Caicco JA: Florid papillomatosis of the nipple. A study of 51 patients, including nine with mammary carcinoma. *Am J Surg Pathol* 1986;10:87–101.

73. Shapiro L, Karpas CM: Florid papillomatosis of the nipple. First reported case in a male. *Am J Clin Pathol* 1965;44:155–159.

74. Smith EJ, Kron SD, Gross PR: Erosive adenomatosis of the nipple. *Arch Dematol* 1970;102:330–332.

75. Smith NP, Wilson EJ: Erosive adenomatosis of the nipple. *Clin Exp Dermatol* 1977;2:79–83.

* 76. Taylor HB, Robertson AG: Adenoma of the nipple. *Cancer* 1965;18:995–1002.

77. Waldo ED, Sidhu GS, Hu AW: Florid papillomatosis of male nipple after diethylstibestrol therapy. *Arch Pathol* 1975;99:364–366.


### Syringomatous Lesions


78. Cooper PH, Mills SE, Leonard DD, et al: Sclerosing sweat duct (syringomatous) carcinoma. *Am J Surg Pathol* 1985;9: 422–433.

79. Goldstein DJ, Barr RJ, Santa Cruz DJ: Microcystic adnexal carcinoma. *Cancer* 1982;13:182–184.

* 80. Jones MW, Norris HJ, Snyder RC: Infiltrating syringomatous adenoma of the nipple. A clinical and pathological study of 11 cases. *Am J Surg Pathol* 1989;13:197–291.

81. Lupton GP, McMarlin SL: Microcystic adnexal carcinoma: report of a case with 30-year follow-up. *Arch Dermatol* 1986;122:286–289.

82. Nickolof BJ, Fleischman HE, Carmel J, et al: Microcystic adnexal carcinoma. Immunohistologic observations suggesting dual (pilar and eccrine) differentiation. *Arch Dermatol* 1986;122:290–294.

* 83. Rosen PP: Syringomatous adenoma of the nipple. *Am J Surg Pathol* 1983;7:739–745.

84. Suster S, Moran CA, Hurt MA: Syringomatous squamous tumors of the breast. *Cancer* 1991;67:2350–2355.

85. Ward BE, Cooper PH, Subramony C: Syringomatous tumor of the nipple. *Am J Clin Pathol* 1989;92:692–696.

### Basal Cell Carcinoma

* 86. Bruce S, Tschen J, Goldberg L: Basal cell carcinoma of the nipple: Case report. *J Dermatol Surg Oncol* 1985;11:4.

87. Congdon GH, Dockerty MB: Malignant lesions of the nipple exclusive of Paget's disease. *Surg Gynecol Obstet* 1956;103:185–192.

* 88. Davis AB, Patchefsky AS: Basal cell carcinoma of the nipple. *Cancer* 1977;40:1780–1781.

89. Farrow JH: Benign and malignant lesions of the nipple. *CA* 1958;8:16–19.

* 90. Lupton GP, Goette D: Basal cell carcinoma of the male breast. *Proc Soc Med* 1965;58:509–510.

91. Rahbari H, Mehregan A: Basal cell epitheliomas in unusual and usual sites. *J Cutan Pathol* 1979;6:425–431.

92. Robinson H: Rodent ulcer of the male breast. *Trans Pathol Soc London* 1893;44:147–148.

* 93. Sauven P, Roberts A: Basal cell carcinoma of the nipple. *J R Soc Med* 1983;76:699.

* 94. Shertz WT, Balogh K: Metastasizing basal cell carcinoma of the nipple. *Arch Pathol Lab Med* 1986:110:761–762.

95. Wainwright J: Carcinoma of the male breast. *Arch Surg* 1927;14:836–859.

* 96. Wyatt AP: Basal cell carcinoma of the male breast. *Proc Soc Med* 1965;58:509–510.

### Miscellaneous Lesions of the Nipple

97. Andersen JA, Pallesen R: Spread to the nipple and areola in carcinoma of the breast. *Ann Surg* 1979;189:367–372.

98. Andersen JA, Gram JB, Pallesen RM: Involvement of the nipple and areola in breast cancer. Value of clinical findings. *Scand J Plast Reconstr Surg* 1981;15:30–42.

99. Azzopardi JG, Eusebi V: Melanocyte colonization of pigmentation of breast carcinoma. *Histopathology* 1977;1:21–30.

100. Barker JNW, Girling AC: A case of metastatic malignant melanoma masquerading as disseminated mammary carcinoma. *Histopathology* 1989;14:219–221.

* 101. Cuberson JD, Horn RC: Paget's disease of the nipple: Review of 25 cases with special reference to melanin pigmentation of "Paget's cells." *Arch Surg* 1956;72:224–231.

* 102. Hernandez EJ: Leiomyosarcoma of male breast originating in the nipple. *Am J Surg Pathol* 1978;2:299–304.

103. Jacoby R, Roses DF, Valensi Q: Carcinoma of the breast metastatic to the skin and simulating malignant melanoma, in Ackerman AB (ed): *Pathology of Malignant Melanoma*. Chicago, Year Book Medical Publishers Inc, 1981, pp 263–267.

* 104. Nascimento AG, Karas M, Rosen PP, et al: Leiomyoma of the nipple. *Am J Surg Pathol* 1979;3:151–154.

105. Peison B, Benisch B: Paget's disease of the nipple simulating malignant melanoma in a black woman. *Am J Dermatopathol* 1985;7:165–169.

106. Poires-Baptista A, Abreu de Vasconselos A: Cutaneous pigmented metastasis from breast carcinoma simulating malignant melanoma. *Int J Dermatol* 1988;27:124–125.

* 107. Sau P, Solis J, Lupton GP, et al: Pigmented breast carcinoma. A clinical and histopathologic simulator of malignant melanoma. *Arch Dermatol* 1989;125:536–539.

108. Smith J, Payne WS, Carney JA: Involvement of the nipple and areola in carcinoma of the breast. *Surg Gynecol Obstet* 1976;143:546.

* 109. Webber B: Leiomyoma of the nipple. *Afr J Surg* 1975;13: 117–120.

# 15

# Miscellaneous Lesions



## MYOEPITHELIAL LESIONS OF THE BREAST

The myoepithelial cells first appear in the 45 mm embryo at the base of the ectodermal ridge of the mid line (3). They are normally present in the breast as an interrupted layer of stellate cells between the continuous luminal epithelial cell layer and the basement membrane throughout the mammary duct system (1,19). Their appearance is generally uniform within a given lobule, but varies significantly from a naked nuclear appearance surrounded by a clear halo, to a myoid look, or even a delicate spindled cell appearance in different lobules within a single field (see Chapter 1). Because of their contractile abilities, their principal function is to serve as a pump in the process of discharging secretory material into the lumens. Curiously, they appear rather inconspicuous in the lactating breast, but quite prominent and myoid around some metaplastic apocrine cells (Fig. 15.1). Sclerosing adenosis is the most common lesion in which they often assume a prominence. Myoepithelial cells become particularly conspicuous in the nodular variant of sclerosing adenosis, sclerosing adenosis occurring in fibroadenomas, and in long-standing and atrophic lesions in which the epithelial cell atrophy results in a more or less pure myoepithelial lesion that appears to infiltrate the sclerotic stroma and is occasionally mistaken for an invasive carcinoma. Less commonly, they appear focally hyperplastic within a papilloma. Myoepithelial cell hyperplasia has been described by Masson and designated as "myoid hyperplasia," (3). The myoepithelial cell

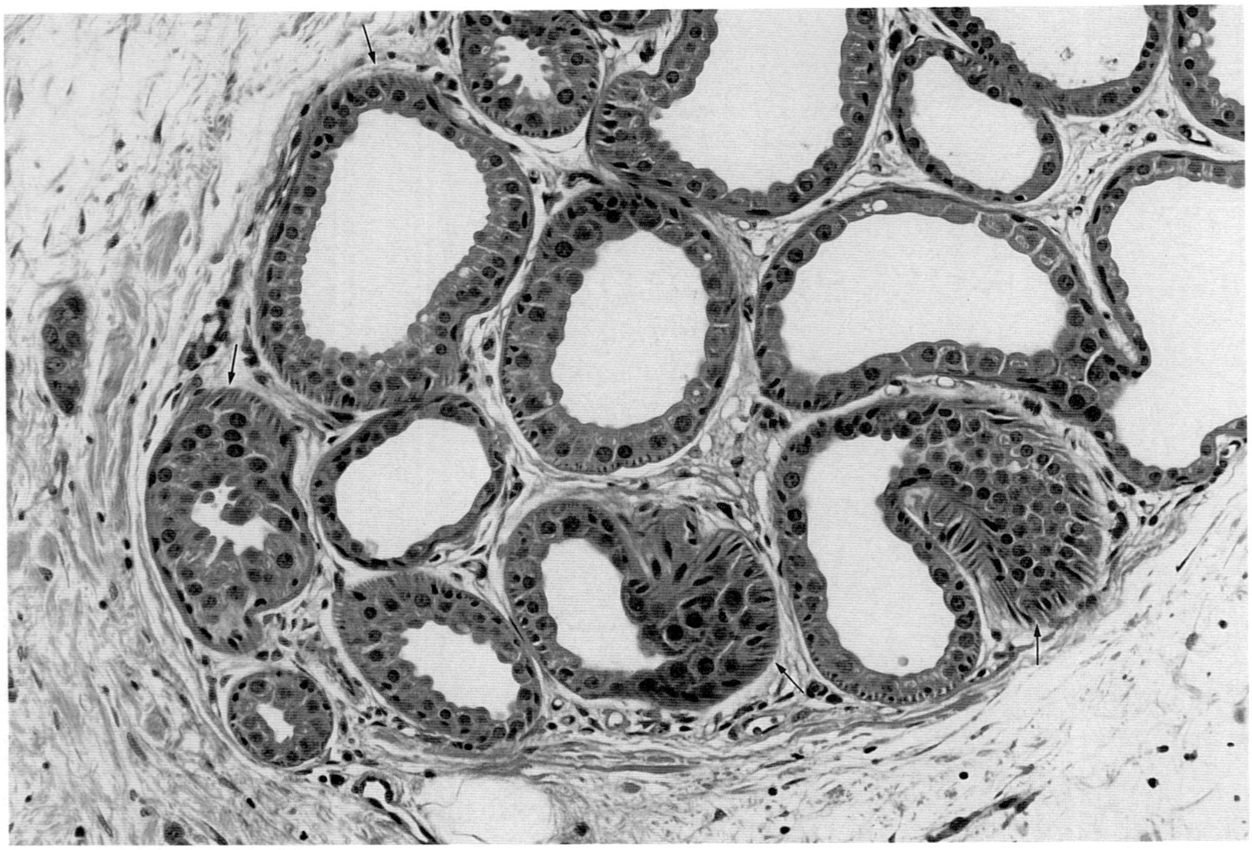

**Figure 15.1** Prominent myoepithelial cells with a myoid appearance (arrows) surround metaplastic apocrine cells. (H&E, X300)

layer persists in many breast lesions. Alterations in the appearance of myoepithelial cells, as well as their immunocytochemical and ultrastructural features in a variety of breast diseases, have been reported (1,2,5, 8,16,18,21,26,30,40).

Tumors composed of, or derived from, the myoepithelial cells have been recognized in the salivary glands for some time (8–11,15,29,36,37,39). In the breast, five types of lesions are either derived from, or composed of, a dominant to pure population of myoepithelial cells. These include adenoid cystic carcinoma, the rare mixed tumor or pleomorphic adenoma (25,26,28,33,38,44,47,48), multifocal myoepitheliosis, adenomyoepithelioma, and malignant myoepithelioma (myoepithelial carcinoma). Although adenoid cystic carcinoma is uncommon and pleomorphic adenoma is actually quite rare in the breast, the morphology of these tumors is so distinctive and well defined in other locations that most pathologists either recognize them immediately, or know where to search for a description and the proper designation. Information regarding myoepitheliosis, adenomyoepithelioma, and malignant myoepithelioma is very limited, with only rare cases reported in the literature prior to the 1980s, (2,6,19, 22,24,43). Subsequently, a surge of reports on myoepithelial tumors has appeared in the literature (3,4, 7,12,13,20,23,31–36,41,45,50,51). A majority of these publications consist of a single case report or fewer than five cases. Because of the paucity of cases in each report, only one early investigator, Hamperl (19), had made an attempt to classify these lesions. He noted myoepithelial hyperplasia in "epimyothelial islands," in fibrosing adenosis (both epimyothelial islands and fibrosing adenosis are generally classified as sclerosing adenosis by current terminology), and as an intraductal hyperplasia. He classified "adeno-myothelioma" among benign tumors containing "myothelia" occurring in several organs, and he described and illustrated a single example of the lesion that he had observed in the breast—the tumor he illustrated would qualify as a tubular adenomyoepithelioma by the recently proposed classification system (41). Based on an evaluation of reports in the literature, Hamperl conceded some variability to "adeno-myotheliomas," and accepted the occurrence of a clear-cell variant of this lesion. He discussed malignant "adeno-myotheliomas" as lesions occurring mainly in the skin and characterized by a clear cell population but noted that some may even appear like

**Table 15.1** Classification of Myoepithelial Lesions of the Breast

I. Myoepitheliosis, multifocal and peripherally located
 A. Intraductal type, with or without a periductal component
 B. Periductal type (associated with sclerosis, it is considered a variant of sclerosing adenosis)
II. Adenomyoepithelioma
 A. Spindle cell type
 B. Tubular type
  Clear or eosinophilic cells
 C. Lobulated type
  Clear or eosinophilic, with or without hyalin cells
 D. Carcinoma arising in adenomyoepithelioma
  Epithelial carcinoma
  Myoepithelial carcinoma
III. Malignant myoepithelioma (myoepithelial carcinoma)
  Spindle cells, invasive

a leiomyosarcoma. He also mentioned that myoepithelial cells participate in the formation of a variety of benign and malignant breast tumors.

Following a review of 31 lesions composed of a dominant to pure population of myoepithelial cells, Tavassoli (41) proposed a classification system for myoepithelial lesions of the breast (Table 15.1) that incorporates the variety of mammary myoepithelial tumors observed in human breast over the past 20 years. In this classification, myoepithelial lesions of the breast are divided into three major categories: myoepitheliosis, adenomyoepithelioma, and malignant myoepithelioma.

Using both animal and human tumors, Baup and de Brux (3) subdivided myoepithelial tumors into myoepithelioma and adenomyoepithelioma, infiltrating myoepithelioma, and malignant myoepithelioma. The main difference between the infiltrating myoepithelioma and malignant myoepithelioma was in the increased degree of atypia and number of mitotic figures in the latter, as well as the presence of areas of hemorrhage and necrosis in the malignant lesions.

## Clinical Features

Except for the absence of a clinically distinct palpable mass in the patients with myoepitheliosis, the clinical presentation of the three categories of myoepithelial lesions does not differ significantly. Patients with myoepitheliosis range in age from 22 to 87 years of age. Patients with adenomyoepithelioma range in age from 38 to 82 years, with a median age of 62 years. Patients with "infiltrating myoepithelioma" or myoepithelial carcinoma range in age from 53 to 81 years. All patients with myoepithelial lesions have been female. The racial origin of 30 patients was known in Tavassoli's series; two were oriental, seven were black, and the remaining were caucasian. Myoepitheliosis generally does not present as a palpable mass when its nodular sclerosing adenosis variant is excluded. All patients with adenomyoepithelioma or myoepithelial carcinoma present with a palpable tumor, which may be massive and rarely fungating. The tumor is tender in a small minority of patients. The lesions are located in either breast with almost equal frequency; one tumor has been reported in the axillary tail of the breast (41). Approximately a fifth of the tumors are centrally located and described as being under the nipple or the areola; about half of these patients have a serous nipple discharge. The duration of the symptoms ranges from several weeks to months. Rarely, an adenomyoepithelioma has been present for 15 years before onset of enlargement shortly prior to the biopsy (41).

## Gross Pathology

**Myoepitheliosis.** These generally present as a firm, irregular area within the biopsy, but a distinct mass is not apparent.

**Adenomyoepithelioma.** Adenomyoepitheliomas range in size from 1 cm to 7 cm in diameter, with a median of cm. The tumors are predominantly sharply-circumscribed, and round to multilobulated nodules. A few have been described as distinct, but ill-defined, incidentally-found lesions in breasts biopsied either for fibrocystic changes or mammographically-detected changes. Cut surfaces of the lesions are uniformly solid with rare, small cystic areas. The tumors are firm to rubbery in consistency, and range in color from pink-white to gray or tan. Focal to diffuse translucency may be present. Hemorrhage is rare, but may be present particularly in larger tumors.

Recurrent tumors may present either as a solitary mass or as multiple nodules. The recurrent nodules

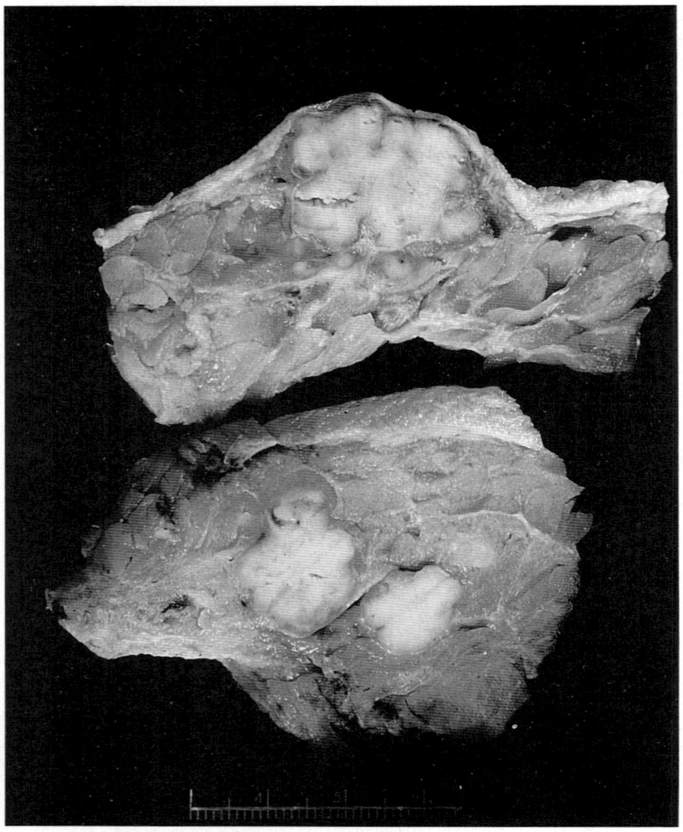

**Figure 15.2** Recurrent adenomyoepithelioma presenting as multiple, discrete, solid nodules. Smaller satellite nodules can be seen below the larger nodule at the top. (From FA Tavassoli: *Am J Surg Pathol* 1991; 15:554–568, with permission)

appear discrete, firm and solid on cut surface (Fig. 15.2).

**Malignant Myoepithelioma.** These tumors range in size from 1 cm to 21 cm. They may have well-defined margins with focal irregularity or they may appear stellate in shape. Satellite nodules may be present adjacent to the main tumor mass. The cut surface appears firm and rubbery, gray-white, and with foci of necrosis and hemorrhage in the larger tumors. Nodular areas of hyalinization are sometimes observed even in smaller tumors.

## Microscopic and Immunohistochemical Features

**Myoepitheliosis.** These are multifocal, microscopic lesions located in the peripheral duct system (mainly in the terminal duct-lobular units). Myoepitheliosis is characterized by a proliferation of spindled to cuboid myoepithelial cells within and sometimes also around (Figs. 15.3–15.5) multiple ducts, variably distending and often occluding the involved ducts, with residual luminal epithelial cells persisting in some of the ducts. The periductal variant, often associated with sclerosis, is generally considered a variant of sclerosing adenosis; this variant was not included among the cases in Tavassoli's study. The involved ducts in the intraductal variant of myoepitheliosis are more or less equally distended, without any one of the ducts becoming a dominant mass. The epithelial cells in the ducts become incorporated in the lesion. A papillary growth pattern is evident in some cases, but atypia and mitotic activity are absent. The spindle cells rarely display a prominent palisading pattern. The early stages in the development of myoepitheliosis are readily apparent in adjacent ducts as a solid proliferation of the myoepithelial cells in small papillae (Fig. 15.4). The cells exhibit a positive reaction for both actin and S-100 protein; the latter is particularly intense and uniform. The spindle cells also show minimal and focally positive reaction for cytokeratin but do not display positivity for GFAP. The epithelial cells, when present, show a positive reaction for cytokeratin.

**Adenomyoepithelioma.** In contrast to myoepitheliosis, the majority of adenomyoepitheliomas present as solitary, centrally-located lesions, except for the rare tumor originating in the axillary tail of the breast. Based on their growth pattern, cell type, or both, the 27 adenomyoepitheliomas in the AFIP series (41) were divided into three categories: spindle-cell (seven cases), tubular (eight cases), and lobulated (12 cases) variants.

The spindle-cell type is composed of a predominant spindle, myoepithelial cell proliferation admixed with a few epithelial-lined spaces. The proliferating cells form a solid mass which distends and almost occludes duct-like structures (Figs. 15.6 a,b). Because of the prominence of the spindle cell proliferation, some sections of the lesion show only the spindle cells. These areas could be confused with a leiomyoma when the epithelial-lined lumens are obliterated by the lesion and become inconspicuous. The spindle cells display a strongly positive reaction for S-100 protein (Fig. 15.7) and a minimal reaction for actin and cytokeratin. Apocrine metaplasia is common in the epithelial cell element. The epithelial cells react strongly for cytokeratin.

The tubular pattern of adenomyoepithelioma is

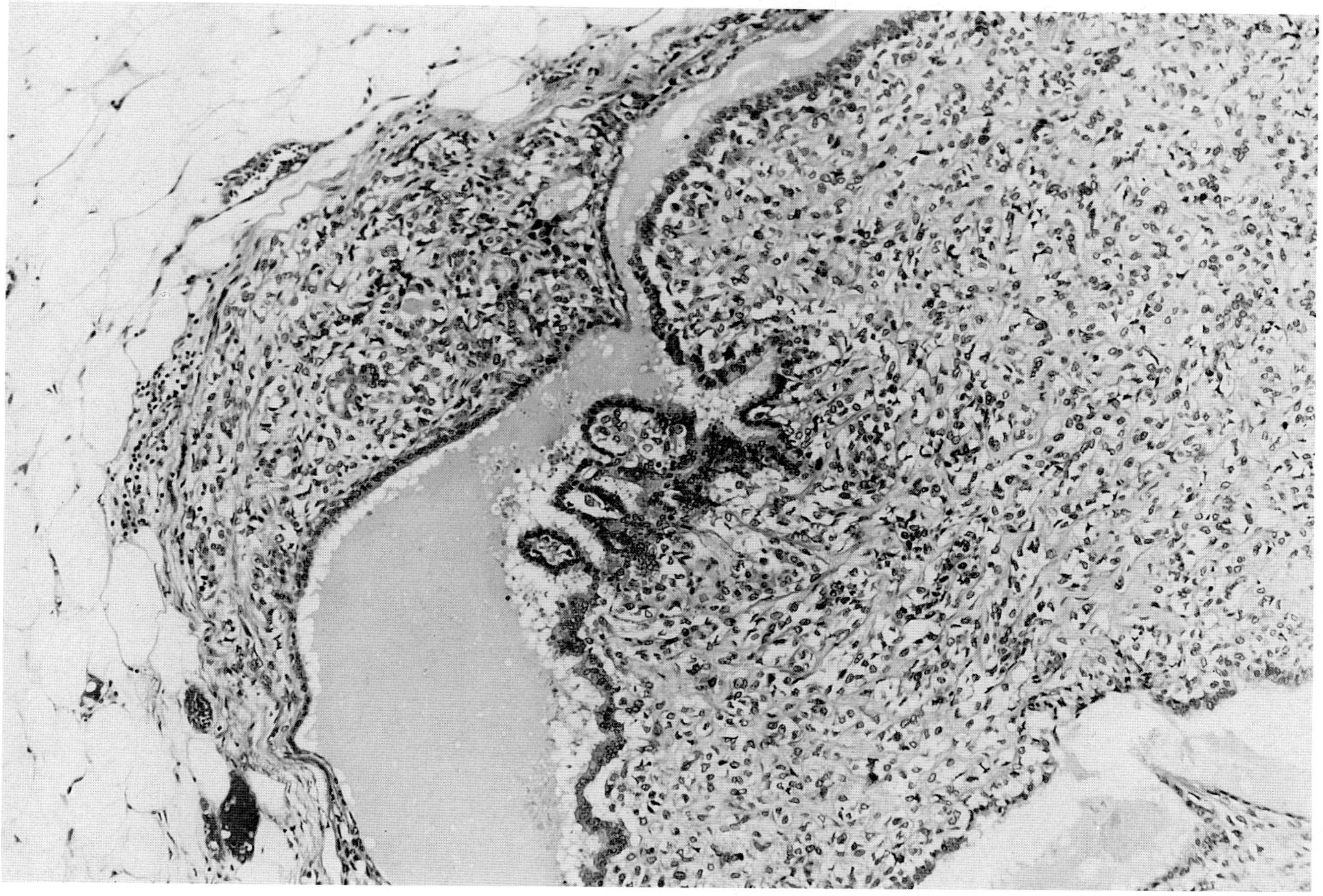

**Figure 15.3** Myoepitheliosis. Intraductal papillary and periductal myoepithelial cell hyperplasia of the clear cell type are readily apparent in and around this duct. (H&E, X350) (From FA Tavassoli: *Am J Surg Pathol* 1991;15:554–568, with permission)

characterized by the proliferation of a collection of rounded tubules lined by both epithelial and myoepithelial cells. While the tumor may be well circumscribed and actually encapsulated (Fig. 15.8), a majority of these lesions display at least focal areas of marginal irregularity where the proliferating tubules extend into, and blend with, the surrounding breast structures. The margins are occasionally quite ill-defined, with no evidence of encapsulation. Superficially reminiscent of tubular and ductal adenomas, as well as some sclerosing papillomas, adenomyoepitheliomas differ from these three lesions, however, by the unusually prominent and actually hyperplastic nature of the myoepithelial cells (Fig. 15.9). The myoepithelial cell hyperplasia is so prominent around some tubules that it causes obliteration of the tubular lumens by compression. Up to three mitotic figures per ten high-power fields (MF/10 HPF) may be seen in the myoepithelial cells. The epithelial cells may also show focal proliferative activity. Mucinous and apocrine metaplasia has been observed in the epithelial cells of several cases (41).

The lobulated adenomyoepithelioma is composed of solid nests of clear, eosinophilic or hyalin (plasmacytoid) myoepithelial cells proliferating around compressed epithelial-lined spaces. A thick fibrous capsule either completely or partially surrounds most tumors. Rounded nests of tumor cells occasionally infiltrate through and beyond the capsule of the tumor (Fig. 15.10). A fibrous connective tissue septa of varying thickness divides the lesion into rounded nests or smaller lobules. In some areas, the acellular septa extend into the cell nests and became so prominent that they replace the cellular component of the tumor. The appearance of the nests within the tumor varies depending on the degree of myoepithelial cell predominance and their morphology. Some tumors are composed of clear myoepithelial cells (Fig. 15.11), while others have myoepithelial cells with pink to amphophilic cytoplasm. Focally, the myoepithelial cells may display a "plasmacytoid" appearance with dense hylin-like eosinophilic cytoplasm and displacement of the nucleus to the periphery, but this cell type never assumes prominence.

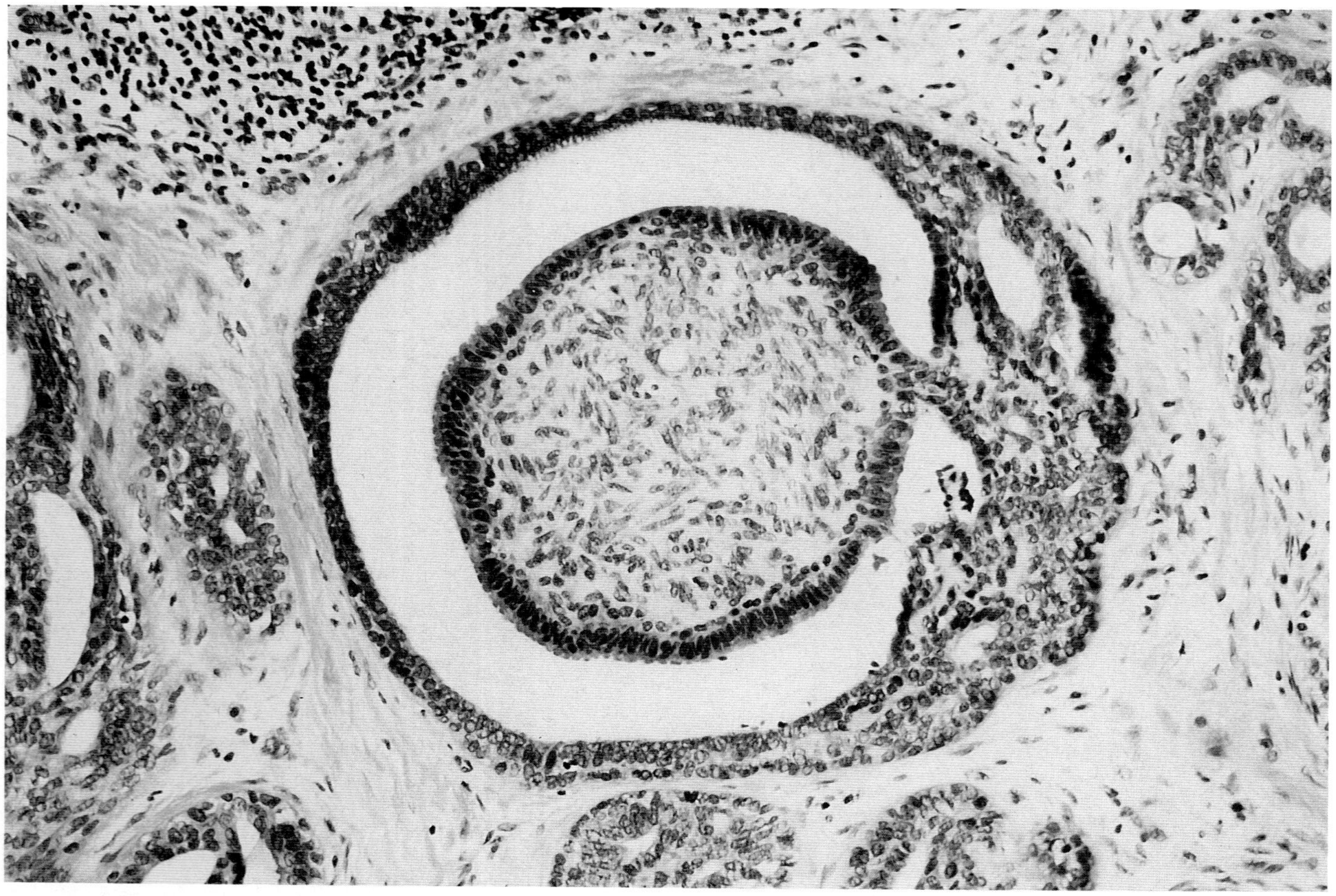

**Figure 15.4** Myoepitheliosis. Early stages in the development of myoepitheliosis. The myoepithelial cell layer is quite distinct in the right side of the papillary proliferation beneath the epithelial cell layer, but it becomes inconspicuous where it gradually becomes spindled and blends with the central mass of proliferating cells. Though not illustrated, the spindle cells displayed positive immunoreaction with actin. (H&E, X150) (From FA Tavassoli: *Am J Surg Pathol* 1991;15:554–568, with permission)

Mitotic activity generally does not exceed one or two MF/10 HPF among the proliferating myoepithelial cells, but in three primary lesions, it exceeded 10 MF/10 HPF. Hyalin degeneration is prominent in many lesions, particularly in the center of the tumor. Massive central infarction is present in a quarter of the tumors, including those with abundant mitotic activity. Calcification occurs in a third of the tumors.

A combination of growth patterns may coexist within the tumors, and the epithelial cell component may demonstrate focal metaplastic changes including apocrine, mucinous, and squamous metaplasia. A sebaceous cell population is seen occasionally. A minor component of the tumor may show a tubular or papillary pattern.

Satellite nodules are seen adjacent to the main tumor mass in some cases. Some of these nodules are morphologically identical to the main tumor mass, while others consist of distended ducts occluded by proliferating myoepithelial cells displacing and undermining the epithelial cell layer in a pagetoid fashion.

The clear cells exhibit a positive reaction for both actin and S-100 protein; however, the positivity is not as strong as that displayed by the spindle cells. The positive reaction for cytokeratin is evident as a thin rim around the cytoplasmic margin of some of the clear cells, while the luminal epithelial cells show a strongly positive cytoplasmic reaction for cytokeratin. In the AFIP experience, the immunoreaction for GFAP has been consistently negative in both neoplastic and non-neoplastic mammary myoepithelial cells.

In my experience, the normal myoepithelial cells show a more uniform and intense reaction with actin, while the proliferative myoepithelial cells, particularly the spindle variant, react more intensely with S-100 protein.

Either the epithelial or the myoepithelial compo-

A

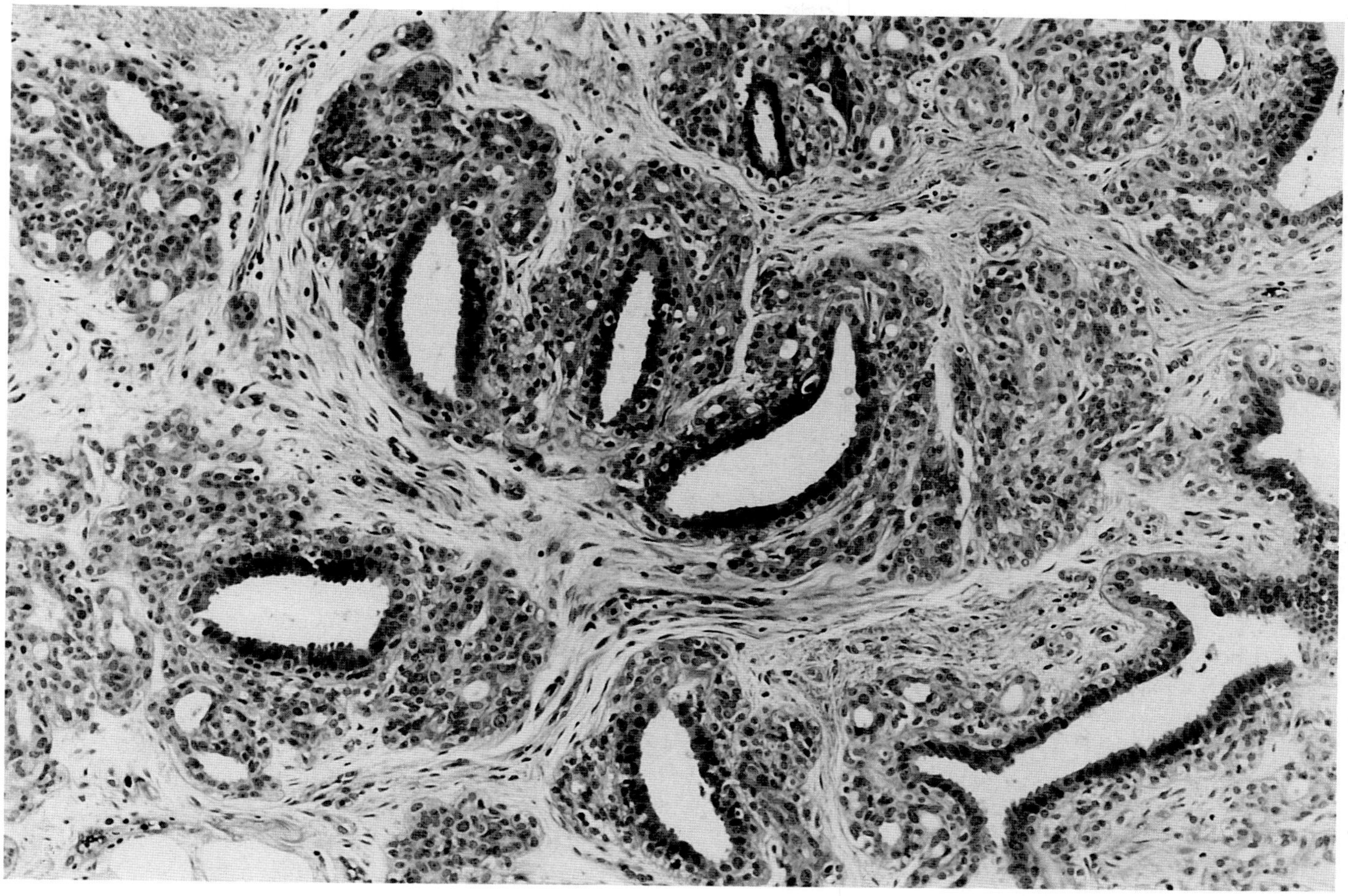

**Figure 15.5(a)** Myoepitheliosis. There is myoepithelial cell proliferation around several ductules. (H&E, X250)

nent of an adenomyoepithelioma may give rise to a carcinoma, while the background lesion retains its adenomyoepithelial appearance. These carcinomas are unequivocally recognizable as malignant. Two of the adenomyoepitheliomas in Tavassoli's study and one additional case in AFIP files since publication of that study harbored a carcinoma. In one lesion, the epithelial cell component displayed a solid pattern of proliferation and significant cytologic atypia. Abundant mitotic activity (more than five mitotic figures in one field at 300 magnification) was evident in the proliferating epithelial cells, with the epithelial/myoepithelial cell pattern persisting at the periphery of the lesion. These areas were interpreted as an epithelial adenocarcinoma arising in the adenomyoepithelioma. The epithelial nature of these areas was confirmed by a positive reaction for cytokeratin and a negative reaction for actin and S-100 protein. The carcinoma appeared as a high grade neoplasm but it was confined to the nodules of the adenomyoepithelioma, displaying a pushing margin without the classic, irregular invasive pattern. Another case showed an adenomyoepithelioma of the lobulated type with focal adenoid cystic carcinoma (Fig. 15.12). The latter was small and confined to the peripheral aspect of the lesion. It consisted of the basaloid-predominant variant of adenoid cystic carcinoma.

In the third tumor, located in the axillary tail of the breast, it was the myoepithelial cell element that displayed mild to moderate atypia, up to four mitotic figures per ten HPF, and formed infiltrating cords and angulated cell clusters composed of cuboid to spindle cells (Fig. 15.13). The epithelial cells lined rare small spaces in the midst of the clusters of myoepithelial cells. This tumor was interpreted as a myoepithelial carcinoma arising in an adenomyoepithelioma based on the presence of infiltrating cords and irregular, angulated clusters of myoepithelial cells. An adjacent axillary lymph node showed "metastatic" tumor composed of epithelial and myoepithelial cell

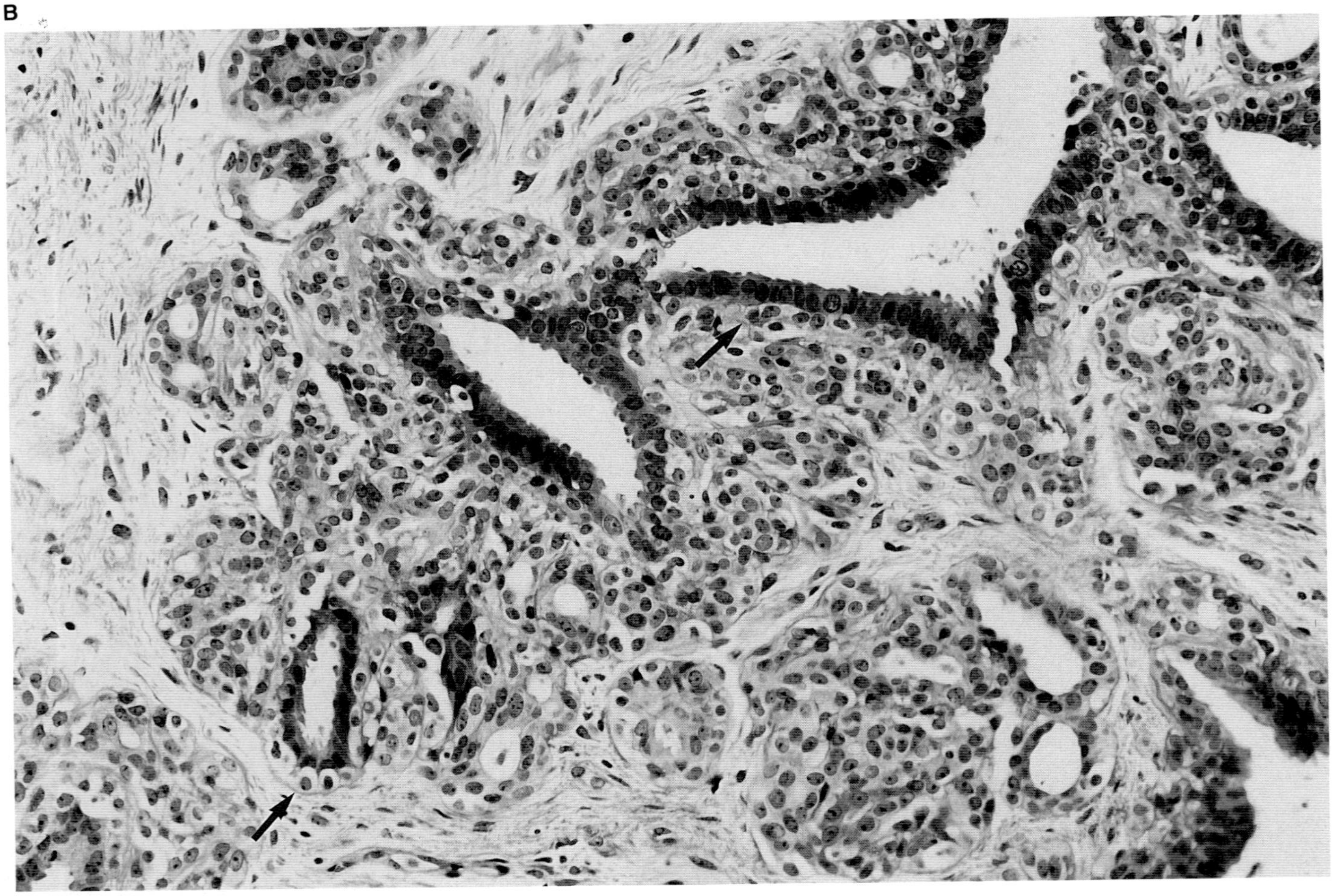

**Figure 15.5(b)** Myoepitheliosis. Note the similarity and continuity of the proliferating cells with the myoepithelial cells (arrows). (H&E, X400)

islands. The appearance of the cell clusters in the node was rather bland, without atypia and only a single mitotic figure; it is possible that this focus reflects extension of the benign portions of the adenomyoepithelioma to an adjacent node rather than true metastasis.

**Malignant Myoepithelioma.** Malignant myoepithelioma is generally a solitary lesion, characterized by an infiltrating proliferation of plump, atypical spindle cells with readily identifiable mitotic figures (Figs. 15.14, 15.15). The tumor is composed purely of spindled myoepithelial cells without any epithelial cell component. It extends with an infiltrating margin into the surrounding tissue. Aggregates of collagen, corresponding to the grossly visible nodules, are evident. The cells displayed a strongly positive reaction for actin and demonstrate a slightly weaker reaction for keratin. Immunoreaction for S-100 protein and actin are at least focally positive.

## Ultrastructural Features

Five malignant (infiltrating) myoepitheliomas (12,31, 35,41,42), as well as one lobulated and one tubular adenomyoepithelioma (41) have been studied at the ultrastructural level. Eosinophilic and/or clear myoepithelial cells were present in both adenomyoepitheliomas. The eosinophilic myoepithelial cells contain myofibrils in prominent aggregates with multiple dense bodies (Fig. 15.16). In the clear myoepithelial cells, much of the expanded clear cytoplasm is empty or electron-lucent, and the myofibrils are aggregated in one focus. The cells are attached to adjacent epithelial and myoepithelial cells by well-developed desmosomes and to the basal lamina by hemidesmosomes. The cell nests and tubules are surrounded by a multilayered basal lamina. In some areas, the tumor cells display arborescent cytoplasmic processes ex-

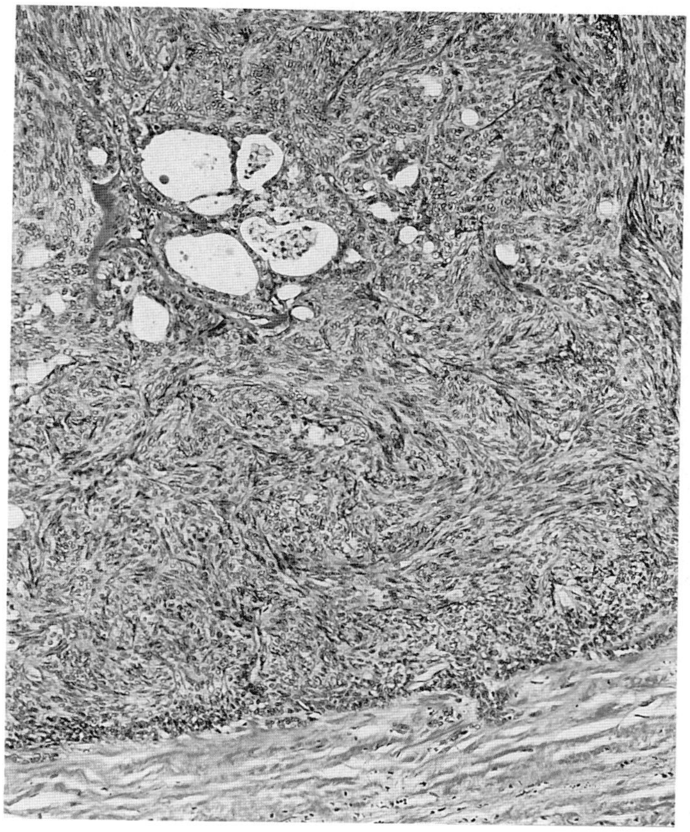

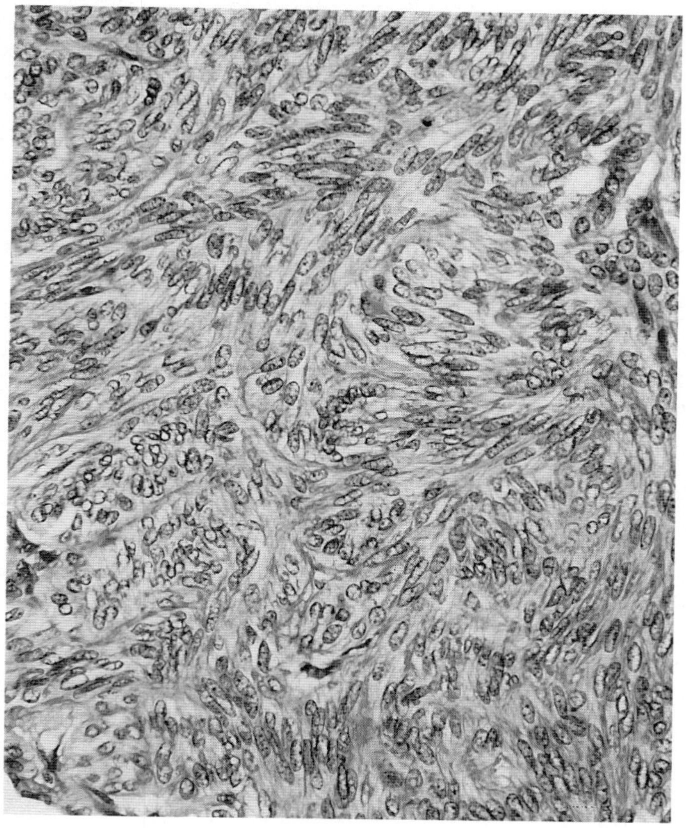

**Figure 15.6** Adenomyoepithelioma, intraductal spindle cell type. (a) Basically, a solitary duct shows proliferation of spindled myoepithelial cells into the duct. (b) The solid areas of spindle cell myoepithelial proliferation appear indistinguishable from a cellular leiomyoma. The myoepithelial cells around the metaplastic apocrine cells blend with the spindle cell proliferation. (H&E, (a) X75; (b) X250)

tending and carrying a complex meshwork of basal lamina into the surrounding stroma. This multilayered basal lamina corresponds to the wide collagenous bands observed by light microscopy. Pinocytotic vesicles are present in all cells but are sparse in the clear myoepithelial cells.

Malignant myoepithelioma is composed purely of elongated or spindle myoepithelial cells dispersed in a collagenous stroma. All cells display pinocytotic vesicles, myofibrils with densities, thick aggregates of tonofilaments, and patchy basal lamina, but the amount and distribution of these varies in different cells (Fig. 15.17). The tonofilaments form thicker and more electron-dense bundles and are located around the nucleus, whereas the myofibrils are located more peripherally. All cells display well-formed pinocytotic vesicles, a feature that invariably distinguishes the myoepithelial from an epithelial cell population. Tight junctions are observed attaching cytoplasmic processes of these cells; true desmosomes are rare.

## Recurrences

While the majority of myoepithelial lesions in the breast have been benign, a few have recurred, and only two tumors are known to have metastasized to an axillary node (41,42), while another patient developed bilateral pulmonary and pleural metastases (35). The three patients with metastases either had a malignant myoepithelioma (two cases) or a carcinoma arising in an adenomyoepithelioma. One of the three patients reported by Young and Clement (49) developed two recurrences, 3 and 4.5 years after the excisional biopsy. Judging from the illustration, this lesion would qualify as the tubular variant of adenomyoepithelioma. The case with multiple recurrences reported by Kiaer et al (23) was noted to have an adenosis pattern by the authors and would also qualify as tubular adenomyoepithelioma. The patient developed four recurrences, which were excised at

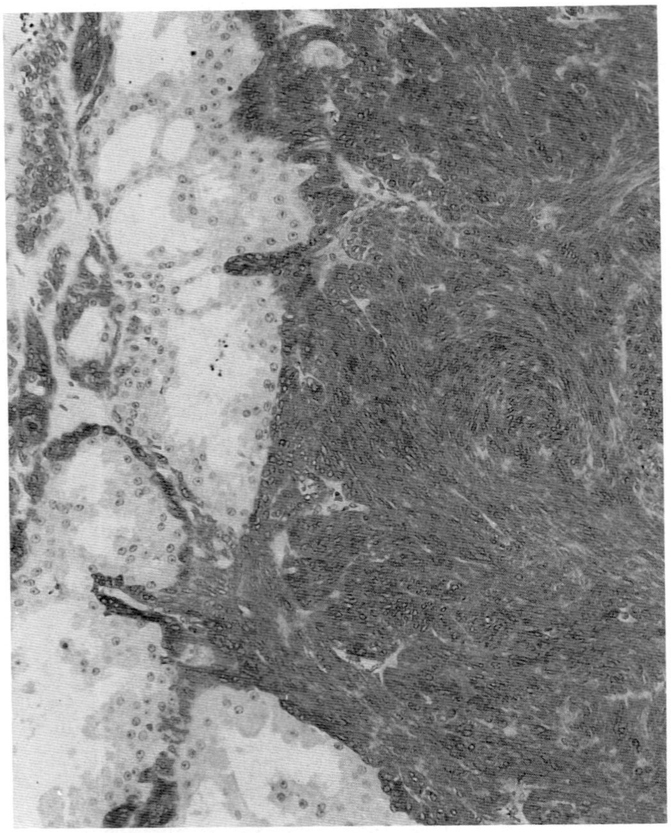

**Figure 15.7** Adenomyoepithelioma, spindle cell type. The spindle cells show a strongly positive reaction for actin, while the epithelial cells fail to react. (Immunoperoxidase reaction for S-100, X160) (From FA Tavassoli: *Am J Surg Pathol* 1991;15:554–568, with permission)

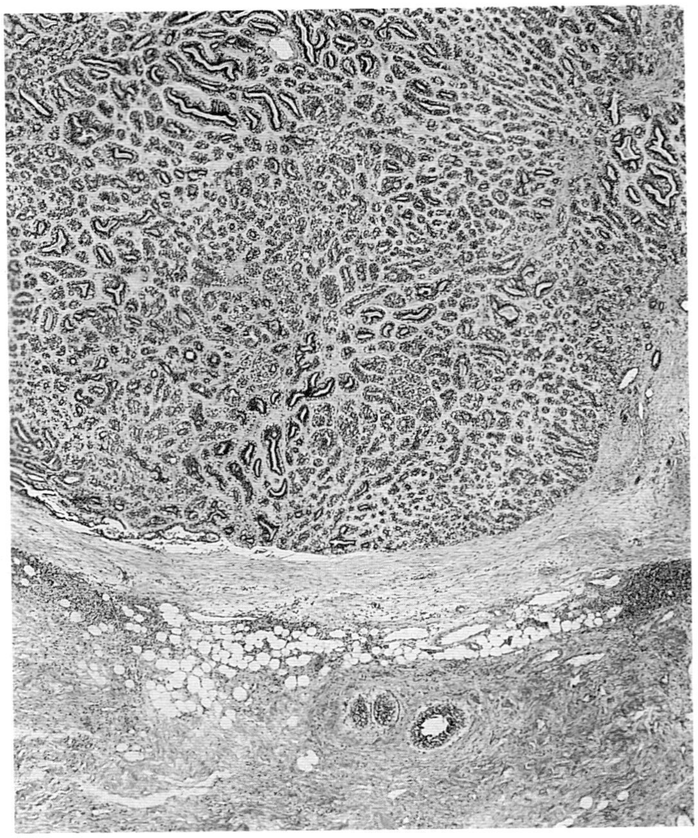

**Figure 15.8** Adenomyoepithelioma, tubular type. The cluster of tubules form a distinct, well-delineated mass separated from the surrounding breast tissue by a capsule. (H&E, X60) (From FA Tavassoli: *Am J Surg Pathol* 1991;15:554–568, with permission)

eight months, eight years, 15 years, and 18 years after the initial excision. One of the three patients who developed recurrences in the AFIP series also had a tubular adenomyoepithelioma. The women, a 41-year-old woman, developed two recurrences. The first recurrence occurred 5.3 years after the biopsy; the second one developed 11 months later. The primary and both recurrent lesions displayed the tubular pattern and were similar in the degree of atypia and mitotic activity. Five months after the second recurrence, she had bilateral total mastectomies. The mastectomy specimen showed no residual tumor. She has had no further recurrences two years following her mastectomies. It appears as if most patients who have developed recurrent adenomyoepitheliomas in the breast have had a tubular type of lesion. Curiously, the eight examples of the tubular variant in the AFIP study (41), including the tumor that recurred, did not have a particularly aggressive morphologic appearance, lacking notable mitotic activity or infiltrating margins. One tumor recurred twice. The recurrent lesions were identical to the original tumor, but the last recurrence had more abundant tubules. One of the characteristics of this variant, however, is an ill-defined boundary or demarcation with the pathologic tubules often extending into and blending with the adjacent normal ducts. This feature could lead to incomplete excision and subsequent recurrence of the tumor.

The second woman who developed recurrence in Tavassoli's study (41) was 80 years of age and had the lobulated variant of adenomyoepithelioma. She developed four simultaneous recurrent nodules eight months after excision of her initial tumor. Two of the recurrent nodules appeared more atypical and displayed more abundant mitotic activity (up to eight mitotic figures per ten HPF) compared to the primary tumor. The original tumor did not display significant atypia, and its mitotic activity did not exceed 3 MF/10 HPF, but it had multiple small satellite nodules and myoepithelial cell proliferation in ducts at a distance from the lesion. Therefore, it is quite likely that the original excision had failed to remove all of the pathologically proliferative ductules which continued

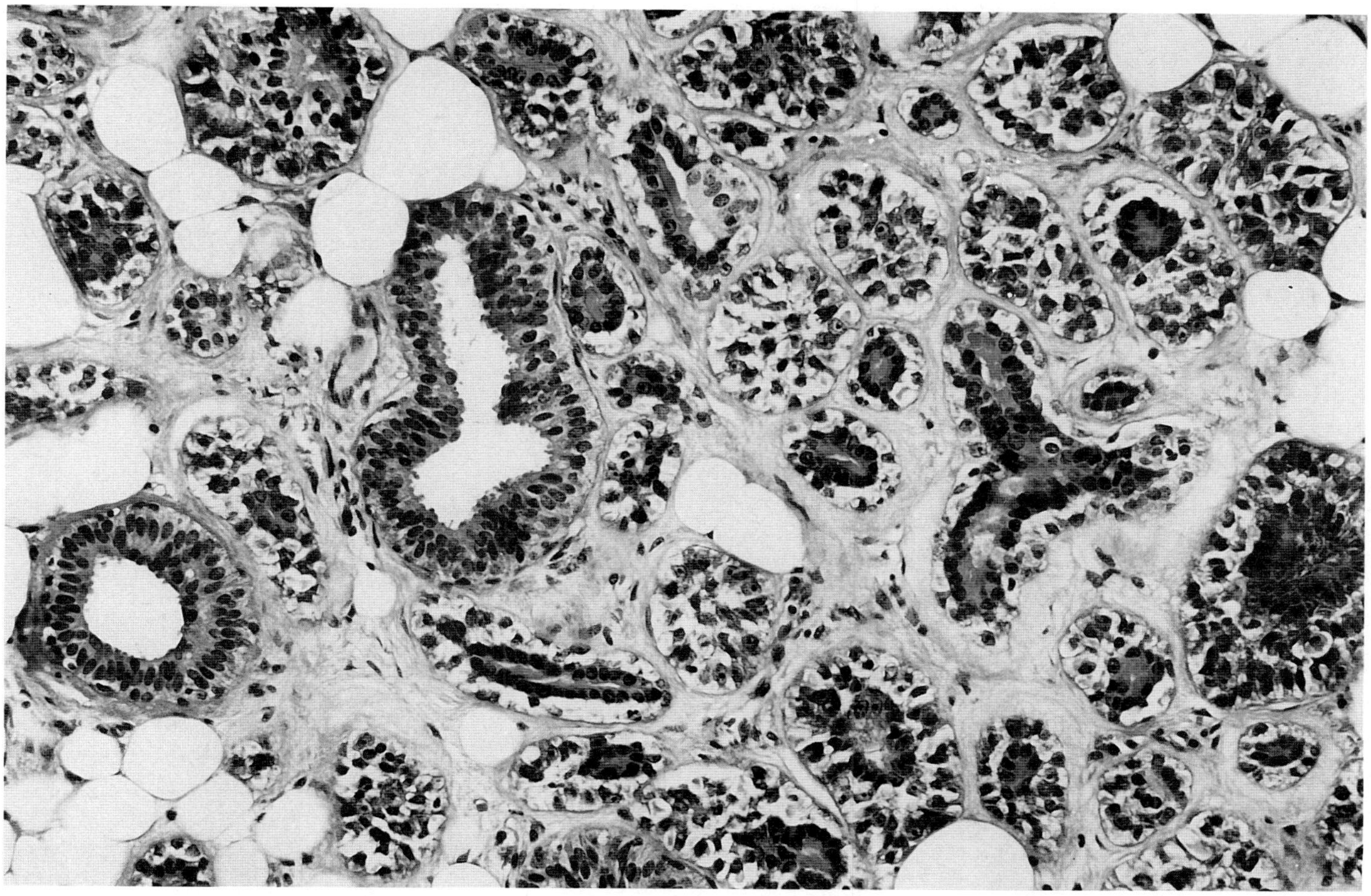

**Figure 15.9** Adenomyoepithelioma, tubular. In some of the ducts, the myoepithelial cells appear merely prominent, but in others, they are hyperplastic. (H&E, X350)

to proliferate and gave rise to new lesions in the vicinity of the original mass. What is interpreted as a recurrence, therefore, may actually reflect a de novo lesion or progression of residual disease. The lobulated variant of adenomyoepithelioma was the lesion most frequently misinterpreted as invasive carcinoma.

The third woman who developed a recurrence was a 61-year-old woman who had a myoepithelial carcinoma arising in an axillary adenomyoepithelioma. She also had axillary node metastasis, composed of both epithelial and myoepithelial cells (Fig. 15.14), at the time of presentation. The tumor in the lymph node was composed of well-differentiated epithelial and myoepithelial cells, and resembled the benign component of the adenomyoepithelioma, while the recurrent lesion which appeared 2.3 years after the initial excision was identical to the malignant myoepithelial carcinoma component of the original tumor. The patient had no evidence of a tumor within the breast proper at the time of presentation, at the time of recurrence, or two years following excision of her recurrent tumor. The ipsilateral breast was not biopsied or removed. The possibility of direct extension of the adenomyoepithelioma to the lymph node cannot be excluded considering the proximity of the node to the primary lesion and the bland appearance of the lesion in the lymph node.

Two examples of metastases from pure myoepithelial carcinomas have been reported (35,42). These two are the best documented cases of malignant behavior by pure myoepithelial carcinomas. It is noteworthy that these tumors were both composed purely of spindle myoepithelial cells. Three other examples of myoepithelial carcinoma composed of spindle cells have been reported (12,31,41), but neither of these three had evidence of metastases at the time of the report; one of these tumors was infiltrating but lacked atypia or mitotic activity (12). In contrast to the myoepitheliosis and adenomyoepithe-

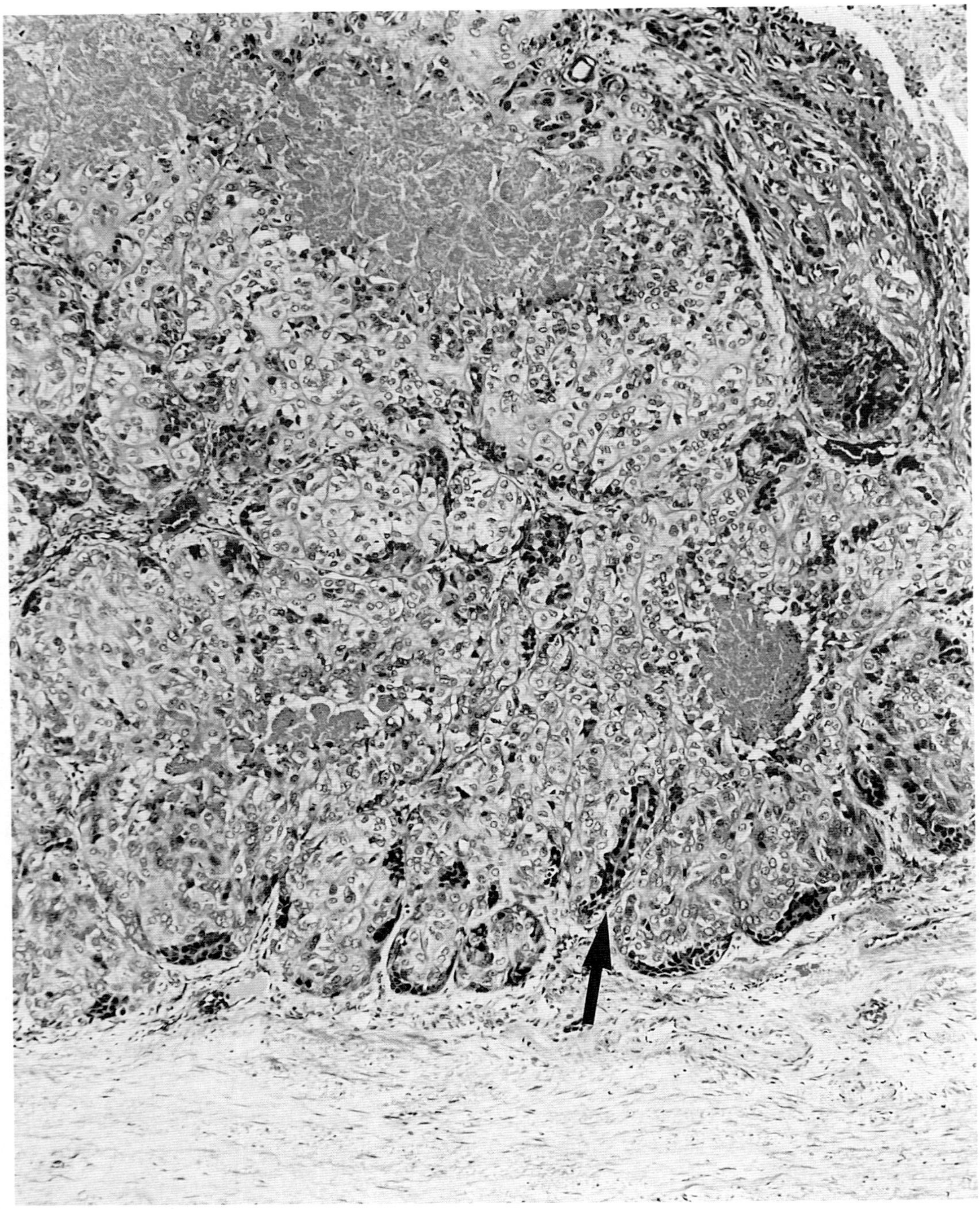

**Figure 15.10** Adenomyoepithelioma, lobulated type. The outline of the nodule is lobulated and there is abundant necrosis. Note compressed tubules lined by epithelial cells (arrow). (H&E, X150)

liomas, the malignant myoepitheliomas reported so far have lacked light microscopic evidence of an epithelial cell population or arrangement and have been composed of spindle cells. At the ultrastructural level, they have all displayed pinocytotic vesicles, in addition to myofibrils (microfilaments), patchy basal lamina and tonofilaments (12,35,41,42). The amount of tonofilaments in their cytoplasm has been variable depending on the degree of differentiation toward the epithelioid aspect of the cell; tight junctions and desmosomes are observed rarely.

## Follow-up

**Myoepitheliosis.** None of the three patients with myoepitheliosis in Tavassoli's series (41) developed

A

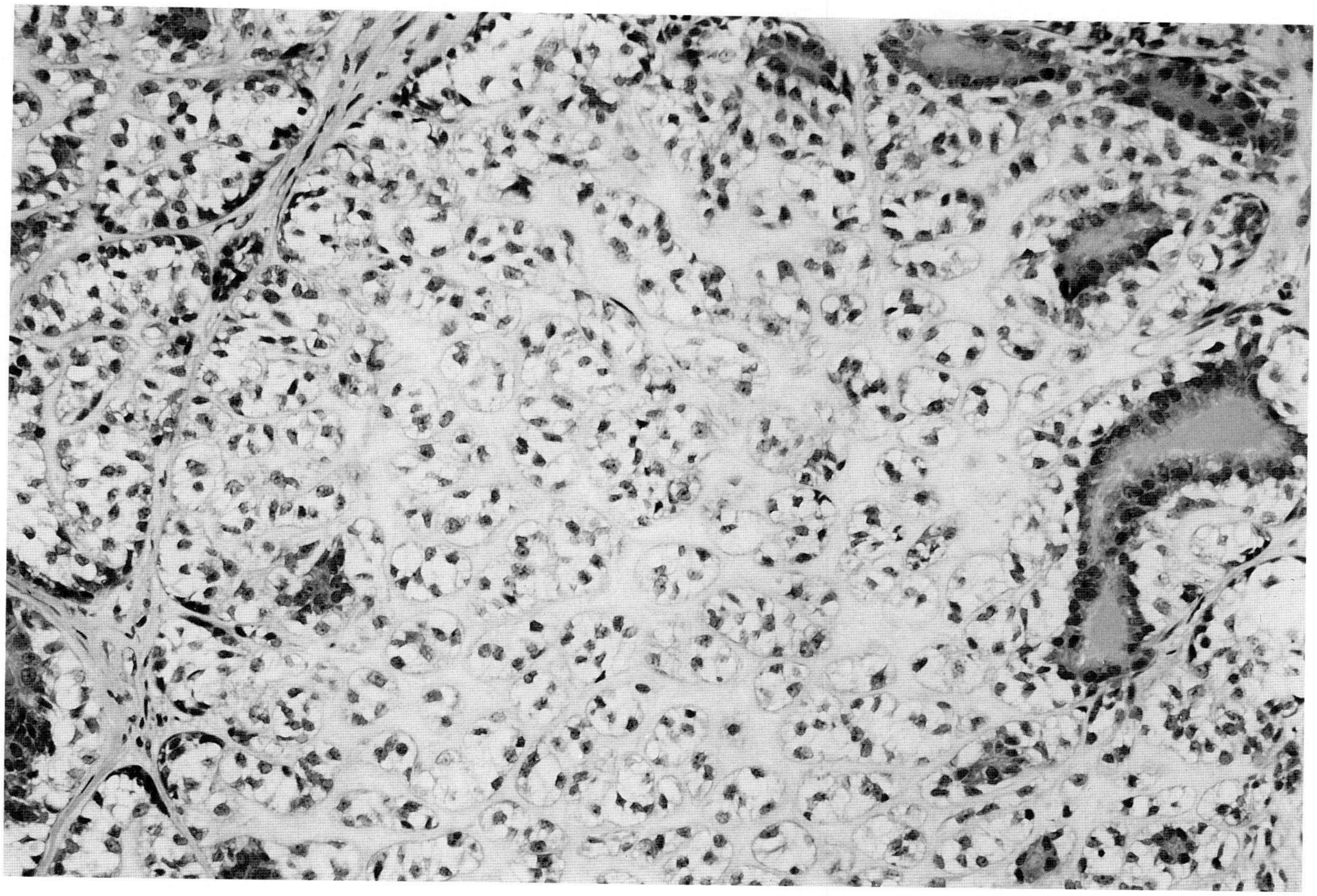

**Figure 15.11(a)** Adenomyoepithelioma, lobulated type. Another lesion composed of clear myoepithelial cells separated by broad collagen bands or a hyalinized matrix. Epithelial cells line the luminal aspect of the tubular structures on the right side. (H&E, X800)

recurrences after the initial biopsy. They were all alive and well 4 to 7.5 years after the tumor resection.

**Adenomyoepithelioma.** Because of initial interpretation of the lesion as carcinoma, nine of the 27 patients in Tavassoli's series (41) had mastectomy, eight with excision of axillary lymph nodes. There was no residual tumor in any of these, and the axillary nodes were negative in all cases. Included among these was the 38-year-old woman with an adenocarcinoma arising in the adenomyoepithelioma; she had 26 lymph nodes excised, and none contained metastatic tumor. She has had no problems as of six months after this procedure. The 61-year-old woman with a myoepithelial carcinoma arising in an axillary adenomyoepithelioma had metastatic tumor in an adjacent lymph node.

Of the remaining patients in the AFIP series (41), one patient died from disseminated pancreatic carcinoma 1.3 years after excision of the breast lesion; no evidence of recurrence was seen at autopsy. Five patients were either lost to follow-up or had less than one year of follow-up. The remaining patients were all alive and well from 1.6 to 17.5 years after their biopsies; the median follow-up was 6.1 years.

**Myoepithelial Carcinoma.** One of the five patients with myoepithelial carcinoma reported in the literature is known to have died with metastatic pulmonary disease six months following radiation therapy and mastectomy for her tumor (35). Another woman died from a cerebrovascular accident two months after the diagnosis of her mammary tumor (42). None of the remaining three patients has died of her myoepithelial carcinoma or developed a recurrence within 3.3, 9, and 19 months after the diagnosis.

B

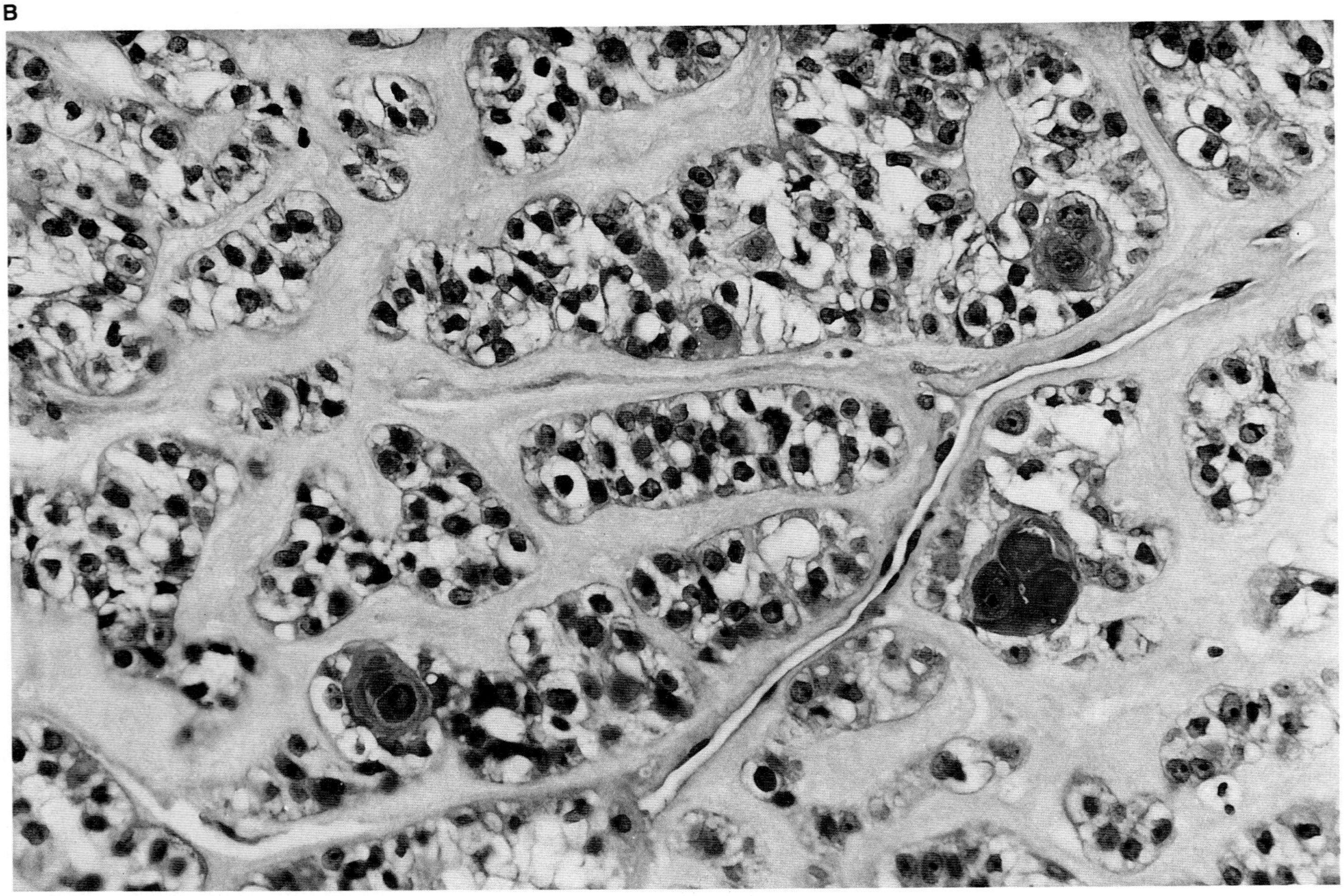

**Figure 15.11(b)** Adenomyoepithelioma, lobulated type. Elsewhere in the same lesion, there are foci of squamous metaplasia. (H&E, X1,000)

## Differential Diagnosis

A spindle cell malignant myoepithelioma should be differentiated from a spindle cell carcinoma (45). Immunohistochemical and often ultrastructural evaluation are necessary to distinguish between these two entities. There has been ultrastructural and immunohistochemical confirmation of the epithelial nature of the cells of spindle carcinomas in several cases and squamous differentiation has been noted in two studies (14,17). While epithelial cells may occasionally coexpress intermediate filaments other than tonofilaments, they have never been shown to develop pinocytotic vesicles. Therefore, the presence of pinocytotic vesicles even with sparse myofibrils and dense bodies would point against a diagnosis of an epithelial tumor. This finding, along with a predominance of cells displaying a positive reaction for actin or S-100 protein rather than cytokeratin-positive cells, would confirm a diagnosis of a malignant myoepithelioma. Predominance of cytokeratin-positive cells and absence of myofibrils with dense bodies, pinocytotic vesicles, and basal laminar investiture, in contrast, would support the diagnosis of a spindle cell carcinoma. The presence of pinocytotic vesicles is a feature that has not been described in epithelial tumors, and therefore its presence at the ultrastructural level would establish the myoepithelial nature of the cells when associated with the other features. The distinction between a metaplastic spindle cell carcinoma and malignant myoepithelioma is simple in most cases as many metaplastic carcinomas have focal, albeit small, areas of epithelial differentiation readily recognizable by light microscopy. Occasionally, however, it becomes very difficult to separate the two lesions. Since both of these tumors are recognized as malignant, mastectomy has been the preferred treatment regardless of the designation in borderline cases.

Another lesion that could be confused with ma-

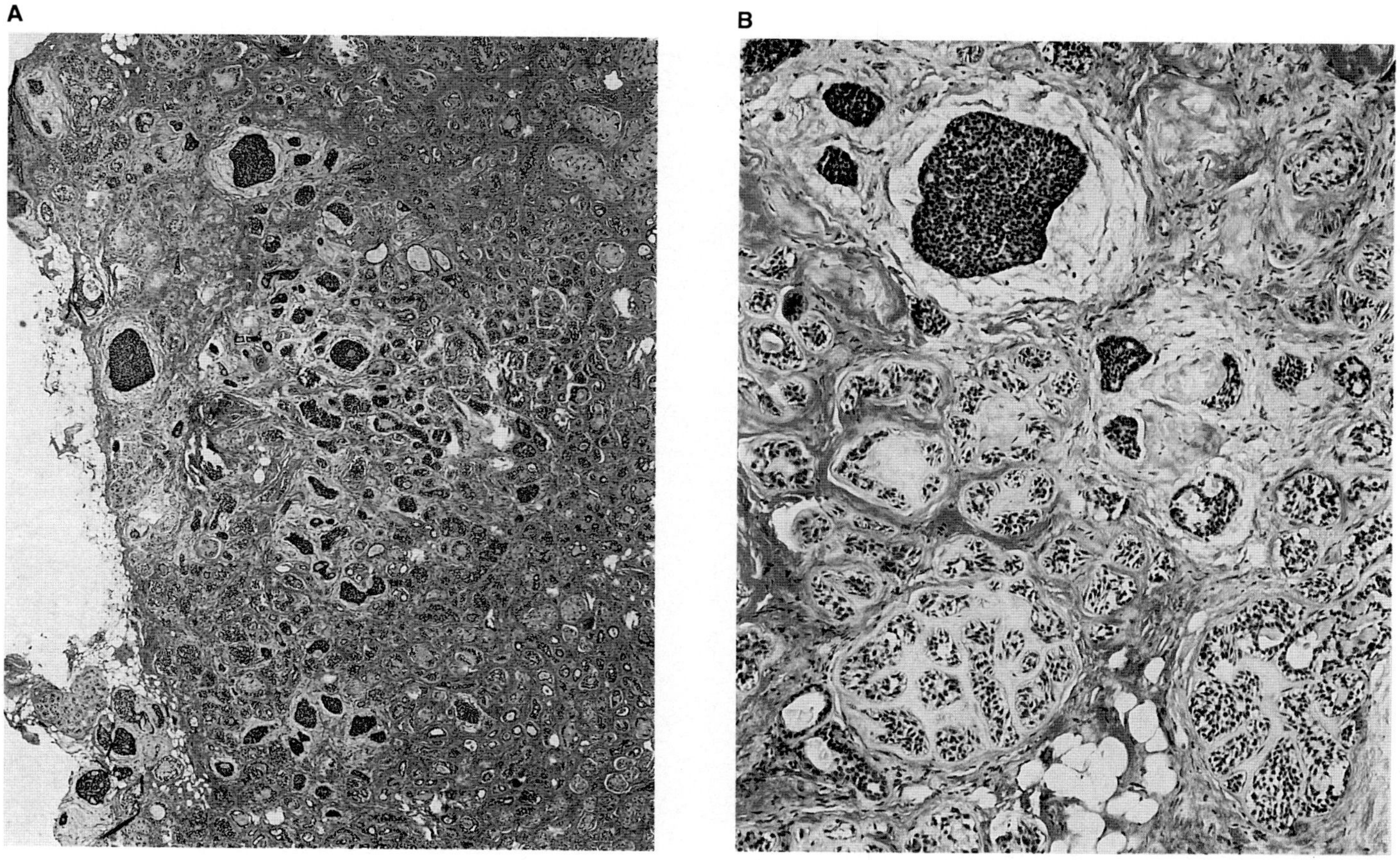


**Figure 15.12** Carcinoma arising in adenomyoepithelioma. (a) At one edge of this adenomyoepithelioma, a basaloid variant of adenoid cystic carcinoma has developed. (b) These areas consist of proliferation of small uniform, basaloid cells in round and angulated clusters admixed with tubules of myoepithelial cells in a hyalinized matrix. (H&E, (a) X30; (b) X120)

lignant myoepithelioma is fibromatosis (49), a lesion composed of myofibroblasts and fibroblasts. At the light microscopic level, the growth pattern of fibromatosis is its most distinctive feature. When compared to malignant myoepithelioma, fibromatosis is a more irregular and ill-defined lesion, displaying an exaggerated infiltrative pattern. The spindle cells in fibromatosis proliferate in fascicles and interlacing bundles with entrapment of normal ducts and lobules in the periphery of the lesion; cytologic atypia is absent or mild. Mitotic figures do not generally exceed two to three per ten HPF and they are normal in appearance. In contrast, malignant myoepithelioma shows a haphazard proliferation of the spindle cells. The proliferating cells display atypia; mitotic figures are readily apparent and may be abnormal. At the ultrastructural level, the fibroblasts and myofibroblasts of fibromatosis lack tonofilaments and tight junctions which are characteristically present in the myoepithelial cells. Furthermore, the myofibrils and pinocytotic vesicles in myofibroblasts are not as well developed as those of myoepithelial cells. Immunohistochemically, a uniformly positive reaction for S-100 protein, a focal positivity for cytokeratin, or both, would exclude the possibility of fibromatosis. Unfortunately, in practice, immunohistochemistry is not always helpful. Immunoreaction for actin is not helpful in this setting since both myoepithelial and myofibroblastic cells show a positive reaction.

Finally, adenomyoepithelioma should be distinguished from mixed tumor or pleomorphic adenoma. The latter always has areas of chondroid, chondromyxoid, or chondro-osseous differentiation.

Sclerosing adenosis with prominent ME cells may be mistaken for an invasive carcinoma (Fig. 15.18).

## *Comparison with Myoepithelial Lesions of the Salivary Glands*

In the salivary glands, myoepithelioma (36), epithelial-myoepithelial carcinoma of intercalated duct origin (9), and malignant myoepitheliomas (10) have been reported. The lesion referred to as epithelial-myoep-

A B

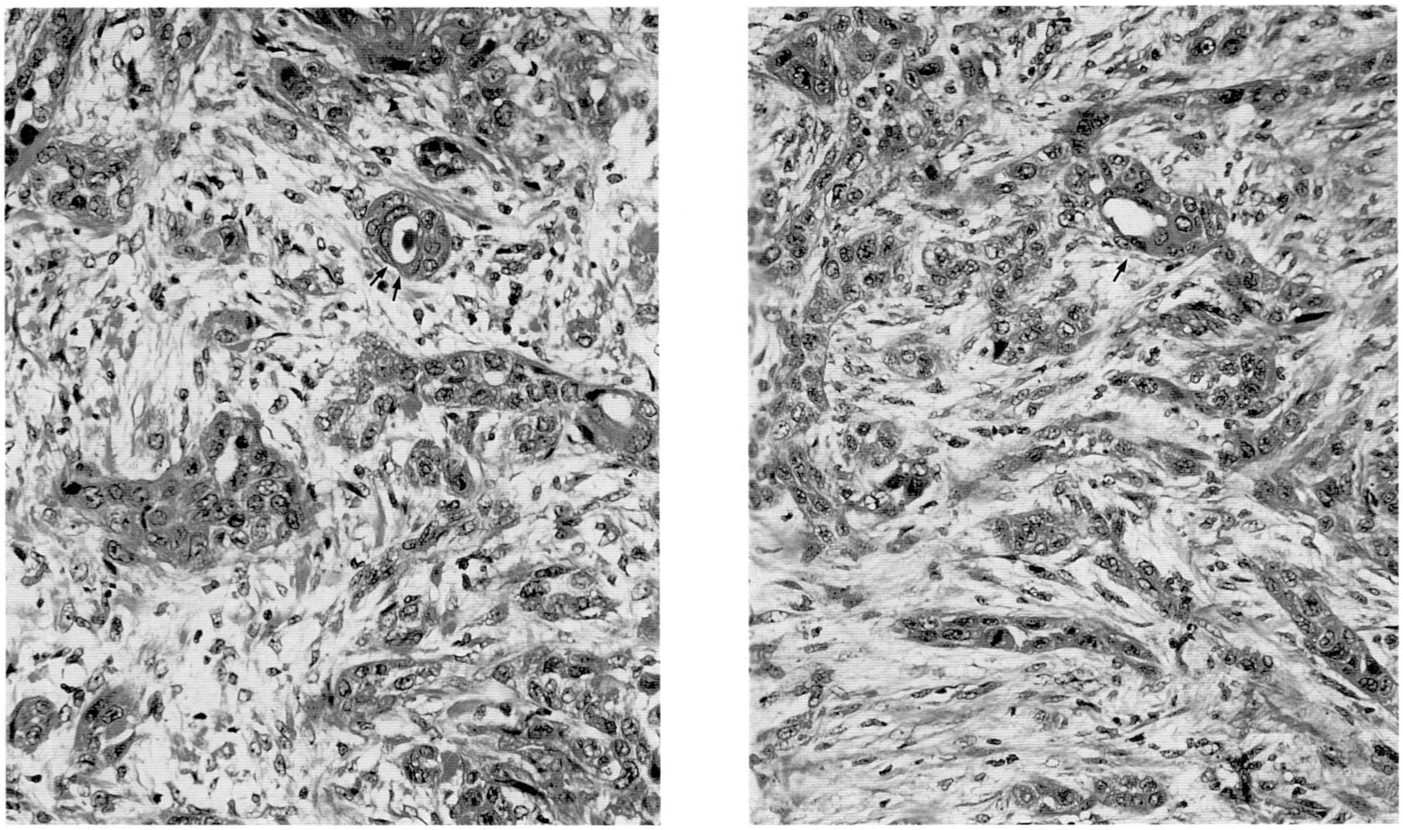

**Figure 15.13** Carcinoma arising in adenomyoepithelioma. (a,b) The malignant component of this tumor was the myoepithelial cell population which assumed a highly epithelioid appearance and infiltrated in cords and irregular clusters. Residual epithelial cells lined the lumen in the center of some of the infiltrating clusters (arrows). (H&E, (a) X200; (b) X240)

ithelial carcinoma of intercalated duct origin or epimyoepithelial carcinoma is considered a low grade carcinoma prone to local recurrences and eventual metastases; morphologically, it is comparable to the lobulated adenomyoepithelioma in the breast. While designated as low grade carcinomas in the salivary glands, cases with documented metastases are uncommon.

The less aggressive behavior manifested by the mammary lesions may be due to the feasibility of a more complete excision of the mammary lesions considering the abundance of breast tissue surrounding these lesions. Also, in this study, seven of the patients with the most mitotically active adenomyoepitheliomas, including the two with infiltrating margins, had mastectomy with axillary node dissection, or basically a cancer treatment. None of these patients had axillary node metastases. While it is possible that follow-up beyond 20 years in patients who had local excision may disclose additional recurrences, judging from the three tumors that recurred in this study and the recurrent case in Young and Clement's study (50) as well as the one reported by Kiaer et al (23), recurrences seem to develop within five to six years after the initial excision.

Another difference noted between mammary myoepithelial cells (normal and neoplastic) and their salivary gland counterparts is in the expression of GFAP. While myoepithelial tumors of salivary gland origin have displayed positivity for GFAP, neither the benign mammary myoepithelial cells nor the neoplastic ones reacted with the GFAP utilized in the AFIP study (41). This may be due to the type of GFAP used at AFIP, but the same GFAP is used for the salivary gland tumors and they do show a positive reaction.

## Treatment

Based on the available data, myoepitheliosis is a benign lesion adequately treated by total excision. Adenomyoepitheliomas have a potential for local

A

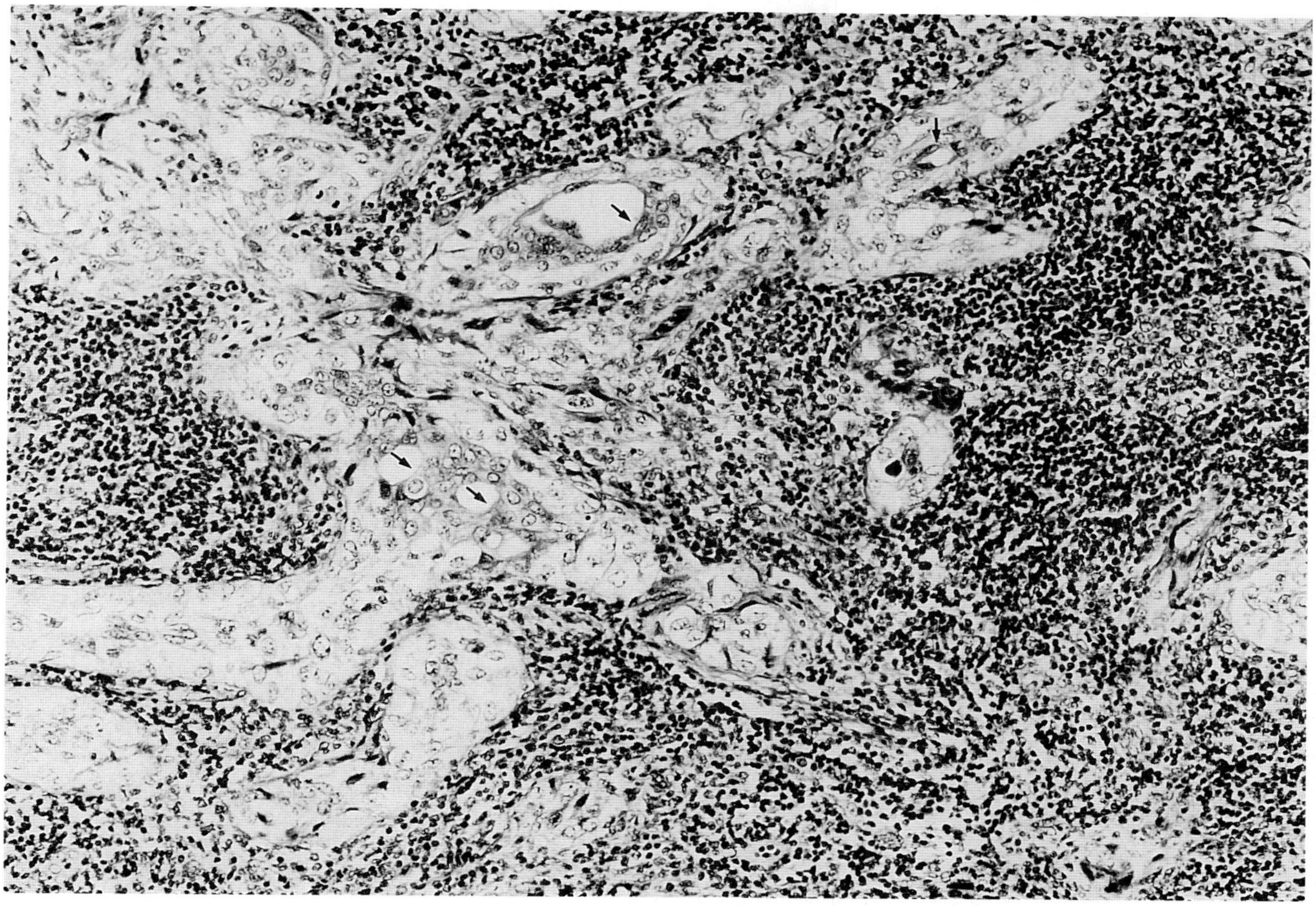

**Figure 15.14(a)** A lymph node adjacent to the axillary myoepithelial tumor illustrated in Fig. 15.12 contained a "metastatic" focus. The nests of metastatic tumor are composed of small epithelial-lined spaces (arrows) surrounded by proliferating myoepithelial cells. (H&E, X300) (From FA Tavassoli: *Am J Surg Pathol* 1991;15:554–568, with permission)

recurrence, but none is known to have metastasized. Therefore, total excision with a margin of uninvolved breast tissue is recommended particularly in case of the tubular variant and the lobulated tumors exhibiting mitotic activity exceeding 3 MF/10 HPF with focally infiltrating margins or satellite nodules. If the lesion recurs, a wider excision would be prudent. Because of the absence of any documented metastases from adenomyoepitheliomas, a mastectomy is not required. When there is a carcinoma (epithelial or myoepithelial) arising in an adenomyopithelioma, however, the lesion is best treated as a carcinoma. The myoepithelial carcinoma (infiltrating malignant myoepithelioma) is unequivocally malignant, with nodal and distant metastases documented in previous reports (35,42). Therefore, management of the lesion as a carcinoma would be justified. It is noteworthy that the only patient in the AFIP (41) series with a malignant myoepithelioma had tylectomy and there has been no evidence of recurrence 1.6 years after the initial excision. The possibility of a metaplastic carcinoma should be excluded, even if it requires both immunohistochemical and ultrastructural evaluation.

## MASTITIS

A variety of reactive and inflammatory changes occur in the breast. These range from acute mastitis associated with lactation which may proceed to the development of an abscess, to more chronic disease and the formation of necrotizing granulomas in tuberculosis. While some of these alterations are known to have an infectious etiology, others are not well understood and may either reflect a local manifestation

B

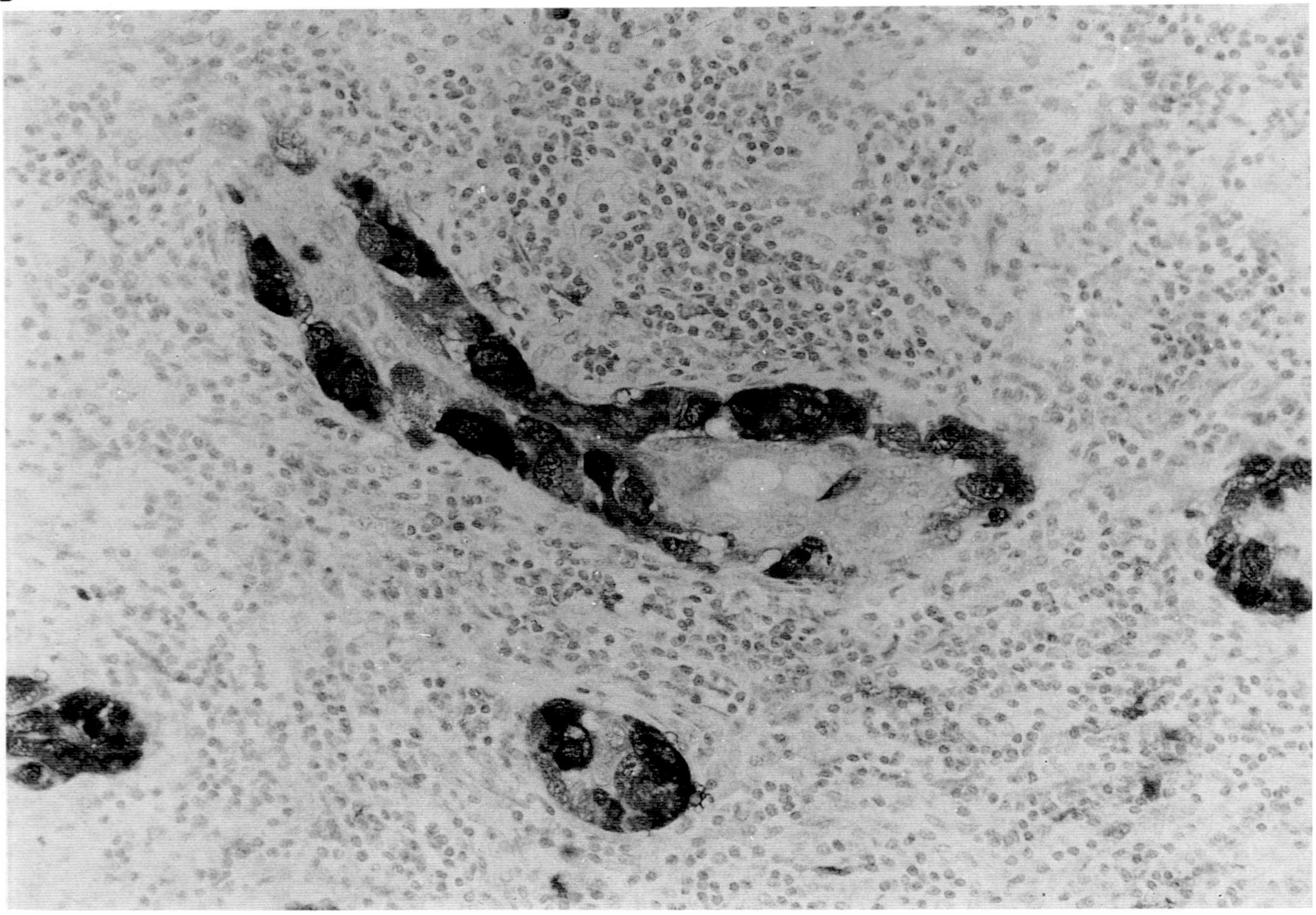

**Figure 15.14(b)** Immunostain for actin decorates the peripheral myoepithelial cells, while the centrally-located epithelial cells fail to react. (X480)

of a systemic disease, a localized antigen-antibody reaction, or an idiopathic process.

## Acute Mastitis

Painful, localized areas of inflammation develop in the breast of lactating women generally as a result of a cracked nipple (73,99) which serves as the portal of entry for bacteria. Haagensen noted that the cracks are the result of changes in the pH of the skin to a more alkaline side, and discussed successful treatment of the problem using a slightly acidic cold cream (74).

Occasionally, the inflammation progresses to the development of an abscess. The overlying skin becomes edematous and red. The abscess may develop a thick fibrous wall which impedes its resolution. Most of these abscesses are due to *Staphylococcus aureus*, a large proportion of which are sensitive to cephalexin (Keflex®). Abscesses caused by organisms resistant to antibiotics are difficult to treat.

## Subareolar Abscess

Subareolar and periareolar abscesses develop in lactating, nonlactating, pre- and postmenopausal women (75,79,82,83,92,95). Patients range in age from 18 to 67 years with a mean of 36 years. The lesions predominates in women of the reproductive age, but may occur in the male breast as well (75). The duration of symptoms ranges from one week to 10 years (75). About 25% of the cases are bilateral and recurrences develop in 92% of the patients (75). Congenital or acquired nipple inversion and retraction were noted in 91 of the 152 patients in Habif's

A

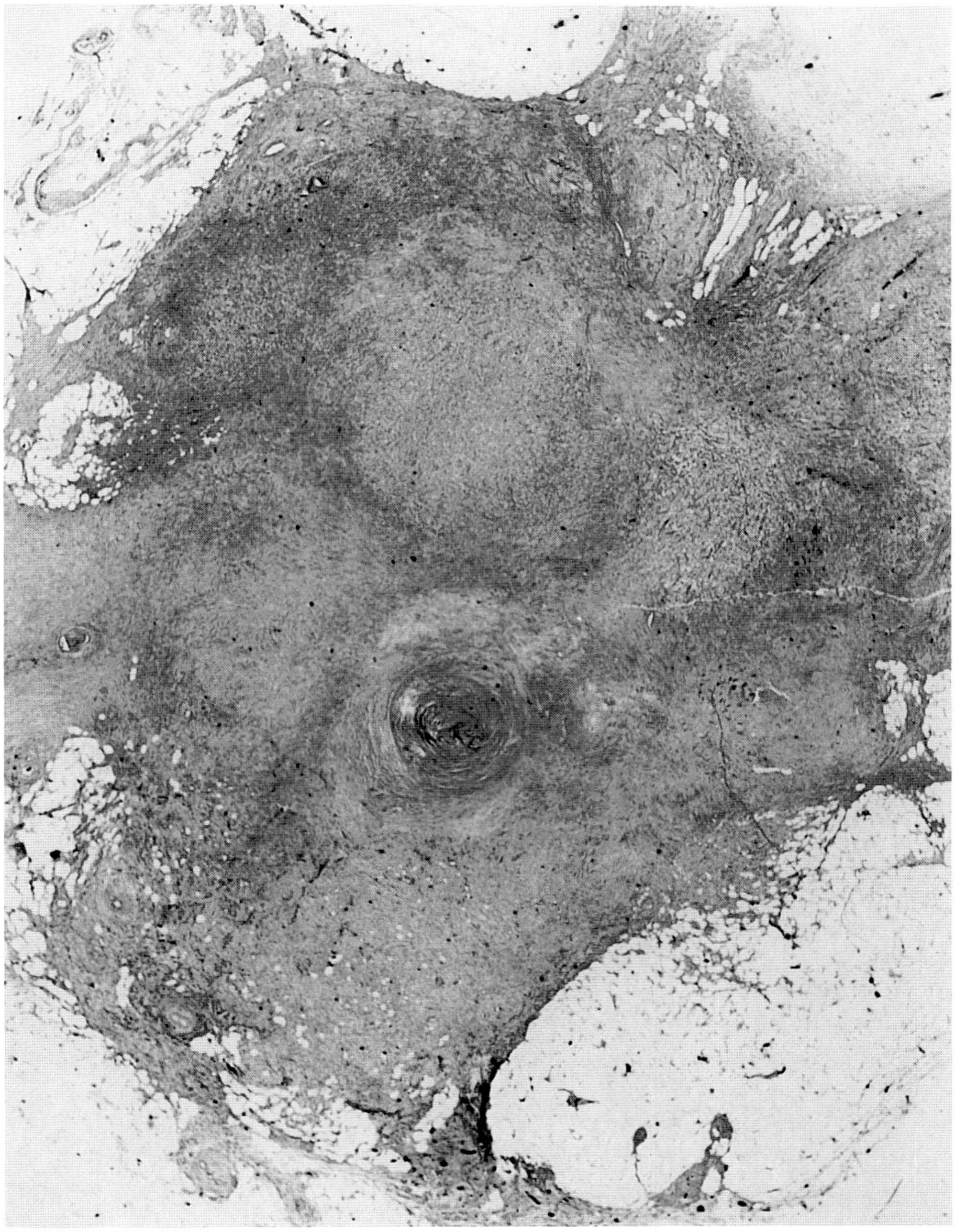

**Figure 15.15(a)** Malignant myoepithelioma. At low magnification, an irregular, infiltrating margin characterized the only tumor in this group. A prominent focus of hyalin degeneration was present in the center of the lesion. (H&E, X25) (From FA Tavassoli: *Am J Surg Pathol* 1991;15:554–568, with permission)

(75) series and in all abscesses caused by anaerobic infections in Leach et al's series (82).

Subareolar abscesses invariably develop in ducts that display complete replacement of the native glandular epithelium by squamous metaplasia (92). Extensive squamous metaplasia of the lactiferous duct(s) and obstruction by keratinous and cellular debris leads to proximal distension of the duct. At some point, the cystically dilated portion of the duct may rupture. Bacterial invasion and the irritating effect of the nonabsorbable keratin can cause a supporative condition and giant cell reaction with eventual development of an abscess. A sinus tract may develop from the abscess to the overlying skin.

The variety of infecting microorganisms include *Staphylococcus* (107), *Proteus* (107), *Bacteroides* (107), and *Streptococcus* (75,96,107,109).

Treatment requires draining the abscess first.

B

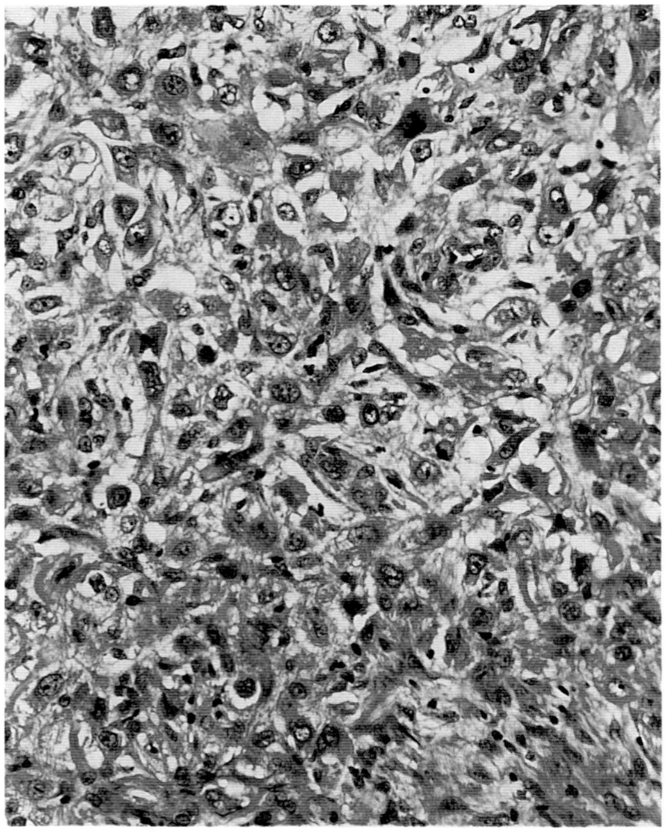

**Figure 15.15(b)** Malignant myoepithelioma. The most cellular area of the lesion was composed of plump, ovoid to spindled cells. (H&E, X200)

Once the inflammation has subsided, the diseased dilated ductal structure can be excised (74,75,111). Relapse in the form of fistulas following incision alone has been reported in 38% of women (108). Removal of the entire nipple and major ducts may be necessary in patients with multiple recurrences and those whose disease fails to resolve by less extensive surgery.

Squamous metaplasia and obstruction of the ducts of the subepidermal areolar glands may lead to the development of similar abscesses in the periareolar region (83). These abscesses are often accompanied by a sinus tract that communicates with the nipple, but are not contiguous with the lactiferous ducts. The tract reflects the pathway of the initial invasive infection and, if allowed to persist, would serve as a nidus for recurrences.

Breast abscesses also develop during the neonatal period in both boys and girls. A majority of these present as a unilateral breast enlargement during the second or third week of life in full term infants. *Staphylococcus aureus* is the most common organism cultured from these abscesses. Drainage of the abscess and antibiotic therapy generally is effective in the management of neonatal breast abscesses (99). The pathogenesis of neonatal mammary abscess is not well established.

## Plasma Cell Mastitis

First described by Adair (52) in 1933, plasma cell mastitis is characterized by a marked infiltration of the breast by plasma cells. The process is diffuse and involves both the duct system and the surrounding stroma (62). In addition, Adair noted proliferation of ductal epithelial cells simulating comedocarcinoma, as well as the presence of giant cells suggestive of tuberculosis. Haagensen (74) believes that the concentration of plasma cells produced by the low grade inflammation associated with duct ectasia is erroneously interpreted as "plasma cell mastitis" by some pathologists. Plasma cells accumulate in the stroma surrounding the ducts as a response to the irritative effect of the intraluminal lipid material reaching the periductal stroma. Patients with plasma cell mastitis are generally older than women with abscesses or granulomatous mastitis; the average age of patients reported by Frantz was 61.7 years (69).

True plasma cell mastitis is indeed a rare disease in which the background stroma is usually richly vascularized. Plasma cells constitute the predominant cellular infiltrate admixed with a few lymphocytes. The ducts, though not always of the typical ectatic type, show various degrees of distension, with inflammatory cells migrating into the epithelial lining and histiocytic collections within the lumens.

A broader definition of plasma cell mastitis has been used by some to include not only the plasma cell infiltration associated with duct ectasia in elderly women, but also a granulomatous reaction that occurs in young women. The latter is now regarded as granulomatous mastitis, five examples of which were described by Kessler and Wolloch (78) who considered an immune reaction as a possible explanation for the granulomatous changes.

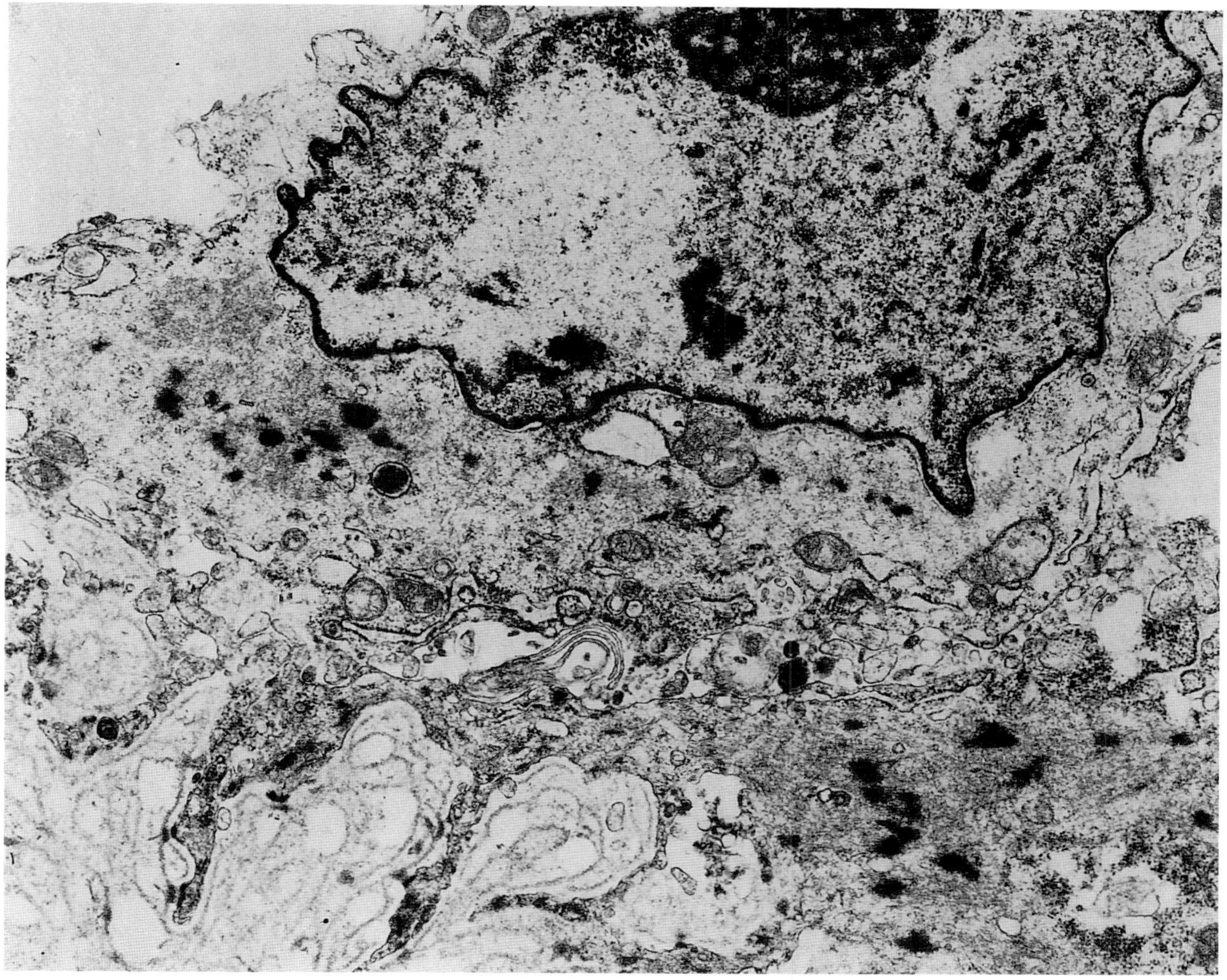

**Figure 15.16** Adenomyoepithelioma, lobulated type with eosinophilic cells. At the ultrastructural level, the myoepithelial cells contain abundant myofibrils with dense bodies. The nucleus of the myoepithelial cell is more electron dense with a different chromatin distribution compared to the adjacent epithelial cell. Note the multilayered basal lamina, a feature typically seen in adenomyoepithelial lesions. (Uranyl acetate-lead citrate, original magnification X3,000)

## Granulomatous Mastitis, Idiopathic

Granulomatous changes occasionally occur around lobules and ducts in the breast in the absence of specific infection, trauma, foreign material or evidence of sarcoidosis. Five patients with such idiopathic granulomatous mastitis were described by Kessler and Wolloch in 1972 (78). Since then many additional cases have been reported (54,58,60,64,65, 68,70,72,75,88,98) and similar cases can be found in the literature prior to 1972 (63,72,86).

### *Clinical Features*

Patients with granulomatous mastitis are generally of reproductive age. The age range is from 17 to 82 years, with an average age of 30 years. Two reports noted an association with recent pregnancy (68,72), with a majority of patients developing granulomatous mastitis within three years of their last pregnancy. No specific relationship to breast feeding or oral contraceptive hormone use has been noted. Two patients in Going's series (72) developed their lesion 15 years after their last pregnancy, however. Hyperprolactinemia, either drug-induced or associated with a pituitary prolactinoma, has been noted in two patients (72,95). All patients present with a palpable nodule which is tender in about a quarter of the patients. Almost a quarter of the patients have bilateral disease. Clinically, half of the published cases were considered malignant or suspicious for carcinoma, and more than half of the published cases describe women who required more than one operation. Nipple inversion and sinus tracts develop in

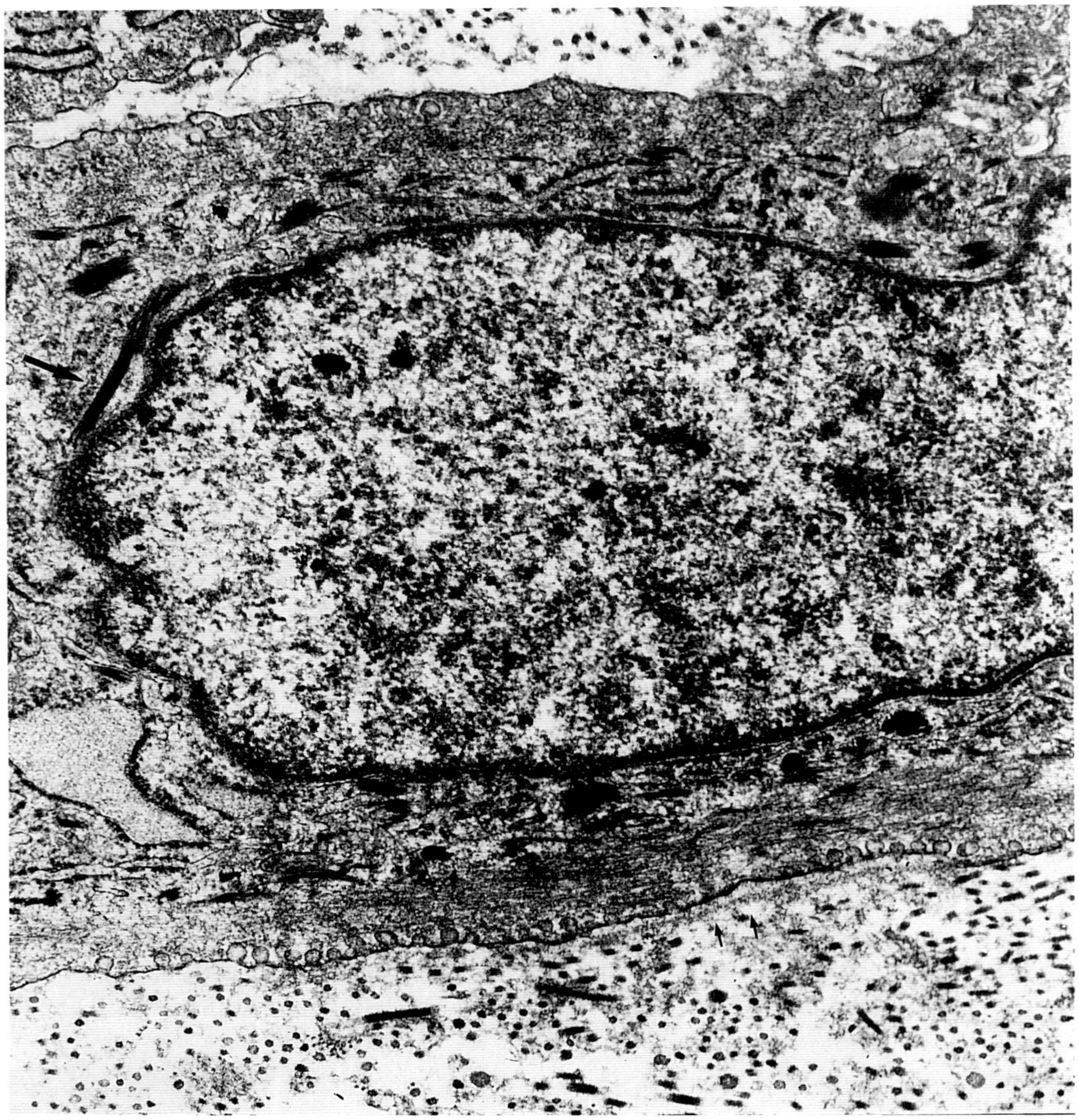

**Figure 15.17** Malignant myoepithelioma. Tumor cells display patchy basal lamina (short arrows), prominent pinocytotic vesicles, myofibrils with dense bodies immediately above the pinocytotic vesicles in the lower field, and bundles of tonofilaments in the perinuclear region (long arrow). (Uranyl acetate-lead citrate, original magnification X2,800) (From FA Tavassoli: *Am J Surg Pathol* 1991;51:554–568, with permission)

some patients. In a few cases, the disease may persist for years; one of the patients reported by Brown and Tang (58) had intermittent problems for 13 years.

### *Pathologic Features*

The lesion varies in size from 0.5 to 8 cm, exceeding 3 cm on the average. The abundance of the lesion is important and quite helpful, providing ample tissue for special studies and cultures.

Microscopically, the hallmark of the lesion is the presence of granulomas involving and often distorting the lobules (Fig. 15.19). The granulomas do extend to the surrounding stroma and adjacent ducts in widespread disease. Varying numbers of giant cells, neutrophilic polymorphs, lymphocytes, plasma cells, and even eosinophils are present. Microabscess formation is not uncommon in advanced disease. Occasionally, squamous metaplasia and foreign body giant cell reaction to keratin have been observed.

In all cases of granulomatous mastitis, proper evaluation of the specimen requires obtaining samples for cultures (aerobic and anaerobic), and special stains to rule out mycobacteria and a variety of other organisms (89,104). The possibility of sarcoidosis should be excluded and Kveim test, chest radiography, as well as measurement of serum angiotensin

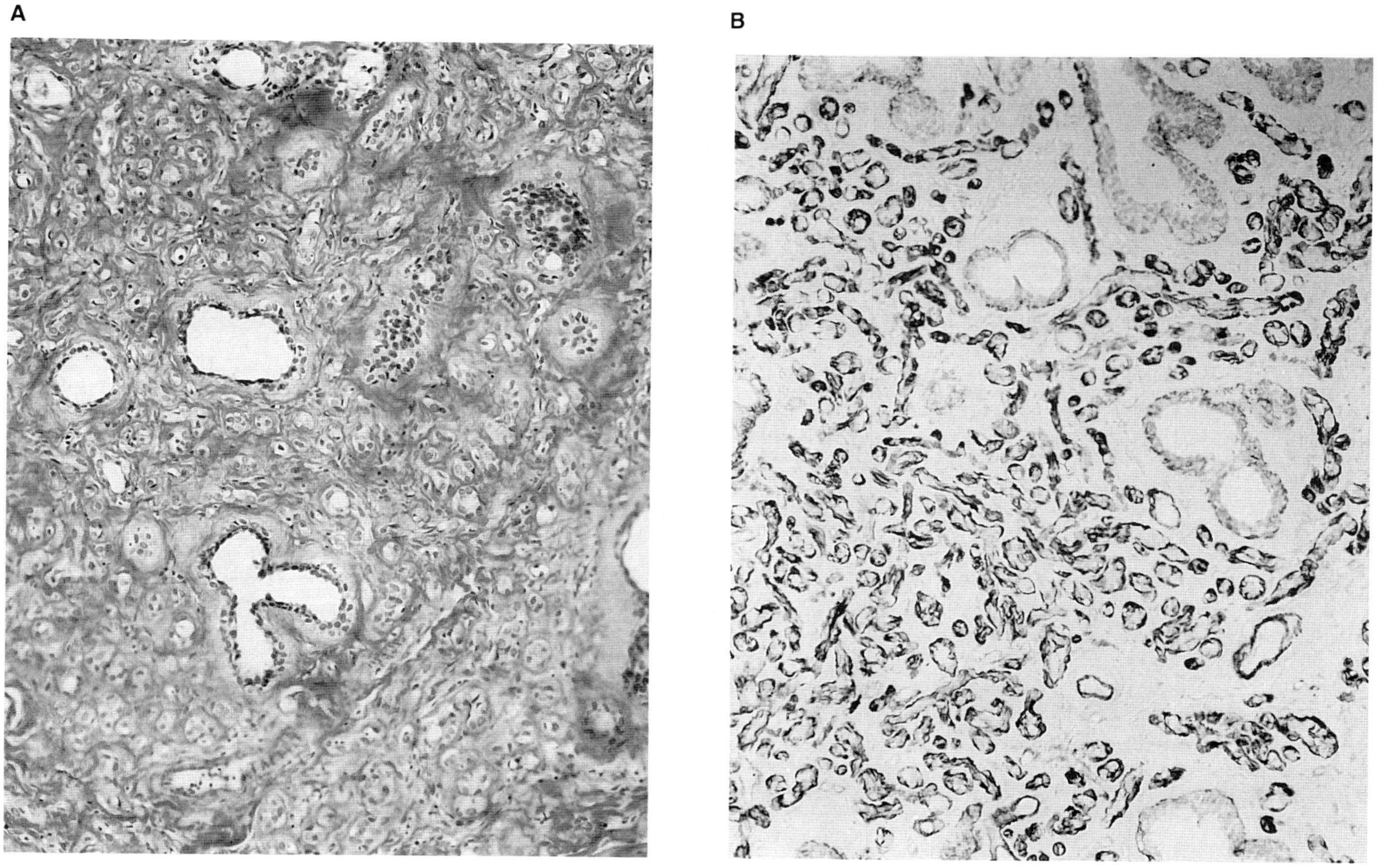

**Figure 15.18** Sclerosing adenosis with myoepithelial cell dominance. (a) The relatively haphazard distribution of small tubules with obliterated lumens around several ducts had led to a misinterpretation of this lesion as an invasive carcinoma. (H&E, X100) (b) Immunostain for actin shows the prominence of myoepithelial cells in this lesion and facilitates recognition of the tubular configuration. (X120) (From FA Tavassoli: *Am J Surg Pathol* 1991;15:554–568, with permission)

converting enzymes (ACE) (142) and lysozyme (134) may be appropriate. The diagnosis of idiopathic granulomatous mastitis should be made after exclusion of all other possibilities.

### *Pathogenesis*

The precise mechanism of the development of granulomatous mastitis is not known. Careful evaluation of the samples in the future with cultures for both aerobic and anaerobic organisms may provide additional information. A plausible explanation offered by Fletcher et al (68) is that damage to the ductular epithelium whether by infection, trauma, or a chemically-induced inflammation would allow luminal secretions to escape into the lobular connective tissue, thereby inducing a granulomatous response, resulting in further damage to the lobular structures.

### *Treatment*

The optimal treatment for idiopathic granulomatous mastitis has not been established. Steroid therapy has been recommended prior to surgery (65). Though used in only rare cases, this approach may be effective and further evaluation is desirable. Radical local excision has been used in refractory cases (80), but could be postponed to follow trials of drug treatment with corticosteroids. It should be emphasized that every effort should be made to exclude the possibility of a specific infection, infestation, or other disease process in granulomatous mastitis before designating it as nonspecific or idiopathic. Appropriate treatment depends on accurate identification of the causative agent or organism.

## Tuberculous Mastitis

While a variety of granulomatous changes occur in the breast, including idiopathic granulomatous mastitis, granulomatous reaction in association with carcinoma (56), and Wegener's granulomatosis (66,91),

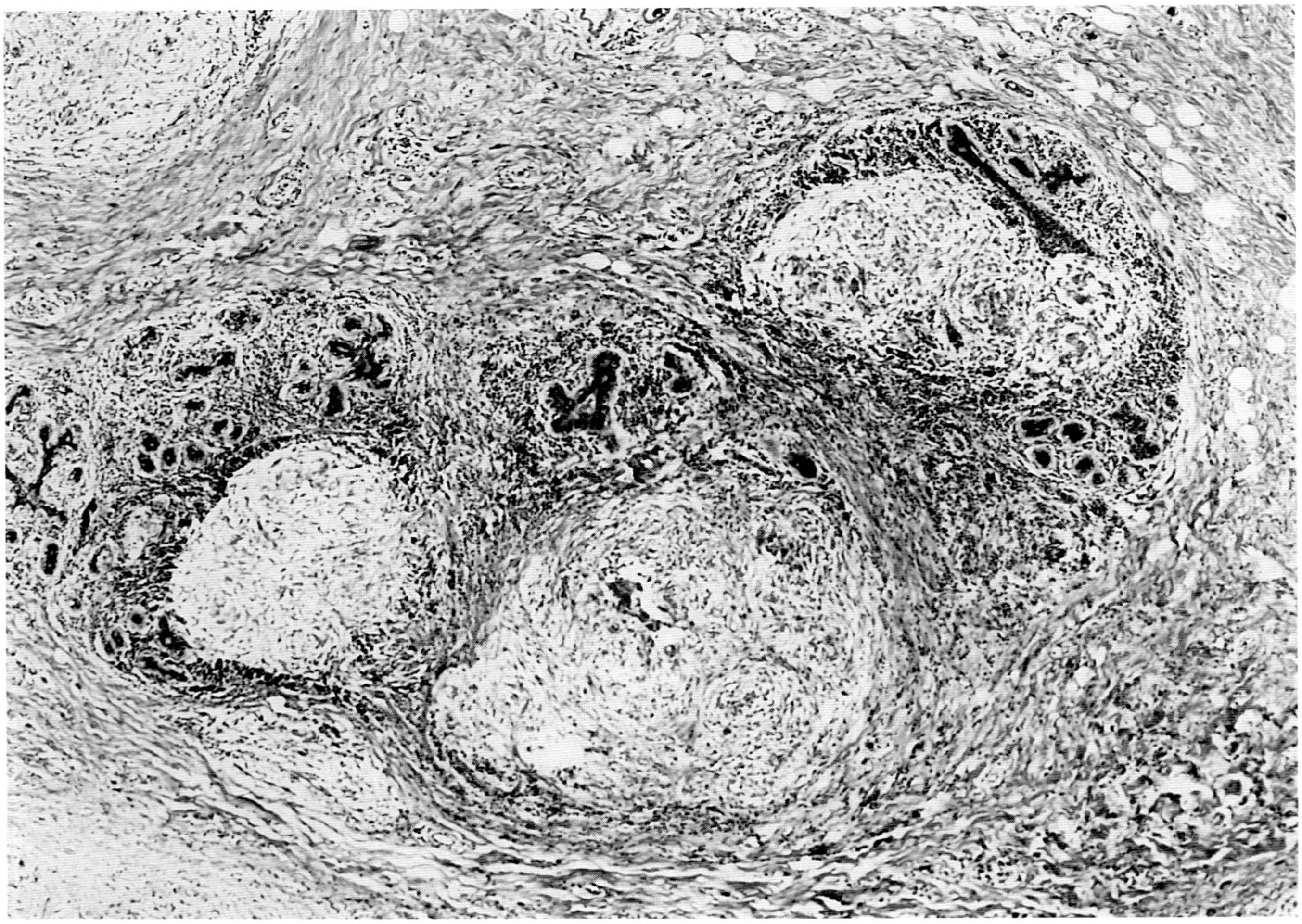

**Figure 15.19** Granulomatous mastitis, idiopathic. The granulomas involve lobules and distort them. (H&E, X75)

mammary tuberculosis is a rare disease in modern medicine and in most western countries (53,55,61,67, 77,100). It accounts for 0.025% of treated breast disease in developed countries (76). Most reports come from the African continent where approximately one case a year has been observed in major medical centers (73). The 28 cases reported by Gottschalk et al (73) occurred in women ranging in age from 20 to 64, but a majority were in their 30s and 40s. More than a third of the women were either pregnant or lactating. The lesion presented as a firm mass (18 cases) or an abscess (10 cases). Clinically, the masses were often mistaken for carcinoma. Half of the patients had axillary lymphadenopathy, though, in another report, Symmers (104) has stated that regional lymph nodes are rarely enlarged. On rare occasions, mammary tuberculosis may actually coexist with carcinoma (84).

Histologically, the granulomas display caseation and may disrupt ductal and lobular architecture (Fig. 15.20). Identification of acid-fast bacilli and preferably isolation of the organism are requisite for a diagnosis of tuberculous mastitis. Acid-fast bacilli were seen in only two of the 28 lesions reported by Gottschulk (73). By the rigid criteria of Symmers (104), which requires isolation of *Mycobacterium tuberculosis*, none of these cases are diagnostic of tuberculosis. In the presence of pulmonary or extrapulmonary tuberculosis, identification of acid-fast bacilli in the mammary lesions could be considered sufficient for a presumptive diagnosis of tuberculous mastitis.

Symmers (104) has emphasized that isolation of *M tuberculosis* is necessary for a definitive interpretation of tuberculous mastitis since a necrotizing granulomatous reaction can be produced by a variety of other conditions. Of 44 cases of caseating granulomatous mastitis initially diagnosed as tuberculous in nature in Symmers' collection, only six were considered as proven examples by isolation of *M tuberculosis*, while five were considered presumptive tuberculosis since *M tuberculosis* was not isolated, but acid-fast bacilli were present in histologic sections of

A

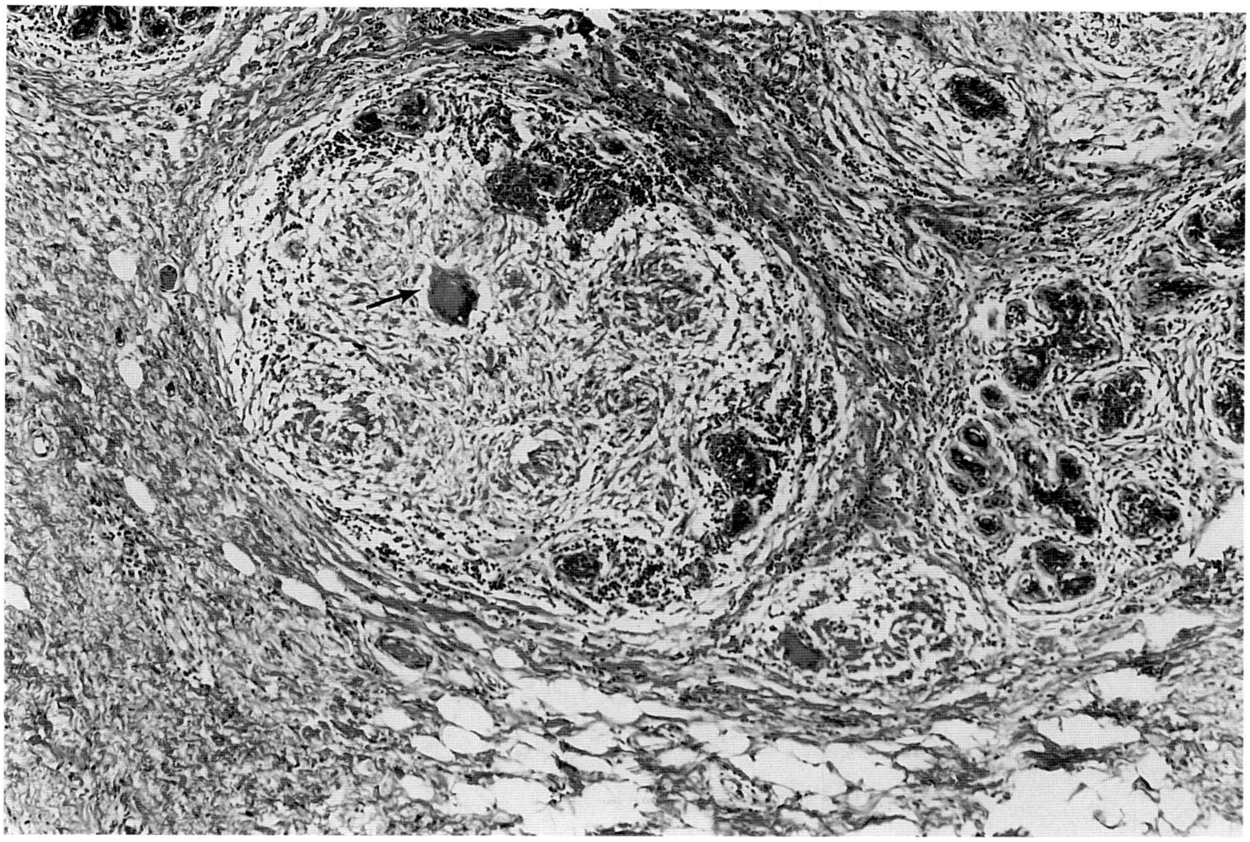

B

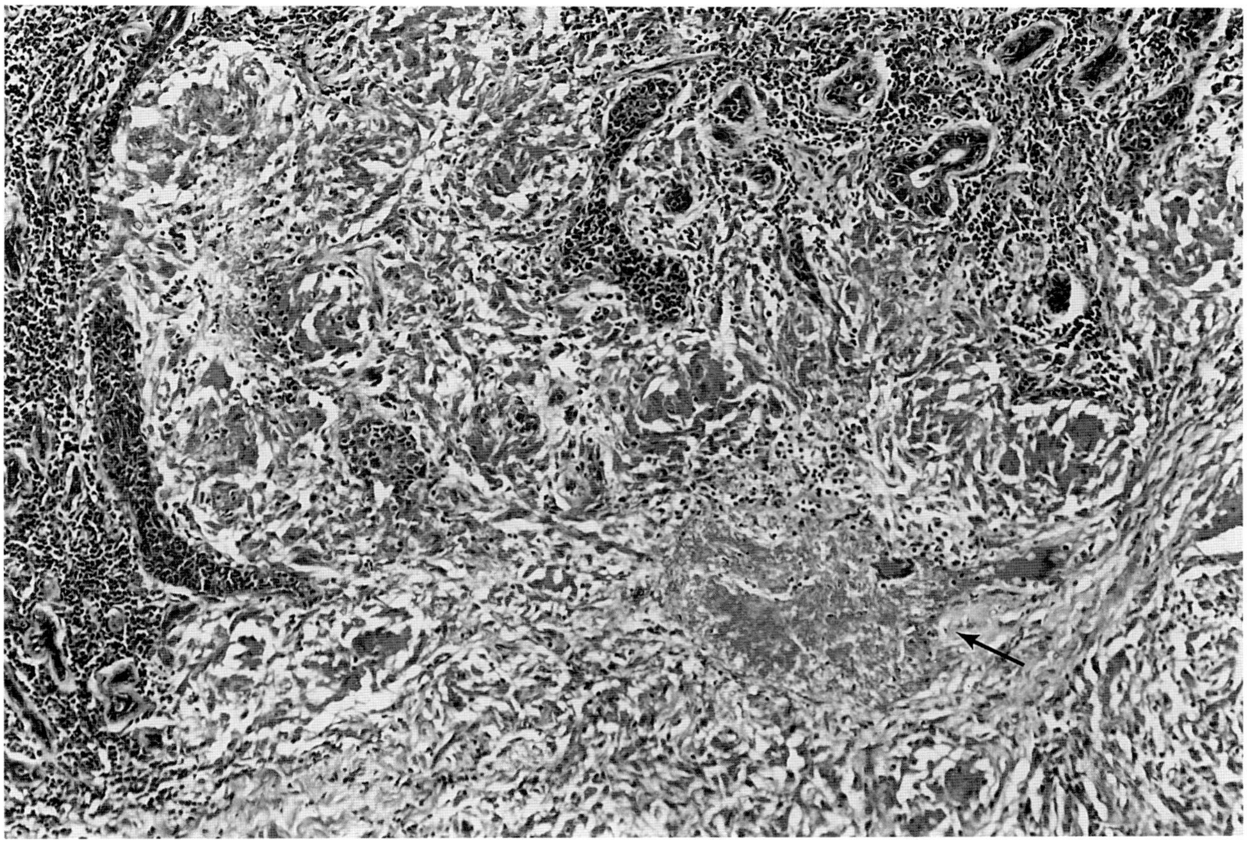

**Figure 15.20** Tuberculous mastitis. The granulomas distort lobules and display giant cells (a, arrow) and caseation (b, arrow). (H&E, (a) X100; (b) X50)

A

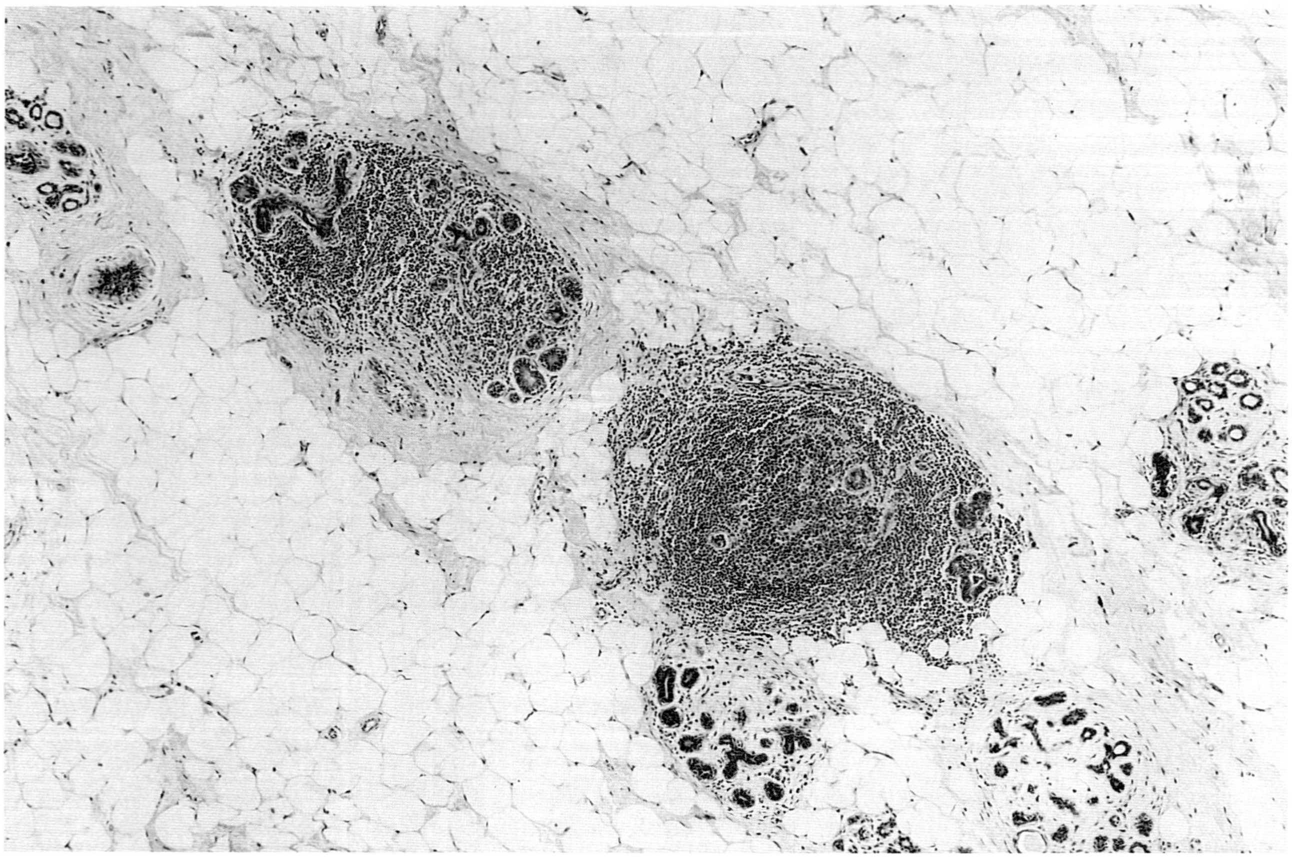

B

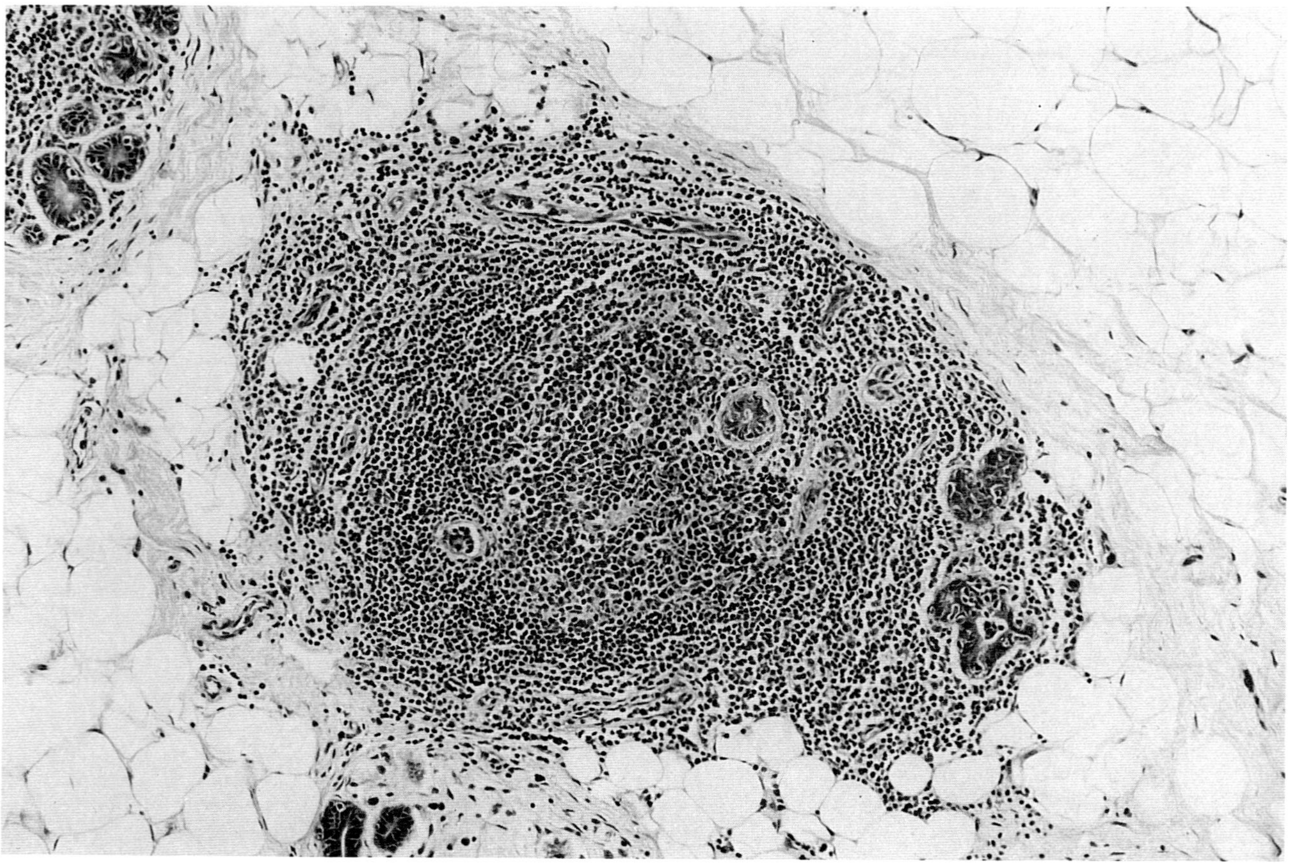

**Figure 15.21** Lymphocytic mastitis. (a) The infiltrate is predominantly lobulocentric, though it may extend to ducts and vessels. (b) The lymphocytes migrate into the epithelial lining of the ductules. (c) Less extensive infiltration is evident in some lobules. (H&E, (a) X200; (b) X400; (c) X400)

C

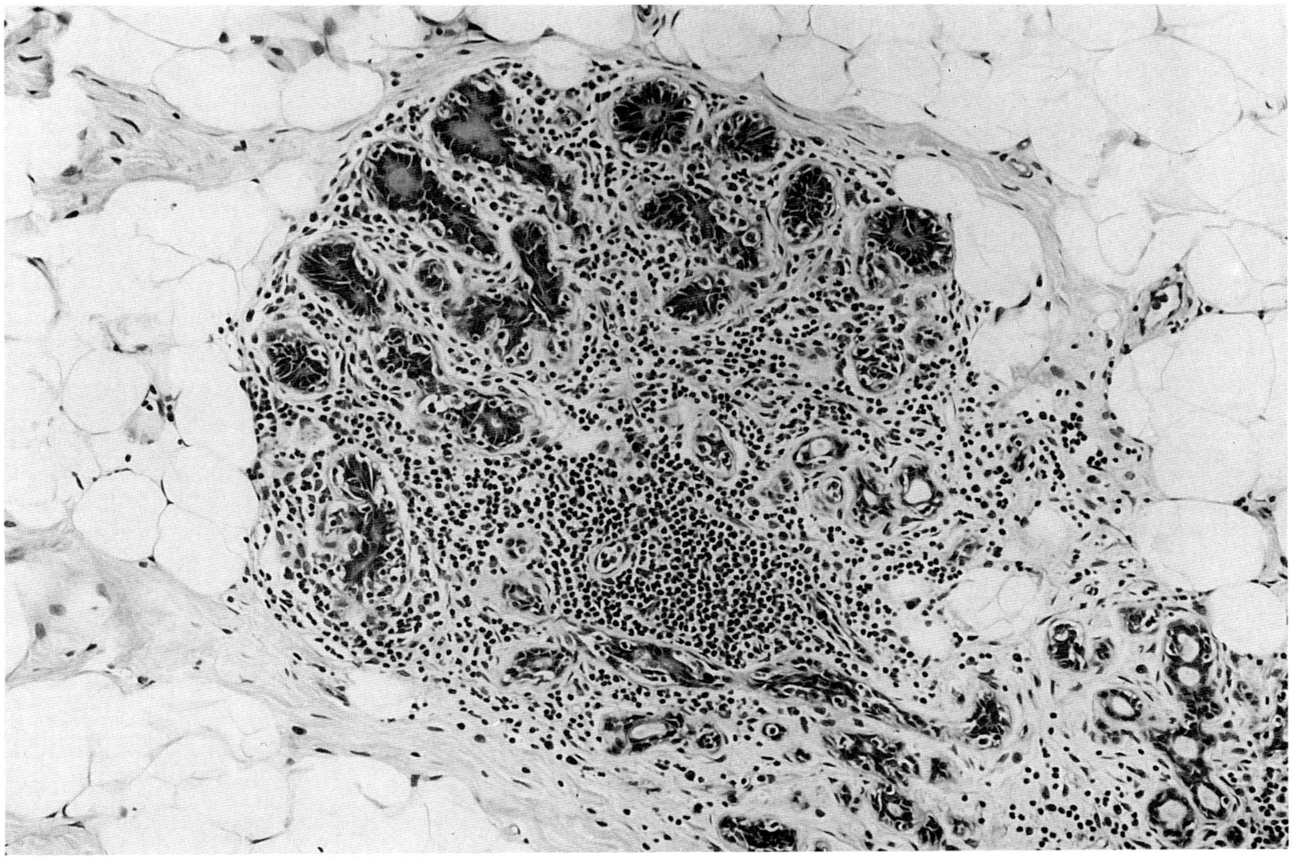

**Figure 15.21(c)** Lymphocytic mastitis. Legend on opposite page.

the lesions. Nine cases were interpreted as of uncertain cause since no acid-fast bacilli were found and the cultures yielded no pathogens. The remaining cases were due to a variety of proven infections (tularemia, syphilis, cryptococcuses, sporotrichosis, etc) and infestations (cystocercosis, hydatid cyst, *Pentosomiasis*), as well as iatrogenic (injection of soft paraffin) or endogenous (post-traumatic) complicating duct ectasia. The development of cholesterol granulomas complicating duct ectasia has been emphasized by Wilhelmus et al (110).

Both hematogenous and lymphatic spread play a role in the development of the mammary disease. Gottschalk et al (73) favored hematogenous spread from an active or occult pulmonary or other focus. Traditionally, however, retrograde lymphatic spread has been regarded as more likely with axillary nodes considered as the source of disease. Curiously, caseous lymphadenitis is rare, with only a few cases reported in the literature (84,106). Cat-scratch disease should be an important consideration as a cause of necrotizing granulomas in the axillary or intramammary lymph nodes (117).

## Lymphocytic Mastitis (Fibrous Mastopathy)

A variety of designations—fibrous mastopathy (87, 90); fibrous disease of the breast (74); fibrosis of the breast (105), fibrous tumor (94), sclerosing lymphocytyic lobulitis (81), and focal fibrous disease of the breast (97)—have been used for this clinically palpable, generally painless, ill-defined mammary lesion characterized by localized, poorly-defined areas of stromal fibrosis (collagenous sclerosis) that may obliterate the ducts and lobules in the affected region and by various degrees of lymphocytic infiltrate which occurs in women 24 to 72 years of age. The lymphocytic infiltrate may be quite intense and form follicular centers; it consists of a polyclonal B-cell population (81,101). In contrast to the periductal distribution of lymphocytes in duct ectasia and in patients with breast cancer (57), the infiltrate in lymphocytic mastitis is generally lobulocentric (Fig. 15.21), though it may involve perivascular and periductal regions as well. The infiltrate is composed predominantly of B-lymphocytes in contrast to the T-cell infiltrate in a variety of other benign and malignant breast lesions (71,81). The affected lobules may also show sclerosis and changes similar to involution. It has been proposed that the lymphocytic cell type involved in autoimmune disease starts with a T-cell infiltration as the primary event, subsequently evolving into a follicular reaction with predominance of B cells and immunoblasts (85).

While for the most part these changes have been thought to be nonspecific, several reports have noted and documented an association with thyroiditis, arthropathy, and diabetes mellitus (81,90,102) and raised the possibility of an autoimmune disease (81,101). Lammie et al (81) carefully checked for the possibility of an autoimmune pathogenesis in 13 young and middle aged women whose breast biopsies displayed these changes. The woman with the most florid lesion subsequently developed Hashimoto's thyroiditis. Three of the women were diabetic. Seven of the women were screened for circulating antibodies, one had smooth muscle antibodies, one had parietal cell antibodies, one had parietal cell and thyroid microsomal antibodies, one had the thyroid antibodies expected in Hashimoto's disease, and three had none. Thirteen of the 17 women whose HLA-status has been determined were HLA-DR3, 4, or 5 positive, either singly or in combination (81,102); HLA-DR3 and 4 are also associated with type 1 diabetes mellitus, while Hashimoto's thyroiditis is associated with HLA-DR5. It appears as if at least some of these cases may have an autoimmune etiology.

Lobular alterations in the form of sclerosis and obliteration have been described in seven of eight cases reported by Schwarz and Strachen (101). The lobule they illustrated as reflecting sclerosis (Fig. 4 of their report), however, could be interpreted as an involuting lobule; a mild degree of lymphocytic infiltrate is not uncommon in involuting lobules. Furthermore, migration of lymphocytes into the epithelial cell layer of the ducts is so common in the breast that I am not convinced that they could be interpreted as a "lymphoepithelial" complex indicative of an autoimmune process in these cases.

Haagensen (74) had seen 156 patients with "fibrous disease" of the breast between 1936 and 1972. Based on the presence of lymphocytic infiltrate of the mammary lobules and their obliteration by fibrosis, Haagensen noted that an inflammatory process is suggested, but the case histories of his patients did not support an inflammatory disease.

While the precise etiology of these changes are not known, I believe there is a subpopulation of these cases in which there is notable association between the mammary alterations and thyroid disease, diabetes, or both. At AFIP, we have collected seven examples of this subgroup from our recent files. In addition to the prominent lymphocytic infiltrate and stromal fibrosis, we also noted the presence of large epithelioid stromal cells that were dispersed as isolated cells or in clusters within the densely collagenous stroma (Fig. 15.22). The cells were so prominent in some cases that the possibility of a carcinoma had been raised by experienced pathologists. Immunostains failed to show a positive reaction for cytokeratin, however, and actually the epithelioid stromal cells contained actin-positive fibrillar material. This constellation of microscopic findings should prompt pathologists to make inquiries regarding the possibility of an autoimmune disease.

## Mycotic and Other Lesions

Though quite rare, a variety of mycotic lesions have been reported in the breast. These may present as an abscess, cyst, a mass, or asymptomatic lesions detected mammographically due to calcifications or cyst formation. The organisms include *Cryptococcus neoformans* (121), *Blastomyces dermatitidis* (112), *Histoplasma capsulatum* (89,119), and *Actinomyces* (120).

The clinical presentation and the morphologic changes induced by these organisms is highly variable. Many of them actually cause necrotizing granulomatous inflammations mimicking tuberculous mastitis (104). Others may mimic carcinoma. Symmers (121) described a 50-year-old woman who had a mastectomy in 1894 for a supposed carcinoma. The specimen had been preserved as an example of colloid carcinoma. The diagnosis was reviewed in 1955 and judged to reflect cryptococcosis; there was no evidence of carcinoma. The patient had died 37 years after her mastectomy at the age of 87 without recurrences.

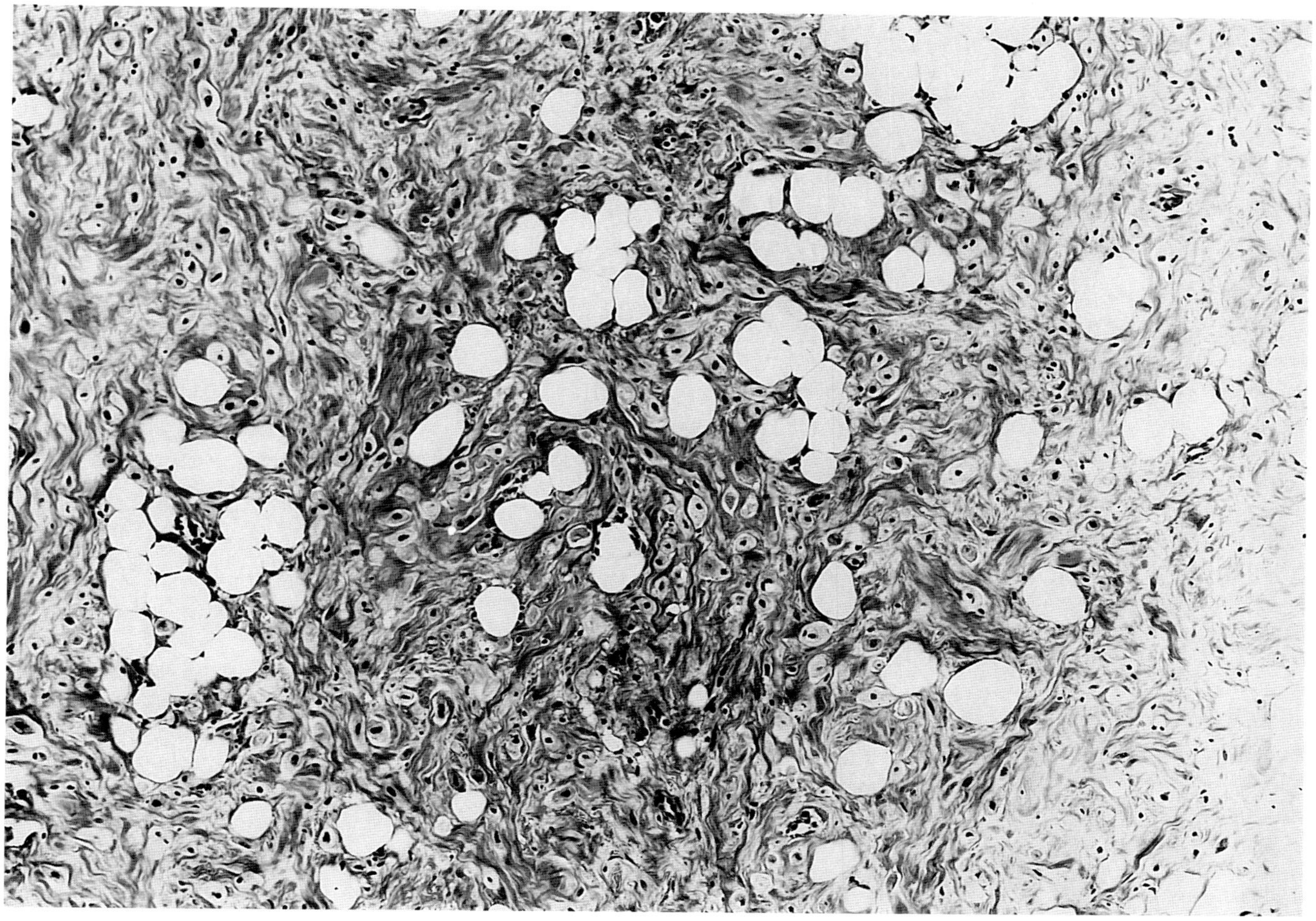

**Figure 15.22** Lymphocytic mastitis. Numerous epithelioid histiocytes infiltrate the collagenous stroma. These cells may be mistaken for infiltrating carcinoma. This patient had a history of "thyroid problems," and diabetes. (H&E, X180)

Approximately 20 examples of parasitic infections of the breast and the overlying skin are in the files of AFIP. These cases were interpreted over a 40-year period. The variety of lesions and organisms include leprosy, histoplasmosis, syphillis, cat-scratch disease (117), molluscum contagiosum, *Demodex follicularum*, and filariasis (*Wuchereria bancrofti*, etc). Filariasis was the most common lesion (12 cases); a majority of the patients with filariasis were native Africans or caucasians who had lived in Africa or Florida.

Among the cases recently reviewed at AFIP, a few were particularly noteworthy in their presentation. An oriental woman in her early 40s and a 35-year-old Filipino woman were found to have areas of microcalcification on routine mammography. The biopsy from both women showed *Schistosoma japonicum* eggs distributed in clusters within the mammary stroma, without inciting an inflammatory reaction (Fig. 15.23). In another woman, a cyst with calcifications in its wall was detected mammographically. Although the cyst was 3 cm in diameter, it could not be palpated clinically. At operation a cyst was identified and excised; a 50 cm coiled worm (*Sparganum*) completely filled the cyst. While some of the exotic parasites diagnosed at AFIP were found in oriental immigrants, others, particularly the microfilaria, are found in patients from Florida and are apparently native to certain regions of the United States.

A large number of cases of mammary microfilarial granulomas have been reported from China where filariasis is common in the eastern provinces (123). Filariasis is also common in the African continent. The *Filaria loa* can present as rows of rod-like or spiral-shaped calcification on mammography, and has been reported in caucasians who have lived in the Congo for many years (118).

Involvement of the breast by syphilis is rare and most reported cases are found in the literature prior to 1950's (113,116).

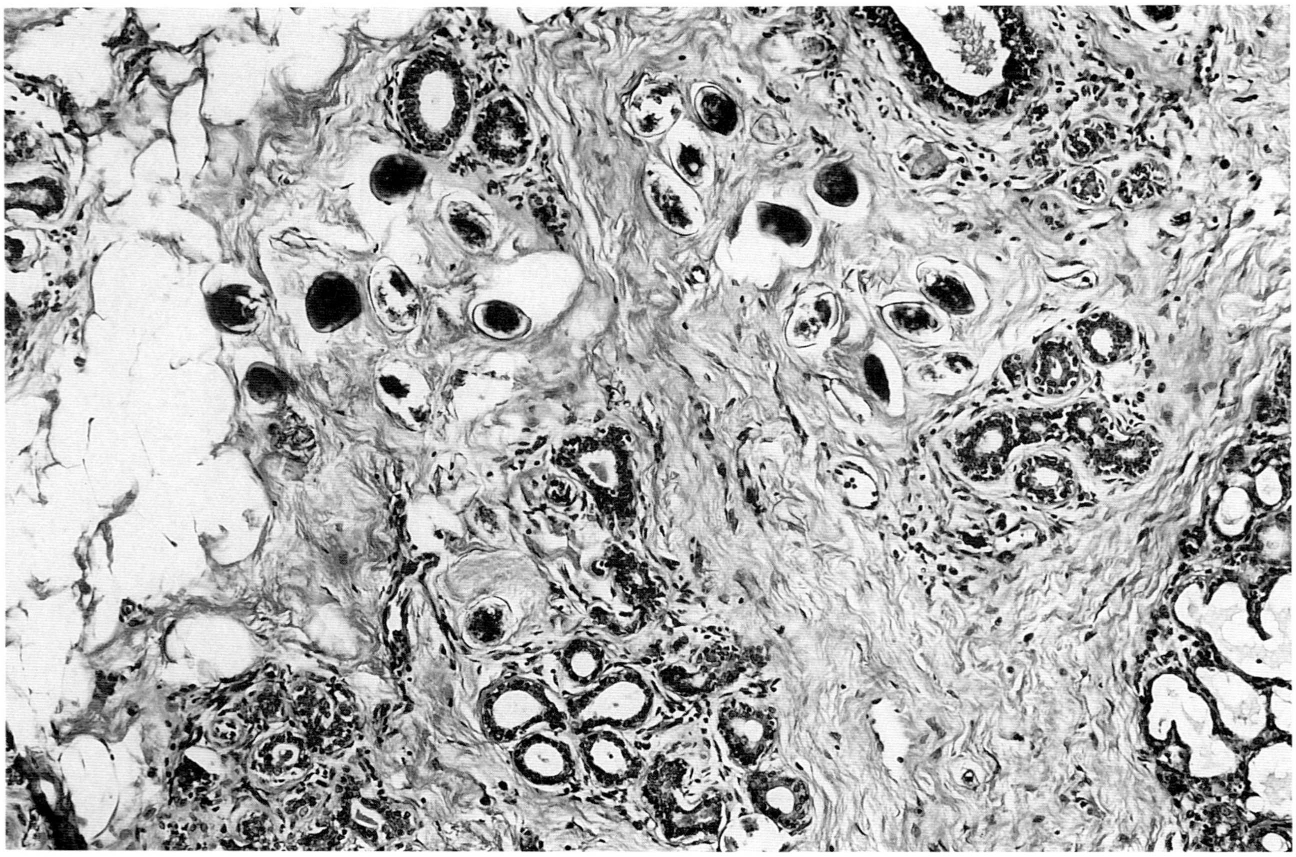

**Figure 15.23** *Schistosoma japonicum* eggs are distributed in clusters within the stroma; notice absence of any inflammatory reaction. The patient was a 35-year-old Filipino woman with microcalcifications on routine mammography. (H&E, X200)

The common skin mite, *Demodex follicularum*, has been observed with a high frequency in the hair follicles and sebaceous ducts of the nipple. Infestation by demodex is generally asymptomatic and the finding is incidental (114). Occasionally, they may be associated with chronic inflammation, but there is little or no pathologic significance to their presence.

It is important to emphasize that Liesegang rings form laminated or microspherular patterns of calcification occasionally with unusual brush borders (Fig. 15.24) that can closely mimic and are sometimes mistaken for a parasitic infestation (122).

## Eosinophilic Mastitis

Eosinophilic mastitis is characterized by an extensive eosinophilic infiltrate around ducts and lobules often admixed with plasma cells and lymphocytes. Eosinophilic mastitis is extremely rare, not associated with peripheral eosinophilia, any known systemic disease or allergic condition. It probably reflects a localized reaction to intraluminal substances that enter the surrounding stroma when a cystically dilated duct disrupts. Reaction to a parasitic infestation should be ruled out in all these lesions.

## SARCOIDOSIS

It is highly unusual for sarcoidosis to involve breast parenchyma (124,125,129,132). In most cases of mammary involvement, there is also evidence of disease elsewhere, therefore, the diagnosis is often facilitated by this information.

Few cases reported in the literature have adequate clinical and histologic documentation (125,129, 130,137,139,140). Two of these reports appear to describe the same 38-year-old patient (139,140). Some of the reported cases lack biopsy documentation of the breast involvement (133,135,141). Other reports

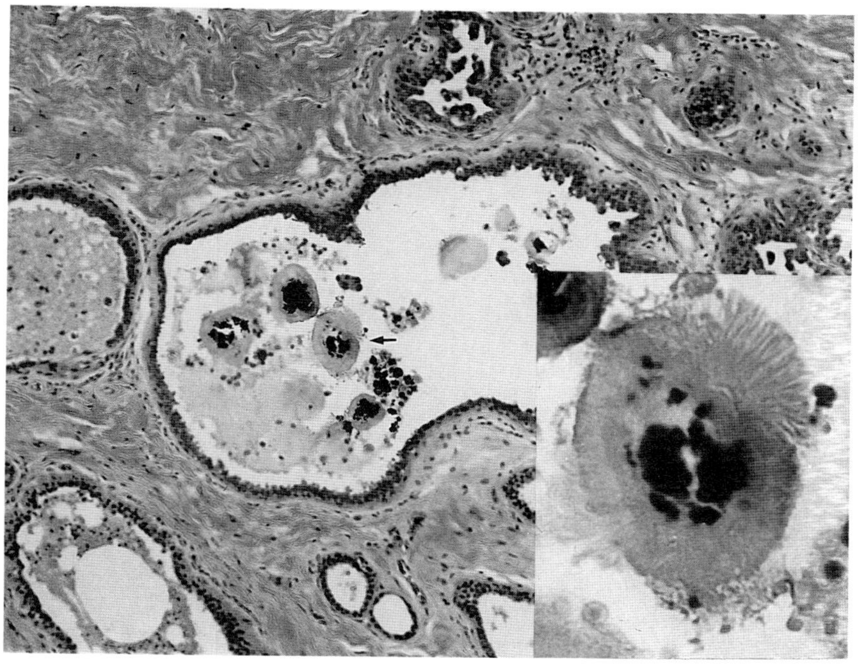

**Figure 15.24** Liesegang rings forming intraluminal calcified structures that may be mistaken for parasites. Inset shows higher magnification of the structure at the end of the arrow with cockscomb type brush borders. (H&E, X100; inset, X400)

have biopsy documentation of a granulomatous mastitis, but lack clinical or radiographic evidence of sarcoidosis elsewhere in the body, or a positive Kveim test (126,127,131,136).

Sarcoidosis may present as a solitary, multiple, or bilateral mammary nodule(s). Microscopically, the granulomas are found in the interlobular stroma, as well as in mammary lobules. The granulomas are typically noncaseating and epithelioid with multinucleated giant cells. Asteroid bodies have been identified in the giant cells.

When there is no known evidence of sarcoidosis elsewhere in the body, other types of granulomatous mastitis should be ruled out. Furthermore, since noncaseating granulomas are also seen in the late stages of duct ectasia, this differential should be kept in mind as well. In the latter, the presence of ectatic ducts in the vicinity of the granulomas is an important helpful feature. To confirm a granulomatous lesion as sarcoidosis presenting primarily in the breast, when there is no evidence of the disease elsewhere and having excluded other granulomatous mastitis, a positive Kveim test, elevated serum concentration of angiotensin converting enzyme (142), and lysozyme (134) should be obtained. If the results of all these tests are negative, the localized mammary granulomatous mastitis most probably reflects idiopathic granulomatous mastitis.

## RHEUMATOID NODULE

Rheumatoid nodule has been reported in a 32-year-old caucasian woman with a 12-year history of rheumatoid arthritis (128). It presented as a breast lump associated with cyclic breast pain and foul smelling nipple discharge.

## AMYLOID TUMOR

Amyloid tumor or amyloid deposition occurs rarely in the breast either in patients with amyloid-related illnesses (patients with long-standing arthritis, multiple myeloma, or systemic amyloidosis), or in the absence of such a clinical background (144,147–151,155,156). The lesion occurs predominantly in elderly women and can be confused with carcinoma clinically and mammographically. Amyloid tumor nodules develop in the breast occasionally along with axillary node involvement (148).

The first and one of the best-documented examples of solitary amyloid tumor of the breast presented as a 3 cm firm, moveable mass in a 62-year-old woman (146). Mammographically, a malignant tumor was suspected. Morphologically, the amyloid nature of the tumor was confirmed by special stains and at the ultrastructural level. The patient had no evidence of predisposing systemic disease.

O'Connor et al (152) suggested that amyloidosis of the breast may be more common than previously recognized. Five of 27 women with primary amyloidosis or multiple myeloma, evaluated retrospectively, were found to have amyloid deposition in their breast tissue either at the time of biopsy or in autopsy specimen. The amyloid deposition was distributed around ducts, vessels, and adipose tissue. It is not quite clear from their paper whether or not all patients had had prior breast biopsies.

Even bilateral breast involvement occurs. Bilateral amyloid tumors of the breast in the absence of a systemic disease has been described in an 82-year-old Australian woman (145). Bilateral massive amyloid infiltrates of the breast along with cutaneous nodules in the abdominal wall were reported in a 60-year-old woman in the course of long-standing rheumatoid arthritis (154).

Grossly, the lesion appears as an indurated area with a granular or waxy cut surface. Microscopically, the amyloid is deposited as a homogeneous, eosinophilic, amorphous material around ducts, lobules, vessels, and in the intervening fibrous and adipose tissue. The deposits are associated with lymphoplasmacytic infiltrate along with giant cells. Intracellular amyloid may be present within plasma cells or in giant cells. Special stain with Congo red shows an intense positivity with green birifringence when viewed under polarizing lenses.

Amyloid should be distinguished from the extensive elastosis that may accompany invasive carcinomas. Azzopardi (143) did not accept the case reported by Patil et al (153) as amyloid deposits, but interpreted the changes as elastosis.

## MASSIVE NECROSIS OF THE BREAST

Several reports have described massive necrosis of the breast as a complication of anticoagulant and coumarin therapy for thromboembolic disorders (157–159,162–165,167). Most patients with breast necrosis have been obese, middle-aged females who had onset of the mammary changes within three to five days following initiation of treatment with oral anticoagulants (161). The hemorrhagic changes usually involve areas with abundant subcutaeous adipose tissue, such as the buttocks, thighs, and breasts. The process starts with onset of pain, rapidly followed by sharply-demarcated ecchymotic discoloration. When the breasts are involved, they may become swollen with a peau d'orange appearance simulating an inflammatory carcinoma. Sometimes, the swelling is followed by development of small blisters which ulcerate. As the lesion progresses, the breast develops a purplish discoloration with dilatation of superficial veins. Clinically and mammographically, an inflammatory carcinoma is often suspected (157).

The histologic appearance of the lesion varies depending on the stage of the process. In some cases, thrombi have been identified in some of the arteries and veins within the breast and in the dermis. In a majority of cases, the breast tissue shows necrosis, interstitial hemorrhage, and various degrees of inflammatory infiltrate. In advanced stages, the breast shows hemorrhagic infarction.

Andersson et al (157) listed the various hypothesis forwarded in the literature regarding the pathogenesis of this complication. These include a toxic effect of the coumarin congeners on the vascular endothelium, arterial thrombosis, venous thrombosis, an allergic-type reaction, and protein C—a vitamin-K-dependent factor with anticoagulant effect (160)—deficiency. The swollen appearance of the breast is probably due to veno-lymphatic stasis, bleeding into the interstitium, and an inflammatory reaction.

While a majority of these cases have required mastectomy, spontaneous healing following discontinuation of Coumadin® therapy has been reported. Early recognition of the nature of changes and its relationship to the anticoagulant therapy is crucial to proper management of the patient.

Rarely, massive necrosis has also been observed in patients with diabetes (168), and in association with lactation and breast abscess (166).

## LYMPHOMA

Occasionally, the breast is the site of a localized, primary lymphoma with no evidence of concurrent widespread or preceding extramammary disease at the time of presentation or within one to six months thereafter. Cases with concurrent or subsequent ipsilateral axillary node involvement have also been accepted as primary lymphomas by some investigators, and such involvement has been observed in 48.5% of the cases (197). More commonly, the breast is involved secondarily by widespread lymphoma. The frequency of primary mammary lymphoma (PML) varies from one per 1,000 (197,211) to one per 1,300 malignant tumors of the breast (186), and has also been expressed as approximately 0.12% to 0.53% of all malignant breast tumors (185,187,202,205,210). In 1990, Hugh et al (202), recorded 257 cases of primary mammary lymphoma in the literature and added 20 cases of their own. Two subsequent reports, one by Cohen and Brooks (180) and the other by Giardini et al (197) added another 18 and 35 cases, respectively, for a total of 330 cases.

The origin of primary lymphomas in the breast is of interest. One possibility is that the cell of origin is a migratory lymphocyte, the other is that the tumors have their origin in an intramammary lymph node. Both sources may contribute to the variety of lymphomas observed in the breast. While recent reports have included breasts among mucosal-associated lymphatic tissue (MALT) sites, it is difficult to accept this concept considering the paucity of lymphocytes in the breast, unless the cellular infiltrate identified as a response to normal "wear and tear" in different tissues is considered sufficient basis for considering that tissue as part of the MALT system. There is no native lymphoid tissue of the type found in the tonsils, ileum, etc, in the breast. As in any other organ, however, lymphocytes and macrophages do migrate into the mammary stroma and the epithelial layers of the duct system, particularly during postpartum involution; some of these cells may remain in the region for a long time. The migration of lymphocytes and macrophages to the breast during gestation, lactation, and the postpartum state is not, in my opinion, a reflection of dependency on sex hormones, but rather a response to the accelerated cellular turnover, involutional changes, and resorption of the secretory material that take place during gestation and lactation. Ferguson found lymphocytes within the epithelial cell layers of the duct system in breast biopsies and concluded that lymphocytes are a normal component of the mammary duct system (189). It is noteworthy that the samples examined by Ferguson (189) cannot be considered as normal "resting" breast if the women who were biopsied had a clinically palpable lesion or a fibroadenoma. On the other hand, the lining cells of the duct system do undergo physiologic cyclic changes during the reproductive years. It is, therefore, not unusual to observe lymphocytes and macrophages infiltrating the duct wall. Also considering the frequency of fibrocystic changes in the female breasts, various types of cellular infiltrates are not uncommon. Another point worthy of consideration is that the ductal epithelium of the breast is not generally considered a mucosal lining. Therefore, it seems more appropriate to consider primary mammary lymphoma as an extranodal lymphoma if one can ascertain that the lesion did not originate in the intramammary lymph node.

A more likely source of primary lymphoma in the breast is the intramammary lymph node. A variety of reactive lesions are observed in the intramammary nodes. While the nodal configuration and capsule of these small lymph nodes may be retained in some lymphomas, others may totally efface the nodal architecture and infiltrate into the surrounding tissue making recognition of a nodal origin impossible.

## *Clinical Features*

Patients with primary mammary lymphoma range in age from 9 to 88 years, with a median of around 50 years. There is a bimodal age distribution curve with a younger group having a mode of 38 years and an older population with a mode of 58 years (202). Adair and Herrmann (170) subdivided mammary lymphomas into a unilateral type which has an age distribution similar to that of primary breast carcinoma, and the bilateral, diffuse type which occurs in younger puerperal women. After analyzing the available information on 257 cases reported in the literature and their own 20 cases, Hugh et al (202) found that a majority of the patients (84%) present with a unilateral mass. A bilateral diffuse variety is rarely reported in North America, with a majority of cases reported in Italian and African literature (202). The latter type affects pregnant or lactating women who present with bilateral enlargement of the breasts followed by rapid dissemination of the disease with notable ovarian and central nervous system (CNS) involvement. Metachronous involvement of the contralateral breast has been reported rarely as a pattern of recurrence (193,205,237). Among women with non-Hodgkin's lymphoma, approximately 7% have metachronous involvement of the contralateral breast, while 10% to 13% have synchronous bilateral disease (173,197).

There appears to be a preponderance of right-sided lesions (180,185,205,230,237).

Clinical symptomatology is highly variable. Most patients complain of pain. About 10% of the patients may have night sweats, fever, and weight loss. Occasionally multiple nodules may be present within the breast. These nodules can cause overlying skin changes similar to those associated with carcinoma. About 30% to 40% of patients with primary mammary lymphoma will have axillary node involvement (199).

Approximately 350 cases of primary and secondary mammary lymphoma were diagnosed at AFIP between 1970 to 1988. About 5% of these cases occurred in male patients. Approximately, half of these had been diagnosed prior to the use of immunohistochemical studies at AFIP. These cases require thorough evaluation to determine the clinical and morphologic features of the primary and secondary lesions.

Mammographically, lymphomas form relatively circumscribed masses, focal or diffuse thickening and densities, and discrete nodules with irregular margins; typically, they lack calcification and retraction (217).

### *Pathologic Features*

Grossly, the tumors range in size from 1 cm to 20 cm, but a majority are around 2 to 3 cm in maximum diameter. The lesions are well-circumscribed, fleshy, and composed of white or gray to tan tissue.

Both non-Hodgkin's and Hodgkin's lymphoma occur in the breast, but the latter is quite infrequent (169,181,198,208,214,231). One of the earliest reports of Hodgkin's disease involving the breast has been attributed to Kuchens who published an example of mammary Hodgkin's disease in the German literature in 1928 (214). A large number of the reports have appeared in the literature prior to 1966 and the introduction of the Lukes-Butler classification scheme. A majority of the cases of Hodgkin's disease occurring in the breast as a primary or secondary tumor have been of the nodular sclerosing type (214). It is believed that the mammary lesion may be due to the involvement of intramammary or internal mammary lymph nodes with extension into the surrounding tissue.

The classification of non-Hodgkin's lymphomas in the breast is similar to that of primary nodal lymphomas. A high proportion of mammary lymphomas occurring in young women who are pregnant or lactating correspond to a Burkitt's type lymphoma (202,226). In the series reported by Cohen and Brooks (180), ten of the 18 primary mammary lymphomas were of the diffuse large cell type, and no specific histologic feature that would distinguish a primary tumor from a secondary one was found. Of 14 cases evaluated immunohistochemically by Cohen and Brooks (180), 13 were of B-cell origin, while one was of T-cell origin. Twelve of the B-cell lymphomas displayed IgM heavy chain reactivity, while only one had IgA reactivity. It is noteworthy that a majority of the secondary lymphomas involving the breast in Cohen's series were also B-cell lymphomas.

The neoplastic cells generally form a mass which may display variable degrees of marginal irregularity or may actually appear well circumscribed. The infiltrating margin often incorporates ducts and lobules into the tumor. The malignant cells migrate into the duct wall and the epithelial cell layers; this feature is observed in benign infiltrates as well, however.

### *Hormone Receptors*

Estrogen and progesterone receptor assays performed on two cases of B-cell lymphoma in Hugh et al's (202) series were both positive. Estrogen receptor activity has also been observed in Hodgkins disease of the breast (231).

### *Differential Diagnosis*

Primary mammary lymphoma should be distinguished from pseudolymphoma (191,209,213), and poorly-differentiated carcinoma, particularly when the latter is poorly fixed. Pseudolymphoma has a mixed cell population that includes plasma cells and histiocytes, a feature that is absent in lymphomas. While pseudolymphomas are characterized by the presence of reactive follicles and germinal centers, this feature is also observed in follicular center cell lymphomas and may not be very helpful in distinguishing the two processes. Cell suspension of a case of pseudolymphoma evaluated for surface markers showed an equal admixture of B and T cells, as well as kappa and lambda light chains in the B cells (191). Distinction from poorly-differentiated carcinoma can be quite difficult; the use of immunostains for cytokeratin and lymphocyte markers are quite valuable in this regard. Clinically, bilaterality has been mentioned occasionally as a feature that would favor lymphoma (175,210,224,227,235,237,238).

### *Behavior and Therapy*

Some investigators have concluded that mammary lymphomas have a poor prognosis (206,216,235). Others, however, feel that when the lymphoma is confined to the breast, it has a prognosis comparable to other localized extranodal lymphomas (175,187, 228). While in the past, radical surgery followed by radiation therapy was advocated (185), more recently, radiotherapy has been used effectively for control of local disease following limited surgery for diagnosis and staging (184). In the series reported from Italy (197), the best results were achieved with combination chemotherapy as primary therapy after debulking surgery with or without regional radiation therapy.

Local recurrences develop in about half of the patients with primary mammary lymphoma, with a tendency for recurrence in other extranodal sites (180).

The survival of patients depends on the stage of the disease at the time of presentation and histologic type of the tumor. The survival of patients treated by biopsy or wedge resection and radiation therapy often with chemotherapy was 49% at five years (210). The five-year survival for the 14 patients in DeCosse et al's study (185) was 64% and it dropped to 54% at ten years. In Schouten et al's study (224) 46% of the patients were free of disease from 11 to 48 months after treatment which included chemotherapy in advanced disease. In the Italian series (197), the overall five-year survival for stages I and II was 43%.

The lymphoblastic type of lymphoma has a tendency to disseminate rapidly and progress to leukemia. Therefore, aggressive chemotherapy has been advocated for this variant (177).

## Atypical Lymphocytic Infiltrate

Occasionally, an unusual amount or pattern of lymphocytic infiltrate is observed in the breast. The infiltrate does not produce a distinct aggregate of pure lymphocytic cells as is generally observed in lymphomas. Rather the infiltrate is closely associated with ducts or lobules, and sometimes it actually appears within areas of adenosis or adenomas (Fig. 15.25). The infiltrate is often composed of lymphocytes and plasma cells. Some of the cells may actually display atypicality. The cell population is polyclonal, however. Often immunostains for monoclonal antibodies are necessary to exclude a diagnosis of malignant lymphoma.

It has not been established whether these lesions may progress to lymphoma locally or systemically.

## Plasmacytoma

Extramedullary plasmacytoma is extremely rare in the breast with less than five cases reported in the literature (182,204,212,219). In the first case reported by Cutler (182), a 39-year-old woman developed multiple recurrences in the same breast, as well as lesions in the lymph nodes, shoulder, and larynx one year following the initial diagnosis of the breast lesion. Plasmacytoma of the breast has also been reported as an unusual presentation of myeloma (174,221,222). Proctor et al (219) and Merino (212) have each described an example of extramedullary plasmacytoma in patients who have remained disease free without progression to multiple myeloma 46 months and nine years, respectively, following the diagnosis of their mammary lesions. The possibility remains that with longer follow-up either one of these patients may develop systemic disease.

Microscopically, mammary plasmacytoma is characterized by proliferation of plasma cells in sheets without an admixture of inflammatory cells and histiocytes. Mitotic figures, atypia, and binucleated cells occur.

Plasmacytomas have been treated by surgery, radiation therapy, and chemotherapy. Follow-up of the patients with serologic and immunologic studies is necessary for early detection of progression to a systemic disease.

## Sinus Histiocytosis with Massive Lymphadenopathy (SHML, Rosai-Dorfman Disease)

A well-defined clinicopathologic entity with a predilection for children, sinus histiocytosis with massive lymphadenopathy (SHML) may present at any time throughout life. About 30% of patients have extranodal manifestations. Two examples of SHML have

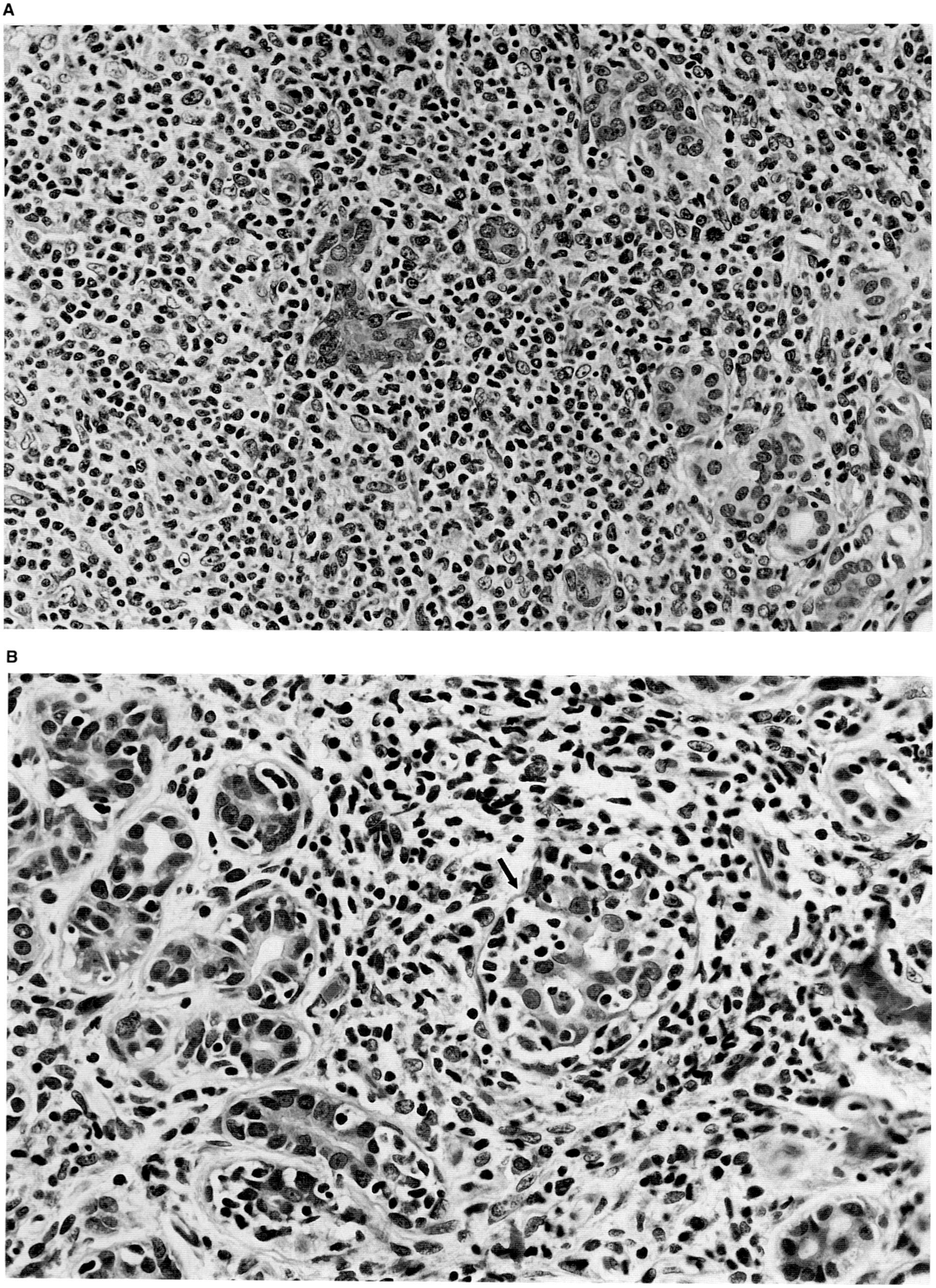


**Figure 15.25** Atypical lymphocytic infiltrate. The patient was a 72-year-old woman with a breast mass which was composed of an adenomatous aggregate of tubules. (a) Within the stroma of this nodule, a massive cellular infiltrate composed of lymphocytes and plasma cells separates the tubules. (b) The lymphocytic cells migrate into the epithelial lining of the tubules, sometimes completely distorting them. The cell population was polyclonal. (H&E, (a) X480; (b) X600)

A

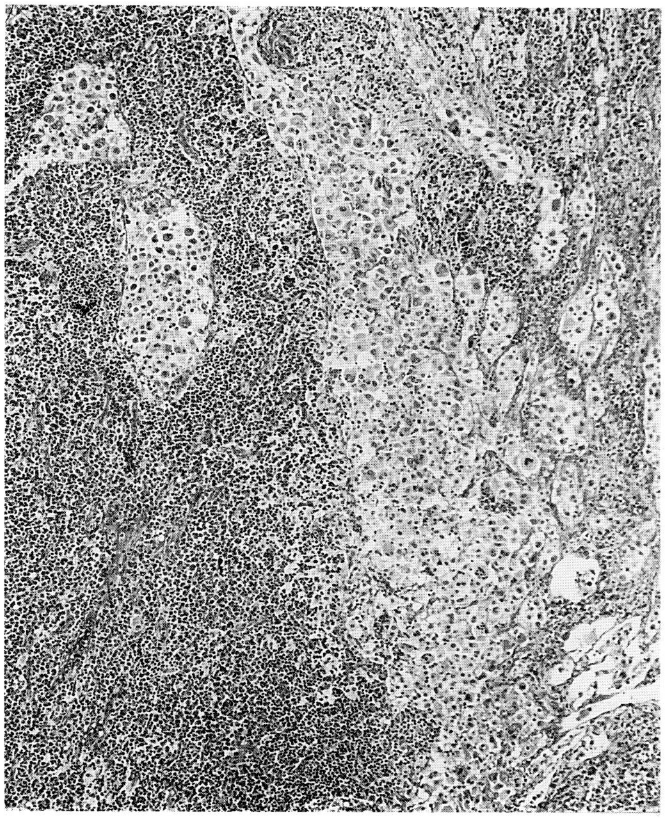

**Figure 15.26** Sinus histiocytosis with massive lymphadenopathy. (a) An intramammary lymph node from a 49-year-old woman showed distended sinuses filled by large histiocytes. (b) Phagocytosis of the lymphocytes by the histiocytic cells (arrows). (H&E, (a) X75; (b) X480)

B

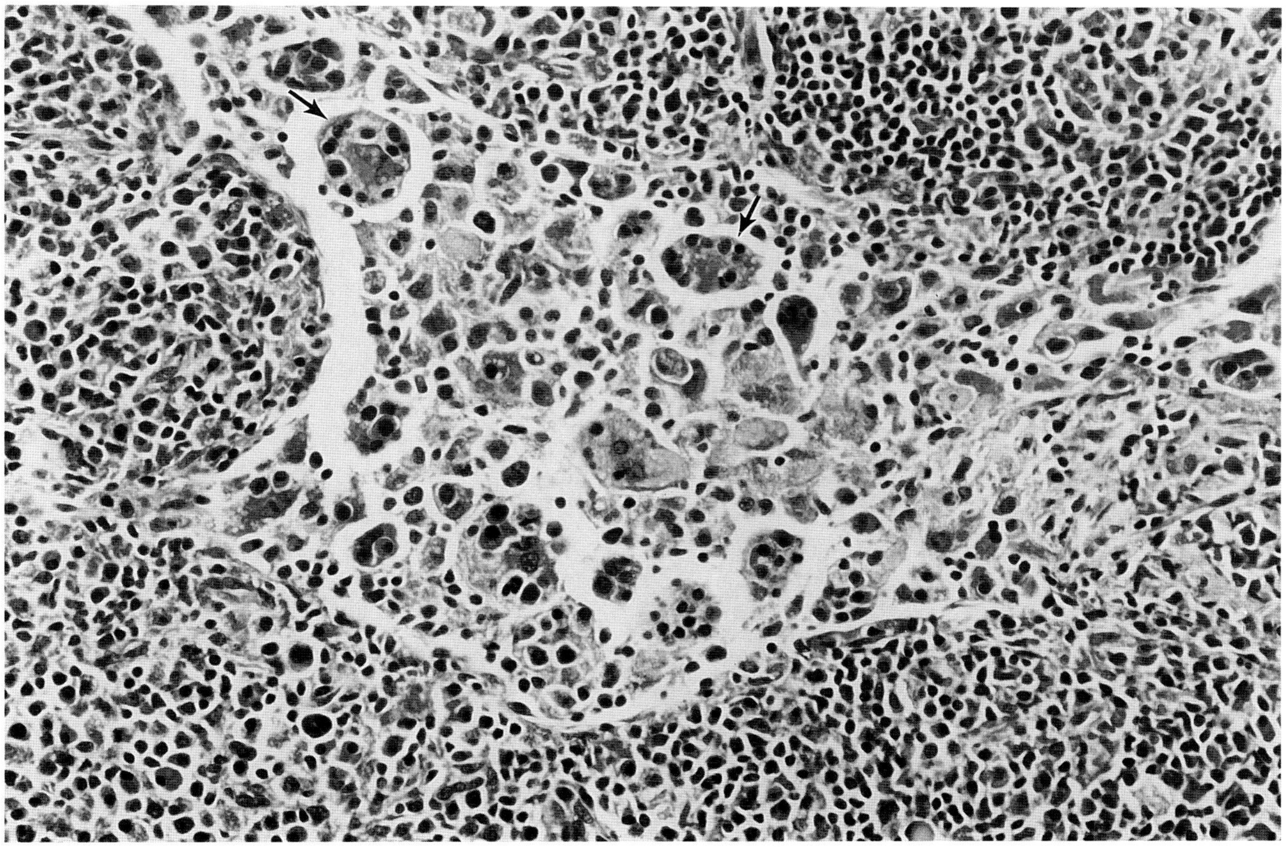

been reported in the breast (192). Both patients were young black women with a mean age of 22; one had involvement of the parotid gland and central nervous system (CNS) as well.

One example of mammary SHML has been diagnosed at AFIP (Fig. 15.26). This case occurred in a 49-year-old caucasian woman who presented with a lump in her breast. She had no palpable lymphadenopathy. Her clinical history indicated splenectomy following trauma and a six-year history of systemic lupus erythematosis. Grossly, the lesion appeared as a 2 cm well-circumscribed, brown-tan, fleshy nodule.

Microscopically, the lesion involved an intramammary lymph node. The sinuses were distended and filled with large histiocytes displaying abundant pink cytoplasm and phagocytized lymphocytes; there was also associated plasmacytosis. Immunostains for S-100 protein showed a strikingly positive reaction in the histiocytes and the plasma cell population was polyclonal confirming the diagnosis of SHML.

## LEUKEMIA

While there are many reports of leukemia induced in patients following radiation or chemotherapy for breast carcinoma (183,190,196), breast involvement by leukemia is not very common and occurs more often in acute leukemias. Breast nodules reflected the initial site of relapse in two children with acute monoblastic leukemia (236). Not infrequently, the lesion presents as bilateral mammary nodules.

## Chloroma (Granulocytic Sarcoma)

Several examples of granulocytic sarcoma have been reported in the breast (178,179,195,218,225,229). Ten examples of granulocytic sarcoma were diagnosed at AFIP between 1970 and 1992. Patients with granulocytic sarcoma range in age from 34 to 56 years.

The tumor generally presents as a unilateral breast mass either without any evidence of systemic disease, or coincident with the development of acute myelogenous leukemia (229). Bilateral metachronous tumors have been reported (195).

Grossly, chloroma has a green color and either presents as a well-circumscribed nodule or an infiltrating mass.

Microscopically, it is characterized by cells with granular eosinophilic cytoplasm. The cells show a positive reaction for esterase. Immunohistochemically, the cells display intracytoplasmic lysozyme (218).

Most patients progress to the development of systemic disease shortly after diagnosis of the breast lesion. The treatment of these tumors is controversial and includes a suggestion to use anti-leukemic drug combinations (179).

## REFERENCES

### Myoepithelial Lesions


1. Ahmed A: The myoepithelium in human breast carcinoma. *J Pathol* 1974;112:121–135.
2. Azzopardi JG: *Problems in Breast Pathology*. Philadelphia, WB Saunders Co, 1979, pp 339–340.
3. * Baup H, de Brux J: La cellule myo-epithelial. *Contracept Fertil Sex* 1991;19:39–44.
4. Bigotti G, DiGiorgio G: Myoepithelioma of the breast: Histologic, immunologic, and electronmicroscopic appearance. *J Surg Oncol* 1986;32:58–64.
5. Bussolati G, Micca B, Eusebi V, et al: Myoepithelial cells in lobular carcinoma in situ of the breast: A parallel immunocytochemical and ultrastructural study. *Ultrastruct Pathol* 1981;2:219–230.
6. * Cameron HM, Hamperl H, Warambo W: Leiomyosarcoma of the breast originating from myothelium (myoepithelium). *J Pathol* 1974;114:263–269.
7. * Cartagena N, Cabello-Inchausti B, Willis I, et al: Clear cell myoepithelial neoplasm of the breast. *Hum Pathol* 1988;19:1239–1243.
8. Caselitz J, Walther B, Wustrow J, et al: A monoclonal antibody that detects myoepithelial cells in exocrine glands, basal cells in other epithelia and basal and suprabasal cells in certain hyperplastic tissues. *Virchows Archiv A* 1986;409:725–738.
9. * Corio RL, Schiubba JJ, Brannon RB, et al: Epithelial-myoepithelial carcinoma of intercalated duct origin. A clinicopathologic and ultrastructural assessment of sixteen cases. *Oral Surg* 1982;53:280–287.
10. Crissman JD, Wirman JA, Harris A: Malignant myoepithelioma of the parotid gland. *Cancer* 1977;40:3042–3049.
11. * Dardick I, Thomas MJ, Van Nostrand AWP: Myoepithelioma—New concepts of histology and classification: A light and electron microscopic study. *Ultrastruct Pathol* 1989;13:187–224.
12. * Erlandson RA, Rosen PP: Infiltrating myoepithelioma of the breast. *Am J Surg Pathol* 1982;6:785–793.
13. * Eusebi V, Casadei GP, Bussolati G, et al: Adenomyoepi-

thelioma of the breast with a distinctive type of apocrine adenosis. *Histopathology* 1987;11:305–315.

14. Eusebi V, Lamovec J, Cattani MG, et al: Acantholytic variant of squamous-cell carcinoma of the breast. *Am J Surg Pathol* 1986;10:855–861.
15. Franke WW, Schmid E, Freudenstein C, et al: Intermediate-sized filaments of the prekeratin type in myoepithelial cells. *J Cell Biol* 1980;84:633–654.
16. Gerald W, Sussman J, True L: Actin-positive myoepitholial cells characterize breast disease. *Lab Invest* 1987;56:27A.
17. Gersell DJ, Katzenstein AA: A spindle cell carcinoma of the breast. *Hum Pathol* 1981;12:550–560.
18. Gould VE, Jao W, Battifora H: Ultrastructural analysis in the differential diagnosis of breast tumors. *Path Res Pract* 1980;167:45–70.
* 19. Hamperl H: The myothelia (myoepithelial cells): Normal state, regressive changes, hyperplasia, tumors. *Curr Top Pathol* 1970;53:194–198.
* 20. Jabi M, Dardick I, Cardigos N: Adenomyoepithelioma of the breast. *Arch Pathol Lab Med* 1988;112:73–76.
21. Joshi K, Smith JA, Perusinghe N, et al: Cell proliferation in the human mammary epithelium. Differential contribution by epithelial and myoepithelial cells. *Am J Pathol* 1986;124: 199–206.
* 22. Kermarec J, Plouvier S, Duplay H, et al: Tumeur mammaire a cellules myoepitheliales. *Arch Anat Pathol* 1973;21: 225–231.
* 23. Kiaer H, Nielsen B, Paulsen S, et al: Adenomyoepithelial adenosis and low-grade malignant adenomyoepithelioma of the breast. *Virchows Archiv (Pathol Anat)* 1984;405:55–67.
* 24. Kuzma JF: Myoepithelial proliferation in the human breast. *Am J Pathol* 1943;19:473–489.
25. Makek M, von Hochstetter AR: Pleomorphic adenoma of the human breast. *J Surg Oncol* 1980;114:281–286.
26. Medina A, Uehlinger K: Das Pleomorphe Adenom der Mamma. *Helv Chir Acta* 1980;47:205–208.
* 27. Murad TM, von Haam E: Ultrastructure of myoepithelial cells in human mammary gland tumour. *Cancer* 1968;21: 1137–1149.
28. Nabert C, Kermanch G, Saout J: Epithelioma a stroma remanie ou tumeur mixte du sein. A propos s'une observation. *J Sci Med Lille* 1969;86:507–510.
29. Nakazato Y, Ishida Y, Takahashi K, et al: Immunohistochemical distribution of S-100 protein and glial fibrillary acidic protein in normal and neoplastic salivary glands. *Virchows Arch A* 1985;405:299–310.
* 30. Ohtani H, Sasano N: Myofibroblasts and myoepithelial cells in human breast carcinoma. *Virchows Arch Pathol Anat Histol (A)* 1980;385:247–261.
* 31. Rode L, Nesland JM, Johannessen JV: Case 6: A spindle cell breast lesion in a 54-year-old woman. *Ultrastruct Pathol* 1986;10:421–425.
* 32. Rosen PP: Adenomyoepithelioma of the breast. *Hum Pathol* 1987;18:421–425.
33. Rettino A, Wilson K: Osseous, cartilaginous and mixed tumors of the human breast. A review of the literature. *Arch Surg* 1945;50:184–193.
34. Saez A, Serrano T, Azpeitia D, et al: Adenomyoepithelioma of the breast. A report of two cases. *Arch Pathol Lab Med* 1992;116:36–38.
* 35. Schurch W, Potvin C, Seemayer TA: Malignant myoepithelioma (myoepithelial carcinoma) of the breast: An ultrastructural and immunohistochemical study. *Ultrastruct Pathol* 1985;8:1–11.
* 36. Sciubba JJ, Brannon RB: Myoepithelioma of salivary glands: report of 23 cases. *Cancer* 1982;49:562–572.
37. Sciubba JJ, Goldstein BH: Myoepithelioma. Review of the literature and report of a case with ultrastructural confirmation. *Oral Surg* 1976;42:328–338.
38. Sheth MT, Hathway D, Petrelli M: Pleomorphic adenoma ("mixed" tumor) of human breast mimicking carcinoma clinico-radiologically. *Cancer* 1978;41:659–665.
39. Stead RH, Qizilbash AH, Kontozouglu T, et al: An immunohistochemical study of pleomorphic adenomas of the salivary gland. Glial fibrillary acidic protein-like immunoreactivity identifies a major myoepithelial component. *Hum Pathol* 1988;19:32–40.
* 40. Sugano I, Nagao K, Matsuzaki O, et al: Immunohistochemical studies on myoepithelial changes in breast tumors. *Acta Pathol Jpn* 1981;31:35–44.
* 41. Tavassoli FA: Myoepithelial lesions of the breast. Myoepitheliosis, adenomyoepithelioma, and myoepithelial carcinoma. *Am J Surg Pathol* 1991;15:554–568.
* 42. Thorner PS, Kahn HJ, Baumal R, et al: Malignant myoepithelioma of the breast. An immunohistochemical study by light and electron microscopy. *Cancer* 1986;57:745–750.
* 43. Toth J: Benign human mammary myoepithelioma. *Virchows Arch (Pathol Anat)* 1977;374:263–269.
44. van der Walt JD, Rohlova B: Pleomorphic adenoma of the human breast: A report of a benign tumour closely mimicking a carcinoma clinically. *Clin Oncol* 1982;8:361–365.
45. Wargotz ES, Deos PH, Norris HJ: Metaplastic carcinomas of the breast. II. Spindle cell carcinomas. *Hum Pathol* 1989;20:732–740.
* 46. Weidner N, Levine JD: Spindle-cell adenomyoepithelioma of the breast. A microscopic, ultrastructural, and immunohistochemical study. *Cancer* 1988;62:1561–1567.
47. Willen R, Uvelius B, Cameron R: Pleomorphic adenoma in the breast of a human female. *Acta Chir Scand* 1986;152:709–713.
48. Williams RW, Leach WB: Mixed tumor of the female breast of unusual duration and size. *South Med J* 1975;68:97–100.
49. Wargotz ES, Norris HJ, Austin RM, et al: Fibromatosis of the breast. A clinical and pathological study of 28 cases. *Am J Surg Pathol* 1987;11:38–45.
* 50. Young RH, Clement PB: Adenomyoepithelioma of the breast: A report of three cases and review of the literature. *Am J Clin Pathol* 1988;89:308–314.
* 51. Zarbo RJ, Oberman HA: Cellular adenomyoepithelioma of the breast. *Am J Surg Pathol* 1983;7:863–870.

## Mastitis and Mastopathy


* 52. Adair FE: Plasma cell mastitis—a lesion simulating mammary carcinoma. A clinical and pathologic study with a report of 10 cases. *Arch Surg* 1933;26:735–749.
53. Alagaratnam TT, Ong GB: Tuberculous disease of the breast. *Br J Surg* 1980;67:125–126.
54. Axelsen RA, Reasbeck P: Granulomatous lobular mastitis: Report of a case with previously undescribed histopathological abnormalities. *Pathology* 1988;20:383–389.
55. Banerjee A, Green B, Burke M: Tuberculous and granulomatous mastitis. *Practitioner* 1989;233:754, 756–757.
* 56. Bassler R, Birke F: Histopathology of tumour associated sarcoid-like stromal reaction in breast cancer. An Analysis of 5 cases with immunohistochemical investigations. *Virchows Arch (A)* 1988;412:231–239.
57. Black MM, Speer FD: Periductal lymphoid infiltrations in mammary tissue. *Arch Pathol* 1955;60:57–91.
58. Brown KL, Tang PHL: Postlactational tumoral granulomatous mastitis: A localised immune phenomenon. *Am J Surg* 1979;138:326–329.
59. Carmalt HL, Ramsey-Stewart G: Granulomatous mastitis. *Med J Aust* 1981;1:356–359.
60. Cohen C: Granulomatous mastitis: A review of 5 cases. *S Afr J Med* 1977;52:14–16.
* 61. Cohen C: Tuberculous mastitis. A review of 34 cases. *S Afr Med J* 1977;52:12–14.
62. Cutler M: Plasma-cell mastitis. Report of a case with bilateral involvement. *Br Med J* 1949;1:94–96.
63. Dalmark G: Lymphogranulomatose benigne. Un cas avec des alterations mammaires comme seul symptome. *Acta Clin Scand* 1942;86:168–178.
64. Davies JD, Burton PA: Postpartum lobular granulomatous mastitis. *J Clin Pathol* 1983;36:363.
* 65. DeHertogh DA, Rossof AH, Harris AA, et al: Prednisone management of granulomatous mastitis. *N Engl J Med* 1980;303:799–800.
66. Deininger HK: Wegener's granulomatosis of the breast. *Radiology* 1985;154:59–60.
67. Dent DM, Webber BL: Tuberculosis of the breast. *S Afr Med J* 1977;51:611–614.
68. Fletcher A, Magrath IM, Riddel RH, et al: Granulomatous mastitis: A report of seven cases. *J Clin Pathol* 1982;35:941–945.
69. Frantz VK, Pickren JW, Melcher GW, et al: Incidence of chronic cystic disease in so-called "normal breasts." A study based on 225 postmortem examinations. *Cancer* 1951;4:762–783.
70. Galea MH, Robertson JF, Ellis IO, et al: Granulomatous lobular mastitis. *Aust NZ J Surg* 1989;59:547–550.
71. Giorno R: Mononuclear cells in malignant and benign human breast tissue. *Arch Pathol Lab Med* 1983;107:415–417.
* 72. Going JJ, Anderson TJ, Wilkinson S, et al: Granulomatous lobular mastitis. *J Clin Pathol* 1987;40:535–540.
* 73. Gottschalk FAB, Decker GAG, Schmaman A: Tuberculosis of the breast. *S Afr J Surg* 1976;14:19–22.
74. Haagensen CD: *Diseases of the Breast*, ed 3. Philadelphia, WB Saunders Co, 1986, Fibrous disease: 125–135; infections: 384–393; plasma cell mastitis: 362.
* 75. Habif D, Perzin K, Lattes R: Subareolar abscess associated with squamous metaplasia. *Am J Surg* 1970;119:523–526.
76. Ikard RW, Perkins D: Mammary tuberculosis: A rare modern disease. *South Med J* 1977;70:208–212.
77. Jayaram G: Cytomorphology of tuberculous mastitis. A report of nine cases with fine needle aspiration cytology. *Acta Cytol* 1985;29:947–948.
78. Kessler E, Wolloch Y: Granulomatous mastitis: A lesion clinically simulating carcinoma. *Am J Clin Pathol* 1972;58:642–646.
79. Knight ICS, Nolan B: Breast abscess. *Br Med J* 1959;1:1224–1231.
80. Koelmeyer TD, MacCormick DEM: Granulomatous mastitis. *Aust NZ J Surg* 1976;46:173–176.
* 81. Lammie GA, Bobrow LG, Staunton MDM, et al: Sclerosing lymphocytic lobulitis of the breast—evidence for an autoimmune pathogenesis. *Histopathology* 1991;19:13–20.
82. Leach RD, Eykyn SJ, Phillips I, et al: Anaerobic subareolar breast abscess. *Lancet* 1979;1(8106):35–37.
83. Maier WP, Berger A, Derrick BM: Periareolar abscess in the nonlactating breast. *Am J Surg* 1982;144:359–361.
* 84. Miller RE, Salomon PF, West JP: The coexistence of carcinoma and tuberculosis of the breast and axillary lymph nodes. *Am J Surg* 1971;121:338–340.
85. Mills SE: Lymphocytic mastopathy, a "new" autoimmune disease? *Am J Clin Pathol* 1990;93:834–835.
86. Milward TM, Gough MH: Granulomatous lesions of the breast presenting as carcinoma. *Surg Gynecol Obstet* 1970;130:478–482.
87. Minkowitz S, Hedayati H, Hiller S, et al: Fibrous mastopathy: A clinical histopathologic study. *Cancer* 1973;32:913–916.
88. Murthy MS: Granulomatous mastitis and lipogranuloma of the breast. *Am J Clin Pathol* 1973;60:432–433.
89. Osborne BM: Granulomatous mastitis caused by histoplasma and mimicking inflammatory breast carcinoma. *Hum Pathol* 1989;20:47–52.
90. Page DL, Anderson TJ: Miscellaneous non-neoplastic conditions, in *Diagnostic Histopathology of the Breast*. New York, Churchill Livingstone, 1987, p 66.
91. Pambakian H, Tishe JR: Breast involvement in Wegener's granulomatosis. *J Clin Pathol* 1971;24:343–347.
92. Petrek J: Postmenopausal breast abscess. *South Med J* 1982;75:1198–1200.
93. Powell BC, Maull KI, Sachatello CR: Recurrent subareolar abscess of the breast and squamous metaplasia of the lactiferous ducts: A clinical syndrome. *South Med J* 1977;70:935–937.
94. Puente JL, Potel J: Fibrous tumor of the breast. *Arch Surg* 1974;109:391–394.

95. Raju GC, Nayarnsingh V, Jankey N: Post-menopausal breast abscess. *Postgrad Med J* 1986;62:1017–1018.
96. Rench MA, Baker CJ: Group B streptococcal breast abscess in a mother and mastitis in her infant. *Obstet Gynecol* 1989;73:875–877.
97. Rivera-Pomar JM, Villanova JR, Burgos-Bretones JJ, et al: Focal fibrous disease of breast: A common entity in young women. *Virchows Arch (A)* 1980;386:59–64.
98. Rowe PH: Granulomatous mastitis associated with a pituitary prolactinoma. *Br J Clin Pract* 1984;38:32–34.
99. Rudoy RC, Nelson JD: Breast abscess during the neonatal period. A review. *Am J Dis Child* 1975;129:1031–1034.
100. Schaeffer G: Tuberculosis of the breast. *Am Rev TB* 1955; 72:810–814.
*101. Schwartz IS, Strauchen AJ: Lymphocytic mastopathy. An autoimmune disease of the breast? *Am J Clin Pathol* 1990; 93:725–730.
102. Soler NG, Khardori R: Fibrous disease of the breast, thyroiditis and cheiroarthropathy in type I diabetes mellitus. *Lancet* 1984;1:193–194.
103. Soltau DHK, Hatcher GW: Some observations on the aetiology of breast abscess in the puerperium. *Br Med J* 1960;1:1603–1607.
*104. Symmers W St C, McKeown KC: Tuberculosis of the breast. *Br Med J* 1984;289:48–49.
105. Vassar PS, Collings CFA: Fibrosis of the breast. *Arch Pathol* 1959;67:128–133.
106. Villard E, Martin JF: Coexistence de cancer et de tuberculose du sein et des ganglions axillaire. *Bull Assoc Franc p. l'etude du Cancer* 1933;22:128–139.
107. Walker AP, Edmiston CE Jr, Krepel CJ, et al: A prospective study of microflora of nonpuerperal breast abscess. *Arch Surg* 1988;123:908–911.
108. Watt-Boolsen S, Rasmussen NR, Blichert-Toft M: Primary periareolar abscess in the nonlactating breast: Risk of recurrence. *Am J Surg* 1987;153:571–573.
109. Weiss RL, Matsen JM: Group B streptococcal breast abscess. *Arch Pathol Lab Med* 1987;111:74–75.
110. Wilhelmus JL, Schrodt GR, Mahaffey LM: Cholesterol granulomas of the breast: A lesion which clinically mimics carcinoma. *Am J Clin Pathol* 1982;77:592–597.
111. Zuska JJ, Crile G, Ayres W: Fistulas of lactiferous ducts. *Am J Surg* 1951;81:312–317.

### Other Infections

112. Azzopardi JG: *Problems in Breast Pathology*. Philadelphia, WB Saunders Co, 1979, p 400.
113. Adair FE: Gumma of the breast: Its differential diagnosis from carcinoma. *Ann Surg* 1924;79:44–54.
114. Fidler WJ: Demodex folliculorum in a nipple imprint. *Acta Cytol* 1978;22:168–169.
115. Haagensen CD: Infections in the breast, in *Diseases of the Breast*, ed 3. Philadelphia, WB Saunders, 1986, pp 384–393.
116. Kampmeier RH: Syphilis of the breast; chancre and gumma. *Am Pract* 1947;1:395–398.
117. Lefkowitz M, Wear DJ: Cat-scratch disease masquerading as a solitary tumor of the breast. *Arch Pathol Lab Med* 1989;113:473–475.
118. Novak R: Calcifications in the breast in *Filaria loa* infection. *Acta Radiol* 1989;30:507–508.
119. Salfelder K, Schwarz J: Mycotic "pseudotumor" of the breast: Report of four cases. *Arch Surg* 1975;110:751–754.
120. Symmers WStC: The breasts, in Payling-Wright G, Symmers WStC (eds): *Systemic Pathology*, Chap 28, Vol 1. London, Longmans Green, 1966, pp 953–955.
121. Symmers WStC: Deep-seated fungal infections currently seen in the histopathologic service of a medical school laboratory in Britain. *Am J Clin Pathol* 1966;46:515–537.
122. Tuur SM, Nelson AM, Gibson DW, et al: Liesegang rings in tissue. How to distinguish Liesegang rings from the giant kidney worm, *Dioctophyma renale*. *Am J Surg Pathol* 1987;11:598–605.
123. Yuehan C, Qun X: Filarial granuloma of the female breast: A histopathological study of 131 cases. *Am J Trop Med Hyg* 1981;30:1206–1210.

### Sarcoidosis and Rheumatoid Nodule

124. Azzopardi JG: *Problems in Breast Pathology*. Philadelphia, WB Saunders Co, 1978, pp 400–401.
125. Banik S, Bishop PW, Ormerod LP, et al: Sarcoidosis of the breast. *J Clin Pathol* 1986;39:446–448.
126. Bodo M, Dobrossy L, Sugar J: Boeck's sarcoidosis of the breast: Cytologic findings with aspiration biopsy cytology. *Acta Cytol* 1978;22:1–2.
127. Bonecchi L, Nanni MR: Sarcoide Di Boeck della mamella. *Radiol Med* 1981;67:656–657.
128. Cooper NE: Rheumatoid nodule in the breast. *Histopathology* 1991;19:193–194.
129. Fitzgibbons PL, Smiley DF, Kern WH: Sarcoidosis presenting initially as breast mass: Report of two cases. *Hum Pathol* 1985;16:851–852.
130. Gansler TS, Wheeler JE: Mammary sarcoidosis. Two cases and literature review. *Arch Pathol Lab Med* 1984;108:673–675.
131. Geschickter CF: *Diseases of the Breast*. Philadelphia, JB Lippincott Co, 1947, pp 164–165.
132. Haagensen CD: *Diseases of the Breast*. Philadelphia, WB Saunders, 1986, pp 357–368.
133. Longcope WT, Freiman DG: A study of sarcoidosis. *Medicine* 1944;31:1–121.
134. Pascual RS, Gee JBL, Finch SC: Usefulness of serum lysozyme in the diagnosis and evaluation of sarcoidosis. *N Engl J Med* 1973;289:1074–1076.
135. Reisner D: Boeck's sarcoid and systemic sarcoidosis: A study of 35 cases. *Am Rev Tuberc* 1944;39:437–462.
136. Rigden B: Sarcoid lesion in breast after probable sarcoidosis in lung. *Br Med J* 1978;2:1533–1534.
137. Ross MJ, Merino MJ: Sarcoidosis of the breast. *Hum Pathol* 1985;16:185–187.

138. Scadding HB: *Sarcoidosis*. London, Eyre and Spottiswoode, 1967, p 335.
139. Scott RB: The sarcoidosis in Boeck. *Br Med J* 1938;2:777–781.
140. Stallard HB, Tait CBV: Boeck's sarcoidosis. *Lancet* 1939;1; 440–442.
141. Strandberg J: Contribution a la question de la clinique et de la pathogenie de la sarcoide de Boeck. *Acta Derm Venerol* 1921;2:253–257.
142. Studdy PR, Lapwork R, Bird R: Angiotensin-converting enzyme and its clinical significance. *J Clin Pathol* 1983;36: 938–947.


### Amyloid Tumor


143. Azzopardi JG: *Problems in Breast Pathology*. Philadelphia, WB Saunders, 1979, p 398.
144. Cetti R, Reuther K, Hansen JPH, et al: Amyloid tumor of the breast. *Dan Med Bull* 1983;30:34–35.
145. Cheung PS, Yan KW, Alagaratnam TT, et al: Bilateral amyloid tumor of the breast. *Aust NZ J Surg* 1986;56:375–377.
*146. Fernandez BB, Hernandez FJ: Amyloid tumor of the breast. *Arch Pathol* 1973;95:102–105.
147. Ganor S, Dollberg L: Amyloidosis of the nipple presenting as pruritis. *Cutis* 1983;31:318.
148. Goonatillake RD, Allsop JR: Amyloid tumour of the breast simulating carcinoma. *Aust NZ J Surg* 1988;58:589–590.
149. Hardy TJ, Myerowitz RL, Bender BL: Diffuse parenchymal amyloidosis of lungs and breast. Its association with diffuse plasmacytosis and kappa chain gammapathy. *Arch Pathol Lab Med* 1979;103:583–585.
150. Lipper S, Kahn LB: Amyloid tumor: a clinicopathologic study of four cases. *Am J Surg Pathol* 1978;2:141–145.
151. McMahon RFT, Waldron D, Given HF, et al: Localized amyloid tumor of the breast—a case report. *Ir J Med Sci* 1984;159:323–324.
152. O'Connor CR, Rubinow A, Cohen AS: Primary (AL) amyloidosis as a cause of breast masses. *Am J Med* 1984;77:981–986.
153. Patil SD, Joshi BG, Datar KG: Amyloid deposit in the carcinoma of breast. Indian J Cancer 1970;7:60–62.
154. Sadeghee SA, Moore SW: Rheumatoid arthritis, bilateral amyloid tumors of the breast and multiple cutaneous amyloid nodules. *Am J Clin Pathol* 1974;62:472–476.
155. Silverman JF, Dabbs DJ, Norris HT, et al: Localized primary (AL) amyloid tumor of the breast. Cytologic, immunohistochemical, and ultrastructural observations. *Am J Surg Pathol* 1986;10:539–545.
156. Walker AN, Fechner RE, Callicott JH Jr: Amyloid tumor of the breast. *Diagn Gynecol Obstet* 1982;4:339–341.


### Anticoagulant Induced Necrosis


157. Andersson I, Adler DD, Ljungberg O: Breast necrosis associated with thromboembolic disorders. *Acta Radiol* 1987;28:517.
158. Banik S, Brun C: Hemorrhagic breast infarction complicating anticoagulant therapy. *Postgrad Med J* 1982;58:41–42.
159. Caldwell EH, Stewart S: Skin necrosis as a consequence of coumadin therapy. *Plast Reconstr Surg* 1983;72:231–233.
160. Clouse LH, Comp PC: The regulation of hemostasis: The protein C system. *N Engl J Med* 1986;314:1298–1304.
161. Kagan RJ, Glassford GH: Coumadin-induced breast necrosis. *Am Surg* 1981;47:509–510.
162. Manstein CH, Steerman PH, Goldstein J: Sodium warfarin-induced gangrene of the breast. *Ann Plast Surg* 1985;15: 161–162.
163. Martin BF, Phillips JD: Gangrene of the female breast with anticoagulant therapy: Report of two cases. *Am J Clin Pathol* 1970;53:622–626.
164. Mason JR: Hemorrhage-induced breast gangrene. *Br J Surg* 1970;57:700–702.
165. Nudelman HL, Kempson RL: Necrosis of the breast: A rare complication of anticoagulant therapy. *Am J Surg* 1966;111: 728–733.
166. Ravina et Jamian. Les Gangrenes de sein pendant la lactation. *Gynec Obst* 1949;48:49–55.
167. Shnider D, D'Souza CR: Cutaneous gangrene: A rare complication of coumarin therapy. *Can J Surg* 1976;19:64–65, 68.
168. Switzer PK: Gangrene of the breast associated with diabetes mellitus. Report of a case. *J SC Med Assoc* 1950;46:42.


### Lymphoma and Leukemia


169. Adair FE, Carver LF, Herrmann JB: Hodgkin's disease of the breast. *Surg Gynecol Obstet* 1945;80:205–210.
170. Adair FE, Herrmann JB: Primary lymphosarcoma of the breast. *Surgery* 1944;16:836–853.
171. Alm P, Brandt L, Osson H: Immunoglobulin-A producing probably primary lymphoma of the breast. *Virchows Arch (A)* 1983;399:355–360.
172. Armitage JO, Geagler JR, Skoog DP: Burkitt's lymphoma during pregnancy with bilateral breast involvement. *JAMA* 1977;237:151.
173. Azzopardi JG: *Problems in Breast Pathology*. Philadelphia, WB Saunders, 1979, pp 371–373.
174. Ben Yehuda A, Steiner-Saltz D, Libson E, et al: Plasmacytoma of the breast. Unusual initial presentation of myeloma: Report of two cases and review of the literature. *Blut* 1989;58:169–170.
*175. Brustein S, Filippa DA, Kimmel M, et al: Malignant lymphoma of the breast: A study of 53 patients. *Ann Surg* 1987;205:144–150.
176. Bucciarelli E, Cavaliere A, Sidoni A, et al: Bilateral primary malignant lymphoma of the breast. A case report. *Tumori* 1988;74:587–591.
177. Carbone A, Volpe R, Tirelli U, et al: Primary lymphoblastic lymphoma of the breast. *Clin Oncol* 1982;8:367–373.
178. Cassi E, Tosi A, De' Poli A, et al: Granulocytic sarcoma without evidence of acute leukemia: 2 cases with unusual

localization (uterus and breast) and 1 case with bone localization. *Haemotologica (Pavia)* 1984;69:464–496.
179. Chua ET: A case of granulocytic sarcoma of the breast and review of the literature. *Singapore Med J* 1989;30:311–312.
180. Cohen PL, Brroks JJ: Lymphomas of the breast. A clinicopathologic and immunohistochemical study of primary and secondary cases. *Cancer* 1991;67:1359–1369.
181. Corrigan C, Sewell C, Martin A: Recurrent Hodgkin's disease in the breast. Diagnosis of a case by fine needle aspiration and immunocytochemistry. *Acta Cytol* 1990;34: 669–672.
182. Cutler C: Plasma cell tumor of the breast with metastases. *Ann Surg* 1934;100:392–395.
183. Curtis RE, Boice JD Jr, Stovall M, et al: Leukemia risk following radiotherapy for breast cancer. *J Clin Oncol* 1989;7:21–29.
184. DeBlasio D, McCormick B, Straus D, et al: Definitive irradiation for localized non-Hodgkin's lymphoma of breast. *Int J Radiat Oncol Biol Phys* 1989;17:843–846.
185. Decosse JJ, Berg JW, Fracchia AA, et al: Primary lymphosarcoma of the breast: A review of 14 cases. *Cancer* 1962; 14:1264–1268.
186. De Leon DM, Villafria L, Crisostomo C: Nonsystemic reticulum cell sarcoma of the breast: A case report. *Philipp J Surg* 1961;16:149–151.
187. Dixon JM, Lumsden AB, Krajewski A, et al: Primary lymphoma of the breast. *Br J Surg* 1987;74:214–217.
188. Elavathil LJ, Kahn HJ, Hanna W: Primary multilobulated B-cell lymphoma of the breast. *Arch Pathol Lab Med* 1989; 113:1081–1084.
189. Ferguson DJP: Intraepithelial lymphocytes and macrophages in the normal breast. *Virchows Archiv (Pathol Anat)* 1985;407:369–378.
190. Fisher B, Rockette H, Fisher ER, et al: Leukemia in breast cancer patients following adjuvant chemotherapy or postoperative radiation: The NSABP experience. *J Clin Oncol* 1985;3:1640–1658.
191. Fisher ER, Palekar AS, Paulson JD, et al: Pseudolymphoma of breast. *Cancer* 1979;44:258–263.
192. Foucar E, Rosai J, Dorfman R: Sinus histiocytosis with massive lymphadenopathy (Rosai-Dorfman disease). Review of the entity. *Sem Diagn Pathol* 1990;7:19–73.
193. Friedman SI, Kagan AR, Friedman JB: Bilaterality in primary lymphosarcoma of the breast. *Am J Clin Pathol* 1971; 55:82–87.
194. Fukutomi T, Makuuchi M, Itabashi M, et al: A rare case of asynchronous bilateral B-cell lymphoma of the breast. *Jpn J Clin Oncol* 1989;19:391–396.
195. Gartenhus WS, Mir R, Pliskin A, et al: Granulocytic sarcoma of breast: A leukemic bilateral metachronous presentation and literature review. *Med Pediatr Oncol* 1985;13:22–29.
196. Geller RB, Boone LB, Karp JE, et al: Secondary acute myelocytic leukemia after adjuvant therapy for early stage breast carcinoma. A new complication of cyclophosphamide, methotrexate, and 5-fluorouracil therapy. *Cancer* 1989;64:629–634.
197. Giardini R, Piccolo C, Rilke F: Primary non-Hodgkin's lymphomas of the female breast. *Cancer* 1992;69:725–735.
198. Graeme-Cook F, Obrian DA, Daly PA: Unusual breast masses. The sequential development of mammary tuberculosis and Hodgkin's disease in a young woman. *Cancer* 1988;61:1457–1459.
199. Haagensen CD: *Diseases of the Breast*, ed 3. Philadelphia, WB Saunders, 1986, pp 346–349.
200. Harrington SW, Miller JM: Lymphosarcoma of the mammary gland. *Am J Surg* 1940;48:346–352.
201. Hoffman WI, Goodman ML: Primary lymphosarcoma of the breast. *Arch Surg* 1968;96:410–413.
202. Hugh JC, Jackson FI, Hanson J, et al: Primary breast lymphoma. An immunohistologic study of 20 new cases. *Cancer* 1990;66:2602–2611.
203. Jernstrom P, Sether JM: Primary lymphosarcoma of the mammary gland. *JAMA* 1967;201:503–506.
204. Kirshenbaum G, Rhone DP: Solitary extramedullary plasmacytoma of the breast with serum monoclonal protein: A case report and review of the literature. *Am J Clin Pathol* 1985;83:230–232.
*205. Lamovec J, Jancar J: Primary malignant lymphoma of the breast: Lymphoma of the MALT. *Cancer* 1987;60:3033–3041.
206. Lattes R: Sarcomas of the breast. *JAMA* 1967;201:121–122.
207. Lawler MR, Richie RE: Reticulum cell sarcoma of the breast. *Cancer* 1967;20:1438–1446.
208. Lawler MR, Riddel DH: Hodgkin's disease of the breast. *Am J Surg* 1960;90:331–334.
209. Lin JJ, Farha GJ, Taylor RJ: Pseudolymphomas of the breast. I. In a study of 8,654 consecutive tylectomies and mastectomies. *Cancer* 1980;45:973–978.
*210. Mambo NC, Burke JS, Butler JJ: Primary malignant lymphomas of the breast. *Cancer* 1977;39:2033–2040.
211. McDivitt RW, Stewart FW, Berg JW: *Tumors of the Breast*, Fasc 2, in Atlas of Tumor Pathology, second series. Washington DC, Armed Forces Institute of Pathology, 1968.
212. Merino MJ: Plasmacytoma of the breast. *Arch Pathol Lab Med* 1984;108:676–678.
213. Merino MJ, Joyner RE, Graham A: Pseudolymphoma of the breast. *Diagn Gynecol Obstet* 1981;3:315–319.
214. Mies JM, Butler JJ, Osborne BM: Hodgkin's disease involving the breast and chest wall. *Cancer* 1986;57:1859–1865.
215. Millis RR, Bobrow LG, Rubens RD, et al: Histiocytic lymphoma of breast responds to tamoxifen. *Br J Cancer* 1988;58:808–809.
216. Oberman HA: Primary lymphoreticular neoplasms of the breast. *Surg Gynecol Obstet* 1966;123:1047–1051.
217. Paulus DD: Lymphoma of the breast. *Radiol Clin North Am* 1990;28:833–840.
218. Pettinato G, De Chiara A, Insabato L, et al: Fine needle aspiration biopsy of a granulocytic sarcoma (chloroma) of the breast. *Acta Cytol* 1988;32:67–71.

219. Proctor R, Shulman G, Graham A: Extramedullary plasmacytoma of the breast. *J Pathol* 1975;116:97–100.

220. Randall KJ, Spalding JE: Primary Hodgkin's disease of the breast: Report of a case and a commentary. *Guy's Hosp Rep* 1945;94:137–141.

221. Rosenberg BM, Attie JM, Mandelbaum HL: Breast tumor as the presenting sign of multiple myeloma. *N Engl J Med* 1963;269:359–363.

222. Ross JS, King TM, Spector JI, et al: Plasmacytoma of the breast: An unusual case of recurrent myeloma. *Arch Int Med* 1987;147:1838.

223. Salvadori B, Cusumano F, DeLellis R: The surgeon's attitude to malignant lymphoma of the breast: Analysis of eight cases. *Eur J Surg Oncol* 1986;12:47–51.

224. Schouten JT, Weese JL, Carbone PP: Lymphoma of the breast. *Ann Surg* 1981;194:749–753.

225. Sears HF, Reid J: Granulocytic sarcoma. *Cancer* 1976;37: 1808–1813.

226. Shepherd JJ, Wright DH: Burkitt's tumor presenting as bilateral swelling of the breast in females of child-bearing age. *Br J Surg* 1967;54:776–780.

227. Shpitz B, Witz M, Kaufman Z, et al: Bilateral primary malignant lymphoma of the breast. *Postgrad Med J* 1985;61: 729–731.

228. Smith MR, Brustein S, Straus DJ: Localized non-Hodgkin's lymphoma of the breast. *Cancer* 1987;59:351–354.

229. Socinski MA, Ersher WB, Belinson JL: Coexistent breast and vaginal granulocytic sarcoma. *Gynecol Oncol* 1983;16: 299–304.

230. Sonnenblick M, Abraham AS: Primary lymphosarcoma of the breast: Review of the literature on occurrence in elderly patients. *J Am Geriatr Soc* 1976;24:225–227.

231. Stark JJ, Lloyd JW, Schellhammer PF: Estrogen receptor activity in a case of Hodgkin's disease. *Ann Int Med* 1981;95:186–187.

232. Stierer M, Rosen HR, Heinz R, et al: Synchrony of malignant lymphoma and breast cancer. *JAMA* 1990;263:2922–2923.

* 233. Tanaka T, Hsueh CL, Hayashi K, et al: Primary malignant lymphoma of the breast: With a review of 73 cases among Japanese subjects. *Acta Pathol Jpn* 1984;34:361–373.

234. Tateno M, Yoshiki T, Itoh T, et al: A case of primary B-cell lymphoma of the breast. *Cancer* 1983;52:671–674.

235. Telesinghe PA, Anthony PP: Primary lymphoma of the breast. *Histopathology* 1985;9:297–307.

236. Weinblatt ME, Kochen J: Breast nodules as the initial site of relapse in childhood leukemia. *Med Pediatr Oncol* 1990;18: 510–512.

237. Wiseman C, Liao KT: Primary lymphoma of the breast. *Cancer* 1972;29:1705–1712.

238. Yoshida Y: Reticulum cell sarcoma of the breast: Case report and review of the Japanese literature. *Cancer* 1970; 26:94–99.

# 16

# Male Breast Lesions



## INTRODUCTION

As a vestigial organ, the shape of the mammary gland in the adult male is almost a miniature of the female breast; it is represented by a broad based, low, conical tissue mass. From birth to puberty, however, there is no difference between the male and female breast (26). Microscopically, a dense connective tissue surrounds ducts lined by two cell layers—epithelial and myoepithelial—but the racemose pattern and lobule formation characteristic of the adult female duct system is absent. The microscopic appearance of the male breast approximates that of the prepubertal girl.

Lesions of the male breast, particularly malignant ones, are far less frequent than those in the female breast. While there is almost as much variety, lesions such as lactating adenoma and in situ or invasive lobular carcinoma generally are not observed in the male breast. Lactating adenomas are not expected in the male breast because their development depends on the state of pregnancy, while lobular disease is extremely rare because lobules are normally absent in the male breast. Under the influence of endogenous or exogenous hormones, however, lobules may develop in the male mammary gland and in such a setting, lobular lesions may develop (155,200). On the other hand, gynecomastia consisting of a simultaneous proliferation of the ducts and stroma is a lesion almost exclusive to the male breast. The only lesion in the female breast that occasionally assumes the microscopic appearance of gynecomastia is one of the variants of juvenile hypertrophy which occurs in the adolescent female. All other lesions that occur in both male and female mammary glands are morphologically indistinguishable. The two most common lesions in the male breast are gynecomastia and carcinoma. Holleb (105) estimated that 65% of breast lesions in elderly men are gynecomastia, 25% are carcinoma and 10% are other benign breast lesions.

## GYNECOMASTIA

Gynecomastia, derived from the Greek words for "woman" and "breast," is defined as a potentially reversible enlargement of the male breast, basically characterized by an unencapsulated proliferation of connective tissue and ducts. It is a common disorder which presents as either a unilateral or bilateral palpable, subareolar mass. Gynecomastia accounted for 71% of all male breast tumors treated between 1928 and 1955 at the National Cancer Institute of Milan (38). The overall prevalence of palpable gynecomastia is about 32% among male veterans (7). Palpable bilateral gynecomastia is present in most older men, and does not require clinical evaluation unless symptomatic or of recent onset (29). Gynecomastia was present in 55% of 100 consecutive, nonselected male autopsies; the peak incidence occurred between 60 and 69 years of age (2,3). While the majority of the symptomatic cases are unilateral and present as a discrete, conical, palpable mass below the nipple, about 20% to 30% are bilateral. Occasionally, gynecomastia presents as diffuse enlargement of the breast.

Gynecomastia reflects mammary response to absolute or relative hyperestrogenism, as well as to medications which either have estrogen-like activity, or which adversely affect testosterone levels. While estrogens appear to have a trophic and stimulatory influence on the mammary duct system (32), androgens may actually exert an inhibitory effect on the development of the duct system (43).

Gynecomastia is common in gonadal dysfunction and Klinefelter's syndrome. A majority of patients with Klinefelter's syndrome (XXY) have gynecomastia (31). The gynecomastia in these patients may even show development of lobules (20). Defective androgen receptors and loss of inhibitory androgenic influences on the development of the breast as in testicular feminization (androgen insensitivity) syndrome may also result in gynecomastia (24).

A variety of benign or malignant neoplasms that produce either estrogens or estrogen precursors (androstenedione) may result in gynecomastia. Neoplasms producing human chorionic gonadotropin (HCG) may also induce gynecomastia since HCG can act as luteinizing hormone stimulating Leydig cells to produce excess estrogens (40).

Aside from estrogens, androgenic hormones, and HCG, a variety of other drugs and cytotoxic agents may cause gynecomastia. These include spironolactone (9,22), cimetidine, and digitalis (19,33,47). It is believed that spironolactone and cimetidine may induce gynecomastia by competitive displacement of dihydrotestosterone from its intracellular receptor (33,47). Cytotoxic agents (Busulfan, Vincristine, and Nitrosourea) may induce gynecomastia by damaging the testes (germ cell depletion) and inducing primary hypogonadism (12,37). Tseng et al (42) observed gynecomastia in patients with testicular carcinomas either following chemotherapy, or due to the production of HCG by the tumor.

**Table 16.1** Conditions and Drugs Associated with Gynecomastia

| | |
|---|---|
| Endogenous hormonal imbalance | |
| | Puberty |
| | Senescence |
| Exogenous hormonal therapy | |
| | Estrogen therapy for prostatic carcinoma |
| Drugs | |
| | Spironolactone, reserpine, digitalis, ergotamine tartrate, thyroid extract, diphenyl hydantoin, chorionic gonadotropin, cytotoxic chemotherapeutic agents |
| Hypogonadism | |
| | Klinefelter's syndrome, gonadal dysfunction, testicular atrophy |
| Neoplasm | |
| | Leydig cell tumor, germ cell tumors, hepatoma, feminizing adrenal tumors, pituitary tumors |
| Systemic Disease | |
| | Hepatic disease, renal disease, hyperthyroidism, recovery phase from malnutrition or any prolonged illness |

Drug-related gynecomastia presents at variable intervals following initiation of therapy and regresses, at least partially, once the offending medication is discontinued. Hormone-related and pubertal gynecomastia tend to be bilateral in contrast to the unilateral presentation as a discrete nodule in gynecomastia due to other factors.

Gynecomastia has also been observed following chronic illness, starvation, or malnutrition (during the refeeding phase), as well as in paraplegic patients. Gynecomastia may develop in patients with renal failure after initiation of hemodialysis (35), in patients recovering from any prolonged illness associated with notable weight loss (8), in patients with hepatic disorders, particularly those with alcoholic cirrhosis, and in association with hyperparathyroidism (8). The various conditions that may be associated with gynecomastia are listed in Table 16.1.

Gynecomastia does not appear to constitute a risk factor for the development of breast carcinoma. Of the 625 men with breast carcinoma studied by Crichlow (74,76), only 17 had gynecomastia in the adjacent breast. An increased incidence of breast cancer has only been observed in patients with Klinefelter's syndrome (160).

## Clinical Presentation

Gynecomastia is observed most commonly during puberty and old age associated with periods of physiologic hormonal alteration. Some degree of gynecomastia is evident in up to 60% to 70% of pubertal boys, typically between ages 12 and 15 years (4). The lesion generally presents as bilateral, diffuse enlargement of the breasts; the two sides are not always equally enlarged, however. There may be associated tenderness. Pubertal gynecomastia regresses spontaneously within one to two years. It may occasionally persist into adult life (44).

In a report of 218 cases from Milan (38), the highest incidence of gynecomastia occurred between ages of 50 and 60 years. In an earlier autopsy study, the maximum frequency of gynecomastia was noted in men between 40 to 50 years of age. In elderly men, particularly those past the age of 65, testicular failure occurs to a varying degree resulting in decrease in serum testosterone levels and relative hyperestrogenism, or increased estrogen to androgen ratio. Obesity may further contribute to the increased estrogen levels by enhancing peripheral aromatization of androgens to estrogens leading to the emergence of gynecomastia. It has been suggested that the gynecomastia present in most elderly men correlates with the amount of body fat and does not require clinical evaluation unless symptomatic, or of recent onset (28). Asymptomatic gynecomastia has been found in 36% of military reservists (29), while 40% of 447 men examined at autopsy have had evidence of gynecomastia (45). According to Andersen and Gram (2), gynecomastia is nearly always bilateral, although clinically it often seems to be a unilateral lesion. If there is no clinical evidence of breast enlargement, however, it is doubtful that a diagnosis of gynecomastia based on microscopic changes is warranted.

About 6% of the patients give a history of antecedent trauma (74). It is generally believed that trauma is coincidental and merely serves to draw attention to an asymptomatic, pre-existing lesion.

## Gross Appearance

When diffuse, gynecomastia appears ill-defined with margins that merge with the surrounding tissues. In the discrete variant, the hyperplastic breast tissue appears well circumscribed, with well-defined margins.

## Microscopic Features

Bannayan and Hajdu (5) divided gynecomastia into three types. The florid type (Fig. 16.1) is characterized by increased number of budding ducts, marked proliferation of ductal epithelium, periductal edema, and a highly cellular fibroblastic stroma accompanied by adipose tissue. The fibrous type (Fig. 16.2) has dilated ducts, slight to moderate epithelial proliferation, absence of adipose tissue, and an almost acellular fibrous stroma. Finally, the intermediate type shows an overlap of the features observed in the other two groups. They found the florid pattern to dominate in gynecomastia of short duration—four months or less. Gynecomastia of one year's duration was usually of the fibrous type and that of five to ten months' duration was most frequently associated with the intermediate pattern. As a result of these findings, Bannayan and Hajdu (5) suggested that gynecomastia goes through a process of maturation proceeding from florid to the fibrous type. More recently, Pages and Ramos (30) also compared three histologic types of gynecomastia with patient's age, duration of illness, and etiologic circumstances. They concluded that the three types are not stages in a progressive process, and their type 2 which corresponds to the fibrous type of Bannayan and Hajdu was the most frequent at any age. They found little correlation between etiology and histology except between the estrogenic therapy and florid gynecomastia.

The ducts in gynecomastia may have the normal bilayered arrangement with epithelial and myoepithelial cell layers, or they may show various degrees of epithelial hyperplasia. The hyperplasia is generally in the form of increased cell layers with superimposed epithelial tufts (Fig. 16.1c). Cystic dilatation of the ducts occurs occasionally. In florid hyperplasia, the ducts show delicate tufts that may undergo squamous metaplasia (Fig. 16.3) (30). Apocrine metaplasia is observed in 5.5%, while squamous metaplasia is found in 2% (5). While Karsner (18) did not observe lobules in any of his cases, lobule formation does occur and is found in approximately 6% of cases (5,36). Lobular development has even been reported

A

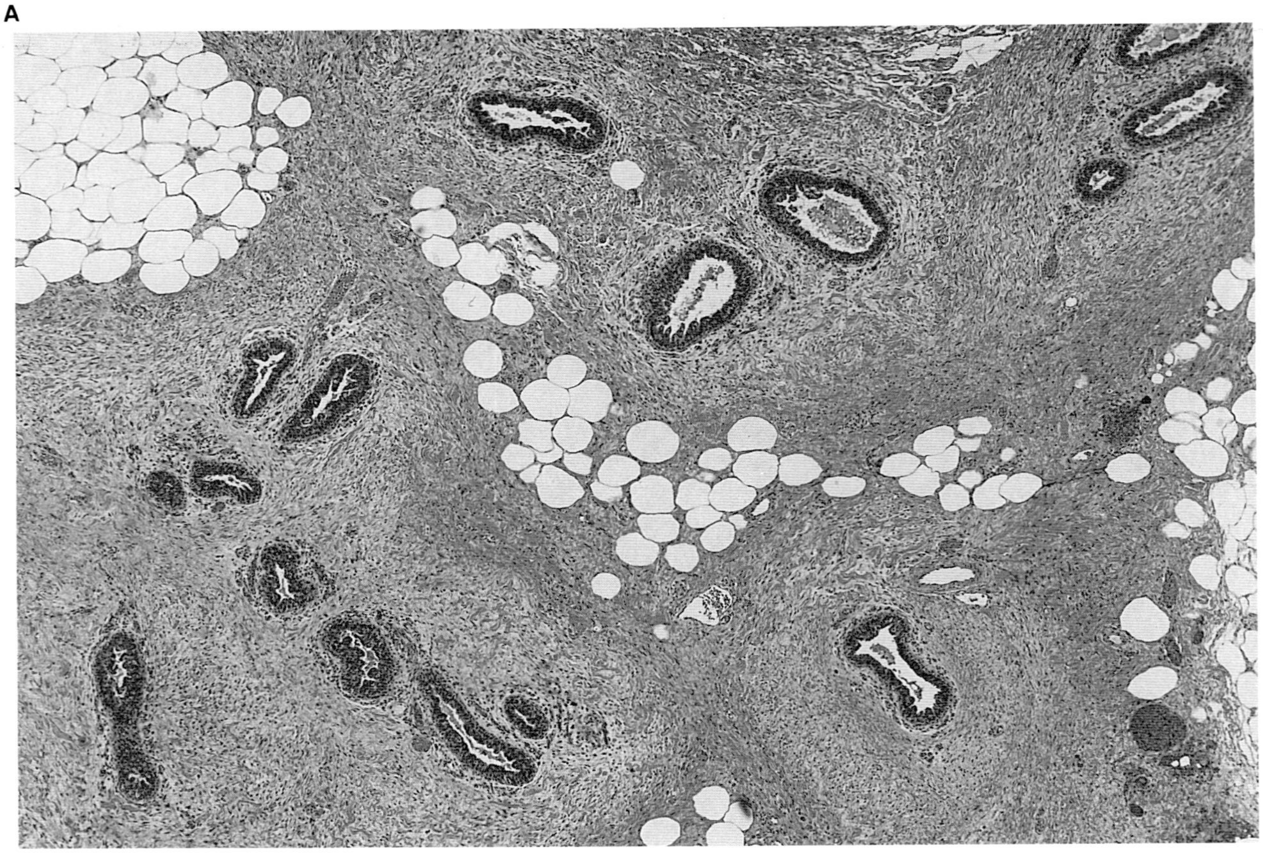

B

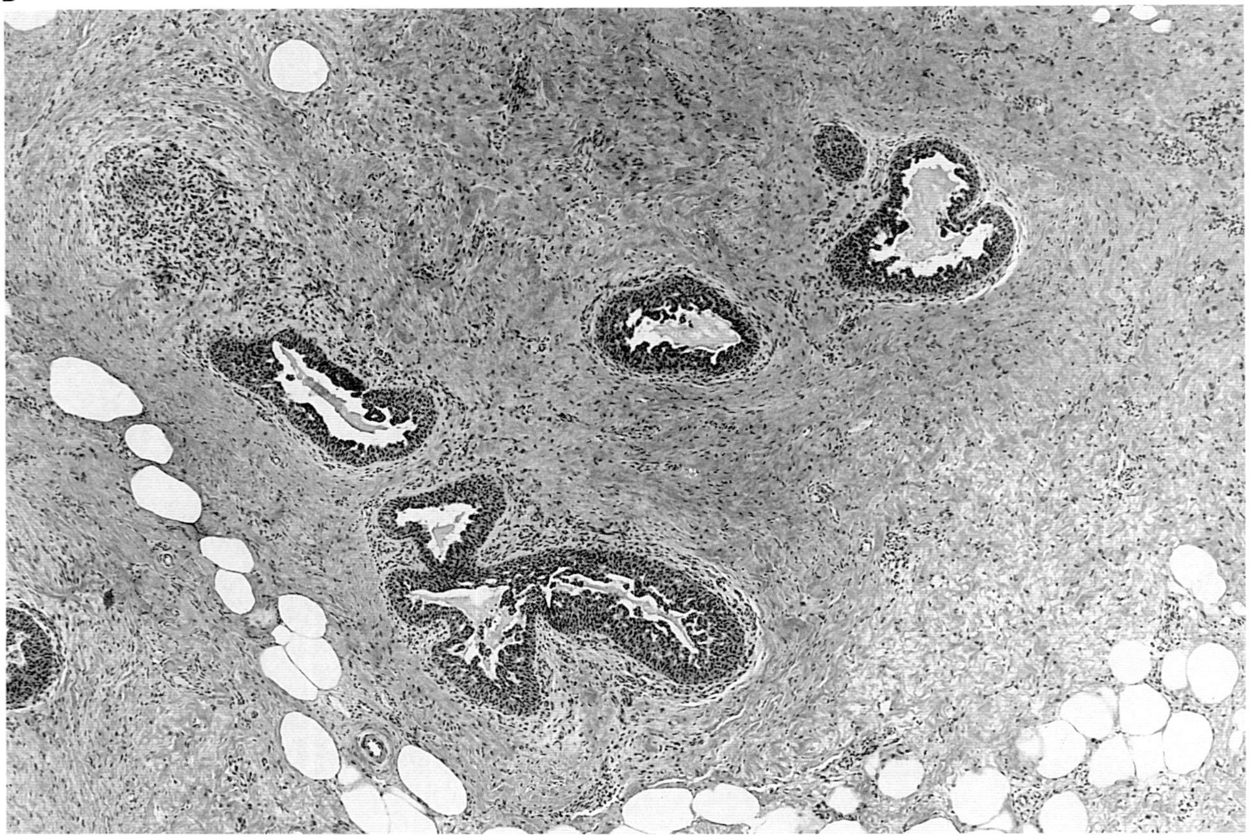

**Figure 16.1(a,b)** Gynecomastia, florid type. (a) The stroma is dense and admixed with adipose tissue; periductal edema is not conspicuous. (H&E, X30) (b) All ducts in this field show epithelial tufting. (H&E, X40)

C

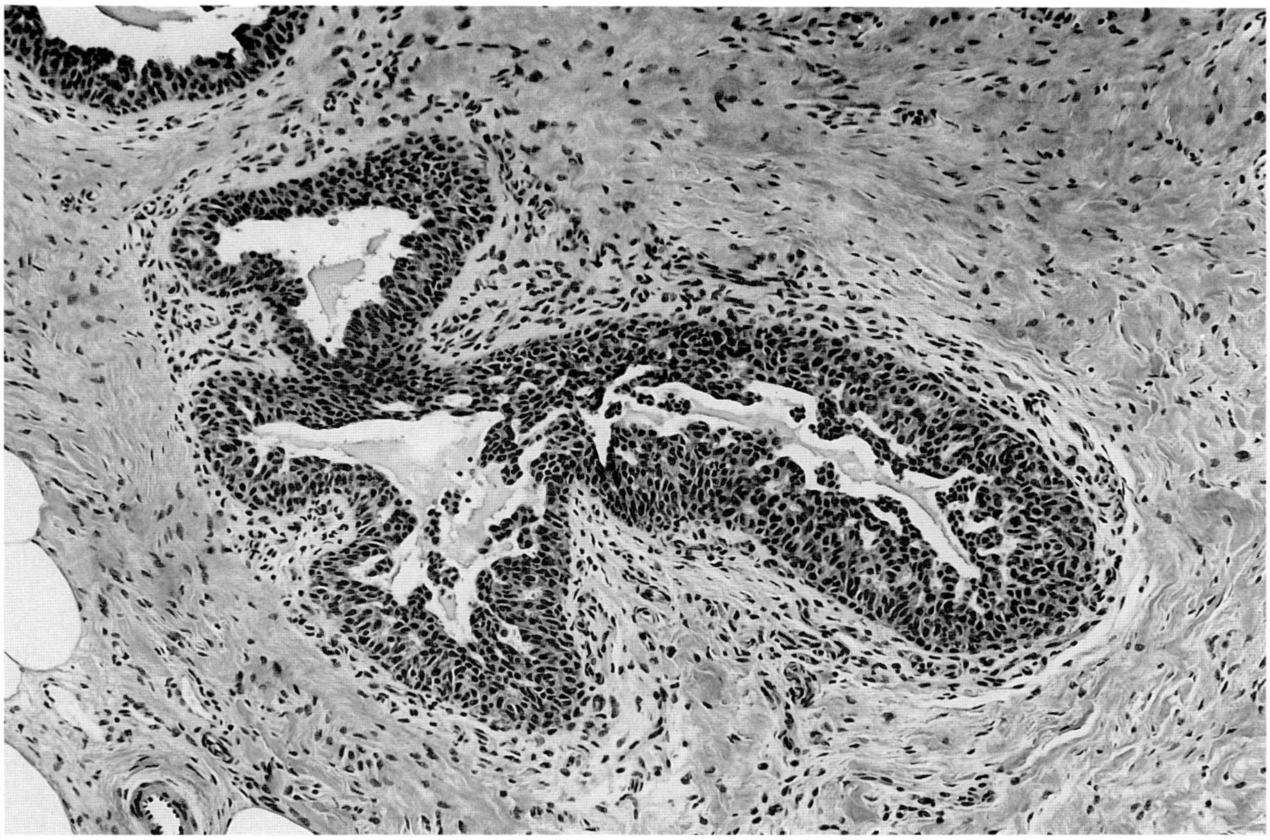

D

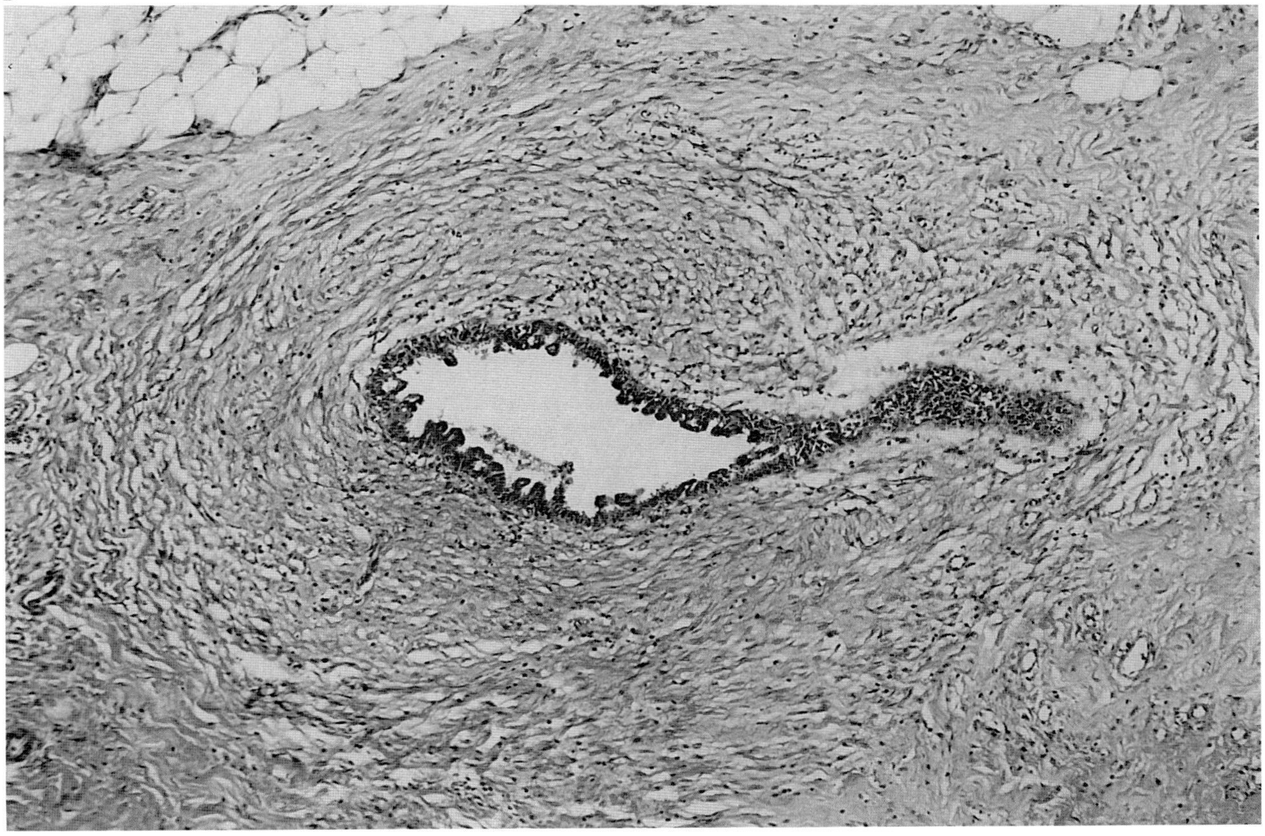

**Figure 16.1(c,d)** Gynecomastia, florid type. (c) The intraductal hyperplasia is characterized by formation of epithelial tufts overlying multiple layers of epithelial proliferation. (H&E, X75) (d) This pattern is often confused with intraductal carcinoma of the micropapillary type; the epithelial tufts are irregularly distributed, however, in contrast to the regular distribution of epithelial tufts in micropapillary carcinoma. (H&E, X60)

A

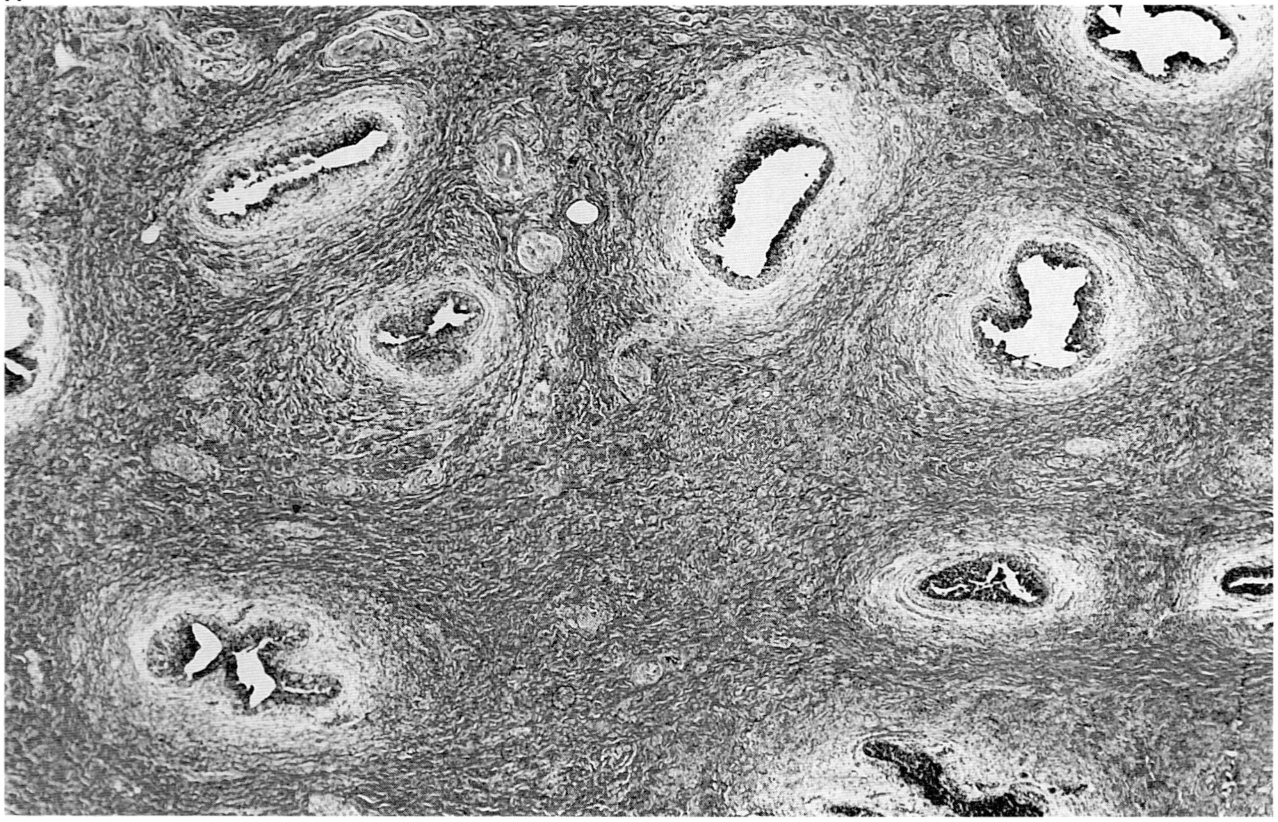

B

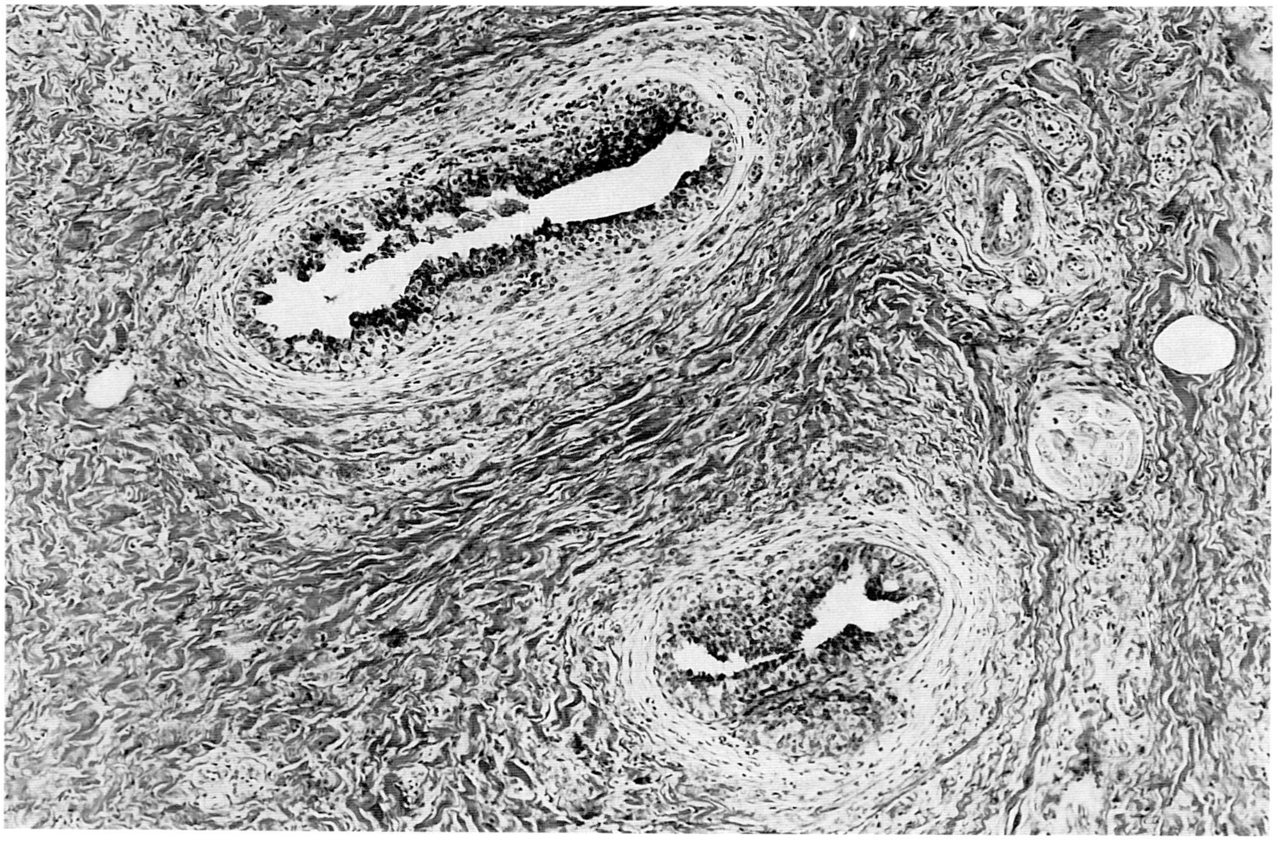

**Figure 16.2** Gynecomastia, fibrous type. (a) The stroma is dense, collagenous and lacks admixture with adipose tissue. The periductal edema is prominent. (b) Mild epithelial hyperplasia (3 to 4 cell layers above the basement membrane) may be seen in this variant. (c) More fibrotic examples. (H&E, (a) X30; (b) X75; (c) X40)

c

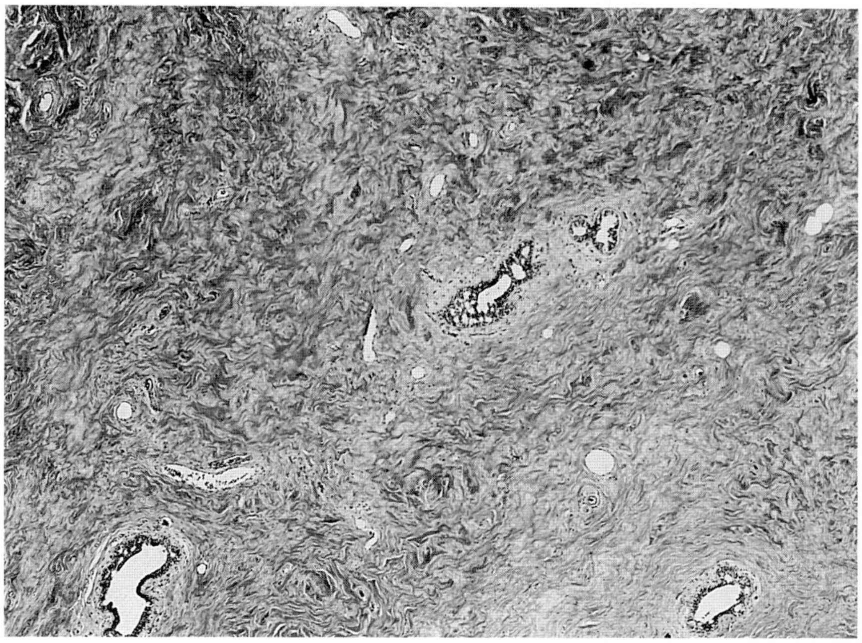

**Figure 16.2(c)** Gynecomastia, fibrous type. Legend on opposite page.

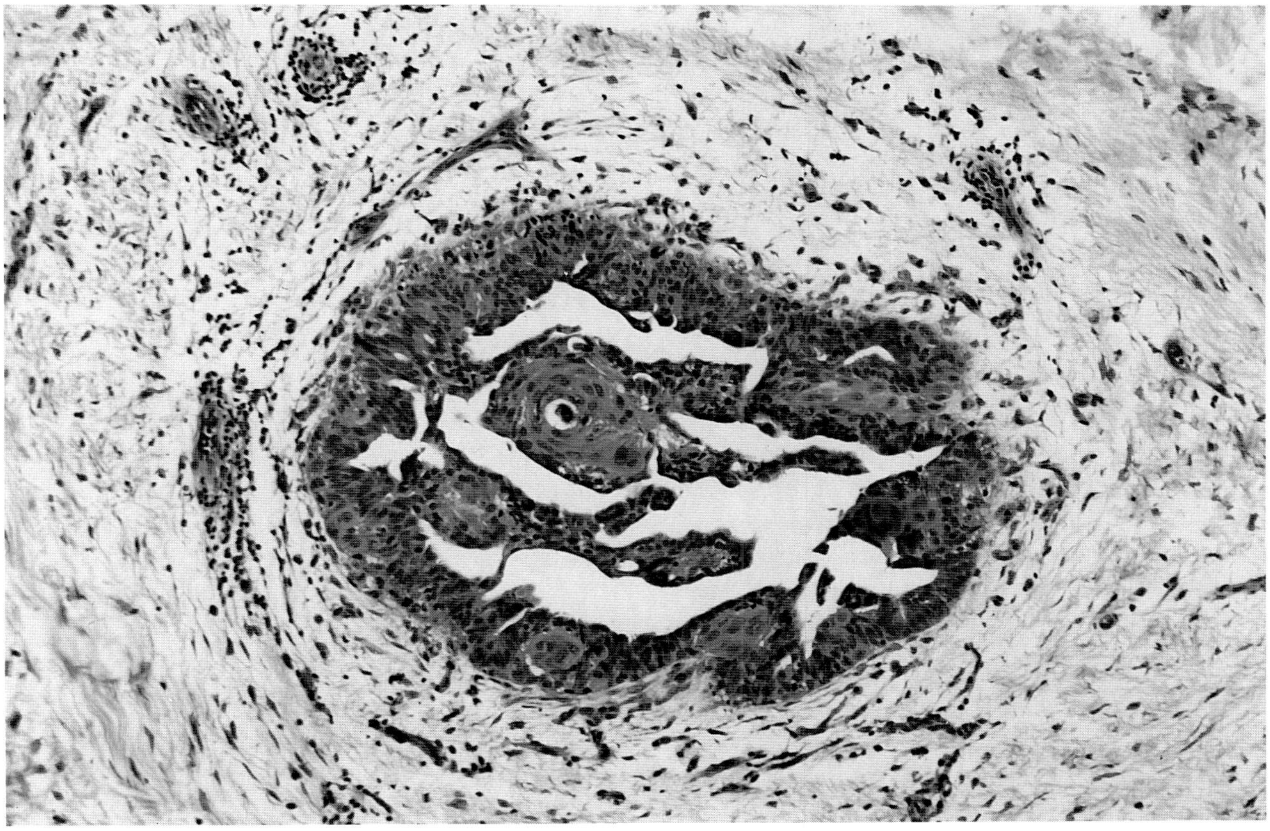

**Figure 16.3** Squamous metaplasia is apparent as small morules of cells with more abundant cytoplasm (arrows) in this hyperplastic duct. (H&E, X100)

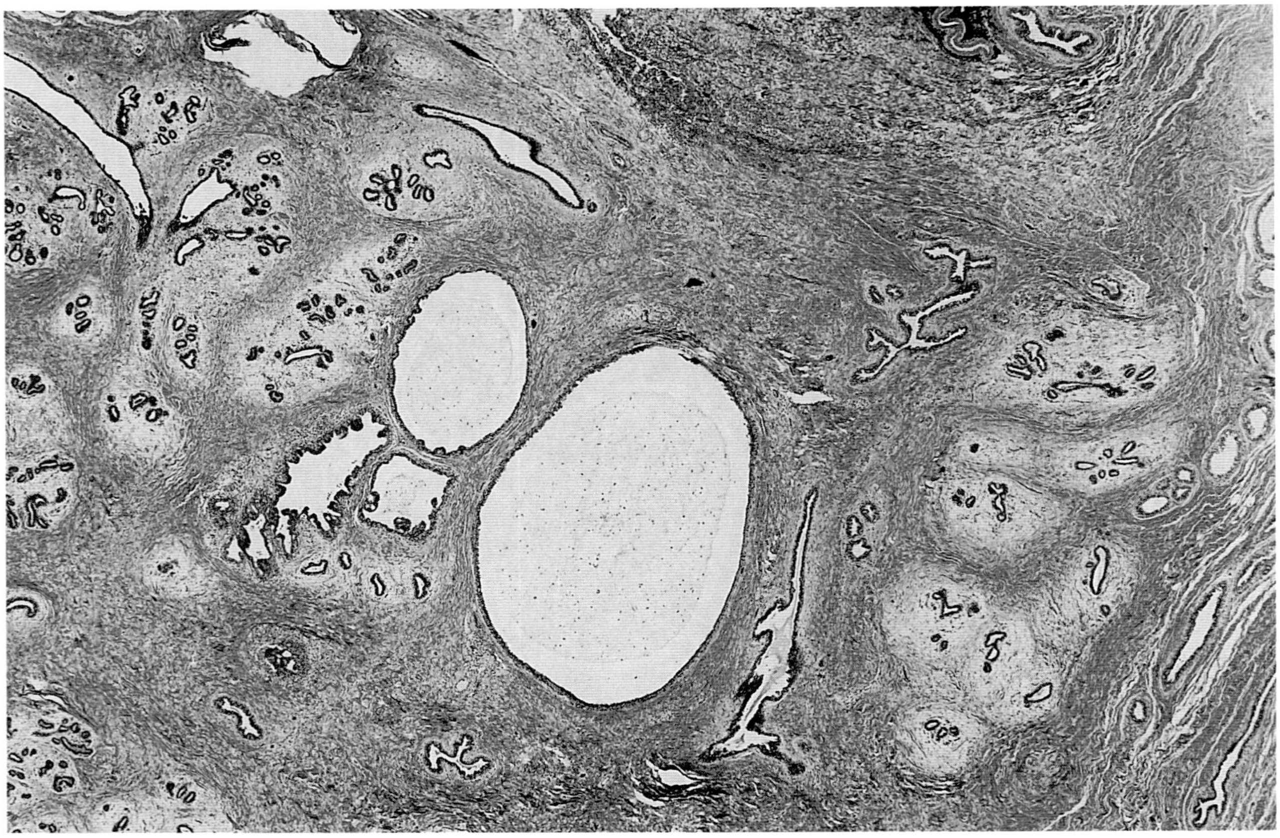

**Figure 16.4** Fibrocystic changes and lobular development are apparent in this case; patient was receiving estrogens for prostatic carcinoma. (H&E, X15)

in an 11-year-old boy with prepubertal gynecomastia (14). Fibrocystic changes (Fig. 16.4) also develop following formation of lobules induced by drugs such as stilbestrol (212). Rarely, atypical intraductal hyperplasia, closely approaching various forms of non-necrotic intraductal carcinoma, also occurs (Fig. 16.5).

## Ultrastructural Features

At the ultrastructural level, the ducts are lined by normal epithelial and myoepithelial cells which are surrounded by a basal lamina which may occasionally show focal interruptions. The periductal connective tissue contains either few collagen fibers dispersed among an abundant, finely granular matrix (30), or it may contain fibroblasts, myofibroblasts, and occasional pericytes (16). Squamous metaplasia (16), abundant centrioles (5), as well as fibroblasts with mature collagen (11) have been described.

## Management of Patients with Gynecomastia

Gynecomastia is a transient disease in the adolescent male. As part of the physiologic process of puberty, it does not require surgical intervention. It generally subsides within one to two years. Asymptomatic gynecomastia of long duration in elderly men does not require treatment and can be safely ignored. Recent or symptomatic gynecomastia is more likely to be clinically significant and requires further investigation.

In patients older than 25 years of age, symptomatic gynecomastia is usually a manifestation of serious underlying disease or reflects a response to hormones or other drugs. In these cases, inquiry into the patient's drug history, careful evaluation of the testicles, adrenal, thyroid, liver, lungs, cardiovascular, renal systems and the nutritional status of the patient is warranted. Anywhere from 10% to 40% of men with hyperthyroidism have gynecomastia which usually regresses when the patient becomes euthy-

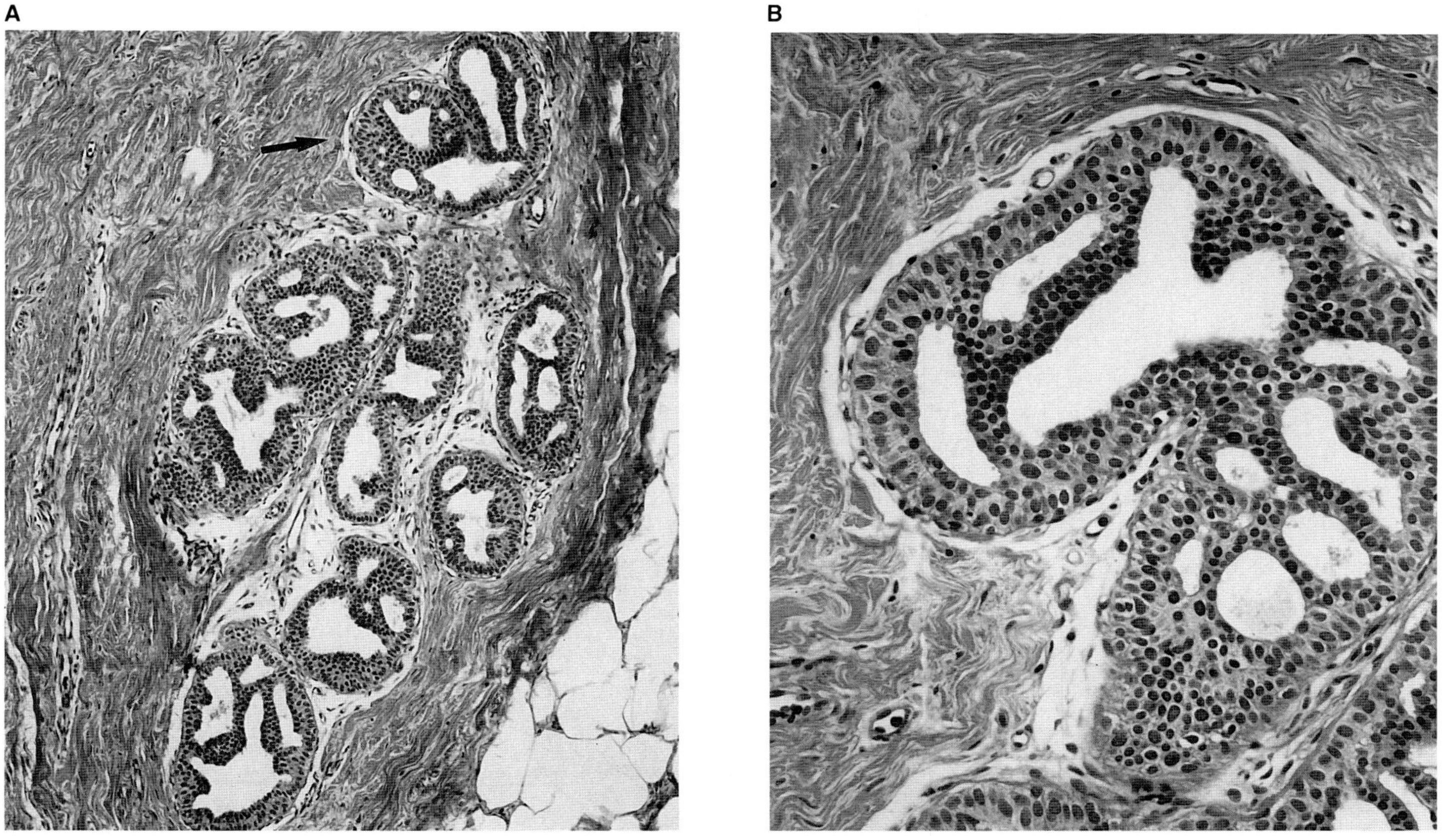


**Figure 16.5** Atypical intraductal hyperplasia. (a) Several small ductules show partial involvement by a proliferation composed of a uniform cell population forming rigid epithelial tufts and bridges. The arrow points at the duct which is depicted in (b). (b) Deeper level of the duct in (a) shows the most advanced lesion in this biopsy which continues to show a partial involvement of the duct by a cribriform growth of uniform cells, qualitatively similar to intraductal cribriform carcinoma. Since not even a single duct shows a complete involvement by this cell population and growth pattern, the lesion falls short of an intraductal carcinoma. (H&E, (a) X100; (b) X250)

roid. In one study (6), 15 of 18 men with hyperthyroidism had histologic evidence of bilateral gynecomastia, but breast enlargement was noted clinically in only six of these men. Medications temporally related to the onset of gynecomastia should be discontinued to determine if they are responsible for the gynecomastia. The value of the drug should weighed against the undesirable side effects such as gynecomastia.

Transient gynecomastia associated with puberty, refeeding, and hemodialysis does not require any treatment. In many other cases, correction of the underlying disorder (hyperthyroidism or tumor) or withdrawal of a drug often leads to gradual regression of the breast enlargement and symptoms. Judicious administration of testosterone in patients with underlying hypogonadism can induce regression of gynecomastia (10). The use of antiestrogens (tamoxifen and clomiphene) has been reported with encouraging results in treatment of gynecomastia (17,39). Because of unpleasant side effects associated with the use of these agents, they should be used in selected patients and the duration of such treatment should not exceed six months (7). In a Chinese study, 80% of 61 men with idiopathic gynecomastia had complete regression when treated with tamoxifen; no adverse effects were observed over a median follow-up of 36 months (1). True gynecomastia must be distinguished from pseudogynecomastia due to the involvement of the breast by neurofibromatosis (215,216,221) or that associated with obesity. The latter is due to increased adipose tissue without the fibroepithelial proliferation typical of gynecomastia.

## CARCINOMA

### Primary Breast Carcinoma

According to the American Cancer Society, each year approximately 300 men die of breast carcinoma while 1,000 cases of male breast carcinoma are diagnosed annually in the United States (61). Mammary cancer constitutes 0.2% to 0.38% of all malignancies in men with an annual sex-specific incidence of 0.58 cases per 100,000 population (85,152). Carcinoma represents only 1% to 2% of all mammary cancers (105,184–187,192). The prevalence of male breast carcinoma is approximately 1% that of the female in the U.S. (26); this prevalence has not changed since 1930. In Denmark, male breast carcinoma comprises 0.8% of all breast carcinomas (158). In contrast, in China and Africa, where the rate of chronic liver disease due to cancer or parasites is relatively high, the incidence of male breast carcinoma appears to be higher (158). In Egypt, the ratio of male breast cancer is 5.1% that of the female population (48); this high percentage is attributed to hyperestrogenism secondary to bilharzial disease. The incidence of gynecomastia is also high in Egypt. In Zambia, where the incidence of female breast cancer is relatively low, the incidence of male breast carcinoma is among the highest in the world accounting for 15% of all breast cancers (60). The high incidence is again due to hyperestrogenism secondary to parasitic liver disease. In both countries, the age of onset is unusually young with a mean age of 41 years in the Egyptian patients and between 40 and 55 years of age for 77% of the Zambian men.

The first documented case report of male breast carcinoma has been accredited to Fabricus Hildanus (1573–1619) (141), but the lesion had been alluded to earlier in writings of John of Arderne (1307) who described what is now recognized as Paget's disease in the nipple of a priest, Franciscus Arcaeus (1493–1573), and in the writings of Ambroise Pare (1510–1590) (98). The rarity of male breast carcinoma was recognized in 1839 when Curveilhier (80) noted that "mammary cancer is as rare among men as it is frequent among women." One of the three cases Curveilhier described, occurred in a 40-year-old man who was cut on the breast by an epee while fighting a duel. The wound did not heal well. The scar tissue persisted around a painful area of induration, while the overlying skin gradually changed color and excoriated. Eventually, an ulcerating cancer became apparent. Recognition of a mammary tumor shortly following injury to the chest wall is not uncommon among men. While a number of series including a report on 406 tumors (86% of which were malignant) in the German literature (165), and another on 100 cases of carcinoma in the English literature (193) appeared subsequently, it was Wainwright's classic study of male breast carcinoma in 1927 that established the salient features which have remained basically unaltered by subsequent studies. Wainwright (192) noted that 1) men develop breast carcinoma at an older age than women; 2) the tumors are frequently centrally located below the nipple; 3) Paget's disease, ulceration, and involvement of the overlying skin are more common in men; 4) axillary metastases occur with about the same frequency as in women; 5) the varieties of carcinoma that occur in the male breast are morphologically indistinguishable from their female counterparts; and 6) men tend to seek treatment after a greater delay than do women. Consequently, men with breast carcinoma had a slightly worse prognosis than women. In both previous and subsequent reports, the age difference has been confirmed; in several studies, the mean age for male breast carcinoma ranged from 63 to 66 which is at least a decade older than that of women (53,106,135,138,149). Norris and Taylor (135) also found a large proportion of male breast carcinomas presenting with central, superficial lesions, and 12 of the 113 patients in their study had microscopic Paget's disease. Visfeldt and Scheike (191) concluded that histologic grade of the tumor influences the prognosis.

## Clinical Features

Patients range in age from 12 to 91 years with an average of around 60 years. In the Middle and Far East, the median age is younger (86,91). Most men with breast carcinoma present with a unilateral, painless subareolar mass which is discoid and sharply circumscribed (105). About 2% to 10% are discovered by physicians during routine physical examinations (161,162,172). Bilateral carcinomas occur and constitute up to 2.5% of cases (62,105). Bloody nipple discharge is more common in malignant lesions than in benign lesions; it was present in 20% of cases in Wolff and Reinin's series (196) and in up to 75% of carcinomas in an older study (187). In Geschickter's (96) experience, a mass was the symptom of the onset of disease in half of the patients, while changes in the nipple were the first noted alteration in the other half. The average duration of symptoms before presentation is approximately 12 months (67,172). The presenting symptoms and distribution into various stages has been more or less similar in various studies on male breast carcinoma (67,76,145,147).

## Gross and Microscopic Features

About half of the carcinomas reported by Scheike were smaller than 3 cm with a range of 1 to 3.8 cm.

The histologic varieties of breast carcinoma corresponds to those found in the female breast. A majority of male breast carcinomas are infiltrating duct carcinomas (105,135). With the notable exception of in situ and invasive lobular carcinoma, only one example of which has been documented in a man with Klinefelter's syndrome (155), all the usual and unusual histologic types (75,64,69,108,129,134,135, 150,156,176,197) including more than 50 examples (at least half of these were confirmed histologically) of Paget's disease (73,83,102,115) and secretory carcinoma (175) also occur in the male patient. The small cell carcinoma reported by Giffler & Kay (97) did not have an associated in situ lobular carcinoma. This case does not qualify as an invasive lobular carcinoma by the AFIP criteria, since we have observed ductal carcinoma composed of a small cell population invade in single files also. There were no lobular carcinomas among the 187 carcinomas reported by Visfeldt and Scheike (191) from Denmark. Thirty of their cases were carcinomas of special types (medullary, mucinous, cribriform, papillary); the remaining cases were infiltrating duct carcinoma. Of the latter, 150 had sufficient tissue for grading. The grade distribution of these cases was 29% grade I, 54% grade II, and 17% grade III. Breast carcinomas with neuroendocrine granules (argyrophilic carcinomas) have also been reported in the male breast (167). Argyrophilic cells have been demonstrated in 20.8% of male breast carcinomas compared to only 5% of female breast carcinomas (167). Inflammatory carcinoma occurs in 2% of men with breast carcinoma and is associated with a poor prognosis (183). In Heller et al's report (104) on 97 cases from the Memorial Hospital in New York, 87% of the cancers were infiltrating duct carcinoma. In Nigeria, papillary carcinoma is more common than in American and Danish males; mucinous carcinoma appears to be more common in Danish men than either Nigerian or American males (51).

In addition to all varieties of infiltrating carcinoma, with the exception of invasive lobular carcinoma, almost the entire range of patterns of intraductal carcinoma has also been observed in the male breast at AFIP.

## Hormone Receptors

The incidence of estrogen receptor positivity in male breast carcinomas appears to be higher than that in women. About 80% to 90% of men have ER+ tumors (71,73,90,94,102,118,148,195). Progesterone receptors (PR) are positive in 26% to 75% of cases (90,102,142, 151). Estrogen receptor positive cases respond to endocrine therapy in 50% to 60% of the cases. Bezwoda et al (59) found that for patients with metastatic disease, hormone receptor status was predictive of response to hormonal manipulation. Measurement of ER appears to be important in men with breast carcinoma as it may have important therapeutic and prognostic implications just as in women with breast carcinoma.

## Epidemiology

Risk factors that may play a role in the development of male breast cancer include hyperthyroidism, Klinefelter's syndrome, radiation, and chest wall trauma (74,76,90,128).

Familial or hereditary factors have not been recognized as major contributing factors in the development of breast carcinoma in men. Schwartz et al (166) reported breast carcinoma in a father and son both of which were of the papillary type. Kozak et al (113) reported breast carcinoma in two related men, an uncle and nephew and reviewed the literature on the subject. They found and tabulated 12 additional reports of breast cancer occurring in two related men (88,103,111,125,157,163,164,166,179,193). Of these, six had occurred in brothers and four in a father and son with or without an additional male family member. Information was available on ten families regarding presence of breast carcinoma in a female relative, and six (60%) had a female with breast carcinoma in the family. Eight (20%) of the patients in Wolff et al's series (196) had a female relative with breast carcinoma.

Hyperestrogenism, absolute or relative, has been implicated as a risk factor. Breast carcinoma occurs in patients with Klinefelter's syndrome (70,77,84,85). This condition is characterized by atrophic testis, hyalinized seminiferous tubules and aspermatogenesis. The buccal epithelium shows a 47 XXY (or mosaic) chromosome pattern. The breasts in this condition are hypertrophic, showing gynecomastia with lobule formation in some cases. Patients with Klinefelter's syndrome have a 6% incidence of mammary cancer (107); the risk for development of breast carcinoma in patients with Klinefelter's syndrome has been reported as almost 20 times that of normal males but it still remains far less than that of a woman (162). Men with the XX chromosome have also developed breast carcinoma (82,95). Breast cancer has been observed in a man with marked testicular atrophy 30 years after mumps orchitis (124,133,164). Baierl (57) reported a breast carcinoma which developed in a 52-year-old man given a total of 45 milligrams of diethystilbestrol over a six-week period for a gastric ulcer. O'Grady and McDivitt (136) also documented the appearance of Paget's disease of the breast in a 77-year-old male after six years of diethylstilbestrol treatment for prostatic carcinoma. In Egypt and Zambia, liver damage caused by *Schistosomiasis* and resulting in hyperestrogenism is associated with a higher frequency of male breast carcinoma (48,86). Two cases of breast carcinoma have been reported in men administered large doses of estrogens for deliberate alteration of secondary sexual characteristics (174).

Studies of estrogen metabolism in men with breast carcinoma have provided conflicting results. Scheike et al (160) noted no difference in the excretion pattern of urinary estrogen metabolites in men with breast carcinoma compared with control patients. Zumoff et al (199) and Dao et al (81) found elevated estriol production and lower levels of estrone, 2-hydroxyestrone, and 2-methoxyestrone in men with breast cancer compared to control patients. In a case control study of 75 men with breast carcinoma, Casagrande et al (68) found that men with a body weight of 80 kg or more at age 30 had twice the risk of developing breast carcinoma compared to a man weighing less than 60 kg at that age.

The association of gynecomastia with breast carcinoma has been variably reported as almost nonexistent (101,126) to being present in up to 20% to 40% of cases (98,104,128,162). The possibility that gynecomastia may even reflect a premalignant lesion was raised by Scheike and Visfeldt (162). Currently, gynecomastia is not considered a risk factor for subsequent development of breast carcinoma. Of 625 men with breast carcinoma gleaned from the literature by Crichlow (76), only 17 had gynecomastia. The high frequency of gynecomastia in the male population and the use of variable diagnostic criteria make determination of its role as a risk factor in the development of breast carcinoma ambiguous and difficult to assess.

Contrary to their expectation of a high rate of breast carcinoma in populations with low rates of prostate carcinoma, Sobin and Sherif noted a fairly direct rather than an inverse relation between the two (171).

Radiation exposure has been reported in men with breast carcinoma (76,79,100,123,137). Crichlow (76) found five cases in which carcinoma followed radiation therapy for eczema, gynecomastia, mediastinal lymphoma and benign breast disease. Thompson et al (180) described a 38-year-old man who developed breast carcinoma 30 years after chest radiation for metastatic osteogenic sarcoma. The risk associated with radiation exposure has not been established but may be similar to that reported previously in women (127,182).

## Recurrence and Metastases

Recurrences are relatively common. Recurrences and metastases have been noted in 25% of patients with stage I disease, rising to 71% of patients with stage II disease (146); Yap et al found almost identical statistics in their series (198). In Ehrlichman et al's series (87), 46 of 89 patients developed recurrence. When local recurrences develop, they generally do so within two years of the mastectomy procedure (146).

Almost half of the patients develop metastases. Forty-five (55.5%) of the 81 men in Spence et al's study (172) developed metastases; 27 (33.3%) metastasized to bone, 14 (17.3%) to the lungs, three (3.7%) to the liver, and one (1.2%) to the brain. Distant metastases occurred in 13 of 40 patients in Wolff et al's series (196) occurring from less than one year to 13 years after the diagnosis. In van Geel et al's (189) study of 104 men from Holland, axillary node metastases were present in 60%; local recurrences developed in 26%, and 16% developed distant metastases. The average time for distant metastases to develop is about three years (172). The most common sites for metastases in Wolff et al's study (196) were the lungs, skeleton, and central nervous system.

## Treatment

Though radical surgery (radical mastectomy or modified radical mastectomy) has been heralded as the treatment of choice and has constituted the standard approach to treatment of primary breast carcinoma in the past, Robison and Montague (147) have suggested that more limited surgery and irradiation controls the disease better than radical surgery, and results in less disability in the arm and shoulder. Conservative therapy of small carcinomas needs to be investigated.

Male breast cancer has a uniquely high frequency of response to endocrine manipulation and ablation (105). Therefore, orchiectomy (85,92,110,117,120,132, 178,184,185,192), and hypophysectomy (110,184) have been used in the management of men with breast carcinoma. Orchiectomy resulted in objective remission of advanced breast carcinoma in 28 of 48 patients reported by Treves (184). Kraybill et al (114) noted objective response to orchiectomy in 48% of the patients; they suggested that estrogen receptor determinations may be useful in selecting patients for orchiectomy and that selective additive hormone therapy may be useful in patients who refuse orchiectomy. Bilateral adrenalectomy has also been utilized as a palliative measure following orchiectomy (117). Chemotherapy may provide palliation in those who fail to respond to orchiectomy and adrenalectomy.

For patients with axillary node metastases, adjuvant chemotherapy similar to that used for female breast cancer with antiestrogen therapy in ER-positive patients has been advised (112). The central location of most male breast carcinomas leads to a high incidence of internal mammary lymph node metastases (58). Therefore, radiation therapy to the internal mammary chain of lymph nodes has been proposed as a reasonable approach by Kinne (112).

Because of the small number of male breast carcinomas treated with adjuvant chemotherapy at any given institution, the role of chemotherapy in advanced stages is yet to be determined. Complete or partial remission was noted in 48% of 31 men who were treated with tamoxifen for advanced breast carcinoma (140). Five of these tumors were ER+; four of them responded to tamoxifen therapy. None of the three patients with ER− tumors responded. Diethystilbestrol was used in another group of men with advanced breast carcinoma with a 38% response rate, and without significant undesirable side effects (146).

Preliminary studies suggest that combination chemotherapy gives a response rate comparable to that seen in women with breast carcinoma (59). Lichter and Lippman (119) were also encouraged by their results of adjuvant chemotherapy in treating men with node-positive breast carcinomas. Bagley et al (56) projected a five-year actuarial survival rate in excess of 80% for 24 men with axillary node metastases who received adjuvant therapy in the form of 12 cycles of cyclophosphamide, methotrexate, 5-fluorouracil (CMF), but no postoperative radiation. Four of these men developed recurrences 15, 45, 61, and 65 months following mastectomy. Lopez et al (122) obtained better results when adriamycin was included in the chemotherapeutic regimen. The overall response rate in their study of 48 patients which included patients with visceral metastases was 32%; the response rate was 50% for patients with less advanced metastatic disease. While these studies are promising, a multi-institutional approach and study of a larger group of men with longer follow-up is needed to better evaluate the value of specific chemotherapeutic agents in the treatment of advanced breast carcinoma.

## Survival and Prognosis

In many studies, particularly those from referral centers, breast cancer in men appears to have a worse prognosis than carcinoma occurring in the female breast with a five-year survival rate of less than 55% in many studies (72,87,120,135,144,146,152,159,172, 182). In Ehrlichman et al's series (87), the actuarial five-year, relapse-free survival was 45%; the median survival after recurrence was 1.16 years. In 1980, Ramantanes et al (144) from Greece reported a five-year survival of 32.5%. In 1985, Spence et al (172) reported overall five- and ten-year survival of 38% and 17% respectively, allowing for all causes of death. When only deaths from breast cancer were considered, corrected five- and ten-year survival was 52% and 29%. The survival was 46% at five years and 29% at ten years in Scheike's series (157). Others have reported five-year survival of 39% (158) and 47.8% (152).

There are a number of studies that do not support a worse prognosis for male breast cancer, however (139,191). The five- and ten-year survival for 29 Finnish men with breast carcinoma was 65% and 47% respectively when death from other causes was excluded from the calculations (54). In another study (50), the five- and ten-year survival was 66% and 52% among 406 Swedish men leading to the conclusion that except for a slightly higher mean age at diagnosis in males, there is a striking similarity in the natural history of breast cancer between men and women. In a study of 104 men from eight hospitals in Holland, van Geel et al (189) also concluded that the prognosis of male breast cancer is no worse than that of women with comparable disease; the five-year survival for the 104 men in the study was 54%, and the disease-free interval was 42%. All patients had at least five years of follow-up. The distribution of the tumors according to the TNM classification was stage I, 25%; stage II, 35%; stage III, 24%; and stage IV, 16%. In a previous study, Brunet et al (63) also provided data in which the prognosis was more favorable in men.

In Axelsson and Andersson's series (55) of 34 patients from Sweden, the overall corrected five-year survival was 54% and the ten-year survival was 37%. The prognosis was inversely related to positive axillary nodes, increasing stage, tumor size, tumor ulceration, fixation to the surrounding tissue, and worsening histologic grade. The histologic grade correlated with prognosis in Visfeldt and Scheike's study (191). The five-year survival was 58% for grade I, 37% for grade II, and 5% for grade III.

It appears that the prognosis can be improved if the disease is detected at an early stage. Vercoutre and O'Connell (190), compared the survival of 45 men from seven community hospitals with that of 2,620 women treated during the same period and found a survival advantage for the men. The five-year survival was 88%, and the disease-free rate was 76% for 17 patients with stage I disease who had five years of follow-up. For the 11 patients with stage II disease followed for five years, the five-year survival rate was 91%, with a disease-free survival rate of 73%. In their study, 55% of the men had stage I disease, 39% had stage II disease, and 6% had stage III disease. The better survival for the men in the study was attributed to the earlier stage of the disease for cases treated at community hospitals. In Heller et al's study (104), the ten-year survival for men with negative nodes was 79%, but it dropped drastically to a low 11% for those with positive nodes. Ouriel et al (136) reported five-year survival for stages I to IV as 80%, 67%, 25%, and 0 respectively. In West Africa, a five-year survival rate of 22% has been reported (52); this is thought to be due to the advanced stage of the tumors at presentation. Based on prolonged survival of 194 and 128 months observed in two of eight patients with stage IV disease, Siddiqui et al suggested that the presence of widespread disease may not indicate an immediately dismal prognosis (169). Yap et al (198) concluded that the size of the primary tumor, status of the axillary nodes, and fixation to either skin or pectoralis muscle constitute important prognostic factors. Cunha et al (78) found tumor size and peritumoral lymphatic permeation to have prognostic significance, but did not find tumor grade, as assessed by Bloom and Richardson's classification, to influence prognosis. A striking sex difference has been noted in the relation between age and relative survival. In males, the relative risk of dying from breast carcinoma is lower in patients less than 40 years of age at diagnosis in contrast to the worse prognosis for women younger than 40 years at diagnosis (49).

## Breast Metastases from Prostatic Carcinoma

The incidence of breast metastases from prostatic carcinoma is 5% (153). Distinction of prostatic carcinoma metastatic to the breast from primary mammary carcinoma can be a difficult task but generally most breast carcinomas appearing in the breast following treatment for prostatic carcinoma have been interpreted as representing metastases from the prostatic carcinoma (66,194). Only seven primary breast carcinomas concurrent with prostatic carcinoma have been reported in the English literature (130,131). The presence of bilaterality and multiple nodules would indicate a metastatic tumor. When the metastatic tumor presents as a solitary nodule, however, the morphologic distinction can sometimes be quite difficult since the tumor cells may proliferate within mammary ducts mimicking an in situ phase of the invasive component. The demonstration of acid phosphatase in the tumor cells would indicate a prostatic primary (168). Also, immunostains for antigens specific to prostatic carcinomas (prostate-specific antigen, PSA) has been proven useful in resolving this problem (99). Moldwin and Orihuela (130) recommended PSA screening on every clinically-evident breast carcinomas in all patients with prostatic carci-

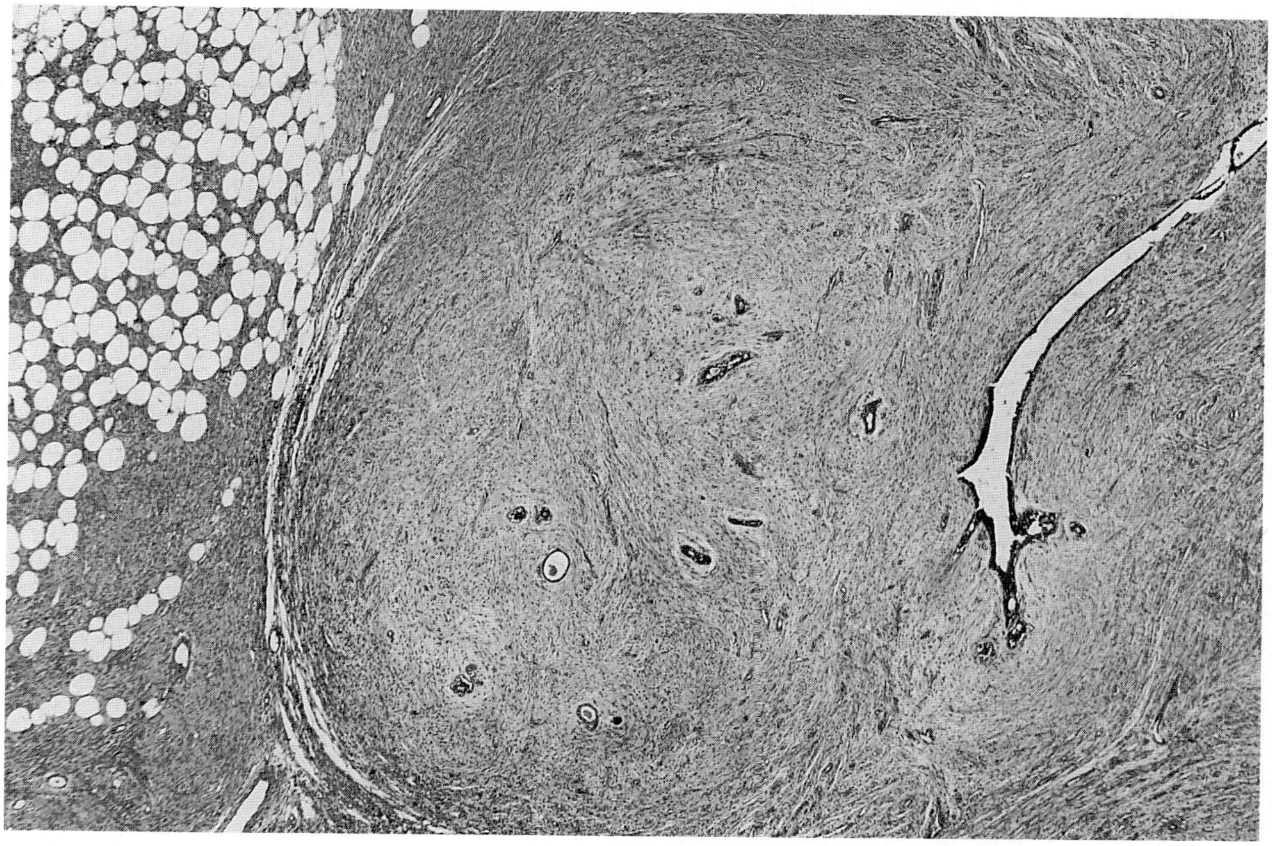

**Figure 16.8** Phyllodes tumor, high grade. This lesion was predominantly a sarcoma invading the adjacent adipose tissue, but the presence of clefts and smaller ducts lined by epithelial and myoepithelial cells focally, indicates a sarcomatous overgrowth within a cystosarcoma phyllodes. (H&E, X25) (Fig. 11.38c on page 465 is from the same patient.)

corded. The patients ranged in age from 19 to 79 with four patients over 50 years of age. Three of the men—19, 56, and 79 years of age—were Japanese, and the cases were contributed to AFIP by the Atomic Bomb Casualty Commission raising the possibility of radiation exposure playing a role in the development of the lesions; it is unclear whether or not the morphology of these cases had been confirmed at AFIP. Another patient, 71 years of age, had prostatic carcinoma. His treatment had included bilateral orchiectomy and estrogen therapy (Tace®, 12 mg daily) for three years prior to the development of the mammary nodule. Well-developed lobules were evident around the fibroadenoma. One other patient also had associated gynecomastia. He was a 61-year-old hypertensive male who had been on Aldomet® for many years followed by about 10 months of Aldoril®; Aldomet® is methyl dopa and Aldoril® is a mixture of methyldopa and chlordiazepoxide. He also had lobular development in the areas of gynecomastia. The seven tumors ranged in size from 1.5 to 4.5 cm. Their gross appearance was similar to that of fibroadenomas in the female breast. Microscopically, a combination of pericanalicular and intracanalicular growth patterns was observed in most lesions (Fig. 16.6).

Several isolated cases of cystosarcoma phyllodes (CP) have been reported as curiosities (205,207–209). All cases have occurred in middle-aged or elderly men. Advanced bilateral gynecomastia was present in the 71-year-old man reported by Nielsen and Andreasen (207). The patient in Reingold's series (209) had gynecomastia with lobule formation in the adjacent breast. There is only one definite cystosarcoma in the male breast in the files of AFIP. This lesion occurred in a 20-year-old boy who had a six year history of gynecomastia. He has had no recurrence of the low grade tumor three years after the diagnosis. Microscopically, the tumor was well delineated with well-developed leaf-like processes, mild to moderate stromal cellularity, focal stromal atypia, and epithelial hyperplasia (Fig. 16.7). A second lesion which probably reflects sarcomatous overgrowth in a cystosarcoma had infiltrating margins and lacked well-formed leaf-like processes (Fig. 16.8). This patient developed multiple recurrences and axillary "node" involvement (see Chapter 11, Biphasic Tumors).

## MISCELLANEOUS LESIONS

A variety of epithelial lesions including papilloma (220), sclerosing adenosis (213), fibrocystic changes (212,218), and nipple duct adenoma have been seen in the male breast (222,223). A papilloma has been described in a 71-year-old man with a ten-year history of phenothiazine therapy (220). Phenothiazine can cause elevation of serum prolactin levels, and the authors discussed the possible role of phenothiazine in the induction of the papilloma. A case of sclerosing adenosis was identified as a palpable 1.8 cm nodule at autopsy in a 41-year-old man who died from oat cell carcinoma of the lung (213). The authors discussed the possibility that lobular development followed by sclerosing adenosis could have been induced by tumor-elaborated hormones from the oat cell carcinoma. The nipple duct adenoma reported by Waldo et al (223) developed ten years after diethylstilbestrol treatment for carcinoma of the prostate. Even secretory, pregnancy-like changes have been reported in two of eight examples of gynecomastia showing lobular formation (36).

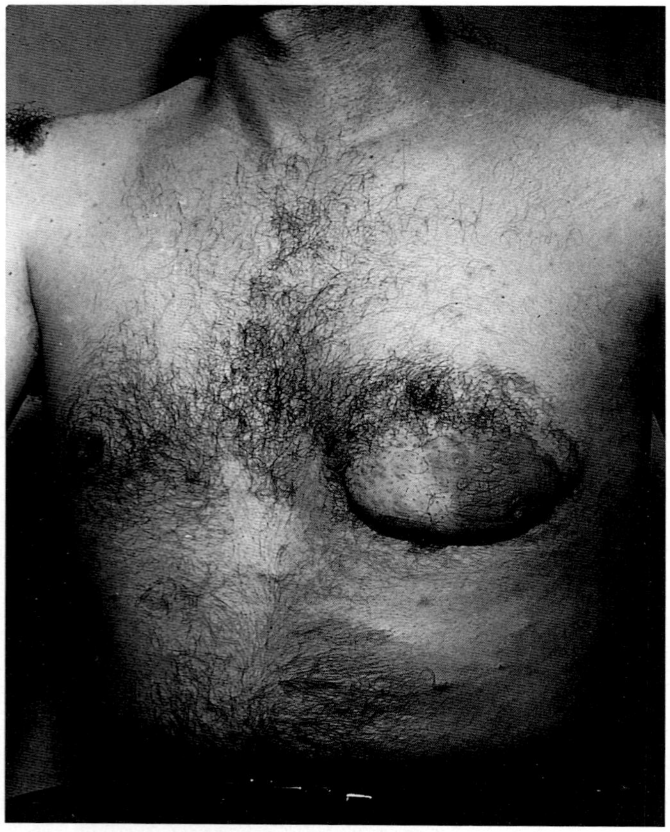

**Figure 16.9** Unilateral pseudogynecomastia secondary to a lymphangioma.

Among mesenchymal lesions, myofibroblastoma (214,224), a benign spindle cell tumor, is observed more frequently in the male breast compared to the female breast (see Chapter 13, Mesenchymal Tumors). Neurofibromatosis can involve the breast parenchyma and present as a unilateral or bilateral enlargement of the breast mimicking gynecomastia (215,216,221). Neal and Simpson (26) have reported a variety of benign lesions in the male breast including lipoma, hemangioma, and lymphangioma (Fig. 16.9). Angiomas and papillary intravascular endothelial proliferation have been observed in the male breast at AFIP, but intramammary angiosarcoma is extremely rare if it truly exists (see Chapter 12, Vascular Tumors). Massive bilateral fat necrosis has been reported in the male breast (207). An unusual giant cell tumor characterized by the proliferation of osteoclastic giant cells in a spindle cell background has been reported (217). The variety of mesenchymal tumors that occurs in the male breast is morphologically indistinguishable from those occurring in the female breast.

## REFERENCES

### Gynecomastia


1. Alagaratnam TT: Idiopathic gynecomastia treated with tamoxifen: a preliminary report. *Clin Ther* 1987;9:483–487.
2. * Andersen JA, Gram JB: Gynecomasty. *Acta Pathol Microbiol Immunol Scand [A]* 1982;90:185–190.
3. * Andersen JA, Gram JB: Male breast at autopsy. *Acta Pathol Microbiol Immunol Scand [A]* 1982;90:191–197.
4. * Bannayan GA, Hajdu SI: Gynecomastia: Clinicopathologic study of 351 cases. *Am J Clin Pathol* 1972;57:431–437.
5. Bassler R, Schafer A: Elektronenmikroskopische Cytomorphologie der Gynakormastie. *Virchows Arch Abt A (Pathol Anat)* 1969;348:356–373.
6. Becker KL, Matthews MJ, Higgins GA, et al: Histologic evidence of gynecomastia in hyperthyroidism. *Arch Pathol* 1974;98:257–260.
7. * Carlson HE: Gynecomastia. *N Engl J Med* 1980;303:795–799.
8. Chopra IJ, Tulchinsky D: Status of estrogen-androgen balance in hyperthyroid men with Graves' disease. *J Clin Endocrinol Metab* 1974;38:269–277.
9. Clark E: Spironolactone therapy and gynecomastia. *JAMA* 1965;163:157–158.
10. * Cole EW: Klinefelter syndrome and breast cancer. *Johns Hopkins Med J* 1976;138:102–108.
11. Fisher ER: Ultrastructure of the human breast and its disorders. *J Clin Pathol* 1979;32:1128–1134.
12. Glass AR, Berenberg J: Gynecomastia after chemotherapy for lymphoma. *Arch Intern Med* 1979;139:1048–1049.

13. Gottfried MR: Extensive squamous metaplasia in gynecomastia. *Arch Pathol Lab Med* 1986;110:971–973.

* 14. Haibech H, Rosenholtz MJ: Prepubertal gynecomastia with lobules and acini: A case report and review of the literature. *Am J Clin Pathol* 1983;80:252–255.

15. Hamilton CR Jr, Henkin RI, Wei G, et al: Olfactory status and response to clomiphene in male gondatrophin deficiency. *Ann Intern Med* 1973;78:47–55.

16. Hassan MO, Olaizola MY: Ultrastructural observations on gynecomastia. *Arch Pathol Lab Med* 1979;103:624–630.

17. Jefferys DB: Painful gynaecomastia treated with tamoxifen. *Br Med J* 1979;1:1119–1120.

18. Karsner HT: Gynecomastia. *Am J Pathol* 1946;22:235–247.

* 19. Lewinn EB: Gynecomastia during digitalis therapy. *N Engl J Med* 1953;248:316–319.

20. Lynch HT, Kaplan AR, Lynch JF: Klinefelter syndrome and cancer: A family study. *JAMA* 1974;229:809–811.

21. MacDonald PC, Madden JD, Brenner PF, et al: Origin of estrogen in normal men and in women with testicular feminization. *J Clin Endocrinol Metab* 1979;49:905–916.

22. Mann NM: Gynecomastia during therapy with spironolactone. *JAMA* 1963;184:778–780.

23. McDivitt RW, Stewart FW, Berg JW: *Tumors of the breast*, Fasc 2. Atlas of Tumor Pathology, second series, Washington, DC, Armed Forces Institute of Pathology, 1968, pp 106–107.

24. Menville JG: Gynecomastia. *Arch Surg* 1933;26:1054–1083.

25. Meyskens FL, Torney DC, Neifeld IP: Male breast cancer: A review. *Cancer Treat Rev* 1976;3:83–93.

26. Neal MP, Simpson BT: Diseases of the male breast. *J Mo State Assoc* 1930;27:565–570.

* 27. Nicolis GL, Modlinger RS, Gabrilone JL: A study of the histopathology of human gynecomastia. *J Clin Endocrinol* 1971;32:173–278.

28. Niewoehner CB, Nuttal FQ: Gynecomastia in a hospitalized male population. *Am J Med* 1984;77:633–638.

29. Nuttal FQ: Gynecomastia as a physical finding in normal men. *J Clin Endocrinol Metab* 1979;48:338–340.

* 30. Pages A, Ramos J: Contribution a l'etude des gynecomasties. A propos de 122 cas. *Ann Pathol* (Paris) 1984;4:137–142.

31. Paulsen CA, Gordon DL, Carpenter RW, et al: Klinefelter's syndrome and its variants: A hormonal and chromosomal study. *Recent Prog Horm Res* 1968;24:321–363.

* 32. Poulsen HS: Demonstration of hormonal sensitivity in gynaecomastic tissue by thymidine incorporation in vitro. *Acta Pathol Microbiol Scand (A)* 1977;85:19–24.

* 33. Rifka SM, Pita JC, Vigersky RA, et al: Interaction of digitalis and spironolactone with human sex steroid receptors. *J Clin Endocrinol Metab* 1977;46:338–344.

* 34. Scheike O, Visfeldt J, Peterson B: Male breast cancer. 3. Breast carcinoma in association with the Klinefelter's syndrome. *Acta Pathol Microbiol Scand (A)* 1973;81:352–358.

35. Schmitt GW, Shehadeh I, Sawin CT: Transient gynecomastia in chronic renal failure during chronic intermittent hemodialysis. *Ann Intern Med* 1968;69:73–79.

* 36. Schwartz CH, Wilens SL: The formation of acinar tissue in gynecomastia. *Am J Pathol* 1963;43:797–807.

37. Sherins RJ, Olweny CLM, Ziegler JL: Gynecomastia and gonadal dysfunction in adolescent boys treated with combination chemotherapy for Hodgkin's disease. *N Engl J Med* 1978;299:12–16.

* 38. Sirtori C, Veronesi U: Gynecomastia. A review of 218 cases. *Cancer* 1957;10:645–654.

39. Stepanas AV, Burnet RB, Harding PE, et al: Clomiphene in the treatment of pubertal-adolescent gynecomastia: a preliminary report. *J Pediatr* 1977;90:651–653.

40. Stepanas AV, Samaan NA, Schultz PN, et al: Endocrine studies in testicular tumor patients with and without gynecomastia: A report of 45 cases. *Cancer* 1978;41:112–118.

41. Sultan CH, Bressot N, Garandeau P, et al: Gynecomasties pubertaires persistantes. Etude biologique. *Sem Hop Paris* 1980;56:1923–1930.

42. Tseng A, Horning SJ, Freiha FS, et al: Gynecomastia in testicular cancer patients. Prognostic and therapeutic implications. *Cancer* 1985;56:2534–2538.

43. Turkington RW, Topper YJ: Androgen inhibition of mammary gland differentiation in vitro. *Endocrinology* 1967;80: 329–336.

* 44. Wheeler CE, Cawley EP, Gray HT, et al: Gynecomastia: A review and analysis of 160 cases. *Ann Intern Med* 1954;40: 985–1004.

* 45. Williams MJ: Gynecomastia: Its incidence, recognition, and host characterization in 447 autopsy cases. *Am J Med* 1963;34:103–112.

* 46. Wilson JD, Aiman J, MacDonald PC: Pathogenesis of gynecomastia. *Adv Intern Med* 1980;25:1–32.

47. Winters SJ, Banks JL, Loriaux DL: Cimetidine is an antiandrogen in the rat. *Gastroenterology* 1979;76:504–508.

### Male Breast Carcinoma

48. Abdel-Aziz MT, Abdel-Kader MM, Khattab M, et al: Urinary oestrogens in normal Egyptian subjects and in patients with bilharzial hepatosplenomegaly. *Acta Med Acad Sci Hung* 1973;30:79–90.

* 49. Adami HO, Hakulinen T, Ewertz M, et al: The survival pattern in male breast cancer. An analysis of 1,429 patients from the Nordic countries. *Cancer* 1989;64:1177–1182.

* 50. Adami HO, Holmberg L, Malker B, et al: Long-term survival in 406 males with breast cancer. *Br J Cancer*, 1985;52:99–103.

51. Aghadiuno PU: Cancer of the male breast: Analysis of forty-three cases in Ibadan, Nigeria. *Afr J Med Med Sci* 1987;16:15–26.

* 52. Ajayi DOS, Osegbe DN, Ademiluyi SA: Carcinoma of the male breast in West Africa and a review of world literature. *Cancer* 1982;50:1664–1667.

53. Alexander LL, Benninghoff DL, Camiel MR, et al: Mammary malignancy in the male. *JAMA* 1978;70:807–810.

* 54. Appelqvist P, Salmo M: Prognosis in carcinoma of the male breast. *Acta Chir Scand* 1982;148:499–502.

* 55. Axelsson J, Andersson A: Cancer of the male breast. *World J Surg* 1983;7:281–287.

* 56. Bagley CS, Wesley MN, Young RC, et al: Adjuvant chemotherapy in males with cancer of the breast. *Am J Clin Oncol* 1987;10:55–60.

57. Baierl W: Zur Frage der Mammacarcinom—Manifestierung nach Cyren-B-Behandlung beim. *Mann Med Klin* 1953;35: 1284.

* 58. Bavafa S, Reyes CV, Choudhury AM: Male breast carcinoma: An updated experience at a veterans administration hospital and review of the literature. *J Surg Oncol* 1983;24: 41–45.

* 59. Bezwoda WR, Hosdorffer C, Dansey R, et al: Breast cancer in men. Clinical features, hormone receptor status, and response to therapy. *Cancer* 1987;60:1337–1340.

60. Bhagwandeen SB: Carcinoma of the male breast in Zambia. *E Afr Med J* 1972;49:89–93.

61. Boring CC, Squires TS, Tong T: Cancer Statistics, 1992. *CA* 1992;42:19–38.

62. Brodie EM, King ER: Histologically different, synchronous, bilateral carcinoma of the male breast (a case report). *Cancer* 1974;34:1276–1277.

63. Brunet M, Jamin ML, Berlie J: Le cancer du sein chez l'homme. *Nouv Presse Med* 1977;6:720–724.

64. Bryant J: Male breast cancer: A case of apocrine carcinoma with psammoma bodies. *Hum Pathol* 1981;12:751–753.

65. Bussolati G, Papotti M, Sapino A, et al: Endocrine markers in argyrophilic carcinomas of the breast. *Am J Surg Pathol* 1987;11:248–256.

66. Campbell JH, Cummins SD: Metastases, simulating mammary cancer, in prostatic carcinoma under estrogenic therapy. *Cancer* 1951;4:303–311.

67. Carlsson G, Haftstrom L, Jonsson PE: Male breast cancer. *Clin Oncol* 1981;7:149–155.

* 68. Casagrande JT, Hanisch R, Pike MC, et al: A case-control study of male breast cancer. *Cancer Res* 1988;48:1326–1330.

69. Cole FM, Qizilbash AH: Carcinoma in situ of the male breast. *J Clin Pathol* 1979;32:1128–1134.

70. Coley GM, Otis RD, Clark WS: Multiple primary tumors including bilateral breast cancers in a man with Klinefelter's syndrome. *Cancer* 1971;27:1476–1481.

* 71. Contesso G, Delarue JC, Guerinot F, et al: Recepteurs aux estrogens et aux progestogenes en pathologie mammaire chez l'homme. *Nouv Presse Med* 1977;6:1951–1963.

72. Cortese AF, Cornell GN: Carcinoma of the male breast. *Ann Surg* 1971;173:275–280.

73. Crews CF, Metropol HJ: Breast cancer in men. *J SC Med Assoc* 1984;80:115–118.

* 74. Crichlow RW: Carcinoma of the male breast. *Surg Gynecol Obstet* 1972;134:1011–1019.

* 75. Crichlow RW, Czernobilsky B: Paget's disease of the male breast. *Cancer* 1969;24:1033–1040.

* 76. Crichlow RW, Kaplan EL, Kearney WH: Male mammary cancer: An analysis of 32 cases. *Ann Surg* 1972;175:489–494.

77. Cuenca CR, Becker KL: Klinefelter's syndrome and cancer of the breast. *Arch Intern Med* 1968;121:159–162.

78. Cunha F, Andre S, Soares J: Morphology of male breast carcinoma in the evaluation of prognosis. *Path Res Pract* 1990;186:745–750.

79. Curtin CT, McHeffy B, Kolarsick AJ: Thyroid and breast cancer following childhood radiation. *Cancer* 1977;40:2911–2913.

* 80. Cruveilhier J: *Anatomie Pathologique de Corps Human*. Paris, JB Bailliere, 1839, pp 1–5.

81. Dao TL, Morreal CE, Nemoto T: Urinary estrogen excretion in men with breast cancer. *N Engl J Med* 1973;289:138–140.

82. Decker JB, Lerner HJ, Schwartz I: Breast carcinoma in a 46XX true hermaphrodite. *Cancer* 1982;49:1481–1484.

83. Ding W, De-Yan W: Paget's disease of the male breast: A report of five cases and a collective review. *Jpn J Clin Oncol* 1981;11:513–516.

84. Dodge OG, Jackson AW, Muldal S, et al: Breast cancer and interstitial-cell tumor in a patient with Klinefelter's syndrome. *Cancer* 1969;22:1027–1032.

* 85. Donegan WL, Perez-Mesa CM: Carcinoma of the male breast. *Arch Surg* 1973;106:273–279.

86. El-Gazayerli MM, Abdel-Aziz AS: On Bilharziasis and male breast cancer in Egypt: A preliminary report and review of literature. *Br J Cancer* 1963;17:566–571.

87. Erlichman C, Murphy L, Elharkin T: Male breast cancer. A 13-year review of 89 patients. *J Clin Oncol* 1984;2:903–909.

* 88. Everson RR, Fraumeni JF, Wilson RE, et al: Familial male breast cancer. *Lancet* 1976;1:9–12.

* 89. Everson RB, Lippman ME: Male breast cancer, in McGuire WL, (ed): *Breast Cancer: Current Topics*, vol 3. New York, Plenum, 1979, pp 239–267.

* 90. Everson RB, Lippman ME, Thompson EB: Clinical correlations of steroid receptors and male breast cancer. *Cancer Res* 1980;40:991–997.

91. Falsafi A: Cancer du sein chez l'homme. *Ann Chir* 1977;31: 957–960.

92. Farrow JH, Adair FE: Effect of orchiectomy on skeletal metastases from cancer of the male breast. *Science* 1942;95: 654.

* 93. Fetissof F, Dubois MP, Arbeille-Brassart B, et al: Argyrophilic cells in mammary carcinoma. *Hum Pathol* 1983;14: 127–134.

94. Friedman MA, Hoffman PG, Dandolos EM, et al: Estrogen receptors in male breast cancer: Clinical and pathologic correlations. *Cancer* 1981;47:134–137.

95. Giammarini A, Rocchi M, Zennaro W, et al: XX male with breast cancer. *Clin Genet* 1980;18:103–108.

* 96. Geschickter CF: *Diseases of the Breast. Diagnosis, Pathology, Treatment*, ed 2. Philadelphia, JB Lippincott Co, 1945, pp 616–633.

97. Giffler RF, Kay S: Small-cell carcinoma of the male mammary gland. A tumor resembling infiltrating lobular carcinoma. *Am J Clin Pathol* 1976;66:715–722.

98. Gilbert JB: Carcinoma of male breast: With special reference to etiology. *Surg Gynecol Obstet* 1933;57:451–466.

* 99. Green LK, Klima M: The use of immunocytochemistry in metastatic prostatic adenocarcinoma to the breast. *Hum Pathol* 1991;22:242–246.

100. Greene MH, Goedert JJ, Bech-Hansen NT, et al: Radiogenic male breast cancer with in vitro sensitivity to ionizing radiation and bleomycin. *Cancer Invest* 1983;1:379–386.

101. Greening WP, Aichroth PM: Cancer of the male breast. *Br J Cancer* 1965;19:92–100.

102. Gupta S, Khanna NN, Khanna S, et al: Paget's disease of the male breast: A clinicopathologic study and a collective review. *J Surg Oncol* 1983;22:151–156.

*103. Haagensen CD: *Diseases of the Breast*, ed 2. Philadelphia, WB Saunders, 1986, pp 776–990.

*104. Heller KS, Rosen PP, Schottenfeld D, et al: Male breast cancer: A clinicopathologic study of 97 cases. *Ann Surg* 1978;188:60–65.

105. Holleb AI, Freeman HP, Farrow JH: Cancer of the male breast. *NY State J Med* 1968;68:544–656.

106. Huggins C, Taylor GW: Carcinoma of male breast. *AMA Arch Surg* 1955;70:303–308.

107. Jackson AW, Muldal S, O'Key C, et al: Carcinoma of male breast in association with the Klinefelter syndrome. *Br Med J* 1965;1:223–225.

108. Jundt G, Schultz A, Heitz Ph U, et al: Small cell neuroendocrine (oat cell) carcinoma of the male breast. *Virchows Archiv (Pathol Anat)* 1984;404:213–221.

109. Kaneko H, Hojo H, Ishikawa S, et al: Norepinephrine-producing tumors of bilateral breast. *Cancer* 1978;14:2002–2007.

110. Kennedy BJ, Kiang DT: Hypophysectomy in the treatment of advanced cancer of the male breast. *Cancer* 1972;29:1606–1612.

111. King R, Arthur D, Lerner I: Familial breast cancer: Affected males and a female in one family (abstr). *Am J Hum Gen* 1983;35;65A.

*112. Kinne DW: Male breast cancer, in Harris JR, Hellman S, Henderson IC, et al (eds): *Breast Disease*. Philadelphia, JB Lippincott, 1987, pp 577–583.

*113. Kozak FK, Hall JG, Baird PA: Familial breast cancer in males. A case report and review of the literature. *Cancer* 1986;58:2736–2739.

114. Kraybill WG, Kaufman R, Kinne D: Treatment of advanced male breast cancer. *Cancer* 1981;47:2185–2189.

115. Lancer HA, Moschella SL: Paget's disease of the male breast. *Am Acad Dermatol* 1982;7:393–396.

116. Langlands AO, Maclean N, Kerr GR: Carcinoma of the male breast: Report of a series of 88 cases. *Clin Radiol* 1976;27:21–25.

117. Li MC, Janelli DE, Kelly EJ, et al: Metastatic carcinoma of the male breast treated with bilateral adrenalectomy and chemotherapy. *Cancer* 1970;25:678–681.

118. Leclercq C, Verhest A, DeBoel MC, et al: Oestrogen receptors in male breast cancer. *Biol Med Exp* 1976;25:327–330.

*119. Lichter AS, Lippman ME: Special situations in the treatment of breast cancer, in Lippman ME, Lichter AS, Danforth DN (eds): *Diagnosis and Management of Breast Cancer*. Philadelphia, WB Saunders Co, 1988, pp 425–438.

120. Leichty RD, Davis J, Gleysteen J: Cancer of the male breast: Forty cases. *Cancer* 1967;20:1617–1624.

121. Lippman ME, Allegra JC, Thompson EB, et al: The relation between estrogen receptors and response rate to cytotoxic chemotherapy in metastatic breast cancer. *N Engl J Med* 1978;298:1223–1228.

*122. Lopez M, Dilauro L, Lazzaro B, et al: Hormonal treatment of disseminated male breast cancer. *Oncology* 1985;42:345–399.

123. Lowell DM, Martineau RC, Luria SB: Carcinoma of the male breast following radiation. *Cancer* 1968;22:581–586.

*124. Mabuchi K, Bross DS, Kessler II: Risk factors for male breast cancer. *J Natl Cancer Inst* 1985;74:371–375.

125. Marger DM, Urdanta N, Fischer JJ: Breast cancer in brothers. *Cancer* 1975;36:458–461.

126. McDivitt RW, Stewart FW, Berg JW: *Tumors of the breast*, Fasc 2. Atlas of Tumor pathology, second series. Washington DC, Armed Forces Institute of Pathology, 1968, pp 105–111.

127. McGregor DH, Land LE, Choi K, et al: Breast cancer incidence among atomic bomb survivors. *J Natl Cancer Inst* 1977;59:799–811.

128. Meyskens FL Jr, Tormey DC, Neifeld JP: Male breast cancer: A review. *Cancer Treat Rev* 1976;3:83–93.

129. Miliauskas JR, Leong A S-Y: Adenoid cystic carcinoma in a juvenile male breast. *Pathology* 1991;23:298–301.

*130. Moldwin RM, Orihuela E: Breast masses associated with adenocarcinoma of the prostate. *Cancer* 1989;63:2229–2233.

131. Mostofi FK, Price EB Jr: *Tumors of the Male Genital System*. Washington DC, Armed Forces Institute of Pathology, 1973, p 239.

132. Neifeld JP, Meyskens F, Tormey DC, et al: The role of orchiectomy in the management of male breast cancer. *Cancer* 1976;37:992–995.

133. Nicolis GL, Sabetghadam R, Hsu CCS, et al: Breast cancer after mumps orchitis. *JAMA* 1973;223:1032–1033.

134. Noguchi M, Miwa K, Miyazaki I: Intracystic carcinoma of the breast in an elderly man. *Jpn J Surg* 1983;13:519–523.

*135. Norris HJ, Taylor HB: Carcinoma of the male breast. *Cancer* 1969;23:1428–1435.

136. O'Grady WP, McDivitt RW: Breast cancer in a man treated with diethylstilbestrol. *Arch Pathol* 1969;88:162–165.

137. Orme SK, Chambers RW, Johnson RH: Postradiation carcinoma of male breast bilaterally. *JAMA* 1967;201(9):137.

*138. Ouriel K, Lotze MT, Hinshaw JR: Prognostic factors of carcinoma of the male breast. *Surg Gynecol Obstet* 1984;159:373–376.

139. Panettiere FJ: Cancer in the male breast. *Cancer* 1974;34:1324–1327.

140. Patterson JS, Battersby LA, Bach BK: Use of tamoxifen in advanced male breast cancer. *Cancer Treat Rep* 1980;64:801–804.

141. Peck ME: Malignant tumors of the male breast. *Surg Clin North Am* 1944;24:1108–1125.

142. Pegaroro RJ, Nirmul D, Joubert SM: Cytoplasmic and nuclear estrogen and progesterone receptors in male breast cancer. *Cancer Res* 1982;42:4812–4814.

143. Ramantanes G, Besbeas S, Garas JG: Breast cancer in the male: A report of 138 cases. *World J Surg* 1980;4:621–624.

144. Ravinsky E, Cavers DJ: Cytology of argyrophilic carcinoma of the breast. *Acta Cytol* 1985;29:1–6.

*145. Ribeiro GG: Carcinoma of the male breast: A review of 200 cases. *Br J Surg* 1977;64:381–383.

146. Ribeiro GG: The result of diethylstilbestrol therapy for recurrent and metastatic carcinoma of the male breast. *Br J Cancer* 1976;33:465–467.

*147. Robison R, Montague ED: Treatment results in males with breast cancer. *Cancer* 1982;49:403–406.

148. Rosen PP, Menendez-Botet CJ, Nisselbaum JS, et al: Estrogen receptor protein in lesions of the male breast. A preliminary report. *Cancer* 1976;37:1866–1868.

149. Roswit B, Edlis H: Carcinoma of the male breast: A thirty year experience and literature review. *Int J Radn Oncol Bio Phys* 1978;4:711–716.

150. Roth JA, Discafani C, O'Malley M: Secretory breast carcinoma in a man. *Am J Surg Pathol* 1988;12:150–154.

151. Ruff SJ, Bauer JE, Keenan EJ, et al: Hormone receptors in male breast carcinoma. *J Surg Oncol* 1981;18:55–59.

*152. Sachs MD: Carcinoma of the male breast. *Radiology* 1941; 37:458–467.

153. Salyer WR, Salyer DC: Metastases of prostatic carcinoma to the breast. *J Urol* 1973;109:671–675.

154. Salzstein EC, Tavaf AM, Latorraca R: Breast carcinoma in a young man. *Arch Surg* 1978;113:880–881.

155. Sanchez AG, Villanueva AG, Redondo C: Lobular carcinoma of the breast in a patient with Klinefelter's syndrome. *Cancer* 1986;57:1181–1183.

156. Satiani N, Powell RW, Mathews WH: Paget's disease of the male breast. *Arch Surg* 1977;112:587–592.

*157. Scheike O: Male breast cancer. *Acta Pathol Microbiol Scand (A)* 1975;251(suppl):1–35.

*158. Scheike O: Male breast cancer. 5. Clinical manifestations in 257 cases in Denmark. *Br J Cancer* 1973;28:552–561.

*159. Scheike O: Male breast cancer. 6. Factors influencing prognosis. *Br J Surg* 1974;39:296–303.

*160. Scheike O, Sventrup B, Frandsen VA: Metabolism of oestradiol-17B in men with breast cancer. *J Steroid Biochem* 1973;4:489–501.

*161. Scheike O, Visfeldt J, Petersen B: Male breast cancer. 3. Breast carcinoma in association with the Klinefelter syndrome. *Acta Pathol Microbiol Scand (A)*. 1973;81:352–358.

*162. Scheike O, Visfeldt J: Male breast cancer. 4. Gynecomastia in patients with breast cancer. *Acta Pathol Microbiol Scand (A)* 1973;8:359–365.

163. Schmitt G, Scheffer J: Das Karzinom der Mannlichen Brustdruse. *Dtsch Med Wochenschr* 1971;96:931–937.

164. Schottenfeld D, Lilienfeld AM, Diamond H: Some observations on the epidemiology of breast cancer among males. *Am J Pub Health* 1963;53:890–897.

165. Schuchardt B: Weiterer fall von Krebs der mannlichen brustdruse. *Arch Klin Chir* 1886;33:529.

166. Schwartz RM, Newell RB, Hauch JF, et al: A study of familial male breast carcinoma and a second report. *Cancer* 1980;46:2697–2701.

167. Scopsi L, Andreola S, Saccozzi R, et al: Argyrophilic carcinoma of the male breast. A neuroendocrine tumor containing predominantly chromogranin B (Secretogranin I). *Am J Surg Pathol* 1991;15:1063–1071.

168. Scott J, Robb-Smith AHT, Burns I: Bilateral breast metastases from carcinoma of the prostate. *Br J Urol* 1974;46:209–214.

169. Siddiqui T, Weiner R, Moreb J, et al: Cancer of the male breast with prolonged survival. *Cancer* 1988;62:1632–1636.

170. Slack RWT: The survival rate of men with carcinoma of the breast. *Br J Surg* 1975;62:963–965.

171. Sobin LH, Sherif M: Relation between male cancer and prostatic cancer. *Br J Cancer* 1980;42:787–790.

172. Spence RAJ, MacKenzie G, Anderson JR, et al: Long-term survival following cancer of the male breast in Northern Ireland. A report of 81 cases. *Cancer* 1985;55:648–652.

173. Stephenson TR, Gordon HE: Primary carcinoma of the male breast. *Arch Surg* 1974;30:261–270.

174. Symmers WS: Carcinoma of breast in transsexual individuals after surgical and hormonal interference with the primary and secondary sex characteristics. *Br Med J* 1968; 2:82–85.

175. Tavassoli FA, Norris HJ: Secretory carcinoma of the breast. *Cancer* 1980;45:2404–2413.

176. Taxy J: Tubular carcinoma in male breast: Report of a case. *Cancer* 1975;36:462–465.

177. Taylor HB: *ASCP Seminar in Breast Pathology*. Chicago, ASCP, 1956.

178. Taylor SG, Li MC, Eckles EJ, et al: Effect of surgical Addison's disease on advanced carcinoma of the breast and prostate. *Cancer* 1953;6:997–1009.

179. Teasdale C, Forbes JF, Baum M: Familial male breast cancer. *Lancet* 1976;1:360–361.

180. Thompson DK, Li FP, Cassady JR: Breast cancer in a man 30 years after radiation for metastatic osteogenic sarcoma. *Cancer* 1979;44:2362–2365.

181. Togoshima S: Mammary carcinoma with argyrophilic cells. *Cancer* 1983;52:2129–2138.

182. Tokunaga M, Norman JE, Asano M, et al: Malignant breast tumors among atomic bomb survivors. *J Natl Cancer Inst* 1979;62:1347–1359.

183. Treves N: Inflammatory carcinoma of the breast in the male patient. *Surgery* 1953;34:810–820.

*184. Treves N: The treatment of cancer, especially inoperable cancer, of the male breast by ablative surgery (orchiectomy, adrenalectomy, and hypophysectomy) and hormone therapy (estrogens and corticosteroids). An analysis of 42 patients. *Cancer* 1959;12:820–832.

*185. Treves N, Abel JC, Woodward HQ, et al: The role of orchiectomy in the management of male breast cancer. *Cancer* 1976;37:992–995.

*186. Treves N, Holleb AI: Cancer of the male breast. *Cancer* 1955;8:1239–1250.

*187. Treves N, Robbins GF, Amoroso WL: Serous and serosanguinous discharge from the male nipple. *Arch Surg* 1956; 73:319–329.

188. Vanderbilt PC, Warren SE: Forty-year experience with carcinoma of the male breast. *Surg Gynecol Obstet* 1971;133: 629.

*189. van Geel AN, van Slooten EA, Mavrunac M, et al: A retrospective study of male breast cancer in Holland. *Br J Surg* 1985;72:724–727.

*190. Vercoutere AL, O'Connell TX: Carcinoma of the male breast. An update. *Arch Surg* 1984;119:1301–1304.

*191. Visfeldt J, Scheike O: Male breast cancer. I. Histologic typing and grading of 187 Danish cases. *Cancer* 1973;32: 985–990.

*192. Wainwright JM: Carcinoma of the male breast. *Arch Surg* 1927;14:836–859.

*193. Williams WR: Cancer of the male breast: Based on the records of one hundred cases; with remarks. *Lancet* 1889; 2:261.

194. Wilson SE, Hutchinson WB: Breast masses in males with carcinoma of the prostate. *J Surg Oncol* 1976;8:105–112.

195. Witliff JL: Specific receptors of the steroid hormones in breast cancer. *Semin Oncol* 1974;1:109–118.

*196. Wolff M, Reinin MS: Breast cancer in the male: Clinicopathological study of 40 patients and review of the literature, in Fenoglio CM, Wolff M (eds): *Progress in Surgical Pathology*, Chap 4, vol III. New York, Masson, 1983, pp 77–109.

197. Yogore MG III, Sahgal S: Small cell carcinoma of the male breast. Report of a case. *Cancer* 1977;39:1748–1751.

198. Yap HY, Tashima CK, Blumenschein GR, et al: Male breast cancer. A natural history study. *Cancer* 1979;44:748–754.

199. Zumoff B, Fishman J, Cassouto J, et al: Estradiol transformation in men with breast cancer. *J Clin Endocr* 1966;26: 960–966.

### Biphasic Tumors

*200. Ansah-Boateng Y, Tavassoli FA: Fibroadenoma and cystosarcoma phyllodes of the male breast. *Mod Pathol* 1992;5: 114–116.

201. Cholnosky T: Benign fibrous tumor of the male breast. *Am J Surg* 1935;30:298–304.

*202. Geschickter CF: *Diseases of the Breast. Diagnosis, Pathology, Treatment*. Philadelphia, JB Lippincott, 1945, pp 617–619.

203. Gurther H: Der organoide character des fibroadenomes der Mamma. *Langenbecks Arch Chir* 1939;194:312–325.

*204. Hilton DA, Jameson JS, Furness PN: A cellular fibroadenoma resembling a benign phyllodes tumor in a young male with gynecomastia. *Histopathology* 1991;18:476–477.

205. Lee BJ, Pack GT: Giant intracanalicular fibroadenomyxoma of the breast. The so-called cystosarcoma phyllodes mammae of Johannes Muller. *Am J Cancer* 1931;15:2583–2609.

*206. Nielsen BB: Fibroadenomatoid hyperplasia of the male breast. *Am J Surg Pathol* 1990;14:774–777.

*207. Nielsen VT, Andreasen C: Phyllodes tumor of the male breast. *Histopathology* 1987;11:761–765.

208. Pantoja E, Llobert RE, Lopez E: Gigantic cystosarcoma phyllodes in a man with gynecomastia. *Arch Surg* 1976;111: 611.

*209. Reingold IM, Ascher GS: Cystosarcoma phyllodes in a man with gynecomastia. *Am J Clin Pathol* 1970;53:852–856.

210. Rud H: Om fibro-adenoma mammae hos maend. *Hospitalstidende* 1922;65:253–266.

211. Rud H: Om fibro-adenoma mammae hos maend. *Hospitalstidende* 1922;65:269–274.

### Miscellaneous

*212. Banik S, Hale R: Fibrocystic disease in the male breast. *Histopathology* 1988;12:214–216.

213. Bigotti G, Kasznica J: Sclerosing adenosis in the breast of a man with pulmonary oat cell carcinoma: Report of a case. *Hum Pathol* 1986;17:861–863.

214. Boger A: Benign spindle cell tumor of the male breast. *J Pathol* 1990;161:1–2.

215. Lacombe MA: Gynecomastia in neurofibromatosis. Report of a case. *J Maine Med Assoc* 1976;67:334–344.

216. Lipper S, Willson CF, Copeland KC: Pseudogynecomastia due to neurofibromatosis—a light microscopic and ultrastructural study. *Hum Pathol* 1981;12:755–759.

217. Lucas J, Sharma HM, O'Toole HV: Unusual giant cell tumor arising in a male breast. *Hum Pathol* 1981;12:840–845.

218. McClure J, Banerjee SS, Sandilands DGD: Female type cystic hyperplasia in a male breast. *Postgrad Med J* 1985;61: 441–443.

219. Nielsen BB, Fenger C, Kjeldsen H: Massive bilateral fat necrosis of the male breast. *Breast* 1984;10:2–4.

220. Sara AS, Gottfried MR: Benign papilloma of the male breast following chronic pheothiazine therapy. *Am J Clin Pathol* 1987;87:649–650.

221. Solomon L, Kim YH, Reiner L: Neurofibromatous pseudogynecomastia associated with prepubertal idiopathic gynecomastia. *NY State J Med* 1976;76:932–935.

222. Taylor HB, Robertson AG: Adenomas of the nipple. *Cancer* 1965;18:995–1002.

223. Waldo ED, Sidhu GS, Hu AW: Florid papillomatosis of male nipple after diethylstilbestrol therapy. *Arch Pathol* 1975;99:364–366.

224. Wargotz ES, Weiss SW, Norris HJ: Myofibroblastoma of the breast. Sixteen cases of a distinctive benign mesenchymal tumor. *Am J Surg Pathol* 1987;11:493–502.

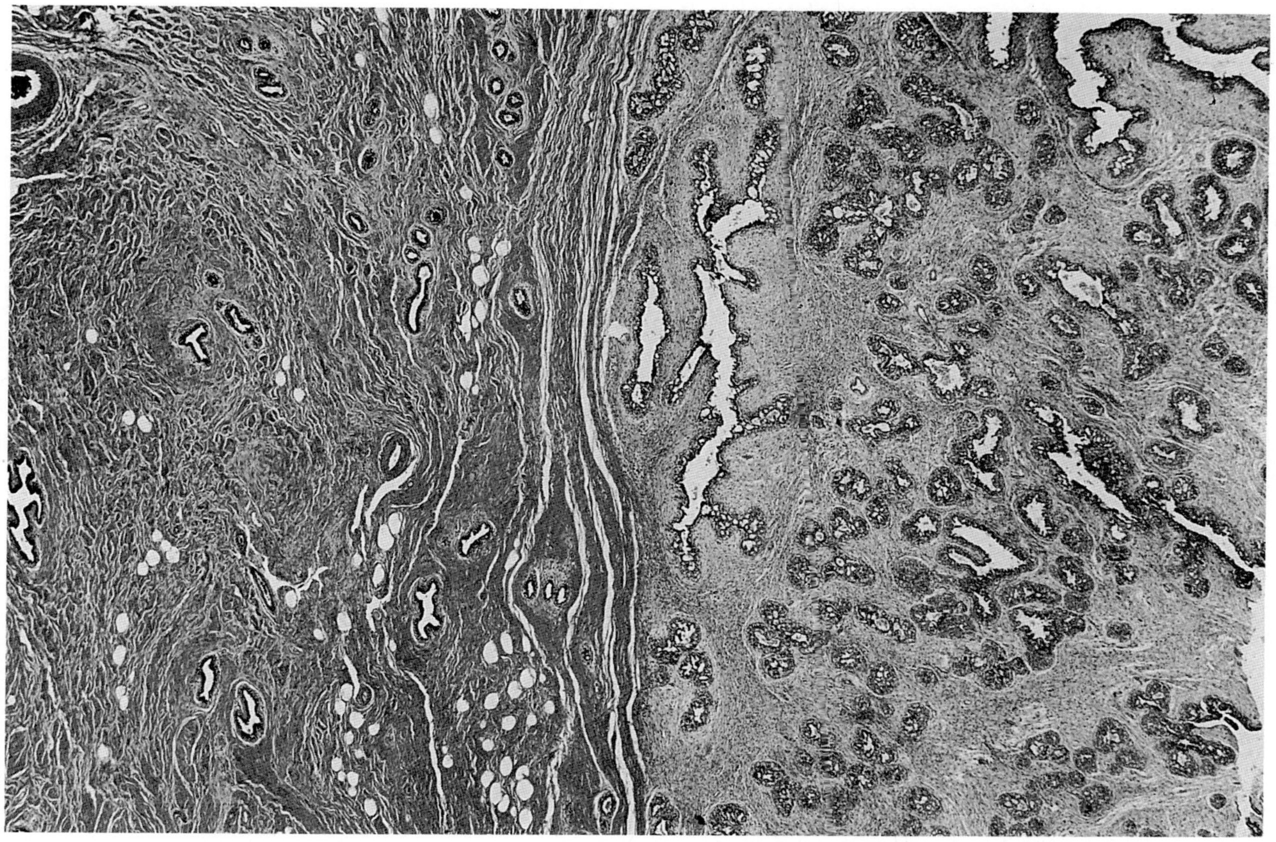

**Figure 16.6** Fibroadenoma in a background of fibrous gynecomastia. The fibroadenoma shows predominance of the pericanalicular growth pattern. (H&E, X30)

noma. This is a small step that can assure proper treatment of the patient. An incorrect diagnosis of metastatic prostate carcinoma in a patient with localized disease while missing a primary breast carcinoma may have disastrous consequences in terms of the patient's management and treatment.

## BIPHASIC TUMORS

Biphasic tumors are rare in the male breast. Reports of either fibroadenoma or cystosarcoma phyllodes (phyllodes tumor) in the breast are scant, sometimes not well documented, and consist of an occasional case report (201–211). Some pathologists have considered the term "fibroadenoma" appropriate for gynecomastia (202). A very interesting case of bilateral, massive fibroadenomatoid hyperplasia of the male breast occurring in a 69-year-old man who had been treated with digoxin for 27 years and spironolactone for four years was reported by Nielsen (206). The breasts had become enlarged and pedunculated measuring 16 cm in diameter. The cut surface showed multiple nodules measuring 0.5 to 3 cm in diameter. Microscopically, some of the nodules had the pericanalicular, while others had the intracanalicular, pattern of fibroadenoma. Well-formed lobules were present elsewhere in the surrounding breast tissue. Since the breast enlargement developed during the four years when spironolactone was added to the patient's medications, Nielsen concluded that spironolactone was the most likely causative agent, with digoxin and liver insufficiency acting as contributing factors.

One of the reasons for the rarity of fibroadenomas in the breast is that fibroadenomas originate in lobules and lobular development is exceedingly rare, even in the hormonally-stimulated male breast. While the origin and mechanism of development of cystosarcomas is not as clearly established, it undoubtedly parallels that of fibroadenomas, except for the more cellular and, at times, clearly sarcomatous appearance of the stromal cells.

In a search of AFIP files, seven examples of fibroadenoma occurring in the male breast were re-

A

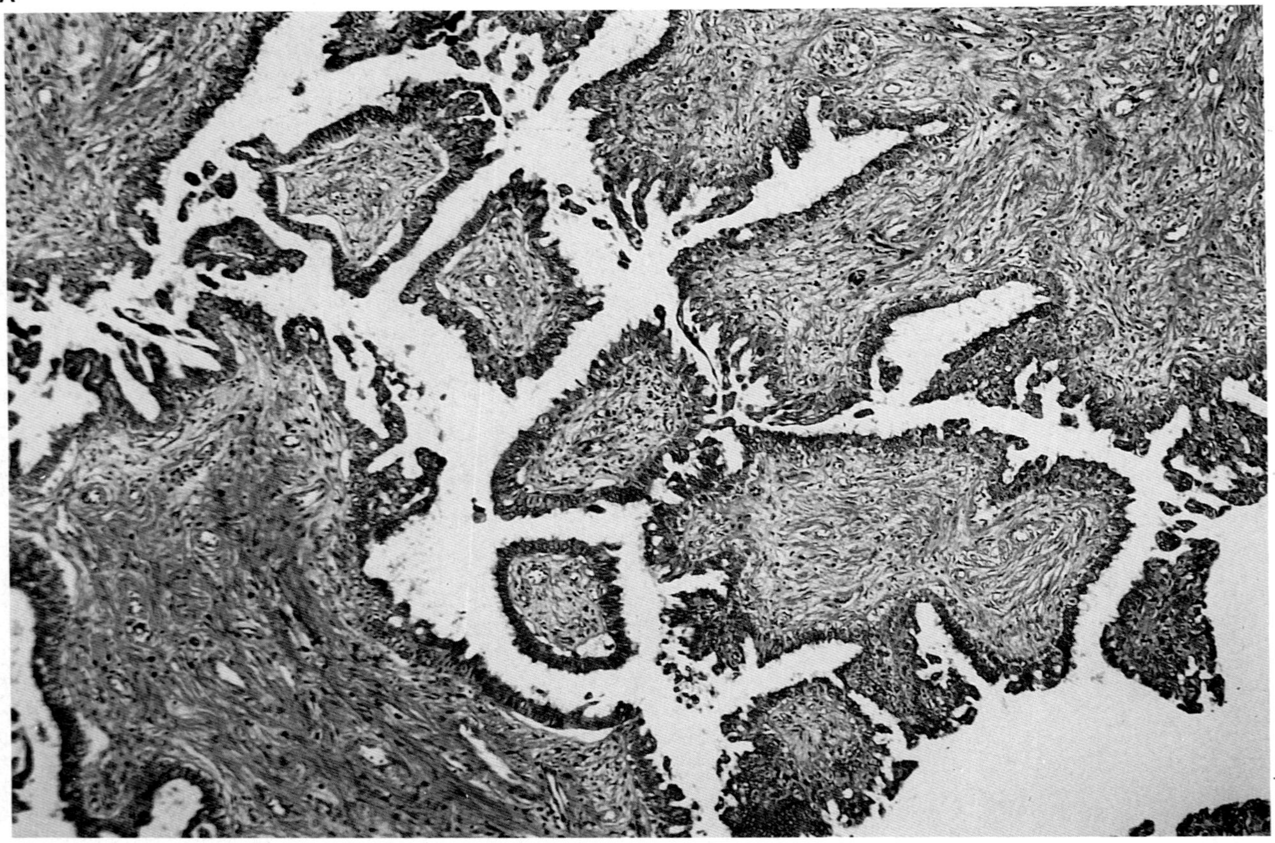

B

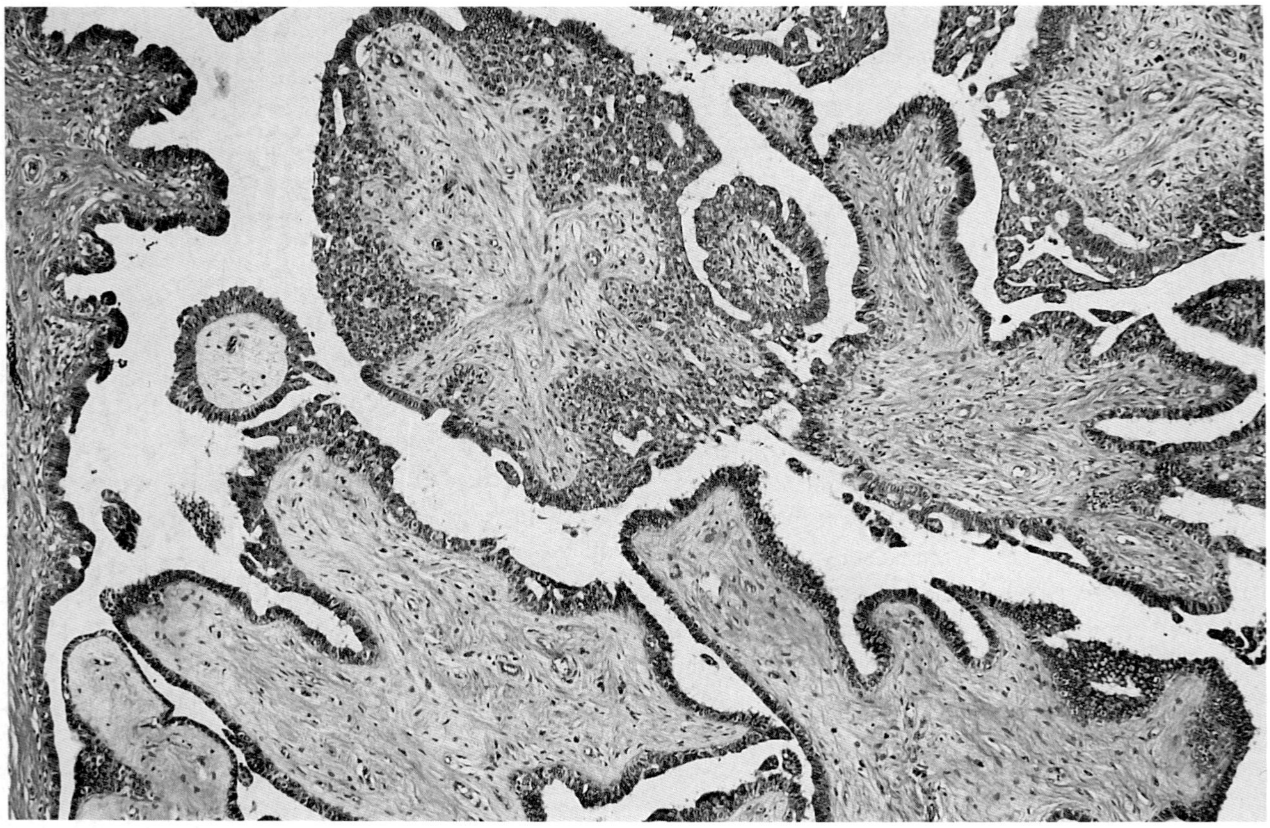

**Figure 16.7** Phyllodes tumor, low grade. (a) Leaf-like processes are abundant. The stroma is mild to moderately cellular and there is epithelial hyperplasia in the form of tufting. (b) The stroma in other parts of the same lesion appear even less cellular, but the leaf-like processes persist. (H&E, (a&b) X60)

# Index

Note: Page numbers in italics refer to figures; page numbers followed by t refer to tables.

**R**



**S**